GRAY'S ANATOMY FOR STUDENTS

GRAY'S ANATOMY FOR STUDENTS

Second South Asia Edition (Volume-01)

Richard L. Drake, PhD, FAAA
Director of Anatomy
Professor of Surgery
Cleveland Clinic Lerner College of Medicine
Case Western Reserve University
Cleveland, Ohio

A. Wayne Vogl, PhD, FAAA
Professor of Anatomy and Cell Biology
Department of Cellular and Physiological Sciences
Faculty of Medicine
University of British Columbia
Vancouver, British Columbia, Canada

Adam W. M. Mitchell, MB BS, FRCS, FRCR
Consultant Radiologist
Director of Radiology
Fortius Clinic
London, United Kingdom

Illustrations by
Richard Tibbitts and **Paul Richardson**

Photographs by
Ansell Horn

Adaptation Editors

Raveendranath Veeramani, MBBS, MD
Associate Professor of Anatomy
Jawaharlal Institute of Postgraduate Medical Education and Research (JIPMER)
Puducherry, India

Sunil Jonathan Holla, MBBS, MS
Professor of Anatomy
Christian Medical College
Vellore, India

ELSEVIER

ELSEVIER

RELX India Pvt. Ltd.
Registered Office: 818, Indraprakash Building, 8thFloor, 21, Barakhamba Road, New Delhi-110001
Corporate Office: 14th Floor, Building No. 10B, DLF Cyber City, Phase II, Gurgaon-122 002, Haryana, India

GRAY'S ANATOMY FOR STUDENTS, 4e, Richard L. Drake, A. Wayne Vogl, Adam W. M. Mitchell

ISBN: 978-0-323-39304-1

This adaptation of chapters 1-5 from **GRAY'S ANATOMY FOR STUDENTS, 4e by Richard L. Drake, A. Wayne Vogl, and Adam W. M. Mitchell** was undertaken by RELX India Private Limited and is published by arrangement with Elsevier Inc.

GRAY'S ANATOMY FOR STUDENTS, Second South Asia Edition (Volume-01)
Adaptation Editors: Raveendranath Veeramani and Sunil Jonathan Holla

Adaptation ISBN: 978-81-312-5574-2 (Set)

Adaptation e-ISBN: 978-81-312-5575-9 (Set)

First Printed in India 2019, Reprinted 2020

Content Strategist: Arvind Koul
Content Project Manager: Ayan Dhar
Cover Designer: Raman Kumar

Printed in India by Sanat Printers, Kundli, Haryana

To my wife, Cheryl, who has supported me; and my parents,
who have guided me.
RLD

To my family, to my professional colleagues and role models,
and to my students—this book is for you.
AWV

To Max, Elsa, and Cathy.
And the man that made us all,
Timothy Ianthor Mitchell!
AWMM

The almighty for the opportunity given and
the capability for the completion of the work.
I would like to thank my wife, Dr Umamageswari and
my son Charvesh who encouraged and supported me in my work.
Raveendranath Veeramani

Jesus Christ, my Lord, who enabled me.
Muriel, my wife, for her inspiration.
Jonathan and David my sons, for their understanding.
Sunil Jonathan Holla

Acknowledgments to the Second South Asia Edition

We acknowledge Dr Nachiket Shankar, St John's Medical College, for his valuable inputs in planning the format of the outlines in the book.

Many thanks to Dr Umamageswari, radiologist at Sri Manakula Vinayagar Medical College, Puducherry, for her opinion and constant support on the radiology content of the book.

We are indebted to Dr Aby S. Charles and Mr Rajkumar of Christian Medical College, Vellore, for their contribution in making the line diagrams (LDs) which will help students understand anatomical concepts and be able to illustrate them. Many thanks to Dr Suganthy Rabi, the head of the Department of Anatomy at CMC Vellore, for giving permission to do this project.

We are thankful to Mr Arvind Kaul, Ms Shabina Nasim, Ms Shivani Pal, and Mr Ayan Dhar, the Elsevier team members, for their assistance and guidance throughout the project.

Raveendranath Veeramani
Sunil Jonathan Holla

Acknowledgments to the Fourth International Edition

First, we collectively thank those who have reviewed drafts of various editions of this book—anatomists, educators, and student members of the editorial review board from around the world. Your input was invaluable.

We also thank Richard Tibbitts and Paul Richardson for their skills in turning our visual ideas into a reality that is not only a foundation for the acquisition of anatomical knowledge but also beautiful.

Thanks must also go to Madelene Hyde, Jeremy Bowes, Bill Schmitt, Rebecca Gruliow, John Casey, and all the team at Elsevier for guiding us through the preparation of this book.

We also thank Professor Richard A. Buckingham of the Abraham Lincoln School of Medicine, University of Illinois, for the provision of Fig. 8.112. Finally, because we worked separately, distanced by, in some cases, thousands of miles, there are various people who gave local support, whom we would like to make mention of individually. We have gratefully listed them here:

Dr Leonard Epp, Dr Carl Morgan, Dr Robert Shellhamer, and Dr Robert Cardell, who profoundly influenced my career as a scientist and an educator.

Richard L. Drake

Dr Sydney Friedman, Dr Elio Raviola, and Dr Charles Slonecker, for their inspiration and support and for instilling in me a passion for the discipline of anatomy.

Dr Murray Morrison, Dr Joanne Matsubara, Dr Brian Westerberg, Laura Hall, and Jing Cui, for contributing images for the chapter on the head and neck.

Dr Bruce Crawford and Logan Lee, for help with images for the surface anatomy of the upper limb.

Professor Elizabeth Akesson and Dr Donna Ford, for their enthusiastic support and valuable critiques.

Dr Sam Wiseman, for contributing surgical and other images in the chapters on abdomen and head and neck.

Dr Rosemary Basson, for writing the "Erectile Dysfunction—In the Clinic" in the chapter on pelvis and perineum.

A. Wayne Vogl

Anatomy changes! We see it through new "glasses"—X-rays, CT, MRI, and now AI ... what's next (I do not know, but it's exciting). We need new eyes and new blood, and I am delighted to have been helped by two inspirational colleagues, Dr Monika Rowe and Dr Rajat Choudhury with the clinical. They are stars of the future.

Dr Justin Lee and Dr Gajan Rajeswaran are the greatest colleagues who challenge me daily with MSK anatomy.

Many thanks for constant support from Mr Andrew Williams, Prof James Calder, and Lucy Ball. They are all awesome!

Adam W.M. Mitchell

Preface to the Second South Asia Edition

The Second South Asia Edition builds on the past and looks to the future. It maintains the goals and objectives of First South Asia Edition. In this new edition, the content has been revised considering the feedback received. New content has been added on the basis of updates in the Fourth International Edition including the addition of a new chapter on neuroanatomy.

The language has been simplified. The use of outlines, as in First South Asia Edition, has been continued. The innovative features of the First South Asia Edition such as Set Inductions, Outlines, and Flowcharts have been improved. Students are encouraged to use online resources available on MedEnact.

The Second South Asia Edition contains a new chapter on neuroanatomy. The addition of this chapter is based on the eFiles of the Fourth International Edition. This chapter is organized in keeping with the pattern of the existing chapters in the First South Asia Edition, with set inductions, specific learning objectives, multimodal approach covering recall, demonstrate structures, analyze concepts, apply and solve problems. Neuroanatomical connections are represented in the form of flowcharts and maps.

A unique feature of this edition is that each chapter contains "line diagrams," abbreviated as LDs. These line diagrams are sketches which are easy to draw during an examination and can help students to acquire anatomical concepts and do well in assessment.

Competencies have been added in all the chapters since the curriculum is becoming competency based.

Based on feedback from students, this book has been split as follows: Volume One—The Body, Upper Limb, Lower Limb, Abdomen, Pelvis and Perineum; and Volume Two— Thorax, Back, Head and Neck, and Neuroanatomy. This division is based on the examination pattern followed in several medical colleges and will enable easy handling and use of the book.

In the outlines in each chapter, the structures to be demonstrated in a prosected specimen are given as Level I, II, and III which represent the Must Know, Desirable to Know, and Nice to Know content, respectively. This helps to emphasize the core content.

The editors are open to and welcome feedback that will help improve this book.

Raveendranath Veeramani
Sunil Jonathan Holla

Preface to the Fourth International Edition

The 4th edition of *Gray's Anatomy for Students* maintains the goals and objectives of the 1st, 2nd, and 3rd editions while at the same time continuing to incorporate input from our readers and adjust the content to align with the evolving educational environment.

One of the major focuses of our attention as we prepared the 4th edition was adjusting print content to accommodate the evolving capacity to move material onto e-learning platforms. We have expanded the number of "In the Clinic" boxes in the printed book but have moved some of the "Clinical Cases" in earlier editions of the book from the print version to the online platform. Moving some of the clinical cases to the e-learning platform has allowed us to add new material to the print version without expanding the size of the book or compromising the basic goals and objectives of the work. New material added has included new imaging to reflect recent advances in the field of radiology and, in response to reader feedback, we have added simple summary line diagrams ("Quick draw sketches") to some of the key figures that can be easily replicated by students.

A new feature in the 4th edition is an accompanying online e-book organized systemically and referred to as *Gray's Systemic Anatomy*. This e-book has chapters on the cardiovascular, respiratory, gastrointestinal, nervous, urogenital, and lymphatic systems. We feel students may find this material useful as many medical school curriculums now use a systems-based, integrated approach.

A second new feature to the 4th edition is the inclusion of a neuroanatomy chapter. We hope that this eChapter will assist students as they advance their knowledge of neuroanatomy.

As was the case in previous editions, review materials/study aids are available on Student Consult as an online resource with the appropriate review materials for each chapter listed at the beginning of that chapter. This information includes an online anatomy and embryology self-study course, medical clinical cases, physical therapy clinical cases, self-assessment questions, an interactive surface anatomy module, and short answer questions. We believe that with these changes the 4th edition of *Gray's Anatomy for Students* is an improved version of the 3rd edition and hope that the book will continue to be a valuable learning resource for students.

Richard L. Drake
A. Wayne Vogl
Adam W. M. Mitchell
October 2018

About the Book

The idea

In the past 20 years or so, there have been many changes that have shaped how students learn human anatomy in medical and dental schools and in allied health programs, with curricula becoming either more integrated or more system based. In addition, instructional methods focus on the use of small group activities with the goals of increasing the amount of self-directed learning and acquiring the skills for the life-long acquisition of knowledge. An explosion of information in every discipline has also been a force in driving curricular change as it increases the amount to be learned without necessarily increasing the time available. With these changes, we felt it was time for a new book to be written that would allow students to learn anatomy within the context of many different curricular designs and within ever-increasing time constraints.

We began in the fall of 2001 by considering the various approaches and formats that we might adopt, eventually deciding upon a regional approach to anatomy with each chapter having four sections. From the beginning, we wanted the book to be designed with multiple entry points, to be targeted at introductory level students in a broad spectrum of fields, and to be a student-oriented companion text for *Gray's Anatomy*, which is aimed at a more professional audience. We wrote the text first and subsequently constructed all the artwork and illustrations to complement and augment the words. Preliminary drafts of chapters, when complete, were distributed to an international editorial board of anatomists, educators, and anatomy students for review. Their comments were then considered carefully in the preparation of the final book.

The text is not meant to be exhaustive in coverage, but to present enough anatomy to provide students with a structural and functional context in which to add further detail as they progress through their careers. *Gray's Anatomy* was used as the major reference, both for the text and for the illustrations during the preparation of this book, and it is the recommended source for acquiring additional detail.

The book

Gray's Anatomy for Students is a clinically oriented, student-friendly textbook of human anatomy. It has been prepared primarily for students in a variety of professional programs (e.g., medical, dental, chiropractic, and physical therapy programs). It can be used by students in traditional, systemic, combined traditional/systemic, and problem-based curricula, and will be particularly useful to students when lectures and laboratories in gross anatomy are minimal.

ORGANIZATION

Using a regional approach, *Gray's Anatomy for Students* progresses through the body in a logical fashion, building on the body's complexities as the reader becomes more comfortable with the subject matter. Each chapter can be used as an independent learning module, and varying the sequence will not affect the quality of the educational experience.

The **Second South Asia Edition** of this book has been split into two volumes: Volume One: The Body, Upper Limb, Lower Limb, Abdomen, Pelvis and Perineum; and Volume Two: Thorax, Back, Head and Neck, and Neuroanatomy. The just-mentioned division is based on the examination pattern followed in several medical colleges and will enable easy handling and best use of the book. We begin with "The Body," which contains an overview of the discipline of gross anatomy and an introduction to imaging modalities and general body systems. We follow this with the "Upper Limb" followed by the "Lower Limb," as they are easy to understand at the beginning of the course. Next begins a progression through the cavities of the body. "Abdomen," "Pelvis and Perineum" followed logically to the "Thorax" and "Back." The last regions discussed are the "Head and Neck" and "Neuroanatomy." These regions contain some of the most difficult anatomy in the body. Covering all the other regions first gives the student the opportunity to build a strong foundation on which to understand these complex regions.

CONTENT

Each regional anatomy chapter consists of four consecutive sections: conceptual overview, regional anatomy, surface anatomy, and clinical cases.

The conceptual overview provides the basis on which information in the later sections is built. This section can be read independently of the rest of the text by students who require only a basic level of understanding and can also be read as a summary of important concepts after the regional anatomy has been mastered.

The regional anatomy section provides more detailed anatomy along with a substantial amount of relevant clinical correlations. It is not an exhaustive discussion but instead provides information to a level that we feel is necessary for understanding the organization of the region. Throughout this section, two levels of clinical material are provided. Clinical hooks are fully integrated with the main anatomical text and function to relate ("hook") the anatomy discussed directly to a clinical application without taking students out of their train of thought and without disrupting the flow of the text. Although fully integrated with the anatomical text, these passages are differentiated from it by the use of green highlighting. Early clinical exposure sections are concise descriptions that provide students with useful and relevant clinical information demonstrating how the application of anatomical knowledge facilitates solving of clinical problems. These are spread throughout the text close to the most relevant anatomical discussion.

Surface anatomy assists students in visualizing the relationship between anatomical structures and surface landmarks. This section also provides students with practical applications of the anatomical information, combining visual inspection with functional assessment, as occurs during any type of patient examination.

The final section of each chapter consists of clinical cases. These cases represent the third level of clinical material in the book. In these cases, a clinical problem is described, and a step-by-step process of questions and answers leads the reader to the resolution of the case. The inclusion of these cases in each chapter provides students with the opportunity to apply an understanding of anatomy to the resolution of a clinical problem.

Illustrations are an integral part of any anatomy text. They must present the reader with a visual image that brings the text to life and presents views that will assist in the understanding and comprehension of the anatomy. The artwork in this textbook accomplishes all of these goals. The illustrations are original and vibrant, and many views are unique. They have been designed to integrate with the text, to present the anatomy in new ways, to deal with the issues that students find particularly difficult, and to provide a conceptual framework for building further understanding. To ensure that the illustrations of the book work together and to enable students to cross-refer from one illustration to another, we have used standard colors throughout the book, except where indicated otherwise. This edition has an additional feature of line diagrams (LDs) along with questions and answers. These will help in acquiring important anatomical concepts and will be useful for students in assessment for learning and assessment of learning.

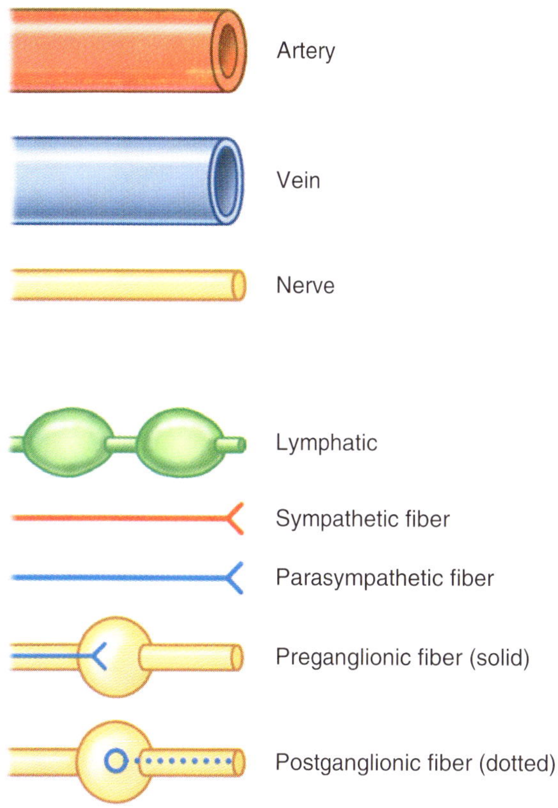

The position and size of the artwork was one of the parameters considered in the overall design of each page of the book.

Clinical images are also an important tool in understanding anatomy and are abundant throughout the text. Examples of state-of-the-art medical imaging, including MRIs, CTs, PETs, ultrasound images, as well as radiographs, provide students with additional tools to increase their ability to visualize anatomy in vivo and, thus, increase their understanding.

What the book does not contain

Gray's Anatomy for Students focuses on gross anatomy. While many curricula around the world are being presented in a more integrated format combining anatomy, physiology, histology, and embryology, we have focused this textbook on understanding only the anatomy and its application to clinical problems. Except for some brief references to embryology where necessary for a better understanding of the anatomy, material from other disciplines is not included. We felt that there are many outstanding textbooks covering these subject areas, and that trying to cover everything in a single book would produce a text of questionable quality and usefulness, not to mention the enormous size!

Terminology

In any anatomical text or atlas, terminology is always an interesting issue. In 1989, the Federative Committee on Anatomical Terminology (FCAT) was formed and was charged with developing the official terminology of the anatomical sciences. The *Terminologia Anatomica* (2nd edition, Thieme, Stuttgart/New York, 2011) was a joint publication by this group and the 56 member associations of the International Federation of Associations of Anatomists (IFAA). We have chosen to use the terminology presented in this publication in the interest of uniformity. Other terminology is not incorrect; we just felt that using terminology from this single, internationally recognized source would be the most logical and straightforward approach.

Although we use anatomical terms for orientation as much as possible, we also use terms such as "behind" or "in front of" occasionally to make the text more readable. In these cases, the context clarifies the meaning.

Anatomical use of adverbs

During the writing of this book, we had many long discussions about how we were going to describe anatomical relationships as clearly as possible but maintain the readability of the text. One issue that arose continually in our discussions was the correct use of the "-ly" adverb form of anatomical orientation terms, such as anterior, posterior, superior, inferior, lateral, and medial. We reached the following consensus:

"-ly" adverbs, *e.g., anteriorly, posteriorly,* have been used to modify (describe) verbs in passages where an action or direction is mentioned. For example, "The trachea passes inferiorly through the thorax."

Circumstantial adverbs, *e.g., anterior, posterior*, have been used to indicate the fixed location of an anatomical feature. For example, "The trachea is anterior to the esophagus."

Furthermore, both usages may occur in the same passage. For example, "The trachea passes inferiorly through the thorax, anterior to the esophagus."

We have very much enjoyed the process of putting this book together. We hope that you enjoy using it to the same degree.

Richard L. Drake
A. Wayne Vogl
Adam W.M. Mitchell
Raveendranath Veeramani
Sunil Jonathan Holla

Contents

Volume I

1 The body

2 Upper limb

Contents

Contents

Contents

Index of Early Clinical Exposure

Volume I

1 The Body

Early Clinical Exposure

Clinical Cases

2 Upper Limb

Early Clinical Exposure

Clinical Cases

Index of Early Clinical Exposure

3 *Lower Limb*

Early Clinical Exposure

Clinical Cases

4 *Abdomen*

Early Clinical Exposure

Clinical Cases

5 *Pelvis and Perineum*

Early Clinical Exposure

Clinical Cases

Volume II

6 *Thorax*

Early Clinical Exposure

Clinical Cases

1

The Body

ADDITIONAL LEARNING RESOURCES for Chapter 1, The Body, on MedEnact (www.MedEnact.com)

- Short Questions—these are questions requiring short responses

THE BODY

Competency: The first-year medical student should be able to apply his or her knowledge about the general features of bones, joints, muscles, vessels, and nerves to effectively perform dissections and comprehend gross anatomy.

What is anatomy?

CONTEXTUAL LEARNING SCENARIO

Two new students joined a medical college who had come from far off places. They were new to the hustle and bustle of the city and need time to settle down into the new environment and schedules of the medical college and the food of the hostel mess.

On the way to their introductory class in Anatomy, they walked past the cadavers lying on steel tables ready for dissection. A senior faculty welcomed them and introduced them to the basics of the subject as well as a new vocabulary of medical terms, which would be necessary to study anatomy. As the first lecture got over, the teacher hoped that the knowledge-thirsty students had absorbed the new terms that had been introduced, as these were essential for the study of anatomy and for the care of patients.

SET INDUCTION—CASE SCENARIO 1: INTERPRETATION OF AN X- RAY

An intern in the emergency department was discussing about a patient who sustained a penetrating injury in the front of the chest. She was given an X-ray and asked to interpret the findings. A sound knowledge of normal anatomy is needed to interpret radiological images.

OUTLINE 1. THE BODY—LEARNING OBJECTIVES
[By the end of this section the student should be able to:]

REMEMBER [Recall Facts]

Anatomical terms
1. Describe the anatomical planes
2. Define and demonstrate terms relative to the anatomical position
3. Define and demonstrate the terms used to describe movements

Imaging
1. Describe the basis of imaging techniques
2. Explain how imaging techniques can be used for diagnosis

Skeletal system
1. Describe the classification of bone based on structure, shape and development
2. Explain some common clinical conditions affecting bone
3. Classify joints based on the shape of the articulating surfaces

Skin
1. Describe the layers of skin and fascia
2. Explain the functions of the skin
3. Explain the importance of the superficial and deep fascia

Muscular system
1. Describe the types of muscle
2. Describe the classification of skeletal muscle based on its structure
3. Describe the classification of skeletal muscle based on its action

Cardiovascular system
1. Describe the types of blood vessels
2. Describe the layers of the walls of blood vessels
3. Explain the common clinical problems affecting arteries and veins

Lymphatic system
1. Describe the parts of the lymphatic system
2. Describe the applied anatomy of lymph nodes
3. Describe the area of the body drained by lymph trunks and the thoracic duct

Nervous system
1. Describe the subdivisions of the nervous system
2. Explain the course of somatic and autonomic nerve fibers
3. Explain the basis of referred pain

DEMONSTRATE AND ANALYZE [Discuss]

Level I

- Anatomical planes:
  Sagittal, coronal, transverse
- Terms used to describe location:
  Anterior, posterior; medial, lateral; superior, inferior; proximal, distal; cranial, caudal, rostral; superficial, deep
- Terms used to describe movements:
  Flexion, extension; abduction, abduction, circumduction; medial rotation, lateral rotation; protraction, retraction; dorsiflexion, plantarflexion; inversion, eversion; supination, pronation
- Imaging
  Plain radiography
  Contrast agents—barium sulfate, iodine
- Intravenous urogram
- Ultrasound
- Doppler ultrasound
- Computed tomography
- Magnetic resonance imaging
- Nuclear medicine imaging
- Skeletal system
  Functions and types of cartilage
  Functions, types, classification, development and ossification of bone; skeletal age
  - Types of joints:
    Synovial joints—description based on shape and movement—plane, hinge, pivot, condylar, saddle, ball and socket
    Fibrous joints—sutures, gomphosis, syndesmoses
    Cartilaginous joints—synchondrosis, symphysis
- Skin and fascias
  Layers of skin—epidermis, dermis
  - Fascia—superficial
  Deep—intermuscular septa, retinacula, extraperitoneal fascia, endothoracic fascia

Level II

Muscular system
- Skeletal muscle—classification based on:
  (a) Arrangement of fasciculi—strap, fusiform, quadrilateral, triangular, pennate (unipennate, bipennate, multipennate, circumpennate)
  (b) Actions—prime mover (agonist), antagonist, synergist, fixator
- Cardiac and smooth muscle
- Cardiovascular system
  Types of blood vessels—arteries, veins, capillaries
  Layers in the walls of blood vessels—tunica intima, tunica media, tunica adventitia

Lymphatic system
  Lymph vessels, lymph nodes
  Sites with palpable lymph nodes; lymphatic trunks and ducts
- Nervous system
  - Parts based on:
    (a) Structure: central nervous system and peripheral nervous system
    (b) Function: Somatic and visceral
  CNS—brain and spinal cord
  Parts—cerebral hemispheres, cerebellum, brainstem
    Cerebrum—gray matter, white matter, ventricles
    Cerebellum—lobes, vermis
    Brainstem—midbrain, pons, medulla, spinal cord
    Meninges—dura mater, arachnoid mater, pia mater
  Somatic part of nervous system:
    Somites, dermomyotome, epaxial muscles, hypaxial muscles
    Motor neurons, sensory neurons
    General somatic afferents and efferents
    Dermatomes, myotomes
  Visceral part of nervous system
    Visceral motor—autonomic part: Sympathetic and parasympathetic
    Visceral sensory neurons—general visceral afferent fibers
    Visceral motor neurons—preganglionic, postganglionic, autonomic ganglia
    Sympathetic and parasympathetic systems
    Enteric system
    Nerve plexuses—somatic and visceral

Level III

Subtraction angiography
Positron emission tomography
Bone fractures
Bone marrow transplant
Avascular necrosis
Epiphyseal fractures

EVALUATE [Explain Concepts]

- Differentiate between regional and systemic anatomy
- Differentiate between arteries and veins
- Drainage areas of lymph nodes
- Explain dermatomes and myotomes

EARLY CLINICAL EXPOSURE [Apply Anatomical Knowledge]

Surgical Anatomy/ Pathology/ Trauma	Imaging/ Surface Anatomy
■ Explain the importance of anatomical terminology ■ Explain the appearance of various tissues in radiographs, CT scans, ultrasound and MRIs ■ Discuss patient safety during imaging ■ Joint replacement ■ Muscle injury, paralysis and atrophy ■ Atherosclerosis ■ Varicose veins	■ Osteoporosis ■ Osteoarthritis ■ Arthroscopy

PROBLEM SOLVING/ CLINICAL CASES [Interpret]

- Describe the terms radiopaque, radiolucent, echogenecity, "weighting" of CT images
- Discuss the role of fascia in limiting spread of infection
- Discuss the role of anastomoses and collateral circulation
- Describe the spread of cancer cells through lymph vessels
- Describe referred pain

Anatomy includes those structures that can be seen grossly (without the aid of magnification) and microscopically (with the aid of magnification). Typically, when used by itself, the term *anatomy* tends to mean gross or macroscopic anatomy—that is, the study of structures that can be seen without using a microscopic. Microscopic anatomy, also called histology, is the study of cells and tissues using a microscope.

Anatomy forms the basis for the practice of medicine. Anatomy leads the physician toward an understanding of a patient's disease, whether he or she is carrying out a physical examination or using the most advanced imaging techniques. Anatomy is also important for dentists, physiotherapists, and all others involved in any aspect of patient treatment that begins with an analysis of clinical signs. The ability to interpret a clinical observation correctly is therefore the end point of a sound anatomical understanding.

Observation and visualization are the primary techniques a student should use to learn anatomy. Anatomy is much more than just memorization of lists of names. Although the language of anatomy is important, the network of information needed to visualize the position of physical structures in a patient goes far beyond simple memorization. Knowing the names of the various branches of the external carotid artery is not the same as being able to visualize the course of the lingual artery from its origin in the neck to its termination in the tongue. Similarly, understanding the organization of the soft palate, how it is related to the oral and nasal cavities, and how it moves during swallowing is very different from being able to recite the names of its individual muscles and nerves. An understanding of anatomy requires an understanding of the context in which the terminology can be remembered.

How can gross anatomy be studied?

The term *anatomy* is derived from the Greek word *temnein*, meaning "to cut." Clearly, therefore, the study of anatomy is linked, at its root, to dissection. Although dissection of cadavers by students is now augmented, or even in some cases replaced, by viewing prosected (previously dissected) material and plastic models, or using computer teaching modules and other learning aids.

Anatomy can be studied following either a regional or a systemic approach.

- With a **regional approach**, each *region* of the body is studied separately and all aspects of that region are studied at the same time. For example, if the thorax is to be studied, all of its structures are examined. This includes the vasculature, the nerves, the bones, the muscles, and all other structures and organs located in the region of the body defined as the thorax. After studying this region, the other regions of the body (i.e., the abdomen, pelvis, lower limb, upper limb, back, head, and neck) are studied in a similar fashion.
- In contrast, in a **systemic approach**, each *system* of the body is studied and followed throughout the entire body. For example, a study of the cardiovascular system looks at the heart and all of the blood vessels in the body. When this is completed, the nervous system (brain, spinal cord, and all the nerves) might be examined in detail. This approach continues for the whole body until every system, including the nervous, skeletal, muscular, gastrointestinal, respiratory, lymphatic, and reproductive systems, has been studied.

Each of these approaches has benefits and deficiencies. The regional approach works very well if the anatomy course involves cadaver dissection but falls short when it comes to understanding the continuity of an entire system throughout the body. Similarly, the systemic approach fosters an understanding of an entire system throughout the body, but it is very difficult to coordinate this directly with a cadaver dissection or to acquire sufficient detail.

Important anatomical terms

The anatomical position

The anatomical position is the standard reference position of the body used to describe the location of structures (Fig. 1.1A). The body is in the anatomical position when standing upright with feet together, hands by the side, and face looking forward. The mouth is closed and the facial expression is neutral. The rim of bone under the eyes is in the same horizontal plane as the top of the opening to the ear, and the eyes are open and focused on something in the distance. The palms of the hands face forward with the fingers straight and together and with the pad of the thumb turned 90° to the pads of the fingers. The toes point forward.

Anatomical planes

Three major groups of planes pass through the body in the anatomical position (Fig. 1.1B).

- **Coronal planes** are oriented vertically and divide the body into anterior and posterior parts.
- **Sagittal planes** also are oriented vertically but are at right angles to the coronal planes and divide the body into right and left parts. The plane that passes through the center of the body dividing it into equal right and left halves is termed the **median sagittal plane**.
- **Transverse, horizontal**, or **axial planes** divide the body into superior and inferior parts.

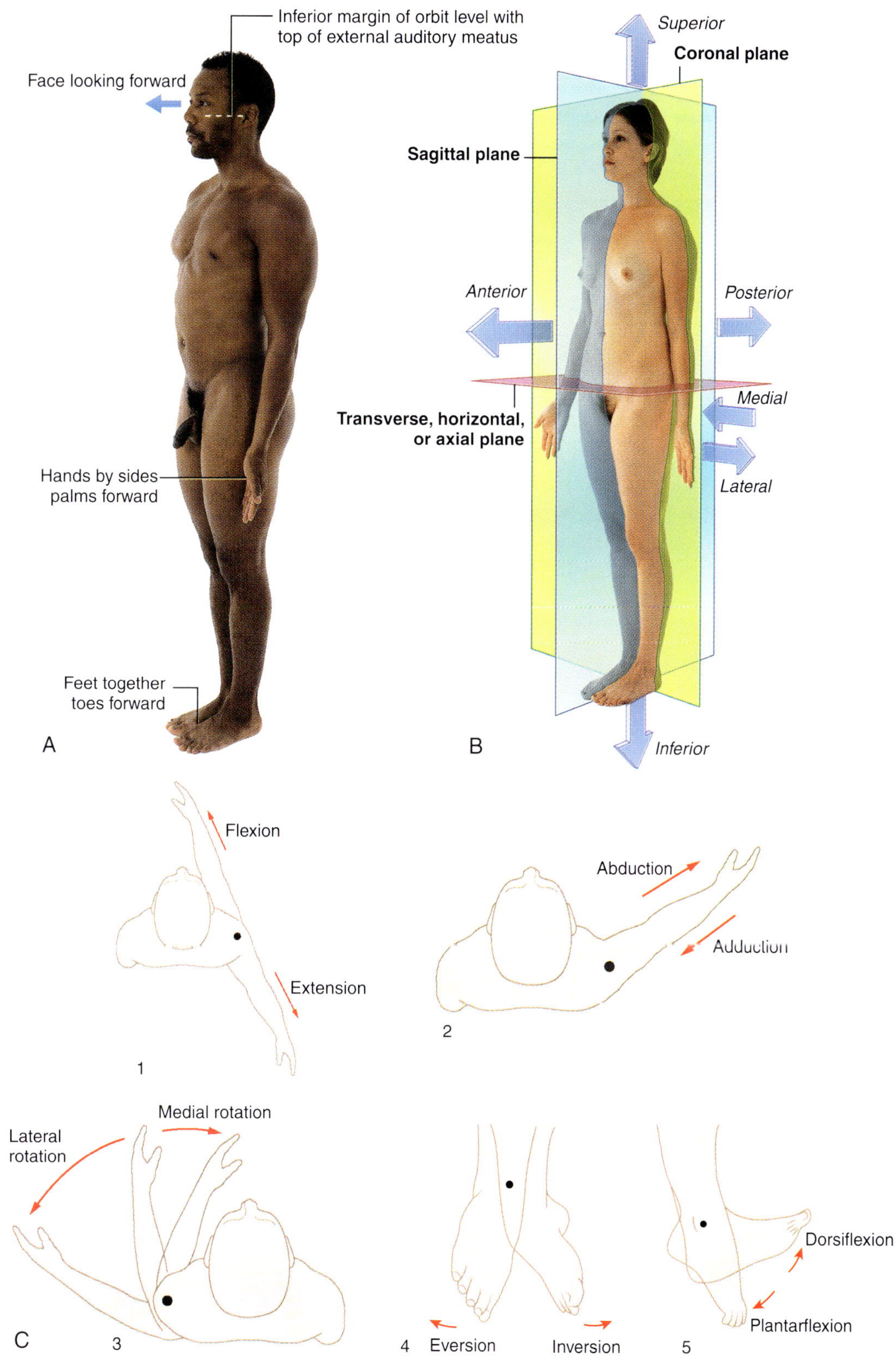

Fig. 1.1 **(A)** The anatomical position. **(B)** Planes, and terms of location and orientation. **(C)** Types of movement. *Source (C):* N. Palastanga, R. Soames. Anatomy and Human Movement: Structure and Function. Churchill Livingstone, 2012: 35-200.

Terms to describe location

Anterior (ventral) and posterior (dorsal), medial and lateral, superior and inferior

Three major pairs of terms are used to describe the location of structures relative to the body as a whole or to other structures (Fig. 1.1B).

- **Anterior** (or **ventral**) and **posterior** (or **dorsal**) describe the position of structures relative to the "front" and "back" of the body. For example, the nose is an anterior (ventral) structure, whereas the vertebral column is a posterior (dorsal) structure. Also, the nose is anterior to the ears and the vertebral column is posterior to the sternum.
- **Medial** and **lateral** describe the position of structures relative to the median sagittal plane and the sides of the body. For example, the thumb is lateral to the little finger. The nose is in the median sagittal plane and is medial to the eyes, which are in turn medial to the external ears.
- **Superior** and **inferior** describe structures with reference to the vertical axis of the body. For example, the head is superior to the shoulders and the knee joint is inferior to the hip joint.

Proximal and distal, cranial and caudal, and rostral

Other terms used to describe positions include proximal and distal, cranial and caudal, and rostral.

- **Proximal** and **distal** are used with reference to being closer to or farther from a structure's origin, particularly in the limbs. For example, the hand is distal to the elbow joint. The glenohumeral joint is proximal to the elbow joint. These terms are also used to describe the relative positions of branches along the course of linear structures, such as airways, vessels, and nerves. For example, distal branches occur farther away toward the ends of the system, whereas proximal branches occur closer to and toward the origin of the system.
- **Cranial** (toward the head) and **caudal** (*caudum*, from the Latin for "tail") are sometimes used instead of superior and inferior, respectively.
- **Rostral** is used, particularly in the head, to describe the position of a structure with reference to the nose. For example, the forebrain is rostral to the hindbrain.

Superficial and deep

Two other terms used to describe the position of structures in the body are **superficial** and **deep**. These terms are used to describe the relative positions of two structures with respect to the surface of the body. For example, the sternum is superficial to the heart, and the stomach is deep to the abdominal wall.

Superficial and deep can also be used in a more absolute fashion to define two major regions of the body. The superficial region of the body is external to the outer layer of deep fascia. Deep structures are enclosed by this layer. Structures in the superficial region of the body include the skin, superficial fascia, and mammary glands. Deep structures include most skeletal muscles and viscera. Superficial wounds are external to the outer layer of deep fascia, whereas deep wounds penetrate through it.

Terms to describe movements

Several pairs of terms are used to describe movements at particular joints (Fig. 1.1C).

Flexion means making a bend, such that two flexor surfaces come closer together, or the position of the fetus just before birth (universal flexion). **Extension** is the opposite movement.

Abduction means moving away from the midline and **adduction** is the opposite movement.

Circumduction is a combination of these movements in a particular sequence such that the distal part of the limb moves in a circle, for example extension, abduction, flexion, and adduction.

Medial rotation means moving the anterior surface of the distal bone toward the midline, and **lateral rotation** is the opposite movement. **Protraction** means moving forward and **retraction** is the opposite movement. **Dorsiflexion** means moving the dorsum of the foot upwards at the ankle joint and **plantarflexion** is the opposite movement. During inversion, the foot is moved so that the sole of the foot turns medially and eversion is the opposite movement. During supination, the forearm is moved so that the palm faces forwards and pronation is the opposite movement.

Imaging

Diagnostic imaging techniques

In 1895, Wilhelm Roentgen used X-rays from a cathode ray tube to expose a photographic plate and produced the first radiographic exposure of his wife's hand. Over the past 35 years, there has been a revolution in body imaging, which has been paralleled by developments in computer technology.

Plain radiography

The basic physics of X-ray generation has not changed.

X-rays are photons (a type of electromagnetic radiation) and are generated from a complex X-ray tube, which is a type of cathode ray tube (Fig. 1.2). The X-rays are then collimated (i.e., directed through lead-lined shutters to stop them from fanning out) to the appropriate area, as determined by the radiographic technician. As the X-rays pass through the body, they are attenuated (reduced in energy) by the tissues. Those X-rays that pass through the tissues interact with the photographic film.

In the body:

- Air attenuates X-rays a little, and is **radiolucent**
- Fat attenuates X-rays more than air but less than water
- Bone attenuates X-rays the most, and is **radiopaque**

These differences in attenuation result in differences in the level of exposure of the film. When the photographic film is developed, bone appears white on the film because this region of the film has been exposed to the least amount of X-rays. Air appears dark on the film because these regions were exposed to the greatest number of X-rays.

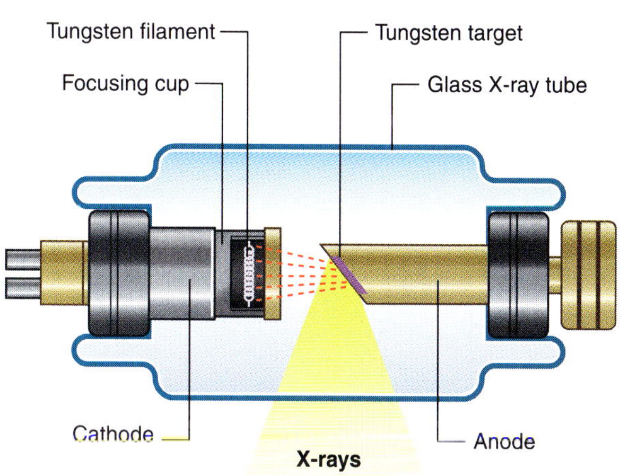

Fig. 1.2 Cathode ray tube for the production of X-rays.

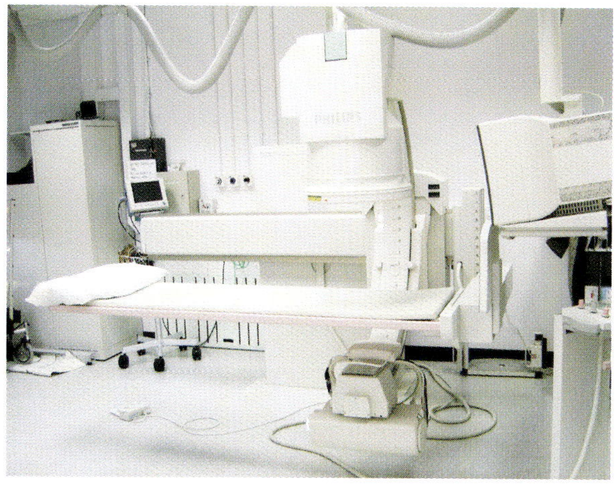

Fig. 1.3 Fluoroscopy unit.

Modifications to this X-ray technique allow a continuous stream of X-rays to be produced from the X-ray tube and collected on an input screen to allow real-time visualization of moving anatomical structures, barium studies, angiography, and fluoroscopy (Fig. 1.3).

Contrast agents

To demonstrate specific structures, such as bowel loops or arteries, it may be necessary to fill these structures with a substance that attenuates X-rays more than bowel loops or arteries do normally. It is, however, extremely important that these substances are nontoxic. Barium sulfate, an insoluble salt, is a nontoxic, relatively high-density agent that is extremely useful in the examination of the gastrointestinal tract. When **barium sulfate suspension** is ingested, it attenuates X-rays and can therefore be used to demonstrate the bowel lumen (Fig. 1.4A). It is common to add air to the barium sulfate suspension, by either ingesting "fizzy" granules or directly instilling air into the body cavity, as in a barium enema. This is known as a double-contrast (air/barium) study.

For some patients, it is necessary to inject contrast agents directly into arteries or veins. In this case, iodine-based molecules are suitable contrast agents. **Iodine** is chosen because it has a relatively high atomic mass and is radiopaque and so markedly attenuates X-rays. It is naturally excreted via the urinary system and hence is not toxic. Intra-arterial and intravenous contrast agents are extremely safe and are well tolerated by most patients. Rarely, some patients have an anaphylactic reaction to intra-arterial or intravenous injections, so the necessary precautions must be taken. Intra-arterial and intravenous contrast agents not only help in visualizing the arteries and veins but because they are excreted by the urinary system, can also be used to visualize the kidneys, ureter, and bladder in a process known as **intravenous urography (IVU) or intravenous pyelography (IVP)** (Fig. 1.4B).

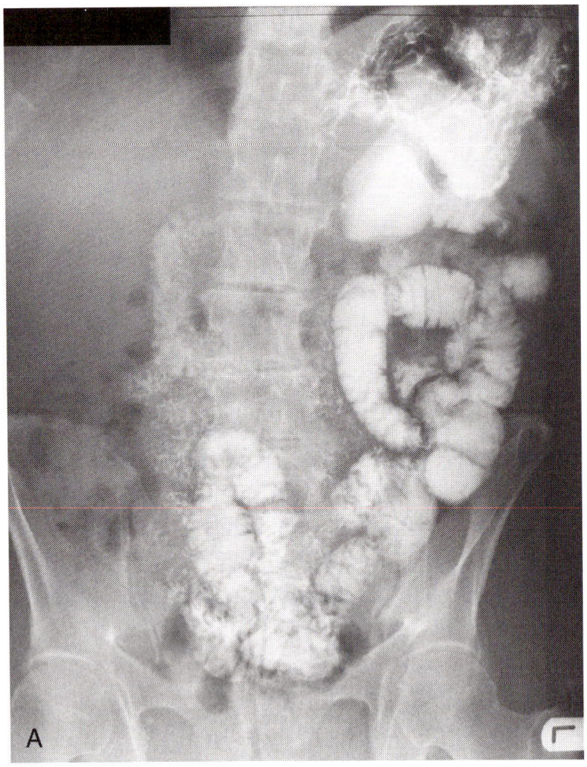

Fig. 1.4 (A) Barium sulfate follow-through.

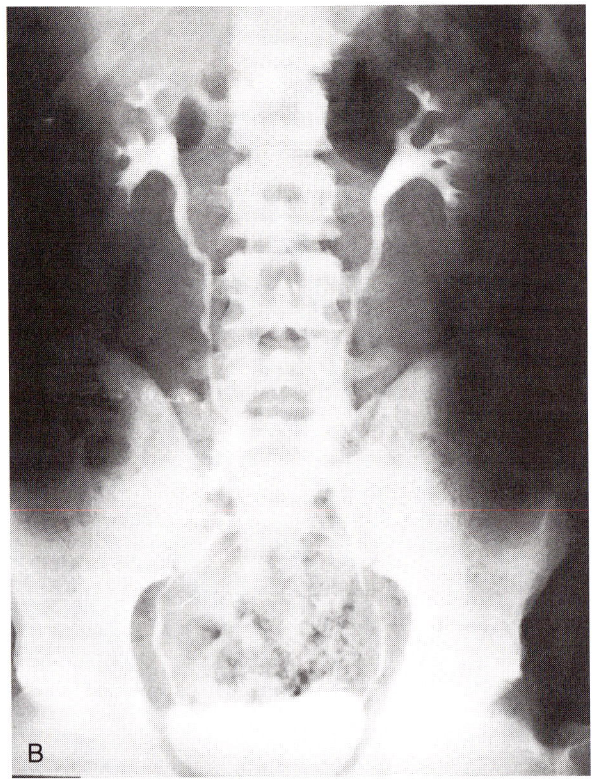

Fig. 1.4 (B) Intravenous urogram. *Source:* James Garden, Andrew W. Bradbury, John L. R Forsythe, Rowan W. Parks, Principles & Practice of Surgery: Urological Surgery. Churchill Livingstone, 2012: 399-423.

Subtraction angiography

During angiography, it is often difficult to appreciate the contrast agent in the vessels through the overlying bony structures. To circumvent this, the technique of subtraction angiography has been developed. Simply, one or two images are obtained before the injection of contrast media. These images are inverted (such that a negative is created from the positive image). After injection of the contrast media into the vessels, a further series of images are obtained, demonstrating the passage of the contrast through the arteries into the veins and around the circulation. By adding the "negative precontrast image" to the positive postcontrast images, the bones and soft tissues are subtracted to produce a solitary image of contrast only. Before the advent of digital imaging, this was a challenge, but now the use of computers has made this technique relatively straightforward and instantaneous (Fig. 1.5).

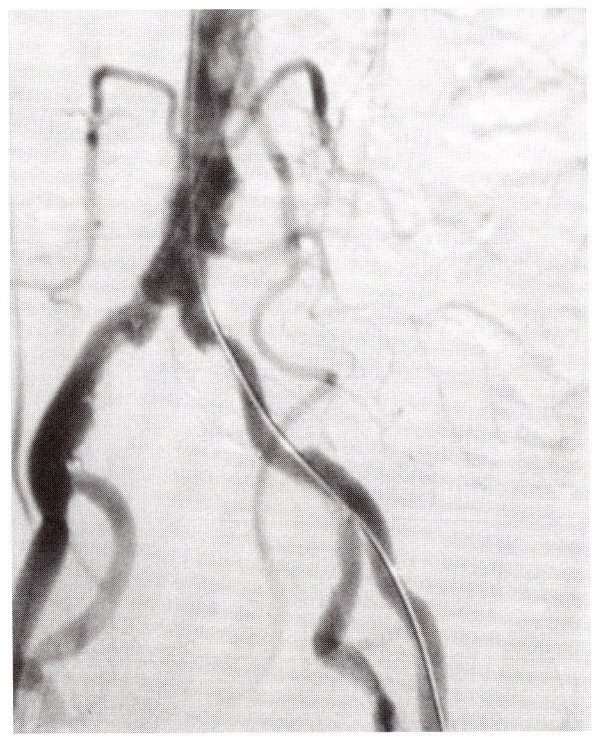

Fig. 1.5 Digital subtraction angiogram.

Ultrasound

Ultrasonography of the body is widely used for all aspects of medicine.

Ultrasound is a very high frequency sound wave (not electromagnetic radiation) generated by piezoelectric materials, such that a series of sound waves is produced. Importantly, the piezoelectric material can also receive the sound waves that bounce back as an echo from the internal organs. The sound waves are then interpreted by a powerful computer, and a real-time image is produced on the display panel (Fig. 1.6A and B). The pattern in which ultrasound waves are reflected from tissue interphases is called its echogenicity. Each tissue has a particular echogenicity. A tissue may be less echogenic (**hypoechoic**) or more echogenic (**hyperechoic**). In diseased states, the echogenicity of a tissue can be altered.

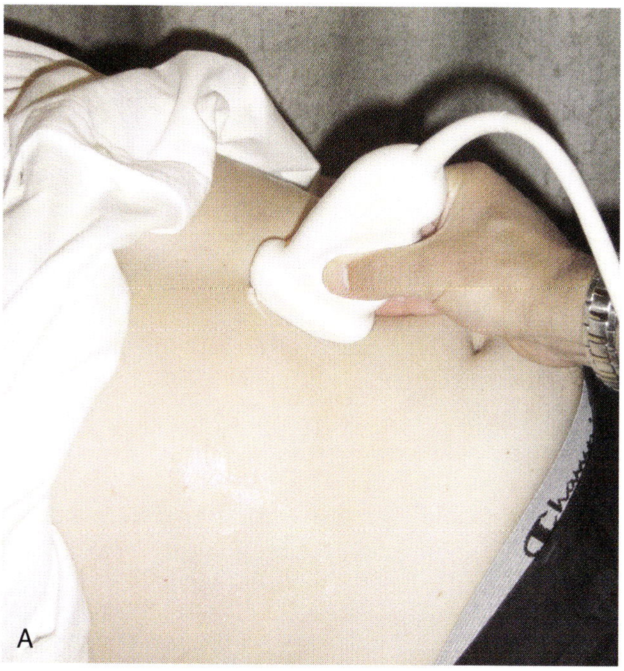

Fig. 1.6 (A) Ultrasound examination of the abdomen.

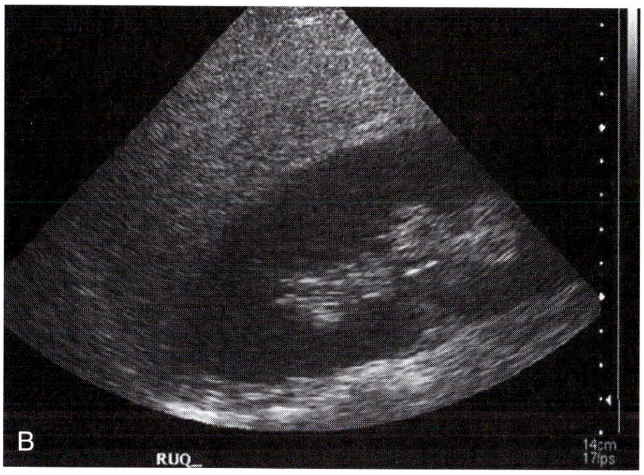

Fig. 1.6 (B) Sonogram of the abdomen. *Source:* Michael M. Henry, Jeremy N. Thompson. Clinical Surgery: Urology, 3rd ed. Saunders, 2012:557-606.

Doppler ultrasound

Developments in ultrasound technology, including the size of the probes and the frequency range, mean that a broad range of areas can now be scanned.

Traditionally ultrasound is used for assessing the abdomen (Fig. 1.6A and B) and the fetus in pregnant women. Ultrasound is also widely used to assess the eyes, neck, soft tissues, and peripheral musculoskeletal system. Probes have been placed on endoscopes, and endoluminal ultrasound of the esophagus, stomach, and duodenum is now routine. Endocavity ultrasound is carried out most commonly to assess the genital tract in women using a transvaginal or transrectal route. In men, transrectal ultrasound is the imaging method of choice to assess the prostate in those with suspected prostate hypertrophy or malignancy.

Doppler ultrasound enables determination of flow, its direction, and its velocity within a vessel using simple ultrasound techniques. Sound waves bounce off moving structures and are returned. The degree of frequency shift determines whether the object is moving away from or toward the probe and the speed at which it is traveling. Precise measurements of blood flow and blood velocity can therefore be obtained, which in turn can indicate sites of blockage in blood vessels.

Computed tomography

Computed tomography (CT) was invented in the 1970s by Sir Godfrey Hounsfield, who was awarded the Nobel Prize in Medicine in 1979. Since this inspired invention, there have been many generations of CT scanners. A CT scanner obtains a series of images of the body (slices) in the axial plane.

The patient lies on a bed, an X-ray tube passes around the body (Fig. 1.7), and a series of images are obtained. A computer carries out a complex mathematical transformation on the multitude of images to produce the final image (Fig. 1.8). Bone is described as **hyperdense** and air as **hypodense**.

Magnetic resonance imaging

Nuclear magnetic resonance imaging (MRI) was first described in 1946 and used to determine the structure of complex molecules. The complexity of the physics necessary to obtain an image is beyond the scope of this textbook, but the reader should be aware of how the image is produced and the types of images typically seen in routine medical practice.

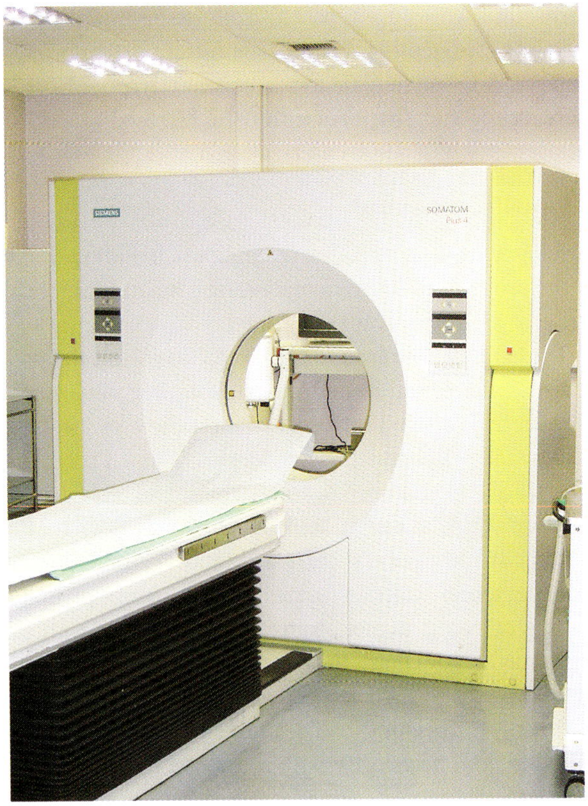

Fig. 1.7 Computed tomography scanner.

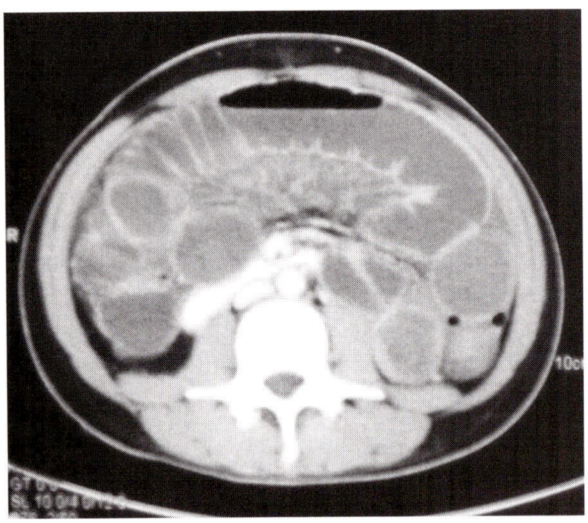

Fig. 1.8 Computed tomography scan of the abdomen at vertebral level L2.

The process of MRI is dependent on the free protons in the hydrogen nuclei in molecules of water (H_2O). Because water is present in almost all biological tissues, the hydrogen proton is ideal. The protons within a patient's hydrogen nuclei can be regarded as small bar magnets, which are randomly oriented in space. The patient is placed in a strong magnetic field, which aligns the bar magnets. When a pulse of radio waves is passed through the patient, the magnets are deflected, and as they return to their aligned position they emit small radio pulses. The strength and frequency of the emitted pulses and the time it takes for the protons to return to their pre-excited state produce a signal. These signals are analyzed by a powerful computer, and an image is created (Fig. 1.9).

By altering the sequence of pulses to which the protons are subjected, different properties of the protons can be assessed. These properties are referred to as the "weighting" of the scan. By altering the pulse sequence and the scanning parameters, T1-weighted images (Fig. 1.10A) and T2-weighted images (Fig. 1.10B) can be obtained. These two types of imaging sequences provide differences in image contrast, which accentuate and optimize different tissue characteristics.

MRI can also be used to assess flow within vessels and to produce complex angiograms of the peripheral and cerebral circulation.

From the clinical point of view:

- Most T1-weighted images show dark fluid and bright fat—for example, the subcutaneous fat in the scalp is bright or hyperintense, and within the brain the cerebrospinal fluid (CSF) is dark or **hypointense**.
- T2-weighted images demonstrate a bright signal from fluid and an intermediate signal from fat—for example, in the brain, the CSF appears white or **hyperintense**.

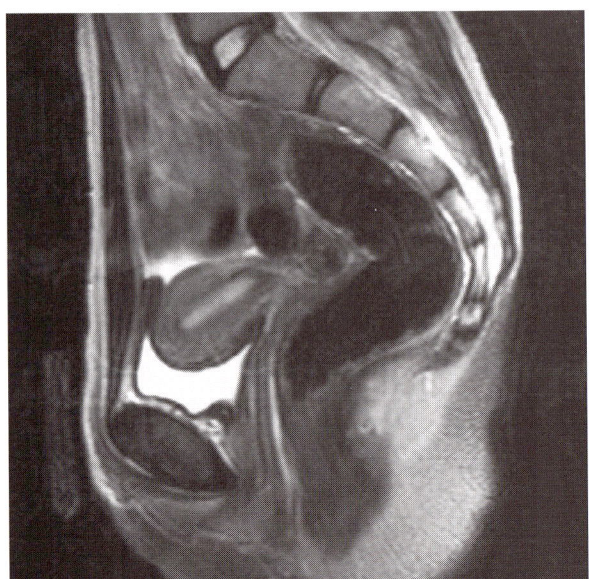

Fig. 1.9 A T2-weighted magnetic resonance image in the sagittal plane of the pelvic viscera in a woman.

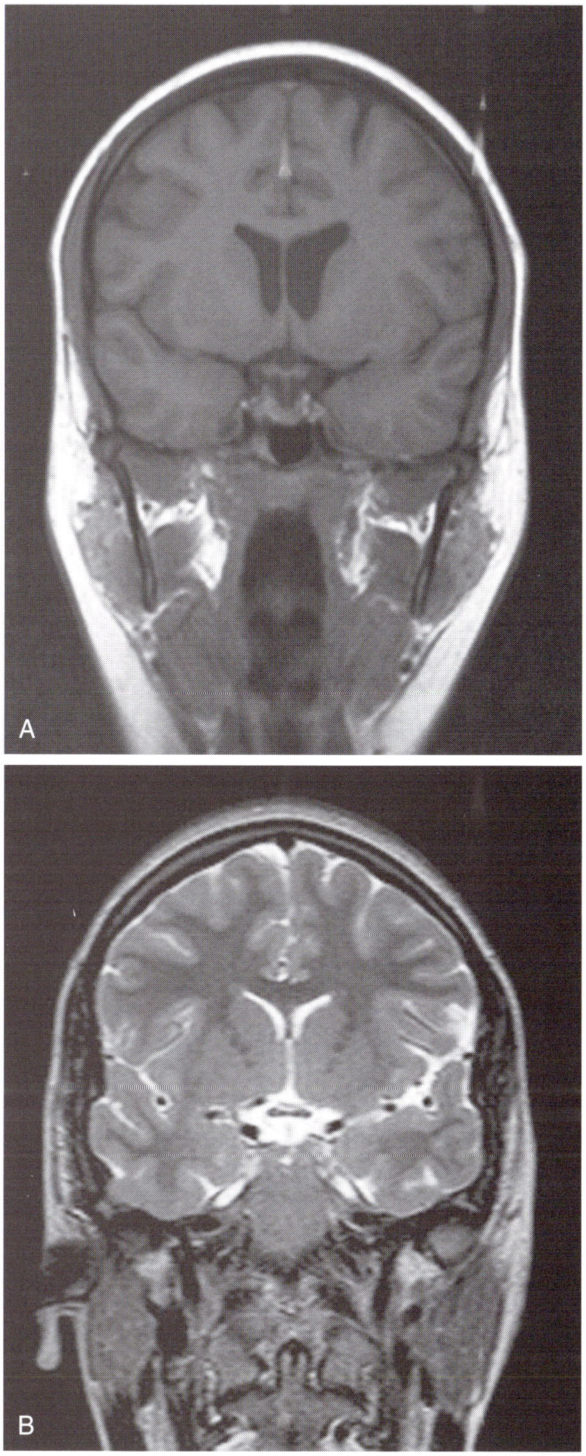

Fig. 1.10 T1-weighted **(A)** and T2-weighted **(B)** magnetic resonance images of the brain in the coronal plane.

Mnemonics

The following abbreviations can be used to recall certain facts:

"ODI," **O**ne **D**ay **I**nternational, stands for the terms **O**paque, **D**ense, and **I**ntense which help to recall the specific words used to describe a bright structure in radiographs, CTs, and MRI, respectively. For X-rays bone is radio-opaque and air is radio-lucent. For CTs bone or acute haemorrhage is hyperdense and CSF or brain ischaemia is hypodense. In T1W MRIs fat is hyperintense and CSF is hypodense. In T2W MRIs CSF is hyperdense and white matter is hypodense. Note that a bright structure in an ultrasound is hyperechoic.
"F1," **F**ormula **1**, helps one remember that Fat is hyperintense in T**1**-weighted images.
"WW2," **W**orld **W**ar **2**, for the fact that **W**ater is "**W**hite" in T**2**-weighted images.

Diffusion weighted imaging

Diffusion weighted imaging provides information about the degree of Brownian motion of water molecules in various tissues. There is relatively free diffusion in extracellular spaces and more restricted diffusion in intracellular spaces. In tumors and infarcted tissue, there is an increase in intracellular fluid water molecules compared with the extracellular fluid environment resulting in overall increased restricted diffusion, and therefore identification of abnormal from normal tissue.

Diffusion tensor imaging

Diffusion tensor imaging (DTI) uses the principle of anisotropic diffusion. Anisotropy denotes the directional dependence of diffusion of water molecules. It permits visualization of white matter tracts.

Tractography

Fiber tractography is a three-dimensional reconstruction method for assessment of the neural tracts. Fibers are color coded according to their directions (Fig. 1.10C).

Functional MRI

Functional MRI (fMRI) is a technique used to obtain functional information by visualizing cortical activity. It is based on the principle of blood-oxygen-level-dependent [BOLD] contrast. The neuronal activity of the brain can be indirectly visualized based on the hemodynamic response referred to as neurovascular coupling. fMRI is limited to visualization of gray matter.

Nuclear medicine imaging

Nuclear medicine involves imaging using gamma rays, which are another type of electromagnetic radiation. The important difference between gamma rays and X-rays is that gamma rays are produced from within the nucleus of an atom when an unstable nucleus decays, whereas X-rays are produced by bombarding an atom with electrons.

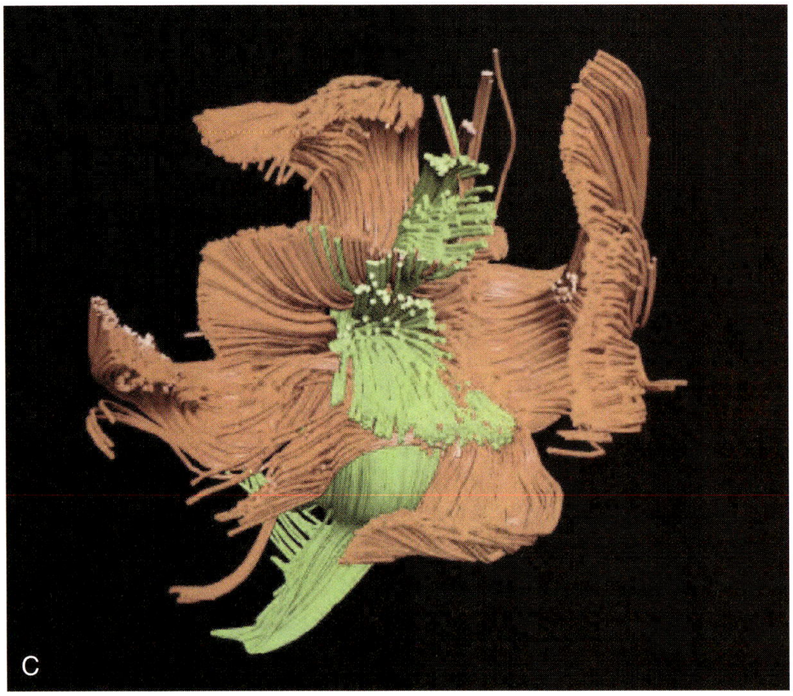

Fig. 1.10 (C) Reconstruction of the short and long connections of the hand region using advanced diffusion tractography. *Source:* Image courtesy of Dr Marco Catani, originally published in Catani M, Dell'Acqua F, Vergani F, et al.; Short frontal lobe connections of the human brain. 2012 *Cortex* 48:273–91.

For an area to be visualized, the patient must receive a gamma ray emitter, which must have a number of properties to be useful, including:

- A reasonable half-life (e.g., 6–24 hours)
- An easily measurable gamma ray
- Energy deposition in as low a dose as possible in the patient's tissues

The most commonly used radionuclide (radioisotope) is technetium-99m. This may be injected as a technetium salt or combined with other complex molecules. For example, by combining technetium-99m with methylene diphosphonate (MDP), a radiopharmaceutical is produced. When injected into the body, this radiopharmaceutical specifically binds to bone, allowing assessment of the skeleton. Similarly, combining technetium-99m with other compounds permits assessment of other parts of the body, for example the urinary tract and cerebral blood flow.

Depending on how the radiopharmaceutical is absorbed, distributed, metabolized, and excreted by the body after injection, images are obtained using a gamma camera (Fig. 1.11).

Positron emission tomography

Positron emission tomography (PET) is an imaging modality for detecting positron-emitting radionuclides. A positron is an anti-electron, which is a positively charged particle of antimatter. Positrons are emitted from the decay of proton-rich radionuclides. Most of these radionuclides are made in a cyclotron and have extremely short half-lives.

The most commonly used PET radionuclide is fluorodeoxyglucose (FDG) labeled with fluorine-18 (a positron emitter). Tissues that are actively metabolizing glucose take up this compound, and the resulting localized high concentration of this molecule compared to background emission is detected as a "hot spot."

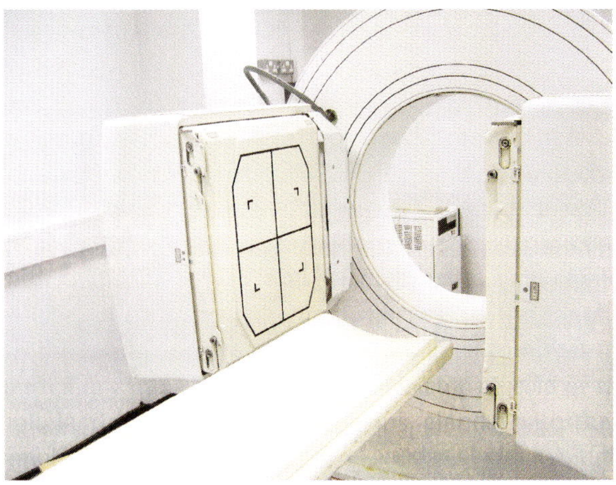

Fig. 1.11 A gamma camera.

PET has become an important imaging modality in the detection of cancer and the assessment of its treatment and recurrence (Fig. 6.49C).

Single photon emission computed tomography

Single photon emission computed tomography (SPECT) is an imaging modality for detecting gamma rays emitted from the decay of injected radionuclides such as technetium-99m, iodine-123, or iodine-131. The rays are detected by a 360-degree rotating camera, which allows the construction of 3D images. SPECT can be used to diagnose a wide range of disease conditions such as coronary artery disease and bone fractures.

Electromyography

Electromyography (EMG) is the recording of electrical activity in muscle. It can distinguish myopathic from neurogenic muscle wasting and weakness. It can detect abnormalities such as chronic denervation or fasciculations in clinically normal muscle. EMG is an obligatory investigation in motor neuron disease to demonstrate the widespread denervation and fasciculation required for secure diagnosis. EMG is a diagnostic procedure to assess the health of muscles and the nerve cells that control them (motor neurons). EMG results can reveal nerve dysfunction, muscle dysfunction, or problems with nerve-to-muscle signal transmission. An EMG uses tiny devices called electrodes to translate these signals into graphs, sounds, or numerical values that are then interpreted by a specialist. During a needle EMG, a needle electrode inserted directly into a muscle records the electrical activity in that muscle. A nerve conduction study, another part of an EMG, uses electrode stickers applied to the skin (surface electrodes) to measure the speed and strength of signals traveling between two or more points.

IMAGE INTERPRETATION

Imaging is necessary in most clinical specialties to diagnose pathological changes to tissues. It is paramount to appreciate what is normal and what is abnormal. An appreciation of how the image is obtained, what the normal variations are, and technical considerations is necessary to obtain a radiological diagnosis. Without understanding the anatomy of the region imaged, it is impossible to comment on the abnormal.

Plain radiography

Plain radiographs are undoubtedly the most common form of image obtained in a hospital or local practice. Before interpretation, it is important to know about the imaging technique and the views obtained as standard.

In most instances (apart from chest radiography), the X-ray tube is 1 m away from the X-ray film. The object in question, for example a hand or a foot, is placed upon the film. When describing subject placement for radiography, the part closest to the X-ray tube is usually referred to as "anterior" and that closest to the film is referred to as "posterior." It is described as an anteroposterior (AP) View.

When X-rays are viewed on a viewing box, the right side of the patient is placed to the observer's left; therefore, the observer views the radiograph as though looking at a patient who is in the anatomical position and facing the observer (Fig. 6.49A).

Chest radiograph

The chest radiograph is one of the most commonly requested plain radiographs. An image is taken with the patient erect and placed postero-anteriorly (PA chest radiograph); that is, with the patient's back closest to the X-ray tube. This reduces the magnification of the heart shadow due to the effect of beam divergence and magnification of structures close to the X-ray tube.

Occasionally, when patients are too unwell to stand erect, films are obtained on the bed in an AP position. These films are less standardized than PA films, and caution should always be taken when interpreting AP radiographs.

The plain chest radiograph should always be checked for quality. Film markers should be placed on the appropriate side. (Occasionally patients have dextrocardia, which may be misinterpreted if the film marker is placed inappropriately.) A good-quality chest radiograph will demonstrate the lungs, cardiomediastinal contour, diaphragm, ribs, and peripheral soft tissues.

Abdominal radiograph

Plain abdominal radiographs are obtained in the AP supine position. Occasionally an erect plain abdominal radiograph is obtained when small bowel obstruction is suspected.

Gastrointestinal contrast examinations

High-density contrast medium is ingested to opacify the esophagus, stomach, small bowel, and large bowel. The bowel is insufflated with air (or carbon dioxide) to provide a double-contrast study. In many countries, endoscopy has superseded upper gastrointestinal imaging, but the mainstay of imaging the large bowel is the double-contrast barium enema. Typically the patient needs to undergo bowel preparation, in which powerful cathartics are used to empty the bowel. At the time of the examination a small tube is placed into the rectum and a barium suspension is run into the large bowel. The patient is made to roll around so that the contrast passes through the entire large bowel. The contrast is emptied and air is passed through the same tube to insufflate the large bowel. A thin layer of barium coats the normal mucosa, allowing mucosal detail to be visualized (see Fig. 1.4A).

Urological contrast studies

Intravenous urography is the standard investigation for assessing the urinary tract. Intravenous contrast medium is injected, and images are obtained as the medium is excreted through the kidneys. A series of films are obtained during this period from immediately after the injection up to approximately 20 minutes later, when the bladder is full of contrast medium.

This series of radiographs demonstrates the kidneys, ureters, and bladder and enables assessment of the retroperitoneum and other structures that may press on the urinary tract.

Computed tomography

Computed tomography is the preferred terminology rather than computerized tomography, though both terms are used interchangeably by physicians.

It is important for the student to understand the presentation of images. Most images are acquired in the axial plane and viewed such that the observer looks from below and upward toward the head (from the foot of the bed). By implication:

- The right side of the patient is on the left side of the image
- The uppermost border of the image is anterior

Many patients are given oral and intravenous contrast media to differentiate bowel loops from other abdominal organs and to assess the vascularity of normal anatomical structures. When intravenous contrast is given, in the initial images there is **arterial enhancement**. As the time is delayed between injection and image acquisition, a **venous phase** and an **equilibrium phase** are also obtained.

The great advantage of CT scanning is the ability to extend and compress the gray scale to visualize the bones, soft tissues, and visceral organs. Altering the window settings and window centering provides the physician with specific information about these structures.

Magnetic resonance imaging

There is no doubt that MRI has revolutionized the understanding and interpretation of the brain and its coverings. Furthermore, it has significantly altered the practice of musculoskeletal medicine and surgery. Images can be obtained in any plane and in most sequences. Typically the images are viewed using the same principles as CT. Intravenous contrast agents are also used to further enhance tissue contrast. Typically, MRI contrast agents contain paramagnetic substances (e.g., gadolinium and manganese).

Nuclear medicine imaging

Most nuclear medicine images are functional studies. Images are usually interpreted directly from a computer, and a series of representative films are obtained for clinical use.

SAFETY IN IMAGING

Whenever a patient undergoes an X-ray or nuclear medicine investigation, a dose of radiation is given (Table 1.1). As a general principle, it is expected that the dose given is as low as reasonably possible for a diagnostic image to be obtained. Numerous laws govern the amount of radiation exposure that a patient can undergo for a variety of procedures, and these are monitored to prevent any excess or additional dosage. Whenever a radiograph is booked, the clinician ordering the procedure must appreciate its necessity and understand the dose given to the patient to ensure that the benefits significantly outweigh the risks.

Imaging modalities such as ultrasound and MRI are ideal because they do not impart significant risk to the patient. Moreover, ultrasound imaging is the modality of choice for assessing the fetus.

Any imaging device is expensive, and consequently the more complex the imaging technique (e.g., MRI) the more expensive the investigation. Investigations must be carried out judiciously, based on a sound clinical history and examination, for which an understanding of anatomy is vital.

Table 1.1 The approximate dosage of radiation exposure as an order of magnitude

Examination	Typical effective dose millisievert (mSv)	Equivalent duration of background exposure
Chest radiograph	0.02	3 days
Abdomen	1.00	6 months
Intravenous urography	2.50	14 months
CT scan of head	2.30	1 year
CT scan of abdomen and pelvis	10.00	4.5 years

Body systems

SKELETAL SYSTEM

The skeleton can be divided into two **subgroups**, the axial skeleton and the appendicular skeleton. The axial skeleton consists of the bones of the skull (cranium), vertebral column, ribs, and sternum, whereas the appendicular skeleton consists of the bones of the upper and lower limbs (Fig. 1.12A).

The skeletal system consists of cartilage and bone.

Cartilage

Cartilage is an avascular form of connective tissue consisting of extracellular fibers embedded in a matrix that contains cells localized in small cavities. The amount and kind of extracellular fibers in the matrix vary depending on the type of cartilage. In heavy weight-bearing areas or areas prone to pulling forces, the amount of collagen is greatly increased and the cartilage is almost inextensible. In contrast, in areas where weight-bearing demands and stress are less, cartilage containing elastic fibers and fewer collagen fibers is common. The **functions** of cartilage are to:

- Support soft tissues
- Provide a smooth, gliding surface for bone articulations at joints
- Enable the development and growth of long bones

There are three **types** of cartilage:

- Hyaline—most common; matrix contains a moderate amount of collagen fibers (e.g., articular surfaces of bones)
- Elastic—matrix contains collagen fibers along with a large number of elastic fibers (e.g., external ear)
- Fibrocartilage—matrix contains a limited number of cells and ground substance amidst a substantial amount of collagen fibers (e.g., intervertebral discs)

Cartilage is nourished by diffusion and has no blood vessels, lymphatics, or nerves.

Bone

Bone is a calcified, living, connective tissue that forms the majority of the skeleton. It consists of an intercellular calcified matrix, which also contains collagen fibers, and several types of cells within the matrix. Bones **function** as:

- Supportive structures for the body
- Protectors of vital organs
- Reservoirs of calcium and phosphorus

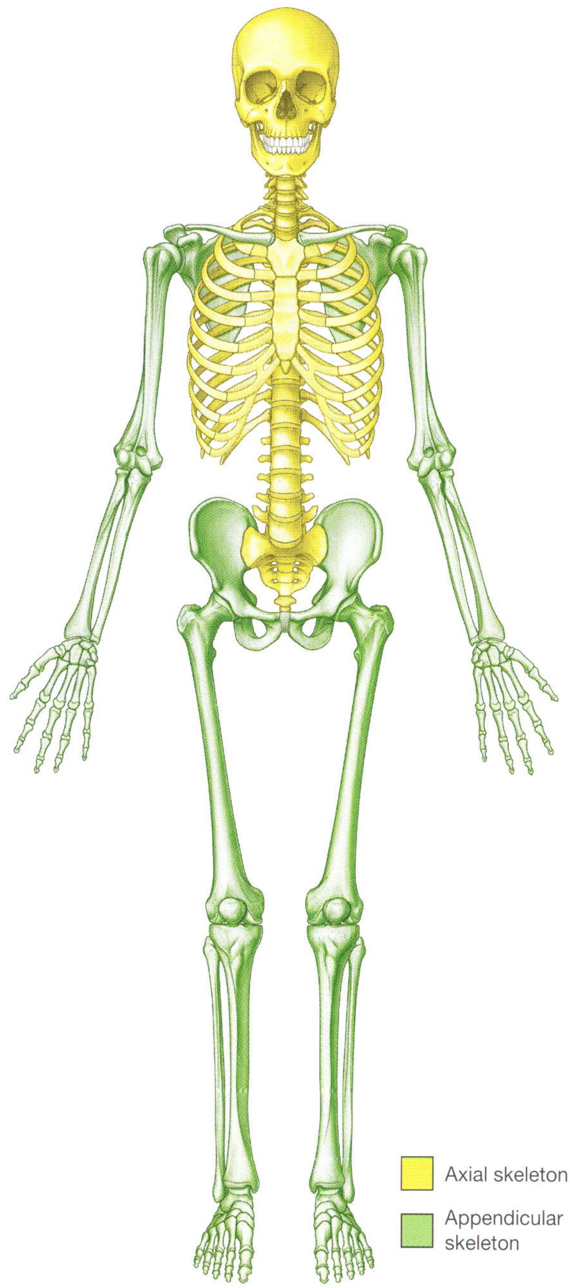

Fig. 1.12 (A) The axial skeleton and the appendicular skeleton.

- Levers on which muscles act to produce movement
- Containers for blood-producing cells

There are two **types** of bone based on structure, compact and spongy (trabecular or cancellous). Compact bone is dense bone that forms the outer shell of all bones including spongy bone. Spongy bone consists of spicules of bone enclosing cavities containing blood-forming cells (marrow). **Classification** of bones is by shape.

- Long bones are tubular (e.g., humerus in upper limb; femur in lower limb).

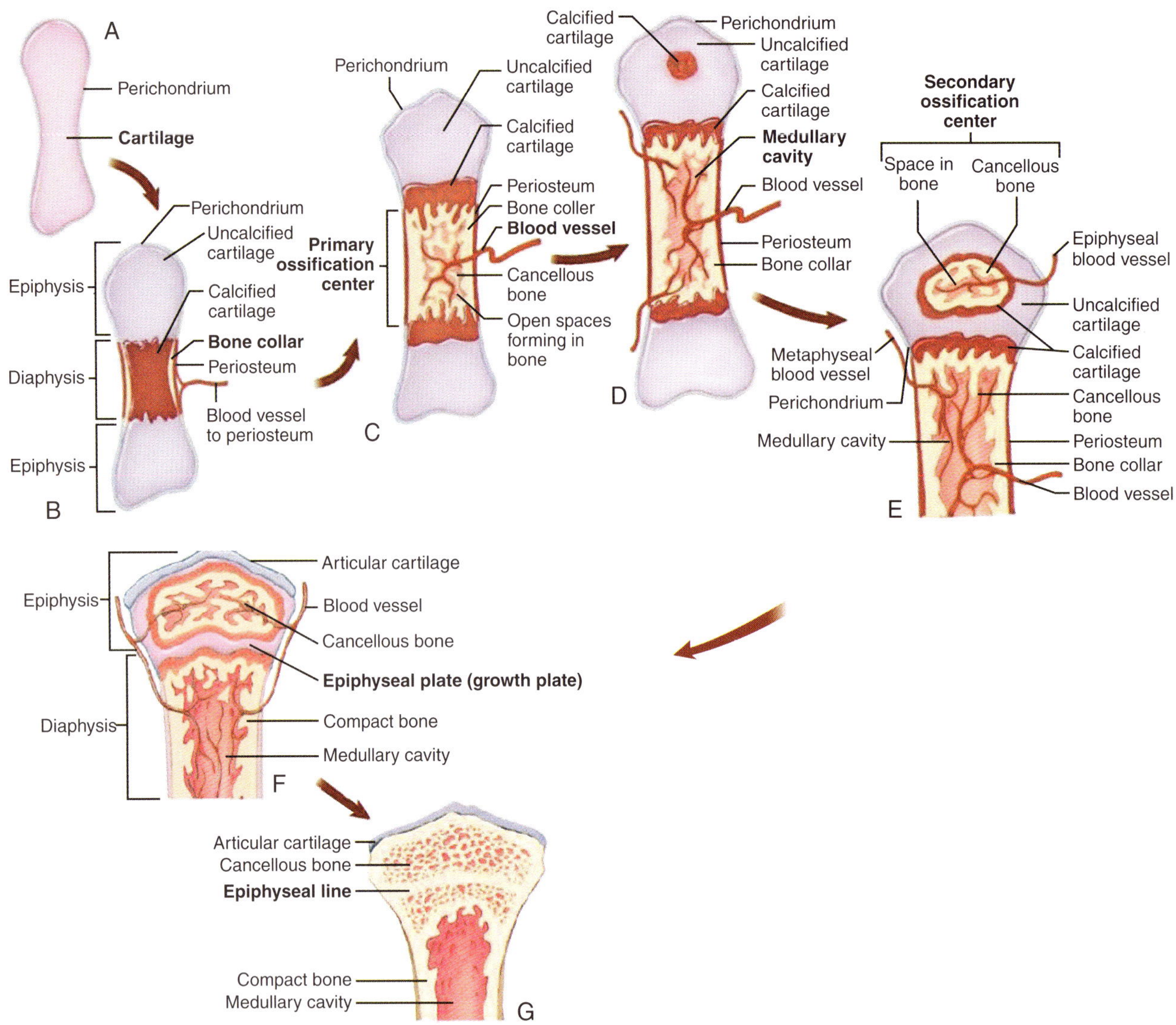

Fig. 1.12 (B) Development of a long bone in sequence from **(A)** to **(G)**. *Source:* Kevin T. Patton , Gary A. Thibodeau, Matthew M. Douglas. Essentials of Anatomy & Physiology: Skeletal Tissues. MOSBY, 2012: 136-151.

- Short bones are cuboidal (e.g., bones of the wrist and ankle).
- Flat bones consist of two compact bone plates separated by spongy bone (e.g., skull).
- Irregular bones are bones with various shapes (e.g., bones of the face).
- Sesamoid bones are round or oval bones that develop in tendons (LD 1.1).

In the clinic

Accessory and sesamoid bones

These are extra bones that are not usually found as part of the normal skeleton, but can exist as a normal variant in many people. They are typically found in multiple locations in the wrist and hands, ankles and feet (Fig. 1.13). These should not be mistaken for fractures on imaging.

Sesamoid bones are embedded within tendons, the largest of which is the patella. There are many other sesamoids in the body particularly in tendons of the hands and feet, and most frequently in flexor tendons of the thumb and big toe.

Degenerative and inflammatory changes of, as well as mechanical stresses on, the accessory bones and sesamoids can cause pain, which can be treated with physiotherapy and targeted steroid injections, but in some severe cases it may be necessary to surgically remove the bone.

Bones are vascular and are innervated. Generally, an adjacent artery gives off a nutrient artery, usually one per bone, which directly enters the internal cavity of the bone and supplies the marrow, spongy bone, and inner layers of compact bone (Fig. 1.12B). In addition, all bones are covered externally, except in the area of a joint where articular

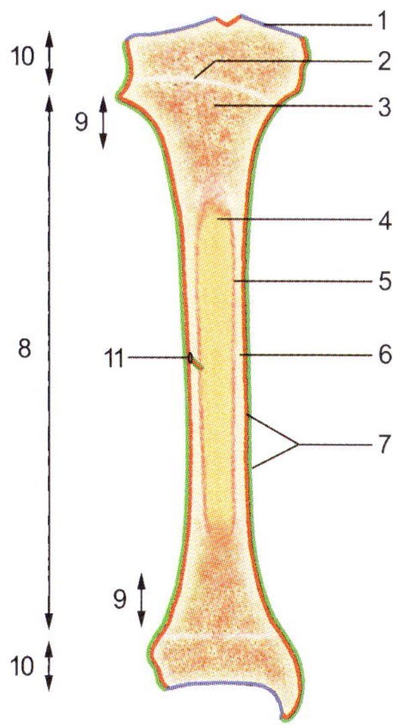

LD 1.1 Parts of a long bone.

Questions

LD 1.1A Name the structures indicated by the labels.

LD 1.1B Name the blood vessels found at numbers 5, 7, 9, 10, and 11.

LD 1.1C What are the ways of classifying bone?

LD 1.1D Which classification of bone is shown by numbers 3 and 6?

Answers:

LD 1.1A The structures indicated by the labels are

1. Articular cartilage
2. Epiphyseal line
3. Spongy bone with red bone marrow
4. Yellow bone marrow
5. Endosteum
6. Compact bone
7. Vascular and fibrous layers of periosteum
8. Diaphysis
9. Metaphysis
10. Epiphysis
11. Nutrient foramen

LD 1.1B The blood vessels found at labels 5, 7, 9, 10, and 11 are

5. Endosteal vessels
7. Periosteal vessels
9. Metaphyseal vessels
10. Epiphyseal vessels
11. Nutrient vessels

LD 1.1C The ways of classifying bone are according to:

i) Shape—long, short, flat, irregular, sesamoid, and pneumatic
ii) Histology— spongy and compact
iii) Development— membranous and cartilaginous
iv) Location—axial and appendicular

LD 1.1D The classification of bone depicted by numbers 3 and 6 is the classification according to histology.

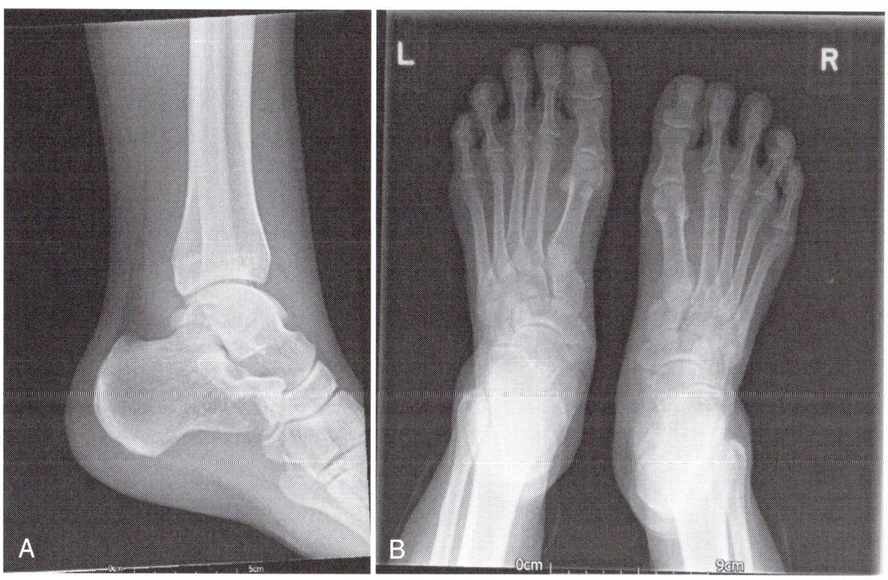

Fig. 1.13 Accessory and sesamoid bones. **(A)** Radiograph of the ankle region showing an accessory bone (os trigonum). **(B)** Radiograph of the feet showing numerous sesamoid bones and an accessory bone (os naviculare).

cartilage is present, by a fibrous connective tissue membrane called the periosteum, which has the unique capability of forming new bone. This membrane receives blood vessels, called periosteal vessels, which supply the outer layers of compact bone. A bone stripped of its periosteum will not survive. Nerves accompany the vessels that supply the bone and the periosteum. Most of the nerves passing into the internal cavity with the nutrient artery are vasomotor fibers that regulate blood flow. Bone itself has few sensory nerve fibers. On the contrary, the periosteum is supplied with numerous sensory nerve fibers and is very sensitive to any type of injury.

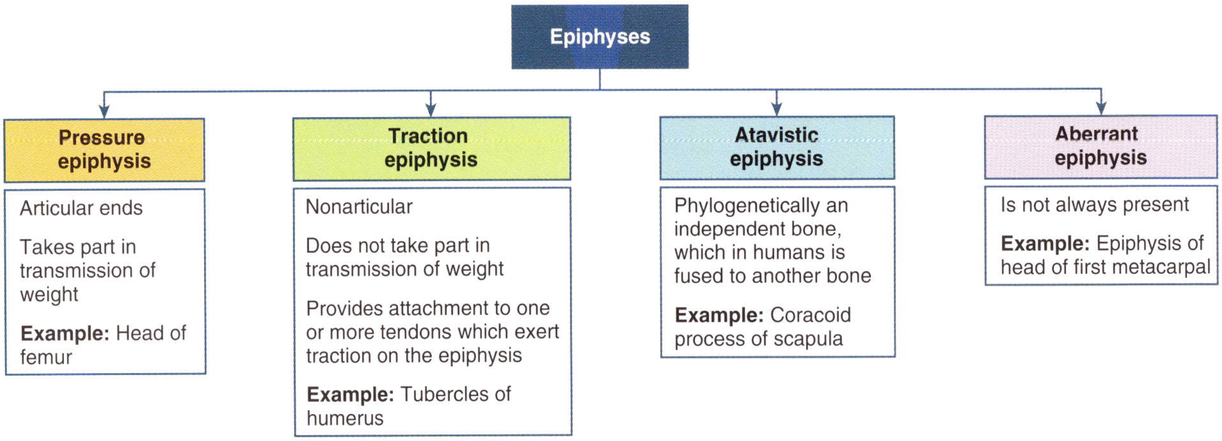

Flowchart 1.1 Types of epiphyses.

Developmentally, all bones come from mesenchyme by either intramembranous ossification, in which mesenchymal models of bones undergo ossification (e.g., cranial vault), or endochondral ossification, in which cartilaginous models of bones develop from mesenchyme and undergo ossification (e.g., long bones, Fig. 1.12).

Ossification

The parts of a long bone are the shaft or diaphysis, and the ends or epiphyses. The metaphysis is the epiphyseal end of the diaphysis. Each of these parts has blood vessels (Fig. 1.12).

The point from where ossification begins is called a center of ossification. A primary ossification center is the first area of the bone to start ossifying and occurs in the diaphysis of long bones. A secondary ossification center is one which appears after the primary ossification center and occurs in the epiphysis of long bones.

The primary ossification center in the diaphysis usually is single (an exception is the clavicle which has two primary ossification centers) and it usually appears before birth (exceptions are the cuneiform and navicular). The secondary ossification centers usually are multiple (an exception is the lower end of femur which has only one) and it usually appears after birth. The **law of ossification** states that the secondary center that appears first fuses last and the center which appears last fuses first. The fibula is one bone that violates the law of ossification. The lower end of fibula appears first and fuses first because it is a pressure epiphysis. The upper end of fibula appears last and fuses last because it is the growing end of the bone.

An epiphysis of a long bone may be classified as a pressure epiphysis, traction epiphysis, atavistic epiphysis, or aberrant epiphysis (Flowchart 1.1).

Early clinical exposure

Determination of skeletal age

Throughout life, the bones develop in a predictable way to form the skeletally mature adult at the end of puberty. In western countries, skeletal maturity tends to occur between the age of 20 and 25 years. However, this may well vary according to geography and socioeconomic conditions. Skeletal maturity will also be determined by genetic factors and disease states.

Up until the age of skeletal maturity, bony growth and development follows a typically predictable ordered state, which can be measured through ultrasound, plain radiographs, or MRI scanning. Typically, the nondominant (left) hand is radiographed, and the radiograph is compared to a series of standard radiographs. From these images, the bone age can be determined (Fig. 1.14).

In certain disease states, such as malnutrition and hypothyroidism, bony maturity may be slow. If the skeletal bone age is significantly less than the patient's true age, urgent treatment may be required. Ossification centers always appear in a specific sequence. A **useful mnemonic** is to correlate the age of a child in years and the number of centers of ossification of carpal bones visible

Early clinical exposure—cont'd

on a radiograph. At 2 years, there are two carpal bones visible; at 3 years, there are three carpals visible; at 4, there are four carpals visible; and at 5, there are five carpals visible (Fig. 1.14).

In the healthy individual, the bone age accurately represents the true age of the patient and can be used to determine the true age of the subject, which may have medicolegal importance.

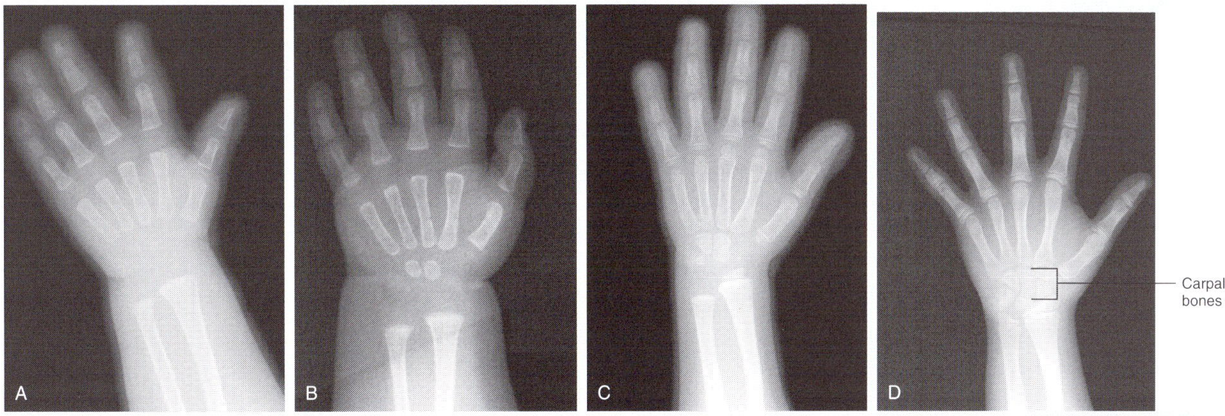

Fig. 1.14 A developmental series of radiographs showing the progressive ossification of carpal (wrist) bones from 3 **(A)** to 10 **(D)** years of age.

Early clinical exposure

Bone marrow transplants

The bone marrow serves an important function. There are two types of bone marrow, the red marrow (otherwise known as myeloid tissue) and the yellow marrow. Red blood cells, platelets, and most white blood cells arise from within the red marrow. In the yellow marrow, a few white cells are made; however, this marrow is dominated by large fat globules (producing its yellow appearance) (Fig. 1.15).

From birth, most of the body's marrow is red; however, as the subject ages, more red marrow is converted into yellow marrow within the medulla of the long and flat bones.

Bone marrow contains two types of stem cells: (1) hemopoietic stem cells give rise to the white blood cells, red blood cells, and platelets, and (2) mesenchymal stem cells differentiate into structures that form bone, cartilage, and muscle.

There are a number of diseases that may involve the bone marrow, including infection and malignancy. In patients who develop a bone marrow malignancy (e.g., leukemia), it may be possible to harvest nonmalignant cells from the patient's bone marrow or cells from another person's bone marrow. The patient's own marrow can be destroyed with chemotherapy or radiation and the new cells infused. This treatment is called bone marrow transplantation.

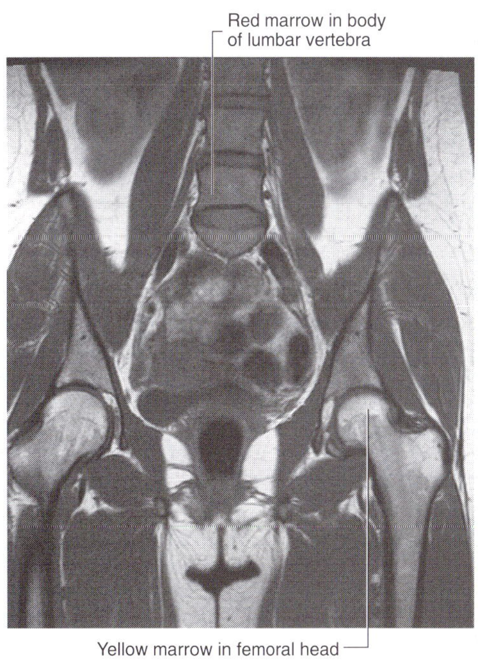

Fig. 1.15 T1-weighted magnetic resonance image in the coronal plane, demonstrating the relatively high signal intensity returned from the femoral heads and proximal femoral necks, consistent with yellow marrow. In this young patient, the vertebral bodies return an intermediate darker signal that represents red marrow. There is relatively little fat in these vertebrae, hence the lower signal return.

Early clinical exposure

Bone fractures

Fractures occur in normal bone because of abnormal load or stress, in which the bone gives way (Fig. 1.16B). Fractures may even occur in bone that is of poor quality (osteoporosis) when subjected to a normal stress.

In children whose bones are still developing, fractures may occur across the growth plate or across the shaft. These shaft fractures typically involve partial cortical disruption, similar to breaking a branch of a young tree; hence, they are termed "greenstick" fractures (Fig. 1.16A).

After a fracture has occurred, the natural response is to heal the fracture. Between the fracture margins, a blood clot is formed into which new vessels grow. A jelly-like matrix is formed, and further migration of collagen-producing cells occurs. On this soft tissue framework, calcium hydroxyapatite is produced by osteoblasts and forms insoluble crystals. Later, bone matrix is laid down. As more bone is produced, a callus can be demonstrated forming across the fracture site.

Treatment of fractures requires a fracture line reduction. If this cannot be maintained in a plaster of Paris cast, it may require internal or external fixation with screws and metal rods Fig. (1.16C).

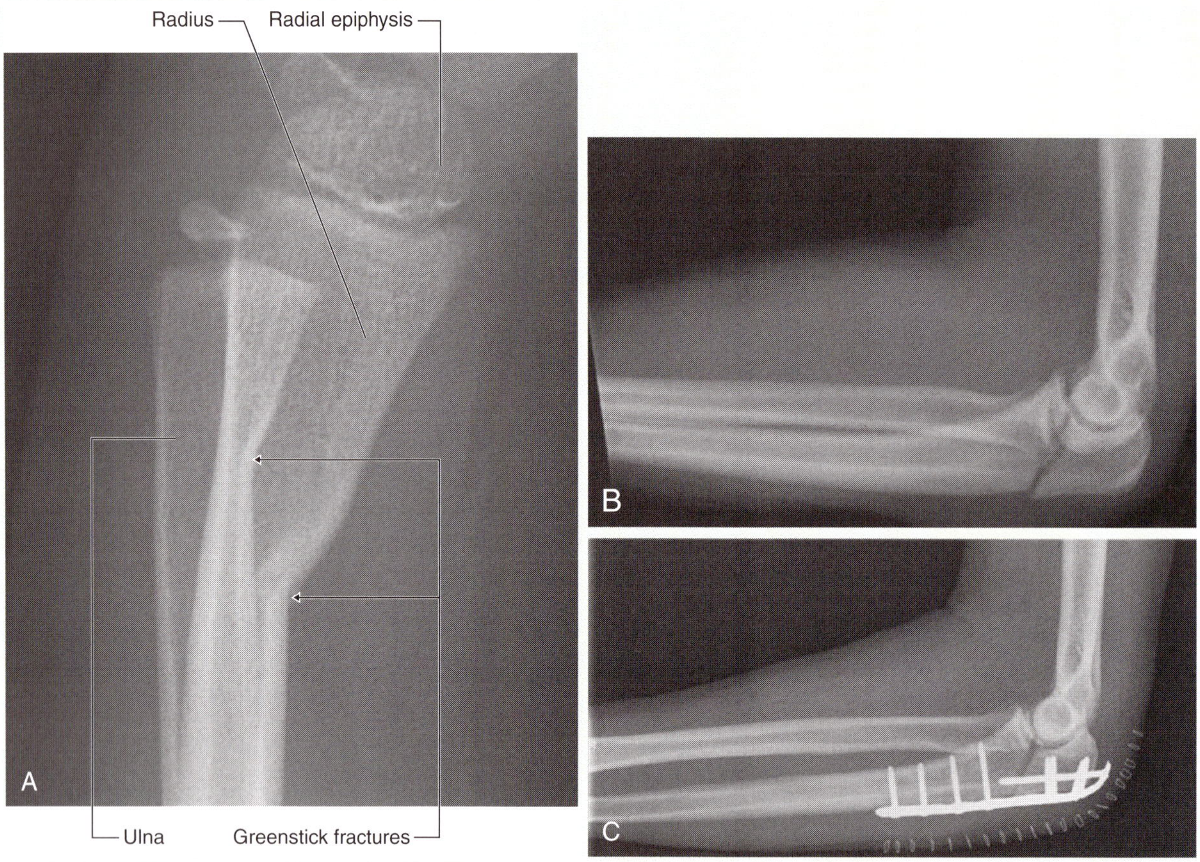

Fig. 1.16 Radiograph, lateral view, showing **(A)** greenstick fractures of the distal radius and distal ulna, **(B)** fracture of the ulna at the elbow joint, and **(C)** repair of this fracture using internal fixation with a plate and multiple screws.

Early clinical exposure

Avascular necrosis

Avascular necrosis is cellular death of bone resulting from a temporary or permanent loss of blood supply to that bone. Avascular necrosis may occur in a variety of medical conditions, some of which have an etiology that is less than clear. A typical cause for avascular necrosis is a fracture across the femoral neck in an elderly patient. In these patients, there is loss of continuity of the cortical and medullary blood flow with loss of blood flow deep to the retinacular fibers. This essentially renders the femoral head bloodless; it subsequently undergoes necrosis and collapses. In these patients, it is necessary to replace the femoral head with a prosthesis (Fig. 1.17).

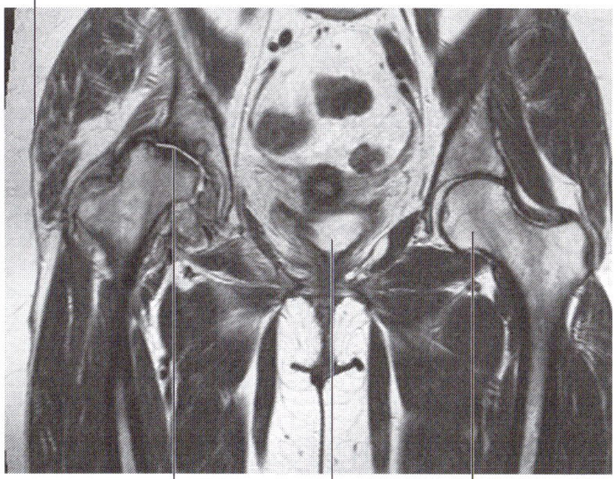

Fig. 1.17 Image of the hip joints demonstrating loss of height of the right femoral head with juxta-articular bony sclerosis and subchondral cyst formation secondary to avascular necrosis. There is also significant wasting of the muscles supporting the hip, which is secondary to disuse and pain.

Early clinical exposure

Osteoporosis

Osteoporosis is a disease in which the bone mineral density is significantly reduced. This renders the bone significantly more at risk of fracture. Typically, osteoporotic fractures occur in the femoral necks, the vertebrae, and the wrist. Although osteoporosis may occur in men, especially elderly men, the typical patients are postmenopausal women. There are a number of risk factors that predispose bones to develop osteoporosis. These factors include poor diet, steroid usage, smoking, and premature ovarian failure. Treatment involves removing underlying potentiating factors, such as improving diet and preventing further bone loss with drug treatment (e.g., vitamin D and calcium supplements; newer treatments include drugs that increase bone mineral density) (Fig. 1.18A and B).

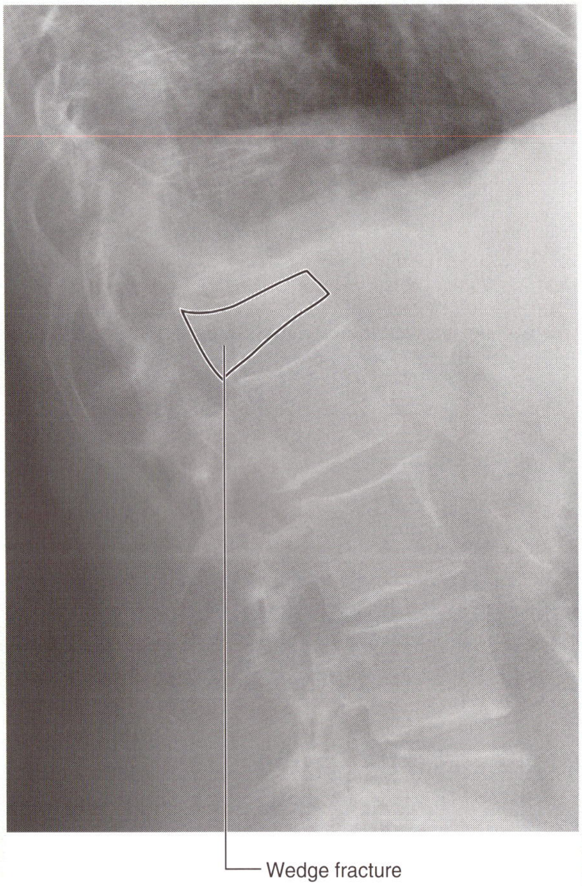

Fig. 1.18 (A) Radiograph of the lumbar region of the vertebral column demonstrating a wedge fracture of the L1 vertebra. This condition is typically seen in patients with osteoporosis.

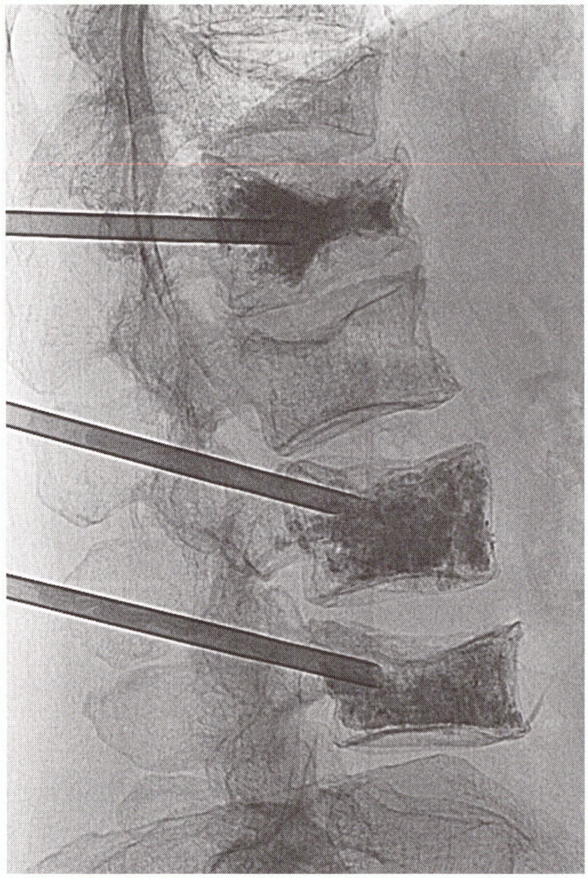

Fig. 1.18 (B) Radiograph of the lumbar region of the vertebral column demonstrating three intrapedicular needles, all of which have been placed into the middle of the vertebral bodies. The high-density material is radiopaque bone cement, which has been injected as a liquid that will harden.

Early clinical exposure

Epiphyseal fractures

As the skeleton develops, there are stages of intense growth typically around the age of 7–10 years and later in puberty. These growth spurts are associated with increased cellular activity around the growth plate and the metaphyseal region. This increase in activity renders the growth plates and metaphyseal regions more vulnerable to injuries, which may occur from dislocation across a growth plate or fracture through a growth plate. Occasionally, an injury may result in growth plate compression, destroying that region of the growth plate, which may result in asymmetrical growth across that joint region. All fractures across the growth plate must be treated with care and expediency, requiring fracture reduction.

Joints

The sites where two skeletal elements come together are termed joints. The two general categories of joints (Fig. 1.19) are those in which:

- The skeletal elements are separated by a cavity (i.e., **synovial joints**)
- There is no cavity and the components are held together by connective tissue (i.e., **solid joints**) (Flowchart 1.2)

Blood vessels that cross a joint and nerves that innervate muscles acting on a joint usually contribute articular branches to that joint.

Synovial joints

Synovial joints are connections between skeletal components where the elements involved are separated by a narrow articular cavity (Fig. 1.20). In addition to containing an articular cavity, these joints have a number of characteristic features.

First, a layer of cartilage, usually **hyaline cartilage**, covers the articulating surfaces of the skeletal elements. In other words, bony surfaces do not normally contact one another directly. As a consequence, when these joints are viewed in normal radiographs, a wide gap seems to separate the adjacent bones because the cartilage that covers the articulating surfaces is more transparent to X-rays than bone.

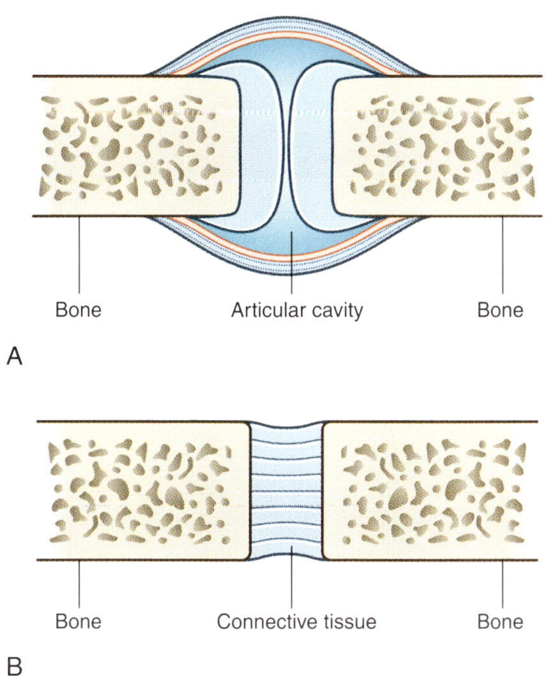

Fig. 1.19 Joints. **(A)** Synovial joint. **(B)** Solid joint.

A second characteristic feature of synovial joints is the presence of a joint capsule consisting of an inner synovial membrane and an outer fibrous membrane.

- The synovial membrane attaches to the margins of the joint surfaces at the interface between the cartilage and bone and encloses the articular cavity. The synovial membrane is highly vascular and produces synovial fluid, which percolates into the articular cavity and lubricates the articulating surfaces. Closed sacs of synovial membrane also occur outside joints, where they form synovial bursae or tendon sheaths. Bursae often intervene between structures, such as tendons and bone, tendons and joints, or skin and bone, and reduce the friction of one structure moving over the other. Tendon sheaths surround tendons and also reduce friction.
- The **fibrous membrane** is formed by dense connective tissue and surrounds and stabilizes the joint. Parts of the fibrous membrane may thicken to form ligaments, which further stabilize the joint. Ligaments outside the capsule usually provide additional reinforcement.

Another common but not universal feature of synovial joints is the presence of additional structures within the area enclosed by the capsule or synovial membrane, such as **articular discs** (usually composed of fibrocartilage), **fat pads**, and **tendons**. Articular discs absorb compression forces, adjust to changes in the contours of joint surfaces during movements, and increase the range of movements that can occur at joints. Fat pads usually occur between the synovial membrane and the capsule and move into and out of regions as joint contours change during movement. Redundant regions of the synovial membrane and fibrous membrane allow for large movements at joints.

Descriptions of synovial joints based on shape and movement

Synovial joints are described based on shape and movement:

- Based on the shape of their articular surfaces, synovial joints are described as plane (flat), hinge, pivot, bicondylar (two sets of contact points), condylar (ellipsoid), saddle, and ball and socket.
- Based on movement, synovial joints are described as uniaxial (movement in one plane), biaxial (movement in two planes), and multiaxial (movement in three planes).

Hinge joints are uniaxial, whereas ball and socket joints are multiaxial (Flowchart 1.2).

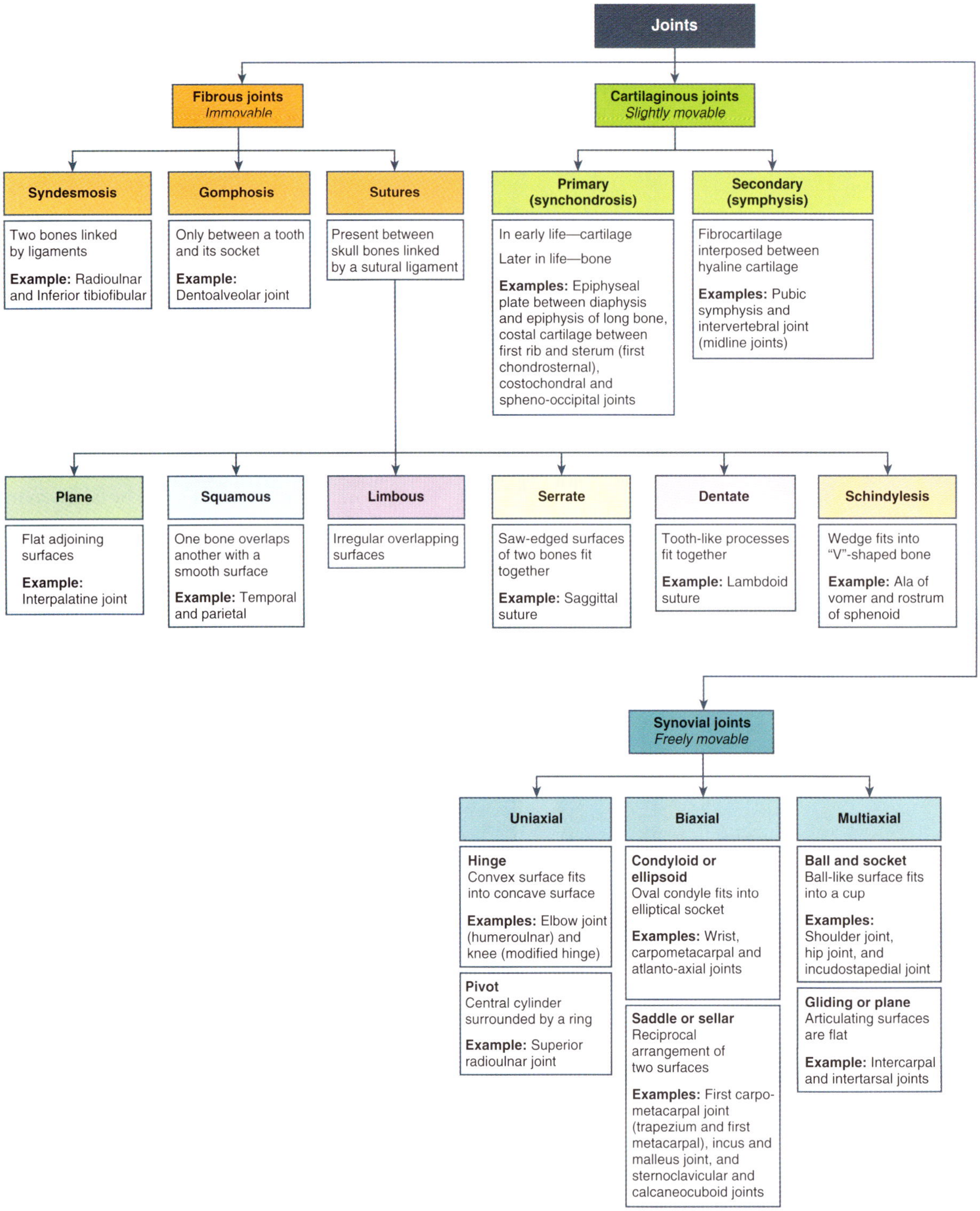

Flowchart 1.2. Types of joints.

Specific types of synovial joints (Fig. 1.21)

- **Plane joints**—allow sliding or gliding movements when one bone moves across the surface of another (e.g., acromioclavicular joint)
- **Hinge joints**—allow movement around one axis that passes transversely through the joint; permit flexion and extension (e.g., elbow [humero-ulnar] joint)
- **Pivot joints**—allow movement around one axis that passes longitudinally along the shaft of the bone; permit rotation (e.g., atlanto-axial joint)
- **Bicondylar joints**—allow movement mostly in one axis with limited rotation around a second axis; formed by two convex condyles that articulate with concave or flat surfaces (e.g., knee joint, Fig. 3.72)

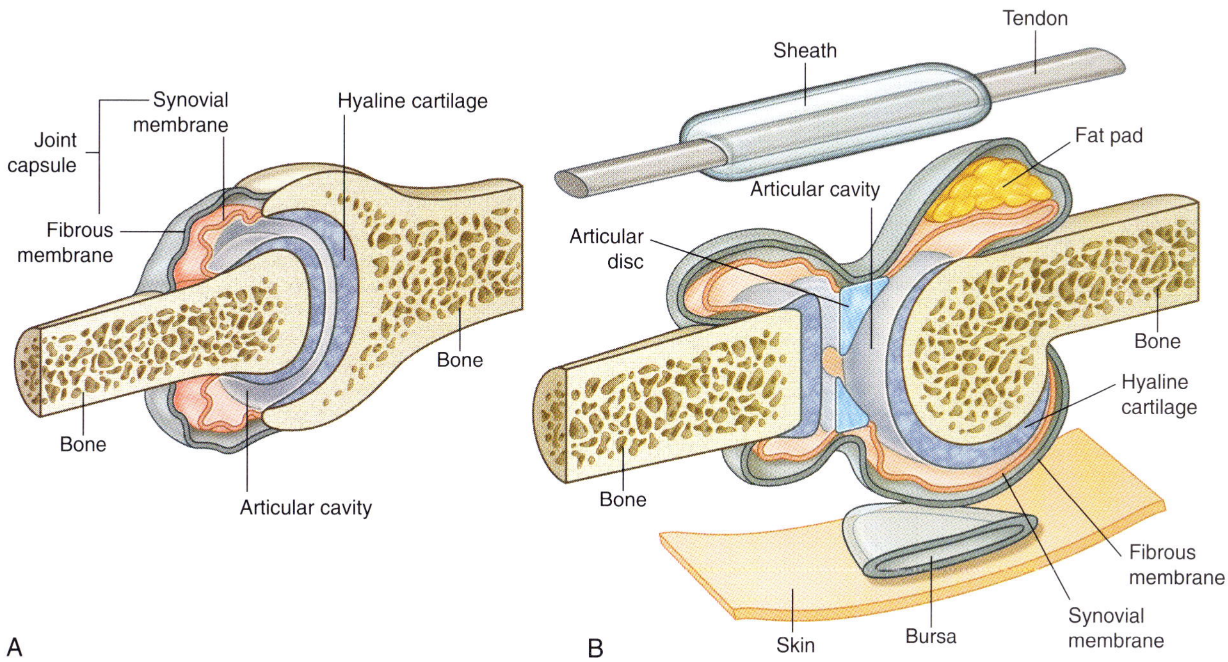

Fig. 1.20 Synovial joints. **(A)** Major features of a synovial joint. **(B)** Accessory structures associated with synovial joints.

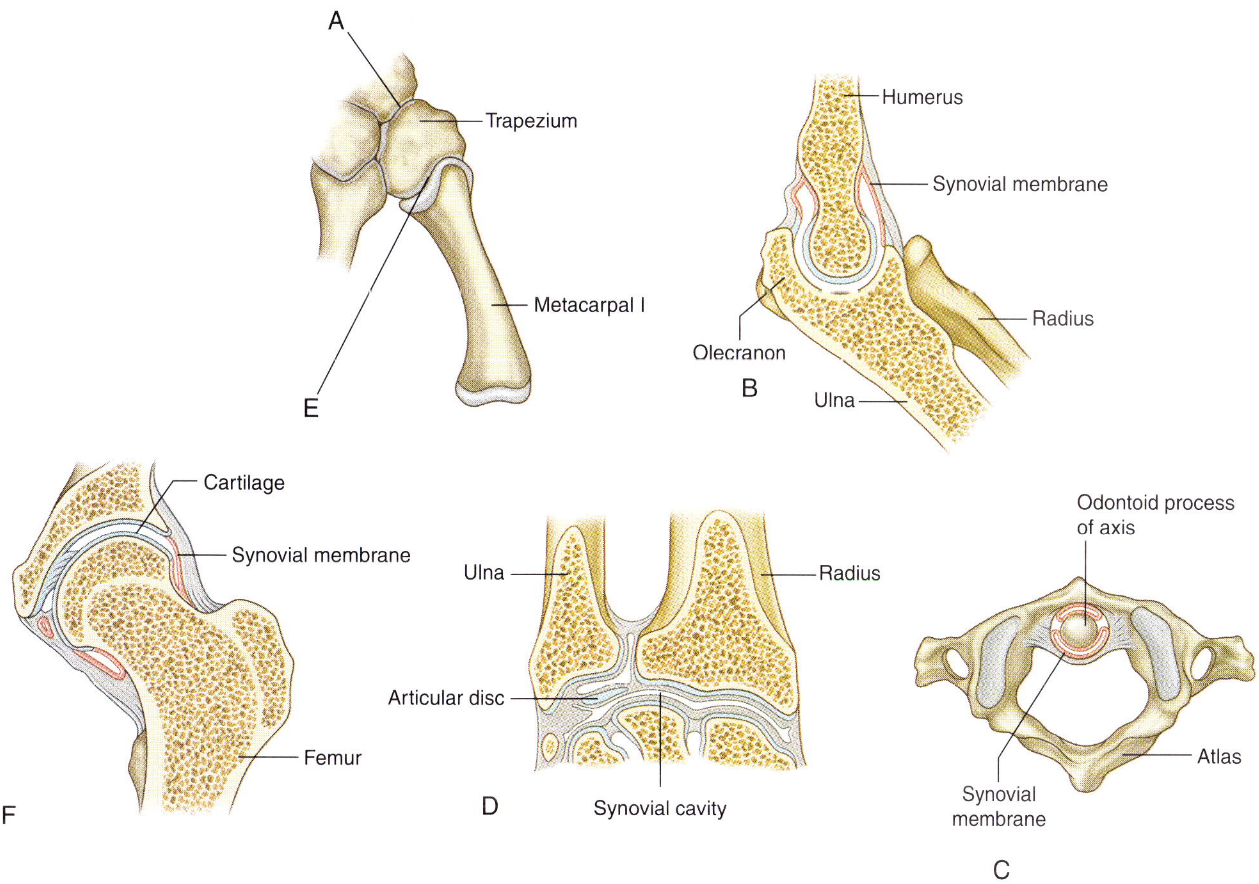

Fig. 1.21 Various types of synovial joints. **(A)** Plane joint (intercarpal joint). **(B)** Hinge or ginglymus (elbow). **(C)** Pivot (atlanto-axial). **(D)** Condylar (wrist). **(E)** Saddle (carpometacarpal of thumb). **(F)** Ball and socket (hip).

- **Condylar (ellipsoid) joints**—allow movement around two axes that are at right angles to each other; permit flexion, extension, abduction, adduction, and circumduction (limited) (e.g., wrist joint)
- **Saddle joints**—allow movement around two axes that are at right angles to each other; the articular surfaces are saddle shaped; permit flexion, extension, abduction, adduction, and circumduction (e.g., carpometacarpal joint of the thumb)
- **Ball and socket joints**—allow movement around multiple axes; permit flexion, extension, abduction, adduction, circumduction, and rotation (e.g., hip joint)

Solid joints

Solid joints are connections between skeletal elements where the adjacent surfaces are linked together either by fibrous connective tissue or by cartilage, usually fibrocartilage (Fig. 1.22). Movements at these joints are more restricted than at synovial joints.

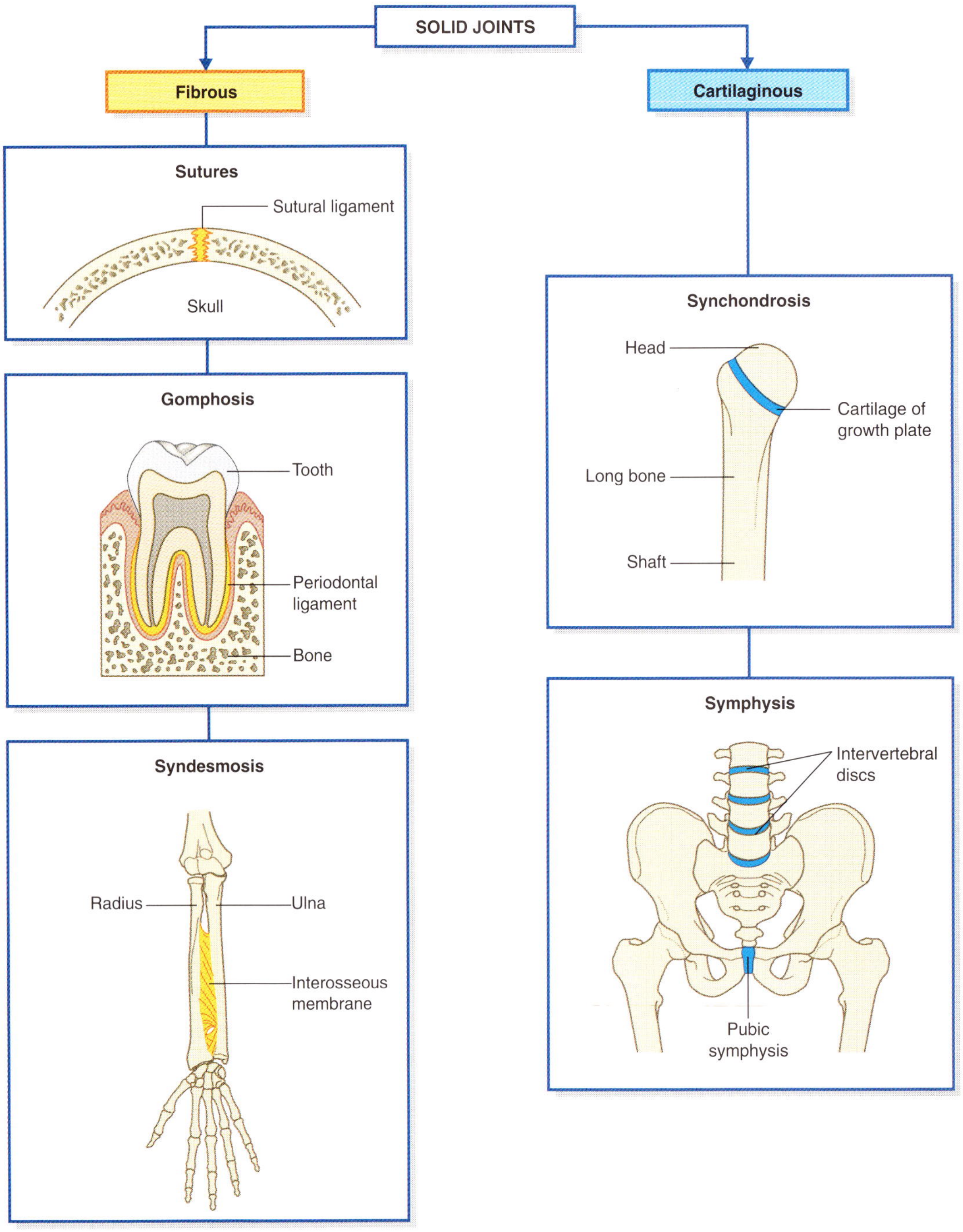

Fig. 1.22 Solid joints.

Fibrous joints include sutures, gomphoses, and syndesmoses (Flowchart 1.2).

- **Sutures** occur only in the skull where adjacent bones are linked by a thin layer of connective tissue termed a *sutural ligament*.
- **Gomphoses** occur only between the teeth and adjacent bone. In these joints, short collagen tissue fibers in the periodontal ligament run between the root of the tooth and the bony socket.
- **Syndesmoses** are joints in which two adjacent bones are linked by a ligament. Examples are the ligamentum flavum, which connects adjacent vertebral laminae, and an interosseous membrane, which links, for example, the radius and ulna in the forearm.

Cartilaginous joints include synchondroses and symphyses.

- **Synchondroses** occur where two ossification centers in a developing bone remain separated by a layer of hyaline cartilage, for example, the growth plate that occurs between the head and shaft of developing long bones. These joints allow bone growth and eventually become completely ossified.
- **Symphyses** occur where two separate bones are interconnected by cartilage, including fibrocartilage. Most of these types of joints occur in the midline and include the pubic symphysis between the two pelvic bones, and intervertebral discs between adjacent vertebrae.

Early clinical exposure

Degenerative joint disease

Degenerative joint disease is commonly known as **osteoarthritis** or osteoarthrosis. The disorder is related to aging but not caused by aging. Typically, there are decreases in water and proteoglycan content within the cartilage. The cartilage becomes more fragile and more susceptible to mechanical disruption (Fig. 1.23). As the cartilage wears, the underlying bone becomes fissured and also thickens. Synovial fluid may be forced into small cracks that appear in the bone's surface, which produces large cysts. Furthermore, reactive juxta-articular bony nodules are formed (osteophytes) (Fig. 1.24). As these processes occur, there is slight deformation, which alters the biomechanical forces through the joint. This in turn creates abnormal stresses, which further disrupt the joint.

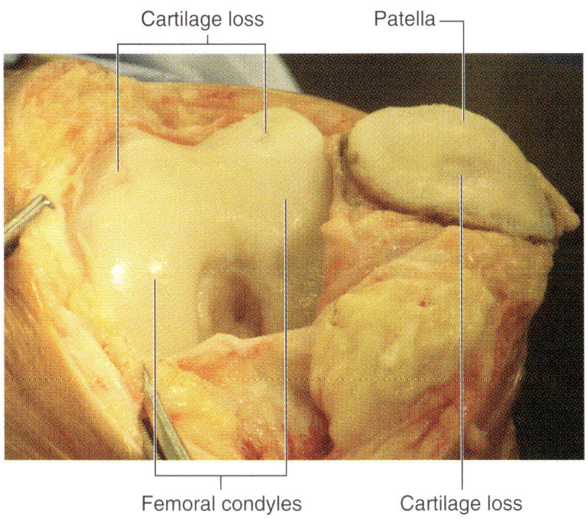

Fig. 1.23 This operative photograph demonstrates the focal areas of cartilage loss in the patella and femoral condyles throughout the knee joint.

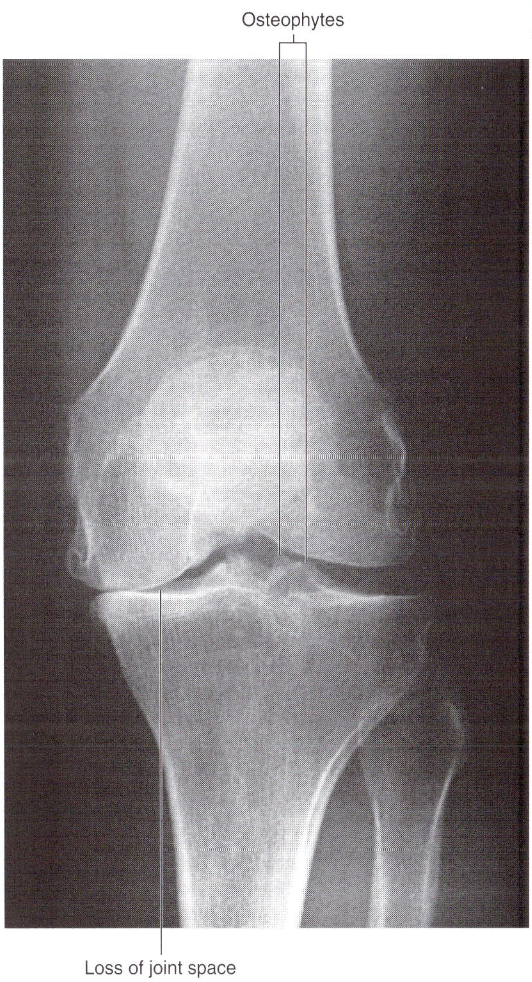

Fig. 1.24 This radiograph demonstrates the loss of joint space in the medial compartment and presence of small spiky osteophytic regions at the medial lateral aspect of the joint.

Continued

Early clinical exposure—cont'd

In the USA, osteoarthritis accounts for up to one-quarter of primary health care visits and is regarded as a significant problem.

The etiology of osteoarthritis is not clear; however, osteoarthritis can occur secondary to other joint diseases, such as rheumatoid arthritis and infection. Overuse of joints and abnormal strains, such as those experienced by people who play sports, often cause one to be more susceptible to chronic joint osteoarthritis.

Various treatments are available, including weight reduction, proper exercise, anti-inflammatory drug treatment, and joint replacement (Fig. 1.25A).

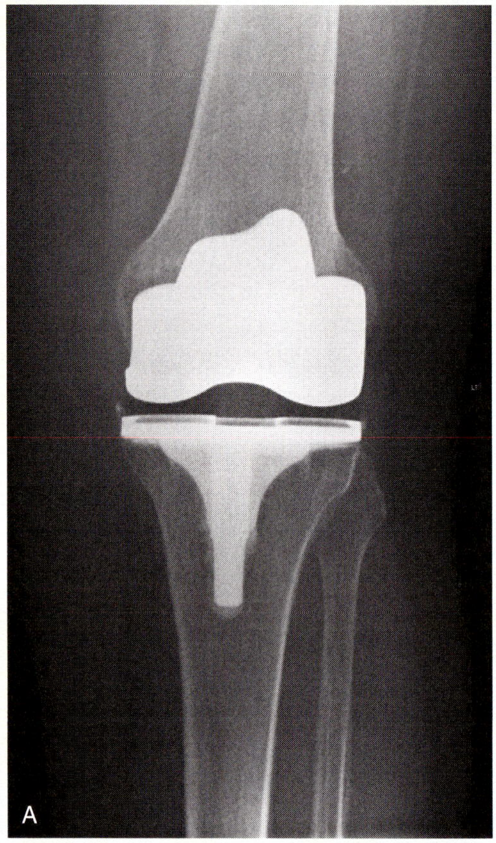

Fig. 1.25 (A) This radiograph shows the position of the prosthesis after knee replacement.

Arthroscopy

Arthroscopy is a technique of visualizing the inside of a joint using a small telescope placed through a tiny incision in the skin. Arthroscopy can be performed in most joints. However, it is most commonly performed in the knee, shoulder, ankle, and hip joints. The elbow joint and wrist joint can also be viewed through the arthroscope.

Arthroscopy allows the surgeon to view the inside of the joint and its contents. Notably, in the knee, the menisci and the ligaments are easily seen, and it is possible using separate puncture sites and specific instruments to remove the menisci and replace the cruciate ligaments. The advantages of arthroscopy are that it is performed through small incisions, it enables patients to quickly recover and return to normal activity, and it only requires either a light anesthetic or regional anesthesia during the procedure (Fig. 1.25B).

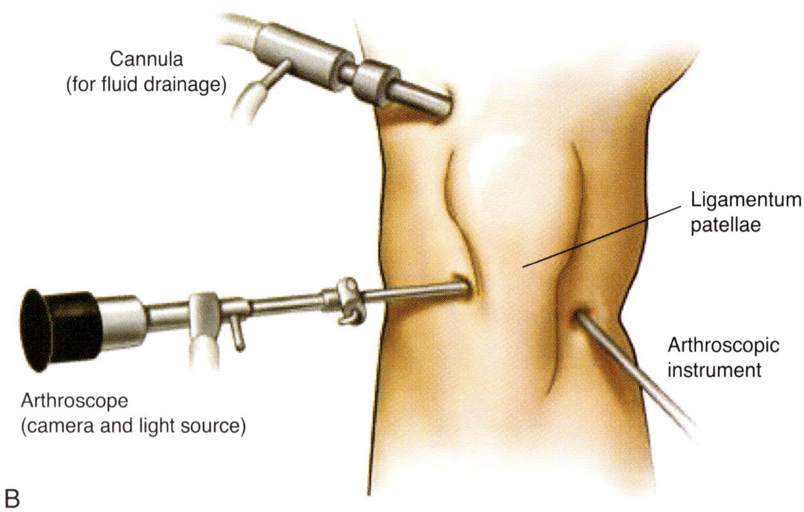

Fig. 1.25 (B) Diagram showing the instruments used for arthroscopy of the knee.

Early clinical exposure

Joint replacement

Joint replacement is undertaken for a variety of reasons. These predominantly include degenerative joint disease and joint destruction. Joints that have severely degenerated or lack their normal function are painful. This can be life limiting, and in otherwise fit and healthy individuals can restrict activities of daily living. In some patients the pain may be so severe that it prevents them from leaving the house and undertaking even the smallest of activities without discomfort.

Large joints are commonly affected, including the hip, knee, and shoulder. However, with ongoing developments in joint replacement materials and surgical techniques, even small joints of the fingers can be replaced.

Typically, both sides of the joint are replaced; in the hip joint the acetabulum will be reamed, and a plastic or metal cup will be introduced. The femoral component will be fitted precisely to the femur and cemented in place (Fig. 1.26).

Most patients derive significant benefit from joint replacement and continue to lead an active life afterward.

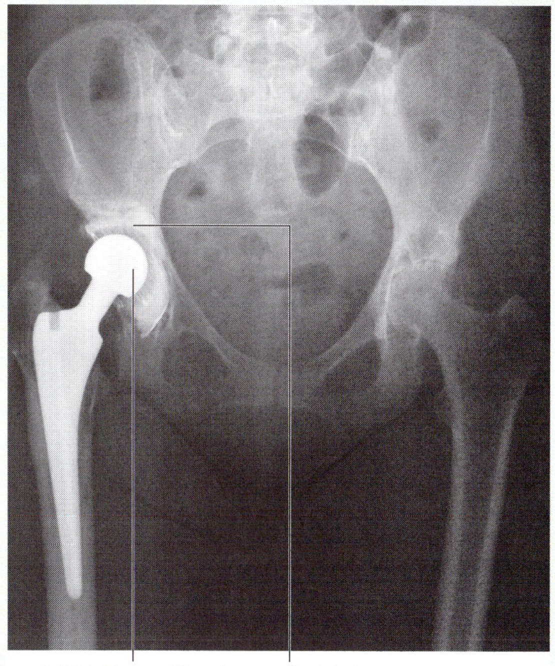

Fig. 1.26 This is a radiograph, anteroposterior view, of the pelvis after a right total hip replacement. There are additional significant degenerative changes in the left hip joint, which will also need to be replaced.

Early clinical exposure

Placement of skin incisions and scarring

Surgical skin incisions are ideally placed along or parallel to Langer's lines, which are lines of skin tension that correspond to the orientation of the dermal collagen fibers. They tend to run in the same direction as the underlying muscle fibers, and incisions that are made along these lines tend to heal better with less scarring. In contrast, incisions made perpendicular to Langer's lines are more likely to heal with a prominent scar and in some severe cases can lead to raised, firm, hypertrophic, or keloid scars.

SKIN AND FASCIAS

Skin

The skin is the largest organ of the body (LD 1.2). It consists of the epidermis and the dermis. The **epidermis** is the outer cellular layer of stratified squamous epithelium, which is avascular and varies in thickness. The **dermis** is a dense bed of vascular connective tissue.

The skin functions as a mechanical and permeability barrier, and as a sensory and thermoregulatory organ. It also can initiate primary immune responses.

Fascia

Fascia is connective tissue containing varying amounts of fat that separate, support, and interconnect organs and structures, enable movement of one structure relative to another, and allow the transit of vessels and nerves from one area to another. There are two general categories of fascia: superficial and deep.

- **Superficial (subcutaneous) fascia** lies just deep to and is attached to the dermis of the skin. It is made up of loose connective tissue usually containing a large amount of fat. The thickness of the superficial fascia (subcutaneous tissue) varies considerably, both from

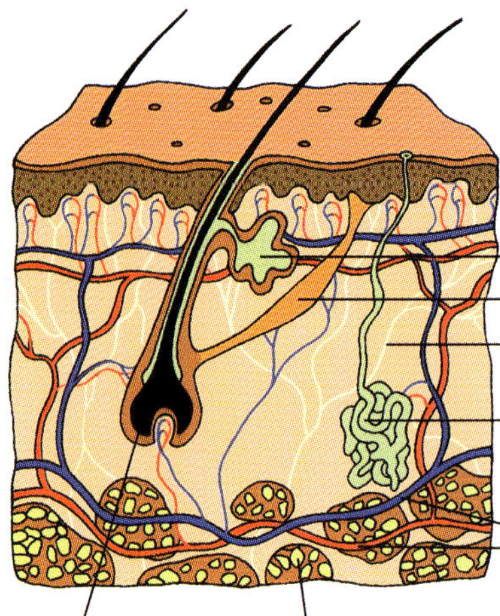

LD 1.2 Hairy skin.
Questions
LD 1.2A What are the subdivisions of the skin?
LD 1.2B What are some structures associated with a hair follicle?

Answers
LD 1.2A The subdivisions of the skin are the epidermis and dermis.
LD 1.2B Some structures associated with a hair follicle are the arrector pilorum and sebaceous glands.

one area of the body to another and from one individual to another. The superficial fascia allows movement of the skin over deeper areas of the body, acts as a conduit for vessels and nerves coursing to and from the skin, and serves as an energy (fat) reservoir.

- **Deep fascia** usually consists of dense, organized connective tissue. The outer layer of deep fascia is attached to the deep surface of the superficial fascia and forms a thin fibrous covering over most of the deeper region of the body. Inward extensions of this fascial layer form **intermuscular septa** that compartmentalize groups of muscles with similar functions and innervations. Other extensions surround individual muscles and groups of vessels and nerves, forming an investing fascia. Near some joints, the deep fascia thickens, forming **retinacula**. These fascial retinacula hold tendons in place and prevent them from bowing during movements at the joints. Finally, there is a layer of deep fascia separating the membrane lining the abdominal cavity (the parietal peritoneum) from the fascia covering the deep surface of the muscles of the abdominal wall (the transversalis fascia). This layer is referred to as **extraperitoneal fascia**. A similar layer of fascia in the thorax is termed the **endothoracic fascia**.

Early clinical exposure

The importance of fascias

A fascia is a thin band of tissue that surrounds muscles, bones, organs, nerves, and blood vessels and often remains uninterrupted as a three-dimensional structure between tissues. It provides important support for tissues and can provide a **boundary** between structures.

Fascias have specific dynamic properties and may be relatively elastic where necessary. They contain small blood vessels and tissue receptors and can respond to injury like any other tissue.

Clinically, fascias are extremely important because they often **limit the spread** of infection and malignant disease. When infections or malignant diseases cross a fascial plain, a primary surgical clearance may require a far more extensive dissection to render the area free of tumor or infection.

A typical example of a fascial layer would be that covering the psoas muscle. Infection within an intervertebral body secondary to tuberculosis can pass laterally into the psoas muscle. Pus fills the psoas muscle but is limited from further spread by the psoas fascia, which surrounds the muscle and extends inferiorly into the groin pointing below the inguinal ligament.

MUSCULAR SYSTEM

The muscular system is generally regarded as consisting of one type of muscle found in the body—skeletal muscle. However, there are two other types of muscle tissue found in the body, smooth muscle and cardiac muscle, that are important components of other systems. These three types of muscle can be characterized by whether they are controlled voluntarily or involuntarily, whether they appear striated (striped) or smooth, and whether they are associated with the body wall (somatic) or with organs and blood vessels (visceral) (LD 1.3).

- **Skeletal muscle** forms the majority of the muscle tissue in the body. It consists of parallel bundles of long, multinucleated fibers with transverse stripes, is capable of powerful contractions, and is innervated by somatic and branchial motor nerves. This muscle is used to move bones and other structures, and provides support and gives form to the body. Individual skeletal muscles are often named on the basis of shape (e.g., rhomboid major muscle), attachments (e.g., sternohyoid muscle), function (e.g., flexor pollicis longus muscle), position (e.g., palmar interosseous muscle), or fiber orientation (e.g., external oblique muscle).

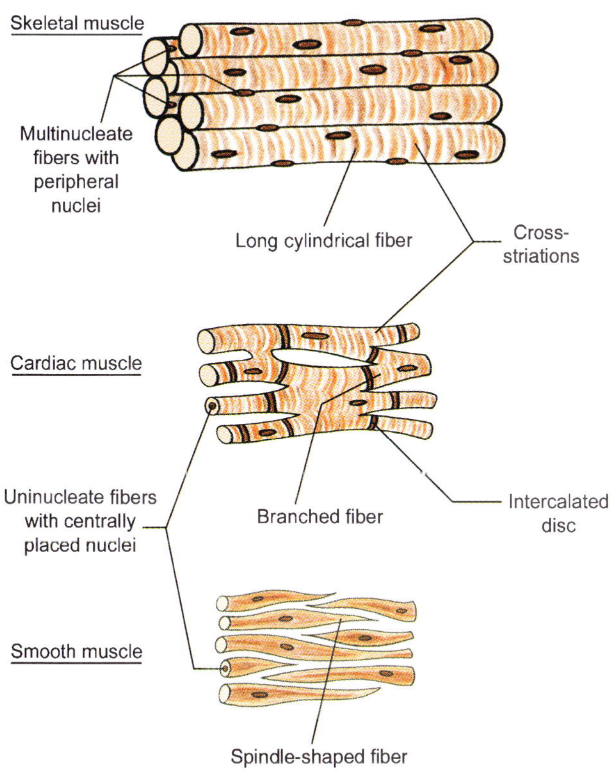

LD 1.3 Types of muscle.

Question

LD 1.3A Describe the three types noting the: (a) number and position of the nuclei, (b) shape of the fibers, and (c) presence of cross-striations.

Answer

LD 1.3A The three types of muscle are: (i) skeletal muscle, which is multinucleated with peripheral nuclei, has cylindrical fibers and cross-striations; (ii) cardiac muscle, which is uninucleated with centrally placed nuclei, has branched fibers, and cross-striations; and (iii) smooth muscle which is uninucleated with centrally placed nuclei, is spindle shaped and does not have cross-striations.

Classification of skeletal muscle: Skeletal muscles may be classified based on the arrangement of fasciculi. A fasciculus is a group of muscle fibers. Fasciculi may be parallel to the line of pull of the muscle, e.g., strap muscles (sternohyoid and sartorius); fusiform muscles (biceps brachii); and quadrilateral muscles (thyrohyoid).

Fasciculi may be oblique to the line of pull of the muscle, e.g., triangular muscles (temporalis); pennate (feather-like)-unipennate muscles (extensor digitorum longus), bipennate muscles (rectus femoris), multipennate muscles (acromial fibers of deltoid), and circumpennate muscles (tibialis anterior). Some muscles exhibit a spiral or twisted arrangement like latissimus dorsi and pectoralis major while some spiral around bone like supinator (LD 1.4).

Skeletal muscle may be classified based on their actions:

- A **prime mover (agonist)** is the main muscle responsible for a particular movement at a joint, for example, brachialis is a prime flexor of the elbow joint.
- An **antagonist** is a muscle that has an action opposite to a prime mover, for example, triceps is an antagonist to the brachialis. It is a prime extensor of the elbow joint.
- A **synergist** helps in the action of the prime movers by stabilizing the intermediate joints or preventing unwanted movements, for example, the deltoid stabilizes the shoulder joint during movements of the elbow.
- A fixator contracts isometrically to stabilize the attachment of the prime movers, so that they contract more effectively, for example, the flexors and extensors of the wrist stabilize this joint while the flexors of the digits contract.
- **Cardiac muscle** is striated muscle found only in the walls of the heart (myocardium) and in some of the large vessels close to where they join the heart. It consists of a branching network of individual cells linked electrically and mechanically to work as a unit. Its contractions are less powerful than those of skeletal muscle and it is resistant to fatigue. Cardiac muscle is innervated by visceral motor nerves.

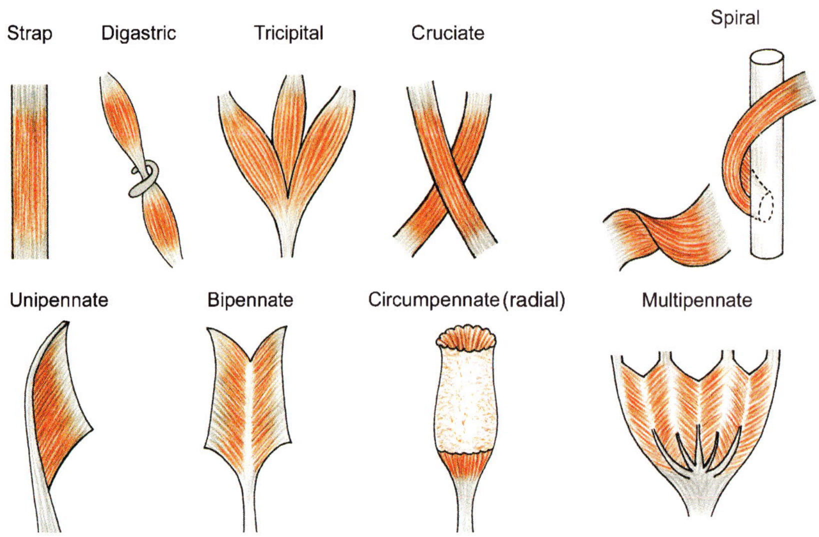

LD 1.4 Classification of skeletal muscle.

Questions

LD 1.4A On what basis is skeletal muscle classified here?

LD 1.4B How does the orientation of the fibers relate to the function of a muscle?

LD 1.4C To what extent can a muscle fiber contract?

Answers

LD 1.4A Skeletal muscle is classified here based on the shape of the muscle and orientation of the fibers.

LD 1.4B The orientation of the fibers relate to the function of the muscle such that muscle fibers which are arranged parallel to the direction of pull of a muscle are for longer and faster contractions, whereas muscle fibers arranged at an angle to the direction of pull of a muscle are for shorter and more powerful contractions.

LD 1.4C The extent to which a muscle fiber can contract is up to half its resting length.

- **Smooth muscle** does not have striations. It consists of elongated or spindle-shaped fibers capable of slow and sustained contractions. It is found in the walls of blood vessels (tunica media), associated with hair follicles in the skin, located in the eyeball, and found in the walls of various structures associated with the gastrointestinal, respiratory, genitourinary, and urogenital systems. Smooth muscle is innervated by visceral motor nerves.

Early clinical exposure

Muscle paralysis

Muscle paralysis is the inability to move a specific muscle or muscle group and may be associated with other neurological abnormalities, including loss of sensation. Paralysis may be due to abnormalities in the brain, the spinal cord, or the nerves supplying the muscles. Major causes include stroke, trauma, poliomyelitis, and iatrogenic factors.

In the long term, muscle paralysis will produce secondary muscle wasting and overall atrophy of the region due to disuse.

Early clinical exposure

Muscle atrophy

Muscle atrophy is a wasting disorder of muscle. It can be produced by a variety of causes, which include nerve damage to the muscle and disuse.

Muscle atrophy is an important problem in patients who have undergone long-term rest or disuse, requiring extensive rehabilitation and muscle building exercises to maintain normal activities of daily living.

Early clinical exposure

Muscle injuries and strains

Muscle injuries and strains tend to occur in specific muscle groups and usually are related to a sudden exertion and muscle disruption. They typically occur in athletes.

Muscle tears may involve a small interstitial injury up to a complete muscle disruption (Fig. 1.27). It is important to identify which muscle groups are affected and the extent of the tear to facilitate treatment and obtain a prognosis, which will determine the length of rehabilitation necessary to return to normal activity.

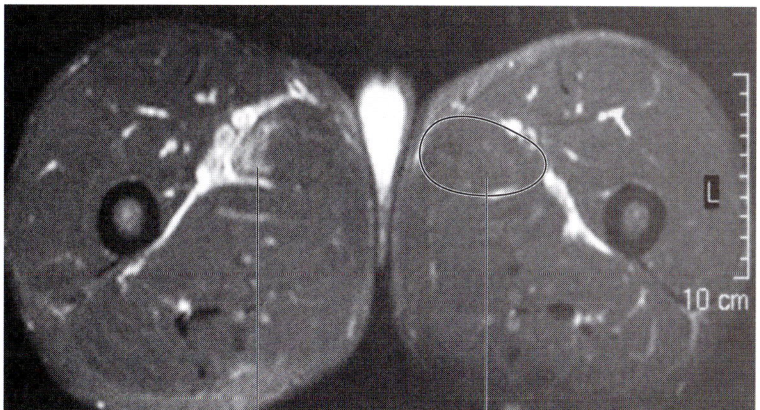

Fig. 1.27 Axial inversion recovery series MRI, which suppresses fat and soft tissue and leaves high signal intensity where fluid is seen. A muscle tear in the right adductor longus with edema in and around the muscle is shown.

CARDIOVASCULAR SYSTEM

The cardiovascular system consists of the heart, which pumps blood throughout the body, and the blood vessels, which are a closed network of tubes that transport the blood. There are three **types of blood vessels**:

- Arteries, which transport blood away from the heart
- Veins, which transport blood toward the heart
- Capillaries, which connect the arteries and veins, are the smallest of the blood vessels and are where oxygen, nutrients, and wastes are exchanged within the tissues

Sinusoids are wide, irregular capillaries which have discontinuous walls formed by fenestrated endothelium. Sinusoids occur in some organs like the liver, spleen, bone marrow, anterior pituitary, and adrenal medulla.

The walls of the blood vessels of the cardiovascular system usually consist of three **layers or tunics**:

- Tunica externa (adventitia)—the outer connective tissue layer
- Tunica media—the middle smooth muscle layer (may also contain varying amounts of elastic fibers in medium and large arteries)
- Tunica intima—the inner endothelial lining of the blood vessels (LD 1.5)

Arteries are usually further subdivided into three types, according to the variable amounts of smooth muscle and elastic fibers contributing to the thickness of the tunica media, the overall size of the vessel, and its function.

- Large elastic arteries contain substantial amounts of elastic fibers in the tunica media, allowing expansion and recoil during the normal cardiac cycle. This helps maintain a constant flow of blood during diastole. Examples of large elastic arteries are the aorta, the brachiocephalic trunk, the left common carotid artery, the left subclavian artery, and the pulmonary trunk.
- Medium muscular arteries are composed of a tunica media that contains mostly smooth muscle fibers. This characteristic allows these vessels to regulate their diameter and control the flow of blood to different parts of the body. Examples of medium muscular arteries are most of the named arteries, including the femoral, axillary, and radial arteries.

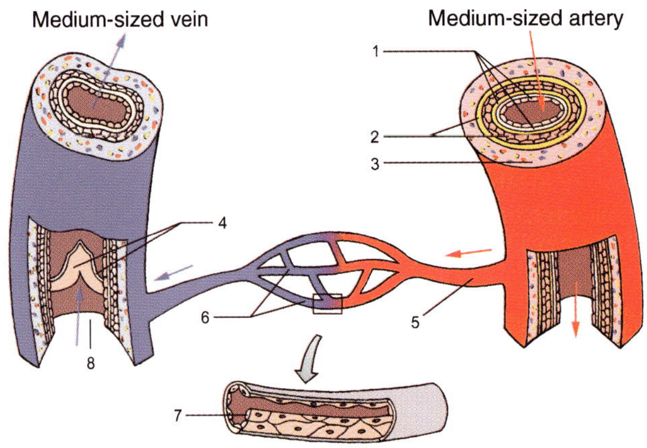

LD 1.5 Structure of blood vessels.
Questions
LD 1.5A Name the structures indicated by the labels.
LD 1.5B Compare elastic and muscular arteries with respect to (a) proportion of the parts, (b) content of the parts, and (c) appearance.

Answers
LD 1.5A The structures indicated by the labels are
1—tunica intima
2—tunica media
3—tunica adventitia
4—valve
5—arteriole
6—capillary
7—endothelium
8—lumen

LD 1.5B Elastic and muscular arteries can be compared based on the
a) Proportion of the parts—the thickness of tunica media in relation to tunica adventitia: it is larger in elastic arteries, and the same size in muscular arteries.
b) Content of the parts—the tunica media is predominantly made up of elastic fibers in large arteries and predominantly made up of smooth muscle fibers in muscular arteries.
c) Appearance—the internal elastic lamina is clearly seen in muscular arteries, but is not clearly seen in elastic arteries.

- Small arteries and arterioles control the filling of the capillaries and directly contribute to the arterial pressure in the vascular system.

Veins also are subdivided into three **types**.

- Large veins contain some smooth muscle in the tunica media, but the thickest layer is the tunica externa. Examples of large veins are the superior vena cava, the inferior vena cava, and the portal vein.
- Small and medium veins contain small amounts of smooth muscle, and the thickest layer is the tunica externa. Examples of small and medium veins are superficial veins in the upper and lower limbs and deeper veins of the leg and forearm.
- Venules are the smallest veins and drain the capillaries.

Although veins are similar in general structure to arteries, they have a number of **distinguishing features.**

- The walls of veins, specifically the tunica media, are thin.
- The luminal diameters of veins are relatively large.
- There often are multiple veins (venae comitantes) closely associated with arteries in peripheral regions.
- Valves often are present in veins, particularly in peripheral vessels inferior to the level of the heart. These are usually paired cusps that facilitate blood flow toward the heart.

More specific information about the cardiovascular system and how it relates to the circulation of blood throughout the body will be discussed, where appropriate, in each of the succeeding chapters of the text.

Early clinical exposure

Atherosclerosis

Atherosclerosis is a disease that affects arteries. There is a chronic inflammatory reaction in the walls of the arteries, with deposition of cholesterol and fatty proteins. This may in turn lead to secondary calcification, with reduction in the diameter of the vessels impeding distal flow. The plaque itself may be a site for attraction of platelets that may "fall off" (embolize) distally. Plaque fissuring may occur, which allows fresh clots to form and occlude the vessel.

The importance of atherosclerosis and its effects depend upon which vessel is affected. If atherosclerosis occurs in the carotid artery, small emboli may form and produce a stroke. In the heart, plaque fissuring may produce an acute vessel thrombosis, producing a myocardial infarction (heart attack). In the legs, chronic narrowing of vessels may limit the ability of the patient to walk and ultimately cause distal ischemia and gangrene of the toes.

Early clinical exposure

Varicose veins

Varicose veins are tortuous, dilated and elongated veins that typically occur in the legs, although they may occur in the superficial veins of the arm and in other organs.

In normal individuals, the contraction of leg muscles pumps the blood in the veins to the heart. Blood is also pumped from the superficial veins through the investing layer of fascia of the leg into the deep veins. Valves in these perforating veins may become damaged, allowing blood to pass in the opposite direction. This increased volume and pressure produces dilatation and tortuosity of the superficial veins (Fig. 1.28). Apart from the unsightliness of larger veins, the skin may become pigmented and atrophic with a poor response to tissue damage. In some patients, even small trauma may produce skin ulceration, which requires elevation of the limb and application of pressure bandages to heal.

Treatment of varicose veins depends on their location, size, and severity. Typically, the superficial varicose veins can be excised and stripped, allowing blood only to drain into the deep system.

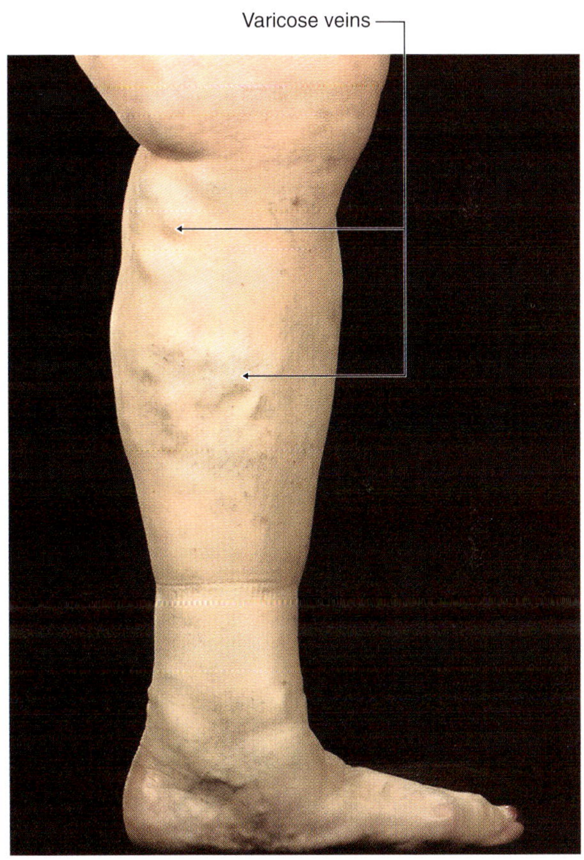

Fig. 1.28 Photograph demonstrating varicose veins.

Early clinical exposure

Anastomoses and collateral circulation

All organs require a blood supply from the arteries and drainage by veins. Within most organs, there are multiple ways of perfusing the tissue such that if the main vessel feeding the organ or vein draining the organ is blocked, a series of smaller vessels (collateral vessels) continue to supply and drain the organ.

In certain circumstances, organs have more than one main vessel perfusing them, such as the hand, which is supplied by the radial and ulnar arteries. Loss of either the radial

Continued

Early clinical exposure—cont'd

or the ulnar artery may not produce any symptoms of reduced perfusion to the hand.

There are circumstances in which loss of a vein produces significant venous collateralization. Some of these venous collaterals become susceptible to bleeding. This is a considerable problem in patients who have undergone portal vein thrombosis or occlusion, where venous drainage from the gut bypasses the liver through collateral veins to return to the systemic circulation.

Normal vascular anastomoses associated with an organ are important. Some organs, such as the duodenum, have a dual blood supply arising from the branches of the celiac trunk and also from the branches of the superior mesenteric artery. Should either of these vessels be damaged, blood supply will be maintained to the organ. The brain has multiple vessels supplying it, derived from the carotid arteries and the vertebral arteries. Vessels within the brain are end arteries and have a poor collateral circulation; hence, occlusion of these end arteries will produce long-term cerebral damage.

LYMPHATIC SYSTEM

Lymphatic vessels

Lymphatic vessels form an extensive and complex interconnected network of channels, which begin as "porous" blind-ended lymphatic capillaries in tissues of the body and converge to form a number of larger vessels, which ultimately connect with large veins in the root of the neck.

Lymphatic vessels mainly collect fluid lost from vascular capillary beds during nutrient exchange processes and deliver it back to the venous side of the vascular system (Fig. 1.29). Also included in this interstitial fluid that drains into the lymphatic capillaries are pathogens, cells of the lymphocytic system, cell products (such as hormones), and cell debris.

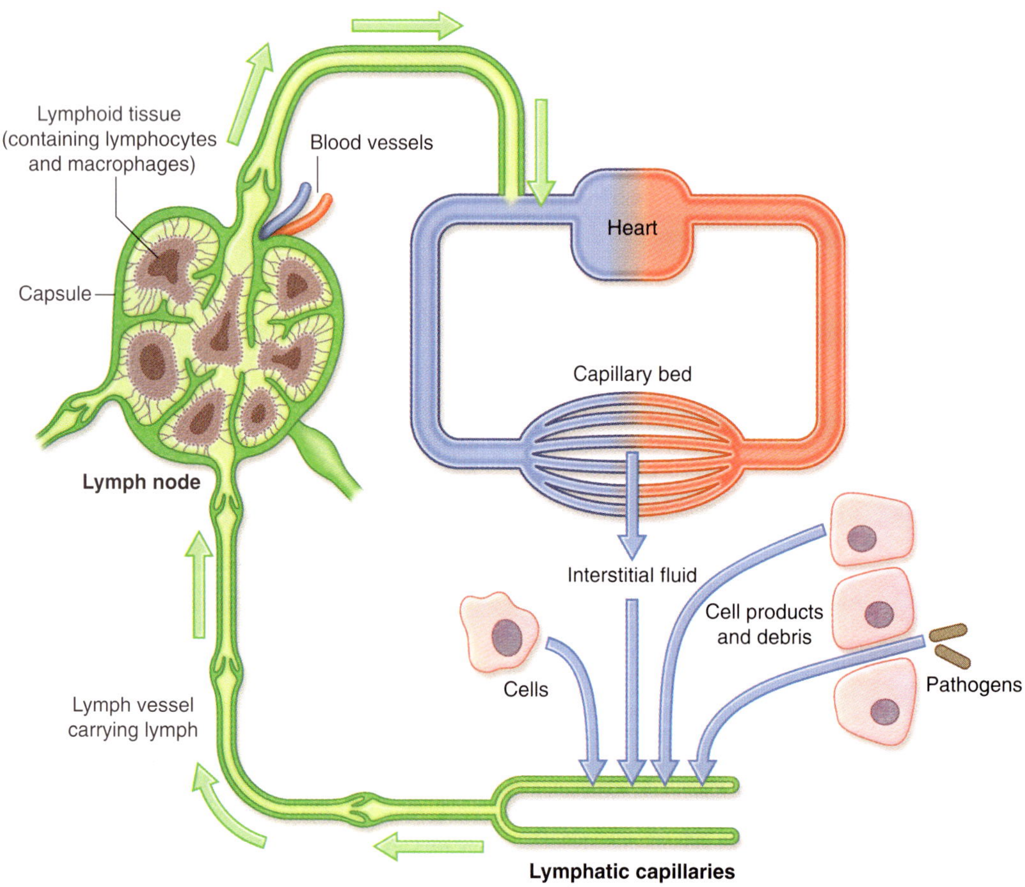

Fig. 1.29 Lymphatic vessels mainly collect fluid lost from vascular capillary beds during nutrient exchange processes and deliver it back to the venous side of the vascular system.

In the small intestine, certain fats absorbed and processed by the intestinal epithelium are packaged into protein-coated lipid droplets (**chylomicrons**), which are released from the epithelial cells and enter the interstitial compartment. Together with other components of the interstitial fluid, the chylomicrons drain into lymphatic capillaries (known as **lacteals** in the small intestine) and are ultimately delivered to the venous system in the neck. The lymphatic system is therefore also a major route of transport for fat absorbed by the gut.

The fluid in most lymphatic vessels is clear and colorless and is known as **lymph**. That carried by lymphatic vessels from the small intestine is opaque and milky because of the presence of chylomicrons and is termed **chyle**.

There are lymphatic vessels in most areas of the body, including those associated with the central nervous system (CNS) (Louveau A et al., *Nature* 2015; 523:337-41; Aspelund A et al., *J Exp Med* 2015; 212:991-9). Exceptions include bone marrow and avascular tissues such as epithelia and cartilage.

The movement of lymph through the lymphatic vessels is generated mainly by the indirect action of adjacent structures, particularly by contraction of skeletal muscles and pulsations in arteries. Unidirectional flow is maintained by the presence of valves in the vessels.

Lymph nodes

Lymph nodes are small (0.1–2.5 cm long) encapsulated structures that interrupt the course of lymphatic vessels and contain elements of the body's defense system, such as clusters of lymphocytes and macrophages. They act as elaborate filters that trap and phagocytose particulate matter in the lymph that percolates through them. In addition, they detect and defend against foreign antigens that are also carried in the lymph (Fig. 1.29).

Because lymph nodes are efficient filters and flow through them is slow, cells that metastasize from (migrate away from) primary tumors and enter lymphatic vessels often lodge and grow as secondary tumors in lymph nodes. Lymph nodes that drain regions that are infected or contain other forms of disease can enlarge and become "tender," or undergo certain physical changes, such as becoming "hard." These changes can be used by clinicians to detect pathologic changes or to track spread of disease.

A number of regions in the body are associated with clusters or a particular abundance of lymph nodes (Fig. 1.30). Not surprisingly, nodes in many of these regions drain the body's surface, the digestive system, or the respiratory system. All three of these areas are high-risk sites for the entry of foreign pathogens.

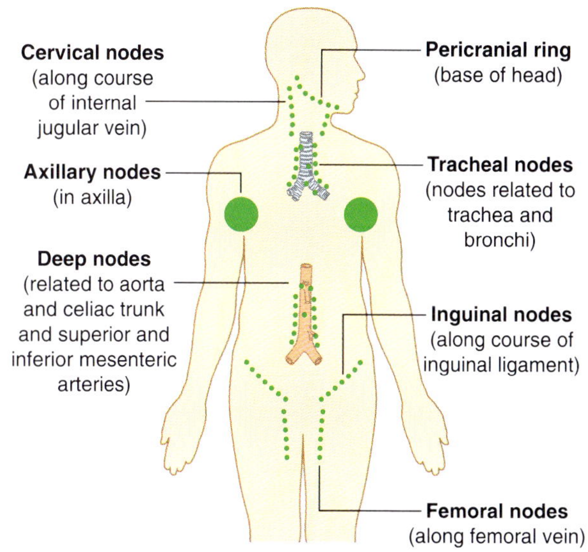

Fig. 1.30 Regions associated with clusters or a particular abundance of lymph nodes.

Lymph nodes are abundant and accessible to palpation in the axilla, the groin and femoral region, and the neck. Deep sites of clusters of lymph nodes that are not palpable include those associated with the trachea and bronchi in the thorax, and with the aorta and its branches in the abdomen.

Lymphatic trunks and ducts

All lymphatic vessels coalesce to form larger trunks or ducts, which drain into the venous system at sites in the neck where the internal jugular veins join the subclavian veins to form the brachiocephalic veins (Fig. 1.31):

- Lymph from the right side of the head and neck, the right upper limb, right side of the thorax, and right side of the upper and more superficial region of the abdominal wall is carried by lymphatic vessels that connect with veins on the right side of the neck.
- Lymph from all other regions of the body is carried by lymphatic vessels that drain into veins on the left side of the neck.

Specific information about the organization of the lymphatic system in each region of the body is discussed in the appropriate chapter.

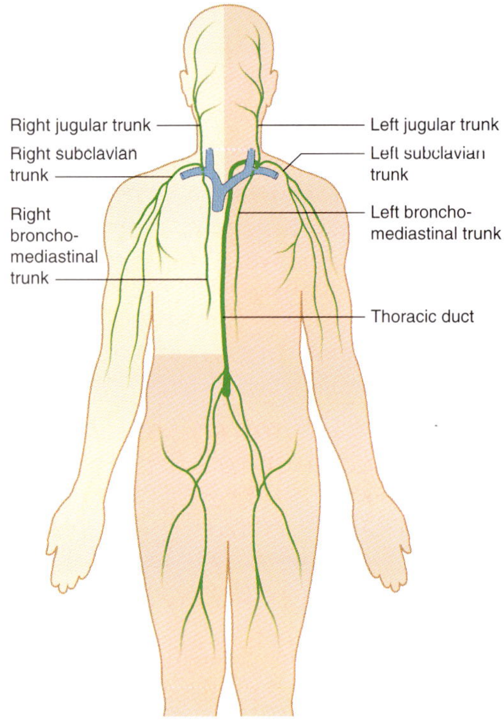

Fig. 1.31 Major lymphatic vessels that drain into large veins in the neck.

Early clinical exposure

Lymph nodes

Lymph nodes are efficient filters and have an internal honeycomb of reticular connective tissue filled with lymphocytes. These lymphocytes act on bacteria, viruses, and other bodily cells to destroy them. Lymph nodes tend to drain specific areas, and if infection occurs within a drainage area, the lymph node will become active. The rapid cell turnover and production of local inflammatory mediators may cause the node to enlarge and become tender. Similarly, in patients with malignancy, the lymphatics may drain metastasizing cells to the lymph nodes. These can become enlarged and inflamed and will need to be removed if clinically symptomatic.

Lymph nodes may become diffusely enlarged in certain systemic illnesses (e.g., viral infection), or local groups may become enlarged with primary lymph node malignancies, such as lymphoma (Fig. 1.32A and B).

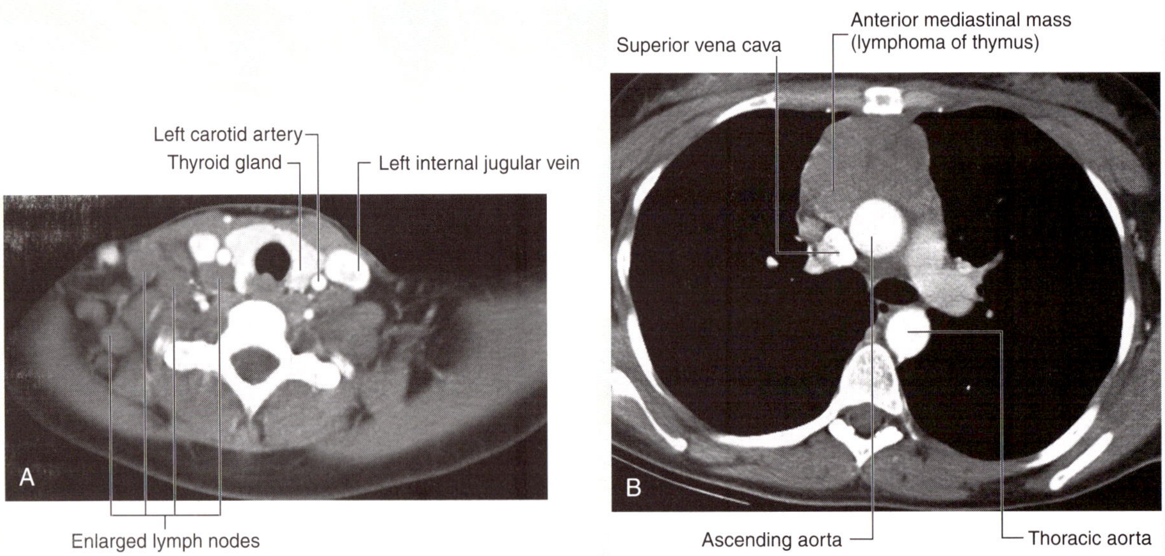

Fig. 1.32 **(A)** This computed tomogram with contrast, in the axial plane, demonstrates the normal common carotid arteries and internal jugular veins with numerous other nonenhancing nodules that represent lymph nodes in a patient with lymphoma. **(B)** This computed tomogram with contrast, in the axial plane, demonstrates a large anterior soft tissue mediastinal mass that represents a lymphoma.

NERVOUS SYSTEM

The nervous system can be separated into parts based on structure and on function:

- **Structurally**, it can be divided into the CNS and the peripheral nervous system (PNS) (Fig. 1.33).
- **Functionally**, it can be divided into somatic and visceral parts.

The CNS is composed of the brain and spinal cord, both of which develop from the neural tube in the embryo.

The PNS is composed of all nervous structures outside the CNS that connect the CNS to the body. Elements of this system develop from neural crest cells and as outgrowths of the CNS. The PNS consists of the spinal and cranial nerves, visceral nerves and plexuses, and the enteric system. The detailed anatomy of a typical spinal nerve is described in Chapter 7, as is the way spinal nerves are numbered. Cranial nerves are described in Chapter 8. The details of nerve plexuses are described in chapters dealing with the specific regions in which the plexuses are located.

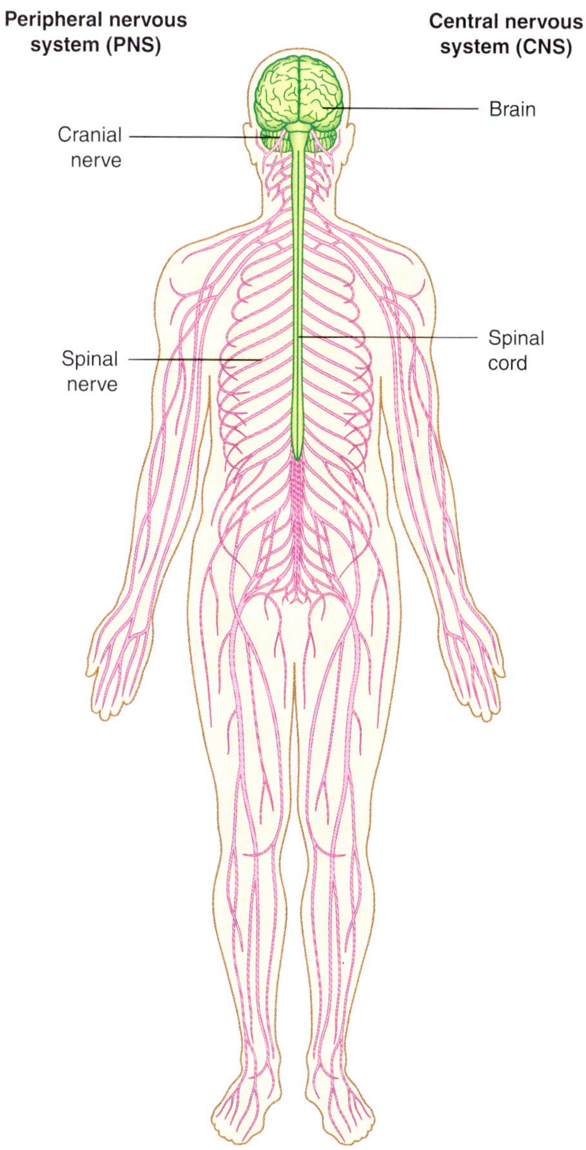

Fig. 1.33 CNS and PNS.

Central nervous system

Brain

The parts of the brain are the cerebral hemispheres, the cerebellum, and the brainstem. The cerebral hemispheres consist of an outer portion, or the **gray matter**, containing cell bodies; an inner portion, or the **white matter**, made up of axons forming tracts or pathways; and the **ventricles**, which are spaces filled with CSF.

The cerebellum has two lateral lobes and a midline portion. In common usage today, the term "brainstem" usually refers to the midbrain, pons, and medulla.

A further discussion of the brain can be found in Chapter 8.

Spinal cord

The spinal cord is the part of the CNS in the superior two-thirds of the vertebral canal. It is roughly cylindrical in shape, and is circular to oval in cross-section with a central canal. A further discussion of the spinal cord can be found in Chapter 7.

Meninges

The meninges (Fig. 1.34) are three connective tissue coverings that surround, protect, and suspend the brain and

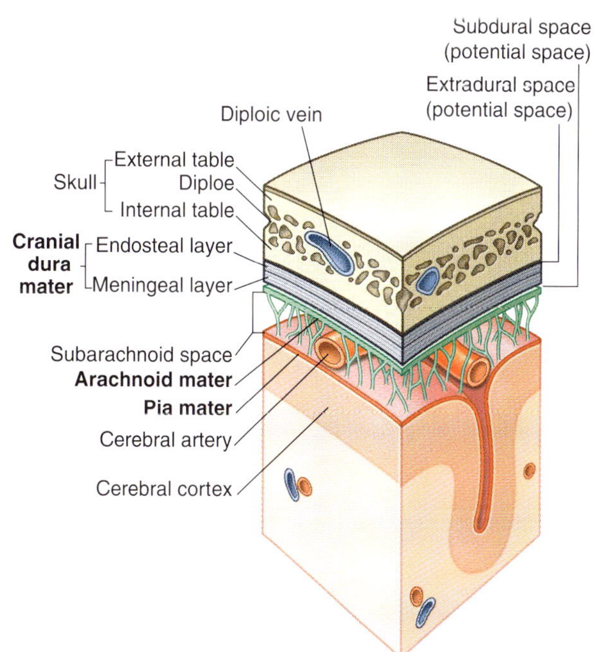

Fig. 1.34 Arrangement of meninges in the cranial cavity.

spinal cord within the cranial cavity and vertebral canal, respectively:

- The dura mater is the thickest and most external of the coverings.
- The arachnoid mater lies on the internal surface of the dura mater.
- The pia mater is adherent to the brain and spinal cord.

Between the arachnoid and pia mater is the subarachnoid space, which contains CSF.

A further discussion of the cranial meninges can be found in Chapter 8 and of the spinal meninges in Chapter 7.

Functional subdivisions of the CNS

Functionally, the nervous system can be divided into somatic and visceral parts.

- The **somatic** part (*soma*, from the Greek for "body") innervates structures (skin and most skeletal muscle) derived from somites in the embryo, and is mainly involved with receiving and responding to information from the external environment.
- The **visceral** part (*viscera*, from the Greek for "guts") innervates organ systems in the body and other visceral elements, such as smooth muscle and glands, in peripheral regions of the body. It is concerned mainly with detecting and responding to information from the internal environment.

Somatic part of the nervous system

The somatic part of the nervous system consists of:

- Nerves that carry conscious sensations from peripheral regions back to the CNS
- Nerves that innervate voluntary muscles

Somatic nerves arise segmentally along the developing CNS in association with **somites**, which are themselves arranged segmentally along each side of the neural tube (Fig. 1.35). Part of each somite (the **dermomyotome**) gives rise to skeletal muscle and the dermis of the skin. As cells of the dermomyotome differentiate, they migrate into

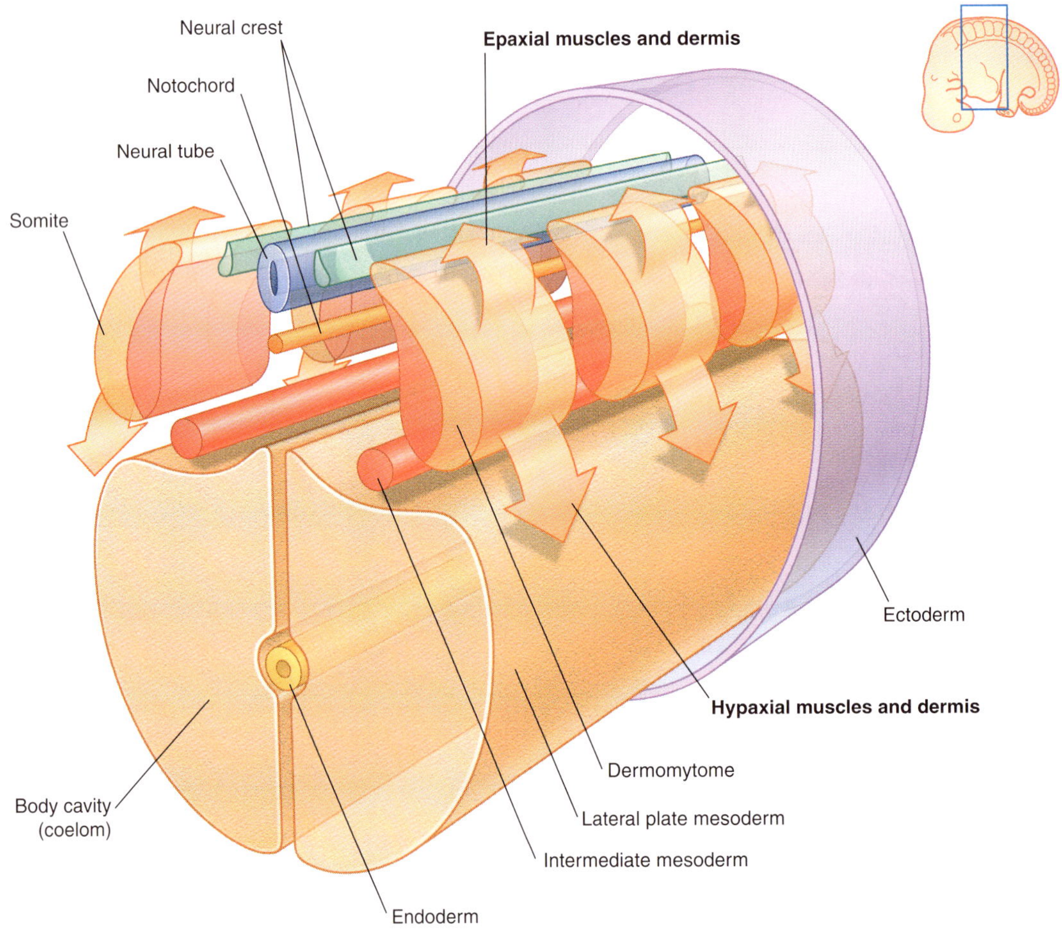

Fig. 1.35 Differentiation of somites in a "tubular" embryo.

posterior (dorsal) and anterior (ventral) areas of the developing body:

- Cells that migrate anteriorly give rise to muscles of the limbs and trunk (**hypaxial muscles**) and to the associated dermis.
- Cells that migrate posteriorly give rise to the intrinsic muscles of the back (**epaxial muscles**) and the associated dermis.

Developing nerve cells within anterior regions of the neural tube extend processes peripherally into posterior and anterior regions of the differentiating dermomyotome of each somite.

Simultaneously, derivatives of neural crest cells (cells derived from neural folds during formation of the neural tube) differentiate into neurons on each side of the neural tube and extend processes both medially and laterally (Fig. 1.36):

- Medial processes pass into the posterior aspect of the neural tube.
- Lateral processes pass into the differentiating regions of the adjacent dermomyotome.

Neurons that develop from cells within the spinal cord are **motor neurons** and those that develop from neural crest cells are **sensory neurons**.

It can be seen that somatic sensory and somatic motor fibers that are organized segmentally along the neural tube become parts of all spinal nerves and some cranial nerves.

The clusters of sensory nerve cell bodies derived from neural crest cells and located outside the CNS form sensory ganglia.

Generally, all sensory information passes into the posterior aspect of the spinal cord, and all motor fibers leave anteriorly.

Somatic sensory neurons carry information from the periphery into the CNS and are also called **somatic sensory afferents** or **general somatic afferents (GSAs)**. The modalities carried by these nerves include temperature, pain, touch, and proprioception. Proprioception is the sense of determining the position and movement of the musculoskeletal system detected by special receptors in muscles and tendons.

Somatic motor fibers carry information away from the CNS to skeletal muscles and are also called **somatic motor efferents** or **general somatic efferents (GSEs)**. Like somatic sensory fibers that come from the periphery, somatic motor fibers can be very long. They extend from cell bodies in the spinal cord to the muscle cells they innervate.

Dermatomes

Because cells from a specific somite develop into the dermis of the skin in a precise location, somatic sensory fibers originally associated with that somite enter the posterior

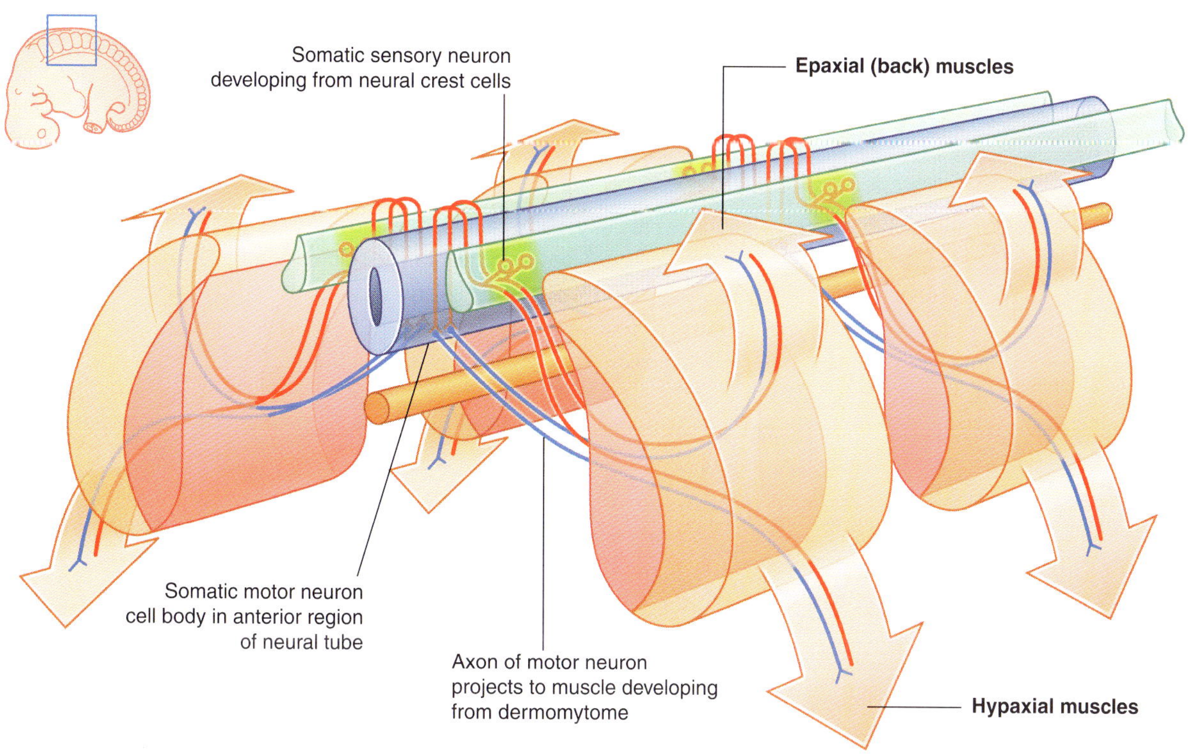

Fig. 1.36 Somatic sensory and motor neurons. Blue lines indicate motor nerves and red lines indicate sensory nerves.

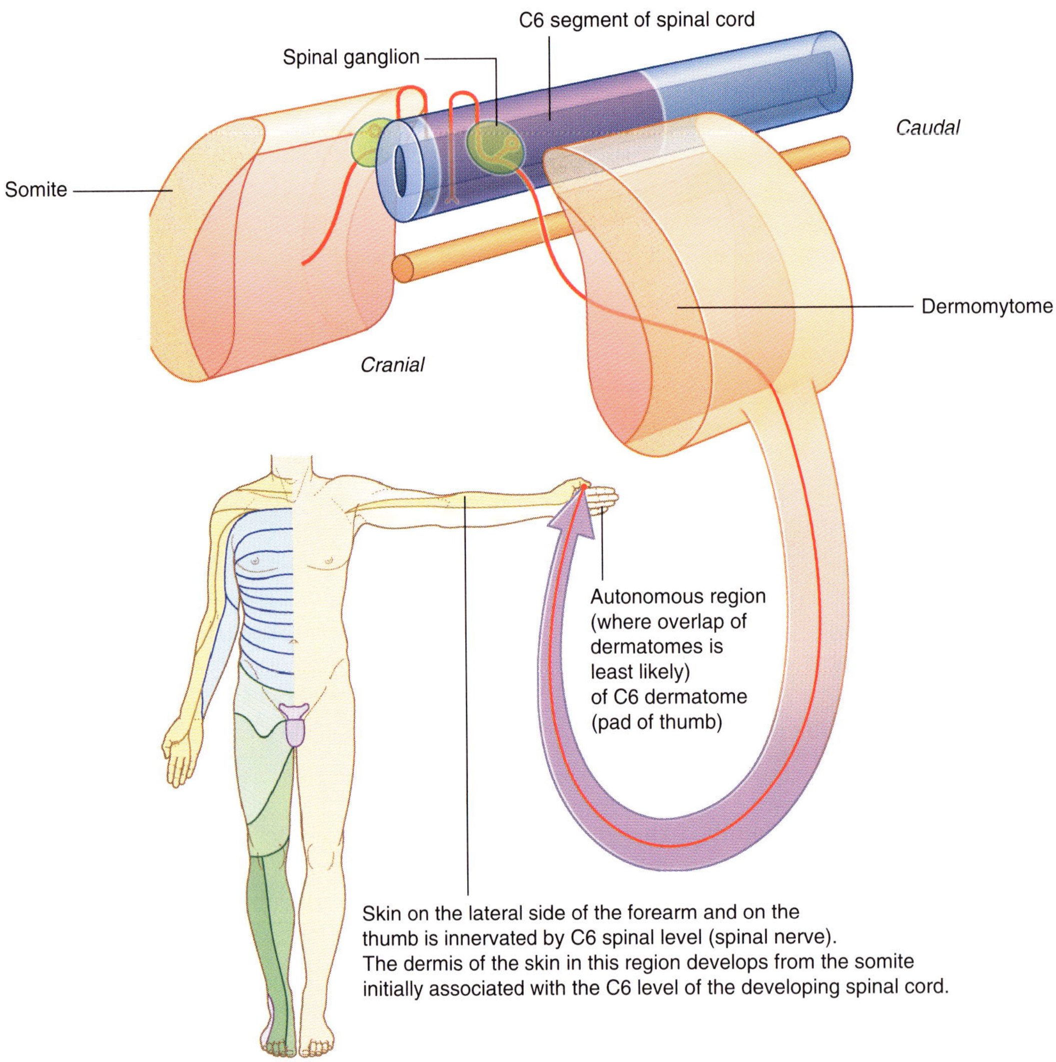

Fig. 1.37 Dermatomes.

region of the spinal cord at a specific level and become part of one specific spinal nerve (Fig. 1.37). Each spinal nerve therefore carries somatic sensory information from a specific area of skin on the surface of the body. A **dermatome** is that area of skin supplied by a single spinal cord level, or on one side, by a single spinal nerve.

There is overlap in the distribution of dermatomes, but usually a specific region within each dermatome can be identified as an area supplied by a single spinal cord level. Testing touch in these autonomous zones in a conscious patient can be used to localize lesions to a specific spinal nerve or to a specific level in the spinal cord.

Myotomes

Somatic motor nerves that were originally associated with a specific somite emerge from the anterior region of the spinal cord and, together with sensory nerves from the same level, become part of one spinal nerve. Therefore, each spinal nerve carries somatic motor fibers to muscles that originally developed from the related somite. A **myotome** is that portion of a skeletal muscle innervated by a single spinal cord level or, on one side, by a single spinal nerve.

Myotomes are generally more difficult to test than dermatomes because each skeletal muscle in the body is usually innervated by nerves derived from more than one spinal cord level (Fig. 1.38).

Testing movements at successive joints can help in localizing lesions to specific nerves or to a specific spinal cord level. For example:

- Muscles that move the shoulder joint are innervated mainly by spinal nerves from spinal cord levels C5 and C6.
- Muscles that move the elbow are innervated mainly by spinal nerves from spinal cord levels C6 and C7.
- Muscles in the hand are innervated mainly by spinal nerves from spinal cord levels C8 and T1.

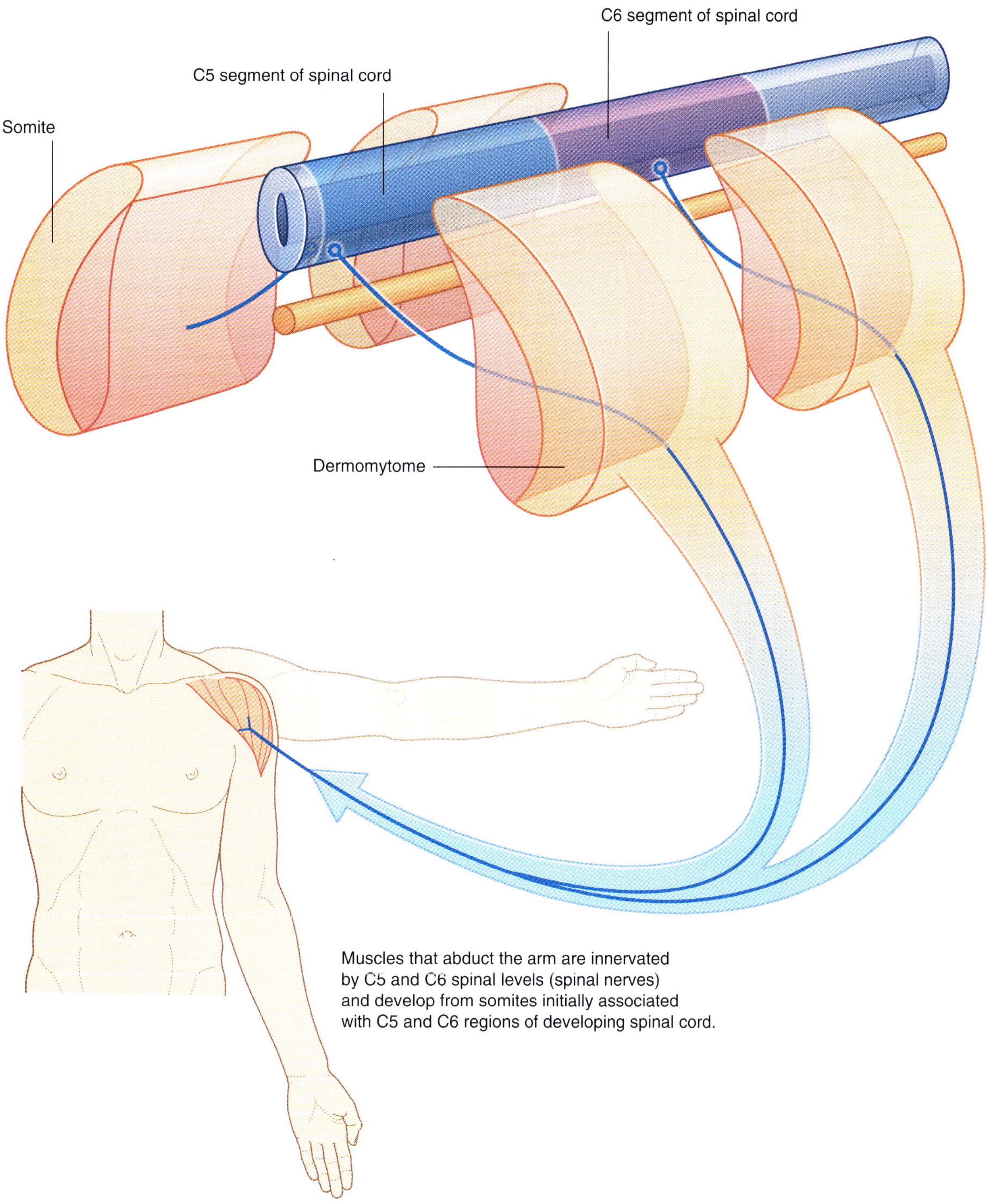

Fig. 1.38 Myotomes.

Early clinical exposure

Dermatomes and myotomes

A knowledge of dermatomes and myotomes is absolutely fundamental to carrying out a neurological examination. A typical dermatome map is shown in Fig. 1.39.

Clinically, a dermatome is that area of skin supplied by a single nerve or spinal cord level. A myotome is that region of skeletal muscle innervated by a single nerve or spinal cord level. Most individual muscles of the body are innervated by more than one spinal cord level, so the evaluation of myotomes is usually accomplished by testing movements of joints or muscle groups.

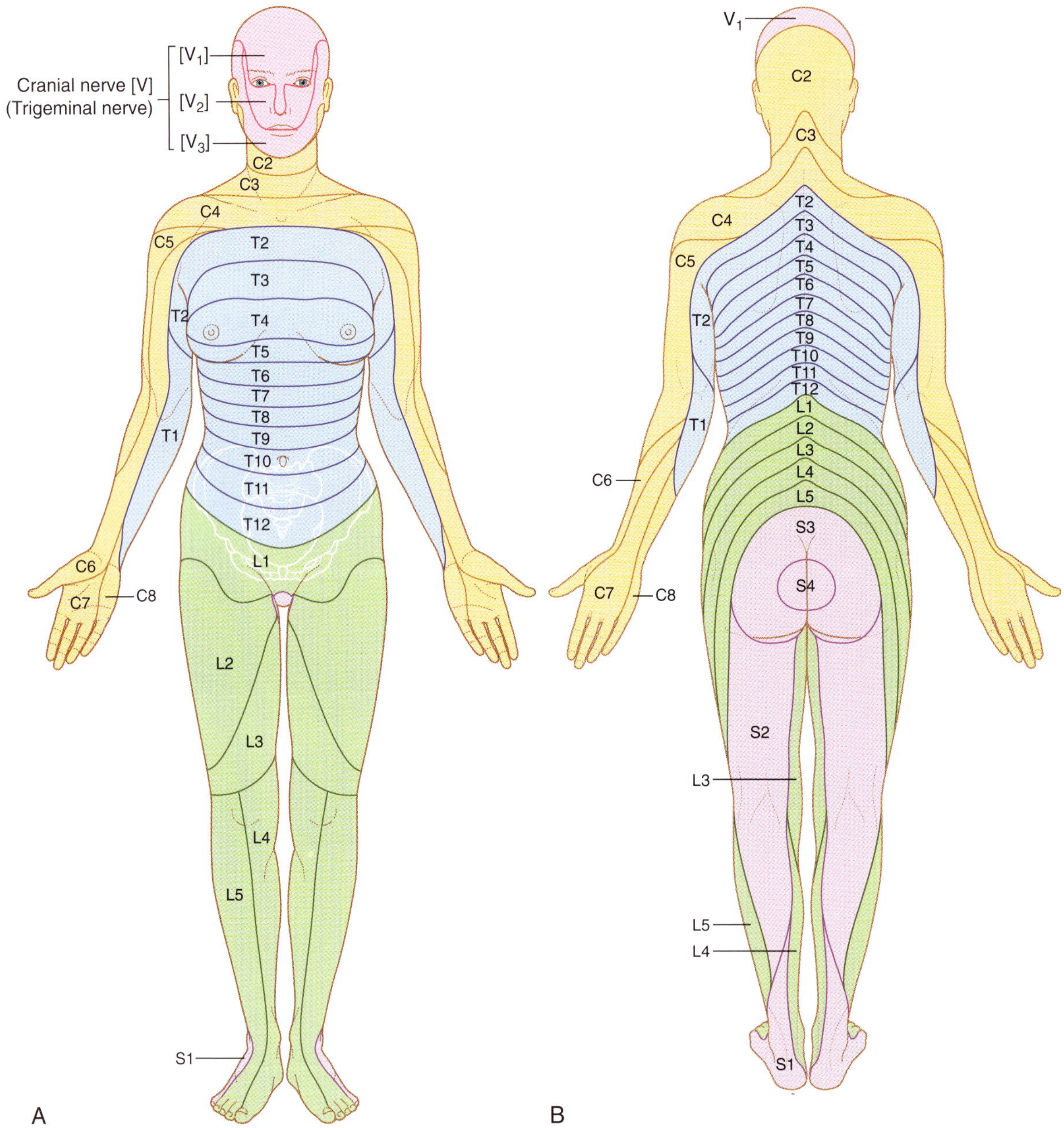

Fig. 1.39 Dermatomes. **(A)** Anterior view. **(B)** Posterior view.

Visceral part of the nervous system

The visceral part of the nervous system, as in the somatic part, consists of motor and sensory components:

- Sensory nerves monitor changes in the viscera.
- Motor nerves mainly innervate smooth muscle, cardiac muscle, and glands.

The visceral motor component is commonly referred to as the **autonomic division of the PNS** and is subdivided into **sympathetic** and **parasympathetic** parts.

Like the somatic part of the nervous system, the visceral part is segmentally arranged and develops in a parallel fashion (Fig. 1.40).

Visceral sensory neurons that arise from neural crest cells send processes medially into the adjacent neural tube and laterally into regions associated with the developing body. These sensory neurons and their processes, referred to as **general visceral afferent fibers (GVAs)**, are associated primarily with chemoreception, mechanoreception, and stretch reception.

Visceral motor neurons that arise from cells in lateral regions of the neural tube send processes out of the

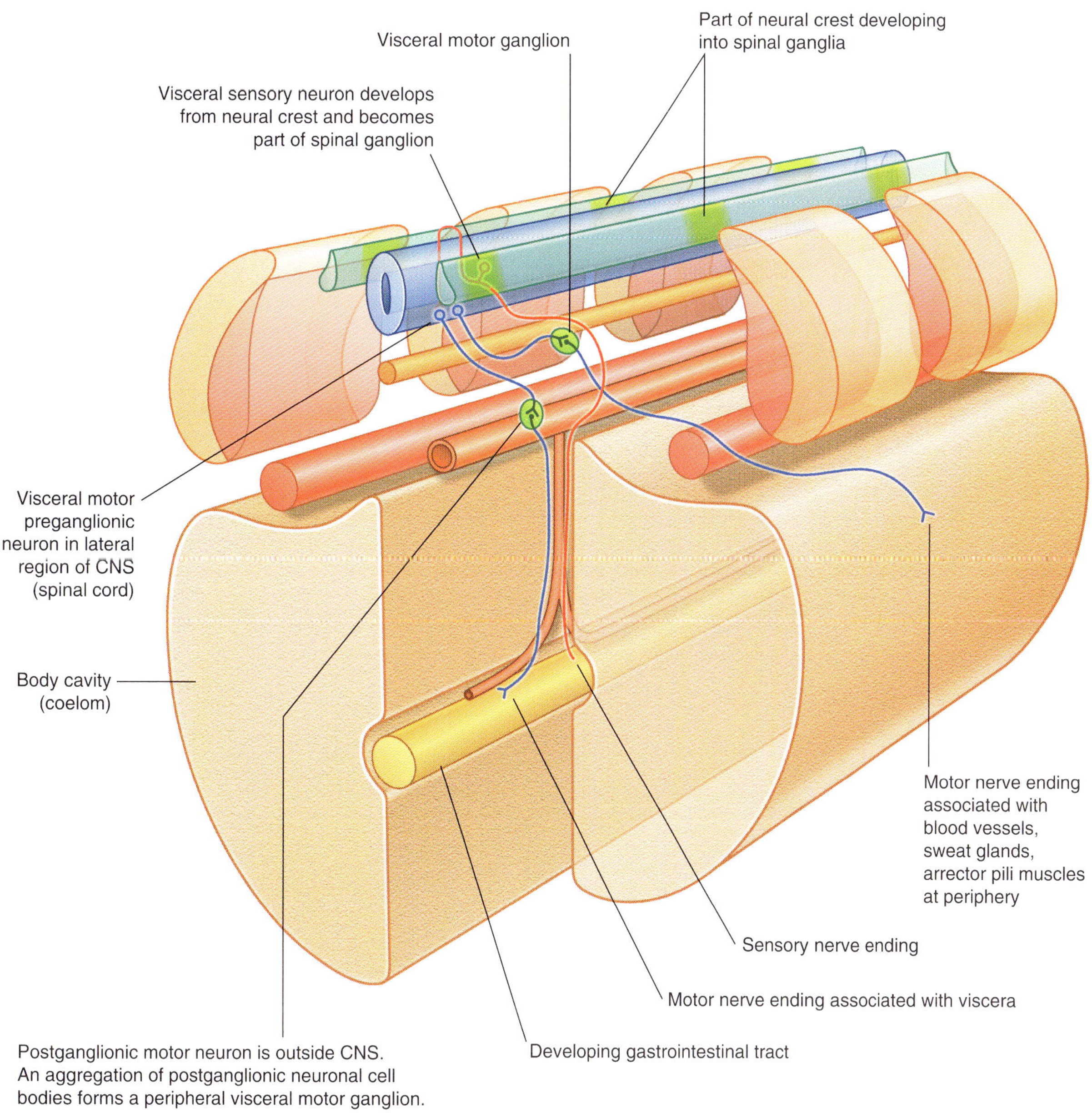

Fig. 1.40 Development of the visceral part of the nervous system.

anterior aspect of the tube. Unlike in the somatic part, these processes, containing **general visceral efferent fibers (GVEs)**, synapse with other cells, usually other visceral motor neurons, that develop outside the CNS from neural crest cells that migrate away from their original positions close to the developing neural tube.

The visceral motor neurons located in the spinal cord are referred to as preganglionic motor neurons and their axons are called **preganglionic fibers**; the visceral motor neurons located outside the CNS are referred to as postganglionic motor neurons and their axons are called **postganglionic fibers**.

The cell bodies of the visceral motor neurons outside the CNS often associate with each other in a discrete mass called an autonomic **ganglion**.

Visceral sensory and motor fibers enter and leave the CNS with their somatic equivalents (Fig. 1.41). Visceral sensory fibers enter the spinal cord together with somatic sensory fibers through posterior roots of spinal nerves. Preganglionic fibers of visceral motor neurons exit the spinal cord in the anterior roots of spinal nerves, along with fibers from somatic motor neurons.

Postganglionic fibers traveling to visceral elements in the periphery are found in the posterior and anterior rami (branches) of spinal nerves.

Visceral motor and sensory fibers that travel to and from viscera form named visceral branches that are separate from the somatic branches. These nerves generally form plexuses from which arise branches to the viscera.

Visceral motor and sensory fibers do not enter and leave the CNS at all levels (Fig. 1.42):

- In the cranial region, visceral components are associated with 4 of the 12 cranial nerves (CN III, VII, IX, and X).

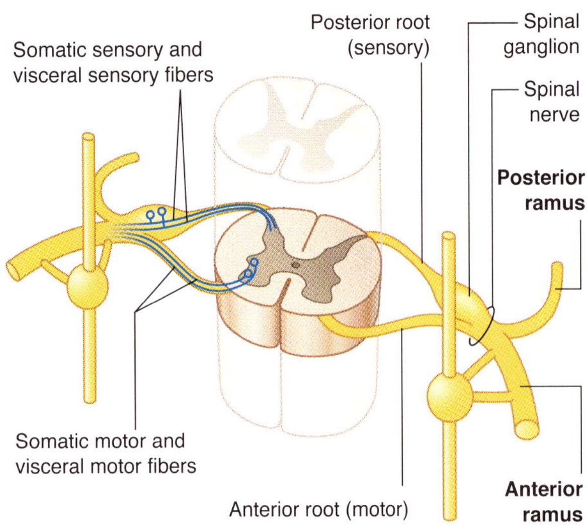

Fig. 1.41 Basic anatomy of a thoracic spinal nerve.

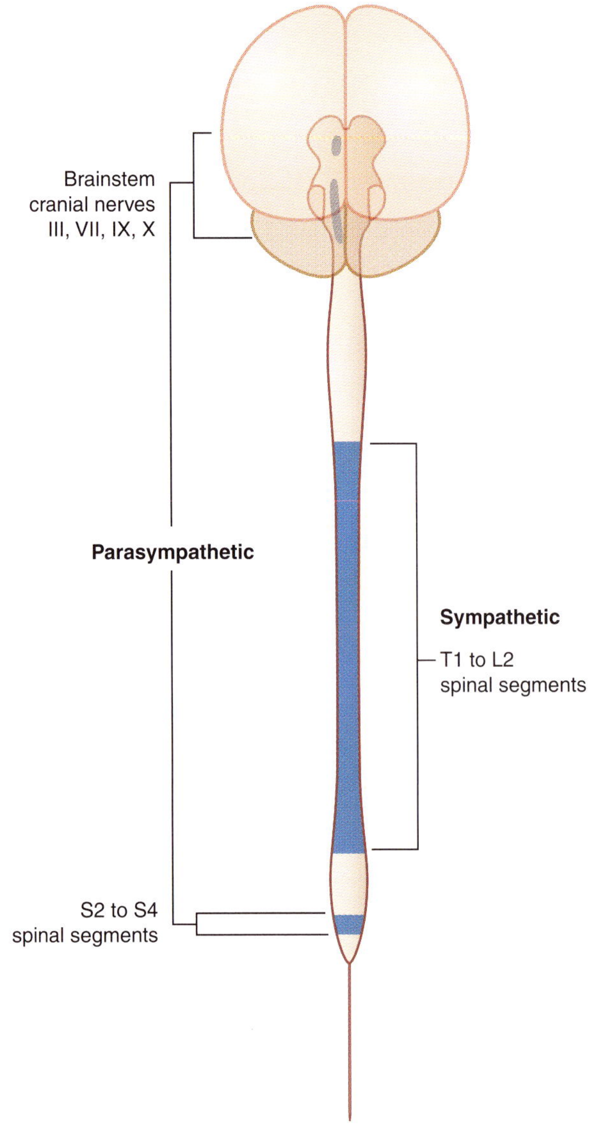

Fig. 1.42 Parts of the CNS associated with visceral motor components.

- In the spinal cord, visceral components are associated mainly with spinal cord levels T1 to L2 and S2 to S4.

Visceral motor components associated with spinal levels T1 to L2 are termed **sympathetic**. Those visceral motor components in cranial and sacral regions, on either side of the sympathetic region, are termed **parasympathetic**:

- The sympathetic system innervates viscera and structures in peripheral regions of the body.
- The parasympathetic system is more restricted to innervation of the viscera only.

Terminology

Spinal sympathetic and spinal parasympathetic neurons share certain developmental and phenotypic features that are different from those of cranial parasympathetic neurons. Based on this, some researchers have suggested reclassifying all spinal visceral motor neurons as sympathetic (Espinosa-Medina I et al., *Science* 2016;354:893-897). Others are against reclassification, arguing that the results only indicate that the neurons are spinal in origin (Neuhuber W et al., *Anat Rec* 2017;300:1369-1370). In addition, sacral nerves do not enter the sympathetic trunk, nor do they have postganglionic fibers that travel to the periphery on spinal nerves, as do T1 to L2 visceral motor fibers. We have chosen to retain the classification of S2, S3, S4 visceral motor neurons as parasympathetic. "Parasympathetic" simply means on either side of the "sympathetic," which correctly describes their anatomy (LD 1.6).

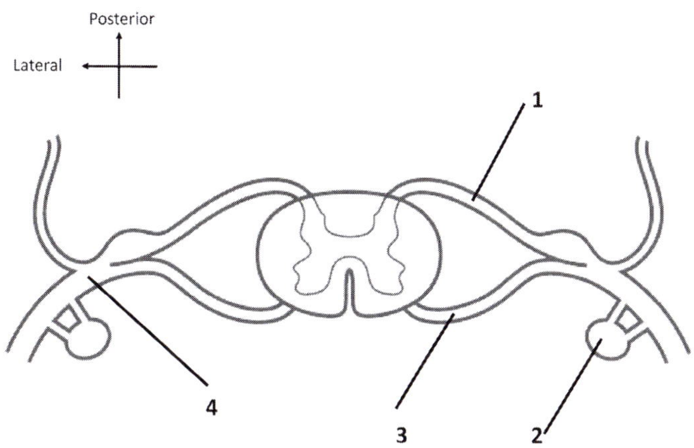

LD 1.6 Structure of a spinal nerve.
Questions
LD 1.6A Name the structures indicated by the labels.
LD 1.6B From which parts of the spinal nerve are the sympathetic and parasympathetic nerve fibers attached?

Answers
LD 1.6A
1. Dorsal root
2. Sympathetic ganglion
3. Ventral root
4. Trunk of spinal nerve

LD 1.6B Sympathetic nerves are attached to all the sympathetic ganglia and parasympathetic nerves are attached to each of the ventral rami of S2, S3, and S4 ventral rami.

Sympathetic system

The sympathetic part of the autonomic division of the PNS leaves thoracolumbar regions of the spinal cord with the somatic components of spinal nerves T1 to L2 (Fig. 1.43). On each side, a paravertebral sympathetic trunk extends from the base of the skull to the inferior end of the vertebral column where the two trunks converge anteriorly to the coccyx at the ganglion impar. Each trunk is attached to the anterior rami of spinal nerves and becomes the route by which sympathetics are distributed to the periphery and all viscera.

Visceral motor preganglionic fibers leave the T1 to L2 part of the spinal cord in anterior roots. The fibers then enter the spinal nerves, pass through the anterior rami and into the sympathetic trunks. One trunk is located on each side of the vertebral column (paravertebral) and positioned anterior to the anterior rami. Along the trunk is a series of segmentally arranged ganglia formed from collections of postganglionic neuronal cell bodies where the preganglionic neurons synapse with postganglionic neurons. Anterior rami of T1 to L2 are connected to the sympathetic trunk or to a ganglion by a **white ramus communicans**, which carries preganglionic sympathetic fibers and appears white because the fibers it contains are myelinated (Fig. 1.44).

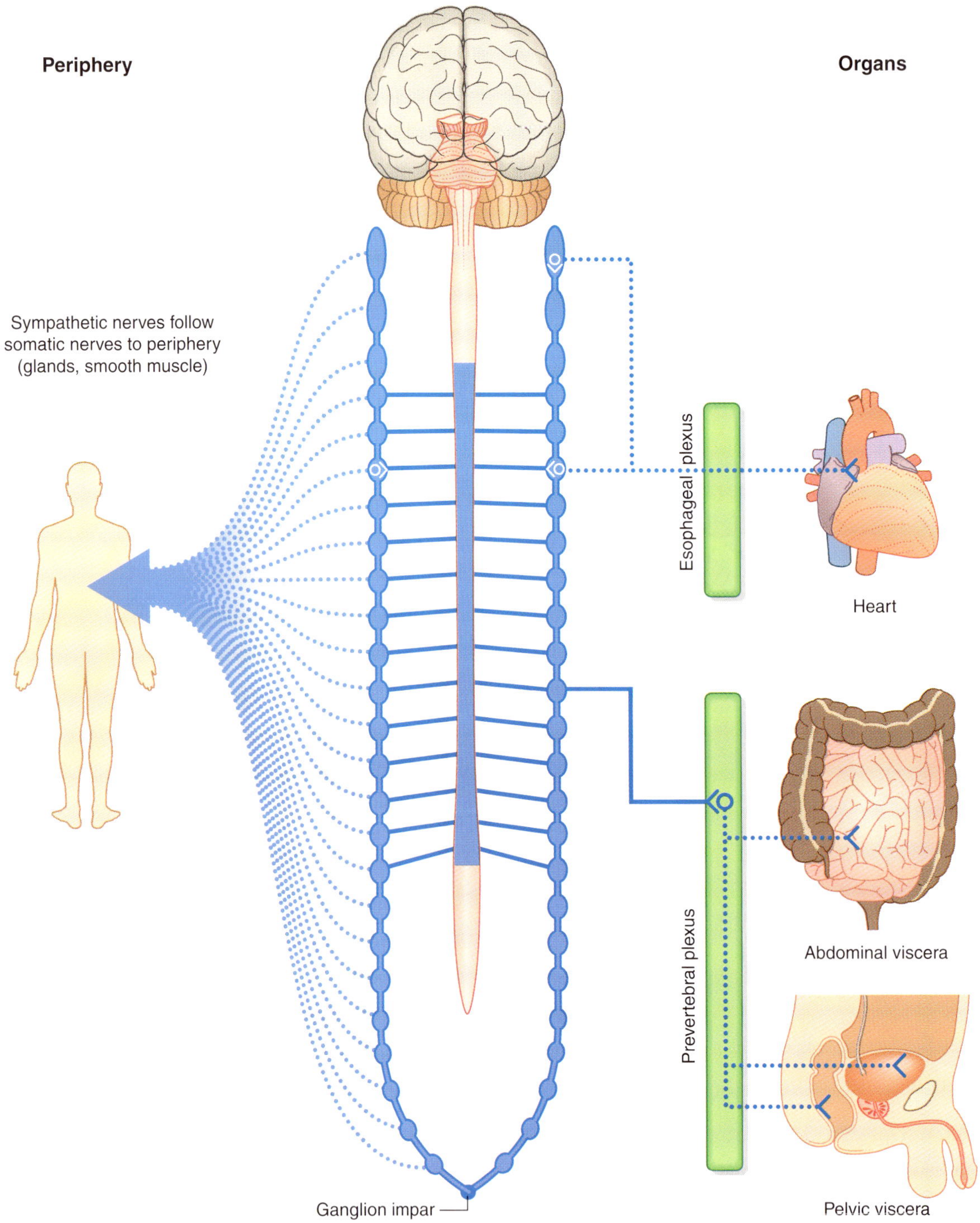

Fig. 1.43 Sympathetic part of the autonomic division of the PNS.

Preganglionic sympathetic fibers that enter a paravertebral ganglion or the sympathetic trunk through a white ramus communicans may take the following four pathways to target tissues:

1. Peripheral sympathetic innervation at the level of origin of the preganglionic fiber

Preganglionic sympathetic fibers may synapse with postganglionic motor neurons in ganglia associated with the sympathetic trunk, after which postganglionic fibers enter the same anterior ramus and are distributed with peripheral branches of the posterior and anterior rami of that spinal nerve (Fig. 1.44). The fibers innervate structures at the periphery of the

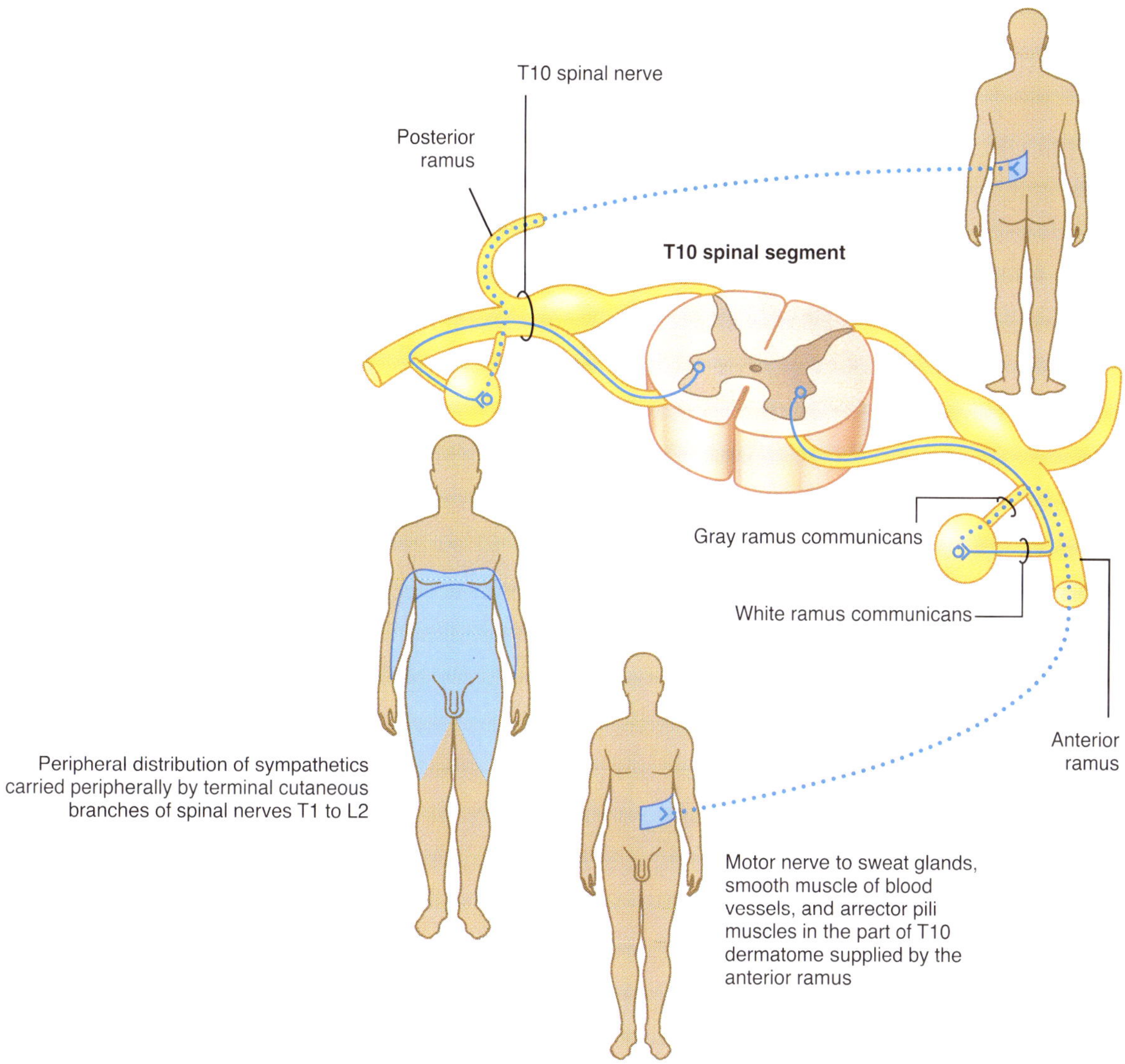

Fig. 1.44 Course of sympathetic fibers that travel to the periphery in the same spinal nerves in which they travel out of the spinal cord.

body in regions supplied by the spinal nerve. The **gray ramus communicans** connects the sympathetic trunk or a ganglion to the anterior ramus and contains the postganglionic sympathetic fibers. It appears gray because postganglionic fibers are nonmyelinated. The gray ramus communicans is positioned medial to the white ramus communicans.

2. Peripheral sympathetic innervation above or below the level of origin of the preganglionic fiber

Preganglionic sympathetic fibers may ascend or descend to other vertebral levels where they synapse in ganglia associated with spinal nerves that may or may not have visceral motor input directly from the spinal cord (i.e., those nerves other than T1 to L2) (Fig. 1.45).

The postganglionic fibers leave the distant ganglia via gray rami communicantes and are distributed along the posterior and anterior rami of the spinal nerves.

The ascending and descending fibers, together with all the ganglia, form the **paravertebral sympathetic trunk**, which extends the entire length of the vertebral column. The formation of this trunk, on each side, enables visceral motor fibers of the sympathetic part of the autonomic division of the PNS, which ultimately emerge from only a small region of the spinal cord (T1 to L2), to be distributed to peripheral regions innervated by all spinal nerves.

White rami communicantes only occur in association with spinal nerves T1 to L2, whereas gray rami communicantes are associated with all spinal nerves.

Fibers from spinal cord levels T1 to T5 pass predominantly superiorly, whereas fibers from T5 to L2 pass inferiorly. All sympathetics passing into the head have preganglionic fibers that emerge from spinal cord level T1 and ascend in the sympathetic trunks

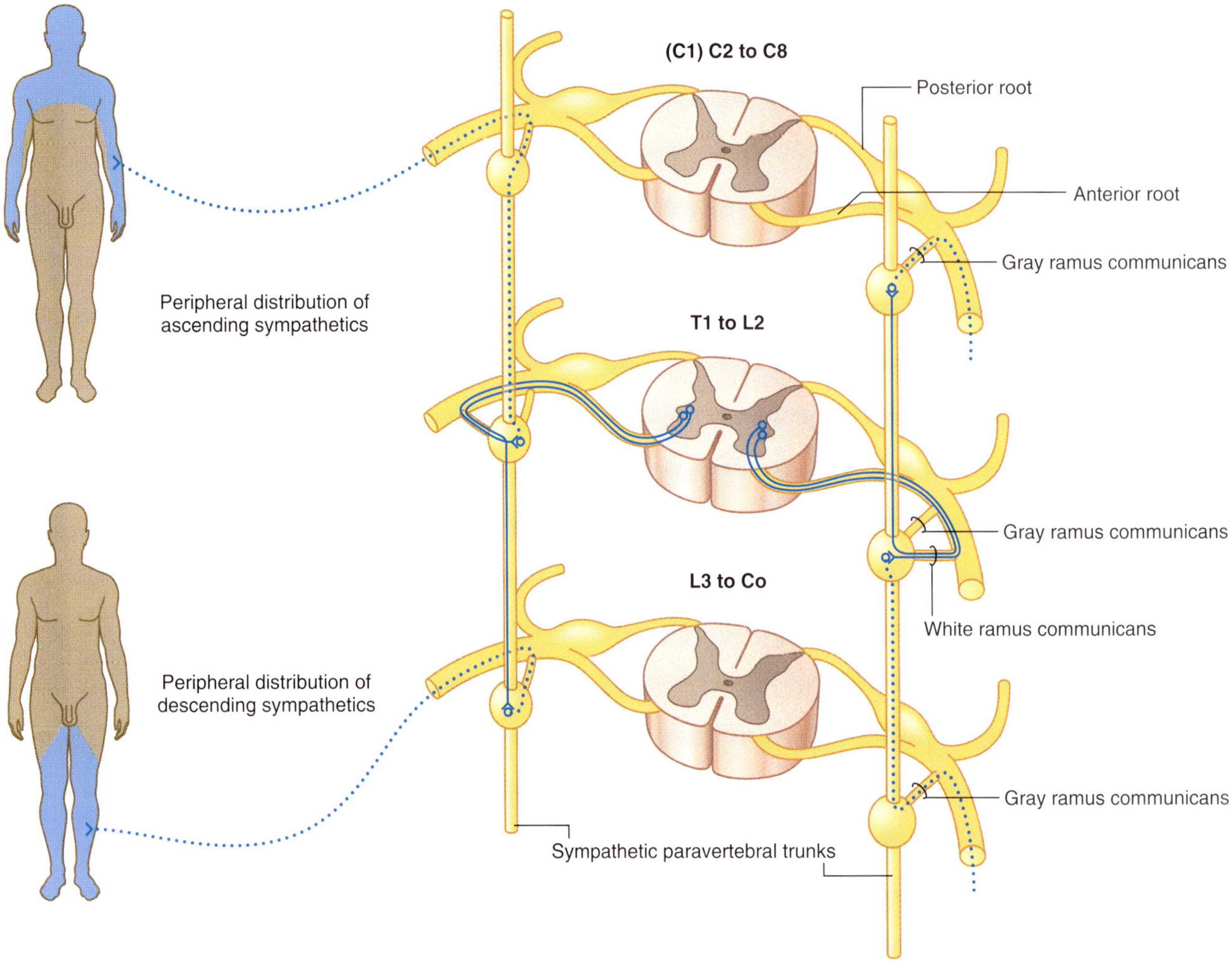

Fig. 1.45 Course of sympathetic nerves that travel to the periphery in spinal nerves that are not the ones through which they left the spinal cord.

to the highest ganglion in the neck (the **superior cervical ganglion**), where they synapse. Postganglionic fibers then travel along blood vessels to target tissues in the head, including blood vessels, sweat glands, small smooth muscles associated with the upper eyelids, and the dilator of the pupil.

3. Sympathetic innervation of thoracic and cervical viscera

Preganglionic sympathetic fibers may synapse with postganglionic motor neurons in ganglia and then leave the ganglia medially to innervate thoracic or cervical viscera (Fig. 1.46). They may ascend in the trunk before synapsing, and after synapsing the postganglionic fibers may combine with those from other levels to form named visceral nerves, such as cardiac nerves. Often, these nerves join branches from the parasympathetic system to form plexuses on or near the surface of the target organ, for example, the cardiac and pulmonary plexuses. Branches of the plexus innervate the organ. Spinal cord levels T1 to T5 mainly innervate cranial, cervical, and thoracic viscera.

4. Sympathetic innervation of the abdomen and pelvic regions and the adrenals

Preganglionic sympathetic fibers may pass through the sympathetic trunk and paravertebral ganglia without synapsing and, together with similar fibers from other levels, form **splanchnic nerves** (**greater, lesser, least, lumbar**, and **sacral**), which pass into the abdomen and pelvic regions (Fig. 1.47). The preganglionic fibers in these nerves are derived from spinal cord levels T5 to L2.

The splanchnic nerves generally connect with sympathetic ganglia around the roots of major arteries that branch from the abdominal aorta. These ganglia are part of a large prevertebral plexus that also

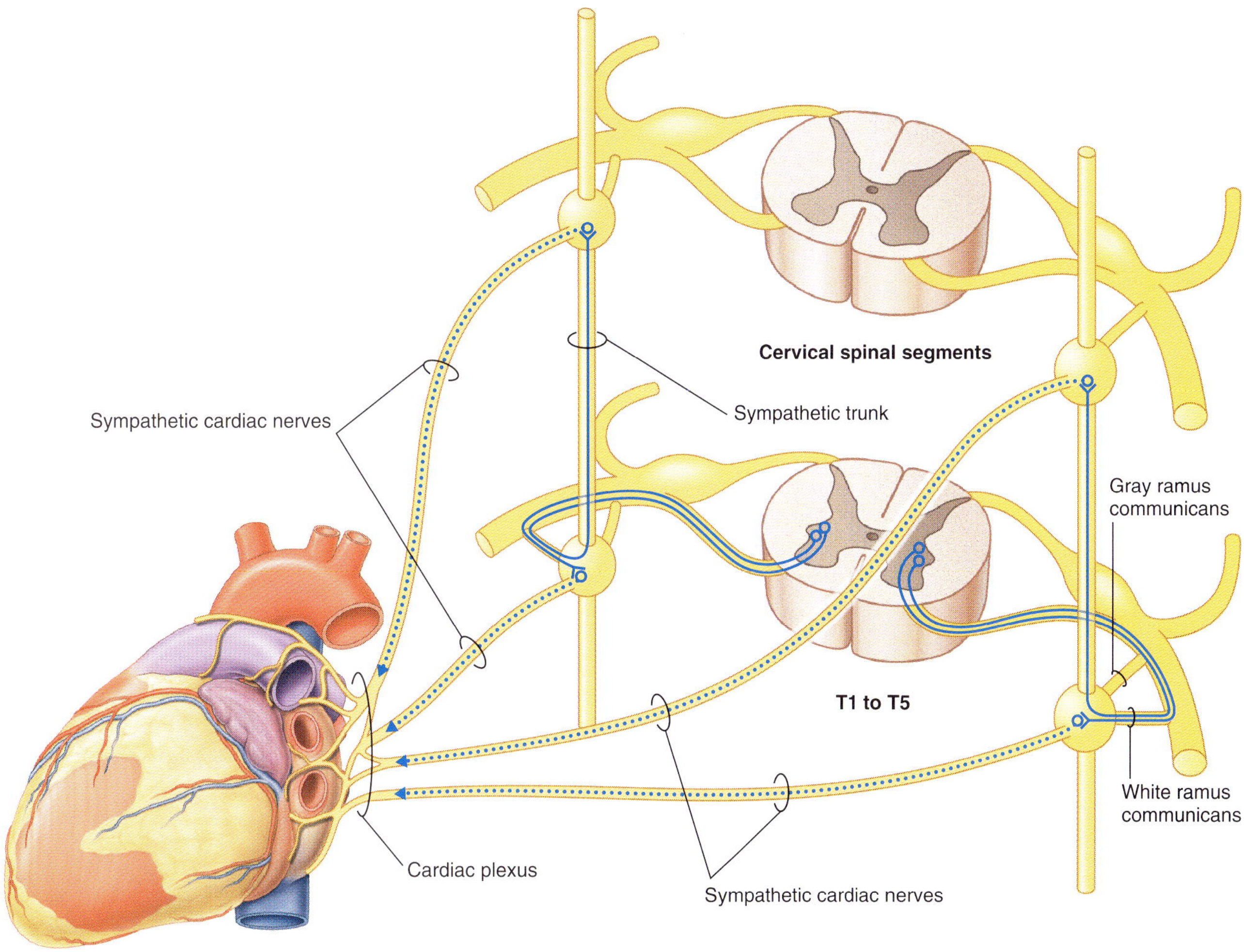

Fig. 1.46 Course of sympathetic nerves traveling to the heart.

has input from the parasympathetic part of the autonomic division of the PNS. Postganglionic sympathetic fibers are distributed in extensions of this plexus, predominantly along arteries, to viscera in the abdomen and pelvis.

Some of the preganglionic fibers in the prevertebral plexus do not synapse in the sympathetic ganglia of the plexus but pass through the system to the adrenal gland, where they synapse directly with cells of the adrenal medulla. These cells are homologues of sympathetic postganglionic neurons and secrete adrenaline and noradrenaline into the vascular system.

Parasympathetic system

The parasympathetic part of the autonomic division of the PNS (Fig. 1.48) leaves cranial and sacral regions of the CNS in association with:

- Cranial nerves III, VII, IX, and X: III, VII, and IX carry parasympathetic fibers to structures within the head and neck only, whereas X (the vagus nerve) also innervates thoracic and most abdominal viscera.
- Spinal nerves S2 to S4: Sacral parasympathetic fibers innervate inferior abdominal viscera, pelvic viscera, and the arteries associated with erectile tissues of the perineum.

Like the visceral motor nerves of the sympathetic part, the visceral motor nerves of the parasympathetic part generally have two neurons in the pathway. The preganglionic neurons are in the CNS, and fibers leave in certain cranial nerves and spinal nerves.

Sacral preganglionic parasympathetic fibers

In the sacral region, the preganglionic parasympathetic fibers form visceral nerves (the **pelvic splanchnic nerves**), which originate from the anterior rami of S2 to S4 and enter pelvic extensions of the large prevertebral plexus formed around the abdominal aorta. These fibers are distributed to pelvic and abdominal viscera mainly along blood vessels. The

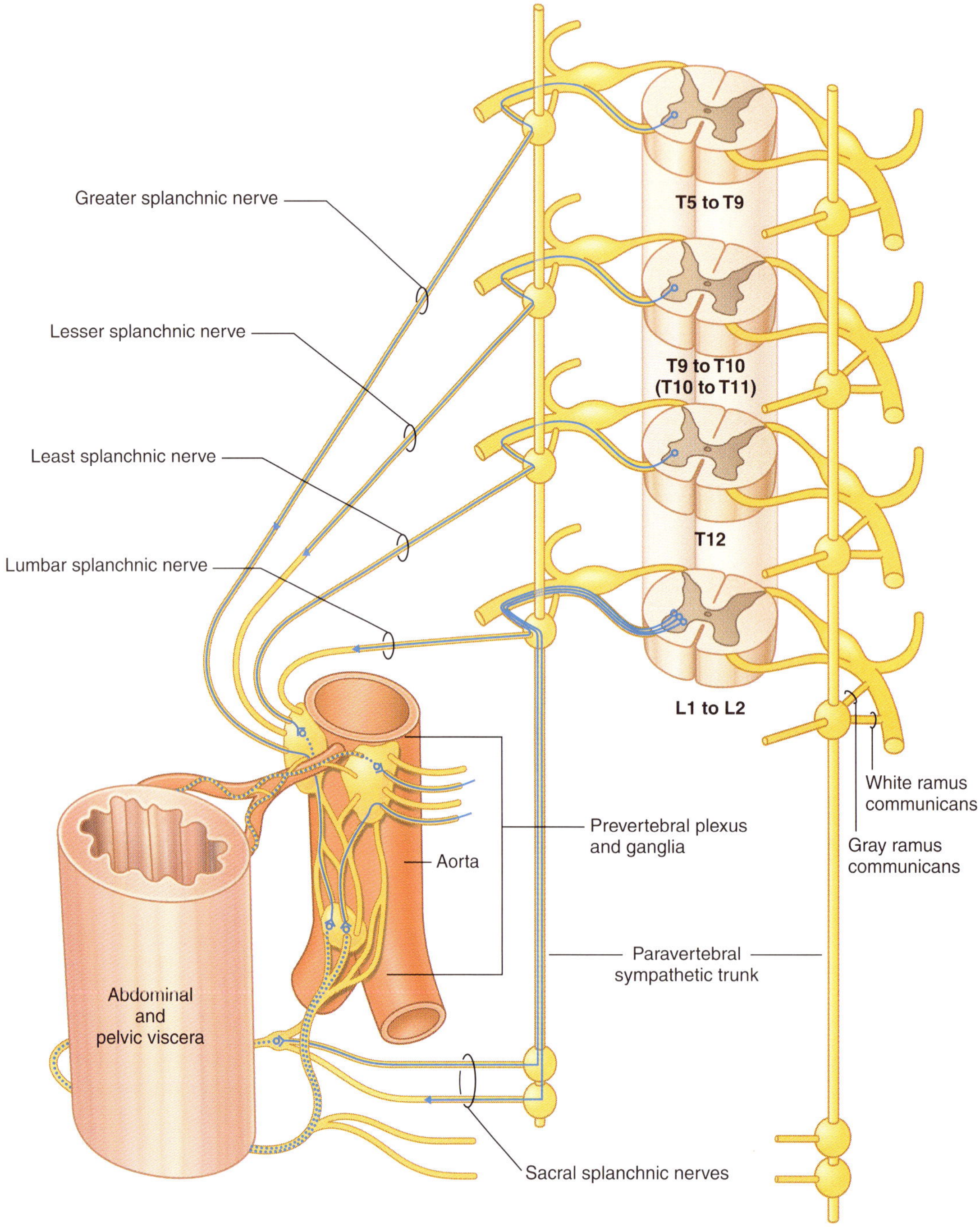

Fig. 1.47 Course of sympathetic nerves traveling to abdominal and pelvic viscera.

postganglionic motor neurons are in the walls of the viscera. In organs of the gastrointestinal system, preganglionic fibers do not have a postganglionic parasympathetic motor neuron in the pathway; instead, preganglionic fibers synapse directly on neurons in the ganglia of the enteric system.

Cranial nerve preganglionic parasympathetic fibers

The preganglionic parasympathetic motor fibers in CN III, VII, and IX separate from the nerves and connect with one of four distinct ganglia, which house postganglionic motor neurons. These four ganglia are near major branches of CN V. Postganglionic fibers leave the ganglia, join the branches of CN V, and are carried to target tissues (ciliary muscle in the eye, constrictor muscle of the pupil; lacrimal, salivary and mucous, glands) with these branches.

The vagus nerve [X] gives rise to visceral branches along its course. These branches contribute to plexuses associated with thoracic viscera or to the large prevertebral

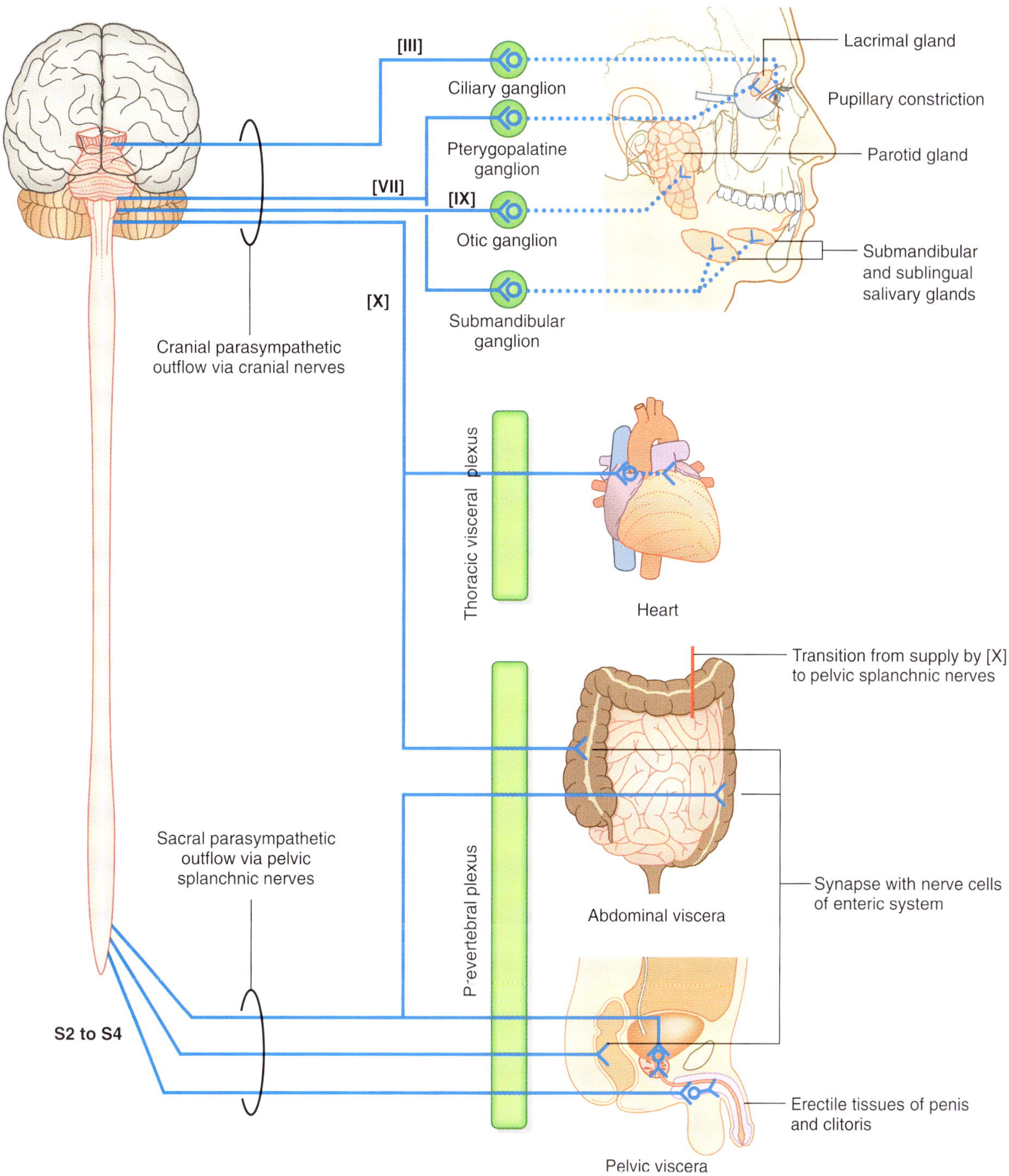

Fig. 1.48 Parasympathetic part of the autonomic division of the PNS.

plexus in the abdomen and pelvis. Many of these plexuses also contain sympathetic fibers.

When present, postganglionic parasympathetic neurons are in the walls of the target viscera (Fig. 1.48).

Visceral sensory innervation (visceral afferents)

Visceral sensory fibers generally accompany visceral motor fibers.

Visceral sensory fibers accompany sympathetic fibers

Visceral sensory fibers follow the course of sympathetic fibers entering the spinal cord at similar spinal cord levels. However, visceral sensory fibers may also enter the spinal cord at levels other than those associated with motor output. For example, visceral sensory fibers from the heart may enter at levels higher than spinal cord level T1.

Visceral sensory fibers that accompany sympathetic fibers are mainly concerned with detecting pain (Fig. 1.46).

Visceral sensory fibers accompany parasympathetic fibers

Visceral sensory fibers accompanying parasympathetic fibers are carried mainly in IX and X and in spinal nerves S2 to S4.

Visceral sensory fibers in IX carry information from chemoreceptors and baroreceptors associated with the walls of major arteries in the neck, and from receptors in the pharynx.

Visceral sensory fibers in X include those from cervical viscera, and major vessels and viscera in the thorax and abdomen.

Visceral sensory fibers from pelvic viscera and the distal parts of the colon are carried in S2 to S4.

Visceral sensory fibers associated with parasympathetic fibers primarily relay information to the CNS about the status of normal physiological processes and reflex activities.

The enteric system

The enteric nervous system consists of motor and sensory neurons and their support cells, which form two interconnected plexuses, the **myenteric** and **submucous nerve plexuses**, within the walls of the gastrointestinal tract (Fig. 1.49). Each of these plexuses is formed by:

- Ganglia, which house the nerve cell bodies and associated cells

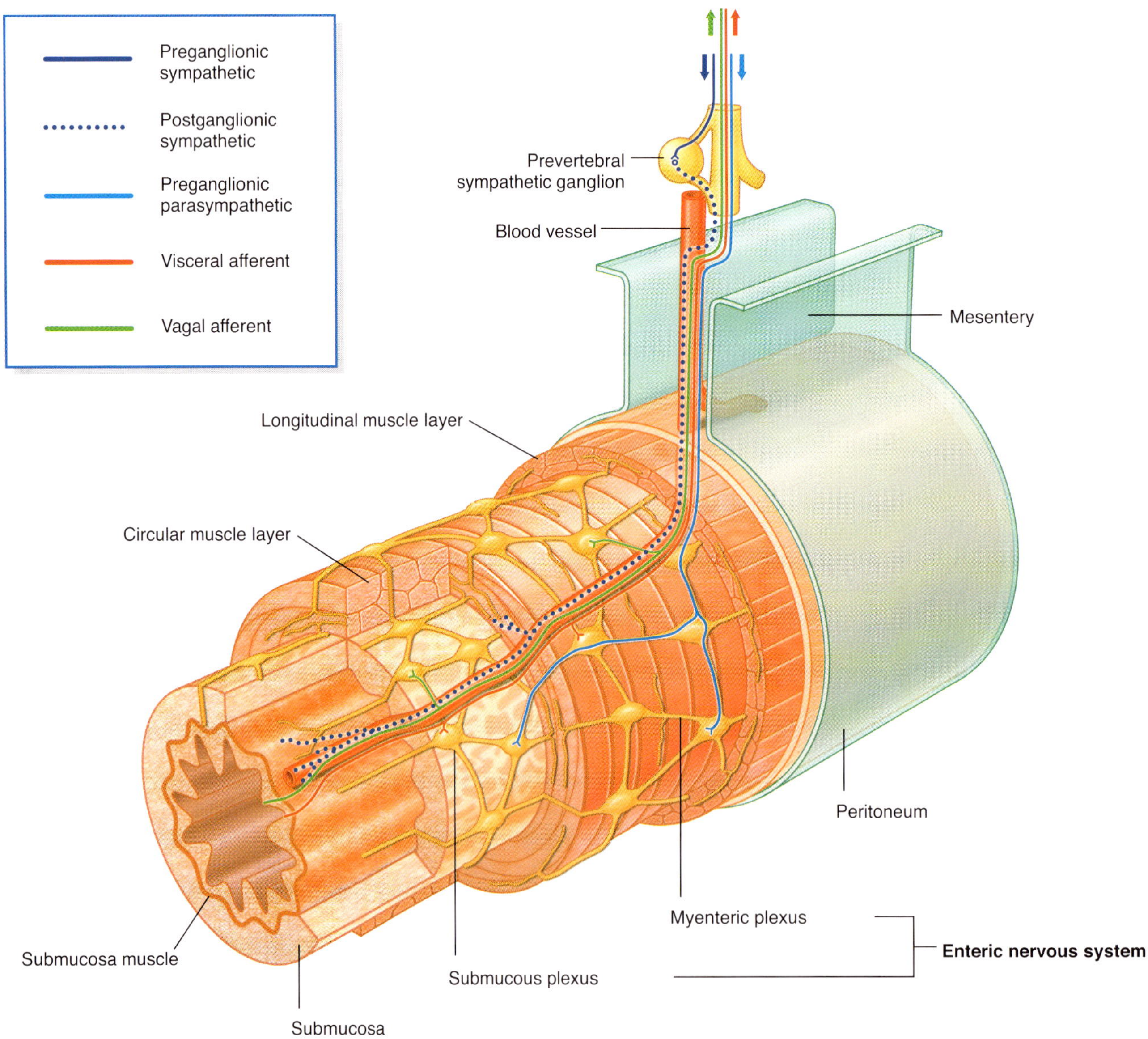

Fig. 1.49 Enteric part of the nervous system.

- Bundles of nerve fibers, which pass between ganglia and from the ganglia into surrounding tissues

Neurons in the enteric system are derived from neural crest cells originally associated with occipitocervical and sacral regions. Interestingly, more neurons are reported to be in the enteric system than in the spinal cord itself.

Sensory and motor neurons within the enteric system control reflex activity within and between parts of the gastrointestinal system. These reflexes regulate peristalsis, secretomotor activity, and vascular tone. These activities can occur independently of the brain and spinal cord, but can also be modified by input from preganglionic parasympathetic and postganglionic sympathetic fibers.

Sensory information from the enteric system is carried back to the CNS by visceral sensory fibers.

Nerve plexuses

Nerve plexuses are either somatic or visceral and combine fibers from different sources or levels to form new nerves with specific targets or destinations (Fig. 1.50). Plexuses of the enteric system also generate reflex activity independent of the CNS.

Somatic plexuses

Major somatic plexuses formed from the anterior rami of spinal nerves are the cervical (C1 to C4), brachial (C5 to T1), lumbar (L1 to L4), sacral (L4 to S3), and coccygeal (S5 to Co) plexuses. Except for spinal nerve T1, the anterior rami of thoracic spinal nerves remain independent and do not participate in plexuses.

Visceral plexuses

Visceral nerve plexuses are formed in association with viscera and generally contain efferent (sympathetic and parasympathetic) and afferent components (Fig. 1.50). These plexuses include cardiac and pulmonary plexuses in the thorax and a large prevertebral plexus in the abdomen anterior to the aorta, which extends inferiorly onto the lateral walls of the pelvis. The massive prevertebral plexus supplies input to and receives output from all abdominal and pelvic viscera.

Early clinical exposure

Referred pain

Referred pain occurs when sensory information comes to the spinal cord from one location but is interpreted by the CNS as coming from another location innervated by the same spinal cord level. Usually, this happens when the pain information comes from a region, such as the gut, which has a low amount of sensory output to the CNS. These afferents converge on neurons at the same spinal cord level that receive information from the skin, which is an area with a high amount of sensory output to the CNS. As a result, pain from the normally low output region is interpreted as coming from the normally high output region.

Pain is most often referred from a region innervated by the visceral part of the nervous system to a region innervated, at the same spinal cord level, by the somatic part of the nervous system.

Pain can also be referred from one somatic region to another. For example, irritation of the peritoneum on the inferior surface of the diaphragm, which is innervated by the phrenic nerve, can be referred to the skin on the top of the shoulder, which is innervated by other somatic nerves arising at the same spinal cord level.

OTHER SYSTEMS

Specific information about the organization and components of the respiratory, gastrointestinal, and urogenital systems will be discussed in each of the succeeding chapters of this text.

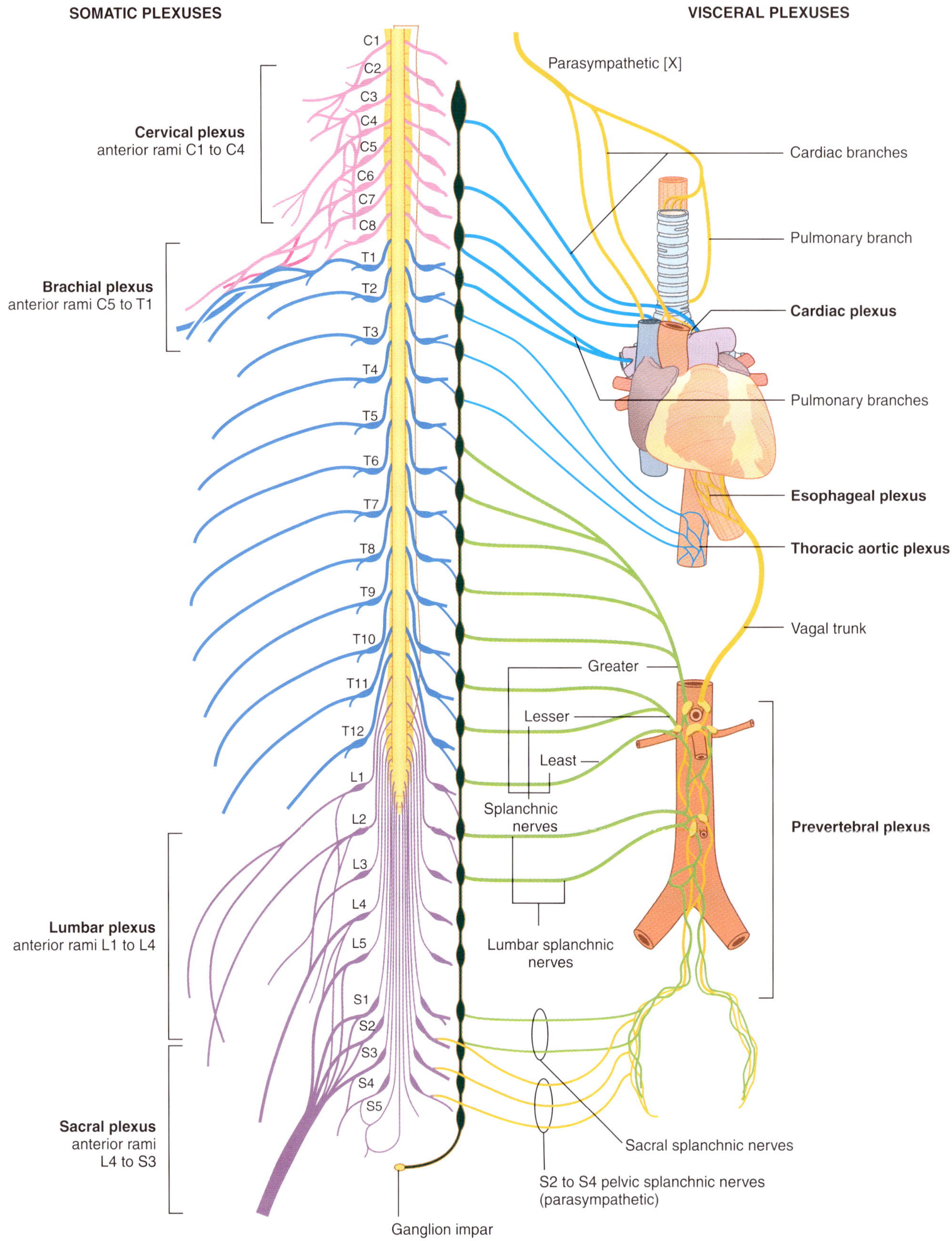

Fig. 1.50 Nerve plexuses.

Clinical cases

Case 1

APPENDICITIS

A young man sought medical care because of central abdominal pain that was diffuse and colicky. After some hours, the pain began to localize in the right iliac fossa and became constant. He was referred to an abdominal surgeon, who removed a grossly inflamed appendix. The patient made an uneventful recovery.

When the appendix becomes inflamed, the visceral sensory fibers are stimulated. These fibers enter the spinal cord at spinal cord level T10. The pain is referred to the dermatome of T10, which is in the umbilical region (Fig. 1.51). The pain is diffuse, not focal; every time a peristaltic wave passes through the ileocecal region, the pain recurs. This intermittent type of pain is referred to as colic.

In the later stages of the disease, the appendix contacts and irritates the parietal peritoneum in the right iliac fossa, which is innervated by somatic sensory nerves. This produces a constant focal pain, which predominates over the colicky pain that the patient felt some hours previously. The patient no longer interprets the referred pain from the T10 dermatome.

Although this is a typical history for appendicitis, it should always be borne in mind that the patient's symptoms and signs may vary. The appendix is situated in a retrocecal position in approximately 70% of patients; therefore, it may never contact the parietal peritoneum anteriorly in the right iliac fossa. It is also possible that the appendix is long and may directly contact other structures. As a consequence, the patient may have other symptoms (e.g., the appendix may contact the ureter, and the patient may then develop urological symptoms).

Although appendicitis is common, other disorders, for example of the bowel and pelvis, may produce similar symptoms.

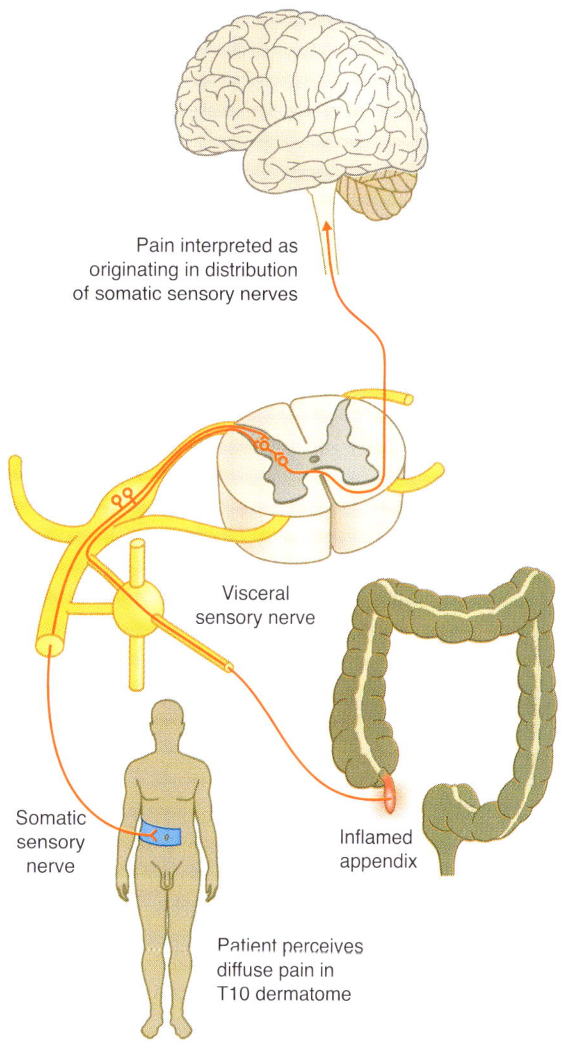

Fig. 1.51 Mechanism for referred pain from an inflamed appendix to the T10 dermatome.

2

Upper Limb

ADDITIONAL LEARNING RESOURCES for Chapter 2, *Upper Limb*, on MedEnact (www.MedEnact.com):

- Multiple-Choice Questions
- Short Questions—these are questions requiring short responses
- Medical Clinical Case Studies
  Clavicular fracture
  Extensor tendon injury of the hand
  Hand infection
  High median nerve palsy
  Radial fracture
  Rotator cuff impingement syndrome
  See more Medical Clinical Case Studies online

FREE Online Anatomy Self-Study Course

- Anatomy modules 32 through 38

Competency: The first-year medical students should be able to apply their knowledge of the course, relations, and distribution of the major arteries and nerves of the upper limb and the actions of the muscles at various joints to explain the anatomical basis of common clinical conditions and procedures.

Conceptual overview

SET INDUCTION—CASE SCENARIO 1: SHOULDER DISLOCATION

A 25-year-old cricketer while bowling had severe pain of sudden onset in the right shoulder region and was unable to move his right shoulder. On examination, a sports physician noted that the normal contour of the right shoulder was lost, with no sensory loss, and a diagnosis of dislocated right shoulder was made.

It is necessary to know the anatomy of the shoulder region before one can manage a patient with dislocation of the shoulder joint.

<table>
<tr><th rowspan="2">REMEMBER
[Recall Facts]</th><th colspan="3">OUTLINE 1. CONCEPTUAL OVERVIEW AND SHOULDER REGION—LEARNING OBJECTIVES
[By the end of this section, the student should be able to:]</th><th colspan="2" rowspan="2">EVALUATE
[Explain Concepts]</th></tr>
<tr><th colspan="3">DEMONSTRATE AND ANALYZE RELATIONSHIPS
[Identify structures in a Prosected Specimen or Figure]</th></tr>
<tr><td rowspan="7">Conceptual overview
1. Explain the divisions of the upper limb
2. Describe the functions of the hand
3. Briefly describe the bones of the upper limb
4. List the groups of muscles in the parts of the upper limb
5. Describe the relation of the upper limb to the neck, back, and thoracic wall
6. Briefly describe the innervations of the upper limb
7. Briefly describe the veins of the upper limb
Shoulder region
1. Mention the bones and joints of the shoulder region
2. Describe in brief the sternoclavicular and acromioclavicular joints
3. Describe in detail the glenohumeral joint
4. Enumerate the muscles of the shoulder region and mention their origin, insertion, action, and nerve supply
5. Enumerate the muscles of the posterior scapular region, and list their origin, insertion, action, and nerve supply
6. Describe the gateways to the scapular region and boundaries and contents of quadrangular and triangular spaces
7. Describe briefly the course and distribution of the axillary nerve and describe the clinical manifestations of its injury</td><td>Level I</td><td>Level II</td><td>Level III</td><td colspan="2" rowspan="2">■ Movements at the shoulder joint and the muscles causing them
■ Boundaries of the spaces
■ Formation of rotator cuff
■ Course of the axillary nerve
■ Scapular arterial anastomosis</td></tr>
<tr><td rowspan="6">■ Deltoid
■ Supraspinatus
■ Infraspinatus
■ Teres major
■ Teres minor
■ Axillary nerve
■ Long head of triceps
Radial nerve</td><td rowspan="6">■ Posterior circumflex humeral vessels
■ Profunda brachii vessels</td><td rowspan="6">■ Upper lateral cutaneous nerve of the arm
■ Circumflex scapular vessels</td></tr>
<tr><th colspan="2">EARLY CLINICAL EXPOSURE
[Apply Anatomical Knowledge]</th></tr>
<tr><th>Surgical Anatomy/ Pathology/ Trauma</th><th>Imaging/ Surface Anatomy</th></tr>
<tr><td>■ Intramuscular injections
■ Fracture of surgical neck of humerus
■ Rotator cuff injuries
■ Quadrangular space syndrome
■ Inflammation of subacromial bursa
■ Fracture of clavicle and dislocation of joints</td><td>■ Radiograph of normal and dislocated joints
■ Radiograph of fracture of clavicle
■ MRI of supraspinatus tendon tear</td></tr>
<tr><th colspan="2">PROBLEM SOLVING/ CLINICAL CASES
[Interpret]</th></tr>
<tr><td colspan="2">■ Shoulder problems after falling on an outstretched hand
■ Torn supraspinatus tendon</td></tr>
</table>

GENERAL DESCRIPTION

The upper limb is suspended from the trunk by muscles and a small skeletal articulation between the clavicle and the sternum—the sternoclavicular joint. Based on the position of its major joints and component bones, the upper limb is divided into shoulder, arm, forearm, and hand (Fig. 2.1A).

The **shoulder** is the area of upper limb attachment to the trunk (Fig. 2.1B).

The **arm** is the part of the upper limb between the shoulder and the elbow joint; the forearm is between the elbow joint and the wrist joint; and the hand is distal to the wrist joint.

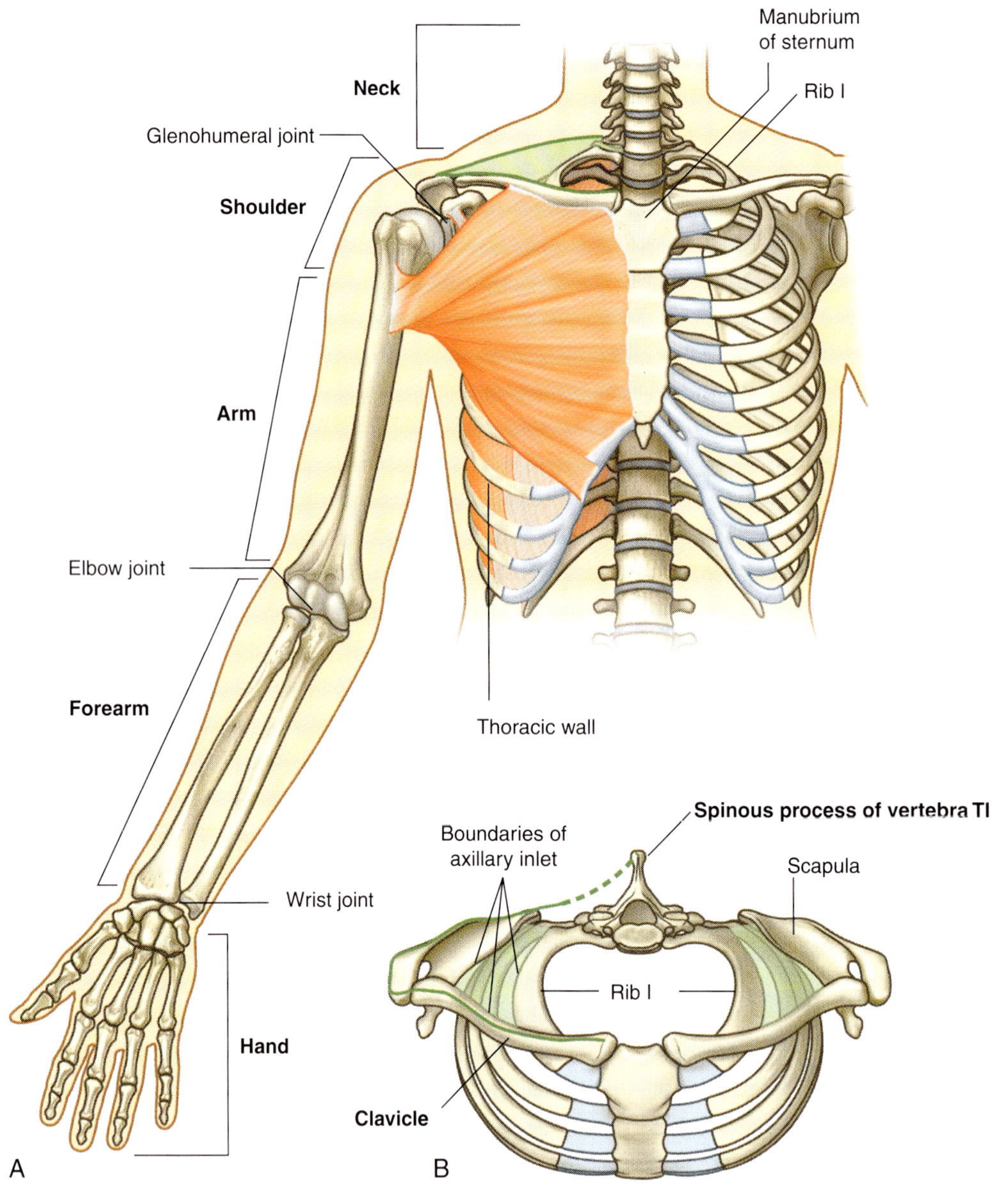

Fig. 2.1 Upper limb. **(A)** Anterior view of the upper limb. **(B)** Superior view of the shoulder.

The axilla, cubital fossa, and carpal tunnel are significant **areas of transition** between the different parts of the limb (Fig. 2.2). Important structures pass through, or are related to, each of these areas.

The **axilla** is an irregularly shaped pyramidal area formed by muscles and bones of the shoulder and the lateral surface of the thoracic wall. The apex or inlet opens directly into the cervicoaxillary canal at the lower portion of the neck. The skin of the armpit forms the floor. All major structures that pass between the neck and arm pass through the axilla.

The **cubital fossa** is a triangularly shaped depression formed by muscles anterior to the elbow joint. The major artery, the brachial artery, passing from the arm to the forearm passes through this fossa, as does one of the major nerves of the upper limb, the median nerve.

The **carpal tunnel** is the gateway to the palm of the hand. Its posterior, lateral, and medial walls form an arch, which is made up of small carpal bones in the proximal region of the hand. A thick band of connective tissue, the flexor retinaculum, spans the distance between each side of the arch and forms the anterior wall of the tunnel. The median nerve and all the long flexor tendons passing from the forearm to the digits of the hand pass through the carpal tunnel.

FUNCTIONS

Positioning the hand

Unlike the lower limb, which is used for support, stability, and locomotion, the upper limb is highly mobile for positioning the hand in space.

The shoulder is suspended from the trunk predominantly by muscles and can therefore be moved relative to the body. Sliding (protraction and retraction) and rotating the scapula on the thoracic wall changes the position of the **glenohumeral joint** (**shoulder joint**) and extends the reach of the hand (Fig. 2.3). The glenohumeral joint allows the arm to move around three axes with a wide range of motion. Movements of the arm at this joint are

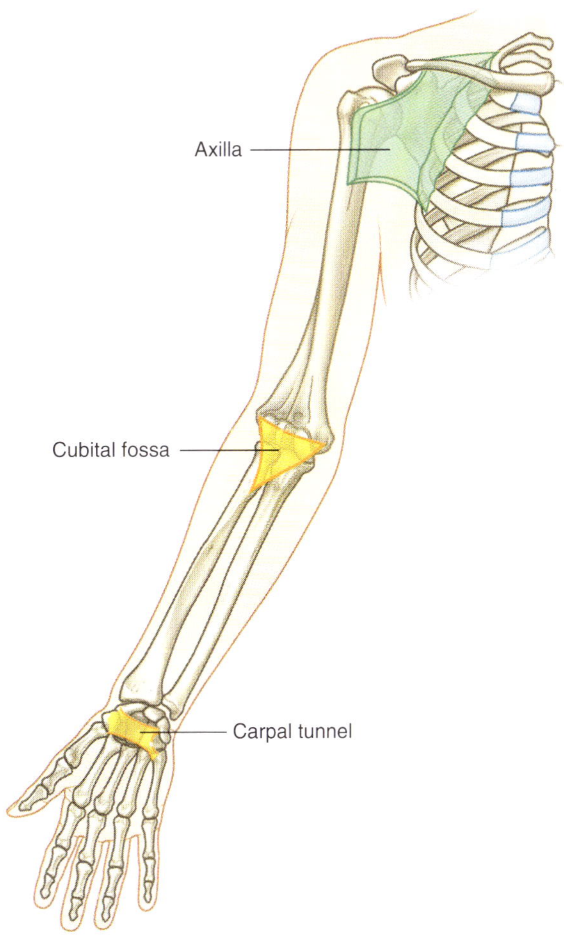

Fig. 2.2 Areas of transition in the upper limb.

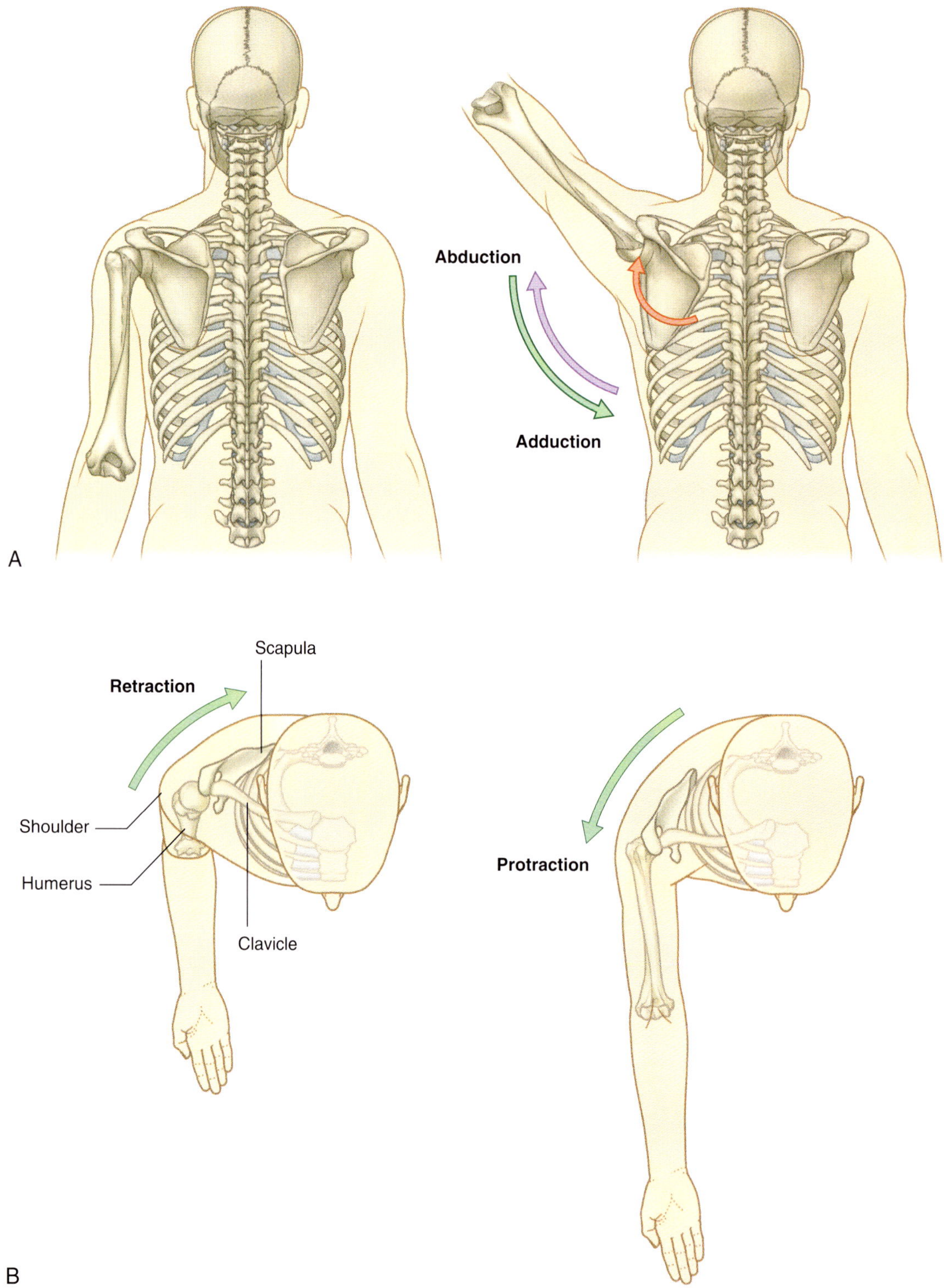

Fig. 2.3 Movements of the scapula. **(A)** Rotation. **(B)** Protraction and retraction.

flexion, extension, abduction, adduction, medial rotation (internal rotation), lateral rotation (external rotation), and circumduction (Fig. 2.4).

The major movements at the **elbow joint** are flexion and extension of the forearm (Fig. 2.5A). At the other end of the forearm, the distal end of the lateral bone, the radius, can be flipped over the adjacent head of the medial bone, the ulna. Because the hand is articulated with the radius, it can be efficiently moved from a palm-anterior position to a palm-posterior position simply by crossing the

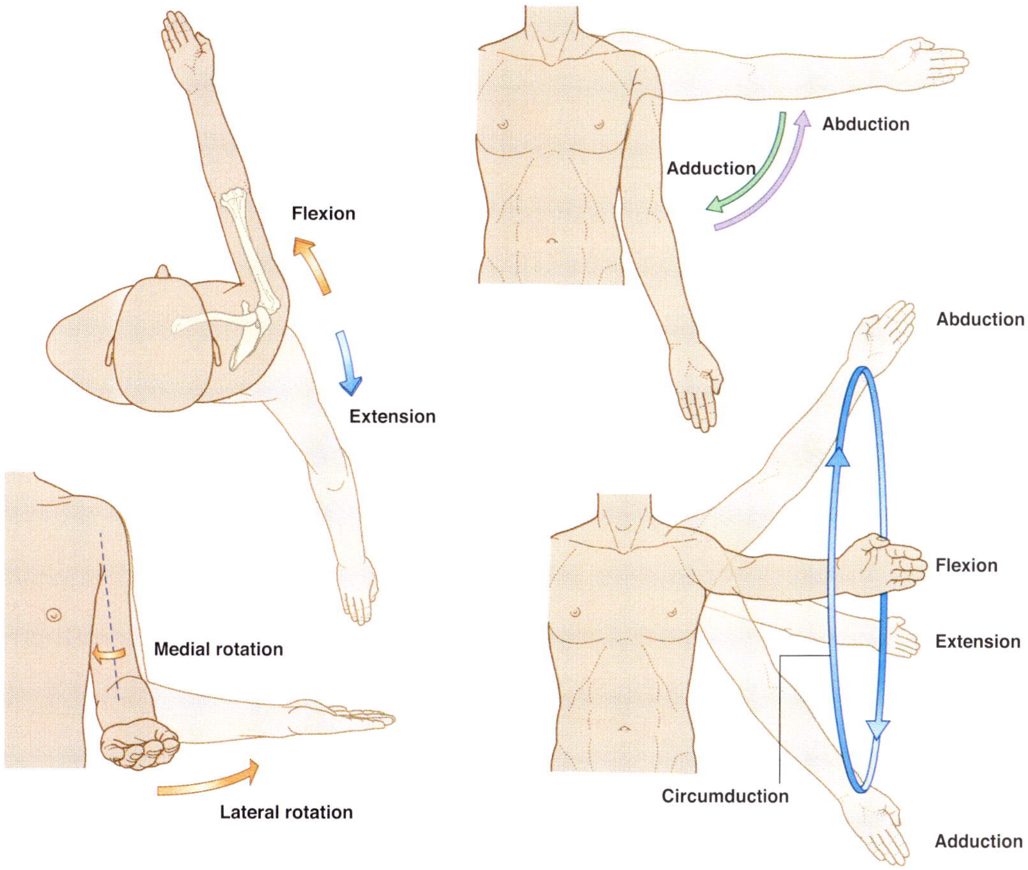

Fig. 2.4 Movements of the arm at the glenohumeral joint.

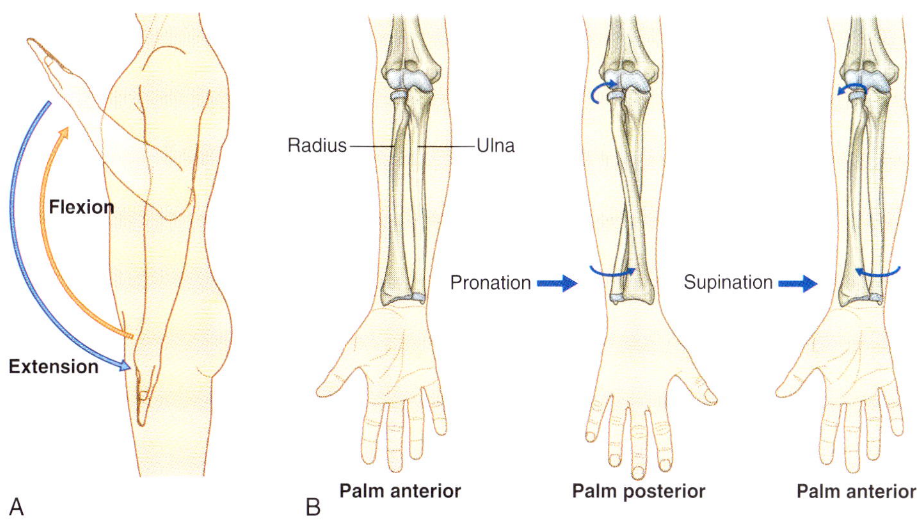

Fig. 2.5 Movements of the forearm. **(A)** Flexion and extension at the elbow joint. **(B)** Pronation and supination.

distal end of the radius over the ulna (Fig. 2.5B). This movement, termed pronation, occurs solely in the forearm. Supination returns the hand to the anatomical position.

At the **wrist joint**, the hand can be abducted, adducted, flexed, extended, and circumducted (Fig. 2.6). These movements, combined with those of the shoulder, arm, and forearm, enable the hand to be placed in a wide range of positions relative to the body.

The hand as a mechanical tool

One of the major functions of the hand is to grip and manipulate objects. Gripping objects generally involves flexing the fingers against the thumb. Depending on the type of grip, muscles in the hand act to:

- Modify the actions of long tendons that emerge from the forearm and insert into the digits of the hand.
- Produce combinations of joint movements within each digit that cannot be generated by the long flexor and extensor tendons alone coming from the forearm.

The hand as a sensory tool

The hand is used to discriminate between objects on the basis of touch. The pads on the palmar aspect of the fingers

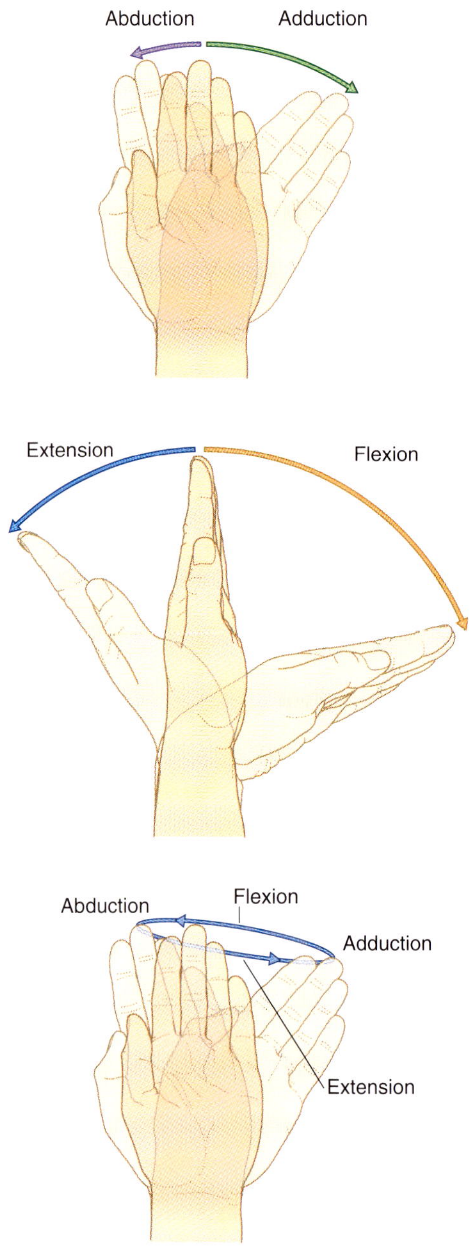

Fig. 2.6 Movements of the hand at the wrist joint.

contain a high density of somatic sensory receptors. Also, the sensory cortex of the brain devoted to interpreting information from the hand, particularly from the thumb, is disproportionately large relative to that for many other regions of skin.

COMPONENT PARTS

Bones and joints

The bones of the shoulder consist of the scapula, clavicle, and proximal end of the humerus (Fig. 2.7).

The clavicle articulates medially with the manubrium of the sternum and laterally with the acromion of the scapula, which arches over the joint between the glenoid cavity of the scapula and the head of the humerus (the glenohumeral joint).

The humerus is the bone of the arm (Fig. 2.7). The distal end of the humerus articulates with the bones of the forearm at the elbow joint, which is a hinge joint that allows flexion and extension of the forearm.

The forearm contains two bones:

- The lateral bone is the radius.
- The medial bone is the ulna (Fig. 2.7)

At the elbow joint, the proximal ends of the radius and ulna articulate with each other as well as with the humerus.

In addition to flexing and extending the forearm, the elbow joint allows the radius to spin on the humerus while sliding against the head of the ulna during pronation and supination of the hand.

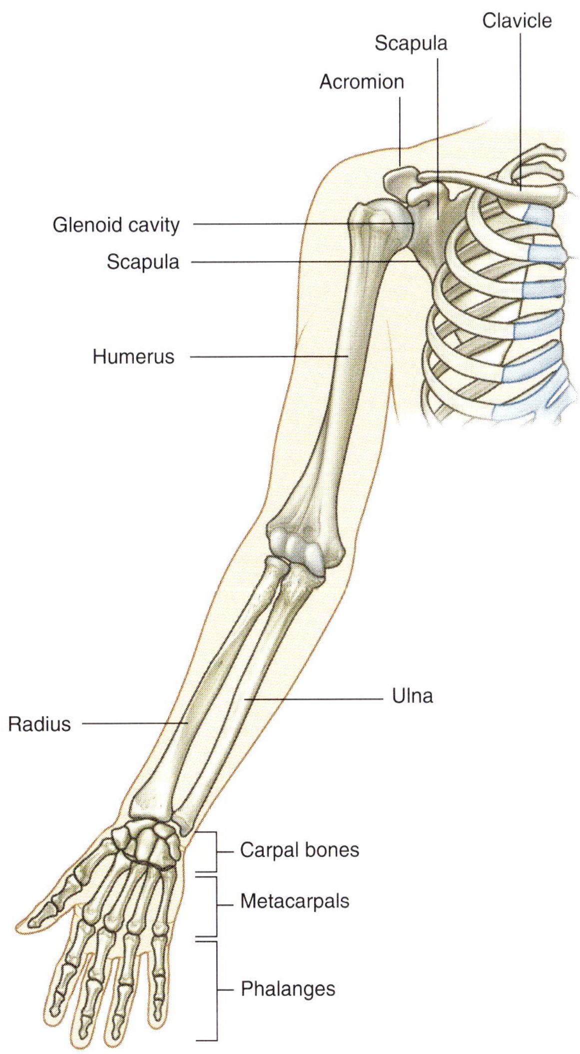

Fig. 2.7 Bones of the upper limb.

The distal portions of the radius and the ulna also articulate with each other. This joint allows the end of the radius to flip from the lateral side to the medial side of the ulna during pronation of the hand.

The wrist joint is formed between the radius and carpal bones of the hand and between an articular disc, distal to the ulna, and carpal bones.

The bones of the hand consist of the carpal bones, the metacarpals, and the phalanges (Fig. 2.7).

The five digits in the hand are the thumb and the index, middle, ring, and little fingers.

Joints between the eight small carpal bones allow only limited amounts of movement; as a result, the bones work together as a unit.

The five metacarpals, one for each digit, are the primary skeletal foundation of the palm (Fig. 2.7).

The joint between the metacarpal of the thumb (metacarpal I) and one of the carpal bones allows greater mobility than the limited sliding movement that occurs at the carpometacarpal joints of the fingers.

Distally, the heads of metacarpals II to V (i.e., except that of the thumb) are interconnected by strong ligaments. Lack of this ligamentous connection between the metacarpal bones of the thumb and index finger together with the biaxial **saddle joint** between the metacarpal bone of the thumb and the carpus provides the thumb with greater freedom of movement than the other digits of the hand.

The bones of the digits are the phalanges (Fig. 2.7). The thumb has two phalanges, while each of the other digits has three.

The metacarpophalangeal joints are biaxial **condylar joints** (**ellipsoid joints**) that allow abduction, adduction, flexion, extension, and circumduction (Fig. 2.8). Abduction and adduction of the fingers is defined in reference to an axis passing through the center of the middle finger in the anatomical position. The middle finger can therefore abduct both medially and laterally and adduct back to the central axis from either side. The interphalangeal joints are primarily **hinge joints** that allow only flexion and extension.

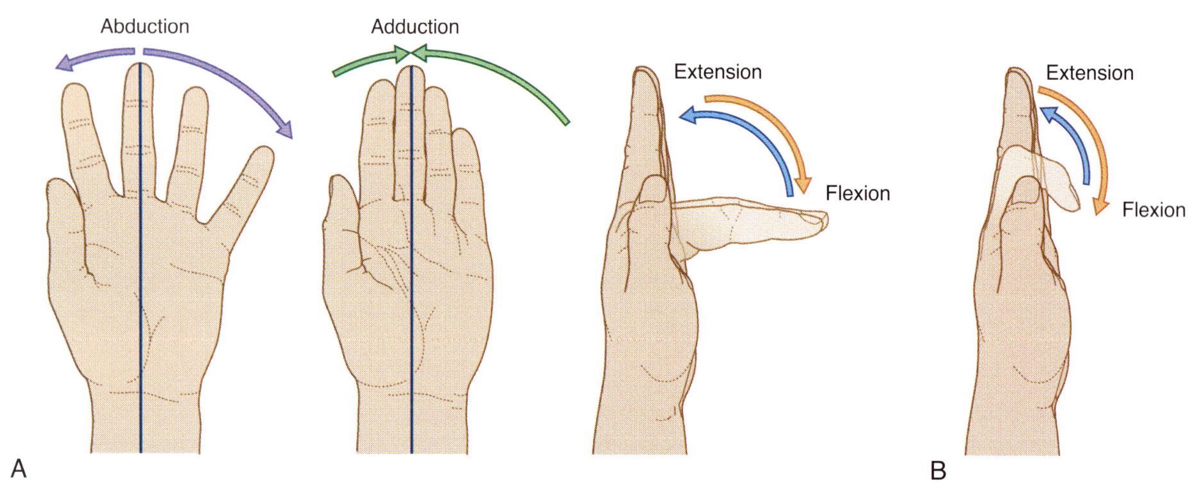

Fig. 2.8 Movements of the metacarpophalangeal (**A**) and interphalangeal (**B**) joints.

Muscles

Some muscles of the shoulder, such as the trapezius, levator scapulae, and rhomboids, connect the scapula and clavicle to the trunk. Other muscles connect the clavicle, scapula, and body wall to the proximal end of the humerus. These include the pectoralis major, pectoralis minor, latissimus dorsi, teres major, and deltoid (Fig. 2.9A and B). The most important of these muscles are the four rotator cuff muscles—the subscapularis, supraspinatus, infraspinatus, and teres minor muscles—which connect the scapula to the humerus and provide support for the glenohumeral joint (Fig. 2.9C).

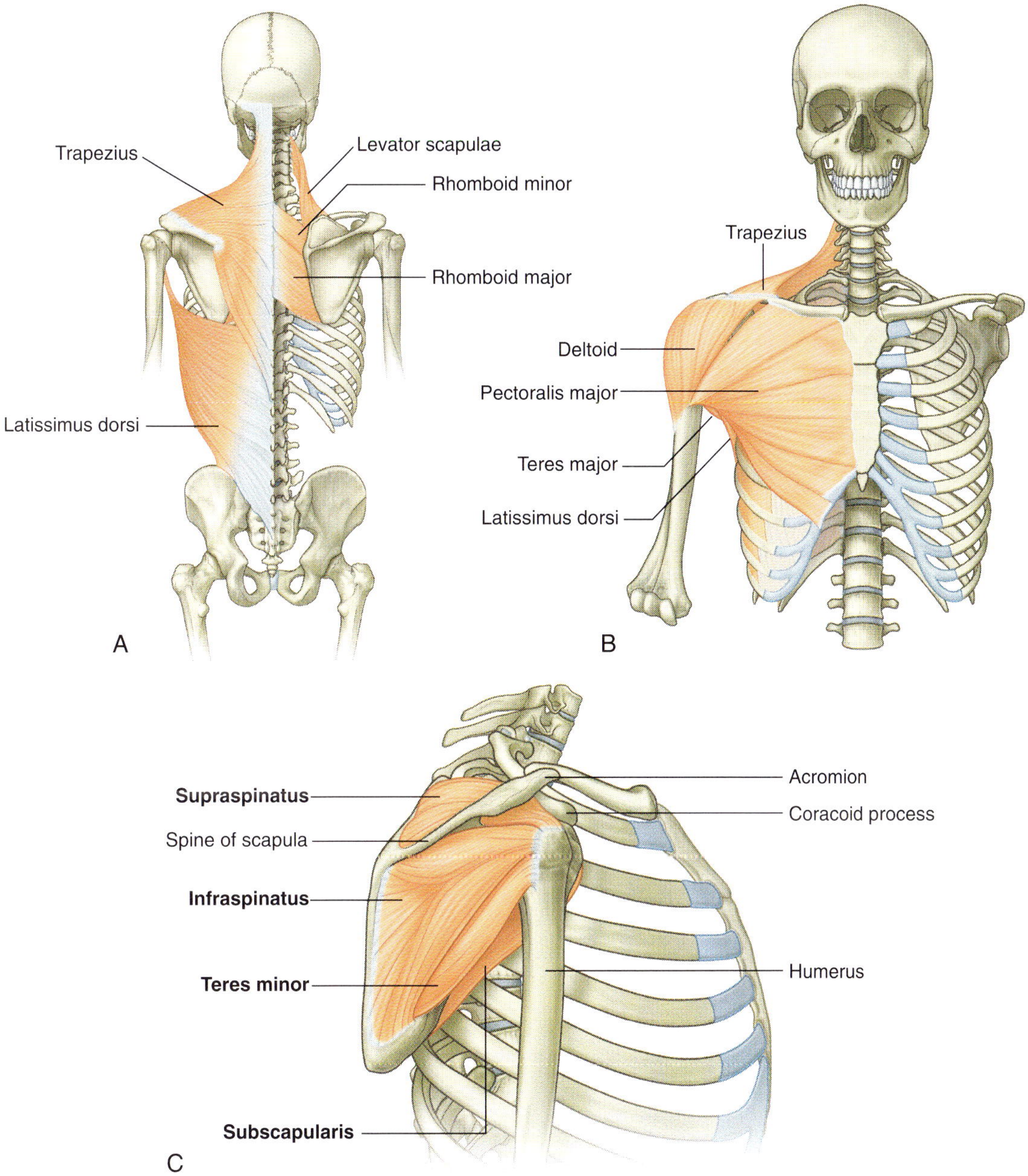

Fig. 2.9 Muscles of the shoulder. **(A)** Posterior shoulder. **(B)** Anterior shoulder. **(C)** Rotator cuff muscles.

Muscles in the arm and forearm are separated into anterior (flexor) and posterior (extensor) compartments by layers of fascia, bones, and ligaments (Fig. 2.10). The upper limb buds during development undergo 90 rotations laterally; hence, the anterior compartment is flexor and posterior is extensor.

The anterior compartment of the arm lies anteriorly in position and is separated from muscles of the posterior compartment by the humerus and by medial and lateral intermuscular septa. These intermuscular septa are continuous with the deep fascia enclosing the arm and attach to the sides of the humerus.

In the forearm, the anterior and posterior compartments are separated by a lateral intermuscular septum, the radius, the ulna, and an interosseous membrane, which joins adjacent sides of the radius and ulna (Fig. 2.10).

Muscles in the arm act mainly to move the forearm at the elbow joint, while those in the forearm function predominantly to move the hand at the wrist joint and the fingers and thumb.

Muscles found entirely in the hand, the intrinsic muscles, generate delicate movements of the digits of the hand and modify the forces produced by tendons coming into the fingers and thumb from the forearm. Included among the intrinsic muscles of the hand are three small thenar muscles, which form a soft tissue mound, called the **thenar eminence**, over the palmar aspect of metacarpal I. The thenar muscles allow the thumb to move freely relative to the other fingers.

RELATIONSHIP TO OTHER REGIONS

Neck

The upper limb is directly related to the neck. Lying on each side of the **superior thoracic aperture** at the base of the neck is an **axillary inlet,** which is formed by:

- The lateral margin of rib I
- The posterior surface of the clavicle
- The superior margin of the scapula

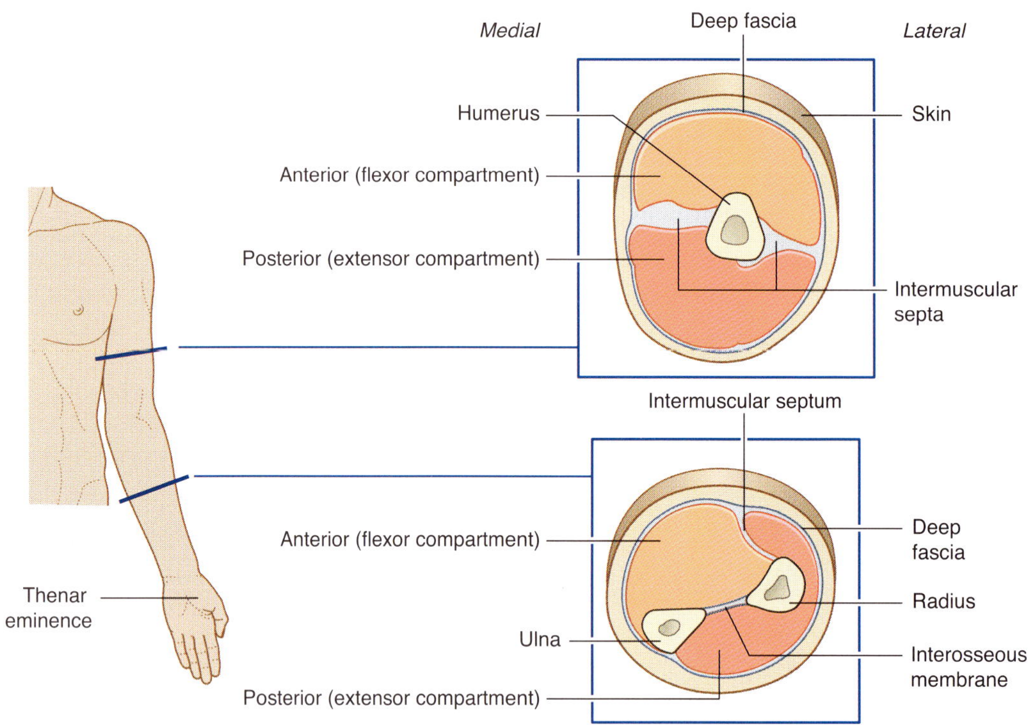

Fig. 2.10 Muscle components in the arm and forearm.

- The medial surface of the coracoid process of the scapula (Fig. 2.11)

The major artery and vein of the upper limb pass between the thorax and the limb by passing over rib I and through the axillary inlet. Nerves, predominantly derived from the cervical portion of the spinal cord, also pass through the axillary inlet and the axilla to supply the upper limb.

Back and thoracic wall

Muscles that attach the bones of the shoulder to the trunk are associated with the back and the thoracic wall and

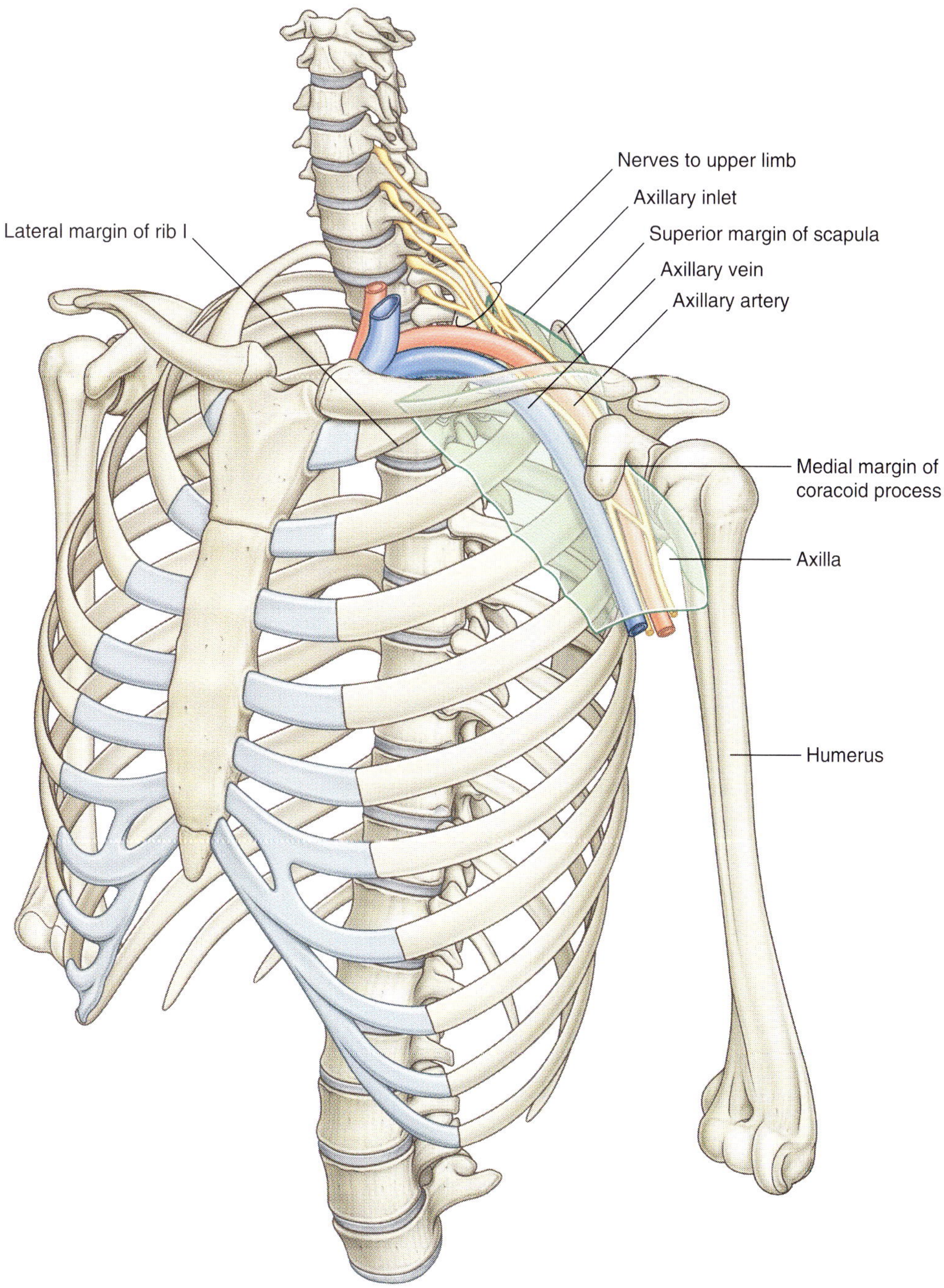

Fig. 2.11 Relationship of the upper limb to the neck.

include the trapezius, levator scapulae, rhomboid major, rhomboid minor, and latissimus dorsi (Fig. 2.12).

The breast on the anterior thoracic wall has a number of significant relationships with the axilla and upper limb. It overlies the pectoralis major muscle, which forms most of the anterior wall of the axilla and attaches the humerus to the chest wall (Fig. 2.13). Often, part of the breast known as the axillary process extends around the lateral margin of the pectoralis major into the axilla.

Lymphatic drainage from lateral and superior parts of the breast is predominantly into lymph nodes in the axilla. Several arteries and veins that supply or drain the gland also originate from, or drain into, major axillary vessels.

KEY POINTS

Innervation by cervical and upper thoracic nerves

Innervation of the upper limb is by the brachial plexus, which is formed by the anterior rami of cervical spinal

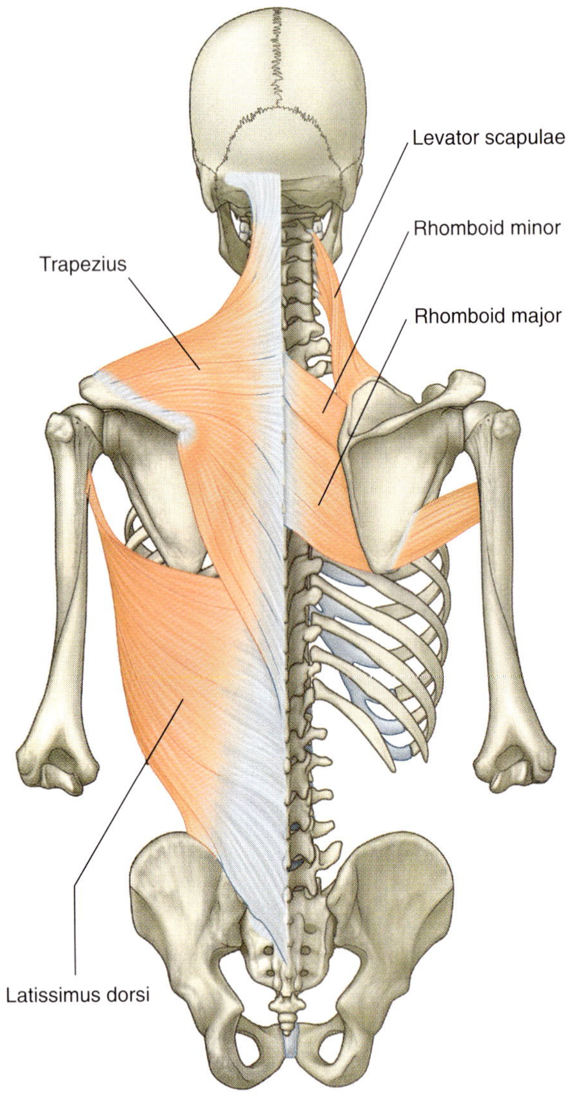

Fig. 2.12 Muscles of the back and thoracic wall.

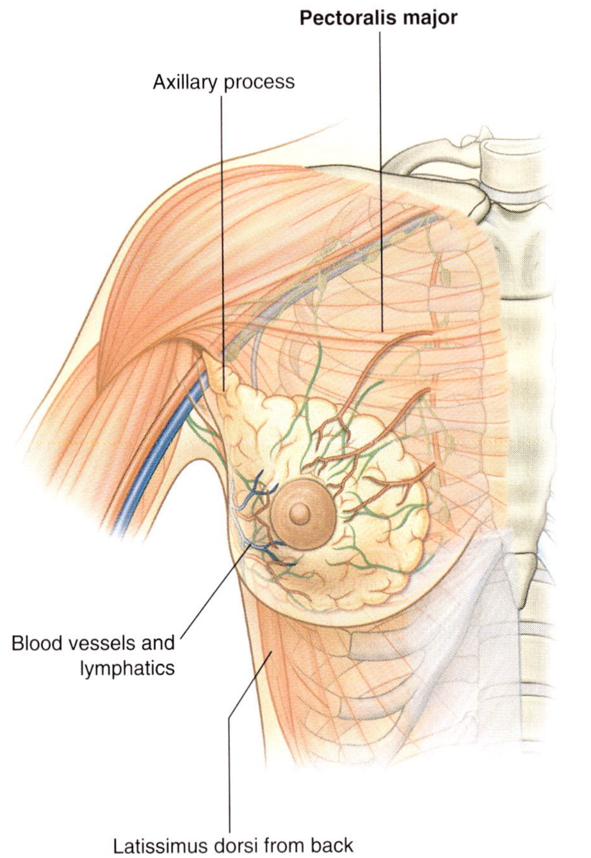

Fig. 2.13 Breast.

nerves C5 to C8, and T1 (Fig. 2.14). This plexus is initially formed in the neck and then continues through the axillary inlet into the axilla. Major nerves that ultimately innervate the arm, forearm, and hand originate from the brachial plexus in the axilla.

As a consequence of this innervation pattern, clinical testing of lower cervical and T1 nerves is carried out by examining dermatomes, myotomes, and tendon reflexes in the upper limb. Another consequence is that the clinical signs of problems related to lower cervical nerves—pain; pins-and-needles sensations, or paresthesia; and muscle twitching—appear in the upper limb.

Dermatomes of the upper limb (Fig. 2.15A) are often tested for sensation. Areas where overlap of dermatomes is minimal include the following:

- Upper lateral region of the arm for spinal cord level C5
- Palmar pad of the thumb for spinal cord level C6
- Pad of the index finger for spinal cord level C7
- Pad of the little finger for spinal cord level C8
- Skin on the medial aspect of the elbow for spinal cord level T1

Selected joint movements are used to test myotomes (Fig. 2.15B):

- Abduction of the arm at the glenohumeral joint is controlled predominantly by C5.
- Flexion of the forearm at the elbow joint is controlled primarily by C6.
- Extension of the forearm at the elbow joint is controlled mainly by C7.
- Flexion of the fingers is controlled mainly by C8.
- Abduction and adduction of the index, middle, and ring fingers is controlled predominantly by T1.

In an unconscious patient, both somatic sensory and motor functions of spinal cord levels can be tested using tendon reflexes:

- A tap on the tendon of the biceps in the cubital fossa tests mainly for spinal cord level C6.
- A tap on the tendon of the triceps posterior to the elbow tests mainly for C7.

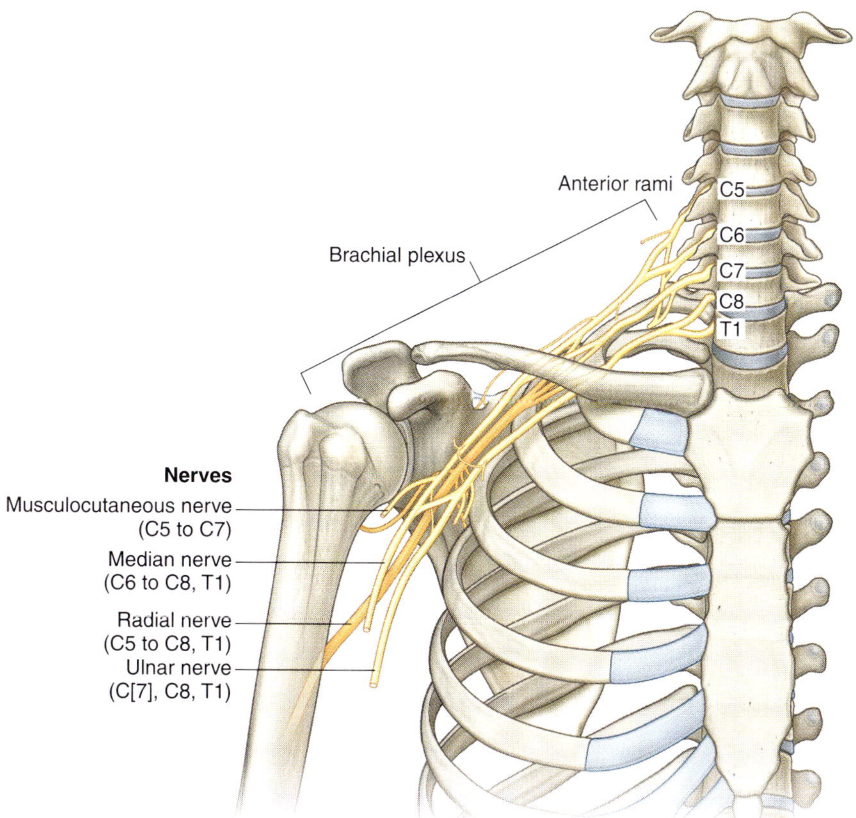

Fig. 2.14 Innervation of the upper limb.

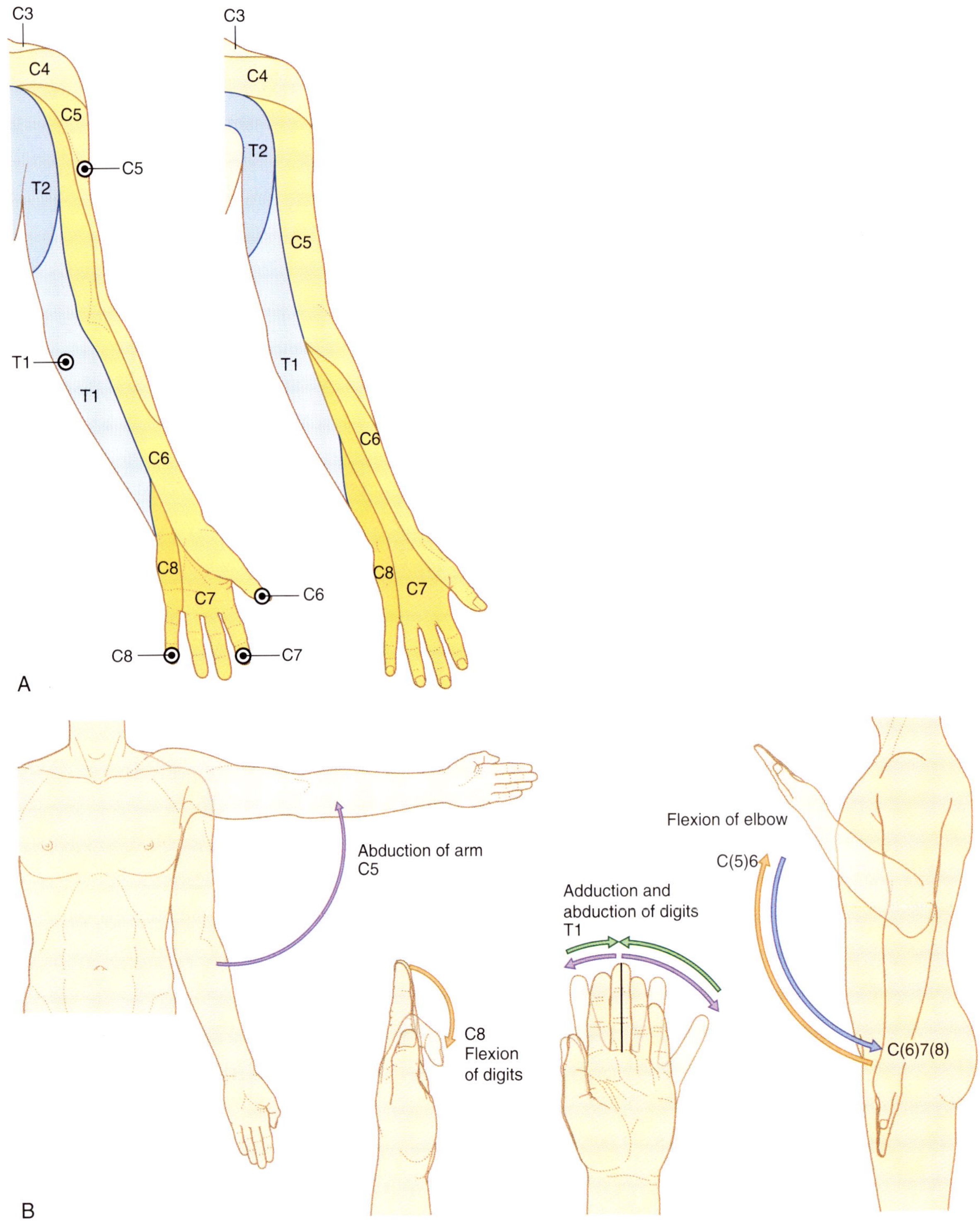

Fig. 2.15 Dermatomes and myotomes in the upper limb. **(A)** Dermatomes. **(B)** Movements produced by myotomes.

The major spinal cord level associated with innervation of the diaphragm, C4, is immediately above the spinal cord levels associated with the upper limb.

Evaluation of dermatomes and myotomes in the upper limb can provide important information about potential breathing problems that might develop as complications of damage to the spinal cord in regions just below the C4 spinal level.

A useful concept while testing joint movements is to note the plane of the movement and the axis around which the movement occurs. For example, abduction at the shoulder (Fig. 2.15B) occurs in the coronal plane around an anteroposterior axis, and flexion of the elbow occurs in the sagittal plane around a transverse axis.

Each of the major muscle compartments in the arm and forearm and each of the intrinsic muscles of the hand are innervated predominantly by one of the major nerves that originate from the brachial plexus in the axilla (Fig. 2.16A):

- All muscles in the anterior compartment of the arm are innervated by the musculocutaneous nerve.

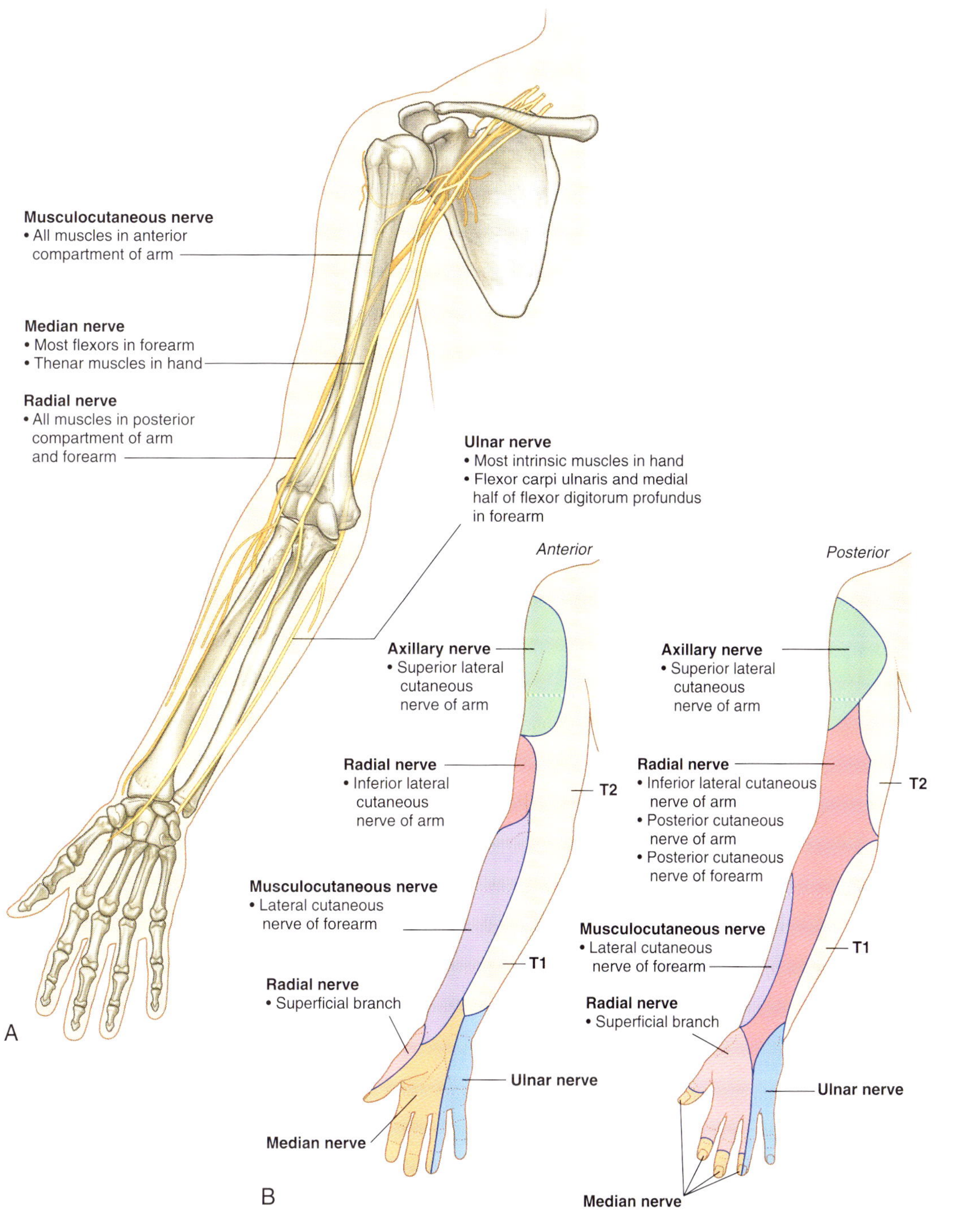

Fig. 2.16 Nerves of the upper limb. **(A)** Major nerves in the arm and forearm. **(B)** Anterior and posterior areas of skin innervated by major peripheral nerves in the arm and forearm.

- The median nerve innervates the muscles in the anterior compartment of the forearm, with two exceptions—one flexor of the wrist (the flexor carpi ulnaris muscle) and part of one flexor of the fingers (the medial half of the flexor digitorum profundus muscle) are innervated by the ulnar nerve.
- Most intrinsic muscles of the hand are innervated by the ulnar nerve, except for the thenar muscles and two lateral lumbrical muscles, which are innervated by the median nerve.
- All muscles in the posterior compartments of the arm and forearm are innervated by the radial nerve.

In addition to innervating major muscle groups, each of the major peripheral nerves originating from the brachial plexus carries somatic sensory information from patches of skin quite different from dermatomes (Fig. 2.16B). Sensation in these areas can be used to test for peripheral nerve lesions:

- The musculocutaneous nerve innervates skin on the anterolateral side of the forearm.
- The median nerve innervates the palmar surface of the lateral three and one-half digits, and the ulnar nerve innervates the medial one and one-half digits.
- The radial nerve supplies skin on the posterior surface of the forearm and the dorsolateral surface of the hand.
- A useful generalization is that an injury of a peripheral nerve causes loss of sensation in the area supplied by it, whereas an injury to a spinal nerve results in loss of sensation in a dermatome.

Nerves related to bone

Three important nerves are directly related to parts of the humerus (Fig. 2.17):

- The axillary nerve, which supplies the deltoid muscle, a major abductor of the humerus at the glenohumeral joint, passes around the posterior aspect of the upper part of the humerus (the surgical neck).

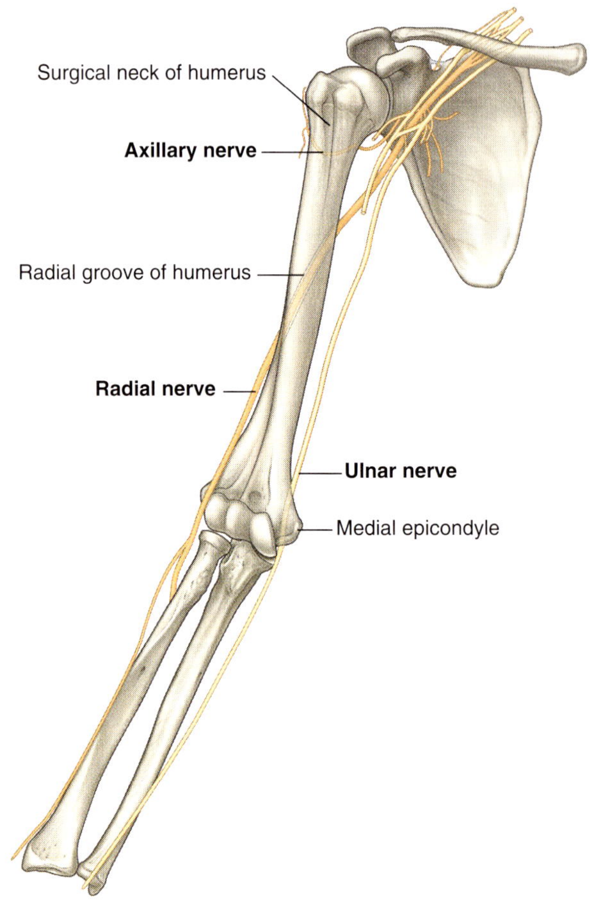

Fig. 2.17 Nerves related to the humerus.

- The radial nerve, which supplies all of the extensor muscles of the upper limb, passes diagonally around the posterior surface of the middle of the humerus in the radial groove.
- The ulnar nerve, which is ultimately destined for the hand, passes posteriorly to a bony protrusion, the medial epicondyle, on the medial side of the distal end of the humerus.

Fractures of the humerus in any one of these three regions can endanger the related nerve.

Superficial veins

Large veins embedded in the superficial fascia of the upper limb are often used to access a patient's vascular system and to withdraw blood. The most significant of these veins are the cephalic, basilic, and median cubital veins (Fig. 2.18).

The **cephalic** and **basilic veins** originate from the **dorsal venous network** on the back of the hand.

The cephalic vein originates over the anatomical snuffbox at the base of the thumb, passes laterally around the distal forearm to reach the anterolateral surface of the limb, and then continues proximally. It crosses the elbow, and then passes up the arm into a triangular depression—the **clavipectoral triangle** (**deltopectoral triangle**)—between the pectoralis major muscle, deltoid muscle, and clavicle. In this depression, the vein passes into the axilla by penetrating deep fascia just inferior to the clavicle.

The basilic vein originates from the medial side of the dorsal venous network of the hand and passes proximally up the posteromedial surface of the forearm. It passes onto the anterior surface of the limb just inferior to the elbow and then continues proximally to penetrate deep fascia about midway up the arm.

At the elbow, the cephalic and basilic veins are connected by the **median cubital vein**, which crosses the roof of the cubital fossa.

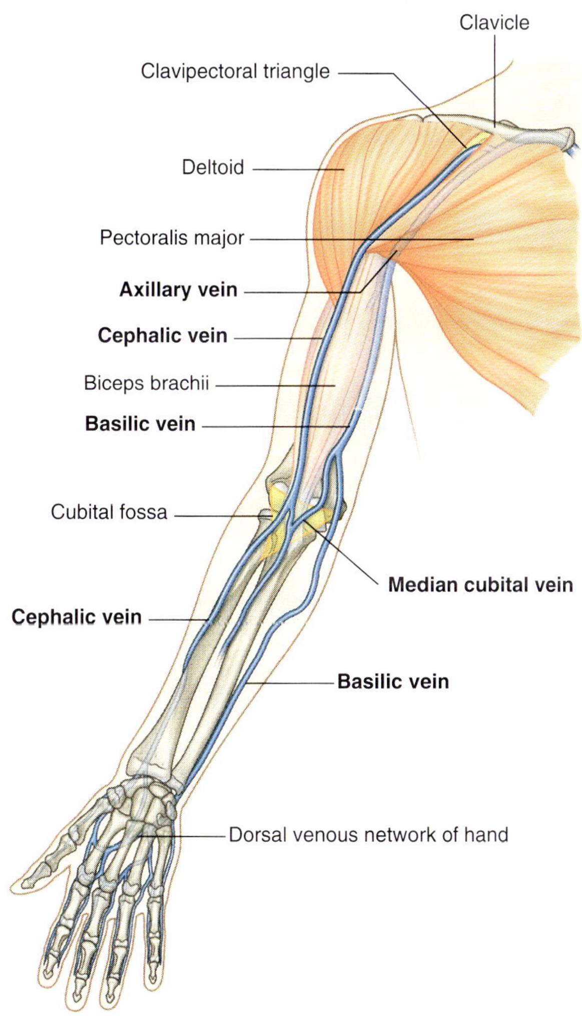

Fig. 2.18 Veins in the superficial fascia of upper limb. The area of the cubital fossa is shown in yellow.

Orientation of the thumb

The thumb is positioned at right angles to the orientation of the index, middle, ring, and little fingers (Fig. 2.19). As a result, movements of the thumb occur at right angles to those of the other digits. For example, flexion brings the thumb across the palm, whereas abduction moves it away from the fingers at right angles to the palm. This movement occurs at the first carpometacarpal joint. The flexor surface of the thumb is the aspect of the thumb toward which flexion is directed. Flexion of the thumb occurs in the coronal place around an anteroposterior axis.

Importantly, with the thumb positioned at right angles to the palm, only a slight rotation of metacarpal I on the wrist brings the pad of the thumb into a position directly facing the pads of the other fingers. This opposition of the thumb is essential for normal hand function.

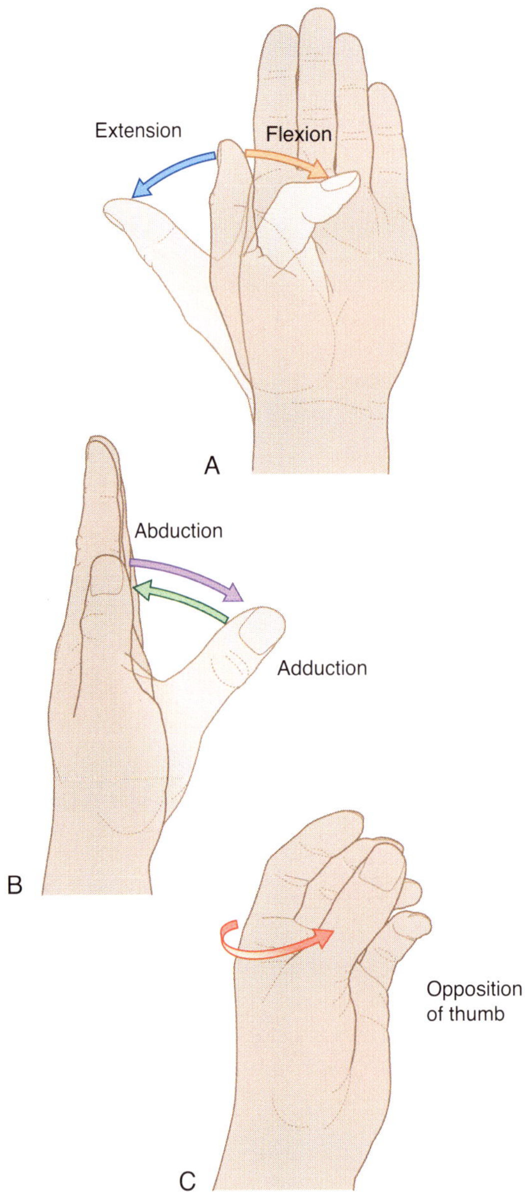

Fig. 2.19 (A–C) Movements of the thumb.

Regional anatomy

SHOULDER

The shoulder is the region of upper limb attachment to the trunk.

The bone framework of the shoulder consists of the following:

- The clavicle and scapula, which form the **pectoral girdle** (**shoulder girdle**)
- The proximal end of the humerus

The superficial muscles of the shoulder consist of the trapezius and deltoid muscles, which together form the smooth muscular contour over the lateral part of the shoulder. These muscles connect the scapula and clavicle to the trunk and to the arm, respectively.

Bones

Clavicle

The clavicle is the only bony attachment between the trunk and the upper limb. It is palpable along its entire length and has a gentle S-shaped contour, with the forward-facing convex part medial and the forward-facing concave part lateral. The acromial (lateral) end of the clavicle is flat, whereas the sternal (medial) end is more robust and somewhat quadrangular in shape (Fig. 2.20).

The acromial end of the clavicle has a small oval facet on its surface for articulation with a similar facet on the medial surface of the acromion of the scapula.

The sternal end has a much larger facet for articulation mainly with the manubrium of the sternum, and, to a lesser extent, with the first costal cartilage.

The inferior surface of the lateral third of the clavicle possesses a distinct tuberosity consisting of a tubercle (the **conoid tubercle**) and lateral roughening (the **trapezoid line**), for attachment of the important coracoclavicular ligament.

In addition, the surfaces and margins of the clavicle are roughened by the attachment of muscles that connect the clavicle to the thorax, neck, and upper limb. The superior surface is smoother than the inferior surface.

Scapula

The scapula is a large, flat triangular bone with:

- Three angles (lateral, superior, and inferior)
- Three borders (superior, lateral, and medial)
- Two surfaces (costal and posterior)
- Three processes (acromion, spine, and coracoid process) (Fig. 2.21)

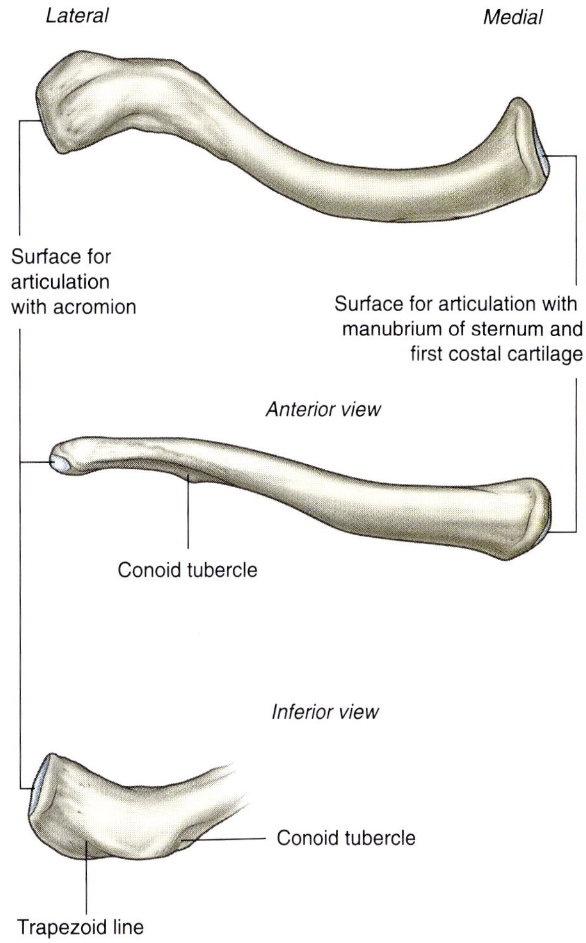

Fig. 2.20 Right clavicle.

The **lateral angle** of the scapula is marked by a shallow, somewhat comma-shaped **glenoid cavity**, which articulates with the head of the humerus to form the glenohumeral joint (Fig. 2.21B and C).

A large triangular-shaped roughening (the **infraglenoid tubercle**) inferior to the glenoid cavity is the site of attachment for the long head of the triceps brachii muscle.

A less distinct **supraglenoid tubercle** is located superior to the glenoid cavity and is the site of attachment for the long head of the biceps brachii muscle.

A prominent **spine** subdivides the **posterior surface** of the scapula into a small, superior **supraspinous fossa** and a much larger, inferior **infraspinous fossa** (Fig. 2.21A).

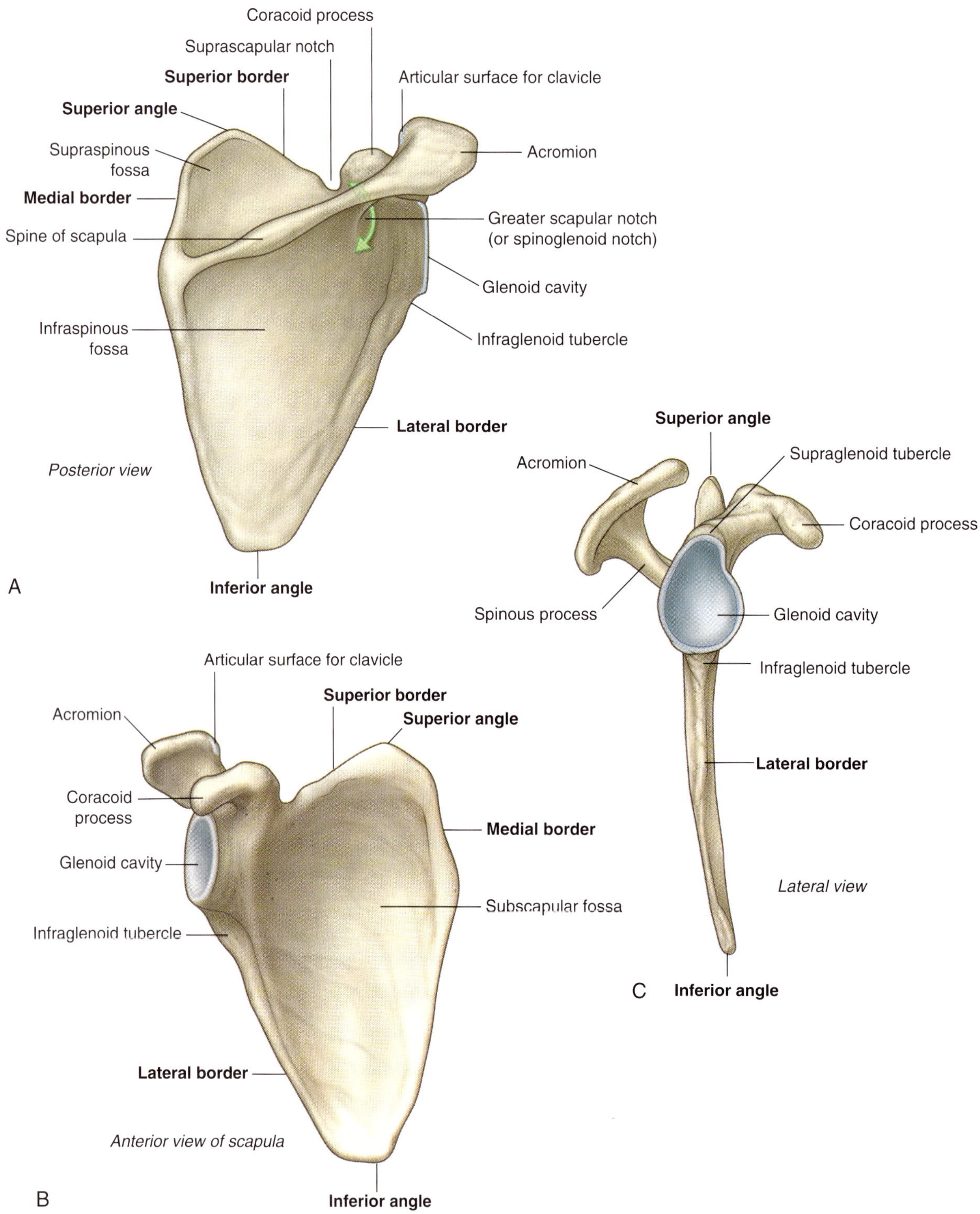

Fig. 2.21 Scapula. **(A)** Posterior view of right scapula. **(B)** Anterior view of costal surface. **(C)** Lateral view.

The **acromion**, which is an anterolateral projection of the spine, arches over the glenohumeral joint and articulates, via a small oval facet on its distal end, with the clavicle.

The region between the lateral angle of the scapula and the attachment of the spine to the posterior surface of the scapula is the **greater scapular notch** (**spinoglenoid notch**).

Unlike the posterior surface, the **costal surface** of the scapula is unremarkable, being characterized by a shallow concave **subscapular fossa** over much of its extent (Fig. 2.21B). The costal surface and margins provide for muscle attachment, and the costal surface, together with its related muscle (**subscapularis**), moves freely over the underlying thoracic wall.

The lateral border of the scapula is strong and thick for muscle attachment, whereas the medial border and much of the superior border is thin and sharp.

The superior border is marked on its lateral end by:

- The **coracoid process**, a hook-like structure that projects anterolaterally and is positioned directly inferior to the lateral part of the clavicle
- The small but distinct **suprascapular notch**, which lies immediately medial to the root of the coracoid process

The spine and acromion can be readily palpated on a patient, as can the tip of the coracoid process, the inferior angle, and much of the medial border of the scapula.

Proximal humerus

The proximal end of the humerus consists of the head, the anatomical neck, the greater and lesser tubercles, the surgical neck, and the superior half of the shaft of the humerus (Fig. 2.22).

The **head** is half-spherical in shape and projects medially and somewhat superiorly to articulate with the much smaller glenoid cavity of the scapula.

The **anatomical neck** is very short and is formed by a narrow constriction immediately distal to the head. It lies between the head and the greater and lesser tubercles laterally, and between the head and the shaft more medially.

Greater and lesser tubercles

The **greater** and **lesser tubercles** are prominent landmarks on the proximal end of the humerus and serve as attachment sites for the four rotator cuff muscles of the glenohumeral joint.

The greater tubercle is lateral in position. Its superior surface and posterior surface are marked by three large smooth facets for muscle tendon attachments:

- The superior facet is for attachment of the supraspinatus muscle.

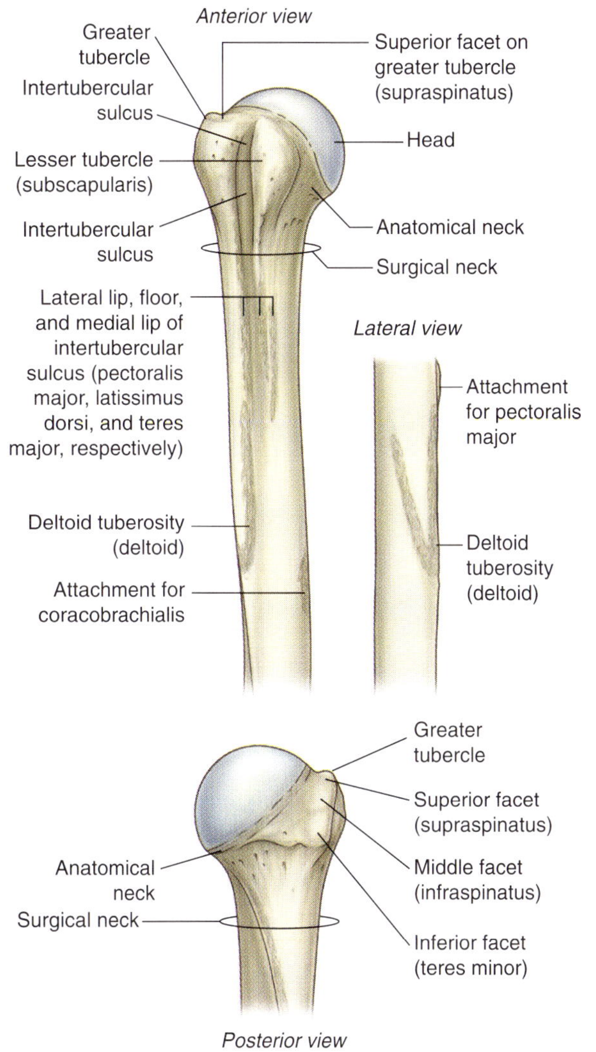

Fig. 2.22 Proximal end of right humerus.

- The middle facet is for attachment of the infraspinatus.
- The inferior facet is for attachment of the teres minor.

The lesser tubercle is anterior in position and its surface is marked by a large smooth impression for attachment of the subscapularis muscle.

A deep **intertubercular sulcus** (**bicipital groove**) separates the lesser and greater tubercles and continues inferiorly onto the proximal shaft of the humerus (Fig. 2.22). The tendon of the long head of the biceps brachii passes through this sulcus.

Roughenings on the lateral and medial lips and on the floor of the intertubercular sulcus mark sites for the attachment of the pectoralis major, teres major, and latissimus dorsi muscles, respectively.

The lateral lip of the intertubercular sulcus is continuous inferiorly with a large V-shaped **deltoid tuberosity** on the lateral surface of the humerus midway along its length (Fig. 2.22), which is where the deltoid muscle inserts onto the humerus.

In approximately the same position, but on the medial surface of the bone, there is a thin vertical roughening for attachment of the coracobrachialis muscle.

Surgical neck

One of the most important features of the proximal end of the humerus is the surgical neck (Fig. 2.22). This region is oriented in the horizontal plane between the expanded proximal part of the humerus (head, anatomical neck, and tubercles) and the narrower shaft. The axillary nerve and the posterior circumflex humeral artery, which pass into the deltoid region from the axilla, do so immediately posterior to the surgical neck. Because the surgical neck is weaker than more proximal regions of the bone, it is one of the sites where the humerus commonly fractures. The associated nerve (axillary) and artery (posterior circumflex humeral) can be damaged by fractures in this region.

Early clinical exposure

Fracture of the proximal humerus

It is extremely rare for fractures to occur across the anatomical neck of the humerus because the obliquity of such a fracture would have to traverse the thickest region of bone. Typically fractures occur around the surgical neck of the humerus. Although the axillary nerve and posterior circumflex humeral artery may be damaged with this type of fracture, this rarely happens. It is important that the axillary nerve is tested before relocation to be sure that the injury has not damaged the nerve and that the treatment itself does not cause a neurological deficit.

Joints

The three joints in the shoulder complex are the sternoclavicular, acromioclavicular, and glenohumeral joints.

The sternoclavicular joint and the acromioclavicular joint link the two bones of the pectoral girdle to each other and to the trunk. The combined movements at these two joints enable the scapula to be positioned over a wide range on the thoracic wall, substantially increasing "reach" by the upper limb.

The glenohumeral joint (shoulder joint) is the articulation between the humerus of the arm and the scapula.

Sternoclavicular joint

The sternoclavicular joint occurs between the proximal end of the clavicle and the **clavicular notch** of the **manubrium of the sternum** together with a small part of the first costal cartilage (Fig. 2.23). It is synovial and saddle shaped. The articular cavity is completely separated into two compartments by an articular disc. The sternoclavicular joint allows movement of the clavicle, predominantly in the anteroposterior and vertical planes, although some rotation also occurs.

The sternoclavicular joint is surrounded by a joint capsule and is reinforced by four ligaments:

- The **anterior** and **posterior sternoclavicular ligaments** are anterior and posterior, respectively, to the joint.
- An **interclavicular ligament** links the ends of the two clavicles to each other and to the superior surface of the manubrium of the sternum.

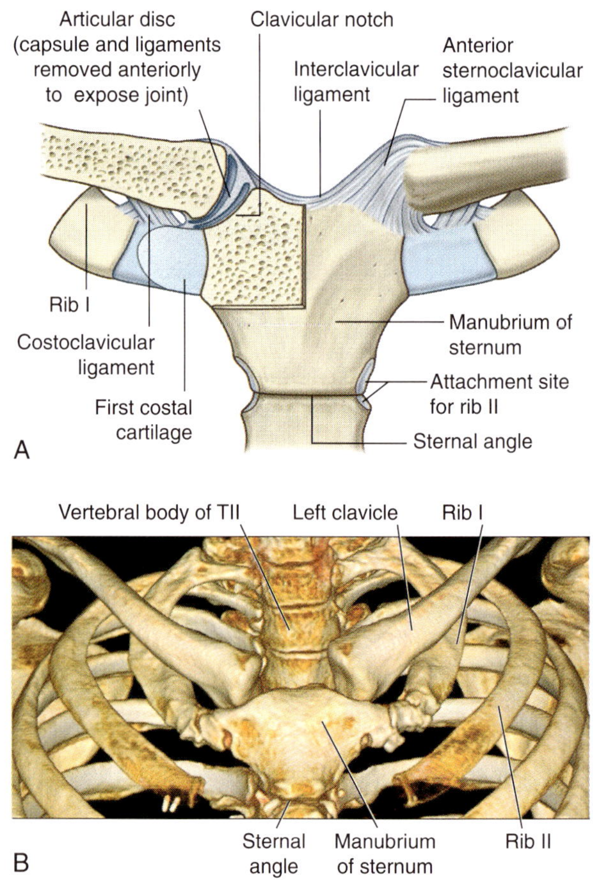

Fig. 2.23 Sternoclavicular joint. **(A)** Bones and ligaments. **(B)** Volume-rendered reconstruction using multidetector computed tomography.

- The **costoclavicular ligament** is positioned laterally to the joint and links the proximal end of the clavicle to the first rib and related costal cartilage.

Acromioclavicular joint

The acromioclavicular joint is a small synovial joint between an oval facet on the medial surface of the acromion and a similar facet on the acromial end of the clavicle (Fig. 2.24; also see Fig. 2.31). It allows movement in the anteroposterior and vertical planes together with some axial rotation.

The acromioclavicular joint is surrounded by a joint capsule and is reinforced by:

- A small **acromioclavicular ligament** superior to the joint and passing between adjacent regions of the clavicle and acromion.
- A much larger **coracoclavicular ligament**, which is not directly related to the joint, but is an important strong accessory ligament, providing much of the weight-bearing support for the upper limb on the clavicle and maintaining the position of the clavicle on the acromion—it spans the distance between the coracoid process of the scapula and the inferior surface of the acromial end of the clavicle and comprises an anterior **trapezoid ligament** (which attaches to the trapezoid line on the clavicle) and a posterior **conoid ligament** (which attaches to the related conoid tubercle).

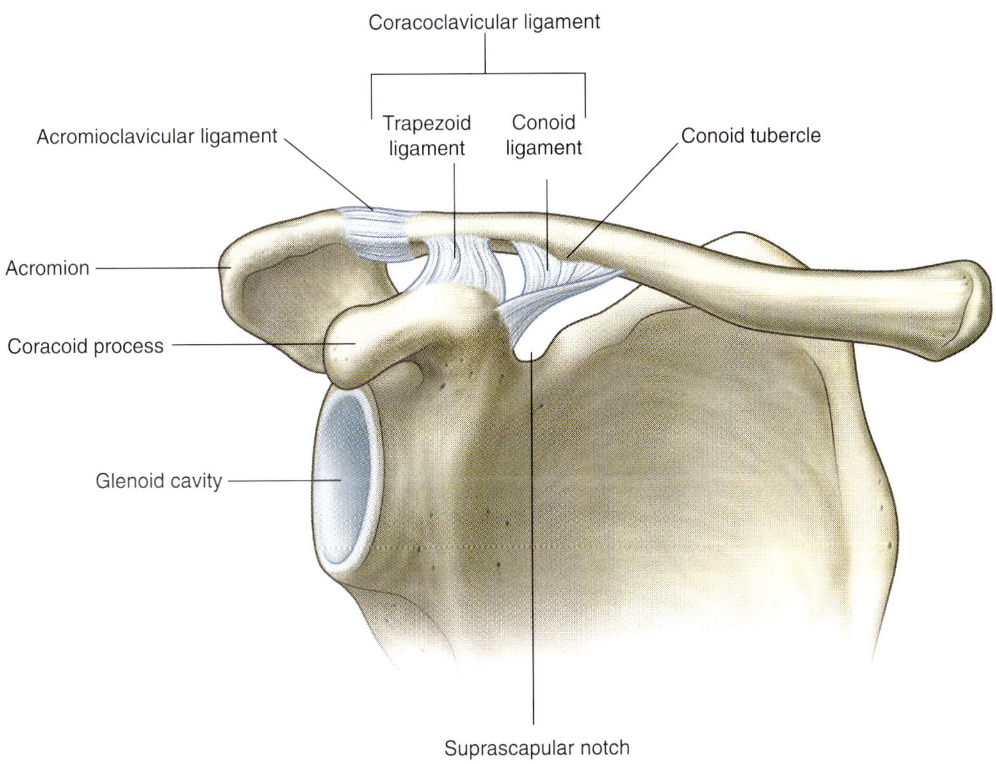

Fig. 2.24 Right acromioclavicular joint.

Glenohumeral joint

The **glenohumeral joint** is a synovial ball and socket articulation between the head of the humerus and the glenoid cavity of the scapula (Fig. 2.25). It is multiaxial with a wide range of movements provided at the cost of skeletal stability. Joint stability is provided, instead, by the rotator cuff muscles, the long head of the biceps brachii muscle, related bony processes, and extracapsular ligaments. Movements at the joint include flexion, extension, abduction, adduction, medial rotation, lateral rotation, and circumduction.

The articular surfaces of the glenohumeral joint are the large spherical head of the humerus and the small glenoid cavity of the scapula (Fig. 2.25). Each of the surfaces is covered by hyaline cartilage.

The glenoid cavity is deepened and expanded peripherally by a fibrocartilaginous collar (the **glenoid labrum**), which attaches to the margin of the fossa. Superiorly, this labrum is continuous with the tendon of the long head of the biceps brachii muscle, which attaches to the supraglenoid tubercle and passes through the articular cavity superior to the head of the humerus.

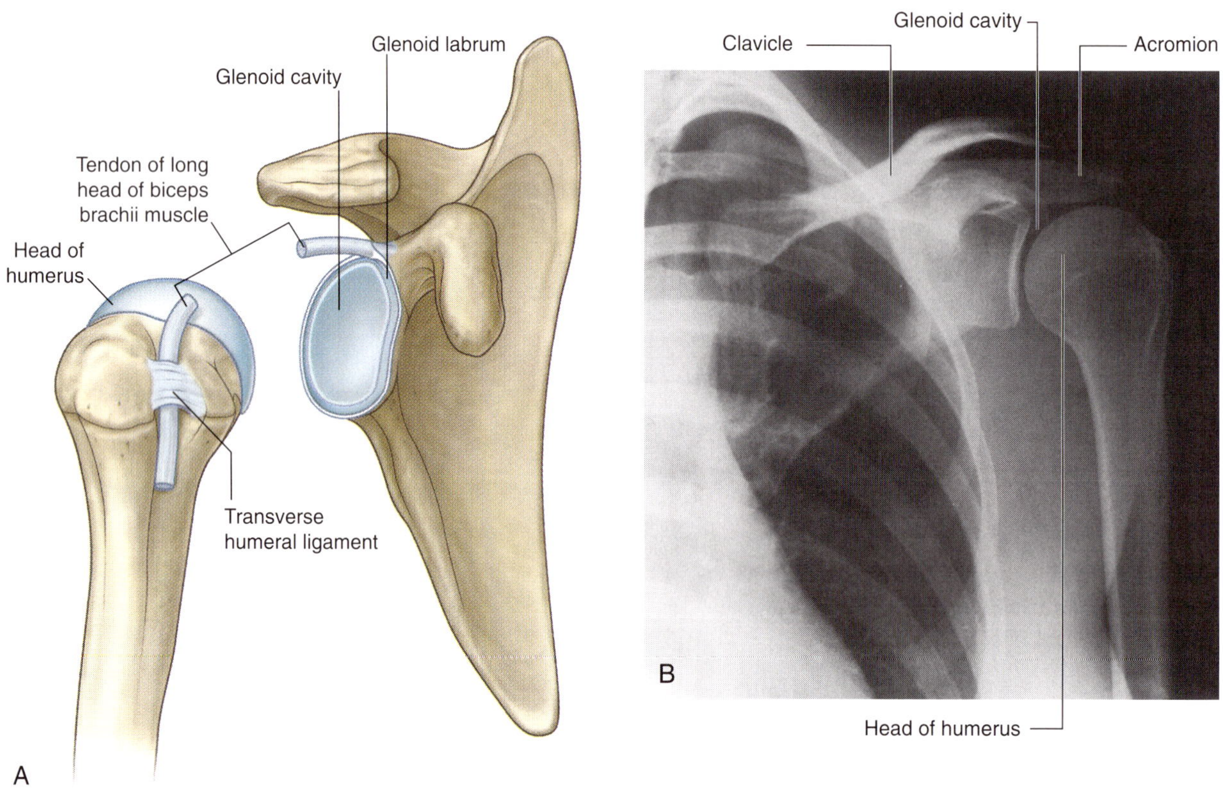

Fig. 2.25 Glenohumeral joint. **(A)** Articular surfaces of right glenohumeral joint. **(B)** Radiograph of a normal glenohumeral joint.

The synovial membrane attaches to the margins of the articular surfaces and lines the fibrous membrane of the joint capsule (Fig. 2.26). The synovial membrane is loose inferiorly. This redundant region of synovial membrane and related fibrous membrane accommodates abduction of the arm.

The synovial membrane protrudes through apertures in the fibrous membrane to form bursae, which lie between the tendons of surrounding muscles and the fibrous membrane. The most consistent of these is the **subtendinous bursa of the subscapularis**, which lies between the subscapularis muscle and the fibrous membrane. The synovial membrane also folds around the tendon of the long head of the biceps brachii muscle in the joint and extends along the tendon as it passes into the intertubercular sulcus. All these synovial structures reduce friction between the tendons and adjacent joint capsule and bone.

In addition to bursae that communicate with the articular cavity through apertures in the fibrous membrane, other bursae are associated with the joint but are not connected to it. These occur:

- Between the acromion (or deltoid muscle) and supraspinatus muscle (or joint capsule) (the **subacromial** or **subdeltoid bursa**)
- Between the acromion and skin
- Between the coracoid process and the joint capsule
- In relationship to tendons of muscles around the joint (coracobrachialis, teres major, long head of triceps brachii, and latissimus dorsi muscles)

The fibrous membrane of the joint capsule attaches to the margin of the glenoid cavity, outside the attachment of the glenoid labrum and the long head of the biceps brachii muscle, and to the anatomical neck of the humerus (Fig. 2.27).

On the humerus, the medial attachment occurs more inferiorly than the neck and extends onto the shaft. In this region, the fibrous membrane is also loose or folded in the anatomical position. This redundant area of the fibrous membrane accommodates abduction of the arm.

Openings in the fibrous membrane provide continuity of the articular cavity with bursae that occur between the joint capsule and surrounding muscles and around the tendon of the long head of the biceps brachii muscle in the intertubercular sulcus.

The fibrous membrane of the joint capsule is thickened:

- Anterosuperiorly in three locations to form **superior**, **middle**, and **inferior glenohumeral ligaments**, which pass from the superomedial margin of the glenoid cavity to the lesser tubercle and inferiorly related anatomical neck of the humerus (Fig. 2.27).

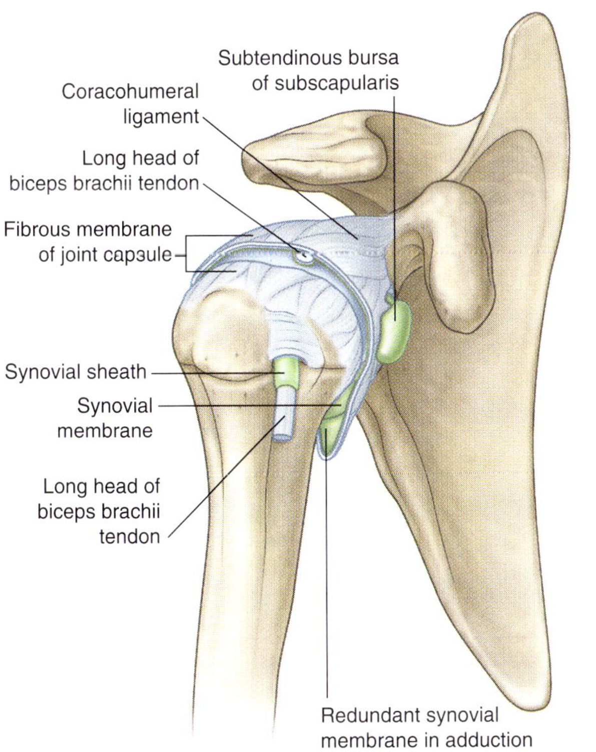

Fig. 2.26 Synovial membrane and joint capsule of right glenohumeral joint.

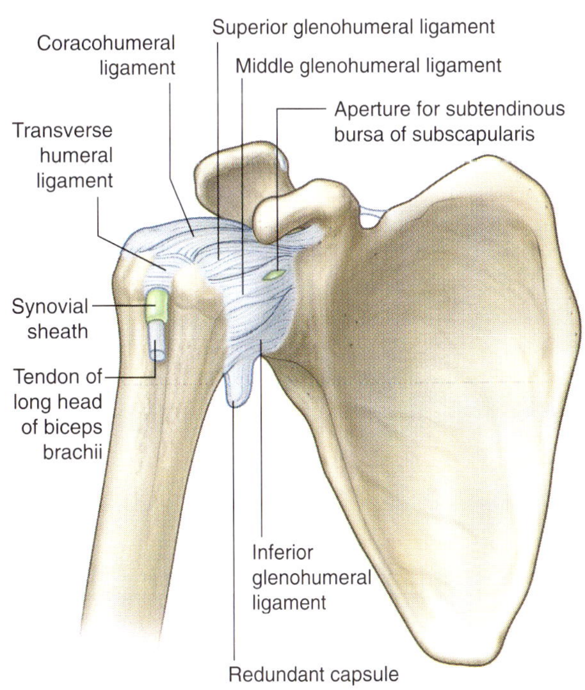

Fig. 2.27 Capsule of right glenohumeral joint.

- Superiorly between the base of the coracoid process and the greater tubercle of the humerus (the **coracohumeral ligament**).
- Between the greater and lesser tubercles of the humerus (**transverse humeral ligament**)—this holds the tendon of the long head of the biceps brachii muscle in the intertubercular sulcus (Fig. 2.27).

Joint stability is provided by surrounding muscle tendons and a skeletal arch formed superiorly by the coracoid process and acromion and the coracoacromial ligament (Fig. 2.28).

Tendons of the rotator cuff muscles (the supraspinatus, infraspinatus, teres minor, and subscapularis muscles) blend with the joint capsule and form a musculotendinous

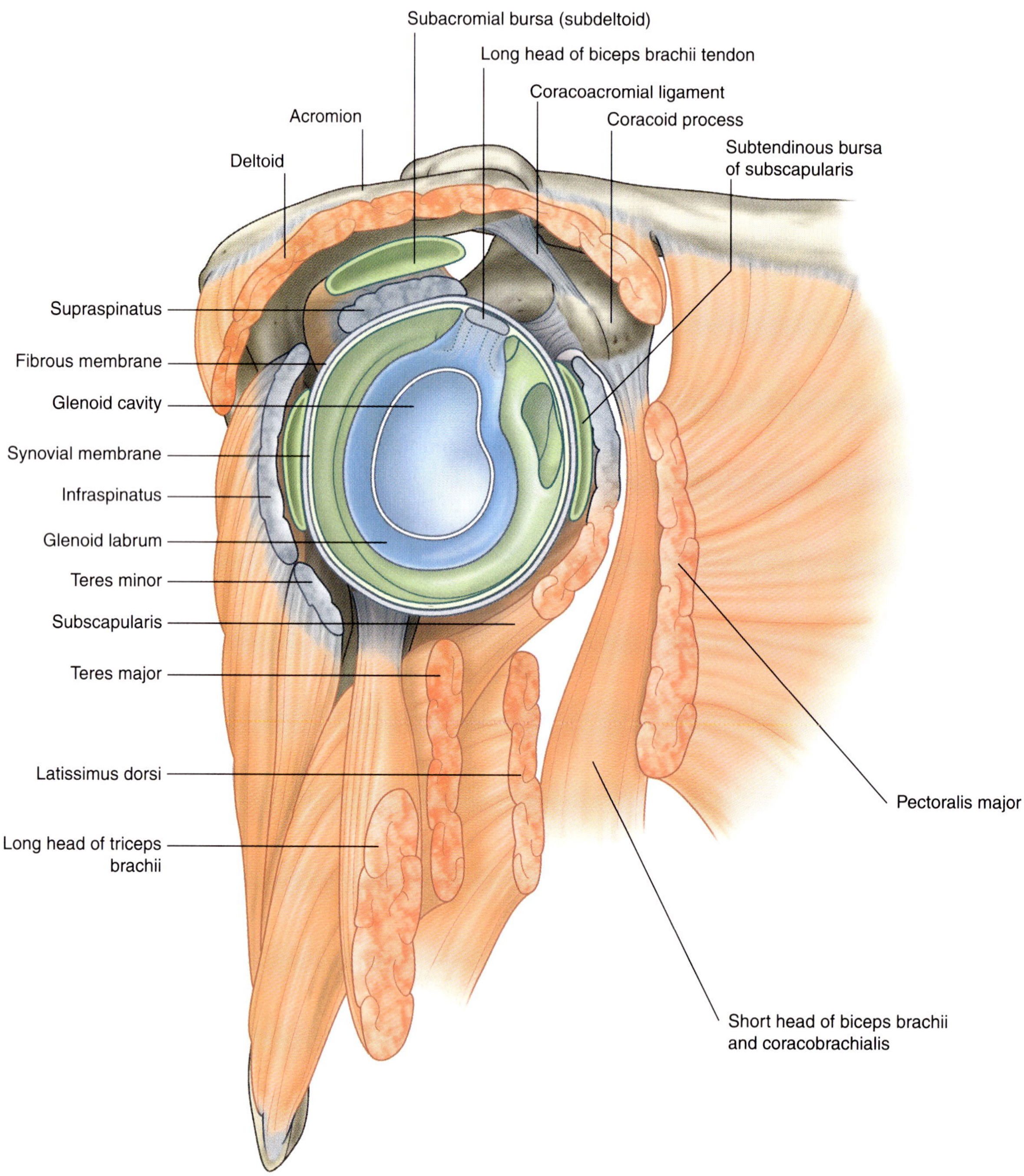

Fig. 2.28 Lateral view of right glenohumeral joint and surrounding muscles with proximal end of humerus removed.

collar that surrounds the posterior, superior, and anterior aspects of the glenohumeral joint (Figs. 2.28 and 2.29). This cuff of muscles stabilizes and holds the head of the humerus in the glenoid cavity of the scapula without compromising the arm's flexibility and range of motion. The tendon of the long head of the biceps brachii muscle passes superiorly through the joint and restricts upward movement of the humeral head on the glenoid cavity.

The glenohumeral joint permits a wide range of movements, namely, flexion, extension, adduction, abduction, lateral, and medial rotation. A combination of all these results in circumduction. Each movement is followed by the names of the muscles producing the movements in parentheses as summarized below:

Flexion (pectoralis major—clavicular part, deltoid—anterior fibers, coracobrachialis)
Extension (deltoid—posterior fibers, teres major)
Abduction (deltoid, supraspinatus—initiation of abduction)
Adduction (pectoralis major, latissimus dorsi)
Medial rotation (subscapularis)
Lateral rotation (infraspinatus, teres minor)

Scapulohumeral rhythm is the movement between the scapula and the humerus, a 2:1 ratio. For every 3° of abduction of the arm, 2° abduction occurs at glenohumeral joint and 1° abduction occurs by rotation of the scapula. Scapulohumeral rhythm is defined as the ratio of the glenohumeral movement to the scapulothoracic movement during arm elevation.

Vascular supply to the glenohumeral joint is predominantly through branches of the anterior and posterior circumflex humeral and suprascapular arteries.

The glenohumeral joint is innervated by branches from the posterior cord of the brachial plexus, and from the suprascapular, axillary, and lateral pectoral nerves.

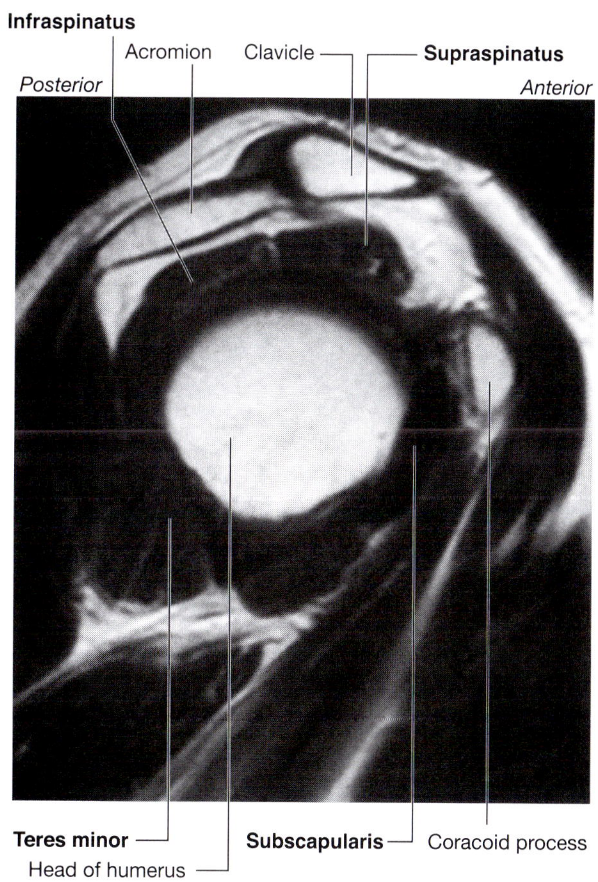

Fig. 2.29 Magnetic resonance image (T1-weighted) of a normal glenohumeral joint in the sagittal plane.

Early clinical exposure

Fractures of the clavicle and dislocations of the acromioclavicular and sternoclavicular joints

The clavicle provides the only bony connection between the upper limb and trunk. Given its relative size and the potential forces that it transmits from the upper limb to the trunk, it is not surprising that it is often fractured. The typical site of fracture is the middle third (Fig. 2.30). The medial and lateral thirds are rarely fractured.

The acromial end of the clavicle tends to dislocate at the acromioclavicular joint with trauma (Fig. 2.31). The outer third of the clavicle is joined to the scapula by the conoid and trapezoid ligaments of the coracoclavicular ligament.

A minor injury tends to tear the fibrous joint capsule and ligaments of the acromioclavicular joint, resulting in acromioclavicular separation on a plain radiograph. More severe trauma will disrupt the conoid and trapezoid ligaments of the coracoclavicular ligament, which results in elevation and upward subluxation of the clavicle.

The typical injury at the medial end of the clavicle is an anterior or posterior dislocation of the sternoclavicular joint. Importantly, a posterior dislocation of the clavicle may impinge on the great vessels in the root of the neck and compress or disrupt them.

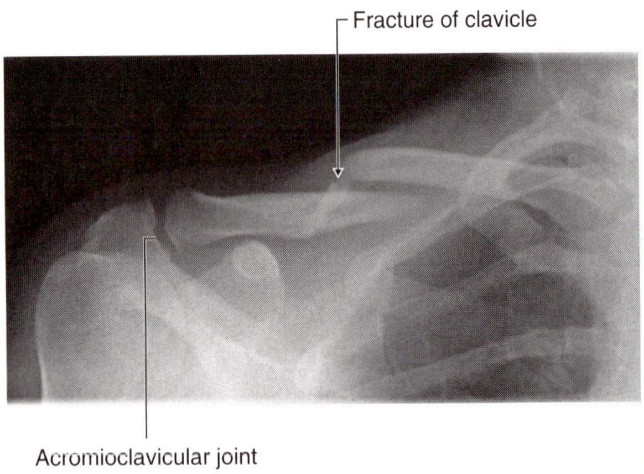

Fig. 2.30 There is an oblique fracture of the middle third of the right clavicle.

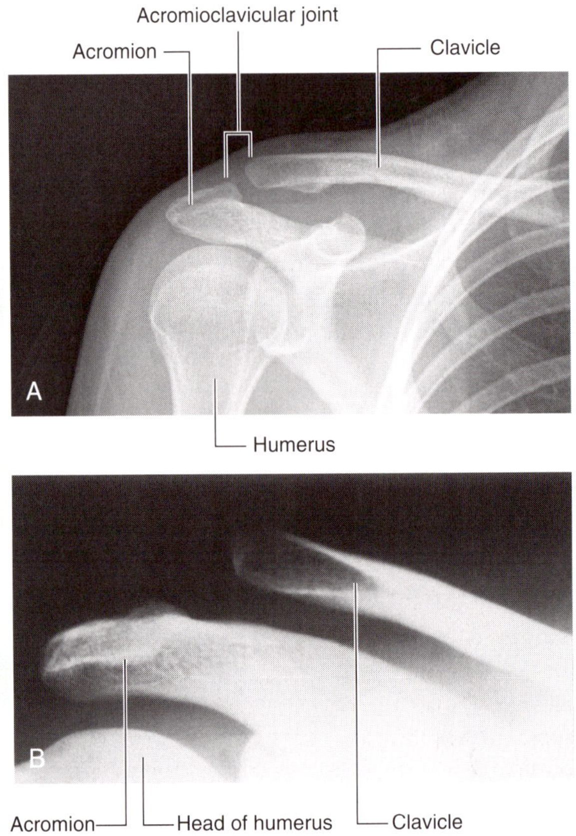

Fig. 2.31 Radiographs of acromioclavicular joints. **(A)** Normal right acromioclavicular joint. **(B)** Dislocated right acromioclavicular joint (shoulder separation).

Early clinical exposure

Dislocations of the glenohumeral joint

The glenohumeral joint is extremely mobile, providing a wide range of movement at the expense of stability. The relatively small bony glenoid cavity, supplemented by the less robust fibrocartilaginous glenoid labrum and the ligamentous support, makes it susceptible to dislocation.

Anterior dislocation (Fig. 2.32) occurs most frequently and is usually associated with an isolated traumatic incident (clinically, all anterior dislocations are anteroinferior). In some cases, the anteroinferior glenoid labrum is torn with or without a small bony fragment. Once the joint capsule and cartilage are disrupted, the joint is susceptible to further (recurrent) dislocations. When an anteroinferior dislocation occurs, the axillary nerve may be injured by direct compression of the humeral head on the nerve inferiorly as it passes through the quadrangular space. Furthermore, the "lengthening" effect of the humerus may stretch the radial nerve, which is tightly bound within the radial groove, and produce a radial nerve paralysis. Occasionally, an anteroinferior dislocation is associated with a fracture, which may require surgical reduction.

Early clinical exposure—cont'd

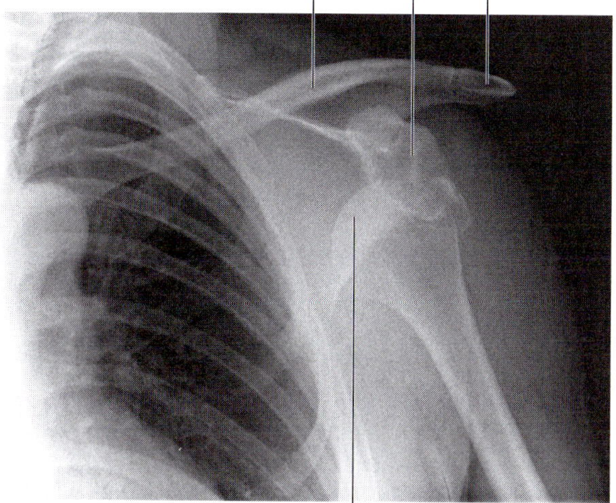

Fig. 2.32 Radiograph showing an anteroinferior dislocation of the shoulder joint.

Posterior dislocation is extremely rare; when seen, the clinician should focus on its cause, the most common being extremely vigorous muscle contractions, which may be associated with an epileptic seizure caused by electrocution. Treatment of recurrent instability can be challenging. The aims of treatment are to maintain function and range of movement while preventing instability (subluxation, dislocation, and the "feeling" of dislocation). This can be achieved through physical therapy and shoulder "re-education." If this fails, capsular tightening and stabilization of the labrum can be achieved arthroscopically. If the problem persists, the coracoid process can be divided at the base, maintaining continuity of the muscular attachments. The process is transferred and a screw fixed to the anterior inferior border of the glenoid to form a buttress to prevent future dislocations.

Early clinical exposure

Rotator cuff disorders

The two main disorders of the rotator cuff are impingement and tendinopathy. The muscle most commonly involved is supraspinatus as it passes beneath the acromion and the acromioclavicular ligament. This space, beneath which the supraspinatus tendon passes, is of fixed dimensions. Swelling of the supraspinatus muscle, excessive fluid within the subacromial/subdeltoid bursa, or subacromial bony spurs may produce significant impingement when the arm is abducted.

The blood supply to the supraspinatus tendon is relatively poor. Repeated trauma, in certain circumstances, makes the tendon susceptible to degenerative change, which may result in calcium deposition, producing extreme pain. The calcium deposits can be extracted through a needle under image guidance and often have the consistency of toothpaste.

When the supraspinatus tendon has undergone significant degenerative change, it is more susceptible to trauma, and partial- or full-thickness tears may develop (Fig. 2.33). These tears are most common in older patients and may result in considerable difficulty in carrying out normal activities of daily living such as combing hair. However, complete tears may be entirely asymptomatic.

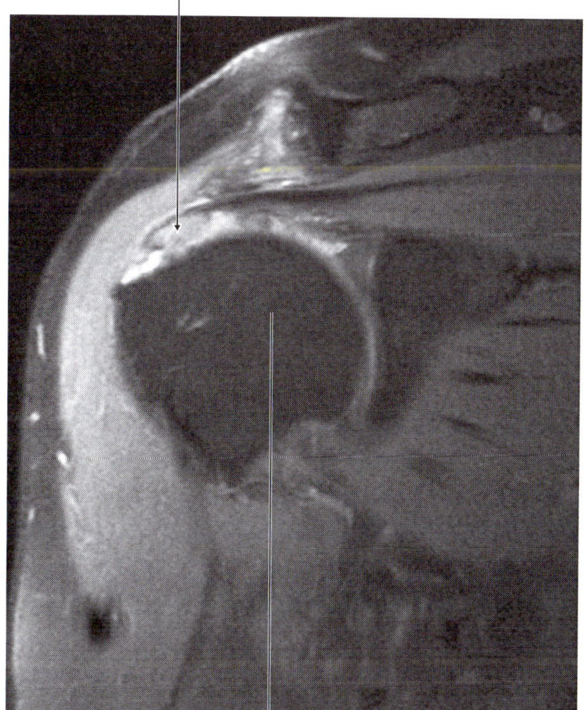

Fig. 2.33 Magnetic resonance image of a full-thickness tear of the supraspinatus tendon as it inserts onto the greater tubercle of the humerus.

Early clinical exposure

Inflammation of the subacromial (subdeltoid) bursa

Between the supraspinatus and deltoid muscles laterally and the acromion medially, there is a bursa referred to clinically as the subacromial or subdeltoid bursa. In patients who have injured the shoulder or who have supraspinatus tendinopathy, this bursa may become inflamed, making movements of the glenohumeral joint painful. These inflammatory changes may be treated by injection of a corticosteroid and local anesthetic agent (Fig. 2.34).

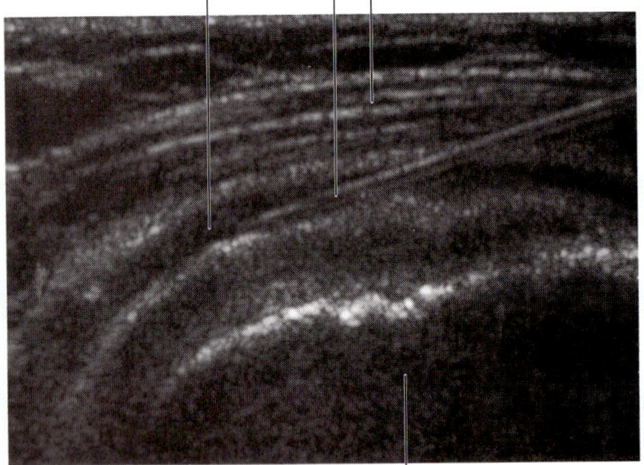

Fig. 2.34 Ultrasound of shoulder showing needle placement into the subdeltoid/subacromial bursa.

Muscles

The two most superficial muscles of the shoulder are the trapezius and deltoid muscles (Fig. 2.35 and Table 2.1). Together, they provide the characteristic contour of the shoulder:

- The trapezius attaches the scapula and clavicle to the trunk.
- The deltoid attaches the scapula and clavicle to the humerus.

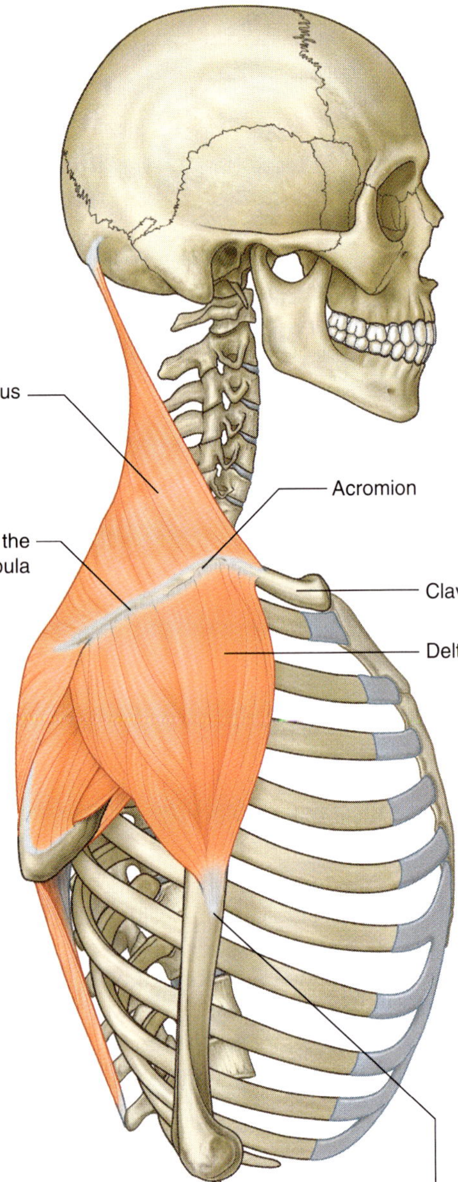

Fig. 2.35 Lateral view of trapezius and deltoid muscles.

Table 2.1 Muscles of the shoulder

Muscle	Origin	Insertion	Innervation	Function
Trapezius	Superior nuchal line, external occipital protuberance, medial margin of the ligamentum nuchae, spinous processes of CVII to TXII and the related supraspinous ligaments	Superior edge of the crest of the spine of the scapula, acromion, posterior border of lateral one-third of clavicle	Motor spinal part of accessory nerve (XI). Sensory (proprioception) anterior rami of C3 and C4	Powerful elevator of the scapula; rotates the scapula during abduction of humerus above horizontal; middle fibers retract scapula; lower fibers depress scapula
Deltoid	Inferior edge of the crest of the spine of the scapula, lateral margin of the acromion, anterior border of lateral one-third of clavicle	Deltoid tuberosity of humerus	Axillary nerve (**C5,** C6)	Major abductor of arm clavicular fibers assist in flexing the arm; posterior fibers assist in extending the arm
Levator scapulae	Transverse processes of CI and CII vertebrae and posterior tubercles of transverse processes of CIII and CIV vertebrae	Posterior surface of medial border of scapula from superior angle to root of spine of the scapula	Branches directly from anterior rami of **C3** and **C4** spinal nerves and by branches (**C5**) from the dorsal scapular nerve	Elevates the scapula
Rhomboid minor	Lower end of ligamentum nuchae and spinous processes of CVII and TI vertebrae	Posterior surface of medial border of scapula at the root of the spine of the scapula	Dorsal scapular nerve (**C4, C5**)	Elevates and retracts the scapula
Rhomboid major	Spinous processes of TII–TV vertebrae and intervening supraspinous ligaments	Posterior surface of medial border of scapula from the root of the spine of the scapula to the inferior angle	Dorsal scapular nerve (**C4, C5**)	Elevates and retracts the scapula

Note: Spinal segments in bold are the major segments innervating the muscle.

Both the trapezius and deltoid are attached to opposing surfaces and margins of the spine of the scapula, acromion, and clavicle. The scapula, acromion, and clavicle can be palpated between the attachments of the trapezius and deltoid.

Deep to the trapezius, the scapula is attached to the vertebral column by three muscles—the levator scapulae, rhomboid minor, and rhomboid major. These three muscles work with the trapezius (and with muscles found anteriorly) to position the scapula on the trunk.

Trapezius

The **trapezius** muscle has an extensive origin from the axial skeleton, which includes sites on the skull and the vertebrae, from CI to TXII (Fig. 2.36A). From CI to CVII, the muscle attaches to the vertebrae through the ligamentum nuchae. The muscle inserts onto the skeletal framework of the shoulder along the inner margins of a continuous U-shaped line of attachment oriented in the horizontal plane, with the bottom of the U directed laterally. Together, the left and right trapezius muscles form a diamond or trapezoid shape, from which the name is derived.

The trapezius muscle is a powerful elevator of the shoulder and also rotates the scapula to extend the reach superiorly.

Innervation of the trapezius muscle is by the accessory nerve (XI) and the anterior rami of cervical nerves C3 and C4 (Fig. 2.36A). These nerves pass vertically along the deep surface of the muscle. The accessory nerve can be evaluated by testing the function of the trapezius muscle. This is most easily done by asking patients to shrug their shoulders against resistance.

Deltoid

The **deltoid** muscle is large and triangular in shape, with its base attached to the scapula and clavicle and its apex attached to the humerus (Fig. 2.36A). It originates along a continuous U-shaped line of attachment to the clavicle and the scapula, mirroring the adjacent insertion sites of the trapezius muscle. It inserts into the deltoid tuberosity on the lateral surface of the shaft of the humerus.

The major function of the deltoid muscle is abduction of the arm.

The deltoid muscle is innervated by the axillary nerve, which is a branch of the posterior cord of the brachial plexus. The axillary nerve and associated blood vessels (the posterior circumflex humeral artery and vein) enter the deltoid by passing posteriorly around the surgical neck of the humerus.

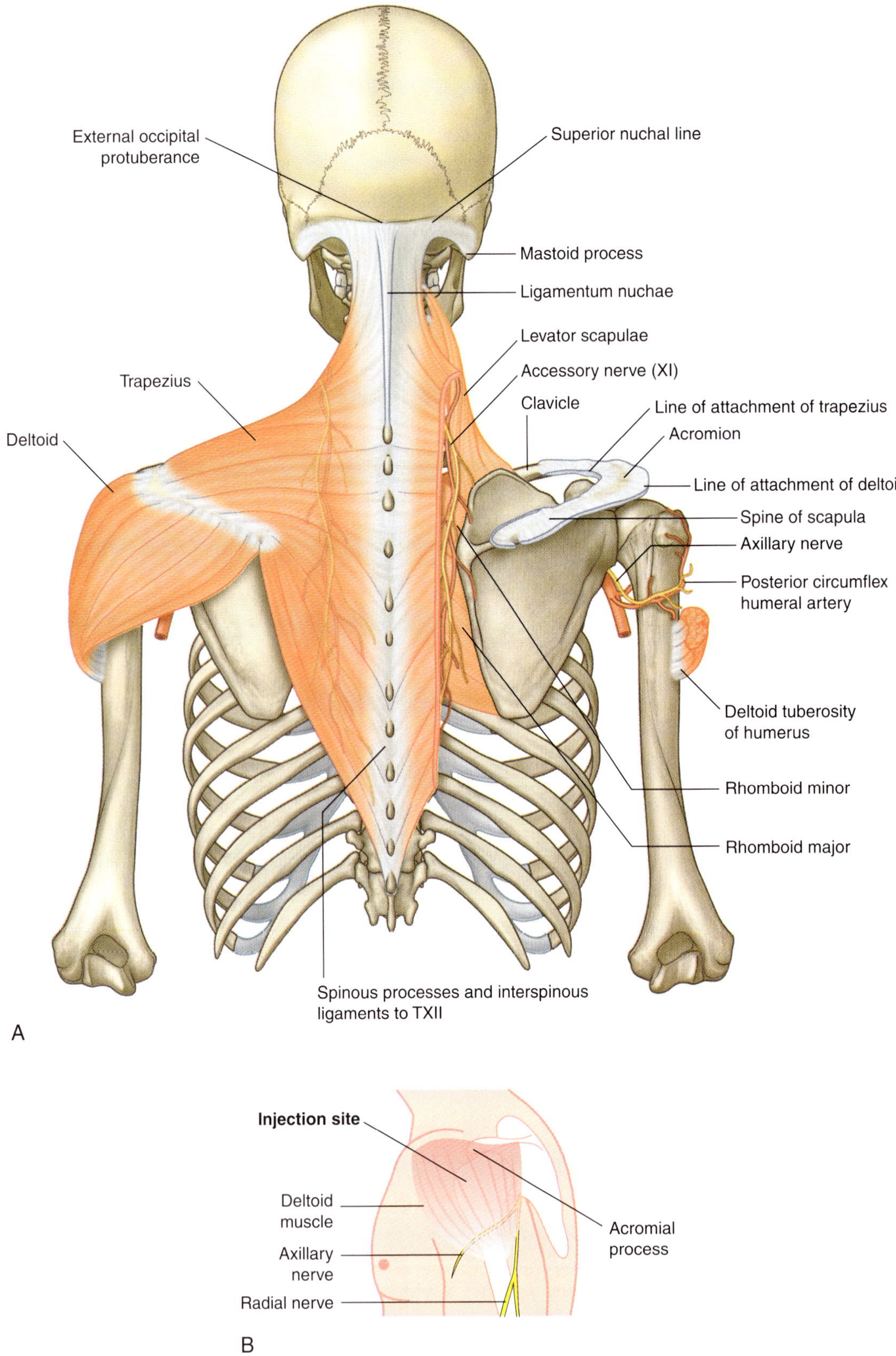

Fig. 2.36 **(A)** Attachments and neurovascular supply of the trapezius and deltoid muscles. **(B)** Intramuscular injection of deltoid. Site for intramuscular injection in the deltoid.

Levator scapulae

The levator scapulae originates from the transverse processes of CI to CIV vertebrae (Fig. 2.36A). It descends laterally to attach to the posterior surface of the medial border of the scapula from the superior angle to the smooth triangular area of bone at the root of the spine.

The levator scapulae muscle is innervated by the dorsal scapular nerve and directly from C3 and C4 spinal nerves.

The levator scapulae elevates the scapula.

Rhomboid minor and major

The rhomboid minor and major muscles attach medially to the vertebral column and descend laterally to attach to the medial border of the scapula inferior to the levator scapulae muscle (Fig. 2.36A).

The rhomboid minor originates from the lower end of the ligamentum nuchae and the spines of CVII and TI vertebrae. It inserts laterally into the smooth triangular area of bone at the root of the spine of the scapula on the posterior surface.

The rhomboid major originates from the spines of vertebrae TII to TV and from the intervening supraspinous ligaments. It descends laterally to insert along the posterior surface of the medial border of the scapula from the insertion of the rhomboid minor to the inferior angle.

The rhomboid muscles are innervated by the dorsal scapular nerve, which is a branch of the brachial plexus.

The rhomboid minor and major retract and elevate the scapula.

Early clinical exposure

Intramuscular injection

The commonest site of intramuscular injection is the deltoid muscle. The axillary nerve winds around the surgical neck of humerus under the cover of deltoid. Care should be taken to avoid axillary nerve injury during intramuscular injections in the deltoid. The landmarks for intramuscular injection are the acromion process and the axillary lines. The needle is inserted two to three finger breadths (1–2 inches) below acromion in the middle of the triangular-shaped deltoid muscle on the lateral aspect of the arm (Fig. 2.36B).

POSTERIOR SCAPULAR REGION

The posterior scapular region occupies the posterior aspect of the scapula and is located deep to the trapezius and deltoid muscles (Fig. 2.37 and Table 2.2). It contains four muscles, which pass between the scapula and proximal end of the humerus: the supraspinatus, infraspinatus, teres minor, and teres major muscles.

The posterior scapular region also contains part of one additional muscle, the long head of the triceps brachii, which passes between the scapula and the proximal end of the forearm. This muscle, along with other muscles of the region and the humerus, participates in forming a number of spaces through which nerves and vessels enter and leave the region.

The supraspinatus, infraspinatus, and teres minor muscles are components of the rotator cuff, which stabilizes the glenohumeral joint.

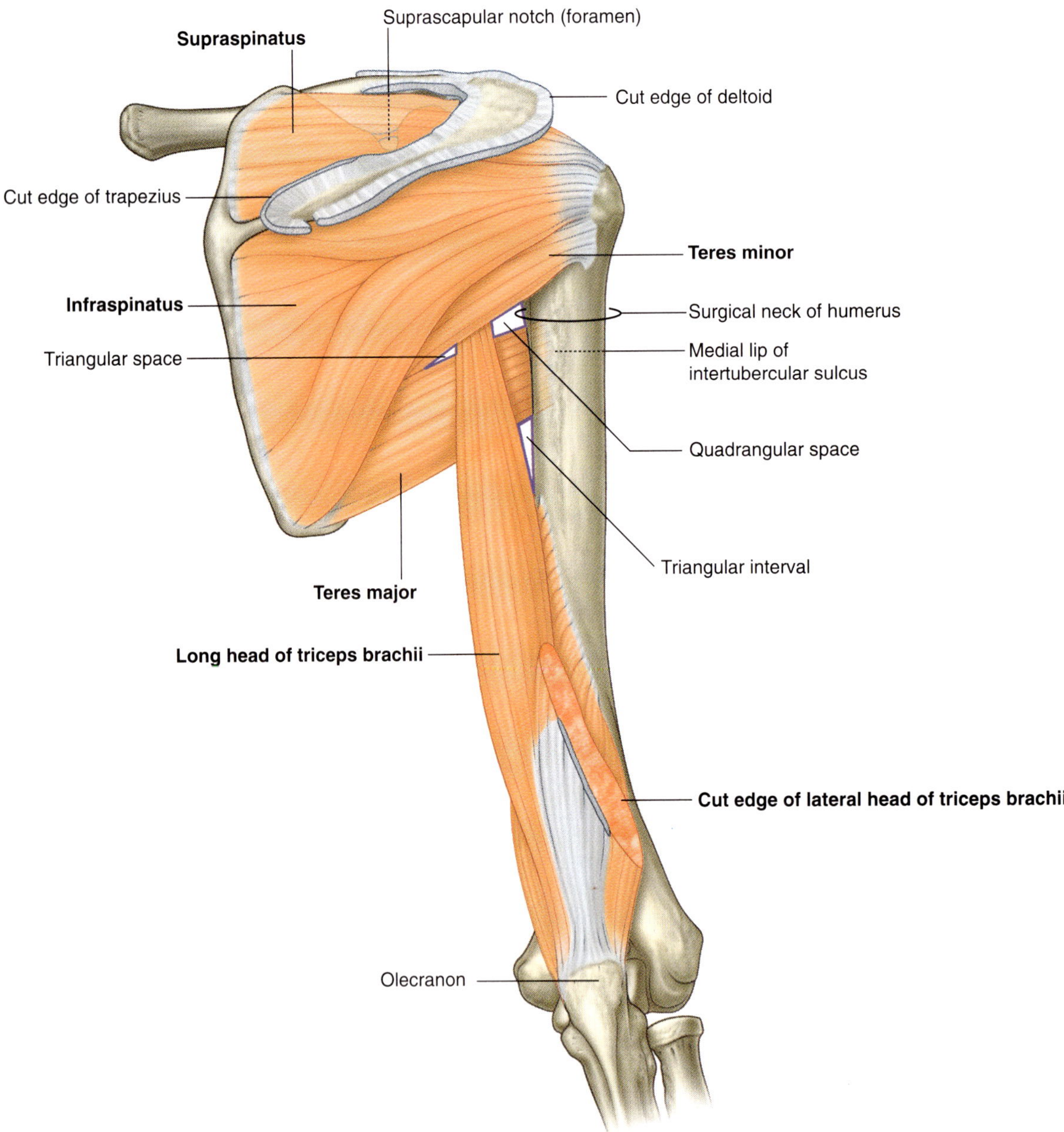

Fig. 2.37 Right posterior scapular region.

Table 2.2 Muscles of the posterior scapular region

Muscle	Origin	Insertion	Innervation	Function
Supraspinatus	Medial two-thirds of the supraspinous fossa of the scapula and the deep fascia that covers the muscle	Most superior facet on the greater tubercle of the humerus	Suprascapular nerve (**C5**, C6)	**Rotator cuff muscle**; participates in abduction of the glenohumeral joint; stabilization of glenohumeral joint
Infraspinatus	Medial two-thirds of the infraspinous fossa of the scapula and the deep fascia that covers the muscle	Middle facet on posterior surface of the greater tubercle of the humerus	Suprascapular nerve (**C5**, C6)	**Rotator cuff muscle**; lateral rotation of arm at the glenohumeral joint; stabilization of glenohumeral joint
Teres minor	Upper two-thirds of a flattened strip of bone on the posterior surface of the scapula immediately adjacent to the lateral border of the scapula	Inferior facet on the posterior surface of the greater tubercle of the humerus	Axillary nerve (**C5**, C6)	**Rotator cuff muscle**; lateral rotation of arm at the glenohumeral joint; stabilization of glenohumeral joint
Teres major	Elongated oval area on the posterior surface of the inferior angle of the scapula	Medial lip of the intertubercular sulcus on the anterior surface of the humerus	Inferior subscapular nerve (**C5**, **C6**, **C7**)	Medial rotation and extension of the arm at the glenohumeral joint
Long head of triceps brachii	Infraglenoid tubercle on scapula	Common tendon of insertion with medial and lateral heads on the olecranon process of ulna	Radial nerve (C6, **C7**, C8)	Extension of the forearm at the elbow joint; accessory adductor and extensor of the arm at the glenohumeral joint

Note: Spinal segments in bold are the major segments innervating the muscle.

Muscles

Supraspinatus and infraspinatus

The **supraspinatus** and **infraspinatus** muscles originate from two large fossae, one above and one below the spine, on the posterior surface of the scapula (Fig. 2.37). They form tendons that insert on the greater tubercle of the humerus.

- The tendon of the supraspinatus passes under the acromion, where it is separated from the bone by a subacromial bursa, passes over the glenohumeral joint, and inserts on the superior facet of the greater tubercle.
- The tendon of the infraspinatus passes posteriorly to the glenohumeral joint and inserts on the middle facet of the greater tubercle.

The supraspinatus participates in abduction of the arm. The infraspinatus laterally rotates the humerus.

Teres minor and teres major

The **teres minor** muscle is a cord-like muscle that originates from a flattened area of the scapula immediately adjacent to its lateral border below the infraglenoid tubercle (Fig. 2.37). Its tendon inserts on the inferior facet of the greater tubercle of the humerus. The teres minor laterally rotates the humerus and is a component of the rotator cuff.

The **teres major** muscle originates from a large oval region on the posterior surface of the inferior angle of the scapula (Fig. 2.37). This broad cord-like muscle passes superiorly and laterally and ends as a flat tendon that attaches to the medial lip of the intertubercular sulcus on the anterior surface of the humerus. The teres major medially rotates and extends the humerus.

Long head of triceps brachii

The **long head of the triceps brachii** muscle originates from the infraglenoid tubercle and passes somewhat vertically down the arm to insert, with the medial and lateral heads of this muscle, on the olecranon of the ulna (Fig. 2.37).

The triceps brachii is the primary extensor of the forearm at the elbow joint. Because the long head crosses the glenohumeral joint, it can also extend and adduct the humerus.

The importance of the triceps brachii in the posterior scapular region is that its vertical course between the teres minor and teres major, together with these muscles and the humerus, forms spaces through which nerves and vessels pass between regions.

Gateways to the posterior scapular region

Suprascapular foramen

The suprascapular foramen is the route through which structures pass between the base of the neck and the posterior scapular region (Fig. 2.37). It is formed by the suprascapular notch of the scapula and the superior transverse scapular (suprascapular) ligament, which converts the notch into a foramen.

The suprascapular nerve passes through the suprascapular foramen; the suprascapular artery and the suprascapular vein follow the same course as the nerve, but normally pass immediately superior to the superior transverse scapular ligament and not through the foramen (Fig. 2.38).

Quadrangular space (from posterior) or space of Velpeau

The quadrangular space provides a passageway for nerves and vessels passing between more anterior regions (the axilla) and the posterior scapular region (Fig. 2.37). In the posterior scapular region, its boundaries are formed by:

- The inferior margin of the teres minor
- The surgical neck of the humerus
- The superior margin of the teres major
- The lateral margin of the long head of the triceps brachii

Viewed from the anterior aspect, the superior boundary is formed by the inferior margin of the subscapularis instead of the teres minor.

The axillary nerve and the posterior circumflex humeral artery and vein pass through this space (Fig. 2.38).

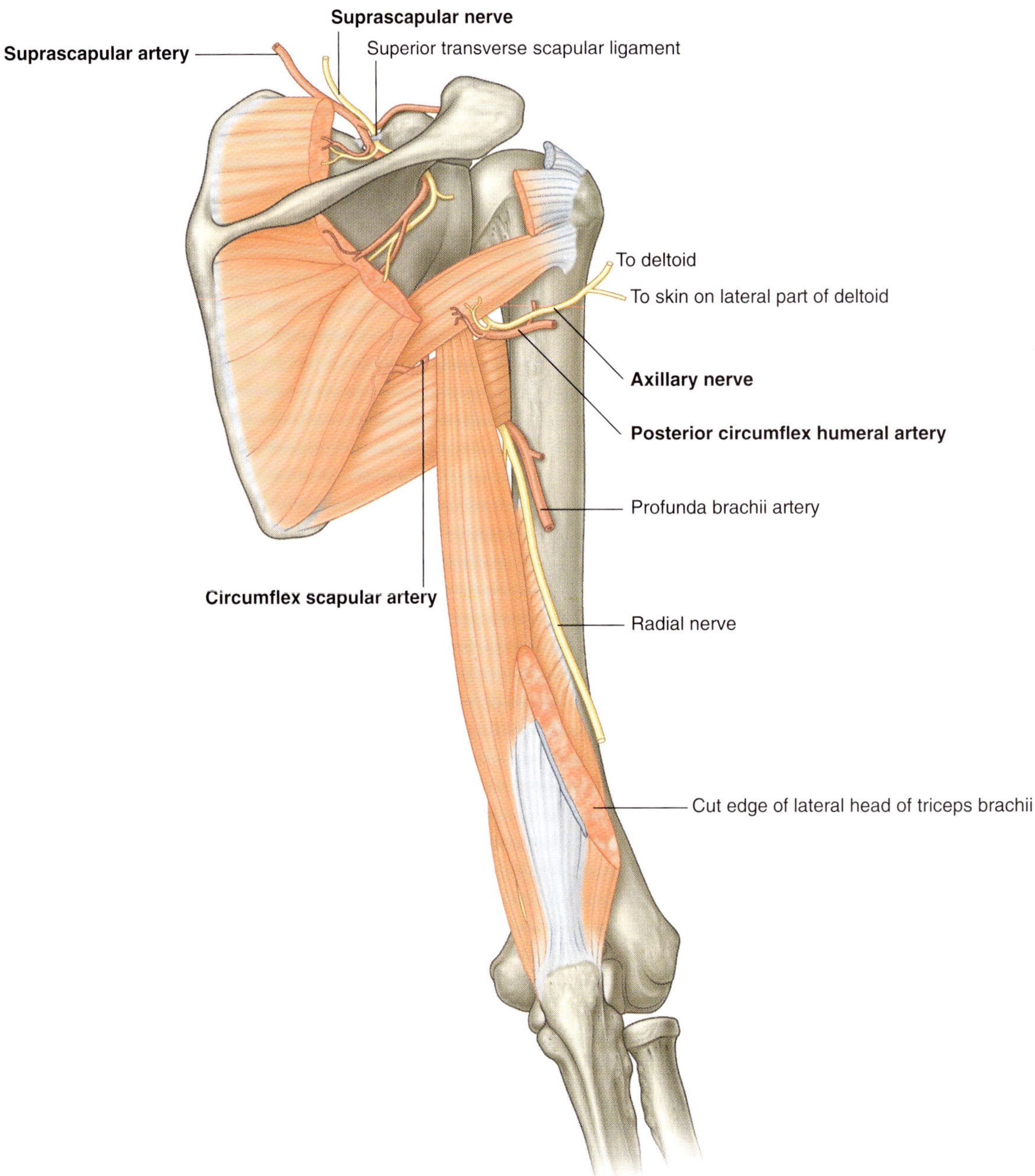

Fig. 2.38 Arteries and nerves associated with gateways in the posterior scapular region.

Triangular space

The triangular space is an area of communication between the axilla and the posterior scapular region (Fig. 2.37). When viewed from the posterior scapular region, the triangular space is formed by:

- The medial margin of the long head of the triceps brachii
- The superior margin of the teres major
- The inferior margin of the teres minor

The circumflex scapular artery and vein pass through this gap (Fig. 2.38).

A useful mnemonic is that both the quadrangular and triangular spaces have three boundaries formed by three muscles whose names begin with the letter "T," the teres minor, triceps brachii, and teres major. In addition, the quadrangular space is bounded by the surgical neck of the humerus.

Triangular interval

The triangular interval is formed by:

- The lateral margin of the long head of the triceps brachii
- The shaft of the humerus
- The inferior margin of the teres major (Fig. 2.37)

Because this space is below the inferior margin of the teres major, which defines the inferior boundary of the axilla, the triangular interval serves as a passageway between the anterior and posterior compartments of the arm and between the posterior compartment of the arm and the axilla. The radial nerve, the **profunda brachii artery (deep artery of arm)**, and associated veins pass through it (Fig. 2.38).

Nerves

The two major nerves of the posterior scapular region are the suprascapular and axillary nerves, both of which originate from the brachial plexus in the axilla (Fig. 2.38).

Suprascapular nerve

The **suprascapular nerve** originates in the base of the neck from the superior trunk of the brachial plexus. It passes posterolaterally from its origin, through the suprascapular foramen to reach the posterior scapular region, where it lies in the plane between bone and muscle (Fig. 2.38).

It innervates the supraspinatus muscle and then passes through the greater scapular (spinoglenoid) notch, between the root of the spine of the scapula and the glenoid cavity, to terminate in and innervate the infraspinatus muscle.

Generally, the suprascapular nerve has no cutaneous branches.

Axillary nerve

The **axillary nerve** originates from the posterior cord of the brachial plexus. It exits the axilla by passing through the quadrangular space in the posterior wall of the axilla, and enters the posterior scapular region (Fig. 2.38). Together with the posterior circumflex humeral artery and vein, it is directly related to the posterior surface of the surgical neck of the humerus.

The axillary nerve innervates the deltoid and teres minor muscles. The branch to teres minor bears a pseudoganglion. In addition, it has a cutaneous branch, the superior lateral cutaneous nerve of the arm to the inferior part of the deltoid muscle (Flowchart 2.1).

Arteries and veins

Three major arteries are found in the posterior scapular region: the suprascapular, posterior circumflex humeral, and circumflex scapular arteries. These arteries contribute to an interconnected vascular network around the scapula (Fig. 2.39). The arterial anastomosis around the scapula permits a collateral pathway between the first part of the subclavian artery and the third part of the axillary artery. This pathway is an alternate pathway to supply the distal part of the axillary artery third besides the direct communication of the subclavian artery with the axillary artery.

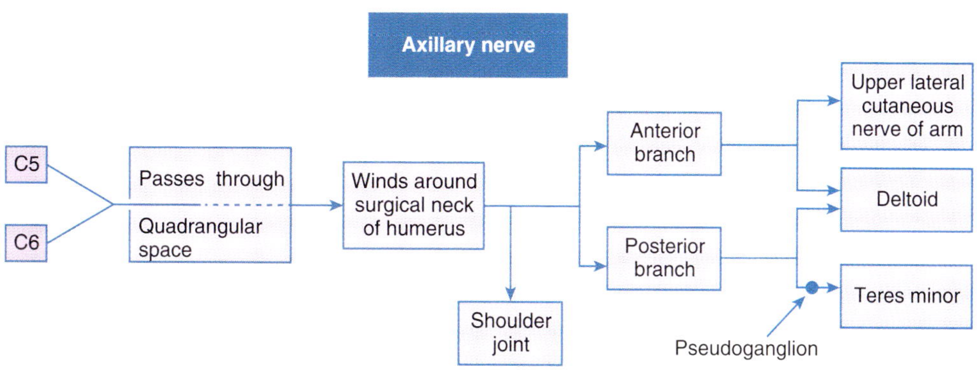

Flowchart 2.1 Course and supply of axillary nerve.

Early clinical exposure

Quadrangular space syndrome (axillary hiatus syndrome)

Hypertrophy of the quadrangular space muscles or fibrosis of the muscle edges may impinge on the axillary nerve. Uncommonly, this produces weakness of the deltoid muscle. Typically it produces atrophy of the teres minor muscle, which may affect the control that the rotator cuff muscles exert on shoulder movement.

Suprascapular artery

The **suprascapular artery** originates in the base of the neck as a branch of the thyrocervical trunk, which, in turn, is a major branch of the subclavian artery (Figs. 2.38 and 2.39). The vessel may also originate directly from the third part of the subclavian artery.

The suprascapular artery normally enters the posterior scapular region superior to the suprascapular foramen, whereas the nerve passes through the foramen. In the posterior scapular region, the vessel runs with the suprascapular nerve.

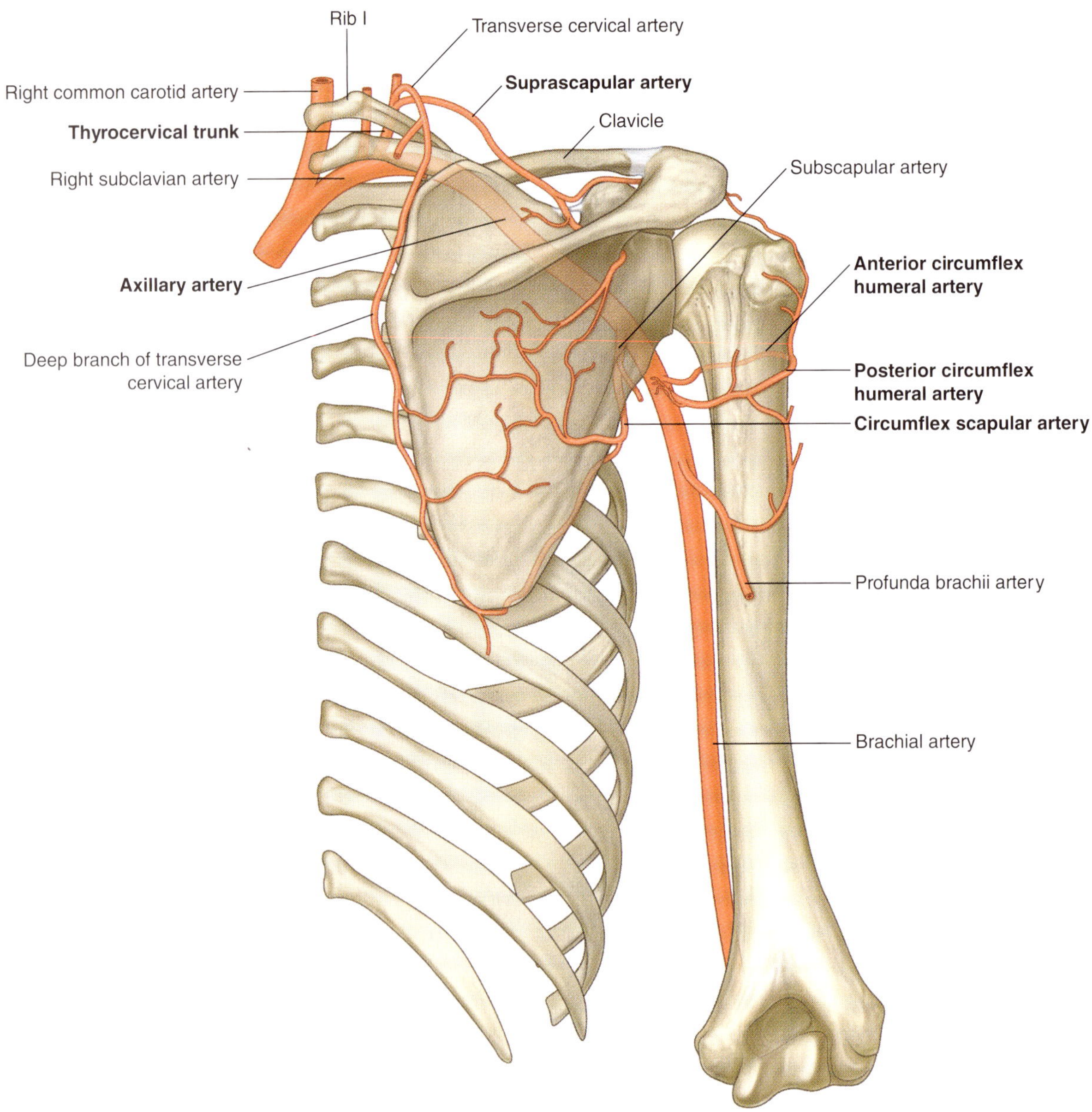

Fig. 2.39 Arterial anastomoses around the shoulder.

In addition to supplying the supraspinatus and infraspinatus muscles, the suprascapular artery contributes branches to numerous structures along its course.

Posterior circumflex humeral artery

The **posterior circumflex humeral artery** originates from the third part of the axillary artery in the axilla (Figs. 2.38 and 2.39).

The posterior circumflex humeral artery and axillary nerve leave the axilla through the quadrangular space in the posterior wall and enter the posterior scapular region. The vessel supplies the related muscles and the glenohumeral joint.

Circumflex scapular artery

The **circumflex scapular artery** is a branch of the subscapular artery that also originates from the third part of the axillary artery in the axilla (Figs. 2.38 and 2.39). The circumflex scapular artery leaves the axilla through the triangular space and enters the posterior scapular region, passes through the origin of the teres minor muscle, and forms anastomotic connections with other arteries in the region.

Veins

Veins in the posterior scapular region generally follow the arteries and connect with vessels in the neck, back, arm, and axilla.

AXILLA

SET INDUCTION—CASE SCENARIO 2: AXILLARY ABSCESS

A 35-year-old man presented to the outpatient department with complaints of pain and swelling in the left axilla. On examination, a swelling was found which was tender and the pus was found to be pointing. A diagnosis of axillary abscess was made and a plan was made for incision and drainage of the abscess under local anesthesia.

It is important to know the anatomy of the axilla to successfully drain an abscess without causing any complications.

<table>
<tr><th rowspan="2">REMEMBER
[Recall Facts]</th><th colspan="3">OUTLINE 2. AXILLA—LEARNING OBJECTIVES
[By the end of this section, the student should be able to:]</th><th rowspan="2" colspan="2">EVALUATE
[Explain Concepts]</th></tr>
<tr><th colspan="3">DEMONSTRATE AND ANALYZE RELATIONSHIPS
[Identify structures in a Prosected Specimen or Figure]</th></tr>
<tr><td rowspan="7">1. Describe the boundaries and contents of the axilla
2. Describe the brachial plexus under the following headings: (a) formation, (b) branches, and (c) lesions of the brachial plexus
3. Describe the axillary artery under the following headings: (a) origin and termination, (b) relations, (c) branches, and (d) clinical anatomy</td><td>Level I</td><td>Level II</td><td>Level III</td><td colspan="2" rowspan="2">■ Formation of axillary sheath
■ Relationship of axillary artery to pectoralis minor
■ Formation and important relations of the brachial plexus
■ Brachial plexus injuries
■ Arrangement of axillary group of lymph nodes</td></tr>
<tr><td rowspan="6">■ Anterior wall of axilla:
  ■ Pectoralis major and minor subclavius
■ Posterior wall of axilla:
  ■ Subscapularis
  ■ Teres major
  ■ Latissimus dorsi
■ Medial wall of axilla: serratus anterior
■ Axillary artery: three parts and branches
■ Cords of the brachial plexus and their main branches:
  ■ Median nerve
  ■ Radial nerve
  ■ Ulnar nerve
  ■ Musculocutaneous nerve
  ■ Axillary nerve
■ Nerve to serratus anterior:
  ■ Axillary lymph nodes</td><td rowspan="6">■ Axillary sheath
■ Axillary vein
■ Other branches of the brachial plexus</td><td rowspan="6">■ Intercostobrachial nerve</td></tr>
<tr><th colspan="2">EARLY CLINICAL EXPOSURE
[Apply Anatomical Knowledge]</th></tr>
<tr><th>Surgical Anatomy/ Pathology/ Trauma</th><th>Imaging/ Surface Anatomy</th></tr>
<tr><td>■ Axillary vein thrombosis
■ Drainage of abscesses in the axilla
■ Trauma to upper limb arteries
■ Subclavian and axillary venous access
■ Lesions of the brachial plexus and its branches:
  ■ Erb's paralysis
  ■ Klumpke's paralysis</td><td>■ Palpation of axillary artery
■ Imaging of blood vessels of the upper limb</td></tr>
<tr><th colspan="2">PROBLEM SOLVING/
CLINICAL CASES
[Interpret]</th></tr>
<tr><td colspan="2">■ Brachial plexus block
■ Winged scapula</td></tr>
</table>

The axilla is the gateway to the upper limb, providing an area of transition between the neck and the arm (Fig. 2.40A). Formed by the clavicle, the scapula, the upper thoracic wall, the humerus, and related muscles, the axilla is an irregularly shaped pyramidal space with:

- Four sides
- An inlet
- A floor (base) (Fig. 2.40A and B)

The axillary inlet is continuous superiorly with the neck, and the lateral part of the floor opens into the arm.

All major structures passing into and out of the upper limb pass through the axilla (Fig. 2.40C). Apertures formed between muscles in the anterior and posterior walls enable structures to pass between the axilla and immediately adjacent regions (the posterior scapular, pectoral, and deltoid regions).

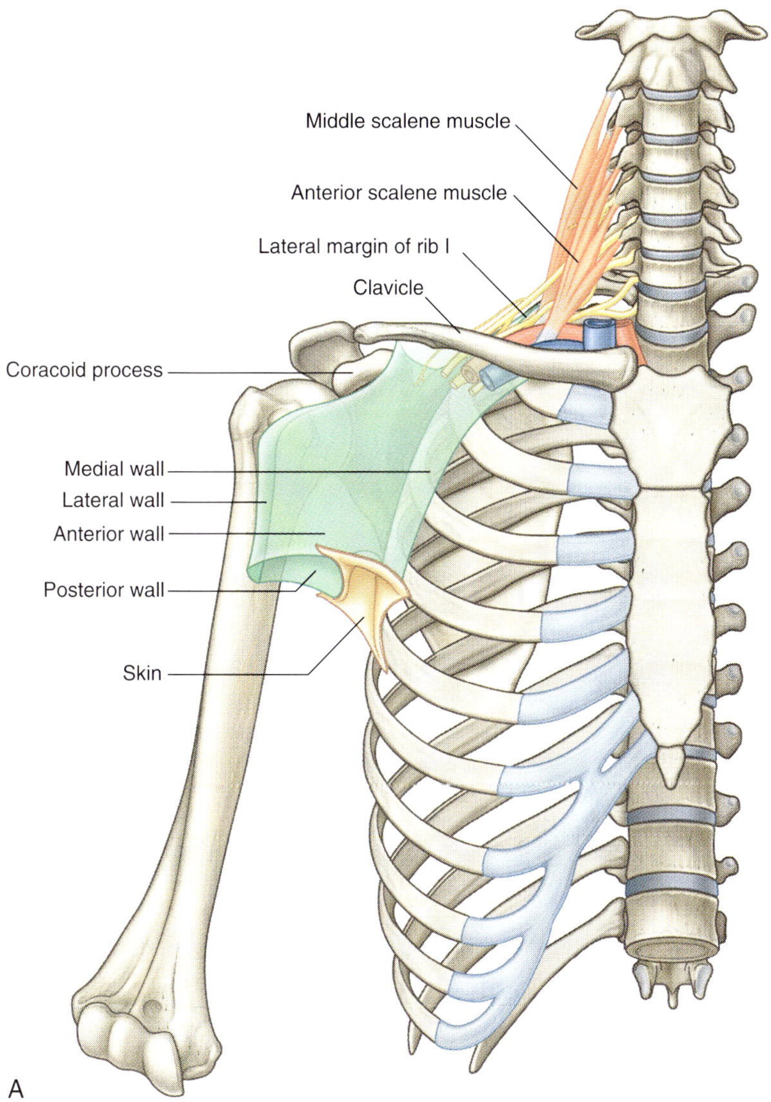

Fig. 2.40 Axilla. **(A)** Walls and transition between neck and arm.

Continued

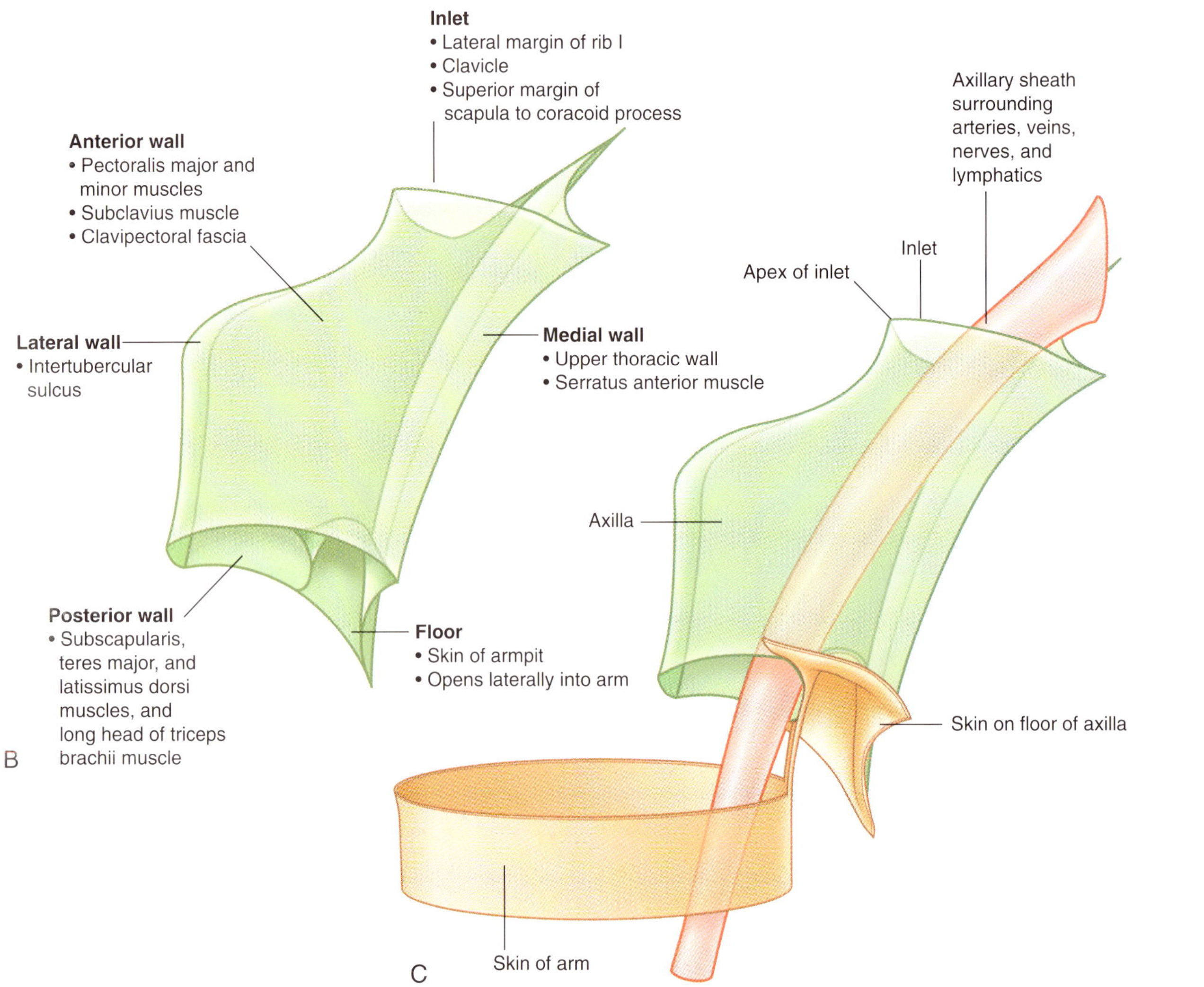

Fig. 2.40, cont'd (B) Boundaries. **(C)** Continuity with the arm.

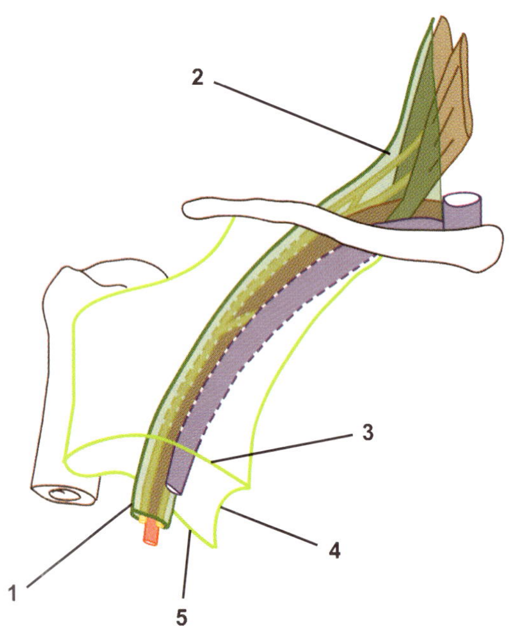

LD Fig. 2.40C.1 Axillary sheath.

Questions

2.40C.1.A Name the structures indicated by the labels, and mention how they are formed.

2.40C.1.B Explain why the contents of the axillary sheath include the axillary artery and brachial plexus, but not the axillary vein.

Answers

2.40C.1.A The structures indicated by the labels and how they are formed

1. Axillary sheath, formed as a continuation of the prevertebral fascia
2. Prevertebral fascia, formed as part of the deep fascia of the neck, in front of the prevertebral muscles
3. Anterior wall of the axilla, formed by the pectoralis major, pectoralis minor, subclavius, and clavipectoral fascia
4. Medial wall of the axilla, formed by the upper four ribs, intercostal muscles, and serratus anterior
5. Posterior wall of the axilla, formed by the subscapularis, teres major, and latissimus dorsi

2.40C.1.B The contents of the axillary sheath include the axillary artery and brachial plexus, but not the axillary vein because the axillary artery and brachial plexus are posterior to the prevertebral fascia as this fascia wraps the structures posterior to it as it gets prolonged into the axilla as the axillary sheath. The axillary vein is anterior to the prevertebral fascia and hence does not become a content of the axillary sheath.

Axillary inlet

The axillary inlet is oriented in the horizontal plane and is somewhat triangular in shape, with its apex directed laterally (Fig. 2.40A and B). The margins of the inlet are completely formed by bone:

- The medial margin is the lateral border of rib I.
- The anterior margin is the posterior surface of the clavicle.
- The posterior margin is the superior border of the scapula up to the coracoid process.

The apex of the triangularly shaped axillary inlet is lateral in position and is formed by the medial aspect of the coracoid process.

Major vessels and nerves pass between the neck and the axilla by crossing over the lateral border of rib I and through the axillary inlet (Fig. 2.40A).

The subclavian artery, the major blood vessel supplying the upper limb, becomes the axillary artery as it crosses the lateral margin of rib I and enters the axilla. Similarly, the axillary vein becomes the subclavian vein as it passes over the lateral margin of rib I and leaves the axilla to enter the neck.

At the axillary inlet, the axillary vein is anterior to the axillary artery, which, in turn, is anterior to the trunks of the brachial plexus.

The inferior trunk (lower trunk) of the brachial plexus lies directly on rib I in the neck, as does the subclavian artery and vein. As they pass over rib I, the vein and artery are separated by the insertion of the anterior scalene muscle (Fig. 2.40A).

Anterior wall

The anterior wall of the axilla is formed by the lateral part of the pectoralis major muscle, the underlying pectoralis minor and subclavius muscles, and the clavipectoral fascia (Table 2.3).

Table 2.3 Muscles of the anterior wall of the axilla

Muscle	Origin	Insertion	Innervation	Function
Pectoralis major	Clavicular head—anterior surface of medial half of clavicle; sternocostal head—anterior surface of sternum; first seven costal cartilages; sternal end of the sixth rib; aponeurosis of external oblique	Lateral lip of intertubercular sulcus of humerus	Medial and lateral pectoral nerves; clavicular head (**C5**, C6); sternocostal head (C6, **C7**, C8, T1)	Flexion, adduction, and medial rotation of arm at glenohumeral joint; clavicular head—flexion of extended arm; sternocostal head—extension of flexed arm
Subclavius	First rib at junction between rib and costal cartilage	Groove on inferior surface of middle one-third of clavicle	Nerve to subclavius (**C5**, **C6**)	Pulls tip of shoulder down; pulls clavicle medially to stabilize sternoclavicular joint
Pectoralis minor	Anterior surfaces and superior borders of ribs III to V, and from deep fascia overlying the related intercostal spaces	Coracoid process of scapula (medial border and upper surface)	Medial pectoral nerve (C5, C6, **C7**, **C8**, T1)	Pulls tip of shoulder down; protracts scapula

Note: Spinal segments in bold are the major segments innervating the muscle.

Pectoralis major

The **pectoralis major** muscle is the largest and most superficial muscle of the anterior wall (Fig. 2.41). Its inferior margin underlies the anterior axillary fold, which marks the anteroinferior border of the axilla. The muscle has two heads:

- The clavicular head originates from the medial half of the clavicle.
- The sternocostal head originates from the medial part of the anterior thoracic wall—often, fibers from this head continue inferiorly and medially to attach to the anterior abdominal wall, forming an additional abdominal part of the muscle.

The muscle inserts into the lateral lip of the intertubercular sulcus of the humerus. The parts of the muscle that have a superior origin on the trunk insert lower and more anteriorly on the lateral lip of the intertubercular sulcus than the parts of the muscle that originate inferiorly.

Acting together, the two heads of the pectoralis major flex, adduct, and medially rotate the arm at the glenohumeral joint. The clavicular head flexes the arm from an extended position, whereas the sternocostal head extends the arm from a flexed position, particularly against resistance.

The pectoralis major is innervated by the lateral and medial pectoral nerves, which originate from the brachial plexus in the axilla.

Subclavius

The **subclavius** muscle is a small muscle that lies deep to the pectoralis major muscle and passes between the clavicle and rib I (Fig. 2.42). It originates medially, as a tendon, from rib I at the junction between the rib and its costal cartilage. It passes laterally and superiorly to insert via a muscular attachment into an elongated, shallow groove on the inferior surface of the middle third of the clavicle.

The function of the subclavius is not entirely clear, but it may act to pull the shoulder down by depressing the

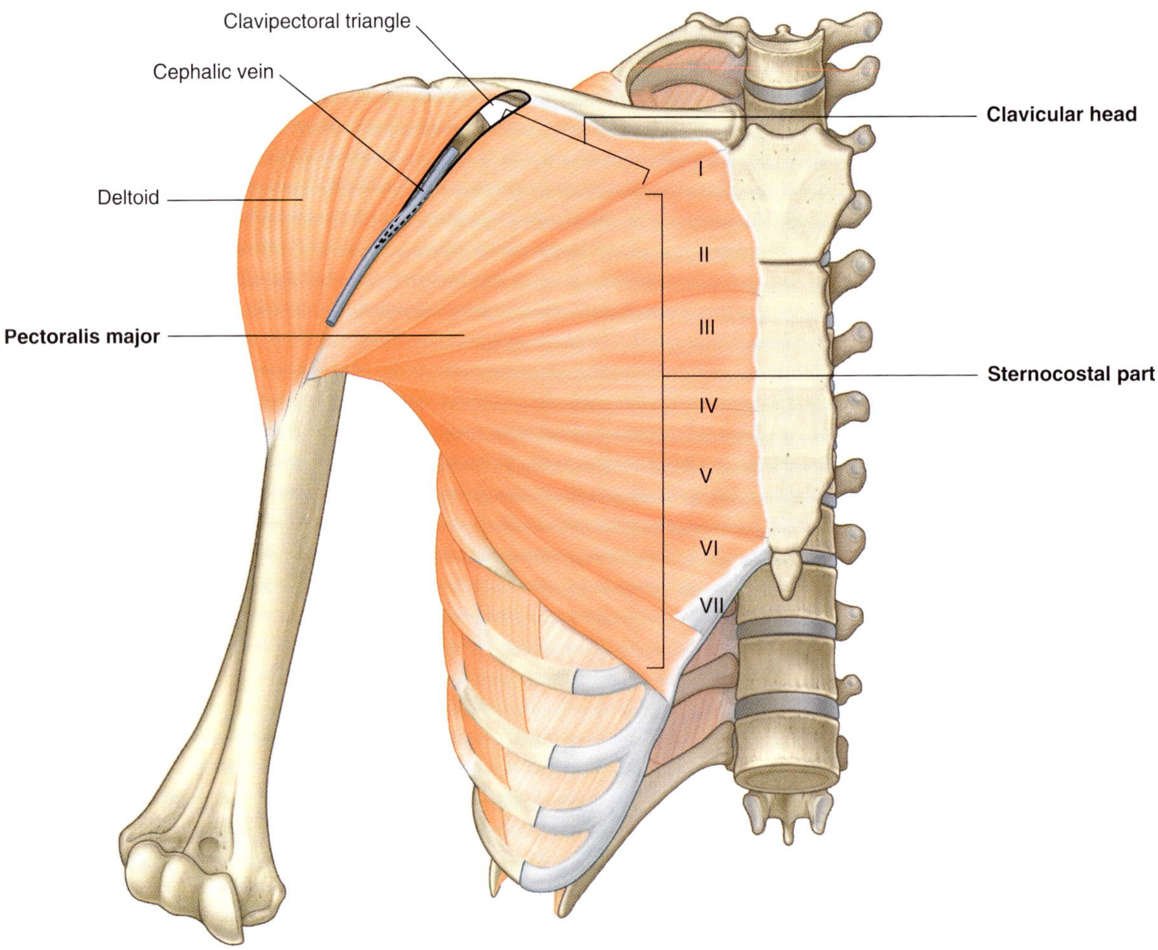

Fig. 2.41 Pectoralis major muscle.

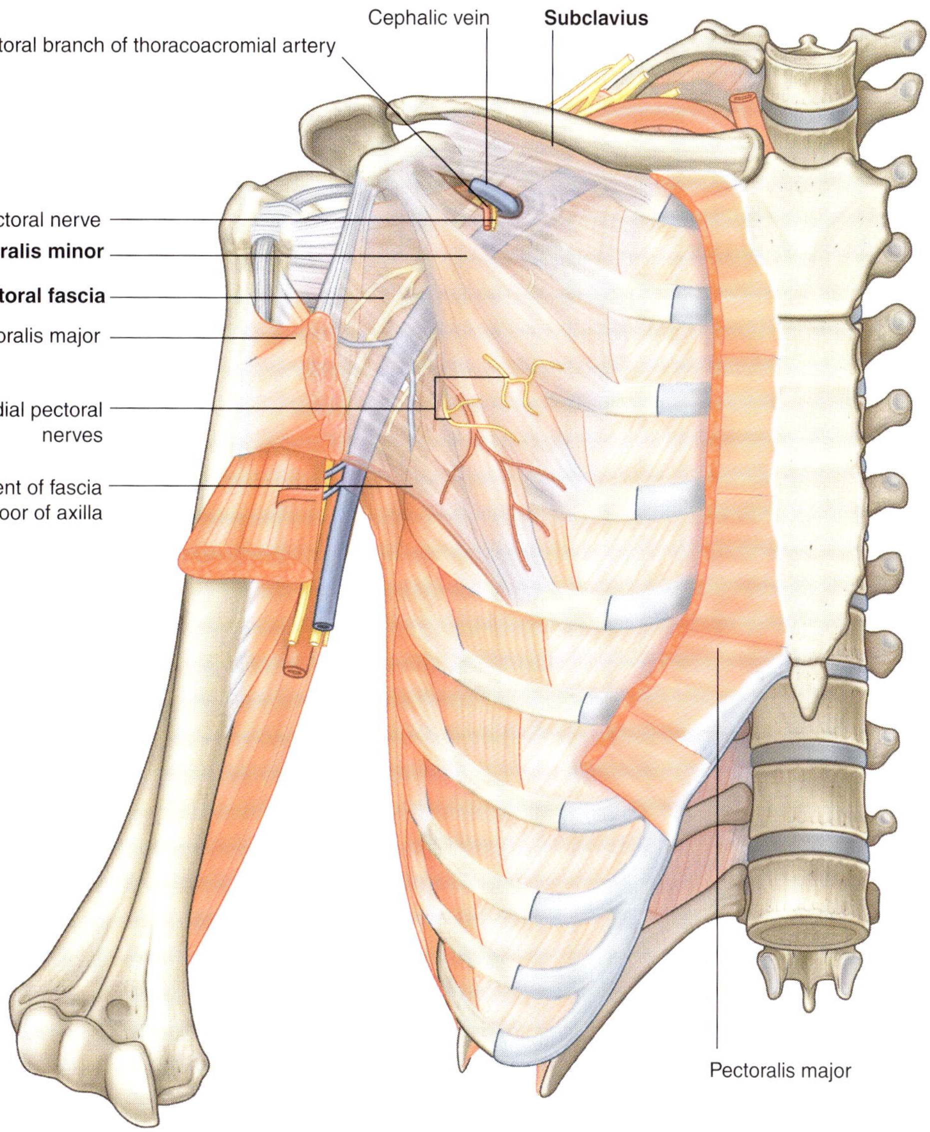

Fig. 2.42 Pectoralis minor and subclavius muscles and clavipectoral fascia.

clavicle and may also stabilize the sternoclavicular joint by pulling the clavicle medially.

The subclavius muscle is innervated by a small branch from the superior trunk of the brachial plexus.

Pectoralis minor

The **pectoralis minor** muscle is a small triangular-shaped muscle that lies deep to the pectoralis major muscle and passes from the thoracic wall to the coracoid process of the scapula (Fig. 2.42). It originates as three muscular slips from the anterior surfaces and upper margins of ribs III to V and from the fascia overlying muscles of the related intercostal spaces. The muscle fibers pass superiorly and laterally to insert into the medial and upper aspects of the coracoid process.

The pectoralis minor muscle protracts the scapula (by pulling the scapula anteriorly on the thoracic wall) and depresses the lateral angle of the scapula.

The pectoralis minor is innervated by the medial pectoral nerve, which originates from the brachial plexus in the axilla.

Clavipectoral fascia

The clavipectoral fascia is a thick sheet of connective tissue that connects the clavicle to the floor of the axilla (Fig. 2.42). It encloses the subclavius and pectoralis minor muscles and spans the gap between them.

Structures travel between the axilla and the anterior wall of the axilla by passing through the clavipectoral

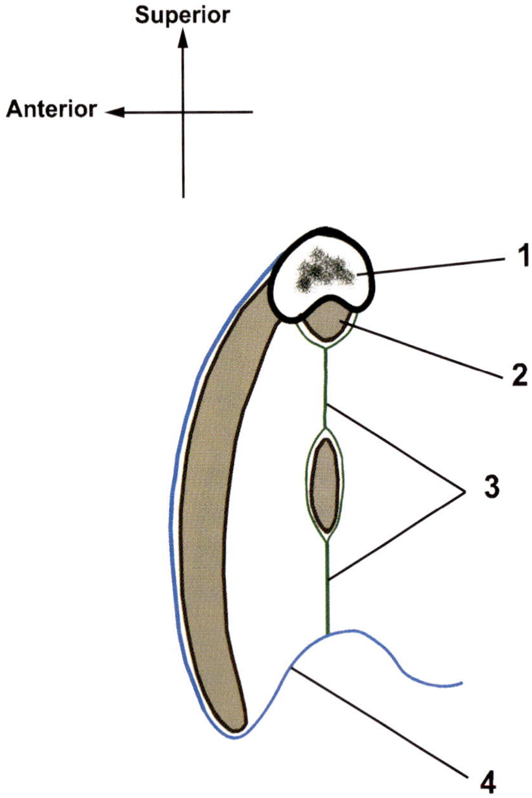

LD Fig. 2.42.1 Clavipectoral fascia.

Question

2.42.1.A Name the structures indicated by the labels.

2.42.1.B Name the parts of the clavipectoral fascia or coracoclavicular fascia.

2.42.1.C Mention a mnemonic for the structures that pierce the clavipectoral fascia.

Answer

2.42.1.A The structures indicated by the labels are

1. Clavicle
2. Subclavius
3. Clavipectoral fascia
4. Floor of axilla

2.42.1.B The parts of the clavipectoral fascia from above downwards include the muscular fascia over the subclavius, the costocoracoid membrane, the muscular fascia over the pectoralis minor and the suspensory ligament of the axilla (Gerdy's ligament).

2.42.1.C A mnemonic for the structures that pierce the clavipectoral fascia are that there is one artery, one vein, one nerve and one lymphatic that pierces the costocoracoid membrane.

fascia either between the pectoralis minor and subclavius muscles or inferior to the pectoralis minor muscle.

Important structures that pass between the subclavius and pectoralis minor muscles include the cephalic vein, the thoracoacromial artery, and the lateral pectoral nerve.

The lateral thoracic artery leaves the axilla by passing through the fascia inferior to the pectoralis minor muscle.

The medial pectoral nerve leaves the axilla by penetrating directly through the pectoralis minor muscle to supply this muscle and to reach the pectoralis major muscle. Occasionally, branches of the medial pectoral nerve pass around the lower margin of the pectoralis minor to reach and innervate the overlying pectoralis major muscle.

Medial wall

The medial wall of the axilla consists of the upper thoracic wall (the ribs and related intercostal tissues) and the serratus anterior muscle (Fig. 2.43A and Table 2.4; a see Fig. 2.40).

Serratus anterior

The **serratus anterior** muscle originates as a number of muscular slips from the lateral surfaces of ribs I to IX and the intervening deep fascia overlying the related intercostal spaces (Fig. 2.43A). The muscle forms a flattened sheet, which passes posteriorly around the thoracic wall to insert primarily on the costal surface of the medial border of the scapula.

The serratus anterior pulls the scapula forward over the thoracic wall and facilitates scapular rotation. It also keeps the costal surface of the scapula closely opposed to the thoracic wall.

The serratus anterior is innervated by the long thoracic nerve, which is derived from the roots of the brachial plexus, passes through the axilla along the medial wall, and passes vertically down the serratus anterior muscle on its external surface, just deep to skin and superficial fascia.

Intercostobrachial nerve

The only major structure that passes directly through the medial wall and into the axilla is the intercostobrachial nerve (Fig. 2.43A). This nerve is the lateral cutaneous branch of the second intercostal nerve (anterior ramus of T2). It communicates with a branch of the brachial plexus (the medial cutaneous nerve of the arm) in the axilla and supplies skin on the upper posteromedial side of the arm, which is part of the T2 dermatome.

Early clinical exposure

"Winging" of the scapula

Because the long thoracic nerve passes down the lateral thoracic wall on the external surface of the serratus anterior muscle, just deep to skin and subcutaneous tissue, it is vulnerable to damage. Loss of function of this muscle causes the medial border, and particularly the inferior angle of the scapula, to elevate away from the thoracic wall, resulting in the characteristic "winging" of the scapula, on pushing forward with the arm. Normal elevation of the arm is no longer possible (Fig. 2.43D–G).

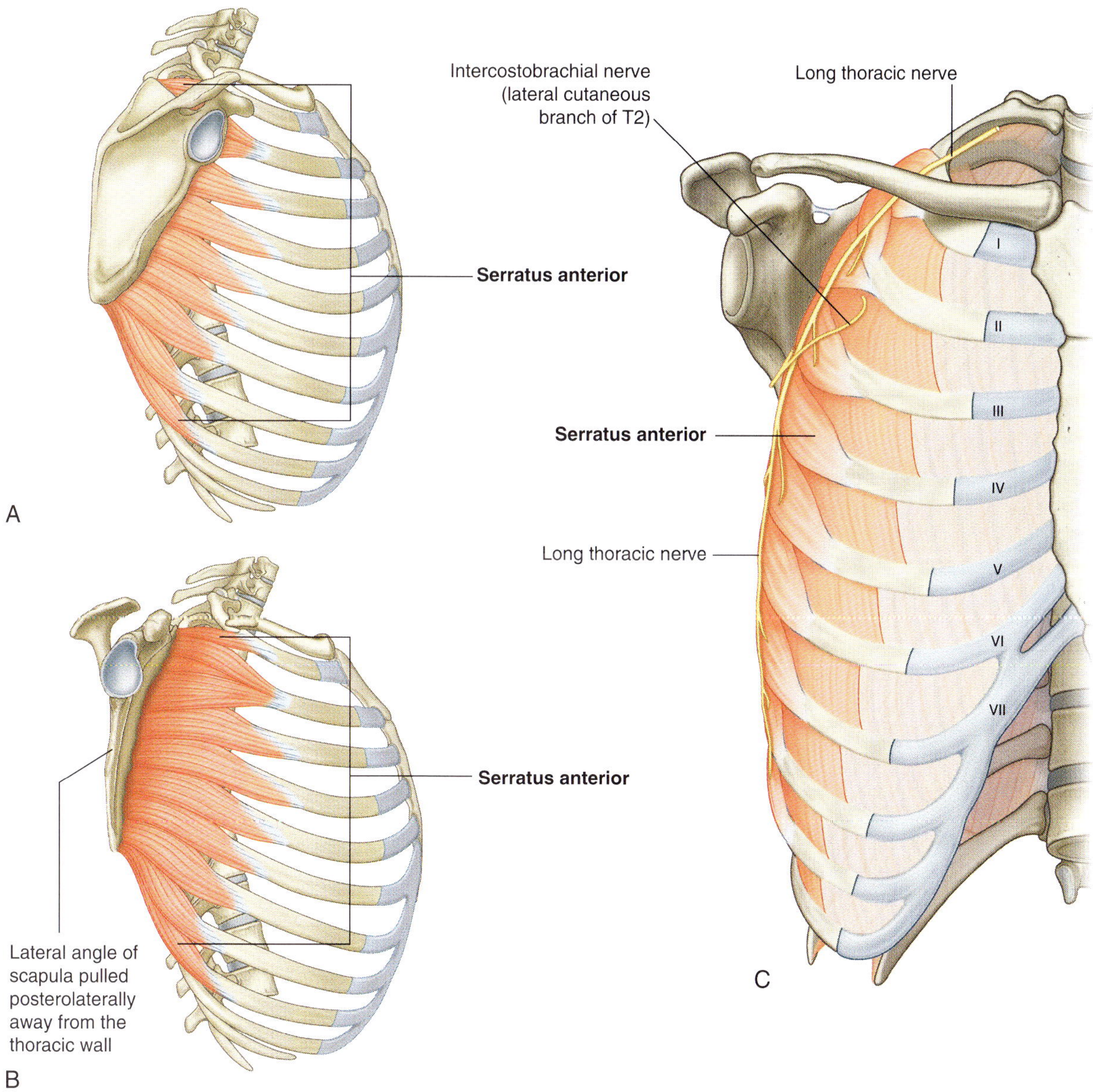

Fig. 2.43 Medial wall of the axilla. **(A)** Lateral view. **(B)** Lateral view with lateral angle of scapula retracted posteriorly. **(C)** Anterior view.

Continued

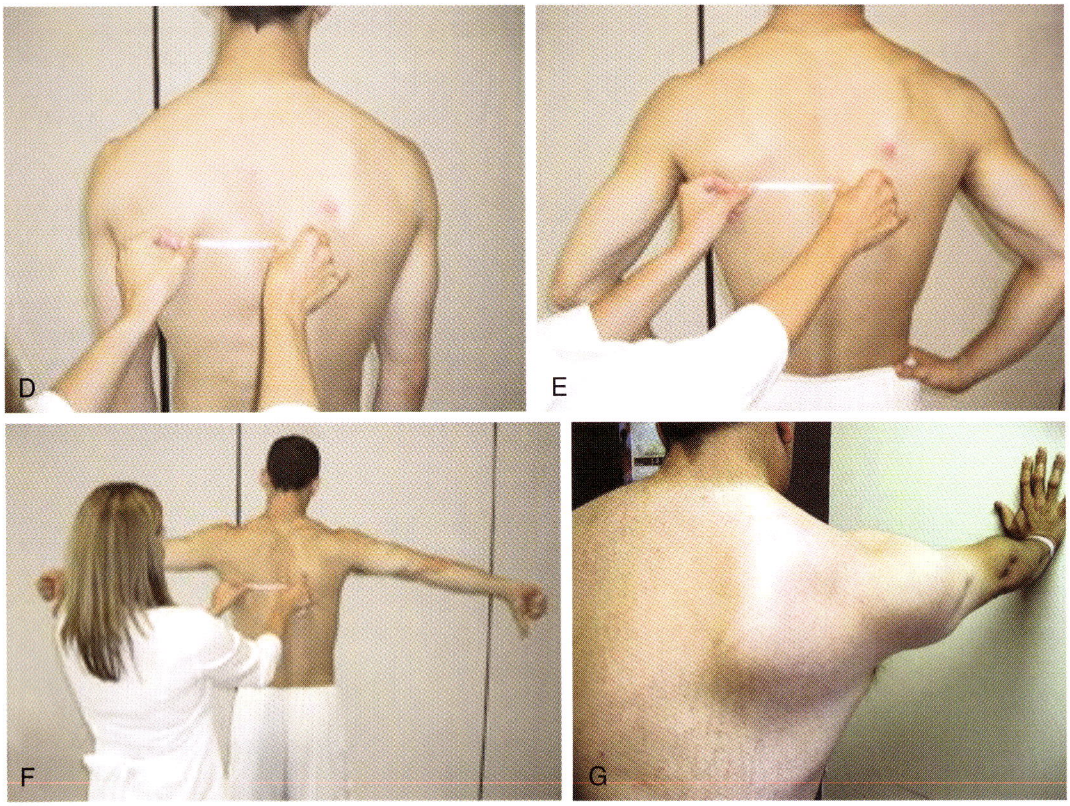

Fig. 2.43, cont'd (D–G) Winging of scapula. Positions for lateral scapular slide test with horizontal linear measurements from inferior angle of scapula to the adjacent spinous process: **(D)** with arms at the side, **(E)** with hands on the hips, and **(F)** with shoulders abducted to 90° and internally rotated. **(G)** Scapular winging is evident on protraction against resistance on the patient's right side secondary to injury of the long thoracic nerve. *Source:* (D and E) TSA Osterman, J Fedorczyk, P Amadio. Rehabilitation of the Hand and Upper Extremity: Examination and Management of Scapular Dysfunction. Mosby, 2011:1209–1224. (G) KC Chung, Lynda J-S Yang, JE McGillicuddy. Practical Management of Pediatric and Adult Brachial Plexus Palsies: Clinical Examination of the Patient with Brachial Plexus Palsy. Saunders, 2012:21–32.

Table 2.4 Muscle of the medial wall of the axilla

Muscle	Origin	Insertion	Innervation	Function
Serratus anterior	Lateral surfaces of upper eight to nine ribs and deep fascia overlying the related intercostal spaces	Costal surface of medial border of scapula	Long thoracic nerve (**C5**, C6, C7)	Protraction and rotation of the scapula; keeps medial border and inferior angle of scapula opposed to thoracic wall

Note: Spinal segment in bold is the major segment innervating the muscle.

Lateral wall

The lateral wall of the axilla is narrow and formed entirely by the intertubercular sulcus of the humerus (Fig. 2.44). The pectoralis major muscle of the anterior wall attaches to the lateral lip of the intertubercular sulcus. The latissimus dorsi and teres major muscles of the posterior wall attach to the floor and medial lip of the intertubercular sulcus, respectively (Table 2.5).

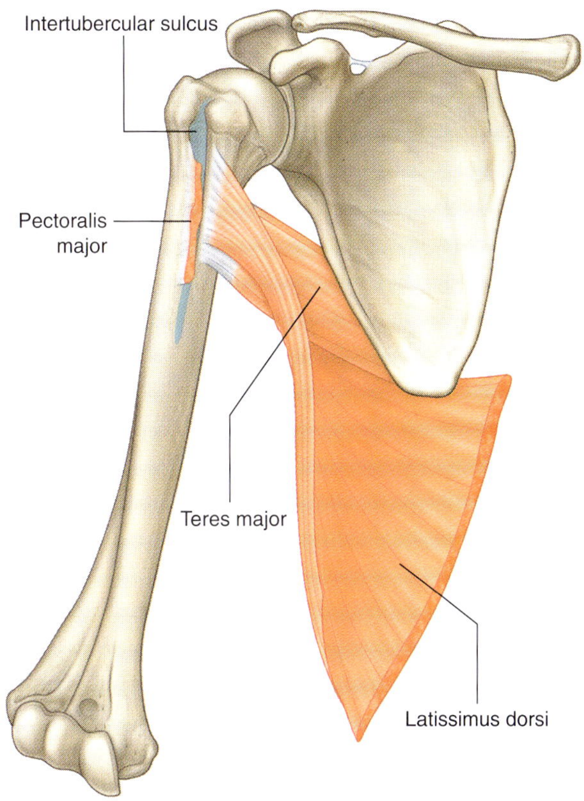

Fig. 2.44 Lateral wall of the axilla.

Table 2.5 Muscles of the lateral and posterior wall of the axilla

Muscle	Origin	Insertion	Innervation	Function
Subscapularis	Medial two-thirds of subscapular fossa	Lesser tubercle of humerus	Upper and lower subscapular nerves (C5, **C6**, (C7))	**Rotator cuff muscle**; medial rotation of the arm at the glenohumeral joint
Teres major	Elongated oval area on the posterior surface of the inferior angle of the scapula	Medial lip of the intertubercular sulcus on the anterior surface of the humerus	Lower subscapular nerve (**C5, C6, C7**)	Medial rotation and extension of the arm at the glenohumeral joint
Latissimus dorsi	Spinous processes of lower six thoracic vertebrae and related interspinous ligaments; via the thoracolumbar fascia to the spinous processes of the lumbar vertebrae, related interspinous ligaments, and iliac crest; lower three to four ribs	Floor of intertubercular sulcus	Thoracodorsal nerve (C6, **C7**, C8)	Adduction, medial rotation, and extension of the arm at the glenohumeral joint
Long head of triceps brachii	Infraglenoid tubercle on scapula	Common tendon of insertion with medial and lateral heads on the olecranon process of ulna	Radial nerve (C6, **C7**, C8)	Extension of the forearm at the elbow joint; accessory adductor and extensor of the arm at the glenohumeral joint

Note: Spinal segments in bold are the major segments innervating the muscle; spinal segments in parentheses do not consistently innervate the muscle.

Posterior wall

The posterior wall of the axilla is complex (Fig. 2.45; also see Fig. 2.50). Its bone framework is formed by the costal surface of the scapula. Muscles of the wall are

- The subscapularis muscle (associated with the costal surface of the scapula)
- The distal parts of the latissimus dorsi and teres major muscles (which pass into the wall from the back and posterior scapular region)
- The proximal part of the long head of the triceps brachii muscle (which passes vertically down the wall and into the arm)

Gaps between the muscles of the posterior wall form apertures through which structures pass between the axilla, posterior scapular region, and posterior compartment of the arm.

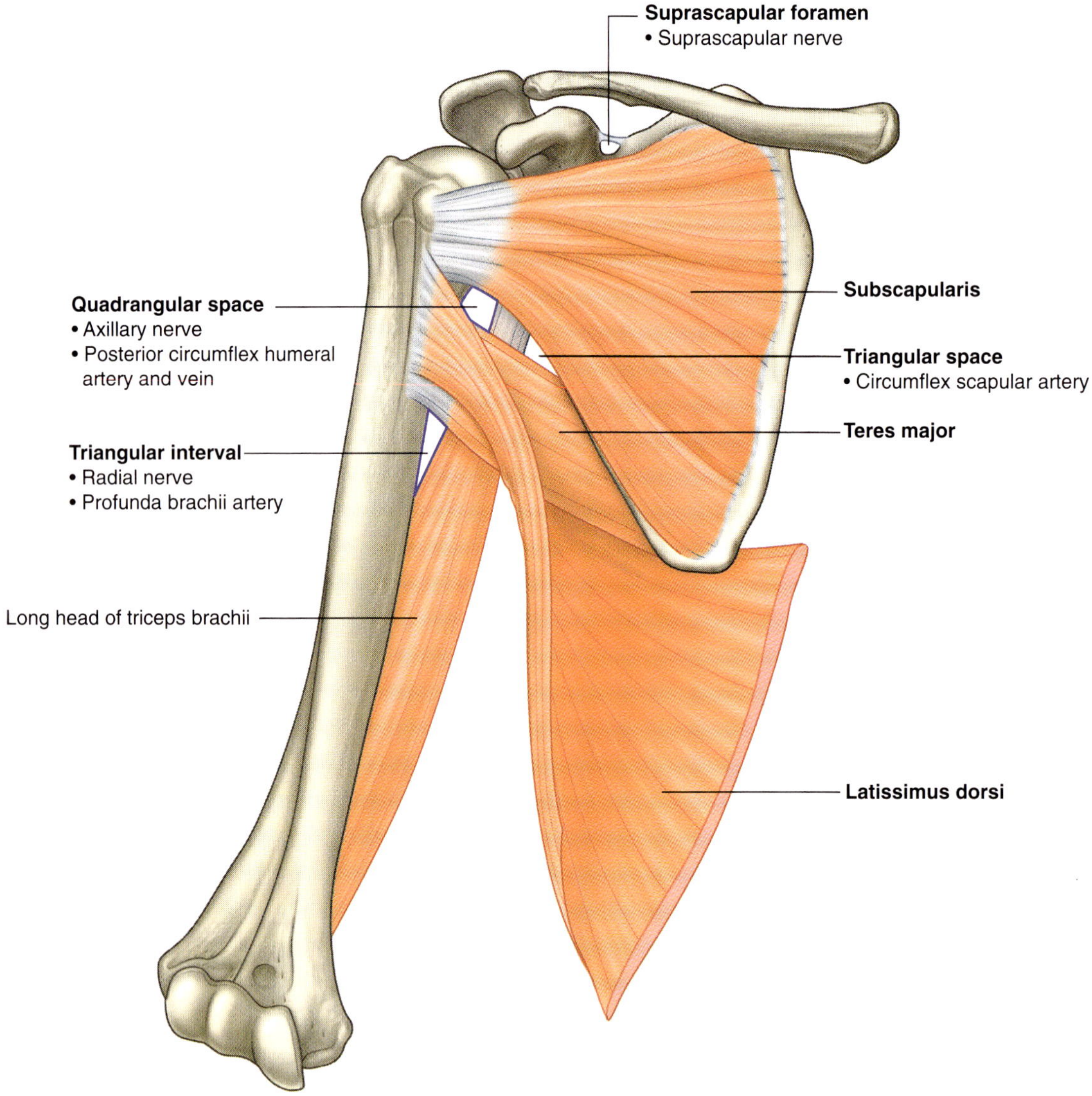

Fig. 2.45 Posterior wall of the axilla.

Subscapularis

The **subscapularis** muscle forms the largest component of the posterior wall of the axilla. It originates from, and fills, the subscapular fossa and inserts onto the lesser tubercle of the humerus (Figs. 2.45 and 2.46). The tendon crosses immediately anterior to the joint capsule of the glenohumeral joint.

Together with three muscles of the posterior scapular region (the supraspinatus, infraspinatus, and teres minor muscles), the subscapularis is a member of the rotator cuff muscle group, which stabilize the glenohumeral joint.

The subscapularis is innervated by branches of the brachial plexus (the **superior** and **inferior subscapular nerves**), which originate in the axilla.

Teres major and latissimus dorsi

The inferolateral aspect of the posterior wall of the axilla is formed by the terminal part of the **teres major** muscle and the tendon of the **latissimus dorsi** muscle (Fig. 2.45). These two structures lie under the posterior axillary fold, which marks the posteroinferior border of the axilla.

The flat tendon of the latissimus dorsi muscle curves around the inferior margin of the teres major muscle on the posterior wall to insert into the floor of the intertubercular sulcus of the humerus. This insertion is anterior to and slightly above the most distal part of the attachment of the teres major muscle to the medial lip of the intertubercular sulcus. As a consequence, the inferior margin of the teres major muscle defines the inferior limit of the axilla laterally.

The axillary artery becomes the brachial artery of the arm as it crosses the inferior margin of the teres major muscle.

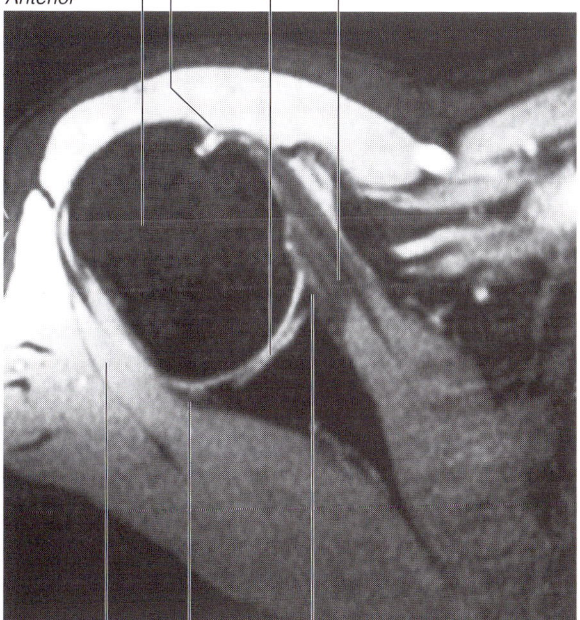

Fig. 2.46 Magnetic resonance image of the glenohumeral joint in the transverse or horizontal plane.

Long head of the triceps brachii

The **long head of the triceps brachii** muscle passes vertically through the posterior wall of the axilla, and, together with surrounding muscles and adjacent bones, results in the formation of three apertures through which major structures pass through the posterior wall:

- The quadrangular space
- The triangular space
- The triangular interval (Fig. 2.45)

Gateways in the posterior wall

Quadrangular space

The quadrangular space provides a passageway for nerves and vessels passing between the axilla and the more posterior scapular and deltoid regions (Fig. 2.45). When viewed from anteriorly, its boundaries are formed by:

- The inferior margin of the subscapularis muscle
- The surgical neck of the humerus
- The superior margin of the teres major muscle
- The lateral margin of the long head of the triceps brachii muscle

Passing through the quadrangular space are the axillary nerve and the posterior circumflex humeral artery and vein.

Triangular space

The **triangular space** is an area of communication between the axilla and the posterior scapular region (Fig. 2.45). When viewed from anteriorly, it is formed by:

- The medial margin of the long head of the triceps brachii muscle
- The superior margin of the teres major muscle
- The inferior margin of the subscapularis muscle

The circumflex scapular artery and vein pass into this space.

Triangular interval

This triangular interval is formed by:

- The lateral margin of the long head of the triceps brachii muscle
- The shaft of the humerus
- The inferior margin of the teres major muscle (Fig. 2.45)

The radial nerve passes out of the axilla traveling through this interval to reach the posterior compartment of the arm.

Floor

The floor of the axilla is formed by fascia and a dome of skin that spans the distance between the inferior margins of the walls (Fig. 2.47 and see Fig. 2.40B). It is supported by the clavipectoral fascia. On a patient, the anterior axillary fold is more superior in position than is the posterior axillary fold.

Inferiorly, structures pass into and out of the axilla immediately lateral to the floor where the anterior and posterior walls of the axilla converge and where the axilla is continuous with the anterior compartment of the arm.

Contents of the axilla

Passing through the axilla are the major vessels, nerves, and lymphatics of the upper limb. The space also contains the proximal parts of two muscles of the arm, the axillary process of the breast, and collections of lymph nodes, which drain the upper limb, chest wall, and breast.

The proximal parts of the biceps brachii and coracobrachialis muscles pass through the axilla (Table 2.6).

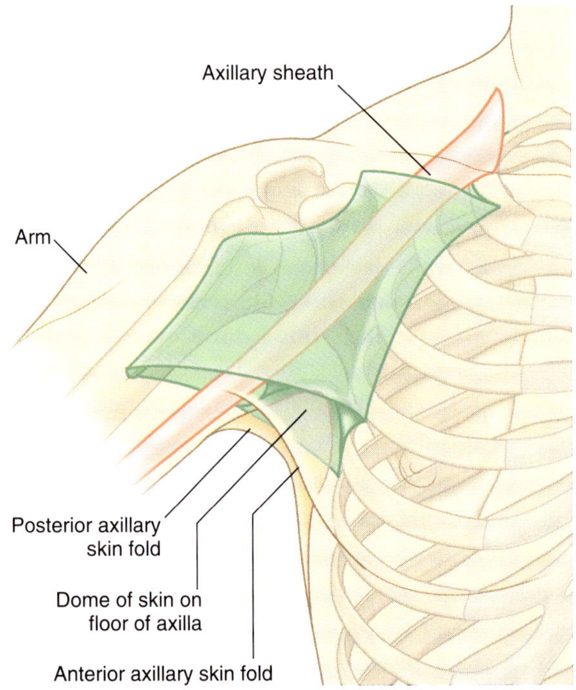

Fig. 2.47 Floor of the axilla.

Table 2.6 Muscles having parts that pass through the axilla

Muscle	Origin	Insertion	Innervation	Function
Biceps brachii	Long head—supraglenoid tubercle of scapula; short head—apex of coracoid process	Tuberosity of radius	Musculocutaneous nerve (**C5, C6**)	Powerful flexor of the forearm at the elbow joint and supinator of the forearm; accessory flexor of the arm at the glenohumeral joint
Coracobrachialis	Apex of coracoid process	Linear roughening on midshaft of humerus on medial side	Musculocutaneous nerve (**C5, C6, C7**)	Flexor of the arm at the glenohumeral joint; adducts arm

Note: Spinal segments in bold are the major segments innervating the muscle.

Biceps brachii

The **biceps brachii** muscle originates as two heads (Fig. 2.48):

- The short head originates from the apex of the coracoid process of the scapula and passes vertically through the axilla and into the arm where it joins the long head.
- The long head originates as a tendon from the supraglenoid tubercle of the scapula, passes over the head of the humerus deep to the joint capsule of the glenohumeral joint, and enters the intertubercular sulcus where it is held in position by a ligament, the transverse humeral ligament, which spans the distance between the greater and lesser tubercles; the tendon passes through the axilla in the intertubercular sulcus and forms a muscle belly in the proximal part of the arm.

The long and short heads of the muscle join in distal regions of the arm and primarily insert as a single tendon into the radial tuberosity in the forearm.

The biceps brachii muscle is primarily a powerful flexor of the forearm at the elbow joint and a powerful supinator in the forearm. Because both heads originate from the scapula, the muscle also acts as an accessory flexor of the arm at the glenohumeral joint. In addition, the long head prevents superior movement of the humerus on the glenoid cavity.

The biceps brachii muscle is innervated by the musculocutaneous nerve.

Coracobrachialis

The **coracobrachialis** muscle, together with the short head of the biceps brachii muscle, originates from the apex of the coracoid process (Fig. 2.48). It passes vertically through the axilla to insert on a small linear roughening on the medial aspect of the humerus, approximately midshaft.

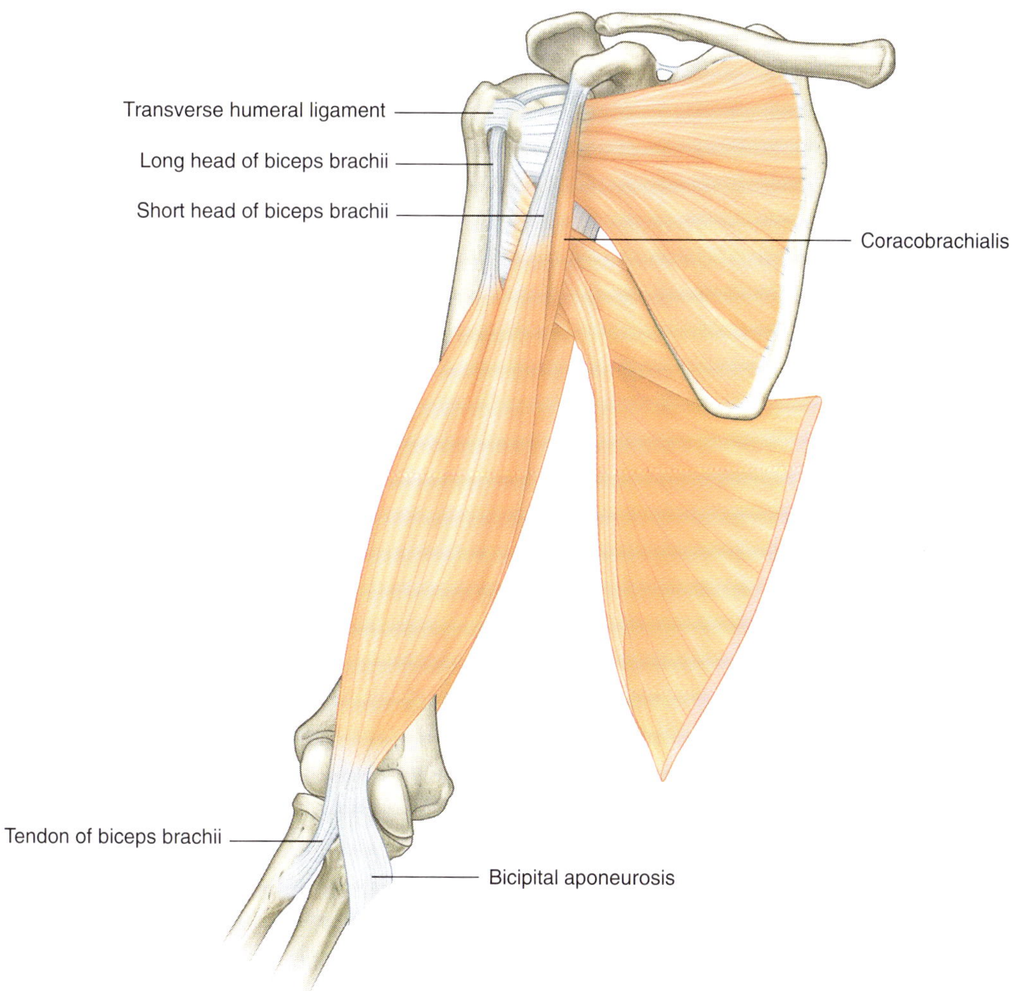

Fig. 2.48 Contents of the axilla: muscles.

The coracobrachialis muscle flexes the arm at the glenohumeral joint.

In the axilla, the medial surface of the coracobrachialis muscle is pierced by the musculocutaneous nerve, which innervates and then passes through the muscle to enter the arm.

Axillary artery

The axillary artery supplies the walls of the axilla and related regions, and continues as the major blood supply to the more distal parts of the upper limb (Fig. 2.49).

The subclavian artery in the neck becomes the axillary artery at the lateral margin of rib I and passes through the axilla, becoming the brachial artery at the inferior margin of the teres major muscle.

The axillary artery is separated into three parts by the pectoralis minor muscle, which crosses anteriorly to the vessel (Fig. 2.49):

- The first part is proximal to the pectoralis minor.
- The second part is posterior to the pectoralis minor.
- The third part is distal to the pectoralis minor.

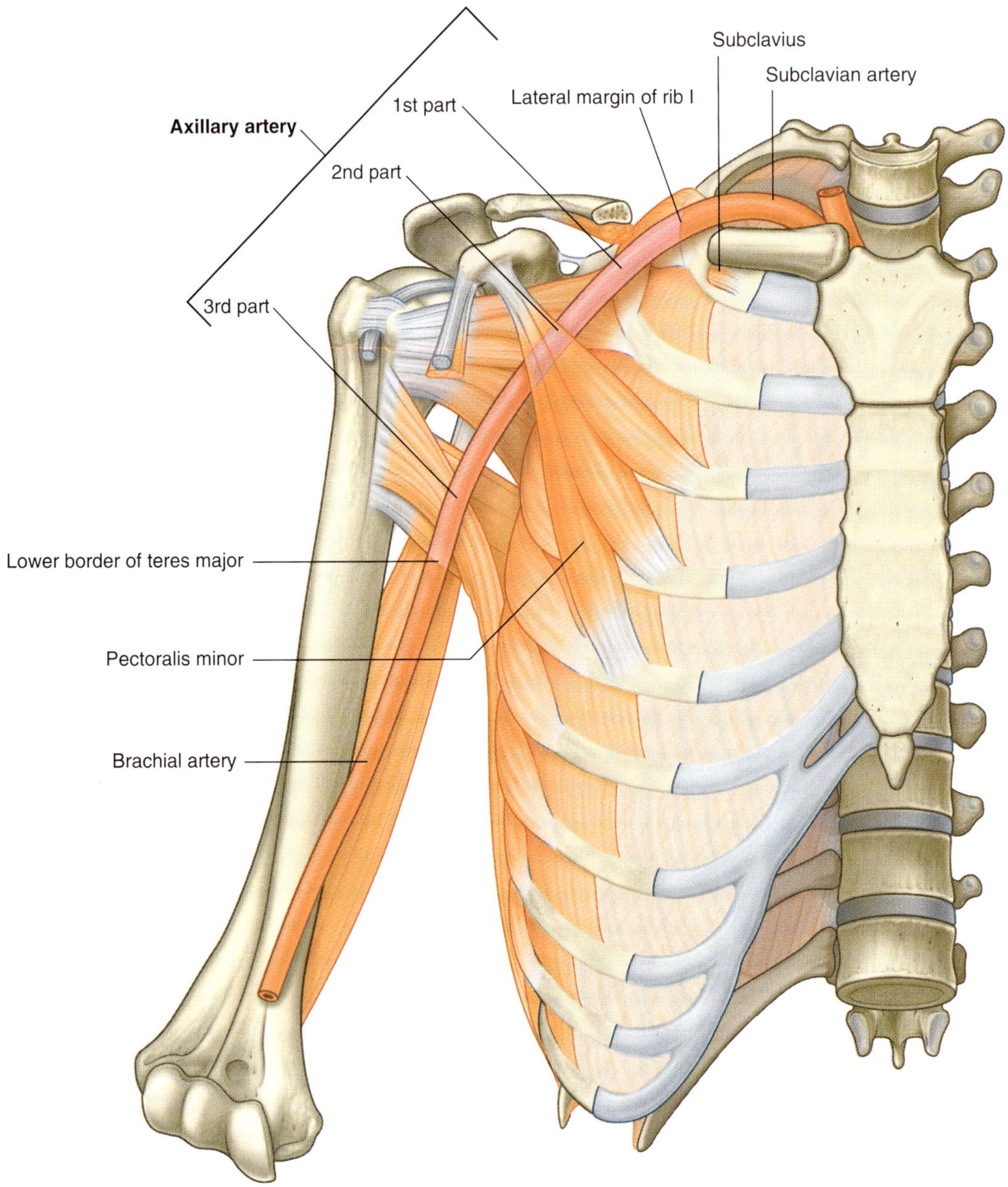

Fig. 2.49 Contents of the axilla: the axillary artery.

Generally, six branches arise from the axillary artery (Flowchart 2.2):

- One branch, the **superior thoracic artery**, takes origin from the first part.
- Two branches, the **thoracoacromial artery** and the **lateral thoracic artery**, take origin from the second part.
- Three branches, the **subscapular artery**, the **anterior circumflex humeral artery**, and the **posterior circumflex humeral artery**, take origin from the third part (Fig. 2.50).

Superior thoracic artery

The superior thoracic artery is small and originates from the anterior surface of the first part of the axillary artery (Fig. 2.50). It supplies upper regions of the medial and anterior axillary walls.

Thoracoacromial artery

The thoracoacromial artery is short and originates from the anterior surface of the second part of the axillary artery just posterior to the medial (superior) margin of the pectoralis minor muscle (Fig. 2.50). It curves around the superior margin of the muscle, penetrates the clavipectoral fascia, and immediately divides into four branches—the pectoral, deltoid, clavicular, and acromial branches, which supply the anterior axillary wall and related regions.

Additionally, the pectoral branch contributes vascular supply to the breast, and the deltoid branch passes into the clavipectoral triangle where it accompanies the cephalic vein and supplies adjacent structures (see Fig. 2.41).

Lateral thoracic artery

The lateral thoracic artery arises from the anterior surface of the second part of the axillary artery posterior to the lateral (inferior) margin of the pectoralis minor (Fig. 2.50). It follows the margin of the muscle to the thoracic wall and supplies the medial and anterior walls of the axilla. In women, branches emerge from around the inferior margin of the pectoralis major muscle and contribute to the vascular supply of the breast.

Subscapular artery

The subscapular artery is the largest branch of the axillary artery and is the major blood supply to the posterior wall of the axilla (Fig. 2.50). It also contributes to the blood supply of the posterior scapular region.

The subscapular artery originates from the posterior surface of the third part of the axillary artery, follows the inferior margin of the subscapularis muscle for a short distance, and then divides into its two terminal branches, the **circumflex scapular artery** and the **thoracodorsal artery**.

- The circumflex scapular artery passes through the triangular space between the subscapularis, teres major, and long head of the triceps muscle. Posteriorly, it passes inferior to, or pierces, the origin of the teres minor muscle to enter the infraspinous fossa. It anastomoses with the suprascapular artery and the **deep branch** (**dorsal scapular artery**) of the transverse cervical artery, thereby contributing to an anastomotic network of vessels around the scapula.
- The thoracodorsal artery approximately follows the lateral border of the scapula to the inferior angle. It contributes to the vascular supply of the posterior and medial walls of the axilla.

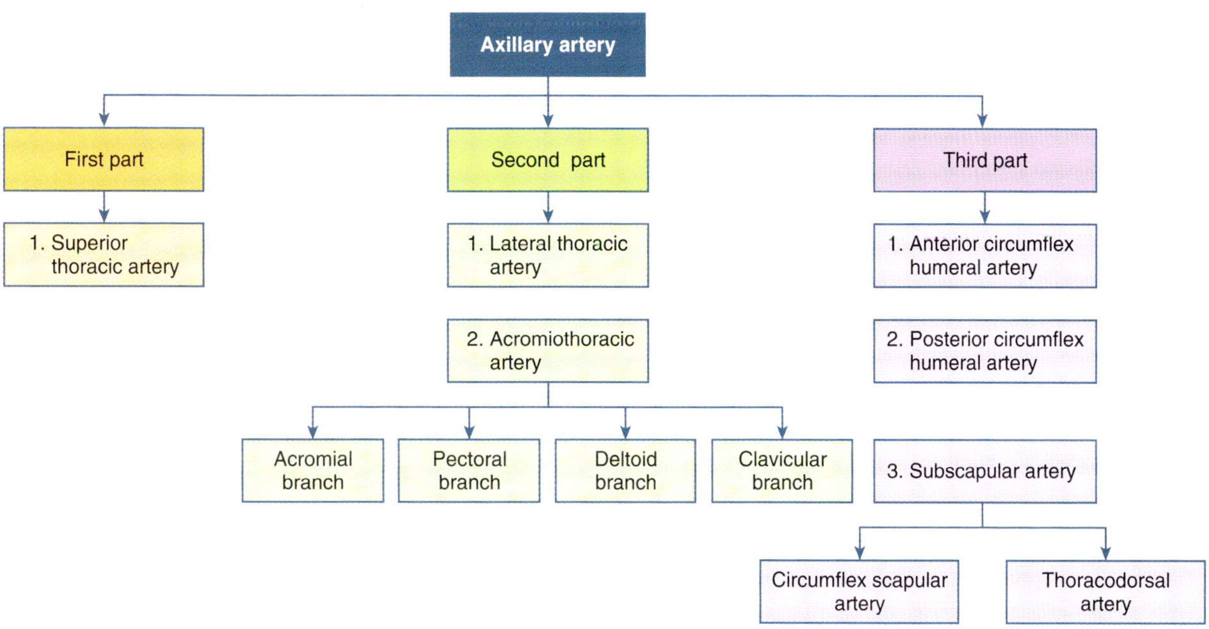

Flowchart 2.2 Branches of the axillary artery.

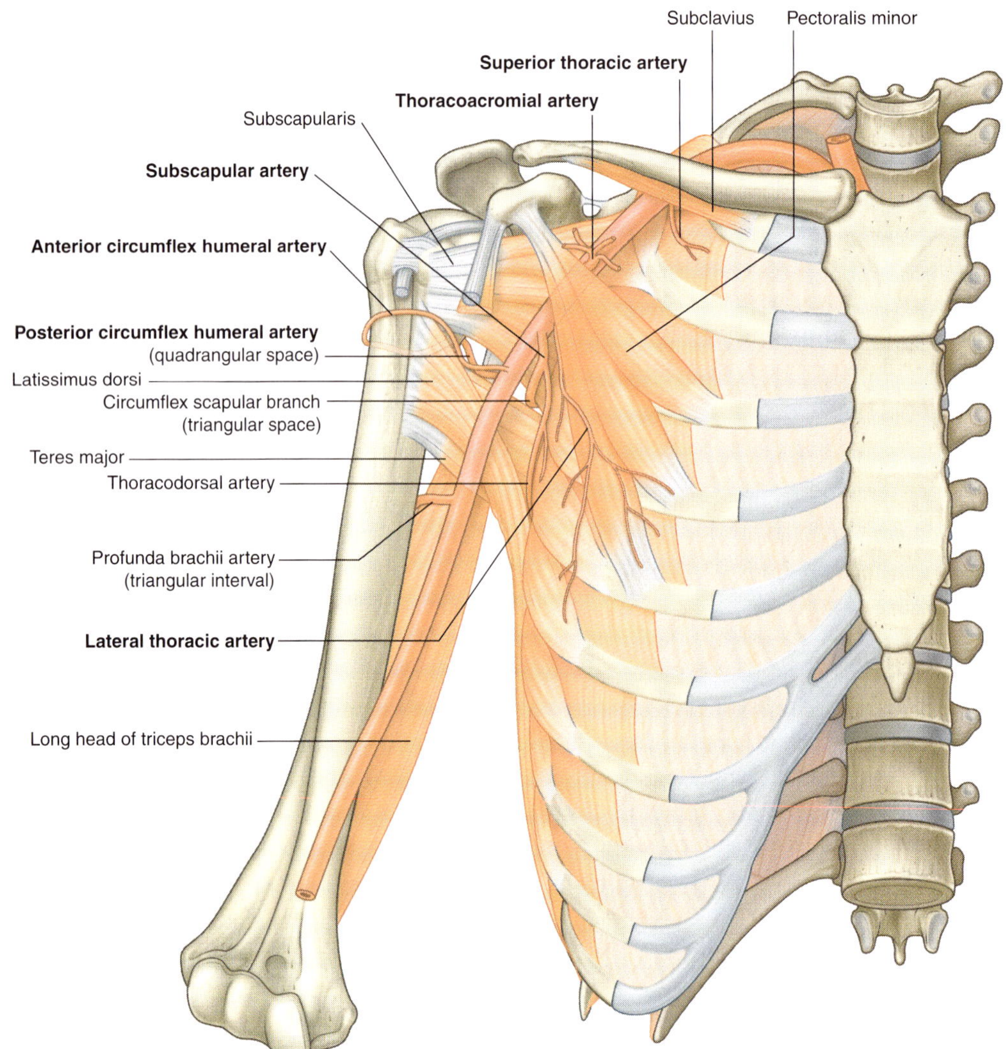

Fig. 2.50 Branches of the axillary artery.

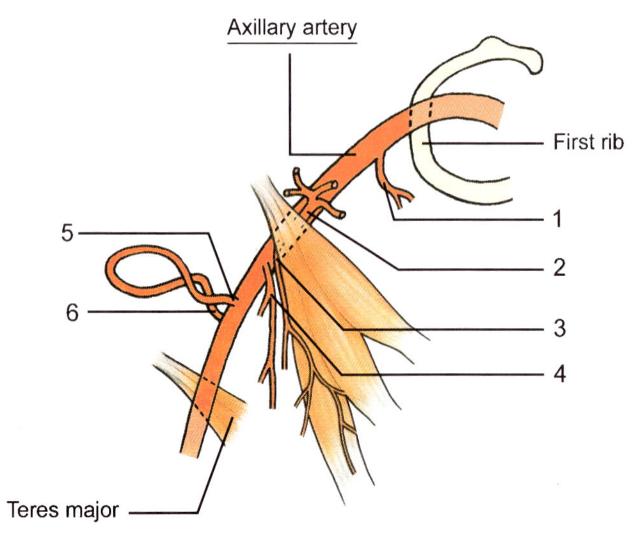

LD Fig. 2.50.1 Axillary artery.

Questions

2.50.1.A How and where does the axillary artery begin and end?

2.50.1.B Name the structures indicated by the labels.

2.50.1.C Mention a mnemonic for the number of branches of each part of the axillary artery, and a mnemonic for the names of these branches.

Answers

2.50.1.A The origin and termination of the axillary artery are

Origin: As a continuation of the subclavian artery at the outer border of the first rib

Termination: By continuing as the brachial artery at the lower border of the teres major

2.50.1.B The structures indicated by the labels are

1. Superior thoracic artery
2. Thoracoacromial artery
3. Lateral thoracic artery
4. Subscapular artery
5. Anterior circumflex humeral artery
6. Posterior circumflex humeral artery

2.50.1.C A mnemonic for the number of branches of each part of the axillary artery is: there is one branch from the first part, two branches from the second part, and three branches from the third part.

A mnemonic for the names of the branches of the axillary artery is: "Save The Lion, Set A Precedent," which stands for Superior thoracic, Thoracoacromial, Lateral thoracic, Subscapular, Anterior circumflex humeral, and Posterior circumflex humeral.

Anterior circumflex humeral artery

The **anterior circumflex humeral artery** is small compared to the posterior circumflex humeral artery, and originates from the lateral side of the third part of the axillary artery (Fig. 2.50). It passes anterior to the surgical neck of the humerus and anastomoses with the posterior circumflex humeral artery.

This anterior circumflex humeral artery supplies branches to surrounding tissues, which include the glenohumeral joint and the head of the humerus.

Posterior circumflex humeral artery

The **posterior circumflex humeral artery** originates from the lateral surface of the third part of the axillary artery immediately posterior to the origin of the anterior circumflex humeral artery (Fig. 2.50). With the axillary nerve, it leaves the axilla by passing through the quadrangular space between the teres major, teres minor, and long head of the triceps brachii muscle and the surgical neck of the humerus.

The posterior circumflex humeral artery curves around the surgical neck of the humerus and supplies the surrounding muscles and the glenohumeral joint. It anastomoses with the anterior circumflex humeral artery and with branches from the profunda brachii, suprascapular, and thoracoacromial arteries.

Axillary vein

The axillary vein begins at the lower margin of the teres major muscle and is the continuation of the basilic vein (Fig. 2.51), which is a superficial vein that drains the posteromedial surface of the hand and forearm and penetrates the deep fascia in the middle of the arm.

The axillary vein passes through the axilla medial and anterior to the axillary artery and becomes the subclavian vein as the vessel crosses the lateral border of rib I at the axillary inlet. Tributaries of the axillary vein generally follow the branches of the axillary artery. Other tributaries include brachial veins that follow the brachial artery, and the cephalic vein.

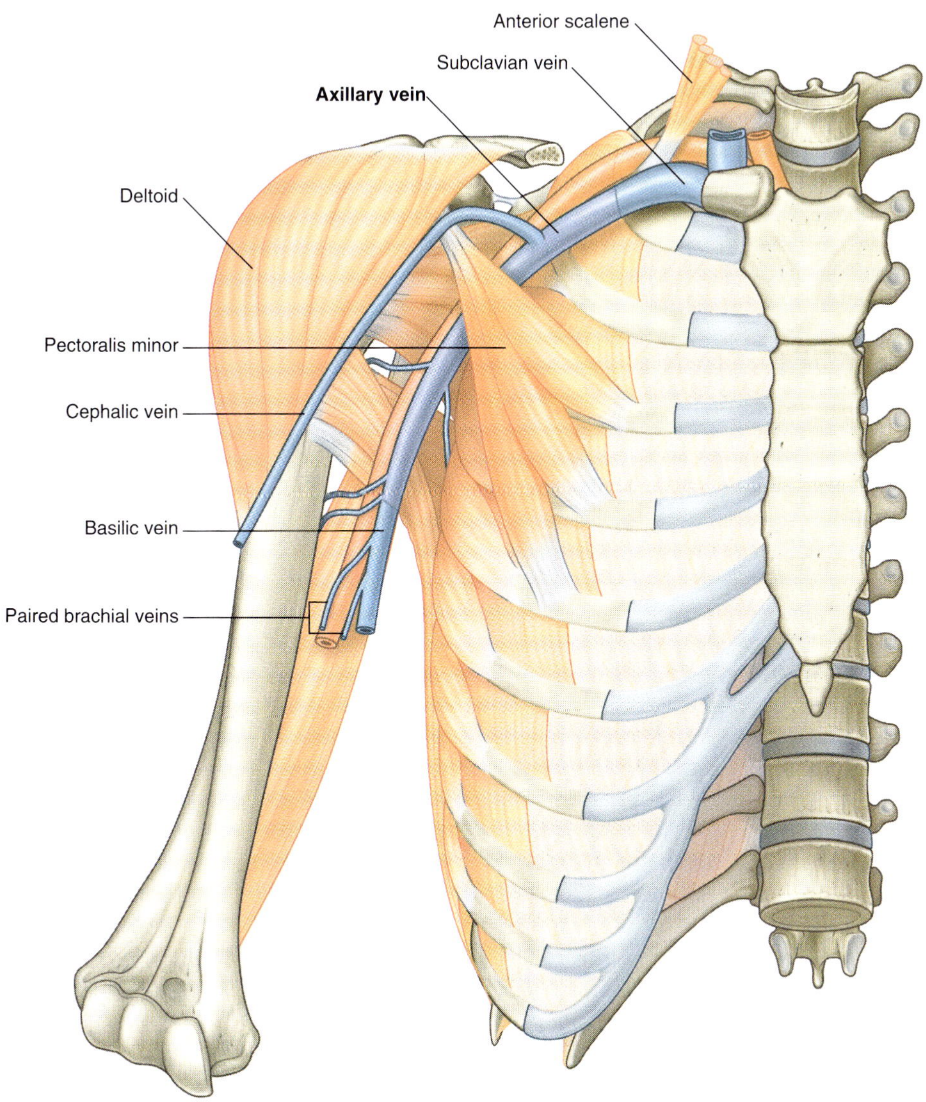

Fig. 2.51 Axillary vein.

The cephalic vein is a superficial vein that drains the lateral and posterior parts of the hand, the forearm, and the arm. In the area of the shoulder, it passes into an inverted triangular cleft (the clavipectoral triangle) between the deltoid muscle, pectoralis major muscle, and clavicle. In the superior part of the clavipectoral triangle, the cephalic vein passes deep to the clavicular head of the pectoralis major muscle and pierces the clavipectoral fascia to join the axillary vein. Many patients who are critically ill have lost blood or fluid, which requires replacement. Access to a peripheral vein is necessary to replace the fluid. The typical sites for venous access are the cephalic vein in the hand or veins that lie within the superficial tissues of the cubital fossa.

Early clinical exposure

Imaging the blood supply to the upper limb

When there is clinical evidence of vascular compromise to the upper limb, or vessels are needed to form an arteriovenous fistula (which is necessary for renal dialysis), imaging is required to assess the vessels.

Ultrasound is a useful tool for carrying out a noninvasive assessment of the vessels of the upper limb from the third part of the subclavian artery to the deep and superficial palmar arteries. Blood flow can be quantified and anatomical variants can be noted.

Angiography is carried out in certain cases. The femoral artery is punctured below the inguinal ligament and a long catheter is placed through the iliac arteries and around the arch of the aorta to enter either the left subclavian artery or the brachiocephalic trunk and then the right subclavian artery. Radiopaque contrast agents are injected into the vessel and radiographs are obtained as the contrast agents pass first through the arteries, then the capillaries, and finally the veins.

Early clinical exposure

Trauma to the arteries of the upper limb

The arterial supply to the upper limb is particularly susceptible to trauma in places where it is relatively fixed or in a subcutaneous position.

Fracture of rib I

As the subclavian artery passes out of the neck and into the axilla, it is fixed in position by the surrounding muscles to the superior surface of rib I. A rapid deceleration injury involving upper thoracic trauma may cause a first rib fracture, which may significantly compromise the distal part of the subclavian artery or the first part of the axillary artery. Fortunately, there are anastomotic connections between branches of the subclavian artery and the axillary artery, which form a network around the scapula and proximal end of the humerus; therefore, even with complete vessel transection, the arm is rarely rendered completely ischemic (ischemia is poor blood supply to an organ or a limb).

Anterior dislocation of the humeral head

Anterior dislocation of the humeral head may compress the axillary artery, resulting in vessel occlusion. This is unlikely to render the upper limb completely ischemic, but it may be necessary to surgically reconstruct the axillary artery to obtain pain-free function. Importantly, the axillary artery is intimately related to the brachial plexus, which may be damaged at the time of anterior dislocation.

Early clinical exposure

Subclavian/axillary venous access

There are a number of routes through which central venous access may be obtained. The "subclavian route" and the jugular routes are commonly used by clinicians. The subclavian route is a misnomer that remains the preferred term in clinical practice. In fact, most clinicians enter the first part of the axillary vein.

There are a number of patients who undergo catheterization of the subclavian vein/axillary vein. Entering the subclavian vein/axillary vein is a relatively straightforward technique. The clavicle is identified and a sharp needle is placed in the infraclavicular region, aiming superomedially. When venous blood is aspirated, access has been obtained. This route is popular for long-term venous access, such as Hickman lines, and for shorter-term access where multiple-lumen catheters are inserted (e.g., intensive care unit).

The subclavian vein/axillary vein is also the preferred site for insertion of pacemaker wires. There is, however, a preferred point of entry into the vein to prevent complications. The vein should be punctured in the midclavicular line or lateral to this line. The reason for this puncture site is the course of the vein and its relationship to other structures. The vein passes anterior to the artery, superior to the first rib, and inferior to the clavicle as it courses toward the thoracic inlet. Beneath the clavicle is situated the subclavius muscle. Should the puncture of the vein enter where the subclavius muscle is related to the axillary vein, the catheter or wire may become kinked at this point. Moreover, the constant contraction and relaxation of this muscle will induce fatigue in the line and wire, which may ultimately lead to fracture. A fractured pacemaker wire or a rupture in a chemotherapy catheter can have severe consequences for the patient.

Brachial plexus

The brachial plexus is a somatic nerve plexus formed by the **anterior rami** of C5 to C8, and most of the anterior ramus of T1 (Fig. 2.52). The plexus originates in the neck, passes laterally and inferiorly over rib I, and enters the axilla.

The parts of the brachial plexus, from medial to lateral, are roots, trunks, divisions, and cords. All major nerves that innervate the upper limb originate from the brachial plexus, mostly from the cords. Proximal parts of the brachial plexus are posterior to the subclavian artery in the neck, while more distal regions of the plexus surround the axillary artery.

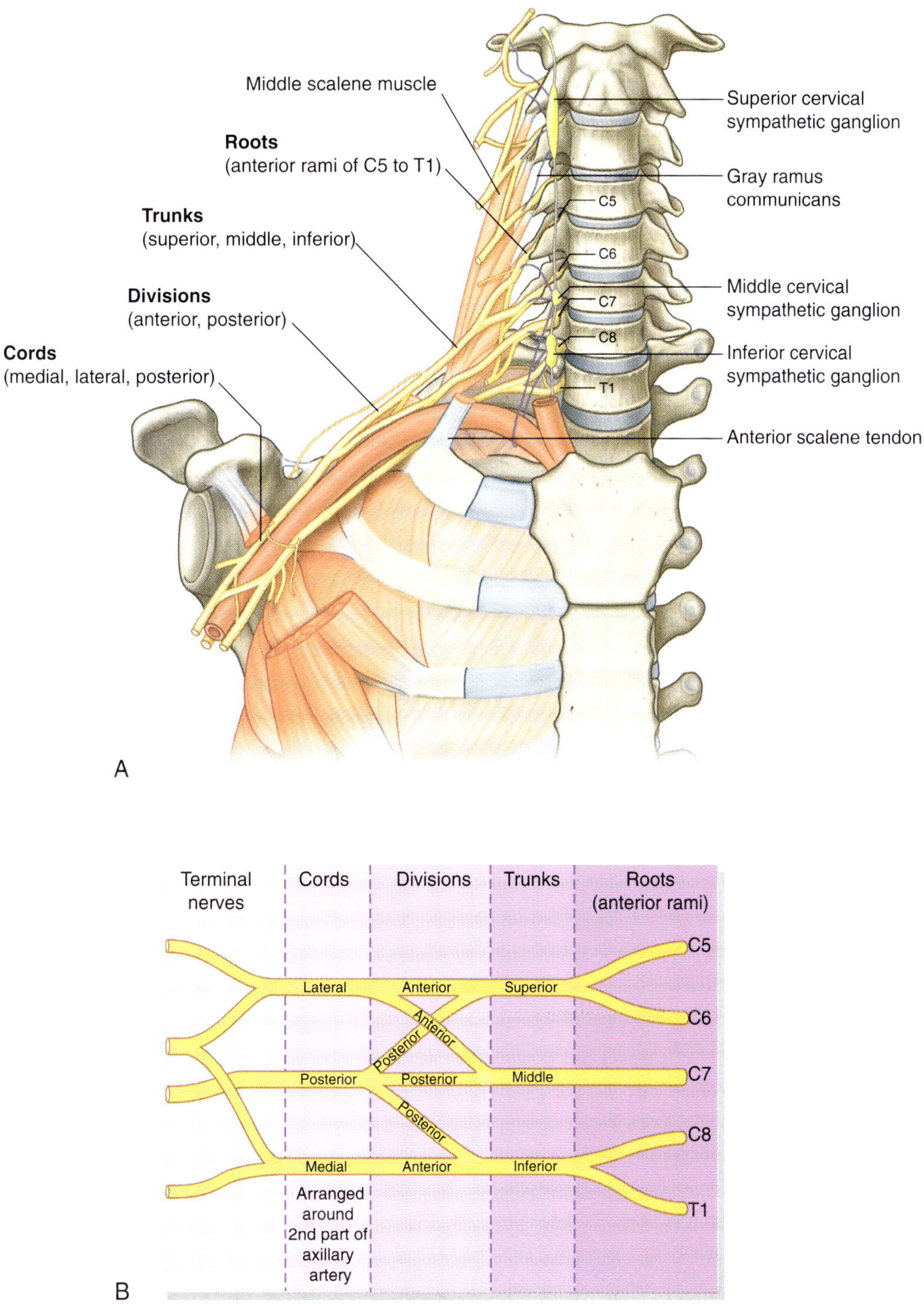

Fig. 2.52 Brachial plexus. **(A)** Major components in the neck and axilla. **(B)** Schematic showing parts of the brachial plexus.

Roots

The roots of the brachial plexus are the anterior rami of C5 to C8, and most of T1. Close to their origin, the roots receive **gray rami communicantes** from the sympathetic trunk (Fig. 2.52). These carry postganglionic sympathetic fibers onto the roots for distribution to the periphery. The roots and trunks enter the **posterior triangle** of the neck by passing between the anterior scalene and middle scalene muscles and lie superior and posterior to the subclavian artery.

Trunks

The three trunks of the brachial plexus originate from the roots, pass laterally over rib I, and enter the axilla (Fig. 2.52):

- The superior trunk is formed by the union of C5 and C6 roots.
- The middle trunk is a continuation of the C7 root.
- The inferior trunk is formed by the union of the C8 and T1 roots.

The inferior trunk lies on rib I posterior to the subclavian artery; the middle and superior trunks are more superior in position.

Divisions

Each of the three trunks of the brachial plexus divides into an **anterior** and a **posterior division** (Fig. 2.52):

- The three anterior divisions form parts of the brachial plexus that ultimately give rise to peripheral nerves associated with the anterior compartments of the arm and forearm.
- The three posterior divisions combine to form parts of the brachial plexus that give rise to nerves associated with the posterior compartments.

No peripheral nerves originate directly from the divisions of the brachial plexus.

Cords

The three cords of the brachial plexus originate from the divisions and are related to the second part of the axillary artery (Fig. 2.52):

- The **lateral cord** results from the union of the anterior divisions of the upper and middle trunks and therefore has contributions from C5 to C7—it is positioned lateral to the second part of the axillary artery.
- The **medial cord** is medial to the second part of the axillary artery and is the continuation of the anterior division of the inferior trunk—it contains contributions from C8 and T1.
- The **posterior cord** occurs posterior to the second part of the axillary artery and originates as the union of all three posterior divisions—it contains contributions from all roots of the brachial plexus (C5 to T1).

Most of the major peripheral nerves of the upper limb originate from the cords of the brachial plexus. Generally, nerves associated with the anterior compartments of the upper limb arise from the medial and lateral cords and nerves associated with the posterior compartments originate from the posterior cord.

Branches (Table 2.7)

Branches of the roots

In addition to small segmental branches from C5 to C8 to muscles of the neck and a contribution of C5 to the phrenic nerve, the roots of the brachial plexus give rise to the dorsal scapular and long thoracic nerves (Fig. 2.53).

The **dorsal scapular nerve**:

- Originates from the C5 root of the brachial plexus.
- Passes posteriorly, often piercing the middle scalene muscle in the neck, to reach and travel along the medial border of the scapula (Fig. 2.54).
- Innervates the rhomboid major and minor muscles from their deep surfaces.

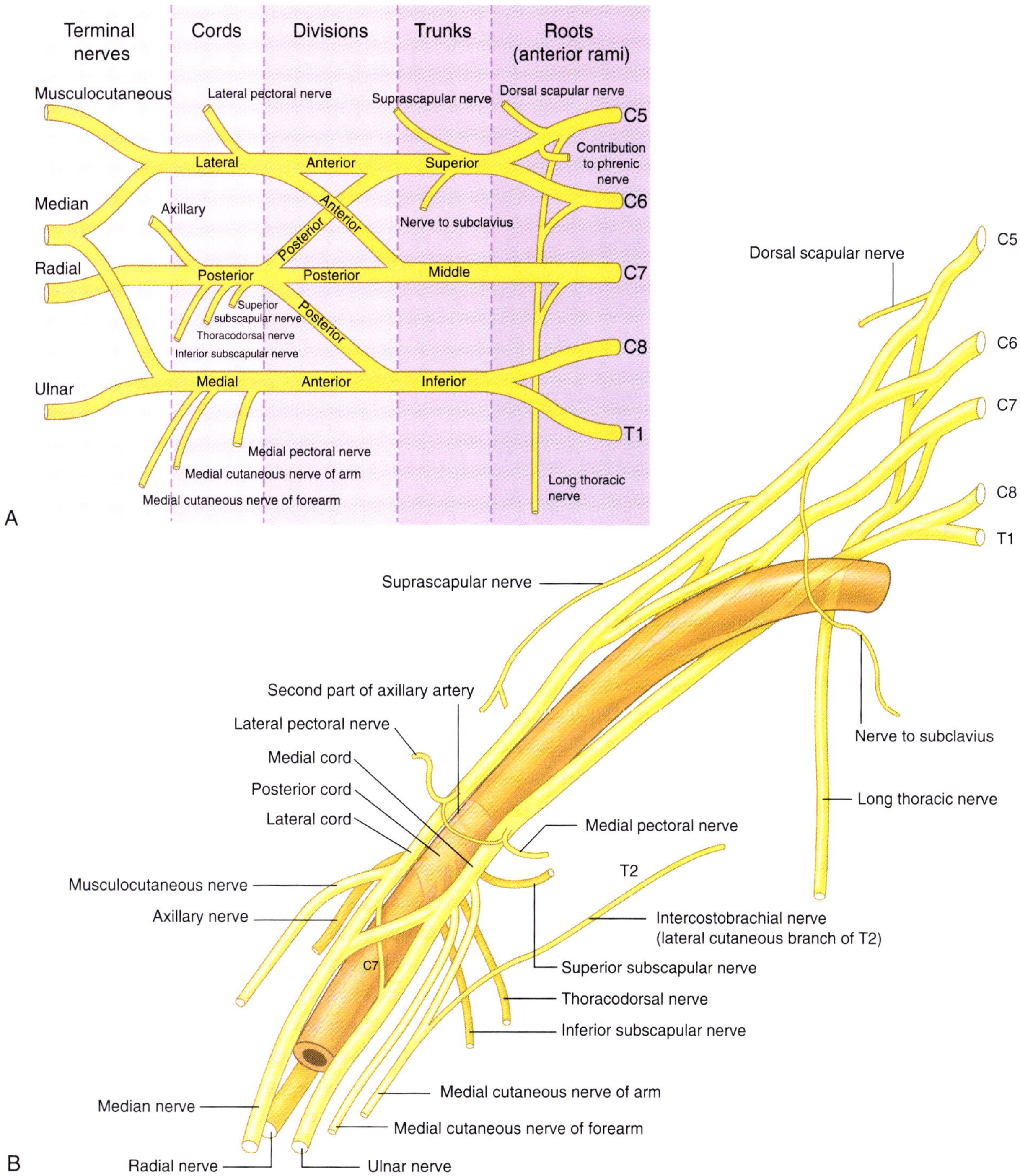

Fig. 2.53 Brachial plexus. **(A)** Schematic showing branches of the brachial plexus. **(B)** Relationships to the axillary artery.

The **long thoracic nerve**:

- Originates from the anterior rami of C5 to C7.
- Passes vertically down the neck, through the axillary inlet, and down the medial wall of the axilla to supply the serratus anterior muscle (Fig. 2.54).
- Lies on the superficial aspect of the serratus anterior muscle.

Branches of the trunks

The only branches from the trunks of the brachial plexus are two nerves that originate from the superior trunk (upper trunk): the suprascapular nerve and the nerve to the subclavius muscle (Fig. 2.53). The upper trunk is called Erb's point. A useful mnemonic is that this trunk is formed by two nerves, ends as two nerves, and has two branches.

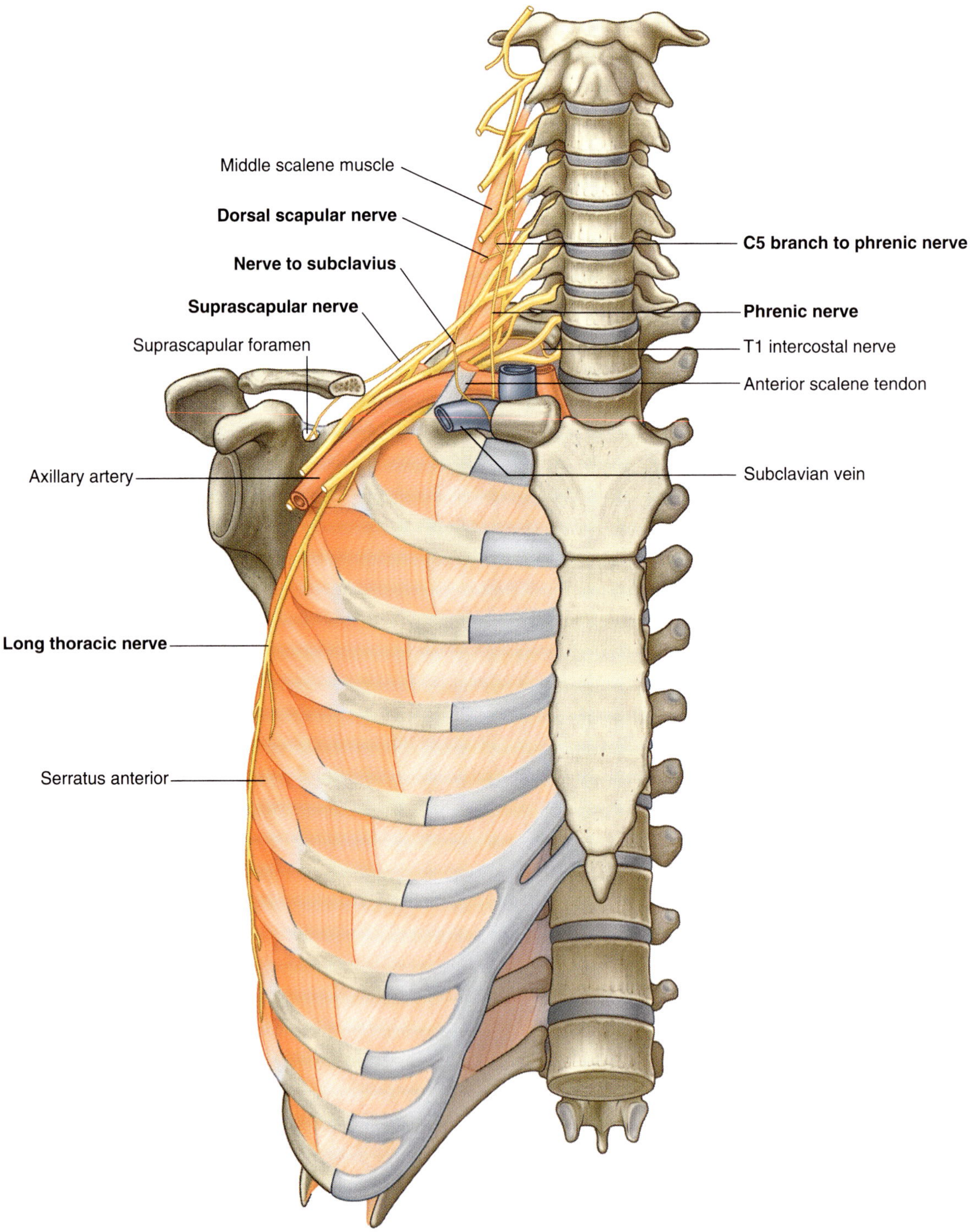

Fig. 2.54 Branches of the roots and trunks of the brachial plexus.

Table 2.7 Branches of brachial plexus

Branch		
Dorsal scapular Origin: C5 root Spinal segment: C5	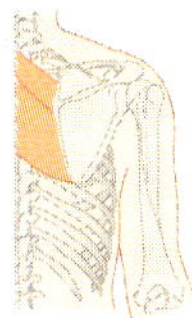	Function: motor Rhomboid major, rhomboid minor
Long thoracic Origin: C5 to C7 roots Spinal segments: C5 to C7	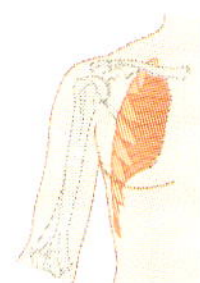	Function: motor Serratus anterior
Suprascapular Origin: superior trunk Spinal segments: C5, C6	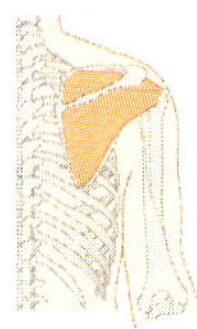	Function: motor Supraspinatus, infraspinatus
Nerve to subclavius Origin: superior trunk Spinal segments: C5, C6	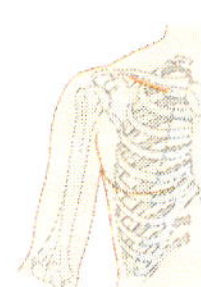	Function: motor Subclavius
Lateral pectoral Origin: lateral cord Spinal segments: C5 to C7	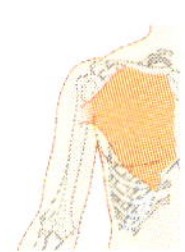	Function: motor Pectoralis major
Musculocutaneous Origin: lateral cord Spinal segments: C5 to C7	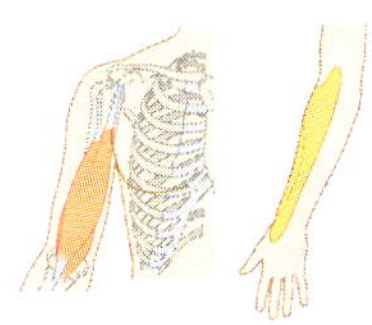	Function: motor All muscles in the anterior compartment of the arm Function: sensory Skin on lateral side of forearm
Medial pectoral Origin: medial cord Spinal segments: C8, T1 (also receives contributions from spinal segments C5 to C7 through a communication with the lateral pectoral nerve)	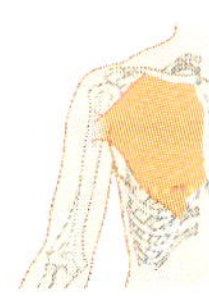	Function: motor Pectoralis major, pectoralis minor
Medial cutaneous of arm Origin: medial cord Spinal segments: C8, T1	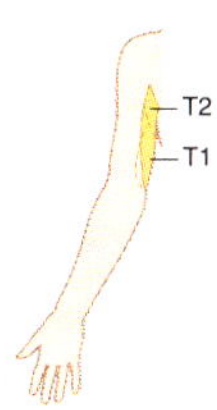	Function: sensory Skin on medial side of distal one-third of arm
Medial cutaneous of forearm Origin: medial cord Spinal segments: C8, T1	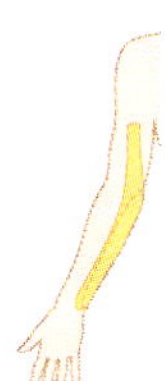	Function: sensory Skin on medial side of forearm

Continued

Table 2.7 Branches of brachial plexus—cont'd

Branch		
Median Origin: medial and lateral cords Spinal segments: (C5), C6 to T1	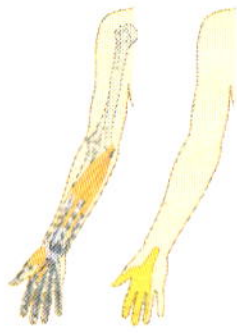	Function: motor All muscles in the anterior compartment of the forearm (except flexor carpi ulnaris and medial half of flexor digitorum profundus), three thenar muscles of the thumb, and two lateral lumbrical muscles Function: sensory Skin over the palmar surface of the lateral three and one-half digits and over the lateral side of the palm and middle of the wrist
Ulnar Origin: medial cord Spinal segments: (C7), C8, T1	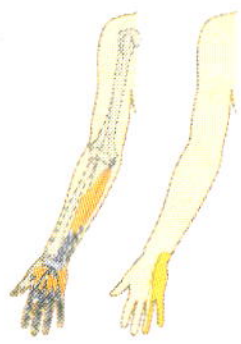	Function: motor All intrinsic muscles of the hand (except three thenar muscles and two lateral lumbricals); also flexor carpi ulnaris and the medial half of flexor digitorum profundus in the forearm Function: sensory Skin over the palmar surface of the medial one and one-half digits and associated palm and wrist, and skin over the dorsal surface of the medial one and one-half digits
Superior subscapular Origin: posterior cord Spinal segments: C5, C6	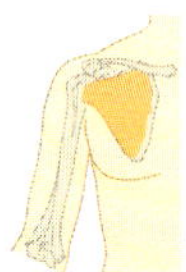	Function: motor Subscapularis
Thoracodorsal Origin: posterior cord Spinal segments: C6 to C8	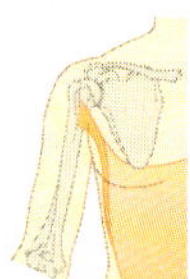	Function: motor Latissimus dorsi
Inferior subscapular Origin: posterior cord Spinal segments: C5, C6	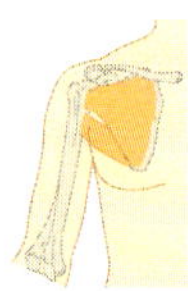	Function: motor Subscapularis, teres major
Axillary Origin: posterior cord Spinal segments: C5, C6	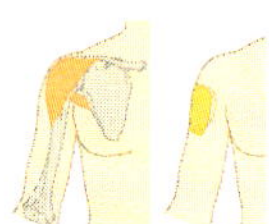	Function: motor Deltoid, teres minor Function: sensory Skin over upper lateral part of arm
Radial Origin: posterior cord Spinal segments: C5 to C8, (T1)	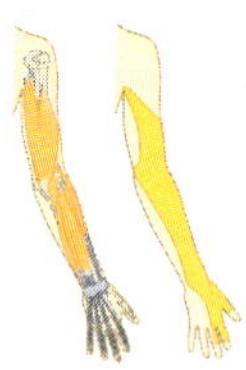	Function: motor All muscles in the posterior compartments of arm and forearm Function: sensory Skin on the posterior aspects of the arm and forearm, the lower lateral surface of the arm, and the dorsal lateral surface of the hand

Note: Parentheses indicate that a spinal segment is a minor component of the nerve or is inconsistently present in the nerve.

The **suprascapular nerve** (C5 and C6):

- Originates from the superior trunk of the brachial plexus.
- Passes laterally through the posterior triangle of the neck (Fig. 2.54) and through the suprascapular foramen to enter the posterior scapular region.
- Innervates the supraspinatus and infraspinatus muscles.
- Is accompanied in the lateral parts of the neck and in the posterior scapular region by the suprascapular artery.

The **nerve to the subclavius muscle** (C5 and C6) is a small nerve that:

- Originates from the superior trunk of the brachial plexus.
- Passes anteroinferiorly over the subclavian artery and vein.
- Innervates the subclavius muscle.

Branches of the lateral cord

Three nerves originate entirely or partly from the lateral cord (Fig. 2.53):

- The **lateral pectoral nerve** is the most proximal of the branches from the lateral cord. It passes anteriorly, together with the thoracoacromial artery, to penetrate the clavipectoral fascia that spans the gap between the subclavius and pectoralis minor muscles (Fig. 2.55), and innervates the pectoralis major muscle.
- The **musculocutaneous nerve** is a large terminal branch of the lateral cord. It passes laterally to penetrate the coracobrachialis muscle and pass between the biceps brachii and brachialis muscles in the arm, and innervates all three flexor muscles in the anterior compartment of the arm, terminating as the **lateral cutaneous nerve of the forearm**.
- The **lateral root of the median nerve** is the largest terminal branch of the lateral cord and passes medially to join a similar branch from the medial cord to form the median nerve (Fig. 2.55).

Branches of the medial cord

The medial cord has five branches (Fig. 2.55):

- The **medial pectoral nerve** is the most proximal branch. It receives a communicating branch from the lateral pectoral nerve which forms a loop called ansa pectoralis, and then passes anteriorly between the axillary artery and axillary vein. Branches of the nerve penetrate and supply the pectoralis minor muscle. Some of these branches pass through the muscle to reach and supply the pectoralis major muscle. Other branches occasionally pass around the inferior or lateral margin of the pectoralis minor muscle to reach the pectoralis major muscle.
- The **medial cutaneous nerve of the arm** (**medial brachial cutaneous nerve**) passes through the axilla and into the arm where it penetrates deep fascia and supplies skin over the medial side of the distal third of the arm. In the axilla, the nerve communicates with the **intercostobrachial nerve** of T2. Fibers of the medial cutaneous nerve of the arm innervate the upper part of the medial surface of the arm and floor of the axilla.
- The **medial cutaneous nerve of the forearm (medial antebrachial cutaneous nerve)** originates just distal to the origin of the medial cutaneous nerve of the arm. It passes out of the axilla and into the arm where it gives off a branch to the skin over the biceps brachii muscle, and then continues down the arm to penetrate the deep fascia with the basilic vein, continuing inferiorly to supply the skin over the anterior surface of the forearm. It innervates skin over the medial surface of the forearm down to the wrist.
- The **medial root of the median nerve** passes laterally to join with a similar root from the lateral cord to form the median nerve anterior to the third part of the axillary artery.
- The **ulnar nerve** is a large terminal branch of the medial cord (Fig. 2.55). However, near its origin, it often receives a communicating branch from the lateral root of the median nerve originating from the lateral cord and carrying fibers from C7. The ulnar nerve passes through the arm and forearm into the hand where it innervates all intrinsic muscles of the hand (except for the three thenar muscles and the two lateral lumbrical muscles). On passing through the forearm, branches of the ulnar nerve innervate the flexor carpi ulnaris muscle and the medial half of the flexor digitorum profundus muscle. The ulnar nerve innervates skin over the palmar surface of the little finger, medial half of the ring finger, and associated palm and wrist, and the skin over the dorsal surface of the medial part of the hand.

Median nerve. The median nerve is formed anterior to the third part of the axillary artery by the union of lateral and medial roots originating from the lateral and medial cords of the brachial plexus (Fig. 2.55). It passes into the arm anterior to the brachial artery and through the arm into the forearm, where branches innervate most of the muscles in the anterior compartment of the forearm (except for the flexor carpi ulnaris muscle and the medial half of the flexor digitorum profundus muscle, which are innervated by the ulnar nerve).

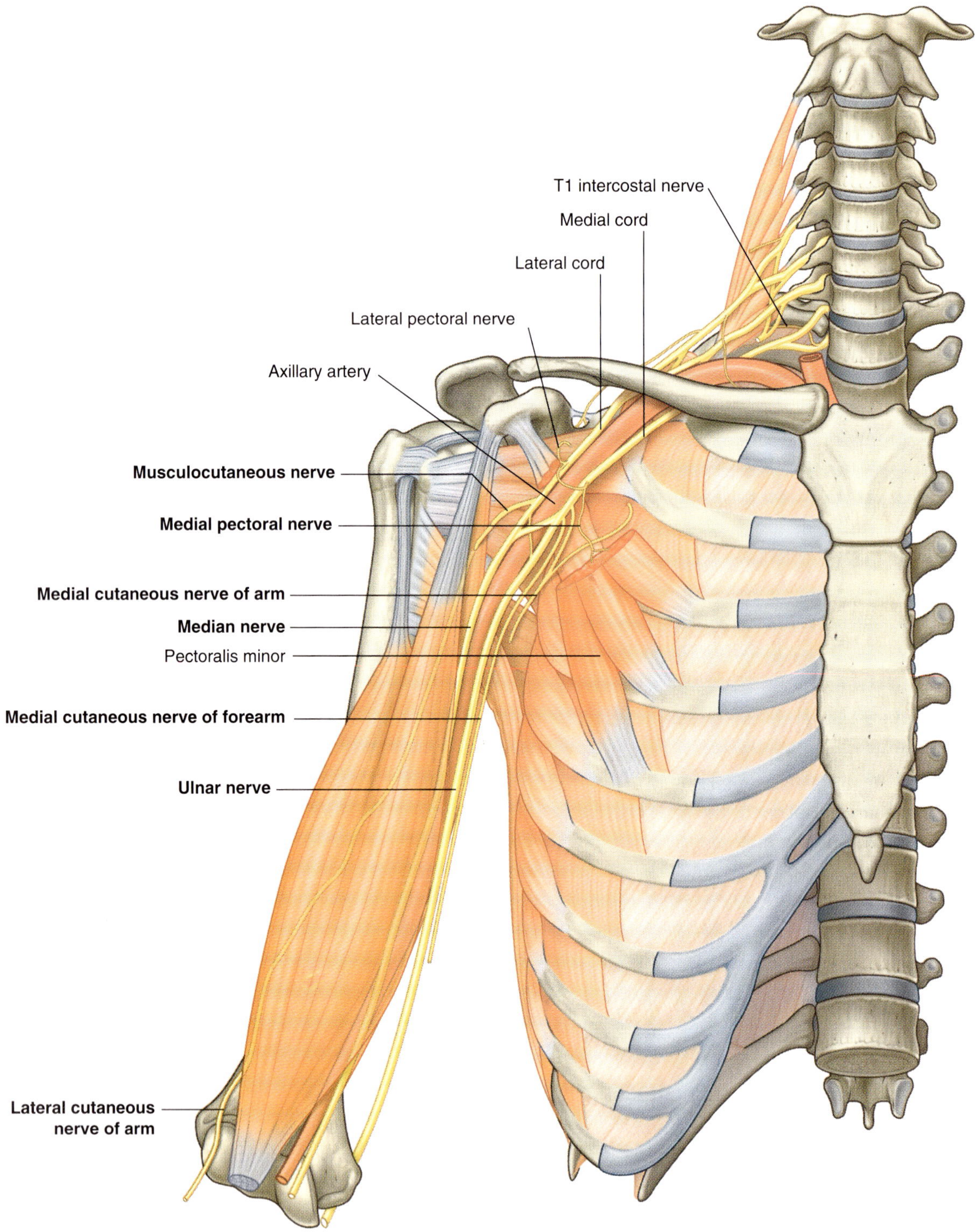

Fig. 2.55 Branches of the lateral and medial cords of the brachial plexus.

The median nerve continues into the hand to innervate:

- The three thenar muscles associated with the thumb
- The two lateral lumbrical muscles associated with movement of the index and middle fingers
- The skin over the palmar surface of the lateral three and one-half digits and over the lateral side of the palm and middle of the wrist

The musculocutaneous nerve, the lateral root of the median nerve, the median nerve, the medial root of the median nerve, and the ulnar nerve form an M over the third part of the axillary artery (Fig. 2.55). This feature, together with penetration of the coracobrachialis muscle by the musculocutaneous nerve, can be used to identify components of the brachial plexus in the axilla.

Branches of the posterior cord

Five nerves originate from the posterior cord of the brachial plexus:

- The superior subscapular nerve
- The thoracodorsal nerve
- The inferior subscapular nerve
- The axillary nerve
- The radial nerve (Fig. 2.53)

All these nerves except the radial nerve innervate muscles associated with shoulder region or the posterior wall of the axilla; the radial nerve passes into the arm and forearm.

The superior subscapular, thoracodorsal, and inferior subscapular nerves originate sequentially from the posterior cord and pass directly into muscles associated with the posterior axillary wall (Fig. 2.56). The **superior subscapular nerve** is short and passes into and supplies the subscapularis muscle. The **thoracodorsal nerve** is the longest of these three nerves and passes vertically along the posterior axillary wall. It penetrates and innervates the latissimus dorsi muscle. The **inferior subscapular nerve** also passes inferiorly along the posterior axillary wall and innervates the subscapularis and teres major muscles.

The **axillary nerve** originates from the posterior cord and passes inferiorly and laterally along the posterior wall to exit the axilla through the quadrangular space (Fig. 2.56). It passes posteriorly around the surgical neck of the humerus and innervates both the deltoid and teres minor muscles. A **superior lateral cutaneous nerve of the arm** originates from the axillary nerve after passing through the quadrangular space and loops around the posterior margin of the deltoid muscle to innervate skin in that region. The axillary nerve is accompanied by the posterior circumflex humeral artery.

The **radial nerve** is the largest terminal branch of the posterior cord (Fig. 2.56). It passes out of the axilla and into the posterior compartment of the arm by passing through the triangular interval between the inferior border of the teres major muscle, the long head of the triceps brachii muscle, and the shaft of the humerus. It is accompanied through the triangular interval by the profunda brachii artery, which originates from the brachial artery in the anterior compartment of the arm. The radial nerve and its branches innervate:

- All muscles in the posterior compartments of the arm and forearm
- The skin on the posterior aspect of the arm and forearm, the lower lateral surface of the arm, and the dorsal lateral surface of the hand

The **posterior cutaneous nerve of the arm** (**posterior brachial cutaneous nerve**) originates from the radial nerve in the axilla and innervates skin on the posterior surface of the arm.

Early clinical exposure

Injuries to the brachial plexus

The brachial plexus is an extremely complex structure. When damaged, it requires meticulous clinical history taking and examination. Assessment of the individual nerve functions can be obtained by nerve conduction studies and electromyography, which assess the latency of muscle contraction when the nerve is artificially stimulated.

Brachial plexus injuries are usually the result of blunt trauma producing nerve avulsions and disruption. These injuries are usually devastating for the function of the upper limb and require many months of dedicated rehabilitation for even a small amount of function to return.

Spinal cord injuries in the cervical region and direct pulling injuries tend to affect the roots of the brachial plexus. Severe trauma to the first rib usually affects the trunks. The divisions and cords of the brachial plexus can be injured by dislocation of the glenohumeral joint.

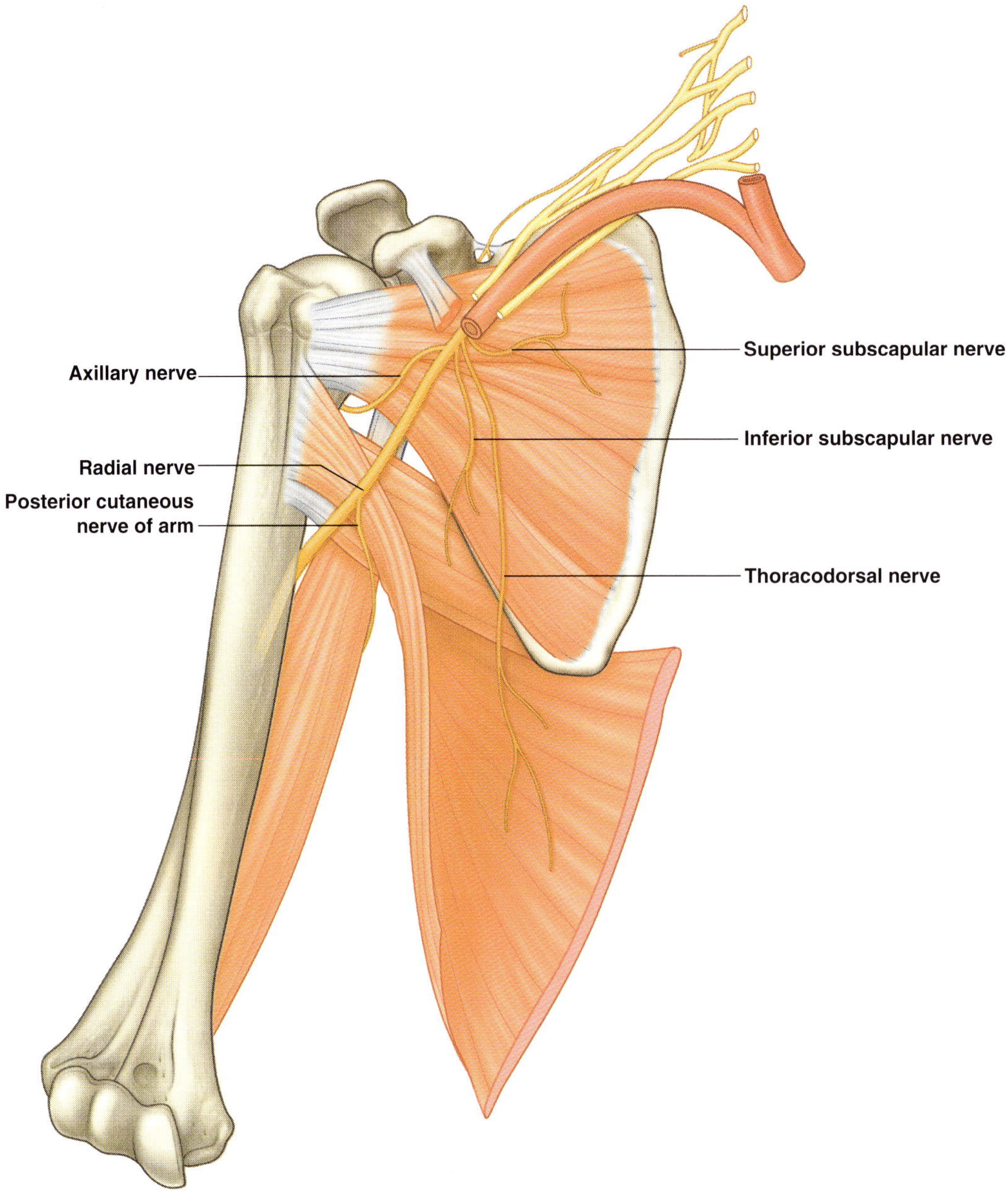

Fig. 2.56 Branches of the posterior cord of the brachial plexus.

Early clinical exposure

Erb's and Klumpke's paralysis

Injury to the superior trunk of the brachial plexus results in Erb's paralysis, where the C5 and C6 roots, suprascapular nerve, and nerve to subclavius along with the anterior and posterior divisions are involved. The resultant deformity is policeman's tip or waiter's tip deformity in which the arm is adducted and medially rotated, elbow extended with the forearm pronated.

Injury to the inferior trunk of the brachial plexus results in Klumpke's paralysis, where the C8 and T1 roots are involved. The resultant deformity is a claw hand. Claw hand refers to hyperextension at metacarpophalangeal joints and flexion at interphalangeal joints. Klumpke's paralysis may be associated with Horner's syndrome.

Nontraumatic lesion

One rare nontraumatic cause of a brachial plexus lesion is idiopathic brachial plexus neuritis.

Lymphatics

All lymphatics from the upper limb drain into lymph nodes in the axilla (Fig. 2.57).

In addition, axillary nodes receive drainage from an extensive area on the adjacent trunk, which includes regions of the upper back and shoulder, the lower neck, the chest, and the upper anterolateral abdominal wall. Axillary nodes also receive drainage from approximately 75% of the mammary gland.

The 20–30 axillary nodes are generally divided into 5 groups on the basis of location:

- **Humeral (lateral) nodes** posteromedial to the axillary vein receive most of the lymphatic drainage from the upper limb.
- **Pectoral (anterior) nodes** occur along the inferior margin of the pectoralis minor muscle along the course of the lateral thoracic vessels and receive drainage from the abdominal wall, the chest, and the mammary gland.

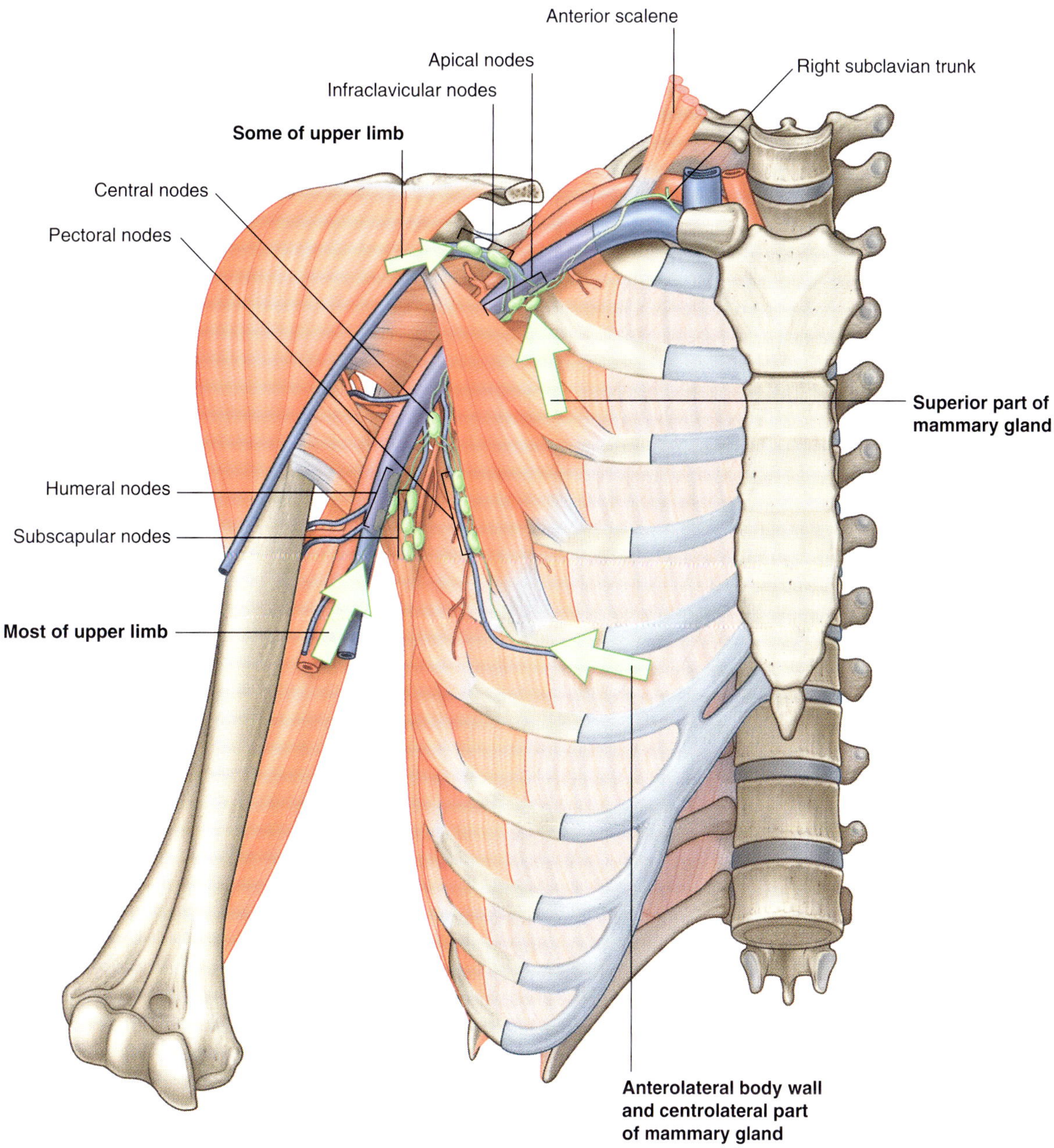

Fig. 2.57 Lymph nodes and vessels in the axilla.

- **Subscapular (posterior) nodes** on the posterior axillary wall in association with the subscapular vessels drain the posterior axillary wall and receive lymphatics from the back, the shoulder, and the neck.
- **Central nodes** are embedded in axillary fat and receive tributaries from humeral, subscapular, and pectoral groups of nodes.
- **Apical nodes** are the most superior group of nodes in the axilla and drain all other groups of nodes in the region. In addition, they receive lymphatic vessels that accompany the cephalic vein as well as vessels that drain the superior region of the mammary gland.

Efferent vessels from the apical group converge to form the subclavian trunk, which usually joins the venous system at the junction between the right subclavian vein and the right internal jugular vein in the neck. On the left, the subclavian trunk usually joins the thoracic duct in the base of the neck.

Early clinical exposure

Breast cancer

Lymphatic drainage from the lateral part of the breast passes through nodes in the axilla. Significant disruption to the normal lymphatic drainage of the upper limb may occur if a mastectomy or a surgical axillary nodal clearance has been carried out for breast cancer. Furthermore, some patients have radiotherapy to the axilla to prevent the spread of metastatic disease, but a side effect of this is the destruction of the tiny lymphatics as well as the cancer cells.

If the lymphatic drainage of the upper limb is damaged, the arm may swell and pitting edema (lymphedema) may develop.

Breast cancer may involve the axillary tail, which may appear like an enlarged axillary lymph node.

The surgical classification of axillary nodes is in three levels, based on their relation to the pectoralis minor muscle: Level 1 refers to nodes located lateral to the pectoralis minor, Level 2 refers to nodes deep to the pectoralis minor, and Level 3 refers to nodes located medial to pectoralis minor.

Axillary process of the mammary gland

Although the mammary gland is in superficial fascia overlying the thoracic wall, its superolateral region extends along the inferior margin of the pectoralis major muscle toward the axilla. In some cases, this may pass around the margin of the muscle to penetrate deep fascia at the foramen of Langer, and enter the axilla (Fig. 2.58). This axillary process, or axillary tail (of Spence), rarely reaches as high as the apex of the axilla.

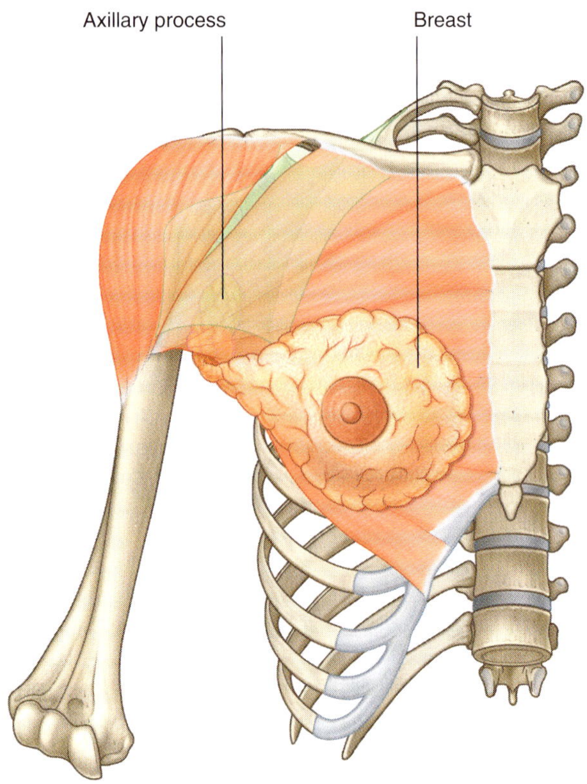

Fig. 2.58 Axillary process of the breast.

ARM

SET INDUCTION—CASE SCENARIO 3: INJURY TO THE ARM

A 25-year-old man was brought by the police after he was involved in a gun fight and was struck by a bullet in the midarm. On examination, severe bleeding and paralysis of muscles of the forearm were noticed, with ape thumb deformity and a feeble radial pulse. He was diagnosed to have brachial artery laceration and median nerve injury.

The relation of nerves and vessels of the anterior compartment of the arm is crucial to come to a diagnosis regarding the affected nerves and vessels in an injury and also to rule out the involvement of other structures.

<table>
<tr><th rowspan="2">REMEMBER
[Recall Facts]</th><th colspan="3">OUTLINE 3. ARM AND CUBITAL FOSSA—LEARNING OBJECTIVES
[By the end of this section, the student should be able to:]</th><th colspan="2" rowspan="2">EVALUATE
[Explain Concepts]</th></tr>
<tr><th colspan="3">DEMONSTRATE AND ANALYZE RELATIONSHIPS
[Identify structures in a Prosected Specimen or Figure]</th></tr>
<tr><td rowspan="6">1. Mention and understand the skeletal support of the arm and the cubital fossa
2. Describe the muscles of the anterior compartment and posterior compartment of the arm with their origin, insertion, actions, and nerve supply
3. Describe the course and branches of the brachial artery
4. Enumerate the muscles of the posterior scapular region
5. Describe the course and distribution of the musculocutaneous nerve
6. Describe the elbow joint in detail
7. Describe in detail the boundaries and contents of the cubital fossa</td><td>Level I</td><td>Level II</td><td>Level III</td><td colspan="2" rowspan="2">■ Division of the arm into compartments
■ Actions of the muscles in this region
■ Relations of the brachial artery and median nerve
■ Course and relations of the musculocutaneous nerve
■ Relationship of structures in the cubital fossa
■ Three heads of triceps
■ Radial nerve in the radial groove</td></tr>
<tr><td rowspan="5">■ Biceps brachii (both heads)
■ Coracobrachialis
■ Brachial artery
■ Median nerve
■ Ulnar nerve
■ Brachialis
■ Musculocutaneous nerve
■ Brachioradialis
■ Extensor carpi radialis longus
■ Triceps
■ Radial nerve
■ Pronator teres
■ Brachialis
■ Supinator
■ Tendon of biceps brachii
■ Median nerve
■ Brachial artery
■ Radial artery
■ Ulnar artery
■ Median cubital vein</td><td rowspan="5">■ Medial cutaneous. Nerves of arm and forearm
■ Branches of the brachial artery in the arm
■ Lateral cutaneous nerve of forearm
■ Bicipital aponeurosis</td><td rowspan="5">■ Branches of the radial nerve in this region</td></tr>
<tr><th colspan="2">EARLY CLINICAL EXPOSURE
[Apply Anatomical Knowledge]</th></tr>
<tr><th>Surgical Anatomy/ Pathology/ Trauma</th><th>Imaging/ Surface Anatomy</th></tr>
<tr><td>■ Rupture of tendon of long head of biceps
■ Auscultatory method of taking blood pressure
■ Venipuncture—median cubital vein
■ Radial nerve and median nerve injury in arm
■ Supracondylar fracture of humerus
■ Pulled elbow
■ Fracture head of radius
■ Tennis elbow and golfer's elbow
■ Elbow arthritis
■ Ulnar nerve injury at elbow
■ Creation of a dialysis fistula</td><td>■ Palpation of brachial artery</td></tr>
<tr><td colspan="2">PROBLEM SOLVING/ CLINICAL CASES
[Interpret]
■ Supracondylar fracture</td></tr>
</table>

The arm is the region of the upper limb between the shoulder and the elbow (Fig. 2.59). The superior aspect of the arm communicates medially with the axilla. Inferiorly, a number of important structures pass between the arm and the forearm through the cubital fossa, which is positioned anterior to the elbow joint.

The arm is divided into two compartments by medial and lateral intermuscular septa, which pass from each side of the humerus to the outer sleeve of deep fascia that surrounds the limb (Fig. 2.59).

The anterior compartment of the arm contains muscles that predominantly flex the elbow joint; the posterior compartment contains muscles that extend the joint. Major nerves and vessels supply and pass through each compartment.

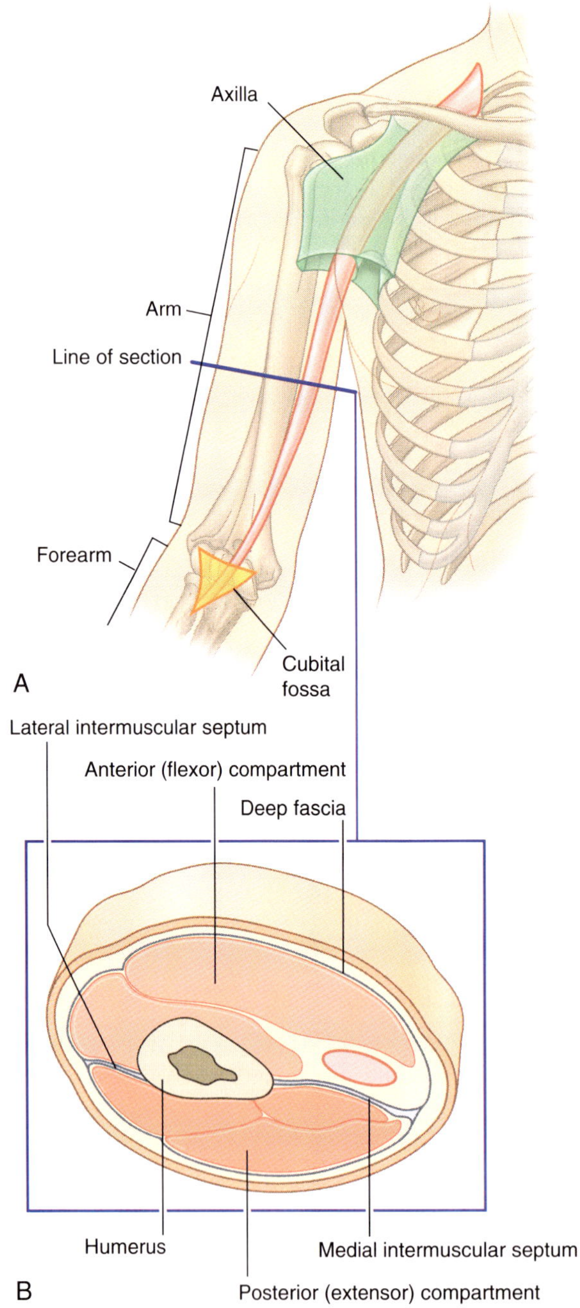

Fig. 2.59 Arm. **(A)** Proximal and distal relationships. **(B)** Transverse section through the middle of the arm.

Bones

The skeletal support for the arm is the humerus (Fig. 2.60). Most of the large muscles of the arm insert into the proximal ends of the two bones of the forearm, the radius and the ulna, and flex and extend the forearm at the elbow joint. In addition, the muscles predominantly situated in the forearm that move the hand originate at the distal end of the humerus.

Shaft and distal end of the humerus

In cross-section, the shaft of the humerus is somewhat triangular with:

- **Anterior, lateral,** and **medial borders**
- **Anterolateral, anteromedial**, and **posterior** surfaces (Fig. 2.60)

The posterior surface of the humerus is marked on its superior aspect by a linear roughening for the attachment of the lateral head of the triceps brachii muscle, beginning just inferior to the surgical neck and passing diagonally across the bone to the **deltoid tuberosity**.

The middle part of the posterior surface and adjacent part of the anterolateral surface are marked by the shallow **radial groove**, which passes diagonally down the bone and parallel to the sloping posterior margin of the deltoid tuberosity. The radial nerve and the profunda brachii artery lie in this groove.

Approximately in the middle of the shaft, the medial border is marked by thin elongate roughening for the attachment of the coracobrachialis muscle.

Intermuscular septa, which separate the anterior compartment from the posterior compartment, attach to the medial and lateral borders (Fig. 2.61).

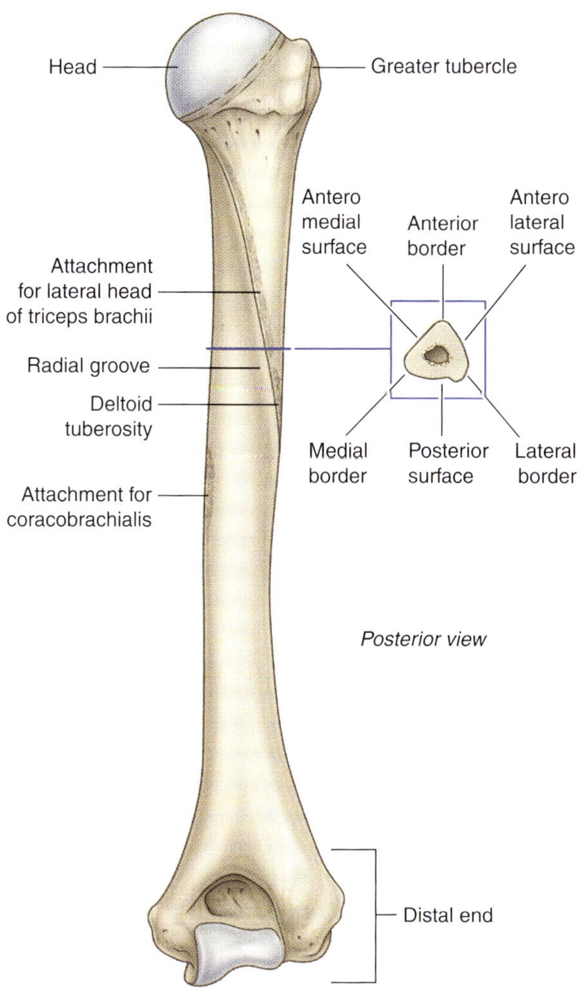

Fig. 2.60 Humerus: posterior view.

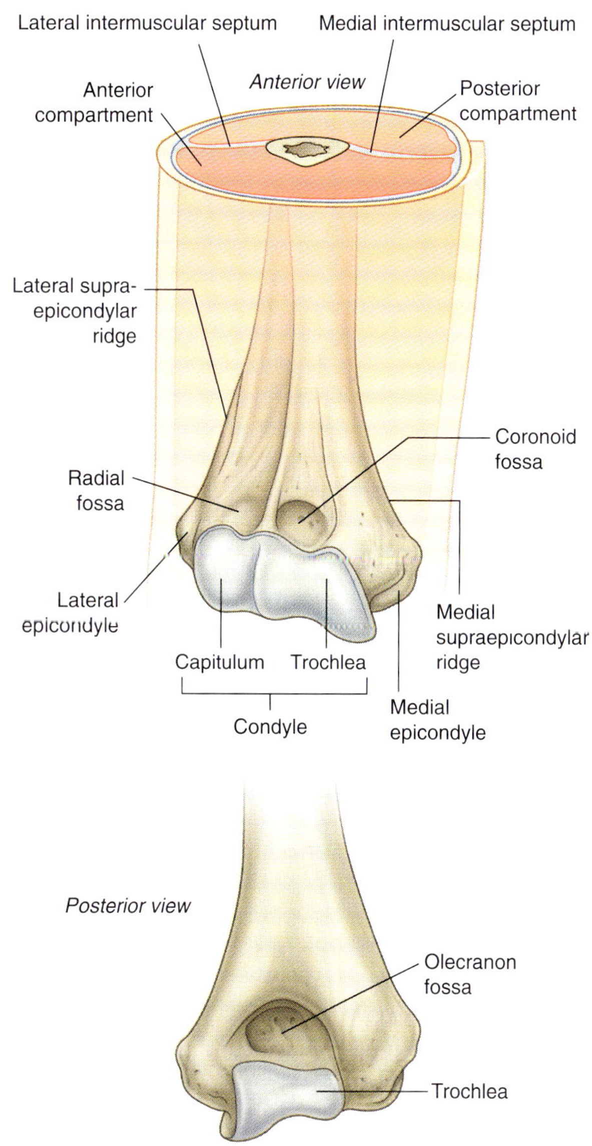

Fig. 2.61 Distal end of the humerus.

Distally, the bone becomes flattened, and these borders expand as the **lateral supraepicondylar ridge** (**lateral supracondylar ridge**) and the **medial supraepicondylar ridge** (**medial supracondylar ridge**). The lateral supraepicondylar ridge is more pronounced than the medial ridge and is roughened for the attachment of muscles found in the posterior compartment of the forearm.

The distal end of the humerus, which is flattened in the anteroposterior plane, bears a condyle, two epicondyles, and three fossae, as follows (Fig. 2.61).

The condyle

The two articular parts of the condyle, the **capitulum** and the **trochlea**, articulate with the two bones of the forearm.

The **capitulum** articulates with the radius of the forearm. Lateral in position and hemispherical in shape, it projects anteriorly and somewhat inferiorly and is not visible when the humerus is viewed from the posterior aspect.

The **trochlea** articulates with the ulna of the forearm. It is pulley shaped and lies medial to the capitulum. Its medial edge is more pronounced than its lateral edge and, unlike the capitulum, it extends onto the posterior surface of the bone.

The two epicondyles

The two epicondyles lie adjacent, and somewhat superior, to the trochlea and capitulum (Fig. 2.61).

The medial epicondyle, a large bony protuberance, is the major palpable landmark on the medial side of the elbow, and projects medially from the distal end of the humerus. On its surface, it bears a large oval impression for the attachment of muscles in the anterior compartment of the forearm. The ulnar nerve passes from the arm into the forearm around the posterior surface of the medial epicondyle and can be palpated against the bone in this location.

The **lateral epicondyle** is much less pronounced than the medial epicondyle. It is lateral to the capitulum and has a large irregular impression for the attachment of muscles in the posterior compartment of the forearm.

The three fossae

Three fossae occur superior to the trochlea and capitulum on the distal end of the humerus (Fig. 2.61).

The **radial fossa** is the least distinct of the fossae and occurs immediately superior to the capitulum on the anterior surface of the humerus.

The **coronoid fossa** is adjacent to the radial fossa and is superior to the trochlea.

The largest of the fossae, the **olecranon fossa**, occurs immediately superior to the trochlea on the posterior surface of the distal end of the humerus.

These three fossae accommodate projections from the bones in the forearm during movements of the elbow joint.

Proximal end of the radius

The proximal end of the radius consists of a head, a neck, and the radial tuberosity (Fig. 2.62A and B).

The **head** of the radius is a thick disc-shaped structure oriented in the horizontal plane. The circular superior surface is concave for articulation with the capitulum of the humerus. The thick margin of the disc is broad medially where it articulates with the radial notch on the proximal end of the ulna.

The **neck** of the radius is a short and narrow cylinder of bone between the expanded head and the radial tuberosity on the shaft.

The **radial tuberosity** is a large blunt projection on the medial surface of the radius immediately inferior to the neck. Much of its surface is roughened for the attachment of the biceps brachii tendon. The oblique line of the radius continues diagonally across the shaft of the bone from the inferior margin of the radial tuberosity.

Proximal end of the ulna

The proximal end of the ulna is much larger than the proximal end of the radius and consists of the olecranon, the coronoid process, the trochlear notch, the radial notch, and the tuberosity of the ulna (Fig. 2.63A and B).

The **olecranon** is a large projection of bone that extends proximally from the ulna. Its anterolateral surface is articular and contributes to the formation of the trochlear notch, which articulates with the trochlea of the humerus. The superior surface is marked by a large roughened impression for the attachment of the triceps brachii muscle. The posterior surface is smooth, shaped somewhat triangularly, and can be palpated as the "tip of the elbow."

The **coronoid process** projects anteriorly from the proximal end of the ulna (Fig. 2.63). Its superolateral surface is articular and participates, with the olecranon, in forming the **trochlear notch**. The lateral surface is marked by the **radial notch** for articulation with the head of the radius.

Just inferior to the radial notch is a fossa that allows the radial tuberosity to change position during pronation and supination. The posterior margin of this fossa is broadened to form the **supinator crest**. The anterior surface of the coronoid process is triangular, with the apex directed distally, and has a number of roughenings for muscle attachment. The largest of these roughenings, the **tuberosity of the ulna**, is at the apex of the anterior surface and is the attachment site for the brachialis muscle.

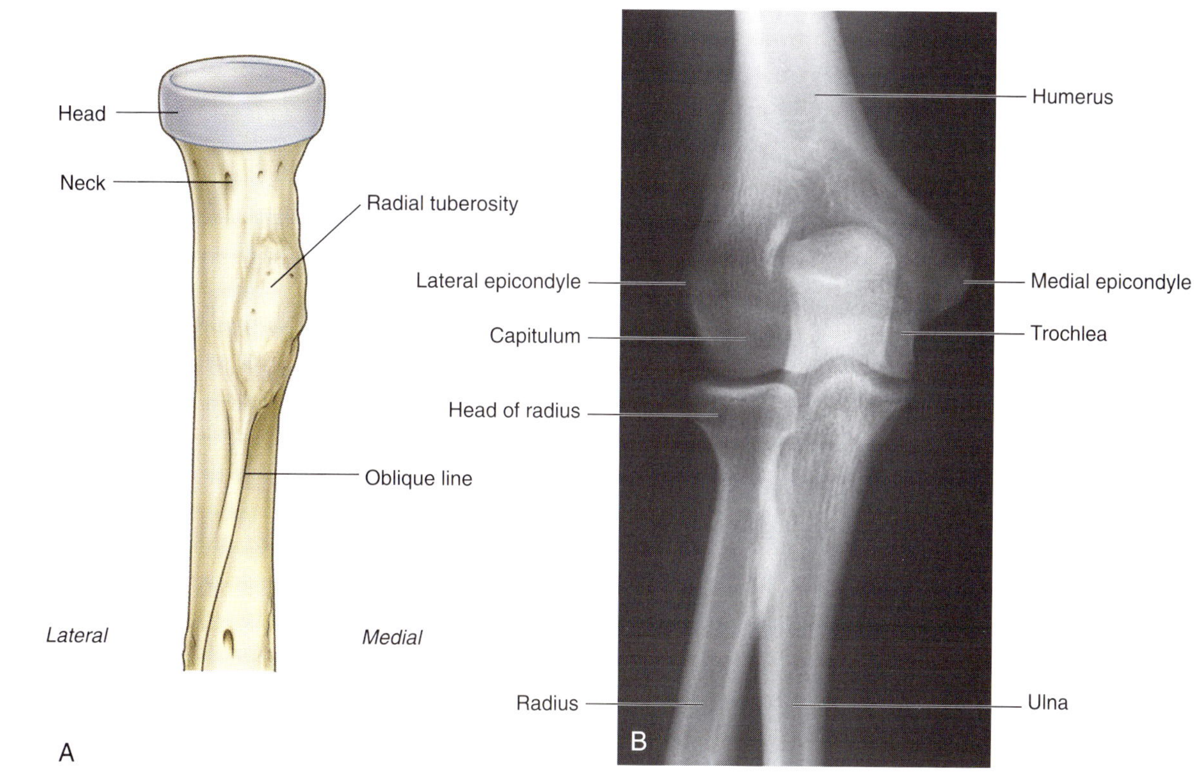

Fig. 2.62 (A) Anterior view of the proximal end of the radius. **(B)** Radiograph of the elbow joint (anteroposterior view).

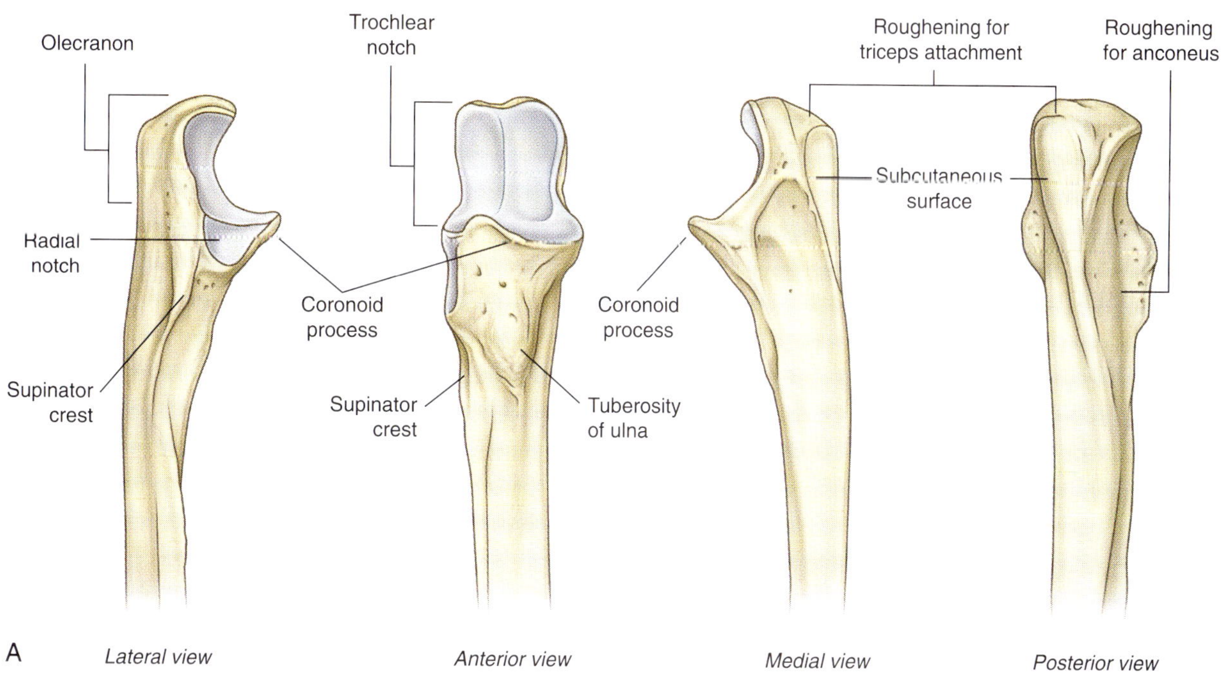

Fig. 2.63 (A) Lateral, anterior, medial, and posterior views of the proximal end of the ulna.

Continued

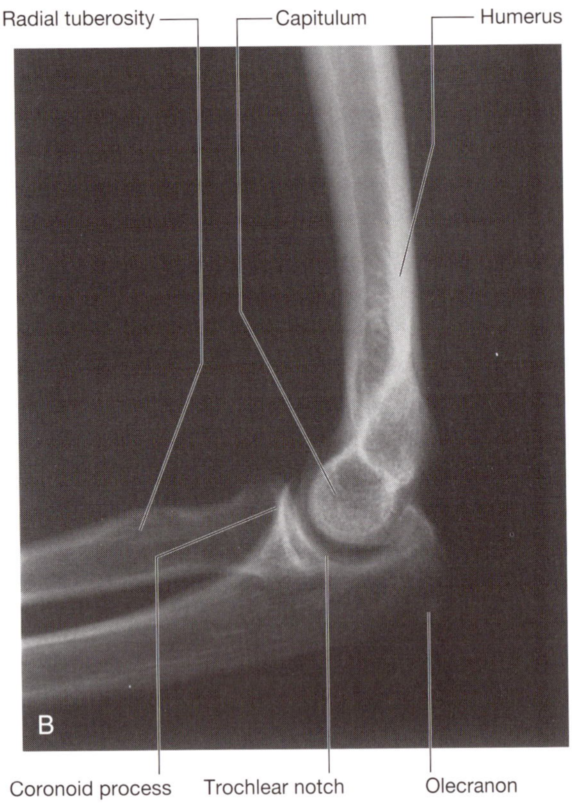

Fig. 2.63, cont'd (B) Radiograph of the elbow joint (lateral view).

Muscles

The anterior compartment of the arm contains three muscles—the coracobrachialis, brachialis, and biceps brachii muscles—which are innervated predominantly by the musculocutaneous nerve.

The posterior compartment contains one muscle—the triceps brachii muscle—which is innervated by the radial nerve.

Coracobrachialis

The **coracobrachialis muscle** extends from the tip of the coracoid process of the scapula to the medial side of the midshaft of the humerus (Fig. 2.64A and Table 2.8). It passes through the axilla and is penetrated and innervated by the musculocutaneous nerve.

The coracobrachialis muscle flexes the arm.

Biceps brachii

The **biceps brachii** muscle has two heads:

- The short head of the muscle originates from the coracoid process in conjunction with the coracobrachialis.
- The long head originates as a tendon from the supraglenoid tubercle of the scapula (Fig. 2.64A and Table 2.8).

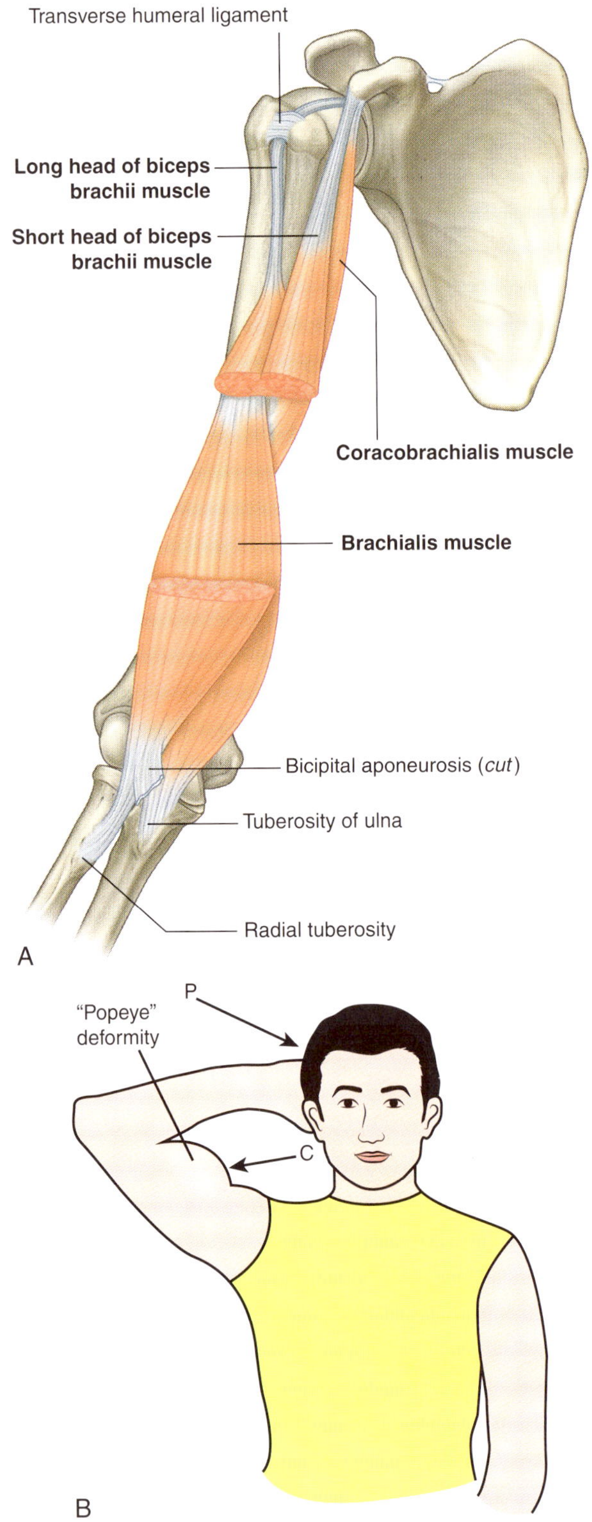

Fig. 2.64 (A) Coracobrachialis, biceps brachii, and brachialis muscles. **(B)** Rupture of biceps brachii tendon. The Ludington's test for ruptured tendon of the long head of the biceps (C, contraction of biceps; P, pressure applied to the back of the head).

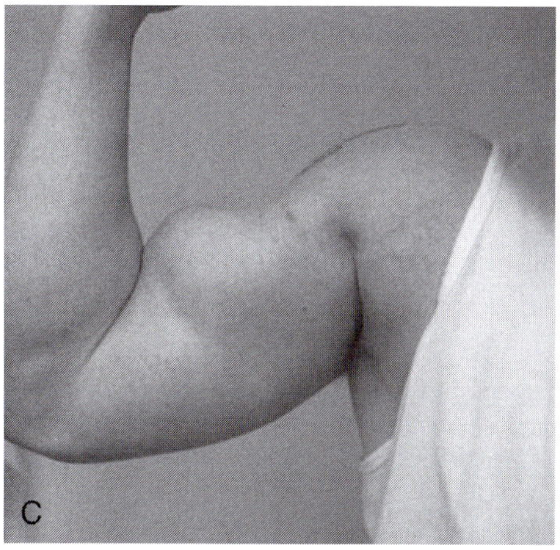

Fig. 2.64, cont'd (C) "Popeye" sign in a patient who sustained a biceps tendon rupture. *Source:* S. Brotzman Robert Manske. Clinical Orthopaedic Rehabilitation: An Evidence-Based Approach. Mosby, 2011:82–210.

The tendon of the long head passes through the glenohumeral joint superior to the head of the humerus and then passes through the intertubercular sulcus and enters the arm. In the arm, the tendon joins with its muscle belly and, together with the muscle belly of the short head, overlies the brachialis muscle.

The long and short heads converge to form a single tendon, which inserts onto the radial tuberosity.

As the tendon enters the forearm, a flat sheet of connective tissue (the **bicipital aponeurosis**) is seen to fan out from the medial side of the tendon. This blends with deep fascia covering the anterior compartment of the forearm.

The biceps brachii muscle is a powerful flexor of the forearm at the elbow joint; it is also the most powerful supinator of the forearm when the elbow joint is flexed. Because the two heads of the biceps brachii muscle cross the glenohumeral joint, the muscle can also flex the glenohumeral joint.

The biceps brachii muscle is innervated by the musculocutaneous nerve. A tap on the tendon of the biceps brachii at the elbow is used to test predominantly spinal cord segment C6.

Early clinical exposure

Rupture of biceps tendon

It is relatively unusual for muscles and their tendons to rupture in the upper limb. However, the tendon that most commonly ruptures is the tendon of the long head of the biceps brachii muscle. In isolation, this has relatively little effect on the upper limb, but it does produce a characteristic deformity—on flexing the elbow, there is an extremely prominent bulge of the muscle belly as its unrestrained fibers contract—the "Popeye" sign (Fig. 2.64B and C). Distal biceps tendon rupture also occurs. It is important to determine the site of the rupture, whether it is at the musculotendinous junction, midtendon, or at the insertion because this will determine the surgical approach for repair.

Brachialis

The **brachialis muscle** originates from the distal half of the anterior aspect of the humerus and from adjacent parts of the intermuscular septa, particularly on the medial side (Fig. 2.64A and Table 2.8). It lies beneath the biceps brachii muscle, is flattened dorsoventrally, and converges to form a tendon, which attaches to the tuberosity of the ulna.

The brachialis muscle flexes the forearm at the elbow joint.

Innervation of the brachialis muscle is predominantly by the musculocutaneous nerve. A small component of the lateral part is innervated by the radial nerve.

Table 2.8 Muscles of the anterior compartment of the arm

Muscle	Origin	Insertion	Innervation	Function
Coracobrachialis	Apex of coracoid process	Linear roughening on midshaft of humerus on medial side	Musculocutaneous nerve (**C5, C6, C7**)	Flexor of the arm at the glenohumeral joint
Biceps brachii	Long head—supraglenoid tubercle of scapula; short head—apex of coracoid process	Radial tuberosity	Musculocutaneous nerve (**C5, C6**)	Powerful flexor of the forearm at the elbow joint and supinator of the forearm; accessory flexor of the arm at the glenohumeral joint
Brachialis	Anterior aspect of humerus (medial and lateral surfaces) and adjacent intermuscular septae	Tuberosity of the ulna	Musculocutaneous nerve (C5, **C6**); small contribution by the radial nerve (C7) to lateral part of muscle	Powerful flexor of the forearm at the elbow joint

Note: Spinal segments in bold are the major segments innervating the muscle.

Posterior compartment

The only muscle of the posterior compartment of the arm is the **triceps brachii muscle** (Fig. 2.65 and Table 2.9). The triceps brachii muscle has three heads:

- The long head originates from the infraglenoid tubercle of the scapula.
- The medial head originates from the extensive area on the posterior surface of the shaft of the humerus inferior to the radial groove.
- The lateral head originates from a linear roughening superior to the radial groove of the humerus.

The three heads converge to form a large tendon, which inserts on the superior surface of the olecranon of the ulna.

The triceps brachii muscle extends the forearm at the elbow joint.

Innervation of the triceps brachii is by branches of the radial nerve. A tap on the tendon of the triceps brachii tests predominantly spinal cord segment C7.

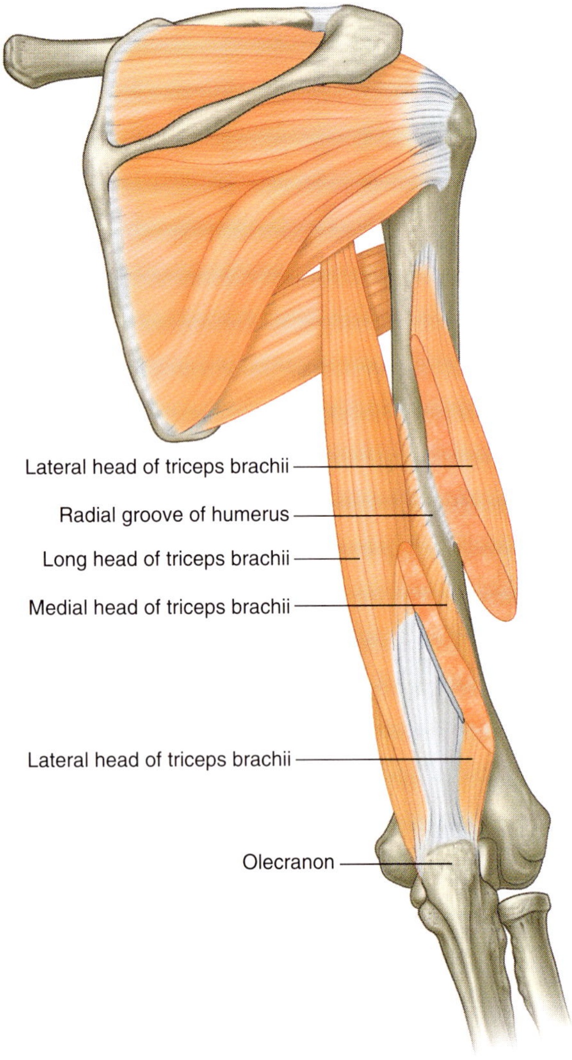

Fig. 2.65 Triceps muscle.

Arteries and veins

Brachial artery

The major artery of the arm, the **brachial artery**, is found in the anterior compartment (Fig. 2.66A). Beginning as a continuation of the axillary artery at the lower border of the teres major muscle, it terminates just distal to the elbow joint where it divides into the radial and ulnar arteries.

In the proximal arm, the brachial artery lies on the medial side. In the distal arm, it moves laterally to assume a position midway between the lateral epicondyle and the medial epicondyle of the humerus. It crosses anteriorly to the elbow joint where it lies immediately medial to the tendon of the biceps brachii muscle. The brachial artery is palpable along its length. In proximal regions, the brachial artery can be compressed against the medial side of the humerus.

Branches of the brachial artery in the arm include those to adjacent muscles and two ulnar collateral vessels, which contribute to a network of arteries around the elbow joint (Fig. 2.66B). Additional branches are the profunda brachii artery and nutrient arteries to the humerus, which pass through a foramen in the anteromedial surface of the humeral shaft.

Table 2.9 Muscle of the posterior compartment of the arm

Muscle	Origin	Insertion	Innervation	Function
Triceps brachii	Long head—infraglenoid tubercle of scapula; medial head—posterior surface of humerus; lateral head—posterior surface of humerus	Olecranon	Radial nerve (C6, **C7**, C8)	Extension of the forearm at the elbow joint; long head can also extend and adduct the arm at the shoulder joint

Note: Spinal segment indicated in bold is the major segment innervating the muscle

Profunda brachii artery

The **profunda brachii artery**, the largest branch of the brachial artery, passes into and supplies the posterior compartment of the arm (Fig. 2.66A and B). It enters the posterior compartment with the radial nerve and together they pass through the triangular interval, which is formed by the shaft of the humerus, the inferior margin of the teres major muscle, and the lateral margin of the long head of the triceps muscle. They then pass along the radial groove on the posterior surface of the humerus deep to the lateral head of the triceps brachii muscle.

Branches of the profunda brachii artery supply adjacent muscles and anastomose with the posterior circumflex humeral artery. The artery terminates as two collateral vessels, which contribute to an anastomotic network of arteries around the elbow joint (Fig. 2.66B).

Early clinical exposure

Blood pressure measurement

Blood pressure measurement is an extremely important physiological parameter. High blood pressure (hypertension) requires treatment to prevent long-term complications such as stroke. Low blood pressure may be caused by extreme blood loss, widespread infection, or poor cardiac output (e.g., after myocardial infarction). Accurate measurement of blood pressure is essential.

Most clinicians use a sphygmomanometer and a stethoscope. The sphygmomanometer is a device that inflates a cuff around the midportion of the arm to compress the brachial artery against the humerus. The cuff is inflated so it exceeds the systolic blood pressure (greater than 120 mm Hg). The clinician places a stethoscope over the brachial artery in the cubital fossa and listens (auscultates) for the pulse. As the pressure in the arm cuff of the sphygmomanometer is reduced just below the level of the systolic blood pressure, the pulse becomes audible as a regular thumping sound. As the pressure in the sphygmomanometer continues to drop, the regular thumping sound becomes clearer. When the pressure in the sphygmomanometer is less than that of the diastolic blood pressure, the audible thumping sound becomes inaudible. Using the simple scale on the sphygmomanometer, the patient's blood pressure can be determined. The normal range is 90–120/60–80 mm Hg (systolic blood pressure/diastolic blood pressure).

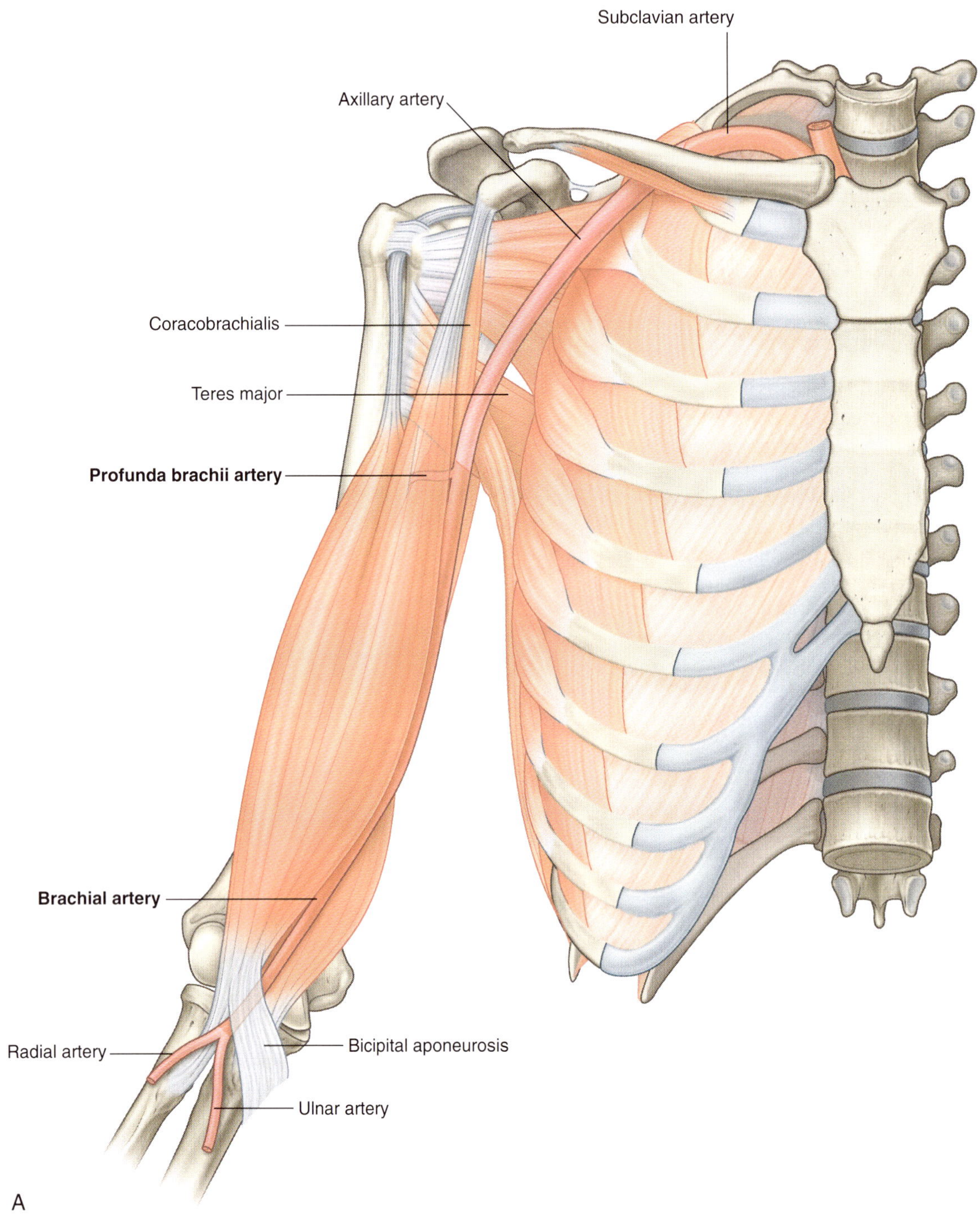

Fig. 2.66 Brachial artery. **(A)** In context.

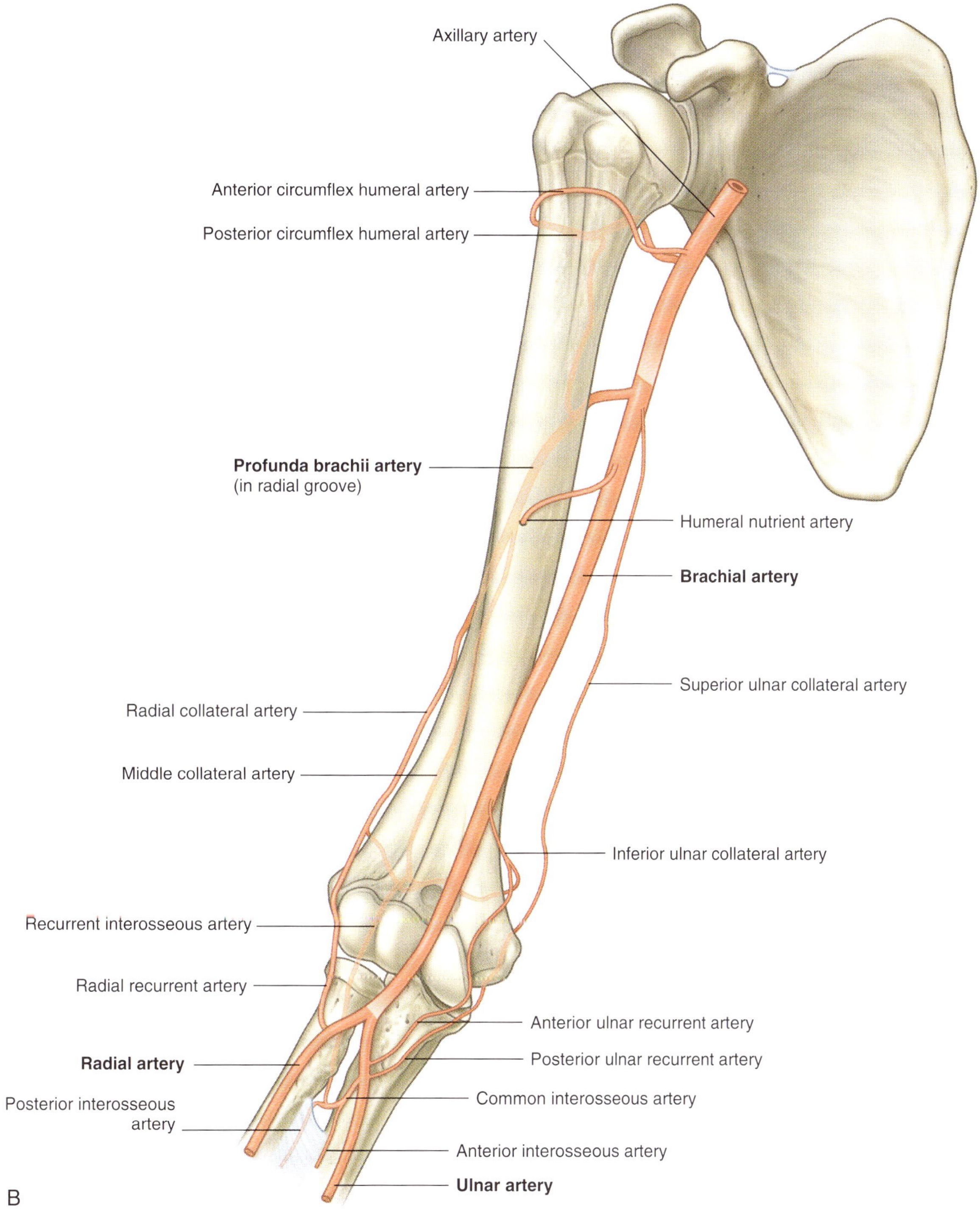

Fig. 2.66, cont'd (B) Branches.

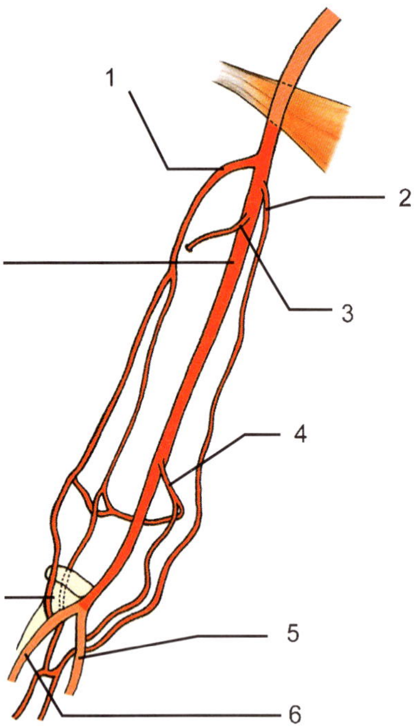

LD Fig. 2.66B.1 Brachial artery.

Questions

2.66.B.1.A How and where does the brachial artery begin and end?

2.66.B.1.B Name the structures indicated by the labels.

2.66.B.1.C Name the branches of the brachial artery which reach the elbow joint and mention which branches they anastomose with.

Answers

2.66.B.1.A The origin and termination of the brachial artery are

Origin: As a continuation of the axillary artery at the lower border of the teres major

Termination: By dividing into the radial and ulnar arteries at the level of the neck of the radius

2.66.B.1.B The structures indicated by the labels are

1. Profunda brachii artery
2. Superior ulnar collateral artery
3. Nutrient artery
4. Inferior ulnar collateral artery
5. Ulnar artery
6. Radial artery

2.66.B.1.C The branches of the brachial artery which reach the elbow joint and the branches they anastomose with are

Profunda brachii artery (divides into the radial collateral artery and the middle collateral artery) anastomoses with the radial recurrent artery and the interosseous recurrent artery.

Superior ulnar collateral artery anastomoses with the posterior ulnar recurrent artery.

Inferior ulnar collateral artery anastomoses with the anterior ulnar recurrent artery.

Veins

Paired brachial veins pass along the medial and lateral sides of the brachial artery, receiving tributaries that accompany branches of the artery (Fig. 2.67).

In addition to these deep veins, two large subcutaneous veins, the basilic vein and the cephalic vein, are located in the arm.

The basilic vein passes vertically in the distal half of the arm, penetrates deep fascia to assume a position medial to the brachial artery, and then becomes the axillary vein at the lower border of the teres major muscle. The brachial veins join the basilic, or axillary, vein.

The cephalic vein passes superiorly on the anterolateral aspect of the arm and through the anterior wall of the axilla to reach the axillary vein.

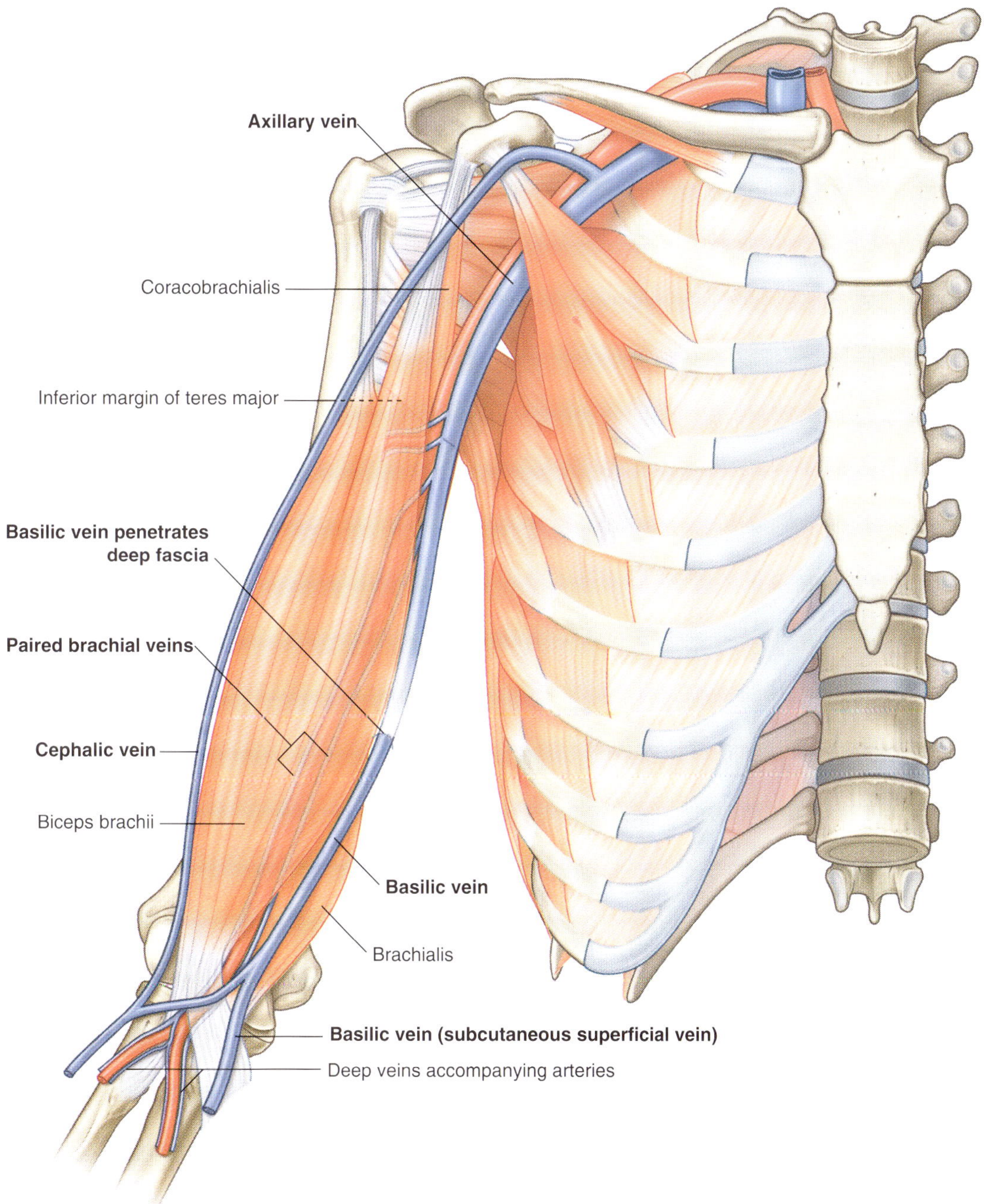

Fig. 2.67 Veins of the arm.

Nerves

Musculocutaneous nerve

The musculocutaneous nerve leaves the axilla and enters the arm by passing through the coracobrachialis muscle (Fig. 2.68). It passes diagonally down the arm in the plane between the biceps brachii and brachialis muscles. After giving rise to motor branches in the arm, it emerges lateral to the tendon of the biceps brachii muscle at the elbow, penetrates deep fascia, and continues as the **lateral cutaneous nerve of the forearm**.

The musculocutaneous nerve provides:

- Motor innervation to all muscles in the anterior compartment of the arm
- Sensory innervation to skin on the lateral surface of the forearm (Flowchart 2.3)

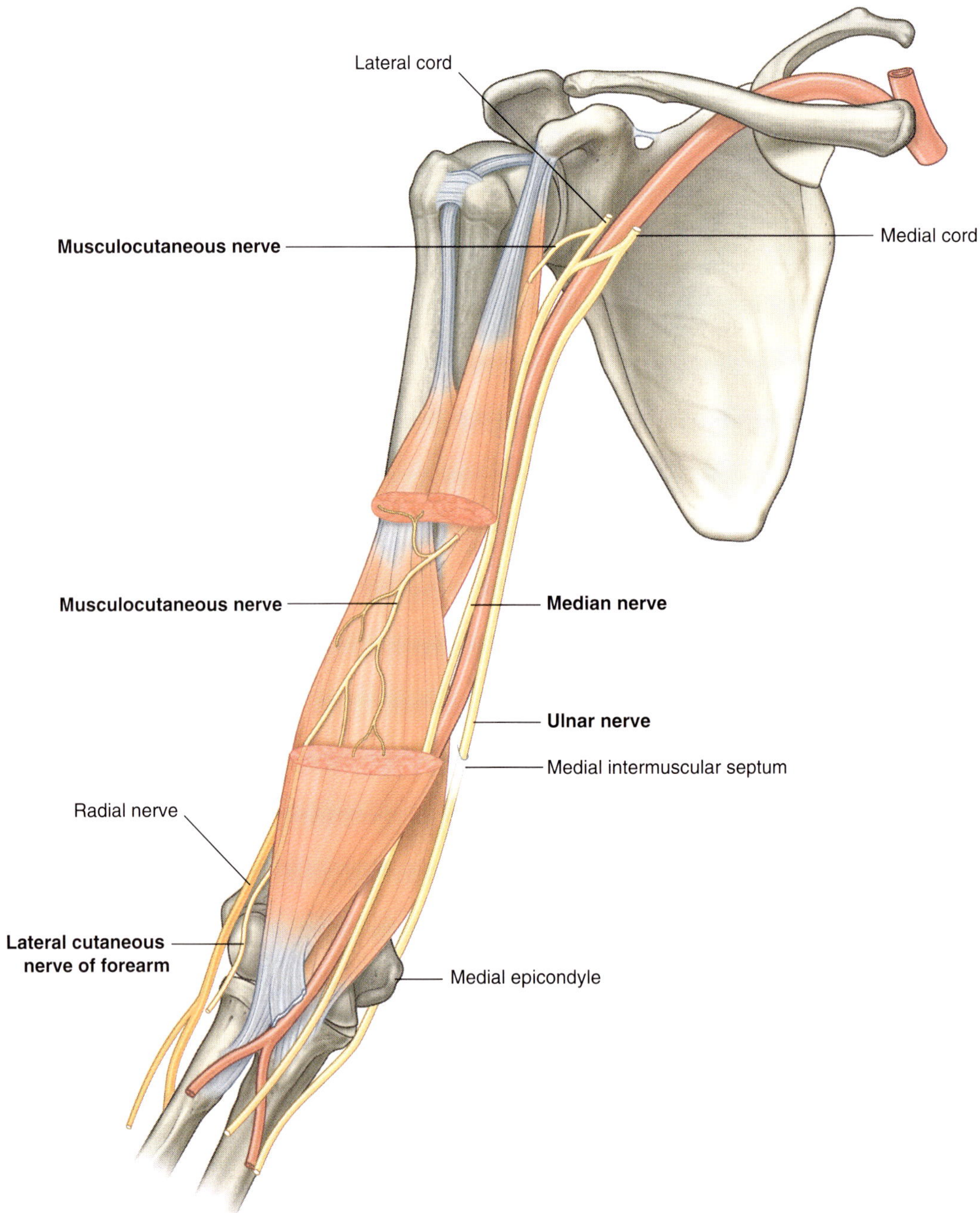

Fig. 2.68 Musculocutaneous, median, and ulnar nerves in the arm.

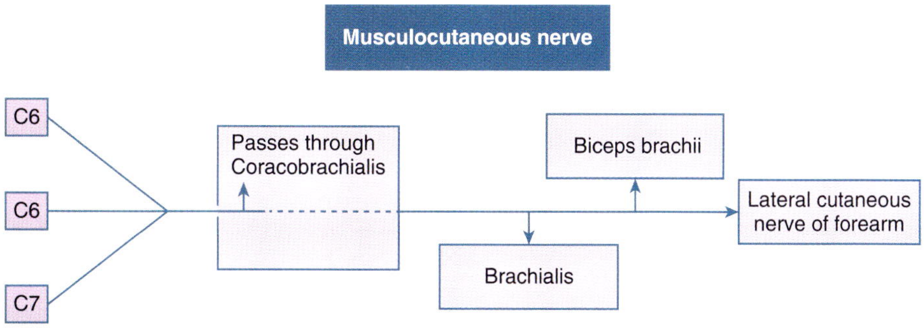

Flowchart 2.3 Course and supply of musculocutaneous nerve.

Median nerve

The median nerve enters the arm from the axilla at the inferior margin of the teres major muscle (Fig. 2.68). It passes vertically down the medial side of the arm in the anterior compartment and is related to the brachial artery throughout its course:

- In proximal regions, the median nerve is immediately lateral to the brachial artery.
- In more distal regions, the median nerve crosses to the medial side of the brachial artery and lies anterior to the elbow joint.

The median nerve has no major branches in the arm, but a branch to one of the muscles of the forearm, the pronator teres muscle, may originate from the nerve immediately proximal to the elbow joint.

Ulnar nerve

The ulnar nerve enters the arm with the median nerve and axillary artery (Fig. 2.68). It passes through proximal regions medial to the axillary artery. In the middle of the arm, the ulnar nerve penetrates the medial intermuscular septum and enters the posterior compartment where it lies anterior to the medial head of the triceps brachii muscle. It passes posterior to the medial epicondyle of the humerus and then into the anterior compartment of the forearm.

The ulnar nerve has no major branches in the arm.

Radial nerve

The radial nerve originates from the posterior cord of the brachial plexus and enters the arm by crossing the inferior margin of the teres major muscle (Fig. 2.69). As it enters the arm, it lies posterior to the brachial artery. Accompanied by the profunda brachii artery, the radial nerve enters the posterior compartment of the arm by passing through the triangular interval.

As the radial nerve passes diagonally, from medial to lateral, through the posterior compartment, it lies in the radial groove directly on bone. On the lateral side of the arm, it passes anteriorly through the lateral intermuscular septum and enters the anterior compartment where it lies between the brachialis muscle and a muscle of the posterior compartment of the forearm—the brachioradialis muscle, which attaches to the lateral supraepicondylar ridge of the humerus. The radial nerve enters the forearm anterior to the lateral epicondyle of the humerus, just deep to the brachioradialis muscle.

In the arm, the radial nerve has muscular and cutaneous branches (Fig. 2.69):

- Muscular branches include those to the triceps brachii, brachioradialis, and extensor carpi radialis longus muscles. In addition, the radial nerve contributes to the innervation of the lateral part of the brachialis muscle. One of the branches to the medial head of the triceps brachii muscle arises before the radial nerve's entrance into the posterior compartment and passes vertically down the arm in association with the ulnar nerve.
- Cutaneous branches of the radial nerve that originate in the posterior compartment of the arm are the **inferior lateral cutaneous nerve of the arm** and the **posterior cutaneous nerve of the forearm**, both of which penetrate through the lateral head of the triceps brachii muscle and the overlying deep fascia to become subcutaneous.

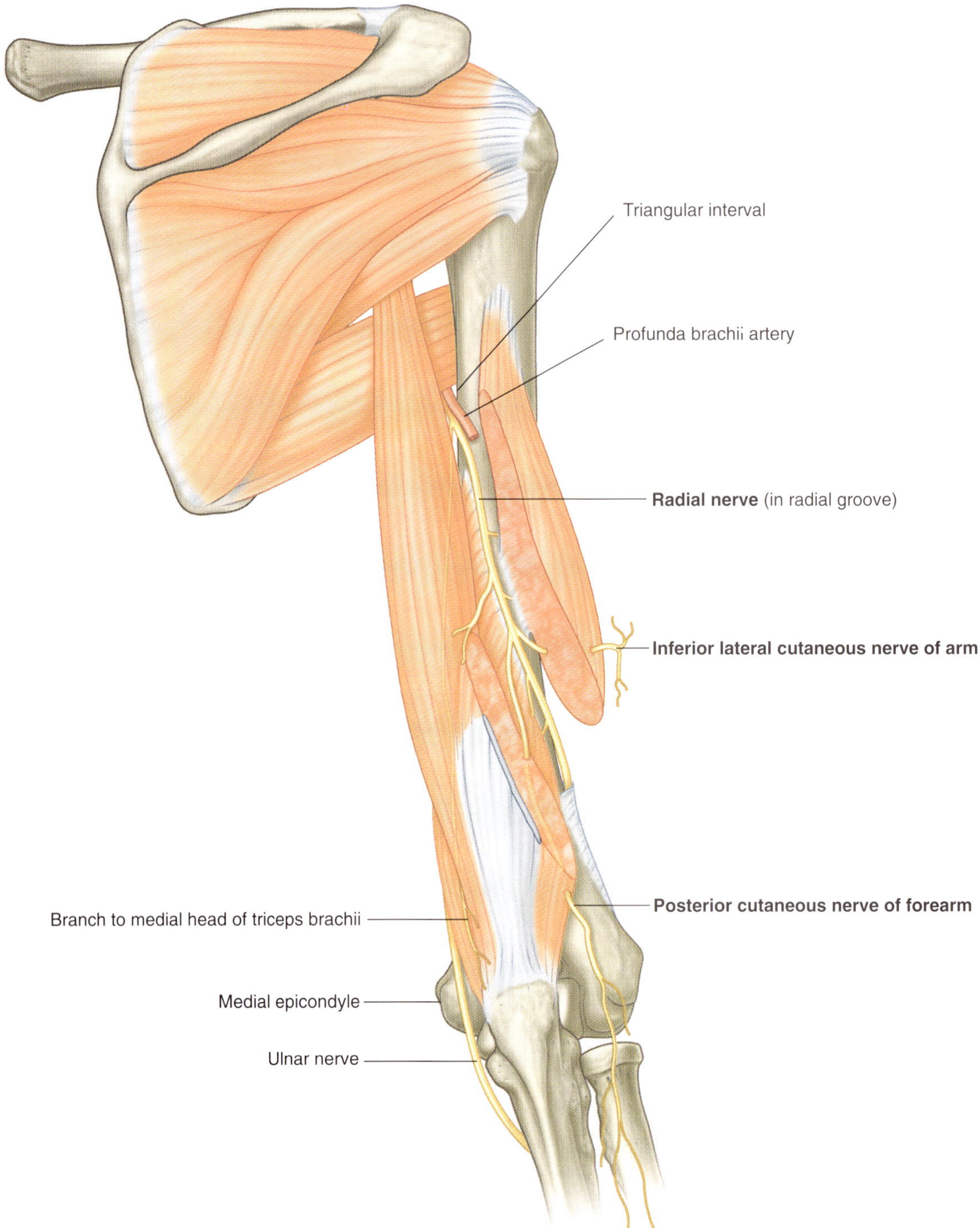

Fig. 2.69 Radial nerve in the arm.

Early clinical exposure

Radial nerve injury in the arm

The radial nerve is tightly bound to the profunda brachii artery between the medial and lateral heads of the triceps brachii muscle in the radial groove. If the humerus is fractured, the radial nerve may become stretched or transected in this region, leading to damage and permanent loss of function. This injury commonly occurs with such a fracture (Fig. 2.70A) and the nerve should always be tested when a fracture of the midshaft of the humerus is suspected. The physical signs usually include sensory changes over the dorsum of the hand and **wrist drop** (due to denervation of the extensor muscles) (Fig. 2.70B and C).

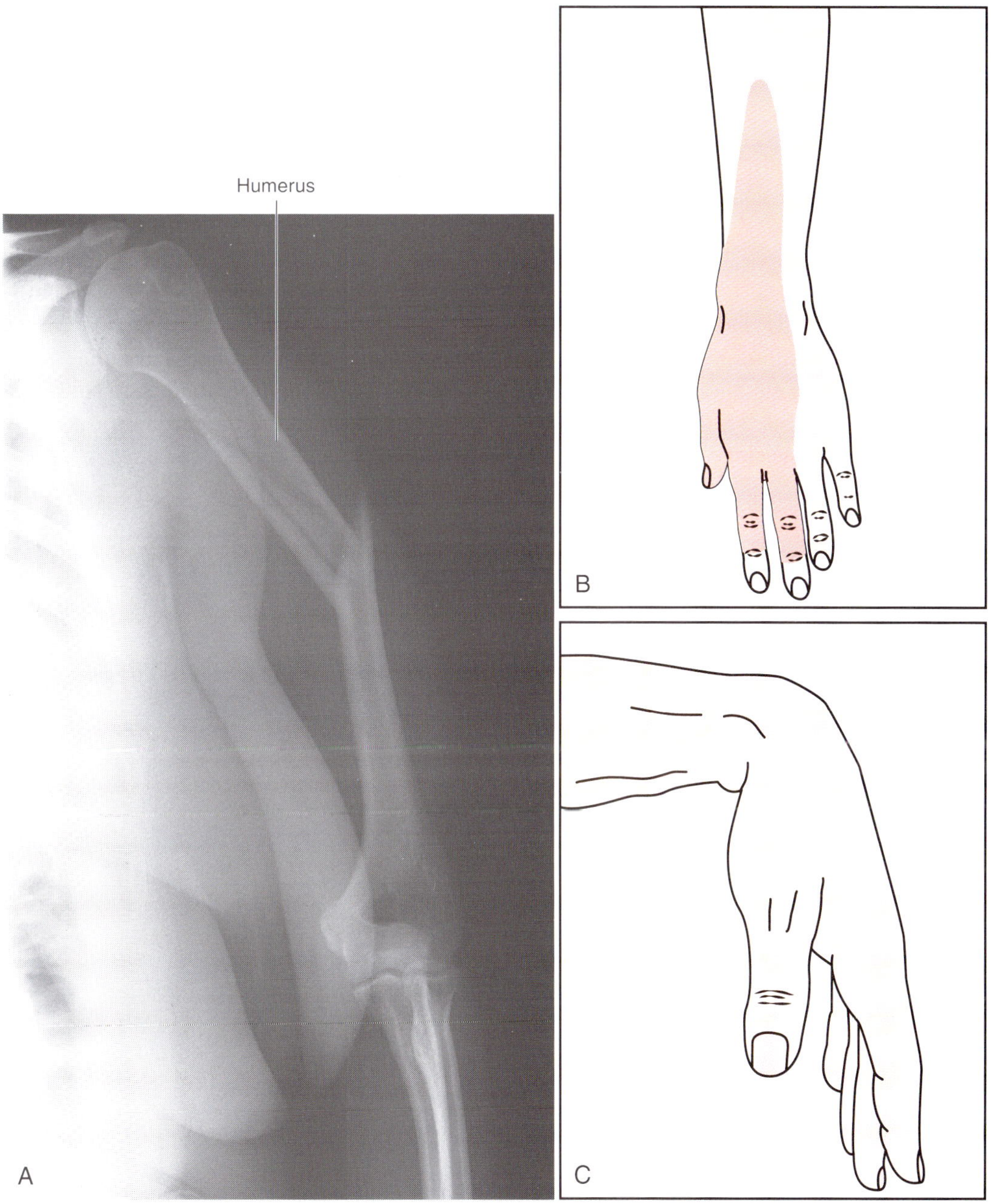

Fig. 2.70 **(A)** Radiograph of the humerus demonstrating a midshaft fracture, which may disrupt the radial nerve. **(B)** Decreased or absent sensation on the radial and dorsal aspect of the hand and wrist. **(C)** Wrist drop: the hand will drop when positioned with the palm facing downwards.

Early clinical exposure

Median nerve injury in the arm

In the arm and forearm, the median nerve is usually not injured by trauma because of its relatively deep position. The commonest neurological problem associated with the median nerve is compression beneath the flexor retinaculum at the wrist (carpal tunnel syndrome).

On very rare occasions, a fibrous band may arise from the anterior aspect of the humerus beneath which the median nerve passes. This is an embryological remnant of the coracobrachialis muscle and is sometimes called the ligament of Struthers; occasionally, it may calcify. This band can compress the median nerve, resulting in weakness of the flexor muscles in the forearm and the thenar muscles. Nerve conduction studies will demonstrate the site of nerve compression.

ELBOW JOINT

The elbow joint is a complex joint involving three separate articulations, which share a common synovial cavity (Fig. 2.71).

- The joints between the trochlear notch of the ulna and the trochlea of the humerus and between the head of the radius and the capitulum of the humerus are primarily involved with hinge-like flexion and extension of the forearm on the arm and, together, are the principal articulations of the elbow joint.
- The joint between the head of the radius and the radial notch of the ulna, the proximal radioulnar joint, is involved with pronation and supination of the forearm.

The articular surfaces of the bones are covered with hyaline cartilage.

The synovial membrane originates from the edges of the articular cartilage and lines the radial fossa, the coronoid fossa, the olecranon fossa, the deep surface of the joint capsule, and the medial surface of the trochlea (Fig. 2.72).

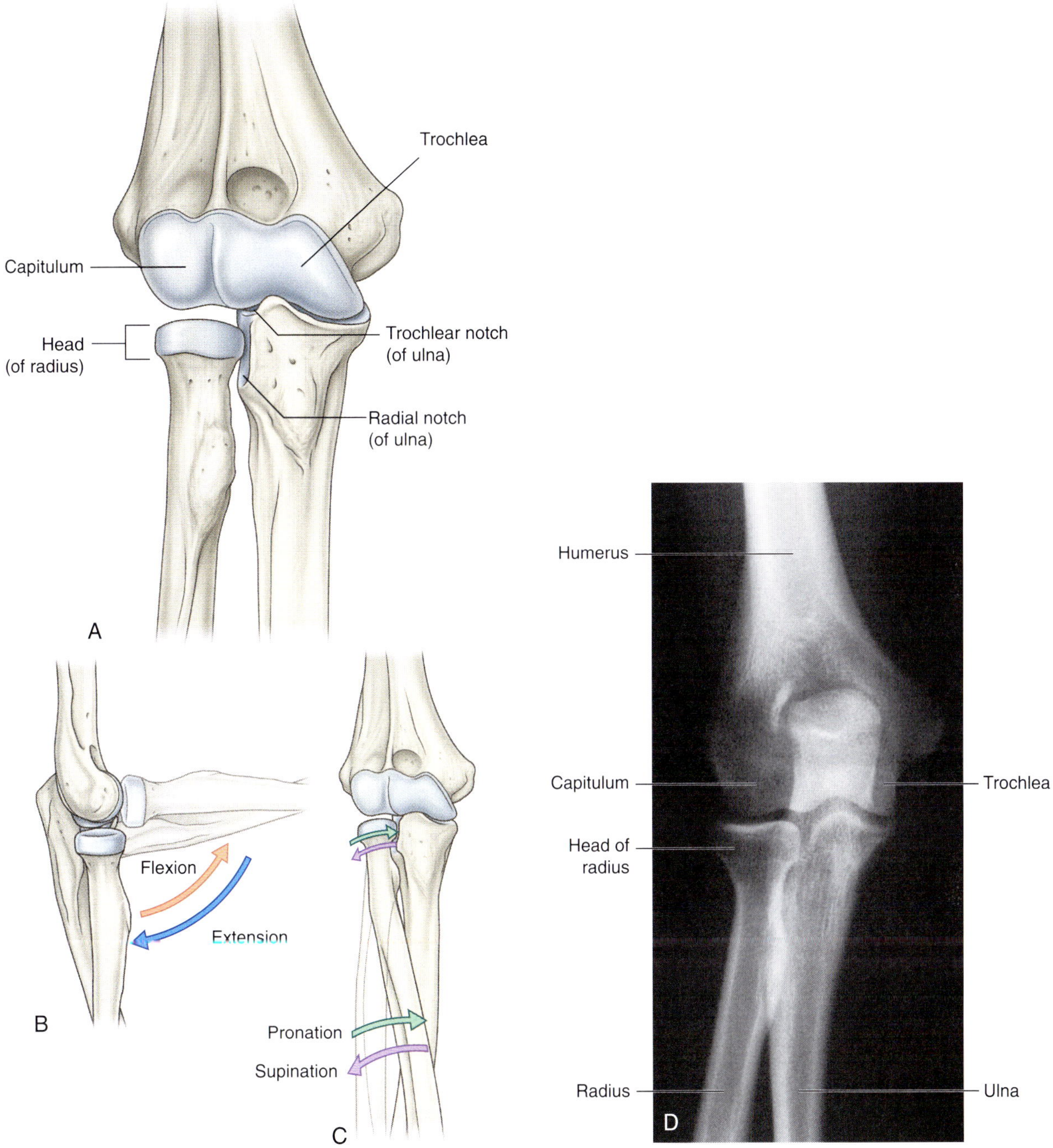

Fig. 2.71 Components and movements of the elbow joint. **(A)** Bones and joint surfaces. **(B)** Flexion and extension. **(C)** Pronation and supination. **(D)** Radiograph of a normal elbow joint (anteroposterior view).

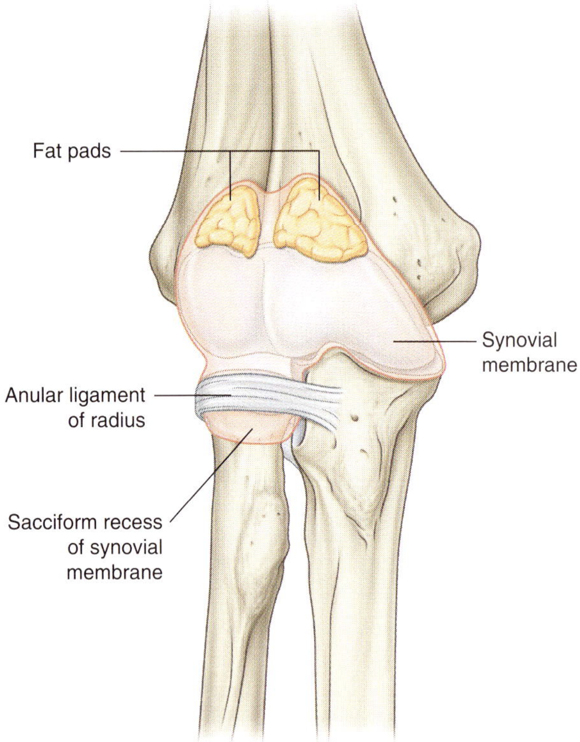

Fig. 2.72 Synovial membrane of elbow joint (anterior view).

The synovial membrane is separated from the fibrous membrane of the joint capsule by pads of fat in regions overlying the coronoid fossa, the olecranon fossa, and the radial fossa. These fat pads accommodate the related bony processes during extension and flexion of the elbow. Attachments of the brachialis and triceps brachii muscles to the joint capsule overlying these regions pull the attached fat pads out of the way when the adjacent bony processes are moved into the fossae.

The fibrous membrane of the joint capsule overlies the synovial membrane, encloses the joint, and attaches to the medial epicondyle and the margins of the olecranon, coronoid, and radial fossae of the humerus (Fig. 2.73). It also attaches to the coronoid process and olecranon of the ulna. On the lateral side, the free inferior margin of the joint capsule passes around the neck of the radius from an anterior attachment to the coronoid process of the ulna to a posterior attachment to the base of the olecranon.

The fibrous membrane of the joint capsule is thickened medially and laterally to form collateral ligaments, which support the flexion and extension movements of the elbow joint (Fig. 2.73).

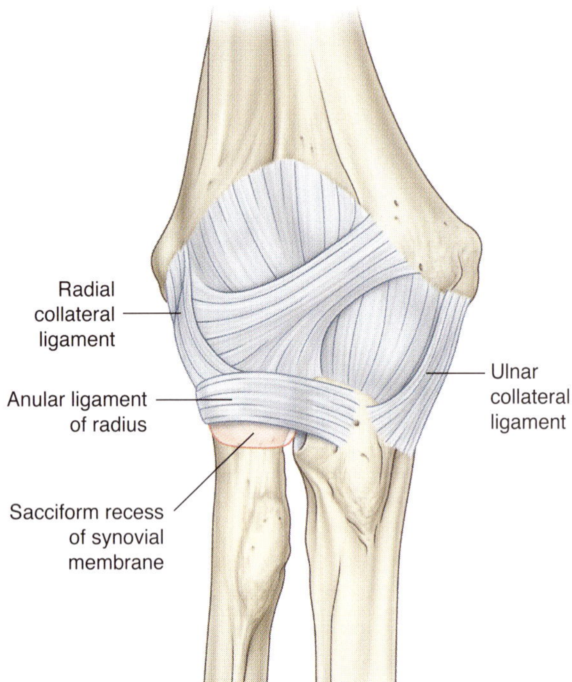

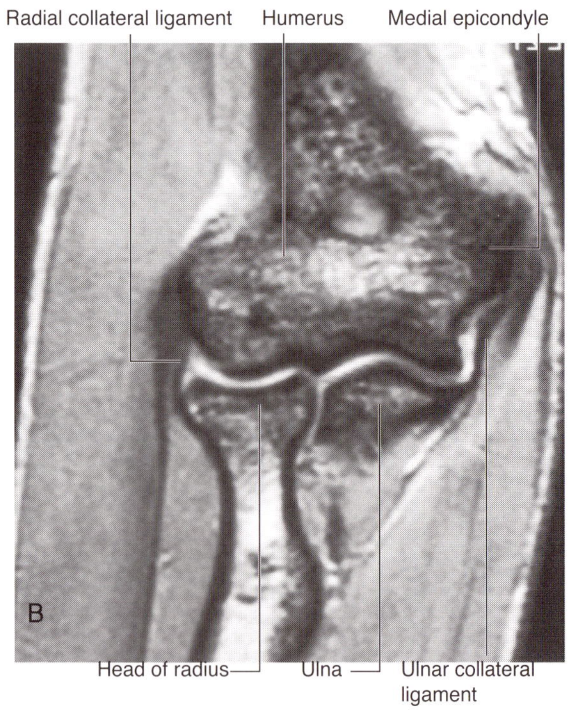

Fig. 2.73 Elbow joint. **(A)** Joint capsule and ligaments of the right elbow joint. **(B)** Magnetic resonance image of the elbow joint in the coronal plane.

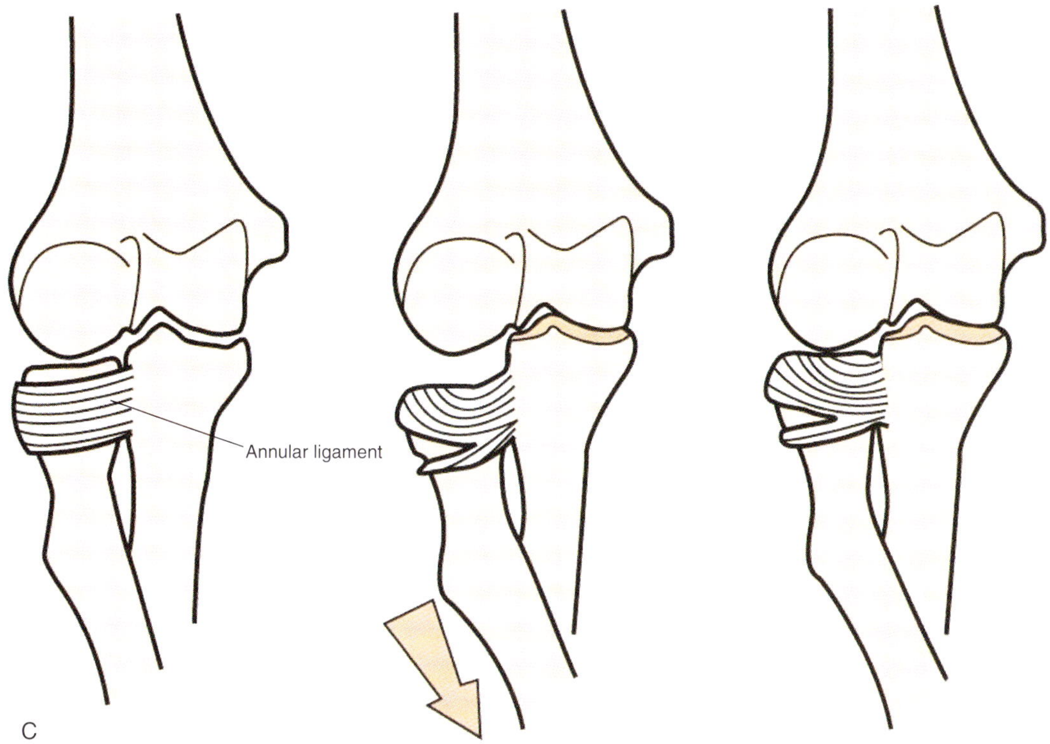

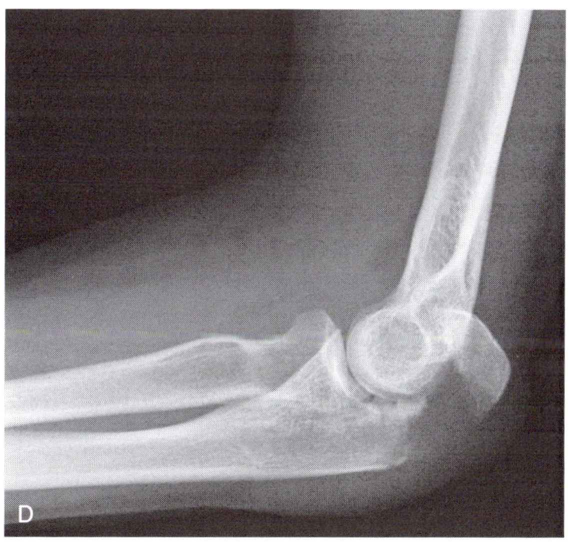

Fig. 2.73, cont'd (C) Pulled elbow, also called nursemaid's elbow. The annular ligament was partially torn and the radial head displaced distally when the forearm was pulled distally, as indicated by the arrow. When the traction was discontinued, the radial head returned into the joint. **(D)** Radiograph of an elbow showing a fracture of the olecranon and involving the insertion of the triceps brachii muscle. *Source:* K Marcdante, RM Kliegman. Nelson Textbook of Pediatrics: The Upper Limb. Saunders, 2011:2383-e673-1. (Original from Rang M. Children's Fractures, 2nd ed. Philadelphia: JB Lippincott, 1983:193.)

In addition, the external surface of the joint capsule is reinforced laterally where it cuffs the head of the radius with a strong **annular ligament of the radius**. Although this ligament blends with the fibrous membrane of the joint capsule in most regions, they are separate posteriorly. The annular ligament of the radius also blends with the **radial collateral ligament**.

The annular ligament of the radius and related joint capsule allow the radial head to slide against the radial notch of the ulna and pivot on the capitulum during pronation and supination of the forearm.

The deep surface of the fibrous membrane of the joint capsule and the related annular ligament of the radius that articulate with the sides of the radial head are lined by cartilage. A pocket of synovial membrane (sacciform recess) protrudes from the inferior free margin of the joint capsule and facilitates rotation of the radial head during pronation and supination.

The movements possible at the elbow joint are flexion and extension. The muscles producing these movements are summarized below:

Flexion (biceps brachii, brachialis, brachioradialis)
Extension (triceps, anconeus)

Vascular supply to the elbow joint is through an anastomotic network of vessels derived from collateral and recurrent branches of the brachial, profunda brachii, radial, and ulnar arteries.

The elbow joint is innervated predominantly by branches of the radial and musculocutaneous nerves, but there may be some innervation by branches of the ulnar and median nerves.

Early clinical exposure

Supracondylar fracture of the humerus

Elbow injuries in children may result in a transverse fracture of the distal end of the humerus, above the level of the epicondyles. This fracture is termed a supracondylar fracture. The distal fragment and its soft tissues are pulled posteriorly by the triceps muscle. This posterior displacement effectively compresses the brachial artery over the irregular proximal fracture fragment. In children, this is a relatively devastating injury: the muscles of the anterior compartment of the forearm are rendered ischemic and form severe contractions, significantly reducing the function of the anterior compartment and flexor muscles (Volkmann's ischemic contracture).

Early clinical exposure

Pulled elbow

Pulled elbow is a disorder that typically occurs in children under 5 years of age. It is commonly caused by a sharp pull of the child's hand. The not-yet-developed head of the radius and the laxity of the annular ligament of the radius allow the head to subluxate from this cuff of tissue. Pulled elbow is extremely painful, but can be treated easily by simple supination and compression of the elbow joint by the clinician. When the radial head is relocated, the pain subsides immediately and the child can continue with normal activity (Fig. 2.73C).

Fracture of the olecranon

Fractures of the olecranon can result from a direct blow to the olecranon or from a fall onto an outstretched hand (Fig. 2.73D). The triceps inserts into the olecranon and injuries can cause avulsion of the muscle.

Early clinical exposure

Developmental changes in the elbow joint

The elbow joint can be injured in many ways; the types of injuries are age dependent. When a fracture or soft tissue trauma is suspected, a plain lateral and an anteroposterior radiograph are obtained. In an adult it is usually not difficult to interpret the radiograph, but in children additional factors require interpretation.

As the elbow develops in children, numerous secondary ossification centers appear before and around puberty. It is easy to mistakenly interpret these as fractures. In addition, it is also possible for the epiphyses and apophyses to be "pulled off" or disrupted. Therefore, when interpreting a child's radiograph of the elbow, the physician must know the child's age (Fig. 2.74). Fusion occurs at around the time of puberty. An understanding of the normal epiphyses and apophyses and their normal relationship to the bones will secure a correct diagnosis. The approximate ages of appearance of the secondary ossification centers around the elbow joint are

- Capitulum—1 year
- Head (of radius)—5 years
- Medial epicondyle—5 years
- Trochlea—11 years
- Olecranon—12 years
- Lateral epicondyle—13 years

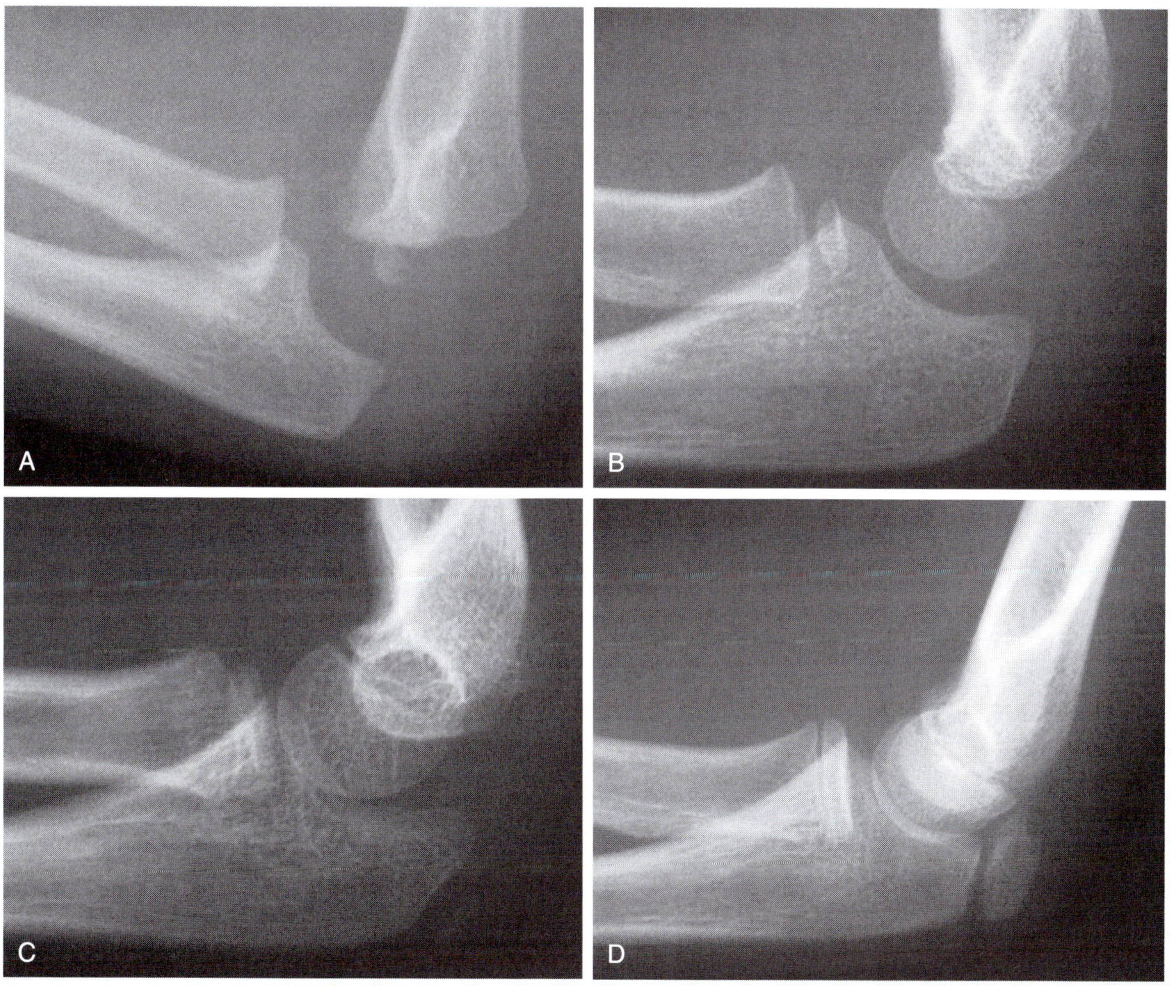

Fig. 2.74 Radiographs of elbow joint development: **(A)** at age 2 years; **(B)** at age 5 years; **(C)** at age 5–6 years; **(D)** at age 12 years. Tennis elbow.

Continued

Early clinical exposure—cont'd

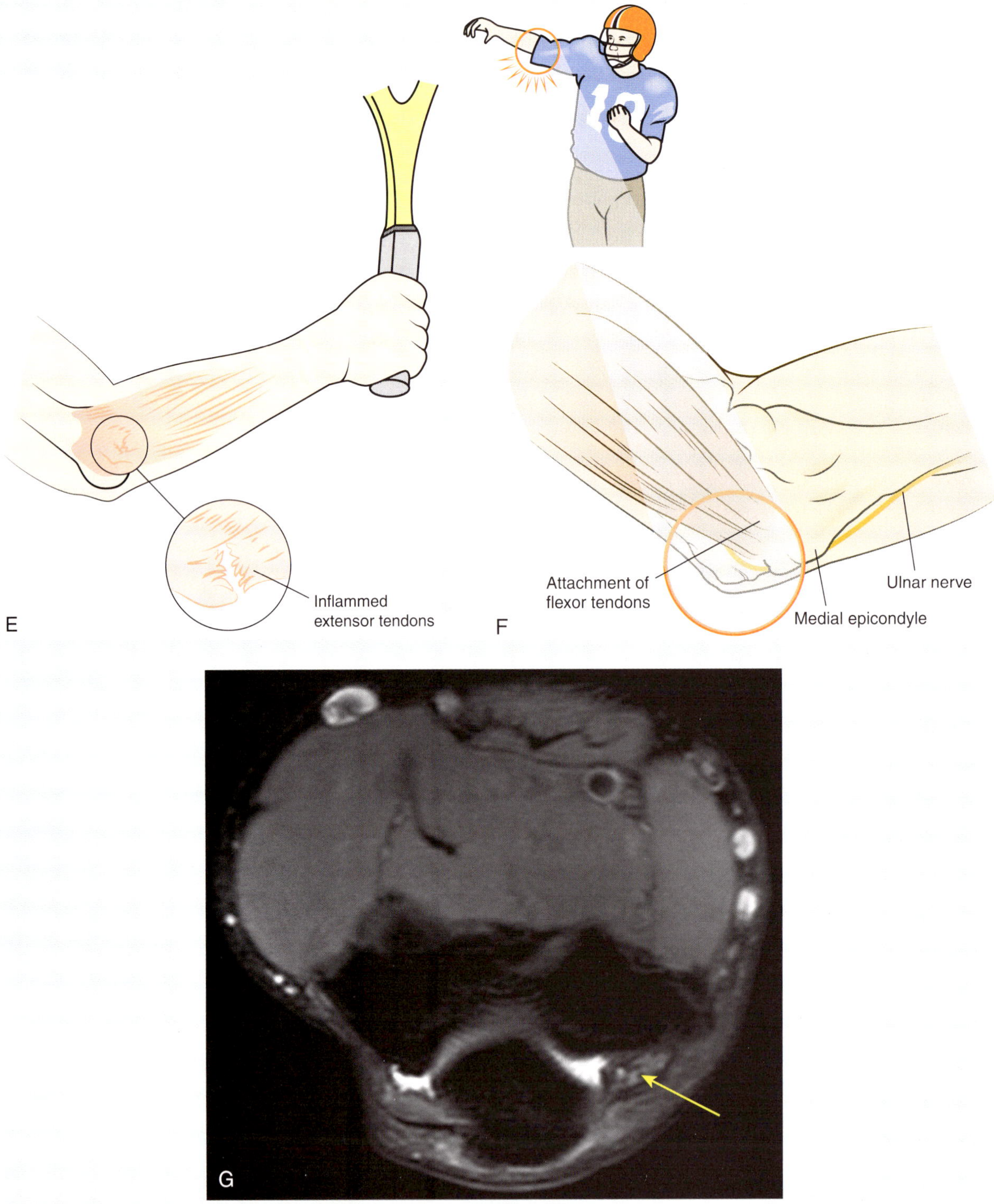

Fig. 2.74, cont'd **(E)** Lateral epicondylitis, or "tennis elbow," affects the common origin of the wrist extensors. **(F)** The pain of medial epicondylitis due to throwing sports or golf (golfer's elbow) occurs at the medial epicondyle. **(G)** MRI of right elbow showing swelling of the ulnar nerve in the cubital tunnel posterior to the medial epicondyle, consistent with nerve compression. *Source:* (E) G Shankman, R Manske. Fundamental Orthopedic Management for the Physical Therapist Assistant: Orthopedic Management of the Elbow, 3rd ed. Mosby, 2011:366–382. (F) SD Waldman, S Waldman. Atlas of Common Pain Syndromes: Golfer's Elbow, 3rd ed. Saunders, 2012:126–128.

Early clinical exposure

Fracture of the head of the radius

A fracture of the head of the radius is a common injury and can cause appreciable morbidity. It is one of the typical injuries that occur with a fall on the outstretched hand. On falling, the force is transmitted to the radial head, which fractures. These fractures typically result in loss of full extension, and potential surgical reconstruction may require long periods of physiotherapy to obtain a full range of movement at the elbow joint.

A lateral radiograph of a fracture of the head of the radius typically demonstrates the secondary phenomenon of this injury. When the bone is fractured, fluid fills the synovial cavity, elevating the small pad of fat within the coronoid and olecranon fossae. These fat pads appear as areas of lucency on the lateral radiograph—the "fat pad" sign. This radiological finding is useful because fracture of the head of the radius is not always clearly visible. If there is an appropriate clinical history, tenderness around the head of the radius, and a positive fat pad sign, a fracture can be inferred clinically even if no fracture can be identified on the radiograph, and appropriate treatment can be instituted.

Early clinical exposure

"Tennis" and "golfer's" elbow (epicondylitis)

It is not uncommon for people who are involved in sports such as golf and tennis to develop an overuse strain of the origins of the flexor and extensor muscles of the forearm. The pain is typically around the epicondyles and usually resolves after rest and physical therapy. It may also be treated with injection of the patient's own plasma, rich in platelets, into the tendon to promote tendon healing and repair. If pain and inflammation persist, surgical division of the extensor or flexor origin from the bone may be necessary. Typically, in tennis players this pain occurs on the lateral epicondyle and common extensor origin (tennis elbow) (Fig. 2.74E), whereas in golfers (and in throwing sports) it occurs on the medial epicondyle and common flexor origin (Fig. 2.74F).

Early clinical exposure

Elbow arthritis

Osteoarthritis is extremely common and is usually most severe in the dominant limb. From time to time an arthritic elbow may undergo such degenerative change that small bone fragments appear in the articular cavity. Given the relatively small joint space, these fragments can result in an appreciable reduction in flexion and extension, and typically lodge within the olecranon and coronoid fossae.

Early clinical exposure

Ulnar nerve injury at the elbow

Posterior to the medial epicondyle of the humerus, the ulnar nerve is bound in a fibro-osseous tunnel (the cubital tunnel) by a retinaculum. Older patients may develop degenerative changes within this tunnel, which compresses the ulnar nerve when flexed. The repeated action of flexion and extension of the elbow may cause local nerve damage, resulting in impaired function of the ulnar nerve. Accessory muscles and localized neuritis in this region secondary to direct trauma may also produce ulnar nerve damage (Fig. 2.74G).

CUBITAL FOSSA

The cubital fossa is an important area of transition between the arm and the forearm. It is located anterior to the elbow joint and is a triangular depression formed between two forearm muscles:

- The brachioradialis muscle originating from the lateral supraepicondylar ridge of the humerus
- The pronator teres muscle originating from the medial epicondyle of the humerus (Fig. 2.75A)

The base of the triangle is an imaginary horizontal line between the medial and lateral epicondyles. The bed or floor of the fossa is formed mainly by the brachialis muscle.

The major contents of the cubital fossa, from lateral to medial, are

- The tendon of the biceps brachii muscle
- The brachial artery
- The median nerve (Fig. 2.75B)

The brachial artery normally bifurcates into the radial and ulnar arteries in the apex of the fossa (Fig. 2.75B), although this bifurcation may occur much higher in the arm, even in the axilla. When taking a blood pressure reading from a patient, the clinician places the stethoscope over the brachial artery in the cubital fossa.

The median nerve lies immediately medial to the brachial artery and leaves the fossa by passing between the ulnar and humeral heads of the pronator teres muscle (Fig. 2.75C).

The brachial artery and the median nerve are covered and protected anteriorly in the distal part of the cubital fossa by the bicipital aponeurosis (Fig. 2.75B). This flat connective tissue membrane passes between the medial side of the tendon of the biceps brachii muscle and deep fascia of the forearm. The sharp medial margin of the bicipital aponeurosis can often be felt.

The radial nerve lies just under the lip of the brachioradialis muscle, which forms the lateral margin of the fossa (Fig. 2.75C). In this position, the radial nerve divides into superficial and deep branches:

- The superficial branch continues into the forearm just deep to the brachioradialis muscle.
- The deep branch passes between the two layers of the supinator muscle (Fig. 2.90) to access the posterior compartment of the forearm.

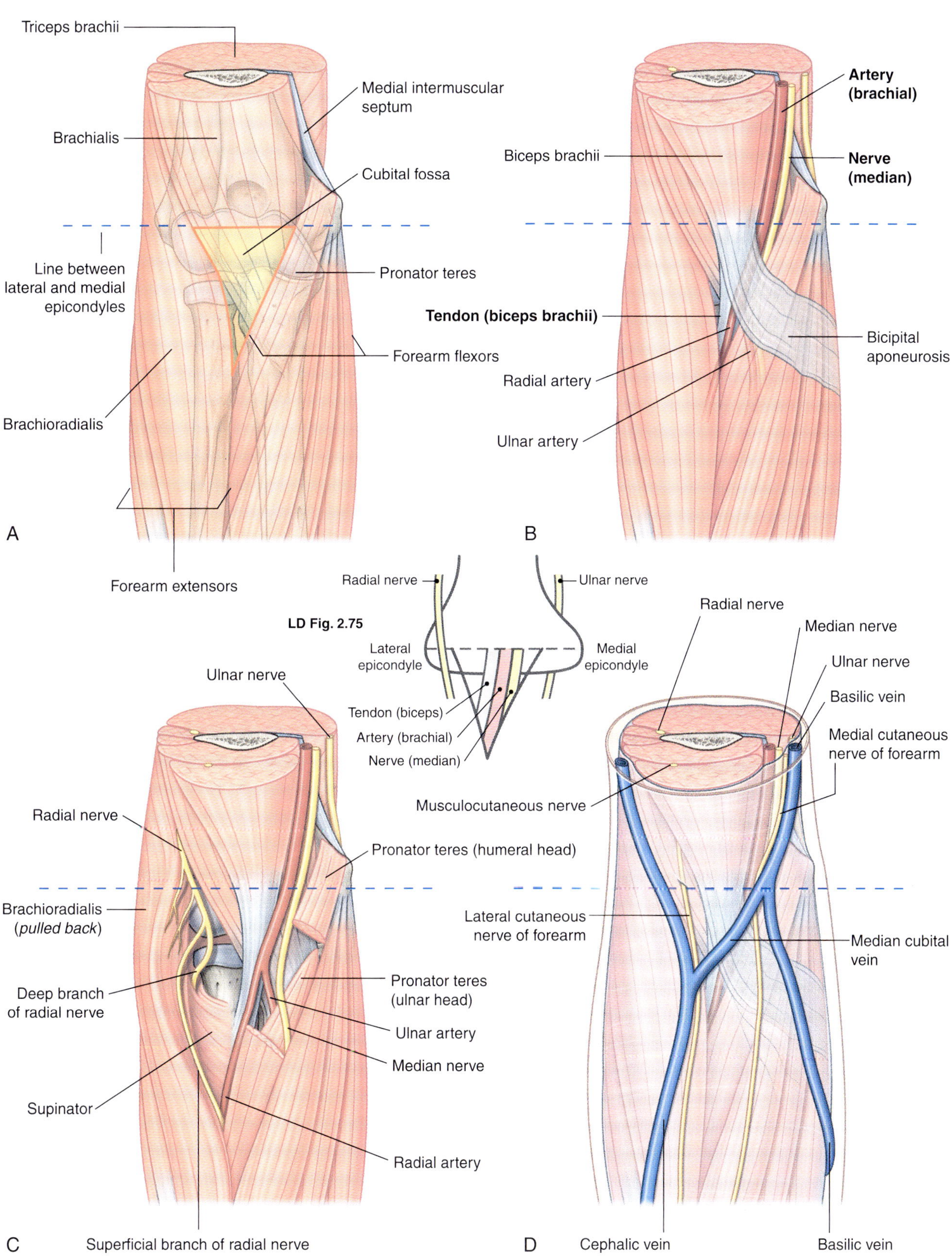

Fig. 2.75 Cubital fossa. **(A)** Margins. **(B)** Contents. **(C)** Position of the radial nerve. **(D)** Superficial structures.
LD Fig. 2.75 Cubital fossa and nerves related to the elbow.

The ulnar nerve does not pass through the cubital fossa. Instead, it passes posterior to the medial epicondyle.

The roof of the cubital fossa is formed by superficial fascia and skin. The most important structure within the roof is the median cubital vein (Fig. 2.75D), which passes diagonally across the roof and connects the cephalic vein on the lateral side of the upper limb with the basilic vein on the medial side. The bicipital aponeurosis separates the median cubital vein from the brachial artery and median nerve. Other structures within the roof are cutaneous nerves—the medial cutaneous and lateral cutaneous nerves of the forearm.

Early clinical exposure

Construction of a dialysis fistula

Many patients throughout the world require renal dialysis for kidney failure. The patient's blood is filtered and cleaned by the dialysis machine. Blood therefore has to be taken from patients into the filtering device and then returned to them. This process of dialysis occurs over many hours and requires considerable flow rates of 250–500 mL/min. To enable such large volumes of blood to be removed from and returned to the body, the blood is taken from vessels that have a high flow. As no veins in the peripheral limbs have such high flow, a surgical procedure is necessary to create such a system. In most patients, the radial artery is anastomosed (joined) to the cephalic vein (Fig. 2.76) at the wrist, or the brachial artery is anastomosed to the cephalic vein at the elbow. Some surgeons place an arterial graft between these vessels.

After 6 weeks, the veins increase in size in response to their arterial blood flow and are amenable to direct cannulation or dialysis.

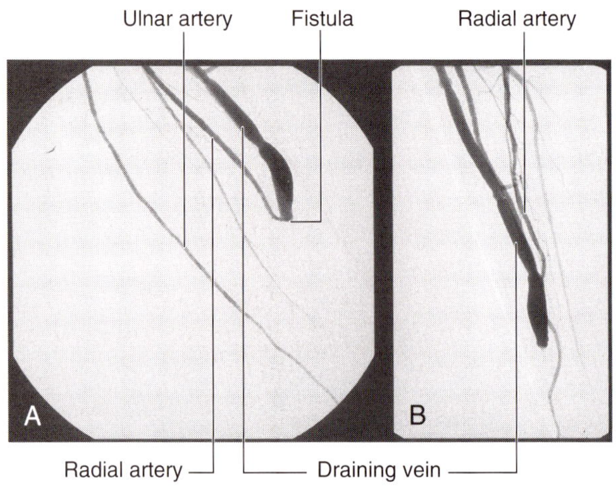

Fig. 2.76 Digital subtraction angiograms of forearm demonstrating a surgically created radiocephalic fistula. **(A)** Anteroposterior view. **(B)** Lateral view.

Early clinical exposure

The median cubital vein is the most commonly used vein for venipuncture because it is large, superficial, anchored by a perforating vein to a deep vein, and separated from the brachial artery by the bicipital aponeurosis.

FOREARM

The forearm is the part of the upper limb that extends between the elbow joint and the wrist joint. Proximally, most major structures pass between the arm and forearm through, or in relation to, the cubital fossa, which is anterior to the elbow joint (Fig. 2.77). The exception is the ulnar nerve, which passes posterior to the medial epicondyle of the humerus.

Distally, structures pass between the forearm and the hand through, or anterior to, the carpal tunnel (Fig. 2.77). The major exception is the radial artery, which passes dorsally around the wrist to enter the hand posteriorly.

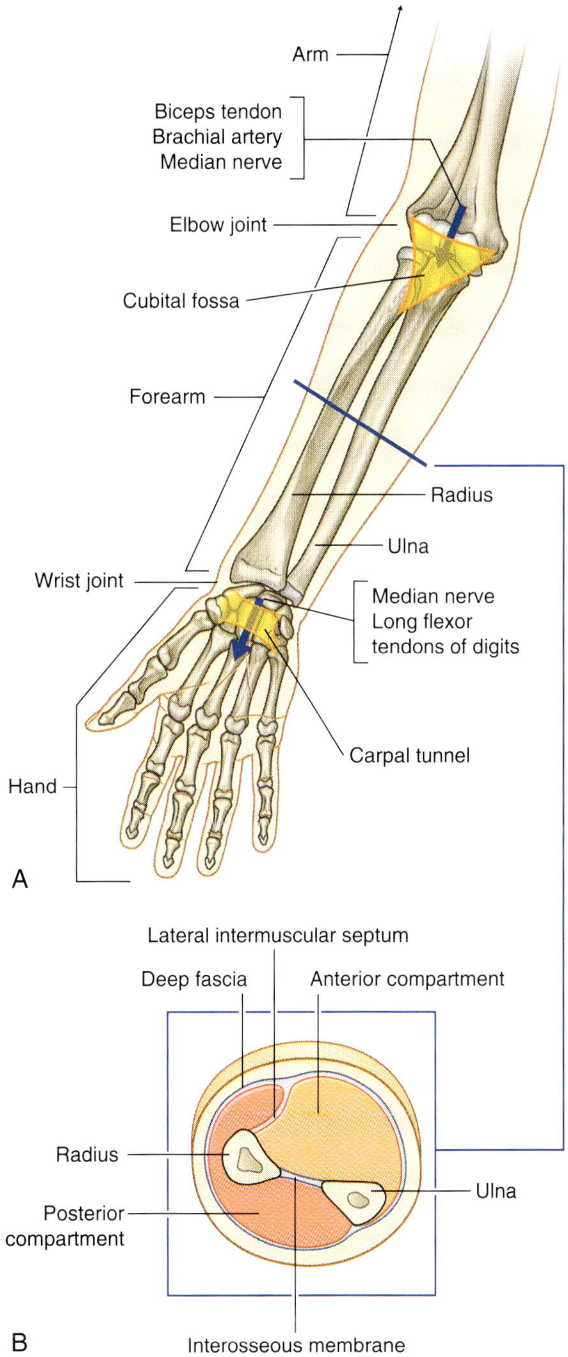

Fig. 2.77 Forearm. **(A)** Proximal and distal relationships of the forearm. **(B)** Transverse section through the middle of the forearm.

The bone framework of the forearm consists of two parallel bones, the radius and the ulna (Figs. 2.77 and 2.78B). The radius is lateral in position and is small proximally, where it articulates with the humerus, and large distally, where it forms the wrist joint with the carpal bones of the hand.

The ulna is medial in the forearm, and its proximal and distal dimensions are the reverse of those for the radius: the ulna is large proximally and small distally. Proximal and distal joints between the radius and the ulna allow the distal end of the radius to swing over the adjacent end of the ulna, resulting in pronation and supination of the forearm.

As in the arm, the forearm is divided into anterior and posterior compartments (Fig. 2.77). In the forearm, these compartments are separated by:

- A lateral intermuscular septum, which passes from the anterior border of the radius to deep fascia surrounding the limb
- An interosseous membrane, which links adjacent borders of the radius and ulna along most of their length
- The attachment of deep fascia along the posterior border of the ulna

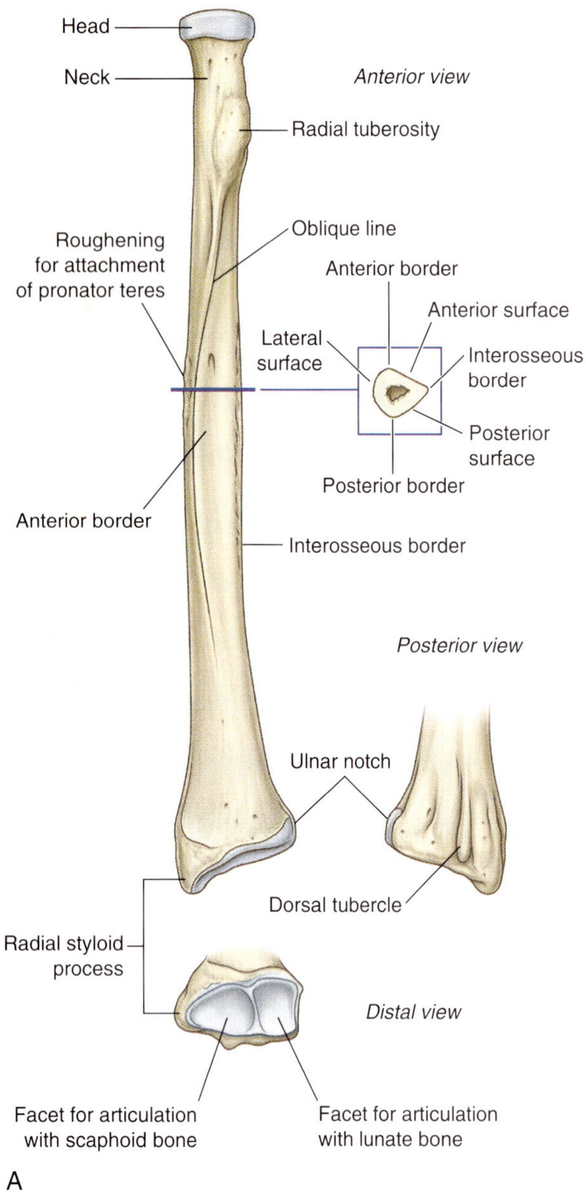

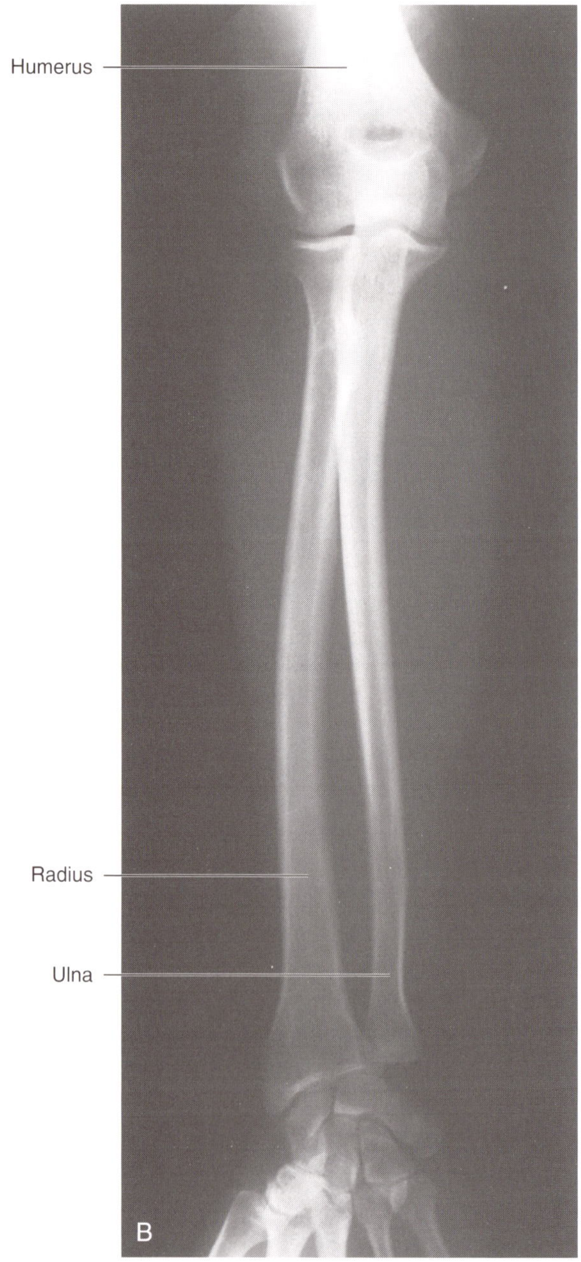

Fig. 2.78 Radius. **(A)** Shaft and distal end of the right radius. **(B)** Radiograph of the forearm (anteroposterior view).

Muscles in the anterior compartment of the forearm flex the wrist and digits and pronate the hand. Muscles in the posterior compartment extend the wrist and digits and supinate the hand. Major nerves and vessels supply or pass through each compartment.

Bones

Shaft and distal end of radius

The shaft of the radius is narrow proximally, where it is continuous with the radial tuberosity and neck, and much broader distally, where it expands to form the distal end (Fig. 2.78).

Throughout most of its length, the shaft of the radius is triangular in cross-section, with:

- Three borders (anterior, posterior, and interosseous)
- Three surfaces (anterior, posterior, and lateral)

The **anterior border** begins on the medial side of the bone as a continuation of the radial tuberosity. In the superior third of the bone, it crosses the shaft diagonally, from medial to lateral, as the oblique line of the radius. The **posterior border** is distinct only in the middle third of the bone. The **interosseous border** is sharp and is the attachment site for the interosseous membrane, which links the radius to the ulna.

The anterior and posterior surfaces of the radius are generally smooth, whereas an oval roughening for the attachment of the pronator teres marks approximately the middle of the lateral surface of the radius.

Viewed anteriorly, the distal end of the radius is broad and somewhat flattened anteroposteriorly (Fig. 2.78). Consequently, the radius has expansive anterior and posterior surfaces and narrow medial and lateral surfaces. Its anterior surface is smooth and unremarkable, except for the prominent sharp ridge that forms its lateral margin.

The **posterior surface** of the radius is characterized by the presence of a large **dorsal tubercle**, which acts as a pulley for the tendon of one of the extensor muscles of the thumb (extensor pollicis longus). The medial surface is marked by a prominent facet for articulation with the distal end of the ulna (Fig. 2.78). The **lateral surface** of the radius is diamond shaped and extends distally as a **radial styloid process**.

The distal end of the bone is marked by two facets for articulation with two carpal bones (the scaphoid and lunate).

Shaft and distal end of ulna

The shaft of the ulna is broad superiorly where it is continuous with the large proximal end and narrow distally to form a small distal head (Fig. 2.79). Like the radius, the shaft of the ulna is triangular in cross-section and has:

- Three borders (anterior, posterior, and interosseous)
- Three surfaces (anterior, posterior, and medial)

The **anterior border** is smooth and rounded. The posterior border is sharp and palpable along its entire length. The **interosseous border** is also sharp and is the attachment

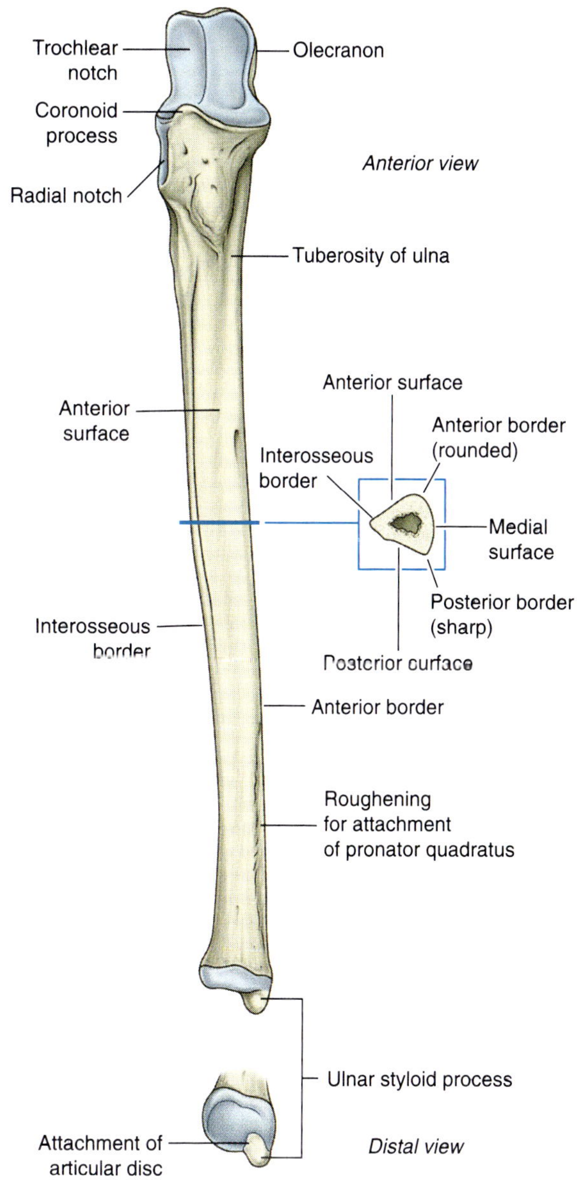

Fig. 2.79 Shaft and distal end of right ulna.

site for the interosseous membrane, which joins the ulna to the radius.

The **anterior surface** of the ulna is smooth, except distally where there is a prominent linear roughening for the attachment of the pronator quadratus muscle. The **medial surface** is smooth and unremarkable. The **posterior surface** is marked by lines, which separate different regions of muscle attachments to bone.

The distal end of the ulna is small and characterized by a rounded head and the **ulnar styloid process** (Fig. 2.79). The anterolateral and distal part of the head is covered by articular cartilage. The ulnar styloid process originates from the posteromedial aspect of the ulna and projects distally.

Early clinical exposure

Fractures of the radius and ulna

The radius and ulna are attached to the humerus proximally and the carpal bones distally by a complex series of ligaments. Although the bones are separate, they behave as one. When a severe injury occurs to the forearm, it usually involves both bones, resulting in either fracture of both bones or more commonly a fracture of one bone and a dislocation of the other. Commonly, the mechanism of injury and the age of the patient determine which of these are likely to occur.

There are three classic injuries to the radius and ulna:

- Monteggia's fracture is a fracture of the proximal third of the ulna and an anterior dislocation of the head of the radius at the elbow.
- Galeazzi's fracture is a fracture of the distal third of the radius associated with subluxation (partial dislocation) of the head of the ulna at the wrist joint.
- Colles' fracture is a fracture, and posterior displacement, of the distal end of the radius.

Whenever a fracture of the radius or ulna is demonstrated radiographically, further images of the elbow and wrist should be obtained to exclude dislocations.

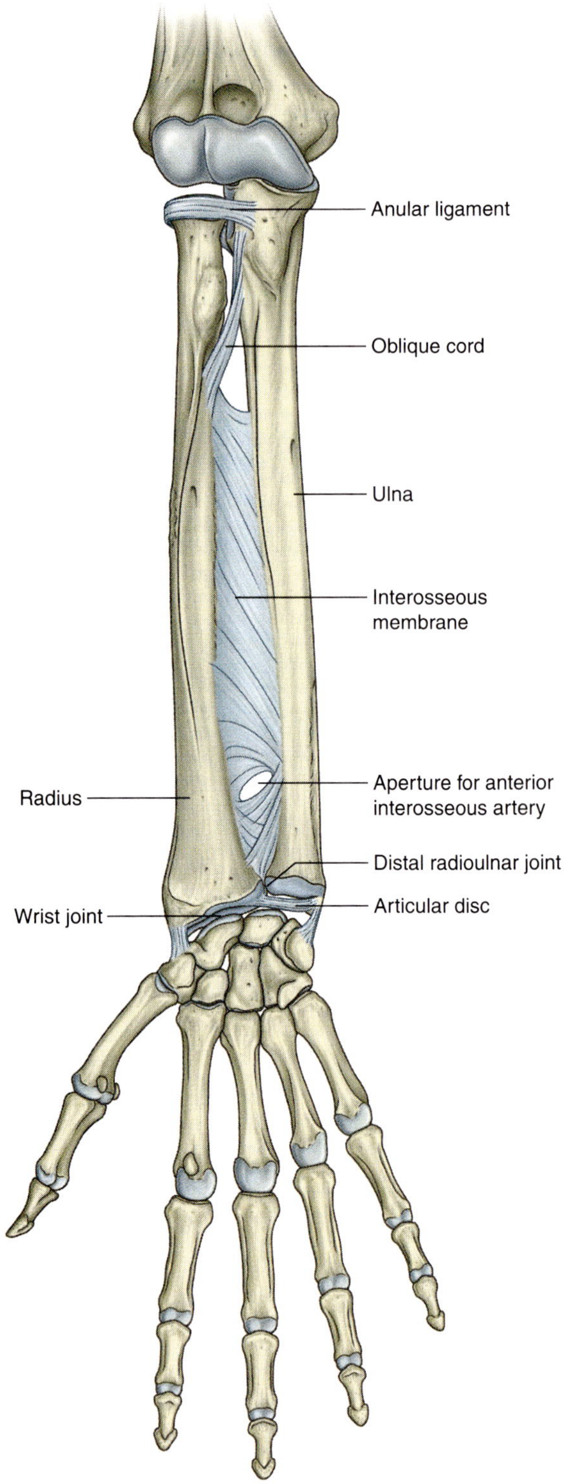

Fig. 2.80 Distal radioulnar joint and the interosseous membrane.

Joints

Distal radioulnar joint

The distal radioulnar joint occurs between the articular surface of the head of the ulna, with the ulnar notch on the end of the radius, and with a fibrous articular disc, which separates the radioulnar joint from the wrist joint (Fig. 2.80).

The triangular-shaped articular disc is attached by its apex to a roughened depression on the ulna between the styloid process and the articular surface of the head, and by its base to the angular margin of the radius between the ulnar notch and the articular surface for the carpal bones.

The synovial membrane is attached to the margins of the distal radioulnar joint and is covered on its external surface by a fibrous joint capsule.

The distal radioulnar joint allows the distal end of the radius to move anteromedially over the ulna.

Interosseous membrane

The interosseous membrane is a thin fibrous sheet that connects the medial and lateral borders of the radius and ulna, respectively (Fig. 2.80). Collagen fibers within the sheet pass predominantly inferiorly from the radius to the ulna.

The interosseous membrane has a free upper margin, which is situated just inferior to the radial tuberosity, and a small circular aperture in its distal third. Vessels pass between the anterior and posterior compartments superior to the upper margin and through the inferior aperture.

The interosseous membrane connects the radius and ulna without restricting pronation and supination and provides attachment for muscles in the anterior and posterior compartments. The orientation of fibers in the membrane is also consistent with its role in transferring forces from the radius to the ulna and ultimately, therefore, from the hand to the humerus.

Pronation and supination

Pronation and supination of the forearm involves movement of the head of the radius at the superior radioulnar joint and movement of the distal end of the radius around the head of the ulna (Fig. 2.81). The axis of this movement is an imaginary line between the head of the radius and the head of the ulna.

At the elbow, the superior articular surface of the radial head spins on the capitulum while, at the same time, the articular surface on the side of the head slides against the radial notch of the ulna and adjacent areas of the joint capsule and annular ligament of the radius. At the distal radioulnar joint, the ulnar notch of the radius slides anteriorly over the convex surface of the head of the ulna. During these movements, the bones are held together by:

- The annular ligament of the radius at the proximal radioulnar joint
- The interosseous membrane along the lengths of the radius and ulna
- The articular disc at the distal radioulnar joint (Fig. 2.81)

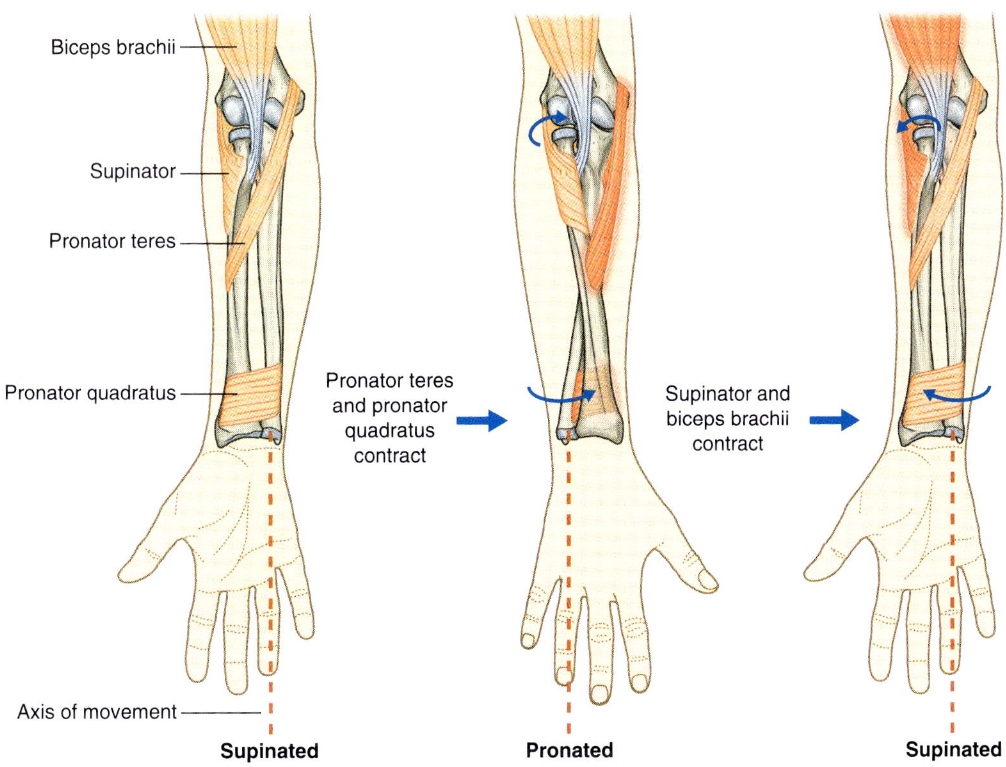

Fig. 2.81 Pronation and supination.

Because the hand articulates predominantly with the radius, the translocation of the distal end of the radius medially over the ulna moves the hand from the palm-anterior (supinated) position to the palm-posterior (pronated) position.

Two muscles supinate and two muscles pronate the hand (Fig. 2.81).

Muscles involved in pronation and supination

Biceps brachii. The biceps brachii muscle, the largest of the four muscles that supinate and pronate the hand, is a powerful supinator as well as a flexor of the elbow joint. It is most effective as a supinator when the forearm is flexed.

Supinator. The second of the muscles involved with supination is the **supinator** muscle. Located in the posterior compartment of the forearm, it has a broad origin, from the supinator crest of the ulna and the lateral epicondyle of the humerus and from ligaments associated with the elbow joint.

The supinator muscle curves around the posterior surface and the lateral surface of the upper third of the radius to attach to the shaft of the radius superior to the oblique line. The arcade between the two layers of supinator that transmit posterior interosseous nerve is known as "arcade of Frohse."

Both the tendon of the biceps brachii muscle and the supinator muscle become wrapped around the proximal end of the radius when the hand is pronated (Fig. 2.81). When they contract, they unwrap from the bone, producing supination of the hand.

Pronator teres and pronator quadratus. Pronation results from the action of the **pronator teres** and **pronator quadratus** muscles (Fig. 2.81). Both these muscles are in the anterior compartment of the forearm:

- The pronator teres runs from the medial epicondyle of the humerus to the lateral surface of the radius, approximately midway along the shaft.
- The pronator quadratus extends between the anterior surfaces of the distal ends of the radius and ulna.

Contraction of these muscles pulls the distal end of the radius ventrally over the ulna, resulting in pronation of the forearm (Fig. 2.81).

Anconeus. In addition to hinge-like flexion and extension at the elbow joint, some abduction of the distal end of the ulna also occurs and maintains the position of the palm of the hand over a central axis during pronation (Fig. 2.82). The muscle involved in this movement is the **anconeus**

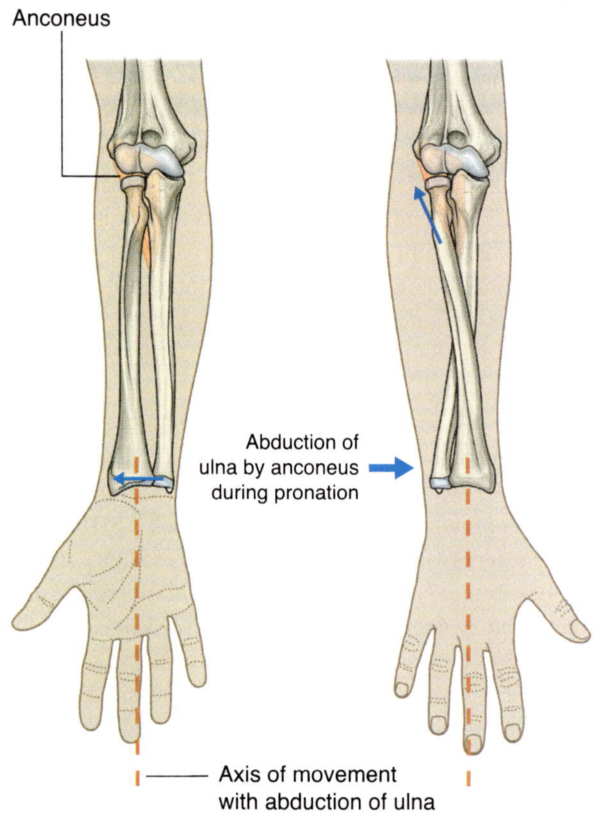

Fig. 2.82 Abduction of the distal end of the ulna by the anconeus during pronation.

muscle, which is a triangular muscle in the posterior compartment of the forearm that runs from the lateral epicondyle to the lateral surface of the proximal end of the ulna.

ANTERIOR COMPARTMENT OF THE FOREARM

SET INDUCTION—CASE SCENARIO 4: WRIST INJURY

A 22-year-old girl was brought to the emergency department with a history of a suicidal cut in her left wrist. On examination she was found to be profusely bleeding from the left wrist and was diagnosed to have ulnar nerve injury and ulnar artery laceration with a partially cut palmaris longus tendon.

Knowledge of the anatomy of the wrist such as relations between tendons of forearm muscles, nerves, and arteries will help the examining doctor to optimally manage the patient.

<table>
<tr><td rowspan="2">REMEMBER
[Recall Facts]</td><td colspan="3">OUTLINE 4. ANTERIOR COMPARTMENT OF FOREARM—LEARNING OBJECTIVES
[By the end of this section the student should be able to:]</td><td colspan="2" rowspan="2">EVALUATE
[Explain Concepts]</td></tr>
<tr><td colspan="3">DEMONSTRATE AND ANALYZE RELATIONSHIPS
[Identify structures in a Prosected Specimen or Figure]</td></tr>
<tr><td rowspan="7">1. Enumerate the muscles of the anterior compartment of forearm and explain their origin, insertion, action, and nerve supply
2. Describe the course and branches of the radial artery
3. Describe the course and branches of the ulnar artery
4. Describe the course and distribution of the median nerve, ulnar nerve, and radial nerve in anterior compartment of the forearm</td><td>Level I</td><td>Level II</td><td>Level III</td><td colspan="2" rowspan="2">■ Attachment and action of these muscles
■ Course of median nerve, ulnar nerve and vessels, superficial branch of radial nerve, and radial vessels in forearm
■ Course of anterior interosseous vessels and nerve</td></tr>
<tr><td rowspan="6">■ Superficial group (in order from lateral to medial):
  ■ Pronator teres
  ■ Flexor carpi radialis
  ■ Palmaris longus
  ■ Flexor carpi ulnaris
■ Middle group:
  ■ Flexor digitorum superficialis
■ Ulnar vessels
■ Ulnar nerve
■ Radial vessels
■ Superficial branch of radial nerve
■ Median nerve
■ Deep group:
  ■ Flexor digitorum profundus
  ■ Flexor pollicis longus
  ■ Pronator quadratus
  ■ Interosseous membrane</td><td rowspan="6">■ Lateral cutaneous nerve of forearm
■ Medial cutaneous nerve of forearm
■ Basilic vein
■ Cephalic vein
■ Common interosseous branch of ulnar artery
■ Anterior interosseous nerve
■ Anterior interosseous artery</td><td rowspan="6">■ Palmar cutaneous branch of ulnar nerve
■ Dorsal branch of ulnar nerve
■ Other branches of ulnar artery
■ Branches of radial artery
■ Palmar branch of median nerve</td></tr>
<tr><td colspan="2">EARLY CLINICAL EXPOSURE
[Apply Anatomical Knowledge]</td></tr>
<tr><td>Surgical Anatomy/ Pathology/ Trauma</td><td>Imaging/ Surface Anatomy</td></tr>
<tr><td>■ Pronator teres syndrome
■ Cubital tunnel syndrome
■ Volkmann's ischemic contracture
■ Transection of radial and ulnar artery</td><td>■ Palpation of radial artery</td></tr>
<tr><td colspan="2">PROBLEM SOLVING/ CLINICAL CASES
[Interpret]</td></tr>
<tr><td colspan="2">■ Median nerve compression</td></tr>
</table>

Muscles

Muscles in the anterior (flexor) compartment of the forearm occur in three layers: superficial, intermediate, and deep. Generally, these muscles are associated with:

- Movements of the wrist joint
- Flexion of the fingers including the thumb
- Pronation

All muscles in the anterior compartment of the forearm are innervated by the median nerve, except for the flexor carpi ulnaris muscle and the medial half of the flexor digitorum profundus muscle, which are innervated by the ulnar nerve.

Superficial layer

All four muscles in the superficial layer—the flexor carpi ulnaris, palmaris longus, flexor carpi radialis, and pronator teres—have a common origin from the medial epicondyle of the humerus, and, except for the pronator teres, extend distally from the forearm into the hand (Fig. 2.83 and Table 2.10).

Flexor carpi ulnaris

The **flexor carpi ulnaris** muscle is the most medial of the muscles in the superficial layer of flexors, having a long linear origin from the olecranon and posterior border of the ulna, in addition to an origin from the medial epicondyle of the humerus (Fig. 2.83A and B).

The ulnar nerve enters the anterior compartment of the forearm by passing through the triangular gap between the humeral and ulnar heads of the flexor carpi ulnaris (Fig. 2.83B). The muscle fibers converge on a tendon that passes distally and attaches to the pisiform bone of the wrist. From this point, force is transferred to the hamate bone of the wrist and to the base of metacarpal V by the **pisohamate** and **pisometacarpal ligaments**.

The flexor carpi ulnaris muscle is a powerful flexor and adductor of the wrist and is innervated by the ulnar nerve (Table 2.10).

Palmaris longus

The **palmaris longus** muscle, which is absent in about 15% of the population, lies between the flexor carpi ulnaris and the flexor carpi radialis muscles (Fig. 2.83A). It is a spindle-shaped muscle with a long tendon, which passes into the hand and attaches to the flexor retinaculum and to a thick layer of deep fascia, the palmar aponeurosis, which underlies and is attached to the skin of the palm and fingers.

In addition to its role as an accessory flexor of the wrist joint, the palmaris longus muscle also opposes shearing forces on the skin of the palm during gripping (Table 2.10).

Flexor carpi radialis

The **flexor carpi radialis** muscle is lateral to the palmaris longus and has a large and prominent tendon in the distal half of the forearm (Fig. 2.83A and Table 2.10). Unlike the tendon of the flexor carpi ulnaris, which forms the medial margin of the distal forearm, the tendon of the flexor carpi radialis muscle is positioned just lateral to the midline. In this position, the tendon can be easily palpated, making it an important landmark for finding the pulse in the radial artery, which lies immediately lateral to it.

The tendon of the flexor carpi radialis passes through a compartment formed by bone and fascia on the lateral side

Table 2.10 Superficial layer of muscles in the anterior compartment of the forearm

Muscle	Origin	Insertion	Innervation	Function
Flexor carpi ulnaris	Humeral head—medial epicondyle of humerus; ulnar head—olecranon and posterior border of ulna	Pisiform bone, and then via pisohamate and pisometacarpal ligaments into the hamate and base of metacarpal V	Ulnar nerve (C7, **C8**, T1)	Flexes and adducts the wrist joint
Palmaris longus	Medial epicondyle of humerus	Palmar aponeurosis of hand	Median nerve (**C7, C8**)	Flexes wrist joint; because the palmar aponeurosis anchors skin of the hand, contraction of the muscle resists shearing forces when gripping
Flexor carpi radialis	Medial epicondyle of humerus	Base of metacarpals II and III	Median nerve (**C6, C7**)	Flexes and abducts the wrist
Pronator teres	Humeral head—medial epicondyle and adjacent supraepicondylar ridge; ulnar head—medial side of coronoid process	Roughening on lateral surface, midshaft of radius	Median nerve (**C6, C7**)	Pronation

Note: Spinal segments indicated in bold are the major segments innervating the muscle.

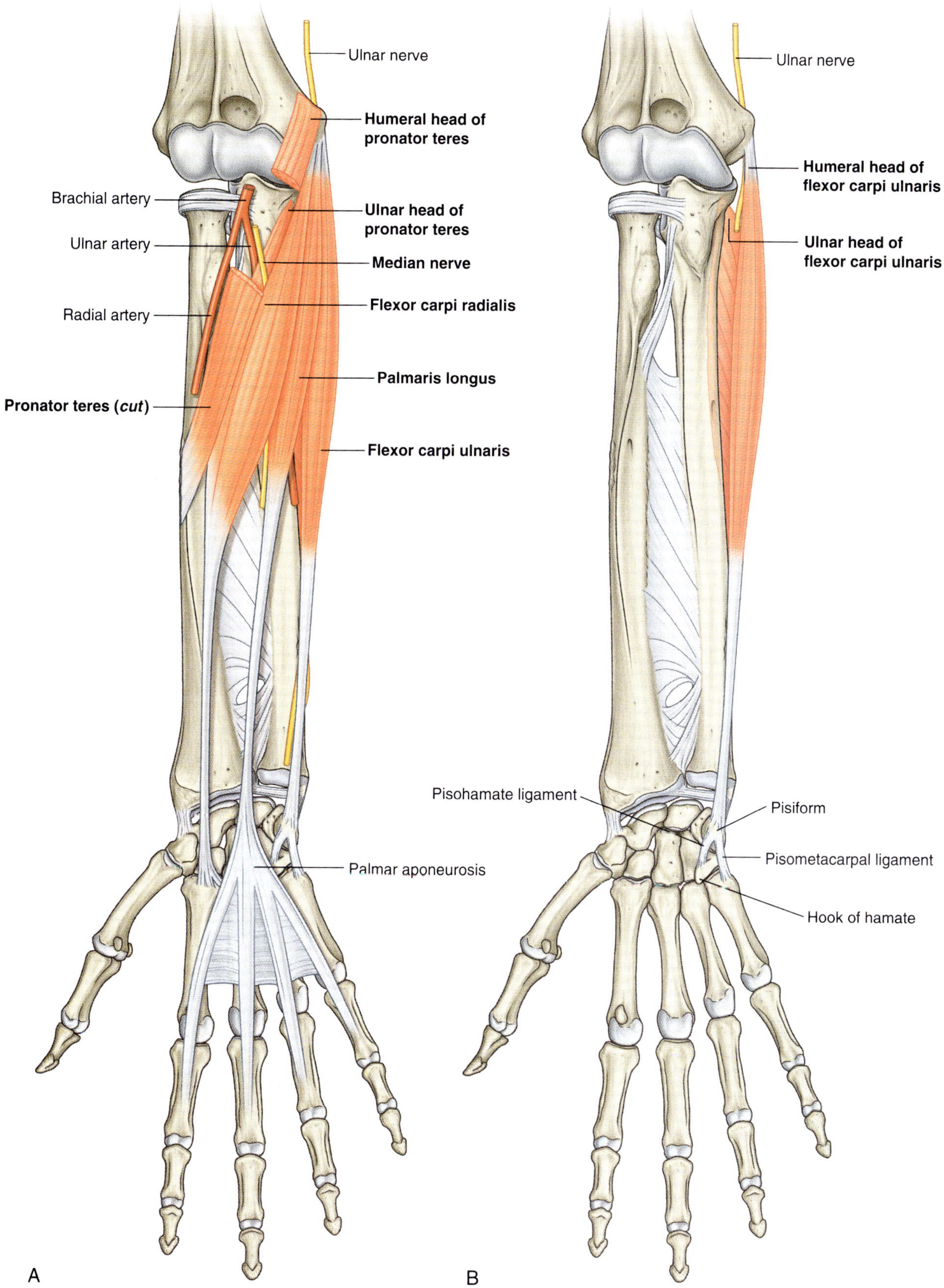

Fig. 2.83 Superficial layer of forearm muscles. **(A)** Superficial muscles (flexor retinaculum not shown). **(B)** Flexor carpi ulnaris muscle.

of the anterior surface of the wrist and attaches to the anterior surfaces of the bases of metacarpals II and III.

The flexor carpi radialis is a powerful flexor of the wrist and can also abduct the wrist.

Pronator teres

The **pronator teres** muscle originates from the medial epicondyle and supraepicondylar ridge of the humerus and from a small linear region on the medial edge of the coronoid process of the ulna (Fig. 2.83A). The median nerve often exits the cubital fossa by passing between the humeral and ulnar heads of this muscle. The pronator teres crosses the forearm and attaches to an oval roughened area on the lateral surface of the radius approximately midway along the bone.

The pronator teres forms the medial border of the cubital fossa and rotates the radius over the ulna during pronation (Table 2.10).

Intermediate layer

Flexor digitorum superficialis

The muscle in the intermediate layer of the anterior compartment of the forearm is the **flexor digitorum superficialis** muscle (Fig. 2.84). This large muscle has two heads:

- The humeroulnar head, which originates mainly from the medial epicondyle of the humerus and from the adjacent medial edge of the coronoid process of the ulna
- The radial head, which originates from the anterior oblique line of the radius

The median nerve and ulnar artery pass deep to the flexor digitorum superficialis between the two heads.

In the distal forearm, the flexor digitorum superficialis forms four tendons, which pass through the carpal tunnel of the wrist and into the four fingers. The tendons for the ring and middle fingers are superficial to the tendons for the index and little fingers.

In the forearm, carpal tunnel, and proximal regions of the four fingers, the tendons of the flexor digitorum superficialis are anterior to the tendons of the flexor digitorum profundus muscle.

Near the base of the proximal phalanx of each finger, the tendon of the flexor digitorum superficialis splits into two parts to pass posteriorly around each side of the tendon of the flexor digitorum profundus and ultimately attach to the margins of the middle phalanx (Fig. 2.84).

The flexor digitorum superficialis flexes the metacarpophalangeal joint and proximal interphalangeal joint of each finger; it also flexes the wrist joint (Table 2.11).

Deep layer

There are three deep muscles in the anterior compartment of the forearm: the flexor digitorum profundus, flexor pollicis longus, and pronator quadratus (Fig. 2.85).

Table 2.11 Intermediate layer of muscles in the anterior compartment of the forearm

Muscle	Origin	Insertion	Innervation	Function
Flexor digitorum superficialis	Humeroulnar head—medial epicondyle of humerus and adjacent margin of coronoid process; radial head—oblique line of radius	Four tendons, which attach to the palmar surfaces of the middle phalanges of the index, middle, ring, and little fingers	Median nerve (**C8**, T1)	Flexes proximal interphalangeal joints of the index, middle, ring, and little fingers; can also flex metacarpophalangeal joints of the same fingers and the wrist joint

Note: Spinal segment indicated in bold is the major segment innervating the muscle.

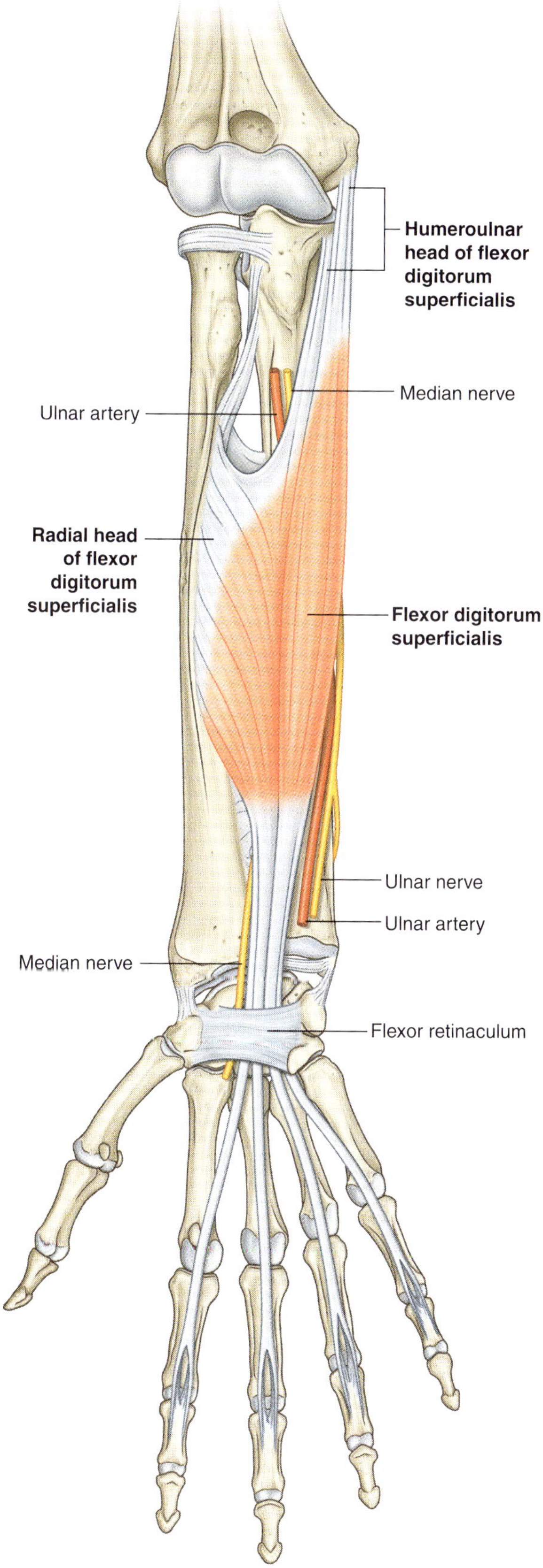

Fig. 2.84 Intermediate layer of forearm muscles.

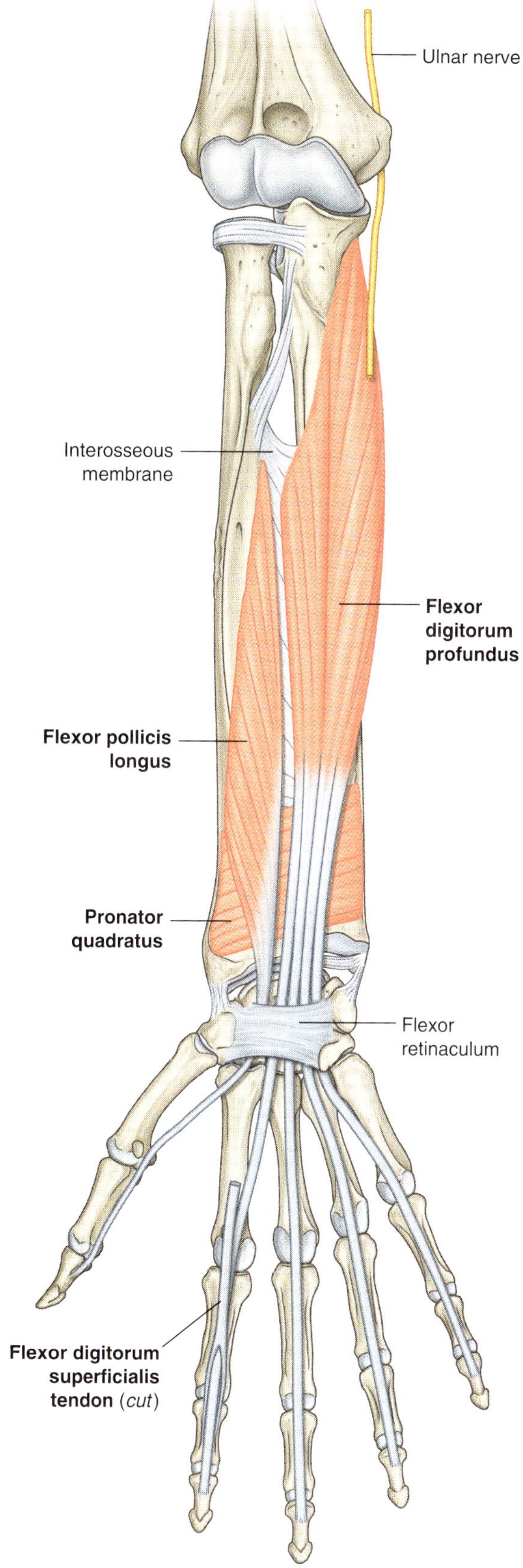

Fig. 2.85 Deep layer of forearm muscles.

Flexor digitorum profundus

The **flexor digitorum profundus** muscle originates from the anterior and medial surfaces of the ulna and from the adjacent half of the anterior surface of the interosseous membrane (Fig. 2.85). It gives rise to four tendons, which pass through the carpal tunnel into the four medial fingers. Throughout most of their course, the tendons are deep to the tendons of the flexor digitorum superficialis muscle.

Opposite the proximal phalanx of each finger, each tendon of the flexor digitorum profundus passes through a split formed in the overlying tendon of the flexor digitorum superficialis muscle and passes distally to insert into the anterior surface of the base of the distal phalanx.

In the palm, the lumbrical muscles originate from the sides of the tendons of the flexor digitorum profundus (see Fig. 2.104).

Innervation of the medial and lateral halves of the flexor digitorum profundus varies as follows:

- The lateral half (associated with the index and middle fingers) is innervated by the anterior interosseous nerve (branch of the median nerve).
- The medial half (the part associated with the ring and little fingers) is innervated by the ulnar nerve.

The flexor digitorum profundus flexes the metacarpophalangeal joints and the proximal and distal interphalangeal joints of the four fingers. Because the tendons cross the wrist, it can flex the wrist joint as well (Table 2.12).

Flexor pollicis longus

The **flexor pollicis longus** muscle originates from the anterior surface of the radius and the adjacent half of the anterior surface of the interosseous membrane (Fig. 2.85). It is a powerful muscle and forms a single large tendon, which passes through the carpal tunnel, lateral to the tendons of the flexor digitorum superficialis and flexor digitorum profundus muscles, and into the thumb where it attaches to the base of the distal phalanx.

Hence, the flexor pollicis longus flexes the thumb and is innervated by the anterior interosseous nerve (branch of the median nerve) (Table 2.12).

Pronator quadratus

The **pronator quadratus** muscle is a flat square-shaped muscle in the distal forearm (Fig. 2.85). It originates from a linear ridge on the anterior surface of the lower end of the ulna and passes laterally to insert onto the flat anterior surface of the radius. It lies deep to, and is crossed by, the tendons of the flexor digitorum profundus and flexor pollicis longus muscles.

The pronator quadratus muscle pulls the distal end of the radius anteriorly over the ulna during pronation and is innervated by the anterior interosseous nerve (branch of the median nerve) (Table 2.12).

Table 2.12 Deep layer of muscles in the anterior compartment of the forearm

Muscle	Origin	Insertion	Innervation	Function
Flexor digitorum profundus	Anterior and medial surfaces of ulna and anterior medial half of interosseous membrane	Four tendons, which attach to the palmar surfaces of the distal phalanges of the index, middle, ring, and little fingers	Lateral half by median nerve (anterior interosseous nerve); medial half by ulnar nerve (**C8**, T1)	Flexes distal interphalangeal joints of the index, middle, ring, and little fingers; can also flex metacarpophalangeal joints of the same fingers and the wrist joint
Flexor pollicis longus	Anterior surface of radius and radial half of interosseous membrane	Palmar surface of base of distal phalanx of thumb	Median nerve (anterior interosseous nerve) (C7, **C8**)	Flexes interphalangeal joint of the thumb; can also flex metacarpophalangeal joint of the thumb
Pronator quadratus	Linear ridge on distal anterior surface of ulna	Distal anterior surface of radius	Median nerve (anterior interosseous nerve) (C7, **C8**)	Pronation

Note: Spinal segments indicated in bold are the major segments innervating the muscle.

Arteries and veins

The largest arteries in the forearm are in the anterior compartment, pass distally to supply the hand, and give rise to vessels that supply the posterior compartment (Fig. 2.86).

The brachial artery enters the forearm from the arm by passing through the cubital fossa. At the apex of the cubital fossa, it divides into its two major branches, the radial and ulnar arteries.

Radial artery

The radial artery originates from the brachial artery at approximately the neck of the radius and passes along the lateral aspect of the forearm (Fig. 2.86). It is:

- Just deep to the brachioradialis muscle in the proximal half of the forearm
- Related on its lateral side to the superficial branch of the radial nerve in the middle third of the forearm
- Medial to the tendon of the brachioradialis muscle and covered only by deep fascia, superficial fascia, and skin in the distal forearm

In the distal forearm, the radial artery lies immediately lateral to the large tendon of the flexor carpi radialis muscle and directly anterior to the pronator quadratus muscle and the distal end of the radius (Fig. 2.86). In the distal forearm, the radial artery can be located using the flexor carpi radialis muscle as a landmark. The radial pulse can be felt by gently palpating the radial artery against the underlying muscle and bone.

The radial artery leaves the forearm, passes around the lateral side of the wrist, and penetrates the posterolateral aspect of the hand between the bases of metacarpals I and II (Fig. 2.86). Branches of the radial artery in the hand often provide the major blood supply to the thumb and lateral side of the index finger.

Branches of the radial artery originating in the forearm include:

- A **radial recurrent artery**, which contributes to an anastomotic network around the elbow joint and to

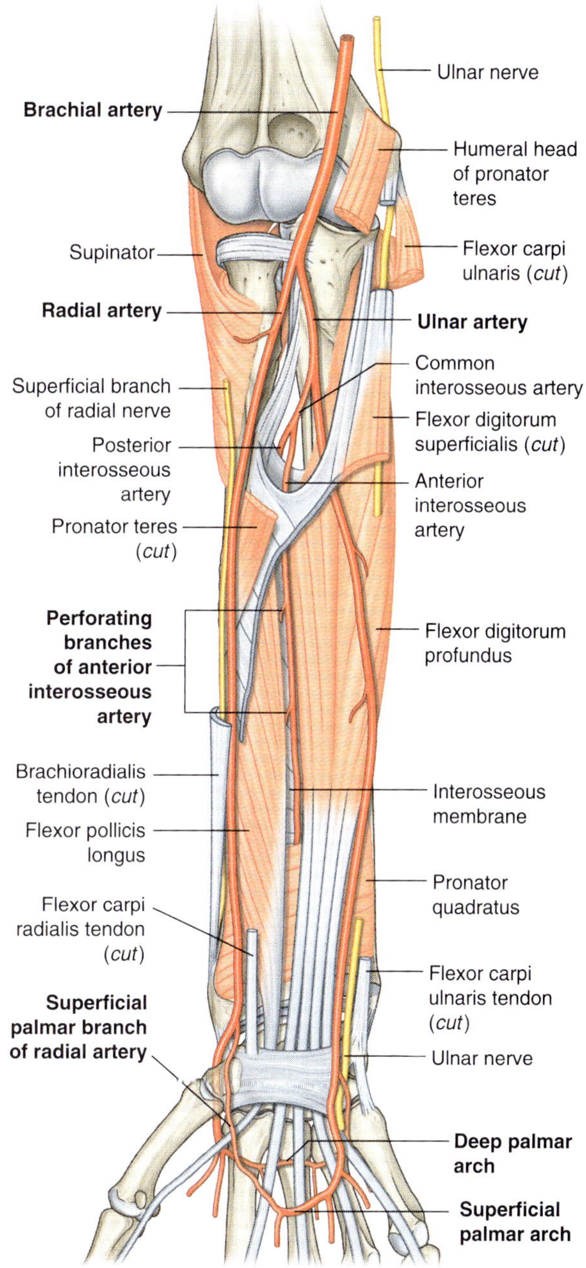

Fig. 2.86 Arteries of the anterior compartment of the forearm.

numerous vessels that supply muscles on the lateral side of the forearm (see Fig. 2.66B)

- A small **palmar carpal branch**, which contributes to an anastomotic network of vessels that supply the carpal bones and joints
- A somewhat larger branch, the **superficial palmar branch**, which enters the hand by passing through, or superficial to, the thenar muscles at the base of the thumb (Fig. 2.86) and anastomoses with the superficial palmar arch formed by the ulnar artery

Ulnar artery

The ulnar artery is larger than the radial artery and passes down the medial side of the forearm (Fig. 2.86). It leaves the cubital fossa by passing deep to the pronator teres muscle, and then passes through the forearm in the fascial plane between the flexor carpi ulnaris and flexor digitorum profundus muscles.

In the distal forearm, the ulnar artery often remains tucked under the anterolateral lip of the flexor carpi ulnaris tendon, and is therefore not easily palpable.

In distal regions of the forearm, the ulnar nerve is immediately medial to the ulnar artery.

The ulnar artery leaves the forearm, enters the hand by passing lateral to the pisiform bone and superficial to the flexor retinaculum of the wrist, and arches over the palm (Fig. 2.86). It is often the major blood supply to the medial three and one-half digits.

Branches of the ulnar artery that arise in the forearm include:

- The **ulnar recurrent artery** with **anterior** and **posterior branches**, which contribute to an anastomotic network of vessels around the elbow joint
- Numerous muscular arteries, which supply surrounding muscles
- The **common interosseous artery**, which divides into anterior and posterior interosseous arteries (Fig. 2.86)
- Two small carpal arteries (**dorsal carpal branch** and **palmar carpal branch**), which supply the wrist

The **posterior interosseous artery** passes dorsally over the proximal margin of the interosseous membrane into the posterior compartment of the forearm.

The **anterior interosseous artery** passes distally along the anterior aspect of the interosseous membrane and supplies muscles of the deep compartment of the forearm and the radius and ulna. It has numerous branches, which perforate the interosseous membrane to supply deep muscles of the posterior compartment; it also has a small branch, which contributes to the vascular network around the carpal bones and joints. Perforating the interosseous membrane in the distal forearm, the anterior interosseous artery terminates by joining the posterior interosseous artery.

Veins

Deep veins of the anterior compartment generally accompany the arteries and ultimately drain into brachial veins associated with the brachial artery in the cubital fossa.

Early clinical exposure

Transection of the radial or ulnar artery

Adult patients may transect the radial or ulnar artery because these vessels are relatively subcutaneous. A typical method of injury is when the hand is forced through a plate glass window. Fortunately, the dual supply to the hand usually enables the surgeon to tie off either the ulnar or the radial artery, without significant consequence. The use of collateral circulation in the hand is also seen when the radial artery is resected as a graft for a coronary artery bypass. The ulnar artery can supply the thumb through the deep and superficial palmar arches which connect the ulnar and radial arteries.

Nerves

Nerves in the anterior compartment of the forearm are the median and ulnar nerves and the superficial branch of the radial nerve (Fig. 2.87).

Median nerve

The median nerve innervates the muscles in the anterior compartment of the forearm except for the flexor carpi ulnaris and the medial part of the flexor digitorum profundus (ring and little fingers). It leaves the cubital fossa by passing between the two heads of the pronator teres muscle and passing between the humeroulnar and radial heads of the flexor digitorum superficialis muscle (Fig. 2.87).

The median nerve continues a straight linear course distally down the forearm in the fascia on the deep surface of the flexor digitorum superficialis muscle. Just proximal to the wrist, it moves around the lateral side of the muscle and becomes more superficial in position, lying between the tendons of the palmaris longus and flexor carpi radialis muscles. It leaves the forearm and enters the palm of the hand by passing through the carpal tunnel deep to the flexor retinaculum.

Most branches to the muscles in the superficial and intermediate layers of the forearm originate medially from the nerve just distal to the elbow joint.

- The largest branch of the median nerve in the forearm is the **anterior interosseous nerve**, which originates between the two heads of the pronator teres, passes distally down the forearm with the anterior interosseous artery, innervates the muscles in the deep layer (the flexor pollicis longus, the lateral half of the flexor digitorum profundus, and the pronator quadratus), and terminates as articular branches to joints of the distal forearm and wrist.
- A small palmar branch originates from the median nerve in the distal forearm immediately proximal to the flexor retinaculum (Fig. 2.87), passes superficial to the flexor retinaculum into the hand, and innervates the skin over the base of the thumb and central palm. This palmar branch is spared in carpal tunnel syndrome because of its course superficial to the flexor retinaculum of the wrist (Flowchart 2.4).

Ulnar nerve

The ulnar nerve passes through the forearm and into the hand, where most of its major branches occur. In the forearm, the ulnar nerve innervates only the flexor carpi ulnaris muscle and the medial part (ring and little fingers) of the flexor digitorum profundus muscle (Fig. 2.87).

The ulnar nerve enters the anterior compartment of the forearm by passing posteriorly around the medial epicondyle

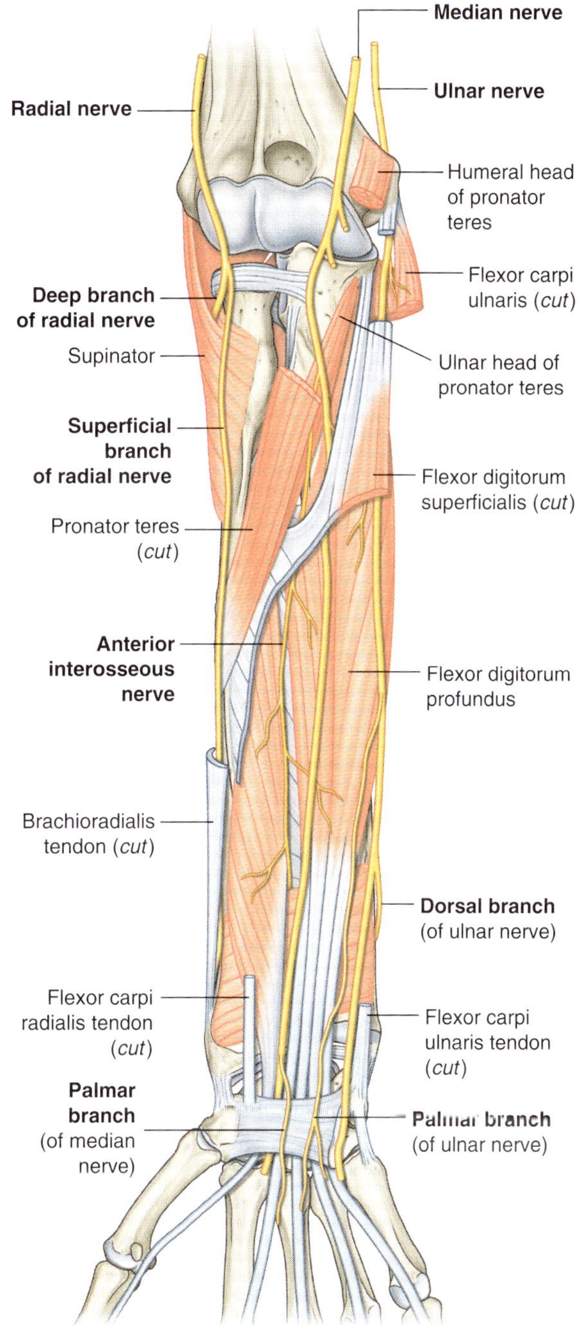

Fig. 2.87 Nerves of anterior forearm.

of the humerus and between the humeral and ulnar heads of the flexor carpi ulnaris muscle. After passing down the medial side of the forearm in the plane between the flexor carpi ulnaris and the flexor digitorum profundus muscles, it lies under the lateral lip of the tendon of the flexor carpi ulnaris proximal to the wrist.

The ulnar artery is lateral to the ulnar nerve in the distal two-thirds of the forearm, and both the ulnar artery and nerve enter the hand by passing superficial to the flexor retinaculum and immediately lateral to the pisiform bone (Fig. 2.87).

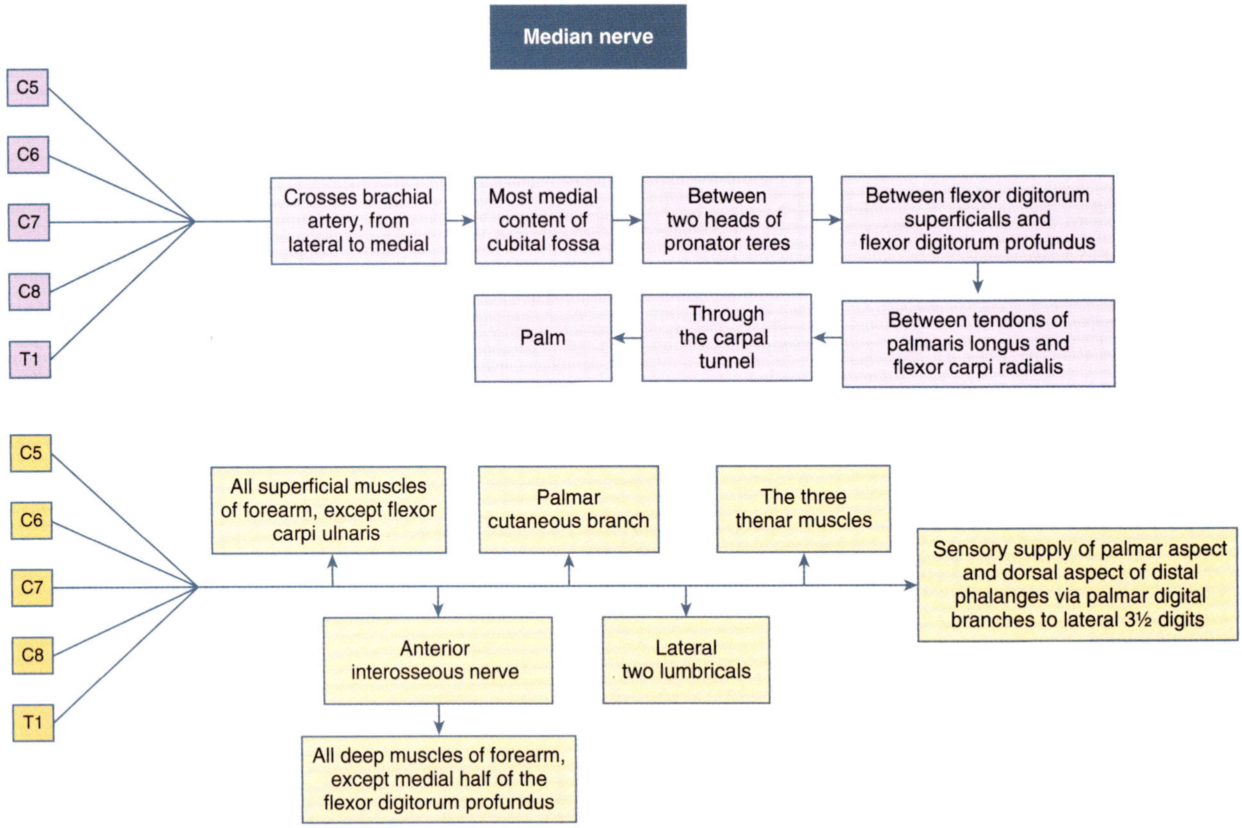

Flowchart 2.4 Course and supply of median nerve.

In the forearm, the ulnar nerve gives rise to:

- **Muscular branches** to the flexor carpi ulnaris and to the medial half of the flexor digitorum profundus that arise soon after the ulnar nerve enters the forearm.
- Two small cutaneous branches—the **palmar branch** originates in the middle of the forearm and passes into the hand to supply skin on the medial side of the palm; the larger **dorsal branch** originates from the ulnar nerve in the distal forearm and passes posteriorly deep to the tendon of the flexor carpi ulnaris and innervates skin on the posteromedial side of the back of the hand and most of the skin on the posterior surfaces of the medial one and a half digits (Flowchart 2.5).

Radial nerve

The radial nerve bifurcates into deep and superficial branches under the margin of the brachioradialis muscle in the lateral border of the cubital fossa (Fig. 2.87).

- The **deep branch** is predominantly motor and passes between the superficial and deep layers of the supinator muscle to access and supply muscles in the posterior compartment of the forearm.
- The **superficial branch** of the radial nerve is sensory. It passes down the anterolateral aspect of the forearm deep to the brachioradialis muscle along with the radial artery. Approximately two-thirds of the way down the forearm, the superficial branch of the radial nerve passes laterally and posteriorly around the radial side of the forearm deep to the tendon of the brachioradialis. The nerve continues into the hand where it innervates skin on the posterolateral surface (Flowchart 2.6 and LD 2.6.1).

Early clinical exposure

Pronator teres syndrome

This is entrapment of the median nerve between the two heads of the pronator teres or entrapment by the ligament of Struthers. The ligament of Struther is a fibrous band connecting the medial epicondyle to a supracondylar spur of bone.

Wartenberg's syndrome/cheiralgia paraesthetica

Gk cheir, hand; algos, pain. This is the entrapment of the superficial branch of radial nerve between brachioradialis and extensor carpi radialis longus.

Cubital tunnel syndrome

This is entrapment of the ulnar nerve between the two heads of flexor carpi ulnaris.

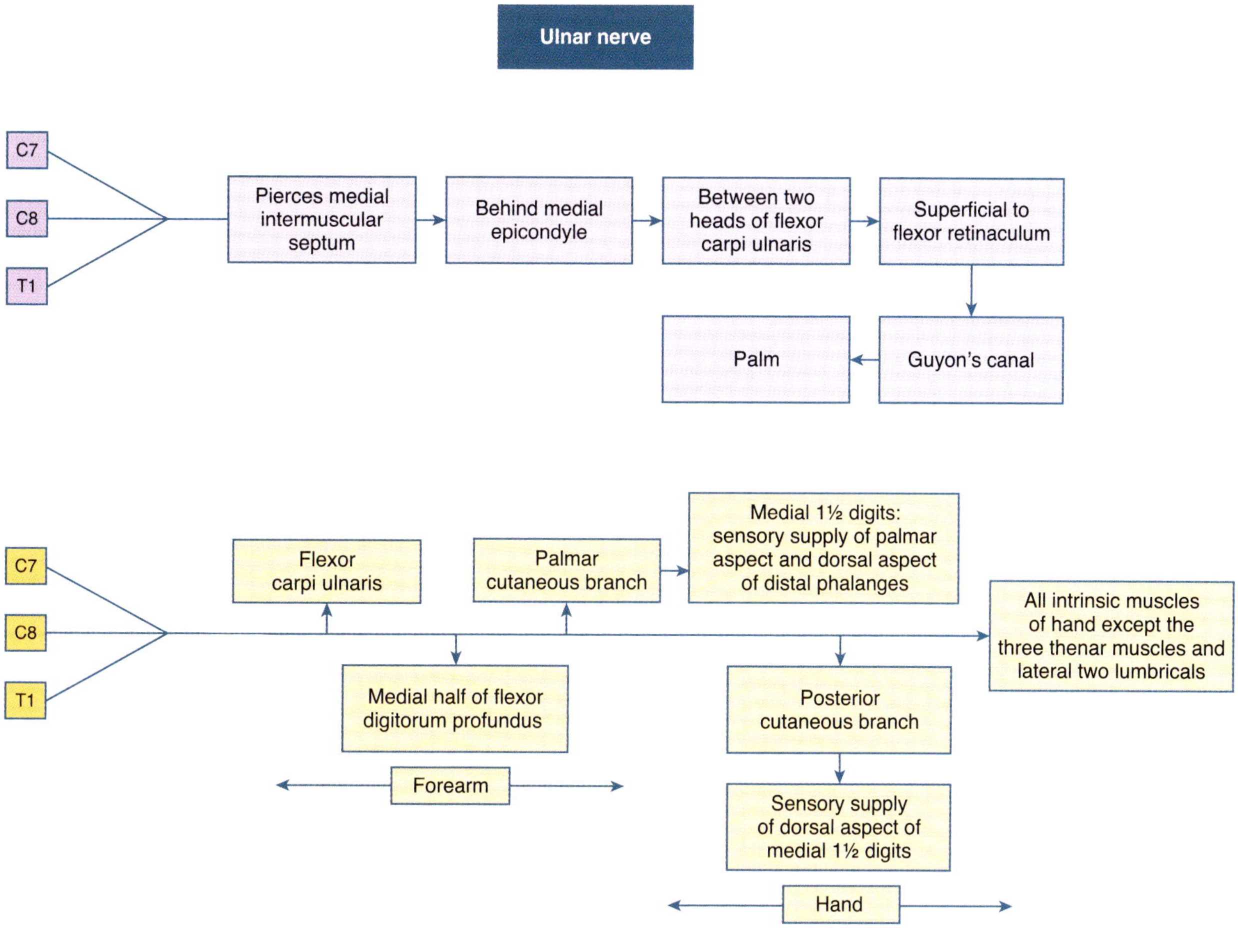

Flowchart 2.5 Course and supply of ulnar nerve.

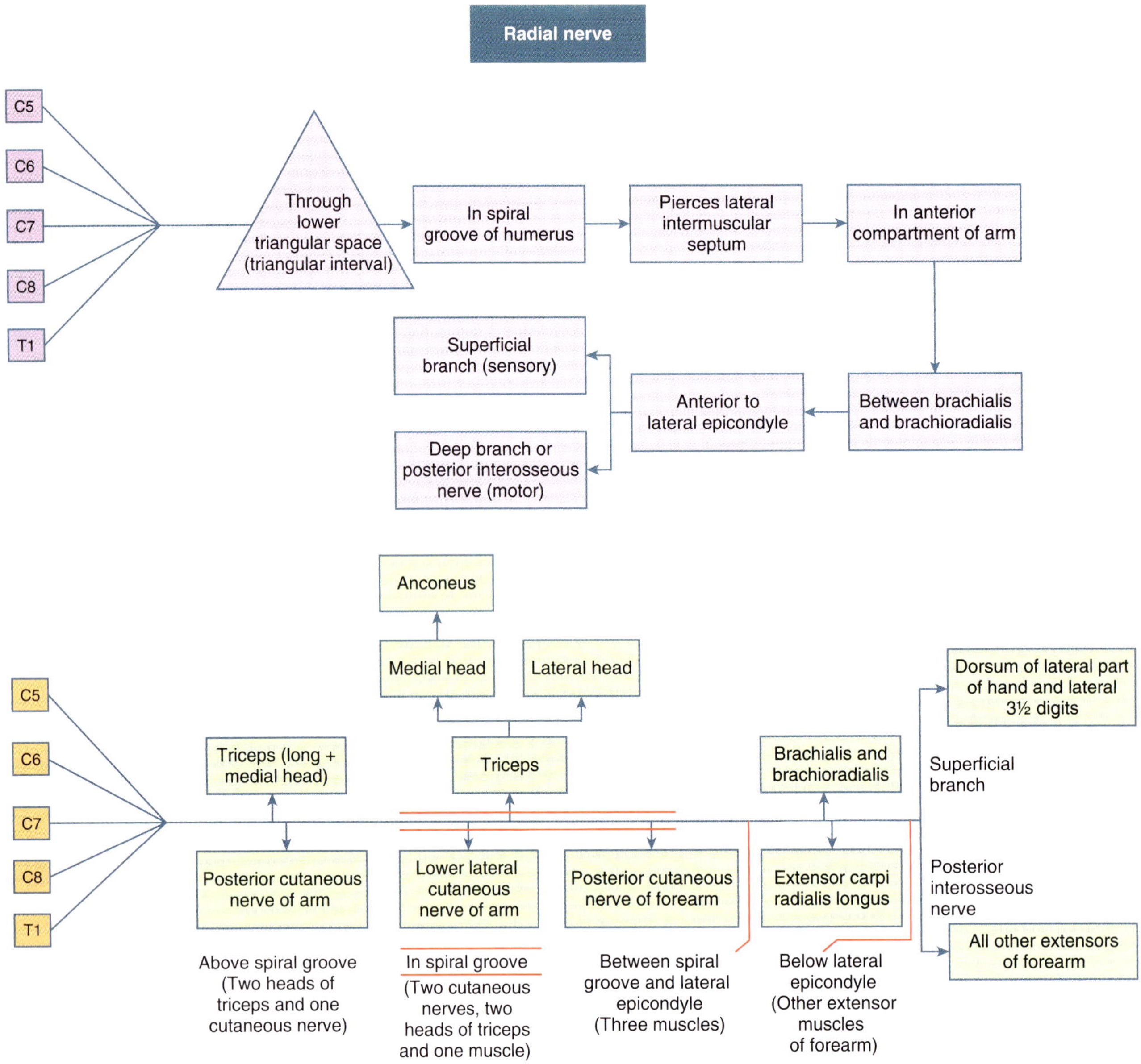

Flowchart 2.6 Course and supply of radial nerve.

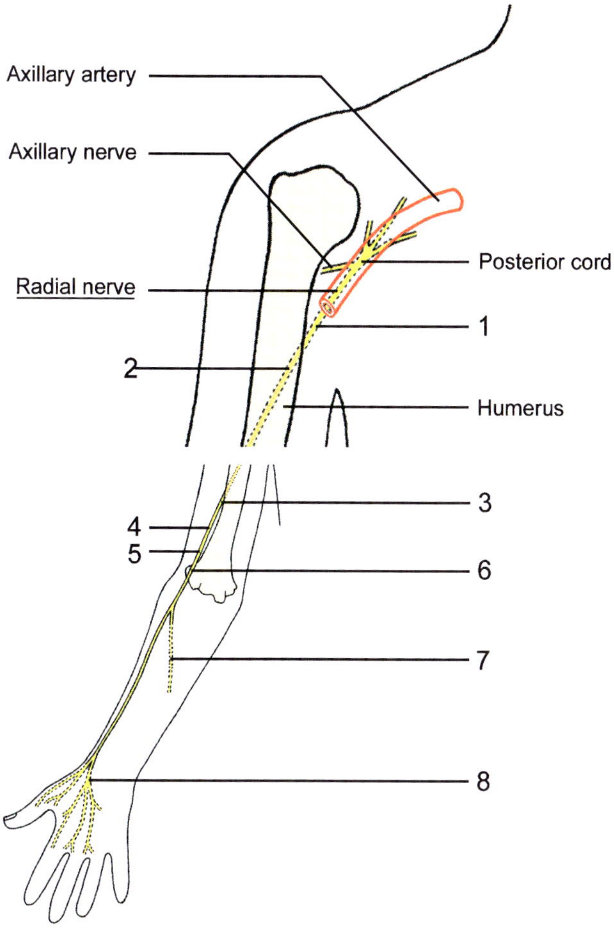

LD 2.6.1 Radial nerve.

Questions

2.6.1A How and where does the radial nerve begin and end?

2.6.1B Name the structures or sites indicated by the labels.

Answers

2.6.1A The origin and termination of the radial nerve are

Origin: As the continuation of the posterior cord after the posterior cord gives off the axillary nerve

Termination: By dividing into the deep and superficial branches of the radial nerve in the lateral wall of the cubital fossa

2.6.1B The structures or sites indicated by the labels are

1. Radial nerve above the spiral groove
2. Radial nerve in the spiral groove
3. Site of the origin of the branch to the brachialis
4. Site of the origin of the branch to the brachioradialis
5. Site of the origin of the branch to the extensor carpi radialis longus
6. Radial nerve in front of the lateral epicondyle
7. Posterior interosseous nerve
8. A terminal branch of the superficial branch of the radial nerve.

POSTERIOR COMPARTMENT OF THE FOREARM

SET INDUCTION—CASE SCENARIO 5: RADIAL NERVE INJURY

A 40-year-old alcoholic fell asleep in his chair with the back of the chair wedged into his right axilla. When he woke up in the morning, he was unable to extend his right wrist and fingers. On examination he was diagnosed to have Saturday night palsy. In this condition, the radial nerve gets compressed and injured in the spiral groove of the humerus resulting in paralysis of all extensor muscles of the forearm.

In order to make such a diagnosis, one must have a detailed anatomical knowledge of the course of the radial nerve. Knowledge of the distribution of the branches of this nerve at different levels enables physicians to localize the site of the lesion and eliminate the presence of other nerve injuries. Assessing the degree of nerve damage by testing the strength of the various muscles is also important.

<table>
<tr><th rowspan="2">REMEMBER
[Recall Facts]</th><th colspan="3">OUTLINE 5. POSTERIOR COMPARTMENT OF FOREARM—LEARNING OBJECTIVES
[By the end of this section the student should be able to:]</th><th rowspan="2" colspan="2">EVALUATE
[Explain Concepts]</th></tr>
<tr><th colspan="3">DEMONSTRATE AND ANALYZE RELATIONSHIPS
[Identify structures in a Prosected Specimen or Figure]</th></tr>
<tr><td rowspan="6">1. Enumerate the muscles of the posterior compartment of forearm and describe their origin, insertion, action, and nerve supply
2. Describe blood supply to posterior compartment of forearm
3. Describe the course and distribution of the radial nerve in the forearm</td><td>Level I</td><td>Level II</td><td>Level III</td><td colspan="2">▪ Actions of the muscles of extensor compartment
▪ Course of posterior interosseous vessels and nerve</td></tr>
<tr><td rowspan="5">▪ Basilic vein
▪ Cephalic vein
▪ Extensor retinaculum of the wrist
▪ Superficial muscles of extensor compartment
▪ Deep muscles of extensor compartment
▪ Posterior interosseous nerve
▪ Posterior interosseous artery
▪ Radial artery</td><td rowspan="5">▪ Superficial branch of radial nerve</td><td rowspan="5">▪ Posterior cutaneous nerve of forearm</td><td colspan="2">EARLY CLINICAL EXPOSURE
[Apply Anatomical Knowledge]</td></tr>
<tr><td>Surgical Anatomy/ Pathology/ Trauma</td><td>Imaging/ Surface Anatomy</td></tr>
<tr><td>▪ Radial nerve injury at the wrist
▪ Wartenberg's syndrome
▪ Supinator syndrome</td><td></td></tr>
<tr><td colspan="2">PROBLEM SOLVING/ CLINICAL CASES
[Interpret]</td></tr>
<tr><td colspan="2">▪ Immobilizing the extensor digitorum brevis</td></tr>
</table>

Muscles

Muscles in the posterior compartment of the forearm occur in two layers: a superficial and a deep layer. The muscles are associated with:

- Movement of the wrist joint
- Extension of the fingers and thumb
- Supination

All muscles in the posterior compartment of the forearm are innervated by the radial nerve.

Superficial layer

The seven muscles in the superficial layer are the brachioradialis, extensor carpi radialis longus, extensor carpi radialis brevis, extensor digitorum, extensor digiti minimi, extensor carpi ulnaris, and anconeus (Fig. 2.88). All have a common origin from the supraepicondylar ridge and lateral epicondyle of the humerus and, except for the brachioradialis and anconeus, extend as tendons into the hand.

Brachioradialis

The **brachioradialis** muscle originates from the proximal part of the supraepicondylar ridge of the humerus and passes through the forearm to insert on the lateral side of the distal end of the radius just proximal to the radial styloid process (Fig. 2.88).

In the anatomical position, the brachioradialis is part of the muscle mass overlying the anterolateral surface of the forearm and forms the lateral boundary of the cubital fossa.

Because the brachioradialis is anterior to the elbow joint, it acts as an accessory flexor of this joint even though it is in the posterior compartment of the forearm. Its action is most efficient when the forearm is midpronated and it forms a prominent bulge as it acts against resistance.

The radial nerve emerges from the posterior compartment of the arm just deep to the brachioradialis in the distal arm and innervates the brachioradialis. Lateral to the cubital fossa, the brachioradialis lies over the radial nerve and its bifurcation into deep and superficial branches. In more distal regions, the brachioradialis lies over the superficial branch of the radial nerve and radial artery (Table 2.13).

Extensor carpi radialis longus

The **extensor carpi radialis longus** muscle originates from the distal part of the supraepicondylar ridge and the lateral epicondyle of the humerus; its tendon inserts on the dorsal surface of the base of metacarpal II (Fig. 2.88). In proximal regions, it is deep to the brachioradialis muscle.

The extensor carpi radialis longus muscle extends and abducts the wrist, and is innervated by the radial nerve before the nerve divides into superficial and deep branches (Table 2.13).

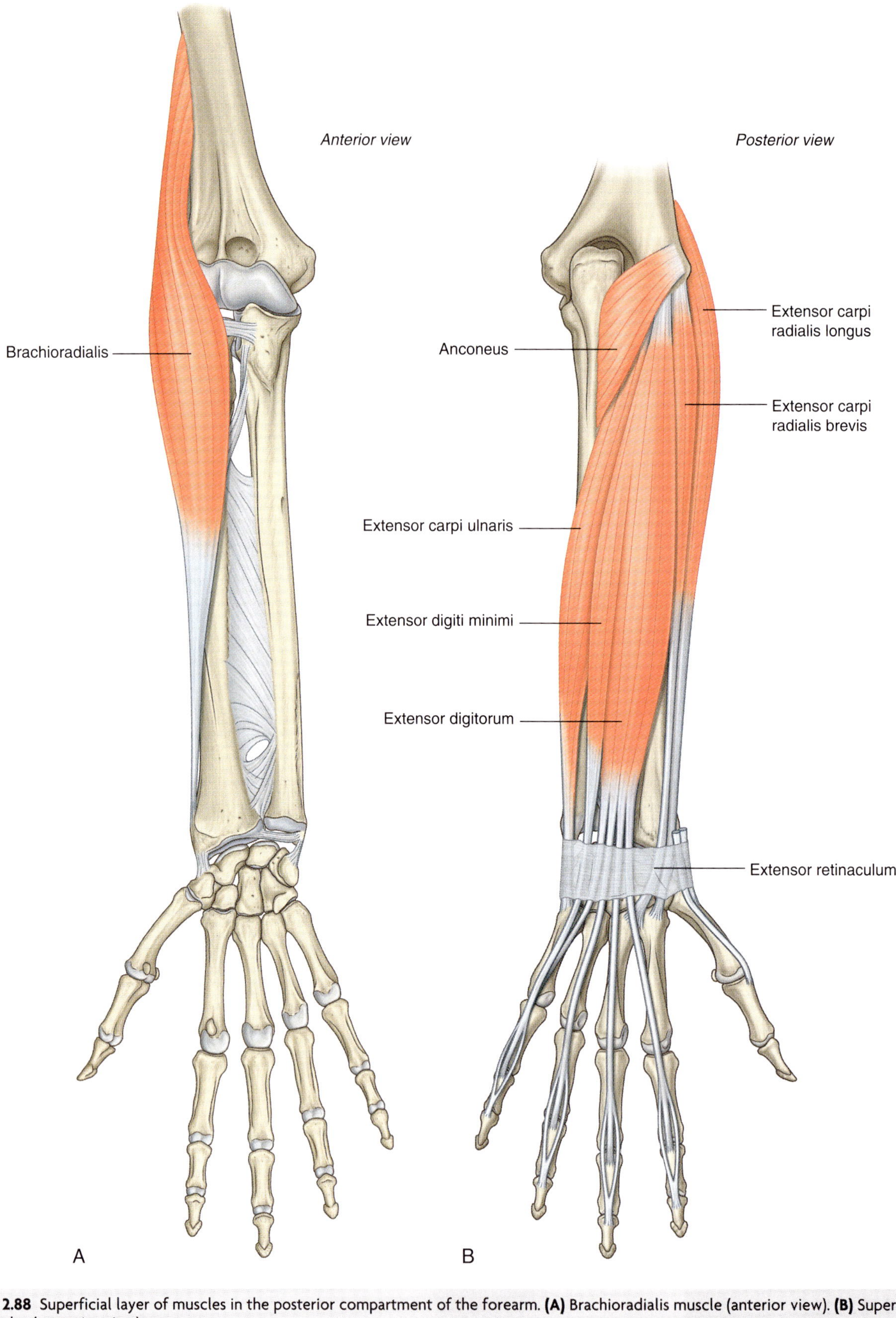

Fig. 2.88 Superficial layer of muscles in the posterior compartment of the forearm. **(A)** Brachioradialis muscle (anterior view). **(B)** Superficial muscles (posterior view).

Table 2.13 Superficial layer of muscles in the posterior compartment of the forearm

Muscle	Origin	Insertion	Innervation	Function
Brachioradialis	Proximal part of lateral supraepicondylar ridge of humerus and adjacent intermuscular septum	Lateral surface of distal end of radius	Radial nerve (C5, **C6**) before division into superficial and deep branches	Accessory flexor of elbow joint when forearm is midpronated
Extensor carpi radialis longus	Distal part of lateral supraepicondylar ridge of humerus and adjacent intermuscular septum	Dorsal surface of base of metacarpal II	Radial nerve (**C6**, C7) before division into superficial and deep branches	Extends and abducts the wrist
Extensor carpi radialis brevis	Lateral epicondyle of humerus and adjacent intermuscular septum	Dorsal surface of base of metacarpals II and III	Deep branch of radial nerve (**C7**, C8) before penetrating supinator muscle	Extends and abducts the wrist
Extensor digitorum	Lateral epicondyle of humerus and adjacent intermuscular septum and deep fascia	Four tendons, which insert via extensor hoods into the dorsal aspects of the bases of the middle and distal phalanges of the index, middle, ring, and little fingers	Posterior interosseous nerve (**C7**, C8)	Extends the index, middle, ring, and little fingers; can also extend the wrist
Extensor digiti minimi	Lateral epicondyle of humerus and adjacent intermuscular septum together with extensor digitorum	Extensor hood of the little finger	Posterior interosseous nerve (**C7**, C8)	Extends the little finger
Extensor carpi ulnaris	Lateral epicondyle of humerus and posterior border of ulna	Tubercle on the base of the medial side of metacarpal V	Posterior interosseous nerve (**C7**, C8)	Extends and adducts the wrist
Anconeus	Lateral epicondyle of humerus	Olecranon and proximal posterior surface of ulna	Radial nerve (**C6, C7, C8**) (via branch to medial head of triceps brachii)	Abduction of the ulna in pronation; accessory extensor of the elbow joint

Note: Spinal segments indicated in bold are the major segments innervating the muscle.

Extensor carpi radialis brevis

The **extensor carpi radialis brevis** muscle originates from the lateral epicondyle of the humerus, and the tendon inserts onto adjacent dorsal surfaces of the bases of metacarpals II and III (Fig. 2.88). Along much of its course, the extensor carpi radialis brevis lies deep to the extensor carpi radialis longus.

The extensor carpi radialis brevis muscle extends and abducts the wrist, and is innervated by the deep branch of the radial nerve before the nerve passes between the two heads of the supinator muscle (Table 2.13).

Extensor digitorum

The **extensor digitorum** muscle is the major extensor of the four fingers (index, middle, ring, and little fingers). It originates from the lateral epicondyle of the humerus and forms four tendons, each of which passes into a finger (Fig. 2.88).

On the dorsal surface of the hand, adjacent tendons of the extensor digitorum are interconnected. In the fingers, each tendon inserts, via a triangular-shaped connective tissue aponeurosis (the extensor hood), into the base of the dorsal surfaces of the middle and distal phalanges.

The extensor digitorum muscle is innervated by the posterior interosseous nerve, which is the continuation of the deep branch of the radial nerve after it emerges from the supinator muscle (Table 2.13).

Extensor digiti minimi

The **extensor digiti minimi** muscle is an accessory extensor of the little finger and is medial to the extensor digitorum in the forearm (Fig. 2.88). It originates from the lateral epicondyle of the humerus and inserts, together with the tendon of the extensor digitorum, into the extensor hood of the little finger.

The extensor digiti minimi is innervated by the posterior interosseous nerve (Table 2.13).

Extensor carpi ulnaris

The **extensor carpi ulnaris** muscle is medial to the extensor digiti minimi (Fig. 2.88). It originates from the lateral epicondyle, and its tendon inserts into the medial side of the base of metacarpal V.

The extensor carpi ulnaris extends and adducts the wrist, and is innervated by the posterior interosseous nerve (Table 2.13).

Anconeus

The **anconeus muscle** is the most medial of the superficial extensors and has a triangular shape. It originates from the lateral epicondyle of the humerus and has a broad insertion into the posterolateral surface of the olecranon and related posterior surface of the ulna (see Fig. 2.82).

The anconeus abducts the ulna during pronation to maintain the center of the palm over the same point when the hand is flipped. It is also considered to be an accessory extensor of the elbow joint.

The anconeus is innervated by the branch of the radial nerve that innervates the medial head of the triceps brachii muscle (Table 2.13).

Deep layer

The deep layer of the posterior compartment of the forearm consists of five muscles: supinator, abductor pollicis longus, extensor pollicis brevis, extensor pollicis longus, and extensor indicis (Fig. 2.89).

Except for the supinator muscle, all these deep layer muscles originate from the posterior surfaces of the radius, ulna, and interosseous membrane and pass into the thumb and fingers.

- Three of these muscles—the abductor pollicis longus, extensor pollicis brevis, and extensor pollicis longus—emerge from between the extensor digitorum and the extensor carpi radialis brevis tendons of the superficial layer and pass into the thumb.
- Two of the three "outcropping" muscles (the abductor pollicis longus and extensor pollicis brevis) form a distinct muscular bulge in the distal posterolateral surface of the forearm.

All muscles of the deep layer are innervated by the posterior interosseous nerve, the continuation of the deep branch of the radial nerve.

Supinator

The **supinator** muscle has two layers, which insert together on the proximal aspect of the radius (Fig. 2.89):

- The more superficial (humeral) layer originates mainly from the lateral epicondyle of the humerus and the related annular ligament and the radial collateral ligament of the elbow joint.
- The deep (ulnar) layer originates mainly from the supinator crest on the posterolateral surface of the ulna.

From their sites of origin, the two layers wrap around the posterior and lateral aspect of the head, neck, and proximal shaft of the radius to insert on the lateral surface of the radius superior to the anterior oblique line and to the insertion of the pronator teres muscle.

The supinator muscle supinates the forearm and hand.

The deep branch of the radial nerve innervates the supinator muscle and passes to the posterior compartment of

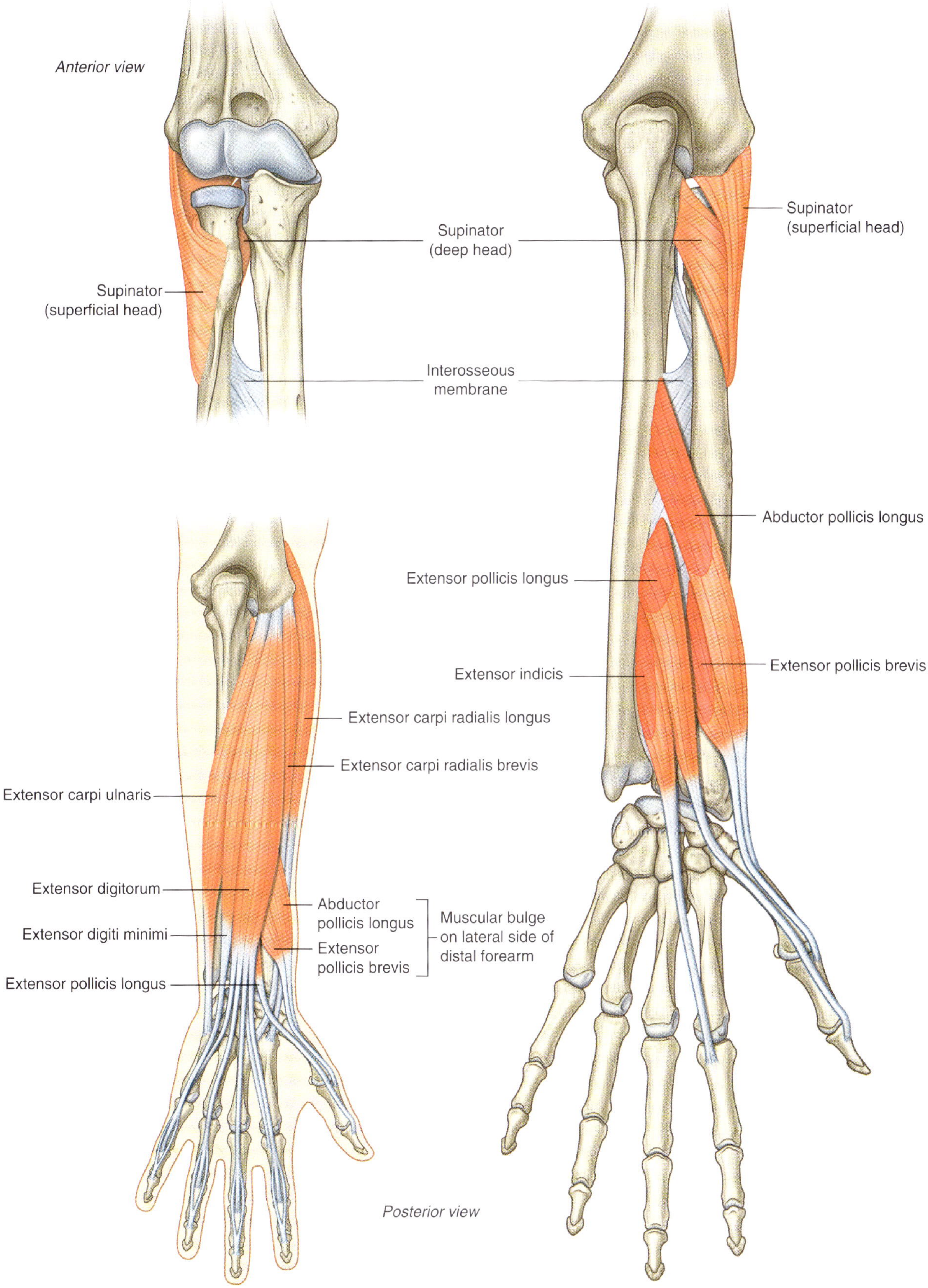

Fig. 2.89 Deep layer of muscles in the posterior compartment of the forearm.

the forearm by passing between the two layers of this muscle (Table 2.14).

Abductor pollicis longus

The **abductor pollicis longus** muscle originates from the proximal posterior surfaces of the radius and the ulna and from the related interosseous membrane (Fig. 2.89). In the distal forearm, it emerges between the extensor digitorum and extensor carpi radialis brevis muscles to form a tendon that passes into the thumb and inserts on the lateral side of the base of metacarpal I. The tendon contributes to the lateral border of the anatomical snuffbox at the wrist.

The major function of the abductor pollicis longus is to abduct the thumb at the joint between the metacarpal I and trapezium bones (Table 2.14).

Extensor pollicis brevis

The **extensor pollicis brevis** muscle arises distal to the origin of the abductor pollicis longus from the posterior surface of the radius and interosseous membrane (Fig. 2.89). Together with the abductor pollicis longus, it emerges between the extensor digitorum and extensor carpi radialis brevis muscles to form a bulge on the posterolateral surface of the distal forearm. The tendon of the extensor pollicis brevis passes into the thumb and inserts on the dorsal surface of the base of the proximal phalanx. At the wrist, the tendon contributes to the lateral border of the anatomical snuffbox.

The extensor pollicis brevis extends the metacarpophalangeal and carpometacarpal joints of the thumb (Table 2.14).

Extensor pollicis longus

The **extensor pollicis longus** muscle originates from the posterior surface of the ulna and adjacent interosseous membrane and inserts via a long tendon into the dorsal surface of the distal phalanx of the thumb (Fig. 2.89). Like the abductor pollicis longus and extensor pollicis brevis, the tendon of this muscle emerges between the extensor digitorum and the extensor carpi radialis brevis muscles. However, it is held away from the other two deep muscles of the thumb by passing medially around the dorsal tubercle on the distal end of the radius. The tendon forms the medial margin of the anatomical snuffbox at the wrist.

The extensor pollicis longus extends all joints of the thumb (Table 2.14).

Extensor indicis

The **extensor indicis muscle** is an accessory extensor of the index finger. It originates distal to the extensor pollicis longus from the posterior surface of the ulna and adjacent interosseous membrane (Fig. 2.89). The tendon passes into the hand and inserts into the extensor hood of the index finger with the tendon of the extensor digitorum (Table 2.14).

Table 2.14 Deep layer of muscles in the posterior compartment of the forearm

Muscle	Origin	Insertion	Innervation	Function
Supinator	Superficial layer—lateral epicondyle of humerus, radial collateral and annular ligaments; deep layer—supinator crest of the ulna	Lateral surface of radius superior to the anterior oblique line	Posterior interosseous nerve (**C6**, C7)	Supination
Abductor pollicis longus	Posterior surfaces of ulna and radius (distal to the attachments of supinator and anconeus), and intervening interosseous membrane	Lateral side of base of metacarpal I	Posterior interosseous nerve (**C7**, C8)	Abducts carpometacarpal joint of thumb; accessory extensor of the thumb
Extensor pollicis brevis	Posterior surface of radius (distal to abductor pollicis longus) and the adjacent interosseous membrane	Dorsal surface of base of proximal phalanx of the thumb	Posterior interosseous nerve (**C7**, C8)	Extends metacarpophalangeal joint of the thumb; can also extend the carpometacarpal joint of the thumb
Extensor pollicis longus	Posterior surface of ulna (distal to the abductor pollicis longus) and the adjacent interosseous membrane	Dorsal surface of base of distal phalanx of thumb	Posterior interosseous nerve (**C7**, C8)	Extends interphalangeal joint of the thumb; can also extend carpometacarpal and metacarpophalangeal joints of the thumb
Extensor indicis	Posterior surface of ulna (distal to extensor pollicis longus) and adjacent interosseous membrane	Extensor hood of index finger	Posterior interosseous nerve (**C7**, C8)	Extends index finger

Note: Spinal segments indicated in bold are the major segments innervating the muscle.

Arteries and veins

The blood supply to the posterior compartment of the forearm occurs predominantly through branches of the radial, posterior interosseous, and anterior interosseous arteries (Fig. 2.90).

Posterior interosseous artery

The posterior interosseous artery originates in the anterior compartment from the common interosseous branch of the ulnar artery and passes posteriorly over the proximal margin of the interosseous membrane and into the posterior compartment of the forearm. It contributes a branch, the **recurrent interosseous artery** (see Fig. 2.66B), to the vascular network around the elbow joint and then passes between the supinator and abductor pollicis longus muscles to supply the superficial extensors. After receiving the terminal end of the anterior interosseous artery, the posterior interosseous artery terminates by joining the dorsal carpal arch of the wrist.

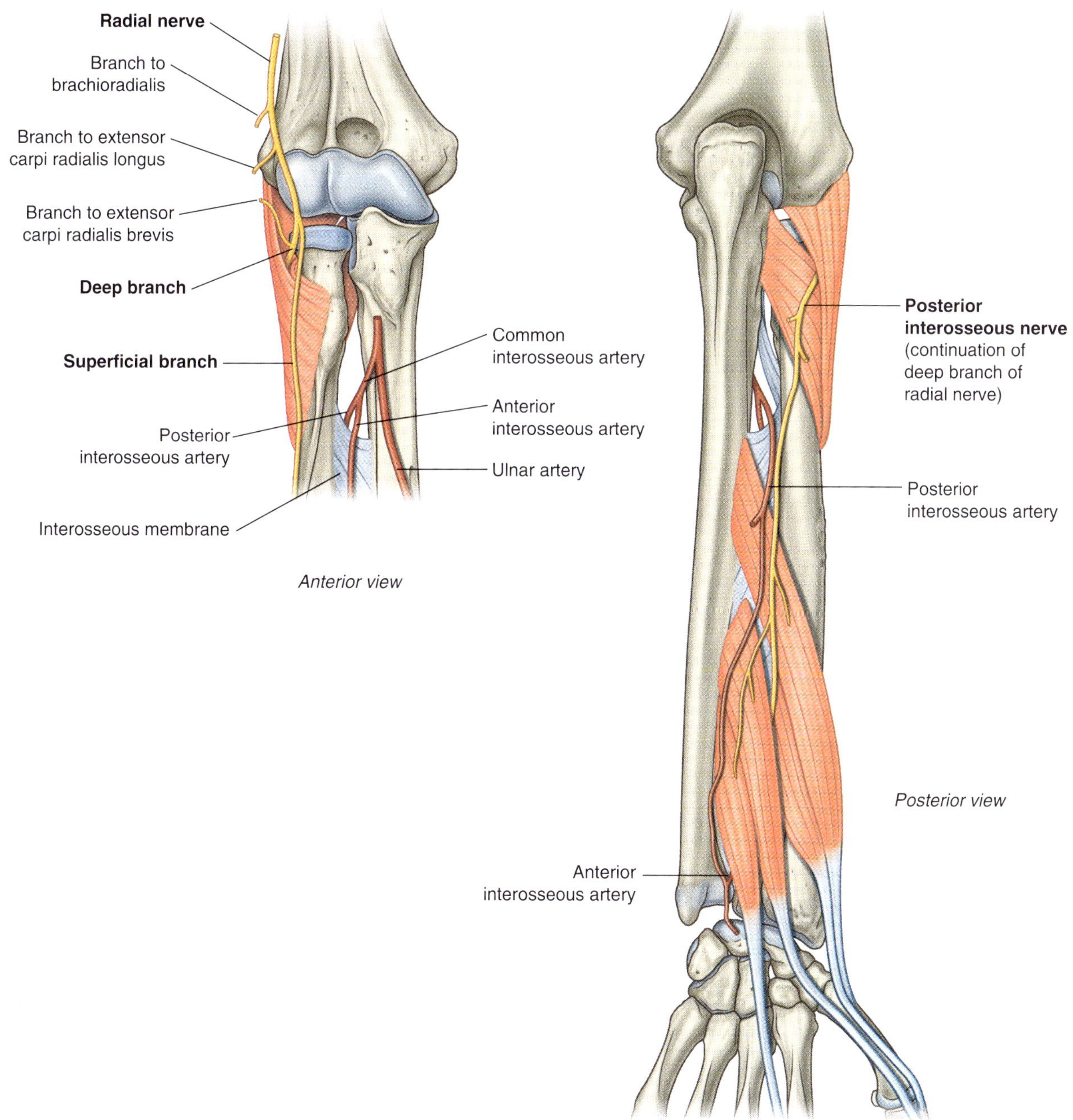

Fig. 2.90 Posterior interosseous artery and radial nerve in posterior compartment of forearm.

Anterior interosseous artery

The anterior interosseous artery, also a branch of the common interosseous branch of the ulnar artery, is situated in the anterior compartment of the forearm on the interosseous membrane. It has numerous perforating branches, which pass directly through the interosseous membrane to supply deep muscles of the posterior compartment. The terminal end of the anterior interosseous artery passes posteriorly through an aperture in the interosseous membrane in distal regions of the forearm to join the posterior interosseous artery.

Radial artery

The radial artery has muscular branches, which contribute to the supply of the extensor muscles on the radial side of the forearm.

Veins

Deep veins of the posterior compartment generally accompany the arteries. They ultimately drain into brachial veins associated with the brachial artery in the cubital fossa.

Nerves

Radial nerve

The nerve of the posterior compartment of the forearm is the radial nerve (Fig. 2.90). Most of the muscles are innervated by the deep branch, which originates from the radial nerve in the lateral wall of the cubital fossa deep to the brachioradialis muscle and becomes the **posterior interosseous nerve** after emerging from between the two layers of the supinator muscle in the posterior compartment of the forearm.

In the lateral wall of the cubital fossa, and before dividing into **superficial** and **deep branches**, the radial nerve innervates the brachioradialis and extensor carpi radialis longus muscles.

The deep branch innervates the extensor carpi radialis brevis, and then passes between the two layers of the supinator muscle and follows the plane of separation between the two layers dorsally and laterally around the proximal shaft of the radius to the posterior aspect of the forearm. It supplies the supinator muscle and then emerges, as the posterior interosseous nerve, from the muscle to lie between the superficial and deep layers of muscles.

The posterior interosseous nerve supplies the remaining muscles in the posterior compartment and terminates as articular branches, which pass deep to the extensor pollicis longus muscle to reach the wrist.

HAND

SET INDUCTION—CASE SCENARIO 6: HAND INFECTION

A 23-year-old martial arts expert accidentally injured the palmar aspect of his fifth digit. In a few days, the wound got infected and the infection spread to the palm. Following this he was diagnosed to have ulnar bursa infection secondary to injury to the fifth digit. His condition was managed after he was informed that the infection could spread to the midpalmar space if untreated.

Knowledge of the anatomy of the synovial sheaths and their continuation to the palm is essential to understand the spread of infection and to manage it effectively.

<table>
<tr><th rowspan="2">REMEMBER
[Recall Facts]</th><th colspan="3">OUTLINE 6. THE HAND—LEARNING OBJECTIVES
[By the end of this section the student should be able to:]</th><th rowspan="2" colspan="2">EVALUATE
[Explain Concepts]</th></tr>
<tr><th colspan="3">DEMONSTRATE AND ANALYZE RELATIONSHIPS
[Identify structures in a Prosected Specimen or Figure]</th></tr>
<tr><td rowspan="7">1. Mention and understand the skeletal support of the hand
2. Describe the wrist joint, carpometacarpal joint, and metacarpal joints of the hand
3. Describe the intrinsic muscles of the hand with their origin, insertion, action, and nerve supply
4. Describe in detail the arterial palmar arches
5. Describe the course and distribution of the median and ulnar nerves in the hand</td><td>Level I</td><td>Level II</td><td>Level III</td><td colspan="2" rowspan="2">■ Structures passing deep to the flexor retinaculum
■ Actions and innervation of thenar and hypothenar muscles
■ Formation of the deep palmar arch
■ Course of the deep branch of the ulnar nerve
■ Attachment, actions, and innervation of lumbricals and interossei
■ Fascial spaces of palm and forearm
■ Extensor retinaculum, with the compartments deep to it and their contents
■ Formation of the dorsal digital expansion
■ Course of the radial artery in the hand
■ Cutaneous innervation of the dorsum of the hand</td></tr>
<tr><td rowspan="6">■ Tendons of flexor digitorum superficialis and profundus, flexor pollicis longus
■ Lumbricals
■ Thenar muscles
■ Hypothenar muscles
■ Dorsal digital expansion
■ Superficial palmar arch</td><td rowspan="6">■ Deep palmar arch
■ Interosseous muscles
■ Dorsal venous arch</td><td rowspan="6">■ Recurrent branch of median nerve
■ Princeps pollicis
■ Radialis indicis</td></tr>
<tr><th colspan="2">EARLY CLINICAL EXPOSURE
[Apply Anatomical Knowledge]</th></tr>
<tr><th>Surgical Anatomy/ Pathology/ Trauma</th><th>Imaging/ Surface Anatomy</th></tr>
<tr><td>■ Claw hand
■ Carpal tunnel syndrome
■ Infection of fascial spaces of palm and their drainage
■ De Quervain's tenosynovitis
■ Tenosynovitis
■ Trigger finger
■ Venipuncture</td><td>■ Position of flexor retinaculum and recurrent branch of median nerve
■ Positions of superficial and deep palmar arches</td></tr>
<tr><th colspan="2">PROBLEM SOLVING/ CLINICAL CASES
[Interpret]</th></tr>
<tr><td colspan="2">■ Examination of the hand</td></tr>
</table>

The hand (Fig. 2.91) is the region of the upper limb distal to the wrist joint. It is subdivided into three parts:

- The wrist (carpus)
- The metacarpus
- The digits (five fingers including the thumb)

The five digits consist of the laterally positioned thumb and, medial to the thumb, the four fingers—the index, middle, ring, and little fingers.

In the normal resting position, the fingers form a flexed arcade, with the little finger flexed most and the index finger flexed least. In the anatomical position, the fingers are extended.

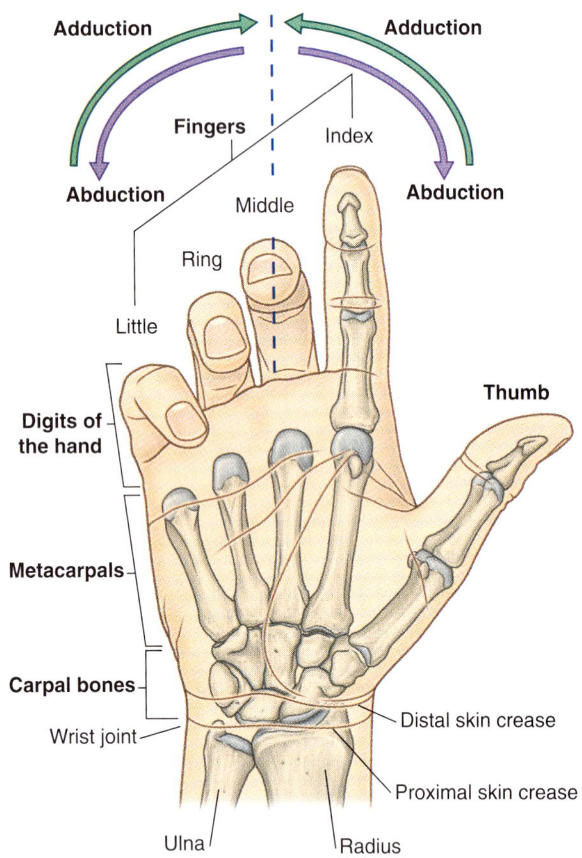

Fig. 2.91 Right hand. The fingers are shown in a normal resting arcade in which they are flexed. In the anatomical position, the digits are straight and adducted.

The hand has an anterior surface (**palm**) and a dorsal surface (**dorsum of hand**). Abduction and adduction of the fingers are defined with respect to the long axis of the middle finger (Fig. 2.91). In the anatomical position, the long axis of the thumb is rotated 90° to the rest of the digits so that the pad of the thumb points medially; consequently, movements of the thumb are defined at right angles to the movements of the other digits of the hand.

The hand is a mechanical and sensory tool. Many of the features of the upper limb are designed to facilitate positioning the hand in space.

Bones

There are three groups of bones in the hand:

- The eight **carpal bones** are the bones of the wrist.
- The five **metacarpals** (**I to V**) are the bones of the metacarpus.
- The **phalanges** are the bones of the digits—the thumb has only two; the rest of the digits have three (Fig. 2.92).

The carpal bones and metacarpals of the index, middle, ring, and little fingers (metacarpals II to V) tend to function as a unit and form much of the bony framework of the palm. The metacarpal of the thumb functions independently and has increased flexibility at the carpometacarpal joint to provide opposition of the thumb to the fingers.

Carpal bones

The small carpal bones of the wrist are arranged in two rows, a proximal and a distal row, each consisting of four bones (Fig. 2.92).

Proximal row

From lateral to medial and when viewed from anteriorly, the proximal row of bones consists of:

- The boat-shaped **scaphoid**
- The **lunate**, which has a crescent shape
- The three-sided **triquetrum** bone
- The pea-shaped **pisiform** (Fig. 2.92)

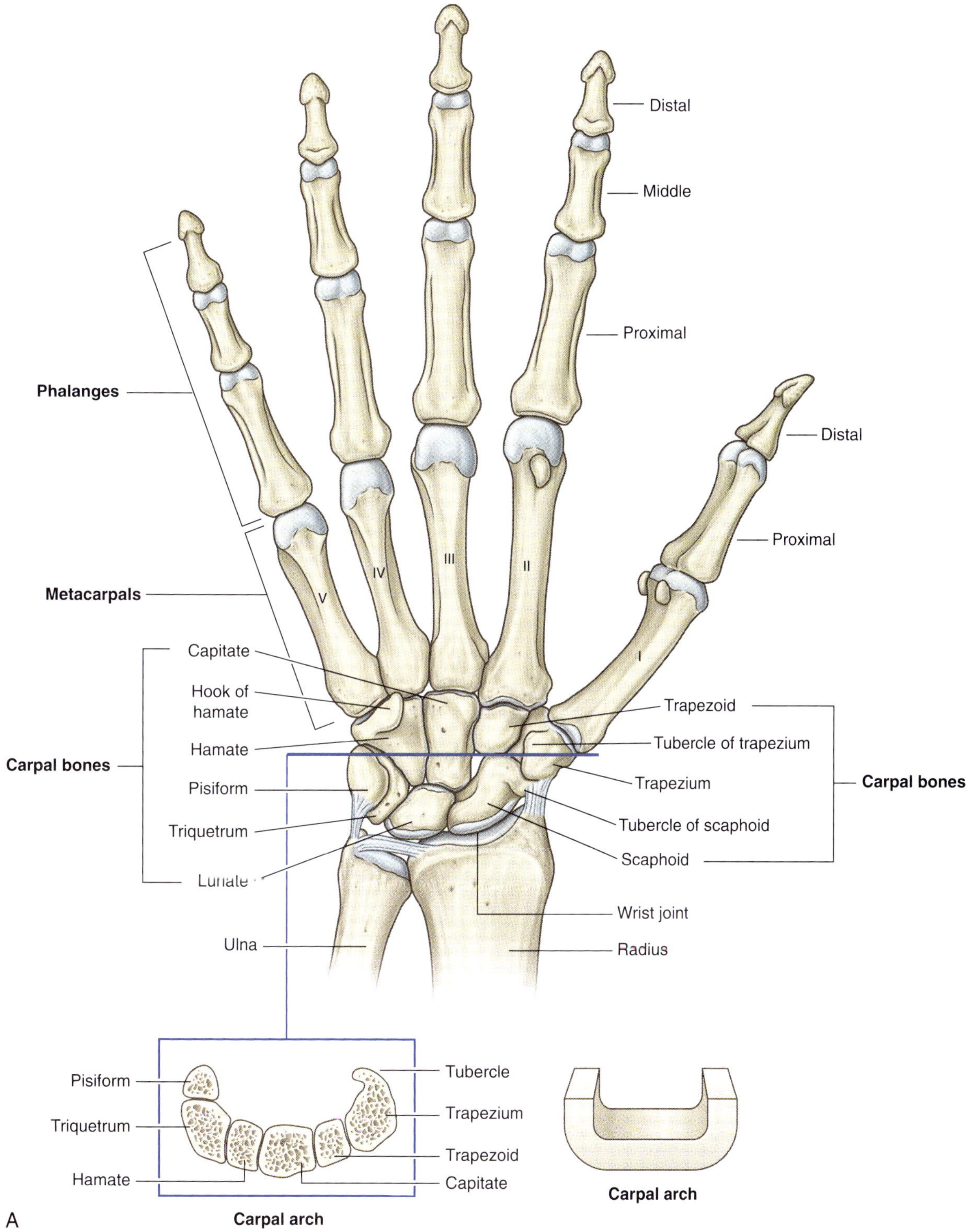

Fig. 2.92 Right hand and wrist joint. **(A)** Bones.

Continued

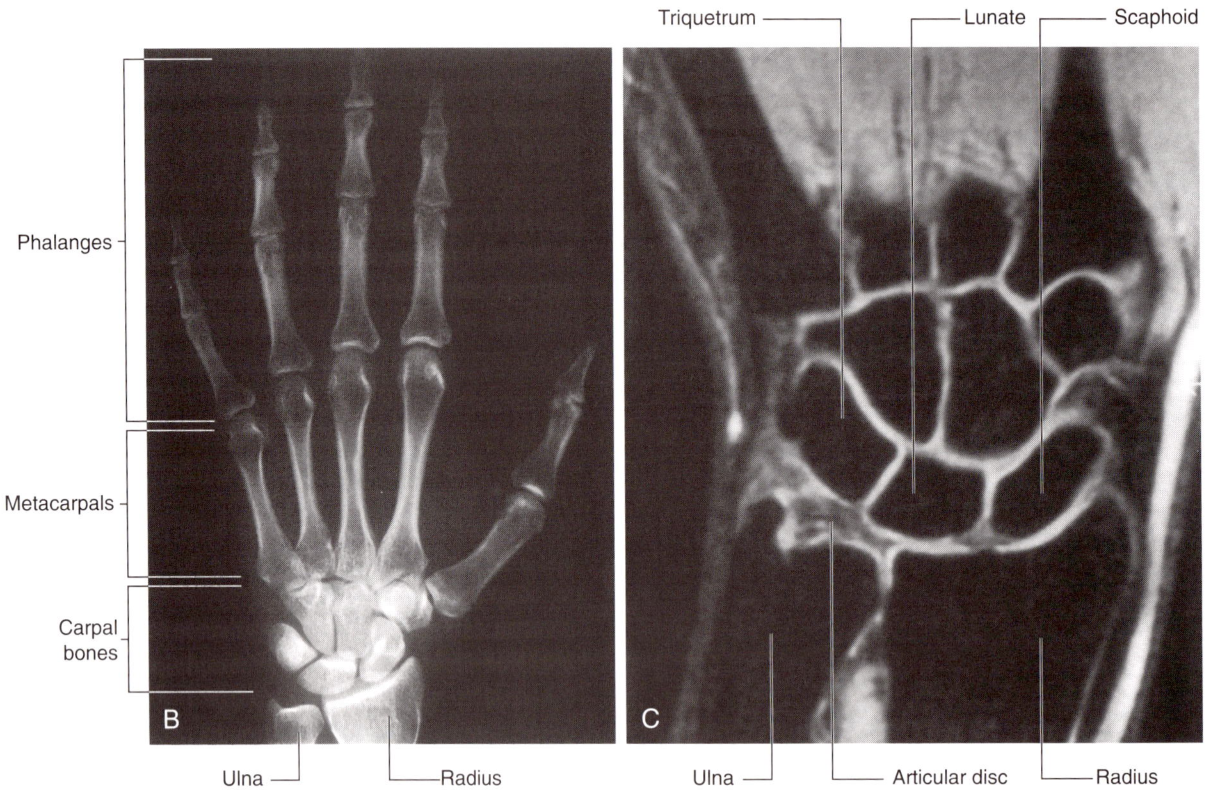

Fig. 2.92, cont'd **(B)** Radiograph of a normal hand and wrist joint (anteroposterior view). **(C)** Magnetic resonance image of a normal wrist joint in the coronal plane.

The **pisiform** is a sesamoid bone in the tendon of the flexor carpi ulnaris and articulates with the anterior surface of the **triquetrum**.

The **scaphoid** has a prominent **tubercle** on its lateral palmar surface that is directed anteriorly.

Distal row

From lateral to medial and when viewed from anteriorly, the distal row of carpal bones consists of:

- The irregular four-sided **trapezium** bone
- The four-sided **trapezoid**
- The **capitate**, which has a head
- The **hamate**, which has a hook (Fig. 2.92)

The **trapezium** articulates with the metacarpal bone of the thumb and has a distinct **tubercle** on its palmar surface that projects anteriorly.

The largest of the carpal bones, the **capitate**, articulates with the base of metacarpal III.

The **hamate**, which is positioned just lateral and distal to the pisiform, has a prominent hook (**hook of hamate**) on its palmar surface that projects anteriorly.

Articular surfaces

The carpal bones have numerous articular surfaces (Fig. 2.92). All of them articulate with each other, and the carpal bones in the distal row articulate with the metacarpals of the digits. With the exception of the metacarpal of the thumb, all movements of the metacarpal bones on the carpal bones are limited.

The expansive proximal surfaces of the scaphoid and lunate articulate with the radius to form the wrist joint.

Carpal arch

The carpal bones do not lie in a flat plane; rather, they form an arch, whose base is directed anteriorly (Fig. 2.92). The lateral side of this base is formed by the tubercles of the scaphoid and trapezium. The medial side is formed by the pisiform and the hook of the hamate.

The flexor retinaculum attaches to, and spans the distance between, the medial and lateral sides of the base to form the anterior wall of the so-called carpal tunnel. The sides and roof of the carpal tunnel are formed by the arch of the carpal bones.

Metacarpals

Each of the five metacarpals is related to one digit:

- Metacarpal I is related to the thumb.
- Metacarpals II to V are related to the index, middle, ring, and little fingers, respectively (Fig. 2.92).

Each metacarpal consists of a **base**, a **shaft** (body), and, distally, a **head**.

All of the bases of the metacarpals articulate with the carpal bones; in addition, the bases of the metacarpal bones of the fingers articulate with each other.

All of the heads of the metacarpals articulate with the proximal phalanges of the digits. The heads form the knuckles on the dorsal surface of the hand when the fingers are flexed.

Phalanges

The phalanges are the bones of the digits (Fig. 2.92):

- The thumb has two—a **proximal** and a **distal phalanx**.
- The rest of the digits have three—a **proximal**, a **middle**, and a **distal phalanx**.

Each phalanx has a **base**, a **shaft** (**body**), and, distally, a **head**.

The base of each proximal phalanx articulates with the head of the related metacarpal bone.

The head of each distal phalanx is nonarticular and flattened into a crescent-shaped palmar tuberosity, which lies under the palmar pad at the end of the digit.

Joints

Wrist joint

The wrist joint is a synovial joint between the distal end of the radius and the articular disc overlying the distal end of the ulna, and the scaphoid, lunate, and triquetrum (Fig. 2.92). Together, the articular surfaces of the carpals form an oval shape with a convex contour, which articulates with the corresponding concave surface of the radius and articular disc.

The wrist joint allows movement around two axes. The hand can be abducted, adducted, flexed, and extended at the wrist joint.

Because the radial styloid process extends further distally than does the ulnar styloid process, the hand can be adducted to a greater degree than it can be abducted.

The capsule of the wrist joint is reinforced by **palmar radiocarpal**, **palmar ulnocarpal**, and **dorsal radiocarpal ligaments**. In addition, **radial** and **ulnar** collateral ligaments of the wrist **joint** span the distance between the styloid processes of the radius and ulna and the adjacent carpal bones. These ligaments reinforce the medial and lateral sides of the wrist joint and support them during flexion and extension.

Carpal joints

The synovial joints between the carpal bones share a common articular cavity. The joint capsule of the joints is reinforced by numerous ligaments.

Although movement at the **carpal joints** (**intercarpal joints**) is limited, the joints do contribute to the positioning of the hand in abduction, adduction, flexion, and, particularly, extension.

Carpometacarpal joints

There are five carpometacarpal joints between the metacarpals and the related distal row of carpal bones (Fig. 2.92).

The saddle joint, between metacarpal I and the trapezium, imparts a wide range of mobility to the thumb that is not a feature of the rest of the digits. Movements at this carpometacarpal joint are flexion, extension, abduction, adduction, rotation, and circumduction.

The carpometacarpal joints between metacarpals II to V and the carpal bones are much less mobile than the carpometacarpal joint of the thumb, allowing only limited gliding movements. Movement of the joints increases medially, so metacarpal V slides to the greatest degree. This can be best observed on the dorsal surface of the hand as it makes a fist.

Metacarpophalangeal joints

The joints between the distal heads of the metacarpals and the proximal phalanges of the digits are condylar joints, which allow flexion, extension, abduction, adduction, circumduction, and limited rotation (Fig. 2.92). The capsule of each joint is reinforced by the **palmar ligament** and by medial and lateral **collateral ligaments**.

Deep transverse metacarpal ligaments

The three deep **transverse metacarpal ligaments** (Fig. 2.93) are thick bands of connective tissue connecting the palmar ligaments of the metacarpophalangeal joints of the fingers to each other. They are important because, by linking the heads of the metacarpal bones together, they restrict the movement of these bones relative to each other. As a result, they help form a unified skeletal framework for the palm of the hand.

Significantly, a deep transverse metacarpal ligament does not occur between the palmar ligament of the metacarpophalangeal joint of the thumb and the palmar ligament of the index finger. The absence of this ligament and the presence of a saddle joint between metacarpal I and the trapezium are responsible for the increased mobility of the thumb relative to the rest of the digits of the hand.

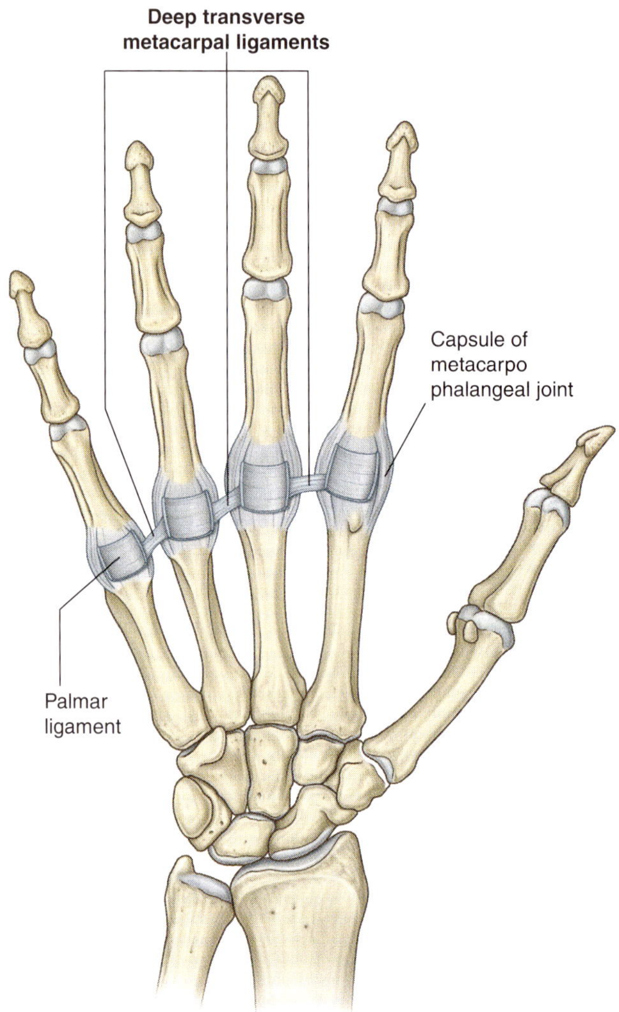

Fig. 2.93 Deep transverse metacarpal ligaments, right hand.

Interphalangeal joints of hand

The **interphalangeal joints of the hand** are hinge joints that allow mainly flexion and extension. They are reinforced by medial and lateral **collateral ligaments** and **palmar ligaments**.

Early clinical exposure

Fracture of the scaphoid and avascular necrosis of the proximal scaphoid

The commonest carpal injury is a fracture across the waist of the scaphoid bone (Fig. 2.94A and B). It is uncommon to see other injuries. In approximately 10% of individuals, the scaphoid bone has a sole blood supply from the radial artery, which enters through the distal portion of the bone to supply the proximal portion. When a fracture occurs across the waist of the scaphoid, the proximal portion therefore undergoes avascular necrosis. It is impossible to predict which patients have this blood supply.

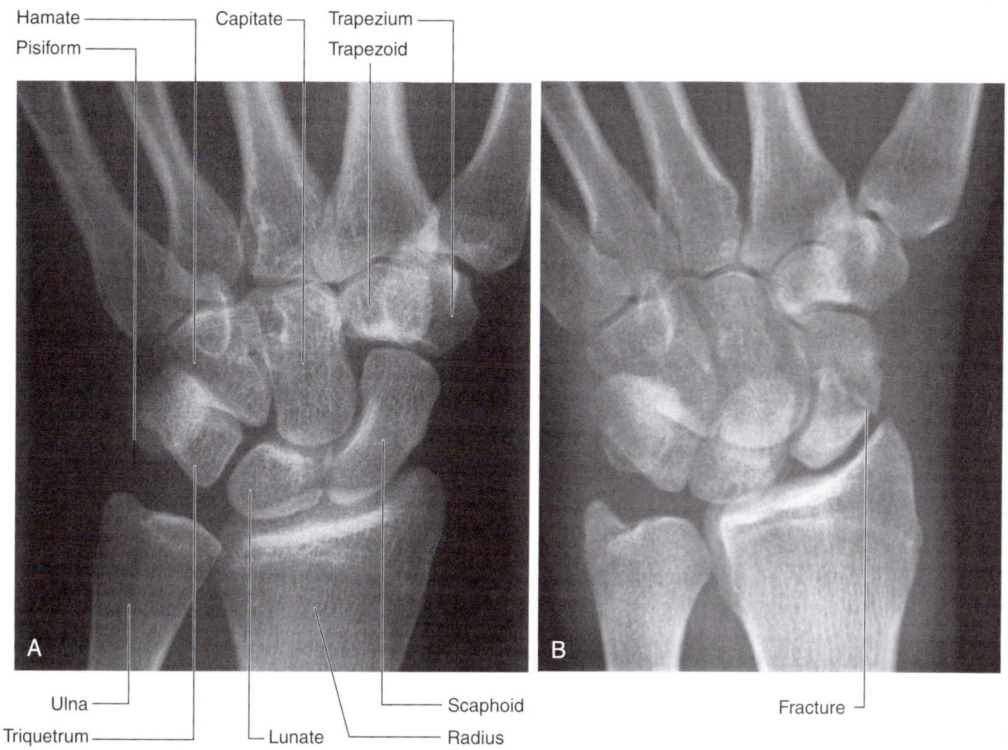

Fig. 2.94 Wrist radiographs (posteroanterior view). **(A)** Normal. **(B)** Scaphoid fracture.

Early clinical exposure

Kienbock's disease

Interruption of the blood supply to the lunate can lead to avascular necrosis of the lunate, known as Kienbock's disease (Fig. 2.94C). This can cause pain and stiffness and arthritis in the longer term.

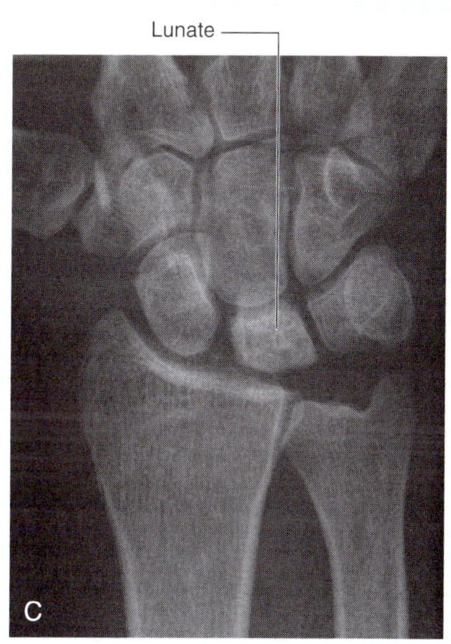

Fig. 2.94, cont'd (C) Radiograph of wrist showing sclerosis in the lunate consistent with avascular necrosis (Kienbock's disease).

Carpal tunnel and structures at the wrist

The carpal tunnel is formed anteriorly at the wrist by a deep arch formed by the carpal bones and the flexor retinaculum (see Fig. 2.92).

The base of the carpal arch is formed medially by the pisiform and the hook of the hamate and laterally by the tubercles of the scaphoid and trapezium.

The flexor retinaculum is a thick connective tissue ligament that bridges the space between the medial and lateral sides of the base of the arch and converts the carpal arch into the carpal tunnel.

The four tendons of the flexor digitorum profundus, the four tendons of the flexor digitorum superficialis, and the tendon of the flexor pollicis longus pass through the carpal tunnel, as does the median nerve (Fig. 2.95).

The flexor retinaculum holds the tendons to the bony plane at the wrist and prevents them from "bowing."

Free movement of the tendons in the carpal tunnel is facilitated by synovial sheaths, which surround the tendons. All the tendons of the flexor digitorum profundus and flexor digitorum superficialis are surrounded by a single synovial sheath; a separate sheath surrounds the tendon of the flexor pollicis longus. The median nerve is anterior to the tendons in the carpal tunnel.

The tendon of the flexor carpi radialis is surrounded by a synovial sheath and passes through a tubular compartment formed by the attachment of the lateral aspect of the flexor retinaculum to the margins of a groove on the medial side of the tubercle of the trapezium.

The ulnar artery, ulnar nerve, and tendon of the palmaris longus pass into the hand anterior to the flexor retinaculum and therefore do not pass through the carpal tunnel (Fig. 2.95). The tendon of the palmaris longus is not surrounded by a synovial sheath.

The radial artery passes dorsally around the lateral side of the wrist and lies adjacent to the external surface of the scaphoid.

The extensor tendons pass into the hand on the medial, lateral, and posterior surfaces of the wrist in six compartments defined by an extensor retinaculum and lined by synovial sheaths (Figs. 2.89 and 2.95):

- The tendons of the abductor pollicis longus and extensor pollicis brevis muscles (first compartment), the extensor carpi radialis longus and extensor carpi radialis brevis muscles (second compartment), and the extensor pollicis longus muscle (third compartment) pass through three compartments on the lateral aspect of the wrist.
- The tendons of the extensor digitorum and extensor indicis share a compartment and synovial sheath on the posterior surface of the wrist, the fourth compartment.
- The tendons of the extensor carpi ulnaris (sixth compartment) and extensor digiti minimi (fifth compartment) have separate compartments and sheaths on the medial side of the wrist.

Early clinical exposure

Carpal tunnel syndrome

Carpal tunnel syndrome is an entrapment syndrome caused by pressure on the median nerve within the carpal tunnel. The etiology of this condition is often obscure, though in some instances the nerve injury may be a direct effect of increased pressure on the median nerve caused by overuse, swelling of the tendons and tendon sheaths (e.g., rheumatoid arthritis), and cysts arising from the carpal joints. Increased pressure in the carpal tunnel is thought to cause venous congestion that produces nerve edema and anoxic damage to the capillary endothelium of the median nerve itself.

Patients typically report pain and pins-and-needles sensations in the distribution of the median nerve. Weakness and loss of muscle bulk of the thenar muscles may also occur. Gently tapping over the median nerve (in the region of the flexor retinaculum) readily produces these symptoms (Tinel's sign).

Initial treatment is aimed at reducing the inflammation and removing any repetitive insults that produce the symptoms. If this does not lead to improvement, nerve conduction studies will be necessary to confirm nerve entrapment, which may require surgical decompression of the flexor retinaculum.

Early clinical exposure

Median artery

A large median artery is an anatomical variant found in some individuals, where a persistent artery runs alongside the median nerve in one or both forearms and through the carpal tunnel. Individuals are at risk from heavy bleeding from deep cuts to the wrist.

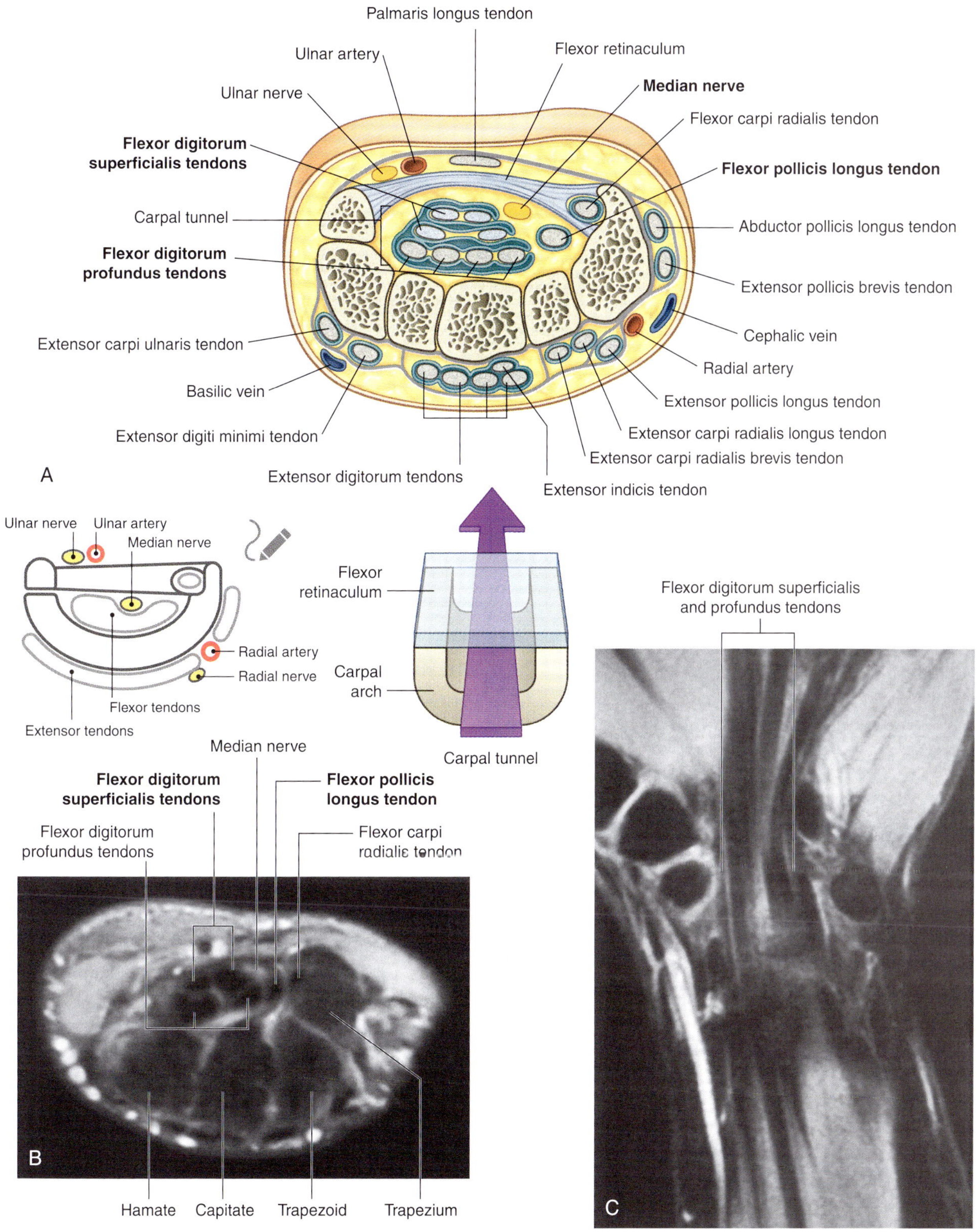

Fig. 2.95 Carpal tunnel. **(A)** Structure and relations. **(B)** Magnetic resonance image of a normal wrist in the axial plane. **(C)** Magnetic resonance image of a normal wrist in the coronal plane.

Palmar aponeurosis

The **palmar aponeurosis** is a triangular condensation of deep fascia that covers the palm and is anchored to the skin in distal regions (Fig. 2.96).

The apex of the triangle is continuous with the palmaris longus tendon, when present; otherwise, it is anchored to the flexor retinaculum. From this point, fibers radiate to extensions at the bases of the digits that project into each of the index, middle, ring, and little fingers and, to a lesser extent, the thumb.

Transverse fibers interconnect the more longitudinally arranged bundles that continue into the digits.

Vessels, nerves, and long flexor tendons lie deep to the palmar aponeurosis in the palm.

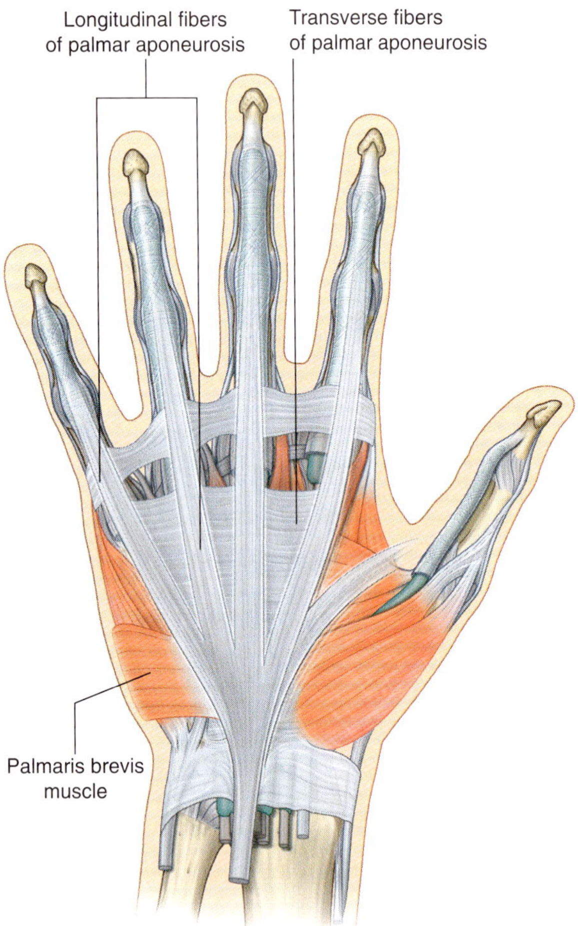

Fig. 2.96 Palmar aponeurosis, right hand.

Early clinical exposure

Dupuytren's contracture

The palmar fascia can become abnormally thickened in certain individuals, causing the fingers to progressively develop a fixed flexion position. This results in loss of dexterity and function, and in severe cases requires surgical removal of the abnormal tissue.

Palmaris brevis

The **palmaris brevis**, a small intrinsic muscle of the hand, is a quadrangular-shaped subcutaneous muscle that overlies the hypothenar muscles, ulnar artery, and superficial branch of the ulnar nerve at the medial side of the palm (Fig. 2.96). It originates from the palmar aponeurosis and flexor retinaculum and inserts into the dermis of the skin on the medial margin of the hand.

The palmaris brevis deepens the cup of the palm by pulling on skin over the hypothenar eminence and forming a distinct ridge. This may improve grip.

The palmaris brevis is innervated by the superficial branch of the ulnar nerve.

Anatomical snuffbox

The "anatomical snuffbox" is a term given to the triangular depression formed on the posterolateral side of the wrist and metacarpal I by the extensor tendons passing into the thumb (Fig. 2.97A). Historically, ground tobacco (snuff) was placed in this depression before being inhaled into the nose. The base of the triangle is at the wrist and the apex is directed into the thumb. The impression is most apparent when the thumb is extended:

- The lateral border is formed by the tendons of the abductor pollicis longus and extensor pollicis brevis.
- The medial border is formed by the tendon of the extensor pollicis longus.
- The floor of the impression is formed by the scaphoid and trapezium, and the distal ends of the tendons of the extensor carpi radialis longus and extensor carpi radialis brevis.

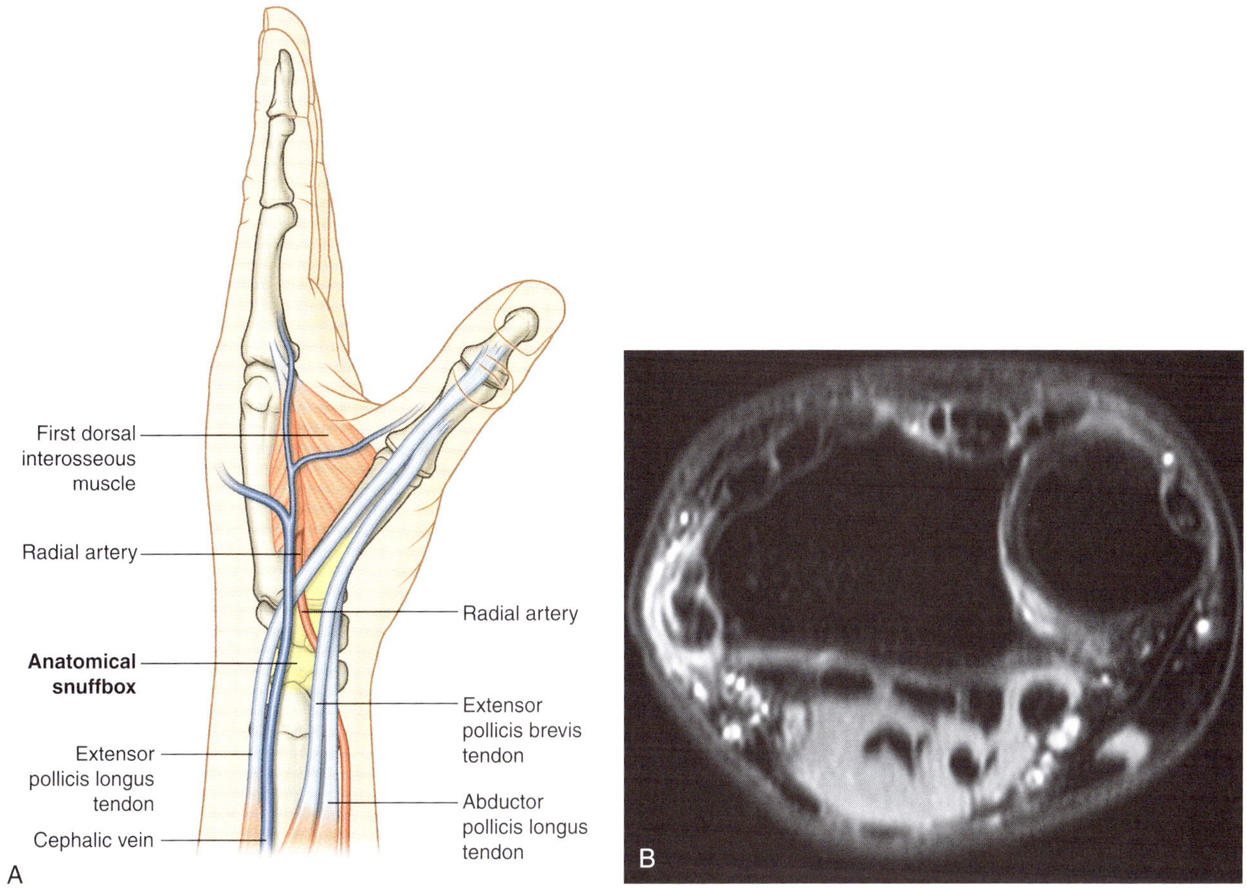

Fig. 2.97 (A) Anatomical snuffbox, left hand. **(B)** MRI of the wrist showing fluid and inflammation associated with the first extensor compartment, consistent with De Quervain's tenosynovitis.

The radial artery passes obliquely through the anatomical snuffbox, deep to the extensor tendons of the thumb, and lies adjacent to the scaphoid and trapezium.

Terminal parts of the superficial branch of the radial nerve pass subcutaneously over the snuffbox as does the origin of the cephalic vein from the dorsal venous arch of the hand.

Early clinical exposure

Snuffbox

The anatomical snuffbox is an important clinical region. When the hand is in ulnar deviation, the scaphoid becomes palpable within the snuffbox. This position enables the physician to palpate the bone to assess for a fracture. The pulse of the radial artery can also be felt in the snuffbox.

Fibrous digital sheaths

After exiting the carpal tunnel, the tendons of the flexor digitorum superficialis and profundus muscles cross the palm and enter fibrous sheaths on the palmar aspect of the digits (Fig. 2.98). These fibrous sheaths:

- Begin proximally, anterior to the metacarpophalangeal joints, and extend to the distal phalanges
- Are formed by fibrous arches and cruciate (cross-shaped) ligaments, which are attached posteriorly to the margins of the phalanges and to the palmar ligaments associated with the metacarpophalangeal and interphalangeal joints
- Hold the tendons to the bony plane and prevent the tendons from bowing when the digits are flexed

Within each tunnel, the tendons are surrounded by a synovial sheath. The synovial sheaths of the thumb and little finger are continuous with the sheaths associated with the tendons in the carpal tunnel (Fig. 2.98).

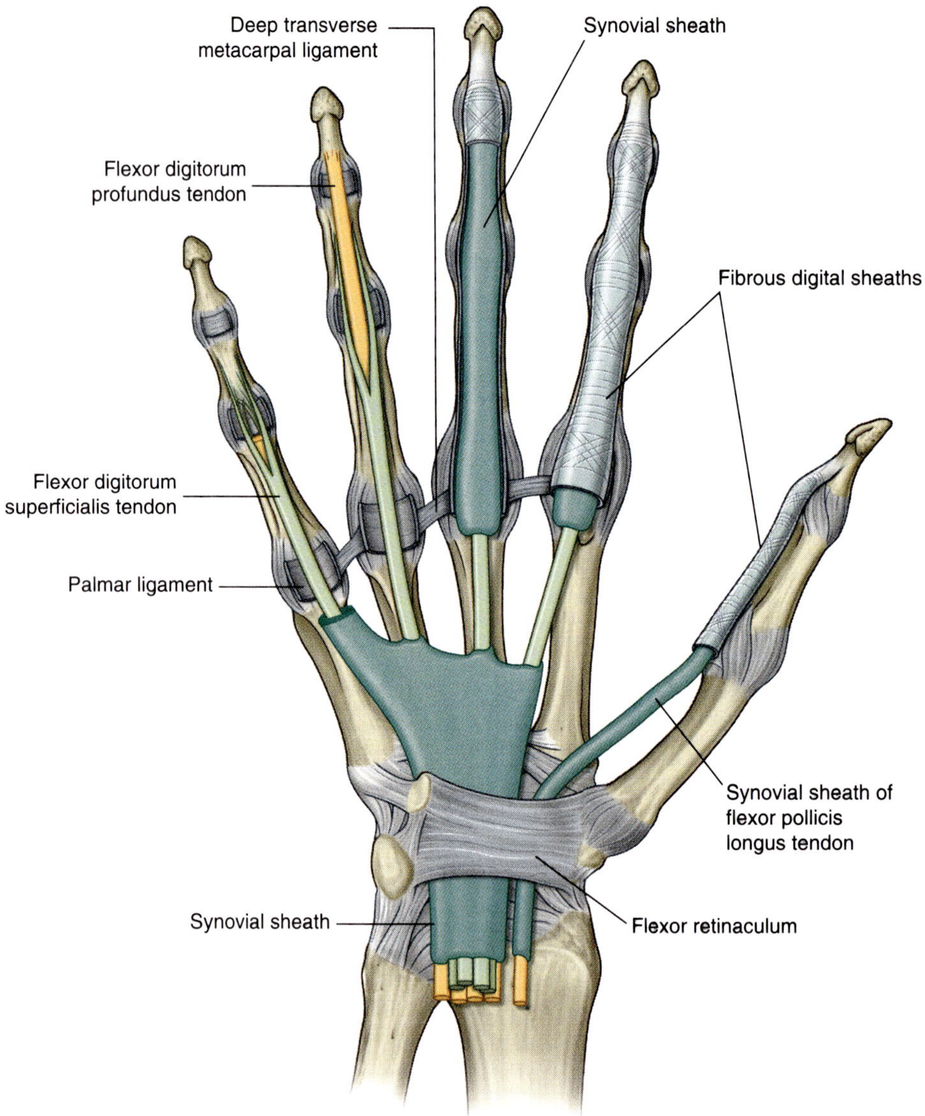

Fig. 2.98 Fibrous digital sheaths and synovial sheaths of the right hand.

Early clinical exposure

De Quervain's syndrome

De Quervain's syndrome or tenosynovitis or gamer's thumb is an inflammatory disorder that occurs within the first dorsal extensor compartment on the lateral aspect of the wrist and involves the extensor pollicis brevis tendon and abductor pollicis longus tendon and their common tendon sheath (Fig. 2.97B). Patients typically present with significant wrist pain preventing appropriate flexion/extension and abduction of the thumb. Pain will occur on the affected area on stretching the involved tendons by flexing the thumb and then attempting to adduct the wrist. The cause of this disorder is often overuse. For example, the syndrome is common in young mothers who are constantly lifting young children. Other causes include inflammatory disorders such as rheumatoid arthritis.

This condition needs to be differentiated from intersection syndrome, which occurs proximal to the wrist due to inflammation of the tendons and sheaths of extensor carpi radialis brevis and longus in the second dorsal extensor compartment (Fig. 2.89). This is due to excess friction of these extensor tendons at their point of intersection with the abductor pollicis longus and extensor pollicis brevis tendons. Flexion of the wrist against resistance (as in weightlifting) will provoke pain in intersection syndrome.

Early clinical exposure

Tenosynovitis

Tenosynovitis is inflammation of a tendon and its sheath. The condition may be caused by overuse; however, it can also be associated with other disorders such as rheumatoid arthritis and connective tissue pathologies. If the inflammation becomes severe and ensuing fibrosis occurs, the tendon will not run smoothly within the tendon sheath, and typically within the fingers the inflamed tendon may temporarily stick (within the stenosed fibrous flexor sheath) or require excess force to fully extend and flex, producing a "triggering" phenomenon.

Early clinical exposure

Trigger finger

Trigger finger is a common disorder of late childhood and adulthood and is typically characterized by catching or snapping and occasionally locking of the flexor tendon(s) in the hand. It can be associated with significant dysfunction and pain. The triggering is usually related to fibrosis and tightening of the fibrous flexor tendon sheath at the level of the metacarpophalangeal joint.

Extensor hoods

The tendons of the extensor digitorum and extensor pollicis longus muscles pass onto the dorsal aspect of the digits and expand over the proximal phalanges to form complex "**extensor hoods**," "**dorsal digital expansions**," or extensor expansions (Fig. 2.99A). The tendons of the extensor digiti minimi, extensor indicis, and extensor pollicis brevis muscles join these hoods.

Each extensor hood is triangular, with:

- The apex attached to the distal phalanx.
- The central region attached to the middle phalanx (index, middle, ring, and little fingers) or proximal phalanx (thumb).
- Each corner of the base wrapped around the sides of the metacarpophalangeal joint—in the index, middle, ring, and little fingers, the corners of the hoods attach mainly to the deep transverse metacarpal ligaments; in the thumb, the hood is attached on each side to muscles.

In addition to other attachments, many of the intrinsic muscles of the hand insert into the free margin of the hood on each side. By inserting into the extensor hood, these intrinsic muscles are responsible for complex delicate movements of the digits that could not be accomplished with the long flexor and extensor tendons alone.

In the index, middle, ring, and little fingers, the lumbrical, interossei, and abductor digiti minimi muscles attach to the extensor hoods. In the thumb, the adductor pollicis and abductor pollicis brevis muscles insert into and anchor the extensor hood.

Because force from the small intrinsic muscles of the hand passes ventral to the transverse axis of the metacarpophalangeal joints and is applied to the extensor hood distal to the fulcrum of these joints, the muscles flex these joints (Fig. 2.99B). Simultaneously, the force is transferred dorsally through the hood to extend the interphalangeal joints. This ability to flex the metacarpophalangeal joints, while at the same time extending the interphalangeal joints, is entirely due to the intrinsic muscles of the hand working through the extensor hoods. This type of precision movement is used in the upstroke when writing a *t* (Fig. 2.99C).

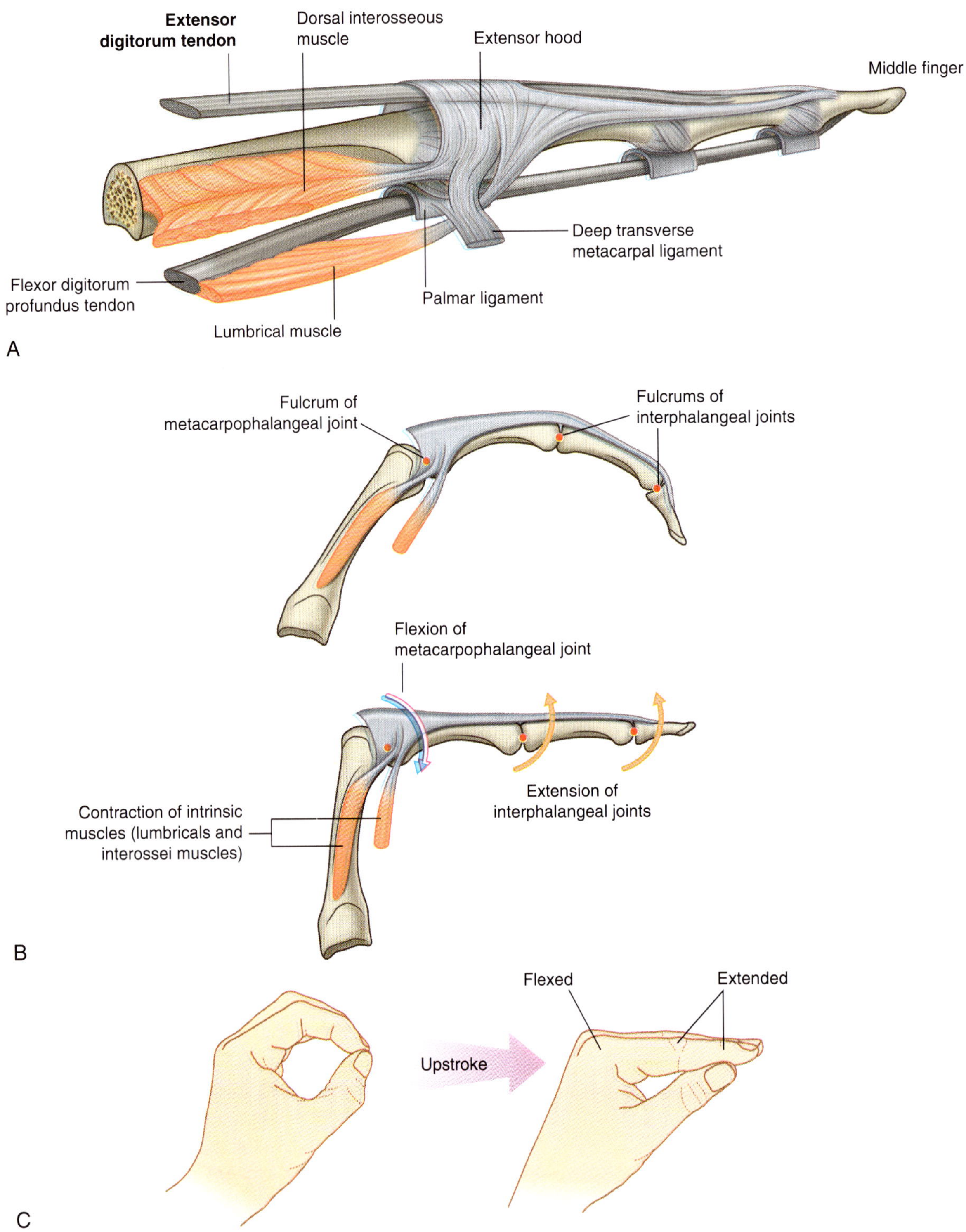

Fig. 2.99 Extensor hood. **(A** and **B)** Middle finger, left hand. **(C)** Function of extensor hoods and intrinsic muscles.

Muscles

The intrinsic muscles of the hand are the palmaris brevis (see Fig. 2.96), interossei, adductor pollicis, thenar, hypothenar, and lumbrical muscles (Figs. 2.100–2.104). Unlike the extrinsic muscles that originate in the forearm, insert in the hand, and function in forcefully gripping ("power grip") with the hand, the intrinsic muscles occur entirely in the hand and mainly execute precision movements ("precision grip") with the fingers and thumb.

All of the intrinsic muscles of the hand are innervated by the deep branch of the ulnar nerve except for the three thenar and two lateral lumbrical muscles, which are innervated by the median nerve. The intrinsic muscles are predominantly innervated by spinal cord segment T1 with a contribution from C8.

The interossei are muscles between and attached to the metacarpals (Figs. 2.100 and 2.101). They insert into the proximal phalanx of each digit and into the extensor hood and are divided into two groups, the dorsal interossei and the palmar interossei. All of the interossei are innervated by the deep branch of the ulnar nerve. Collectively, the interossei abduct and adduct the digits and contribute to the complex flexion and extension movements generated by the extensor hoods.

Dorsal interossei

Dorsal interossei are the most dorsally situated of all of the intrinsic muscles and can be palpated through the skin on the dorsal aspect of the hand (Fig. 2.100). There are four bipennate dorsal interosseous muscles between, and attached to, the shafts of adjacent metacarpal bones (Fig. 2.100). Each muscle inserts both into the base of the

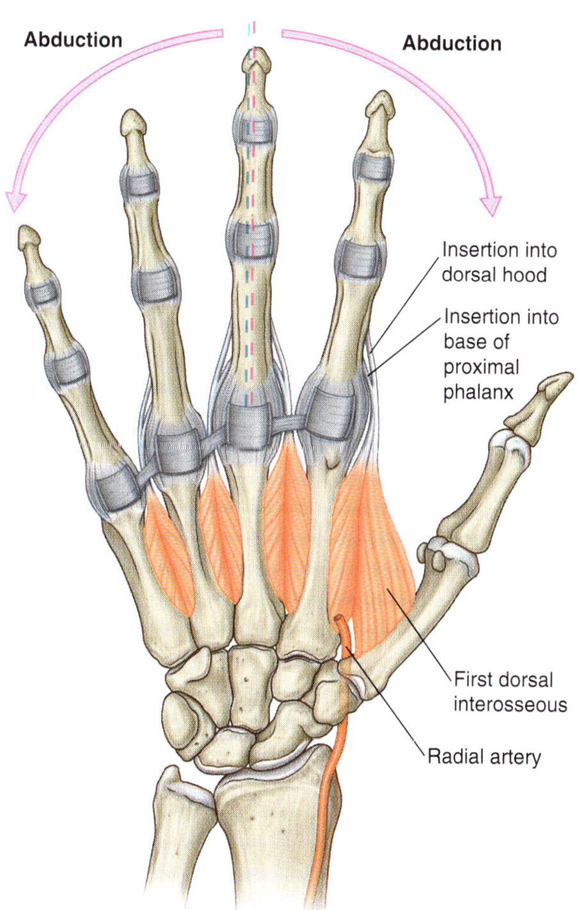

Fig. 2.100 Dorsal interossei (palmar view), right hand.

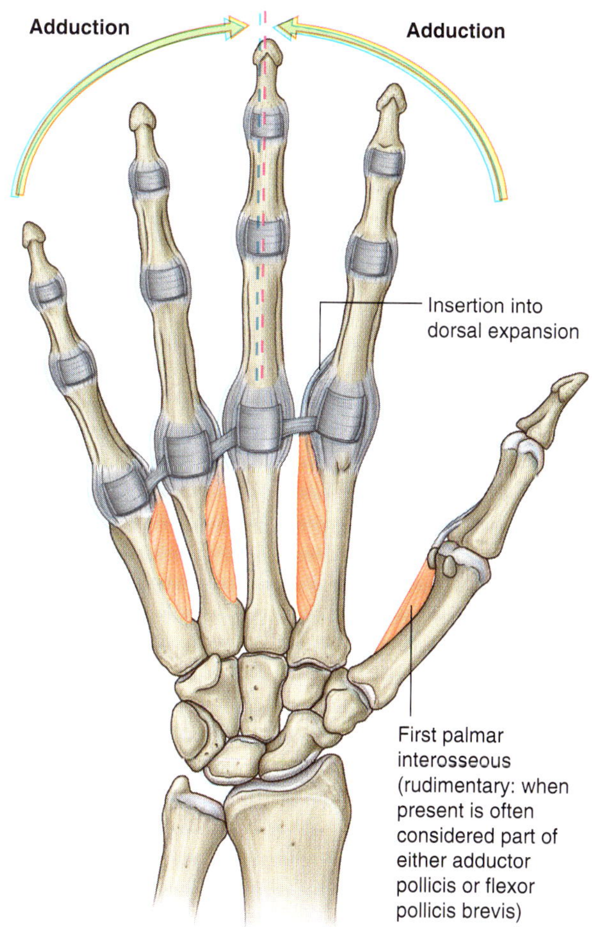

Fig. 2.101 Palmar interossei (palmar view), right hand.

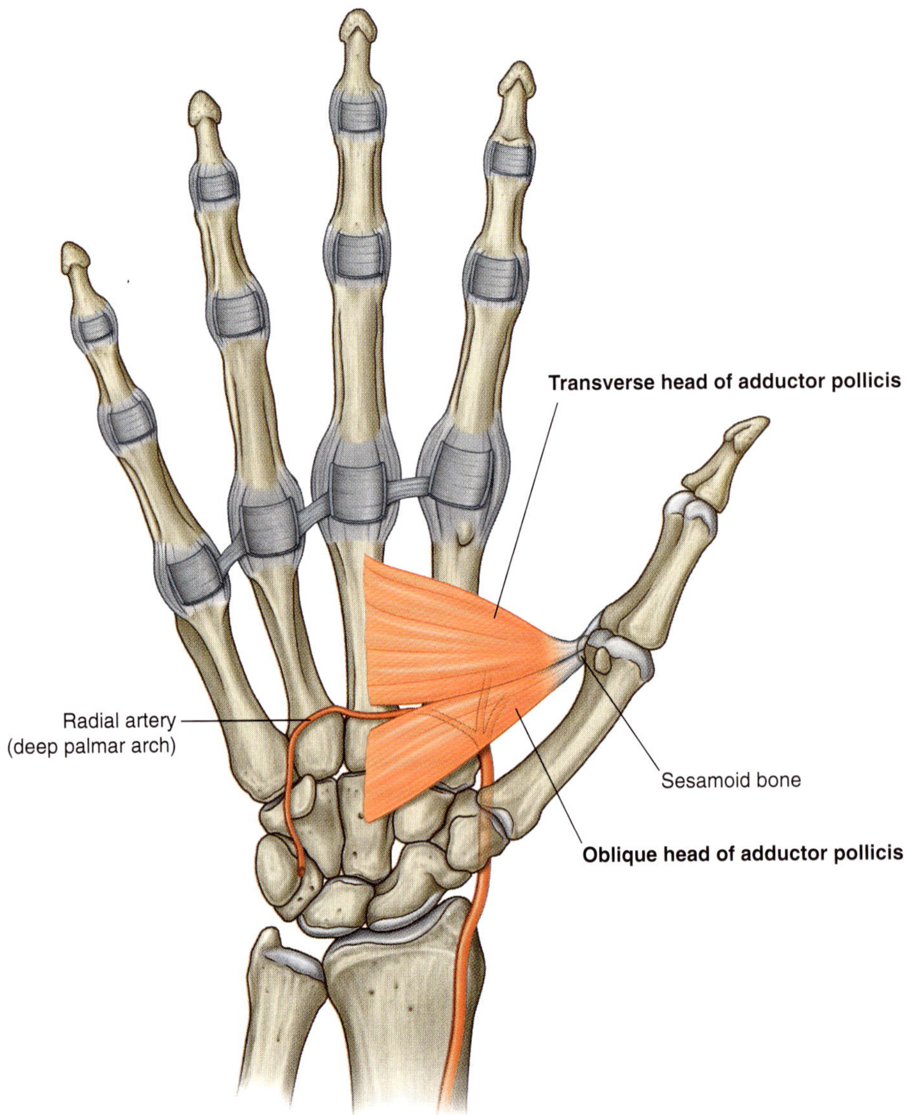

Fig. 2.102 Adductor pollicis, right hand.

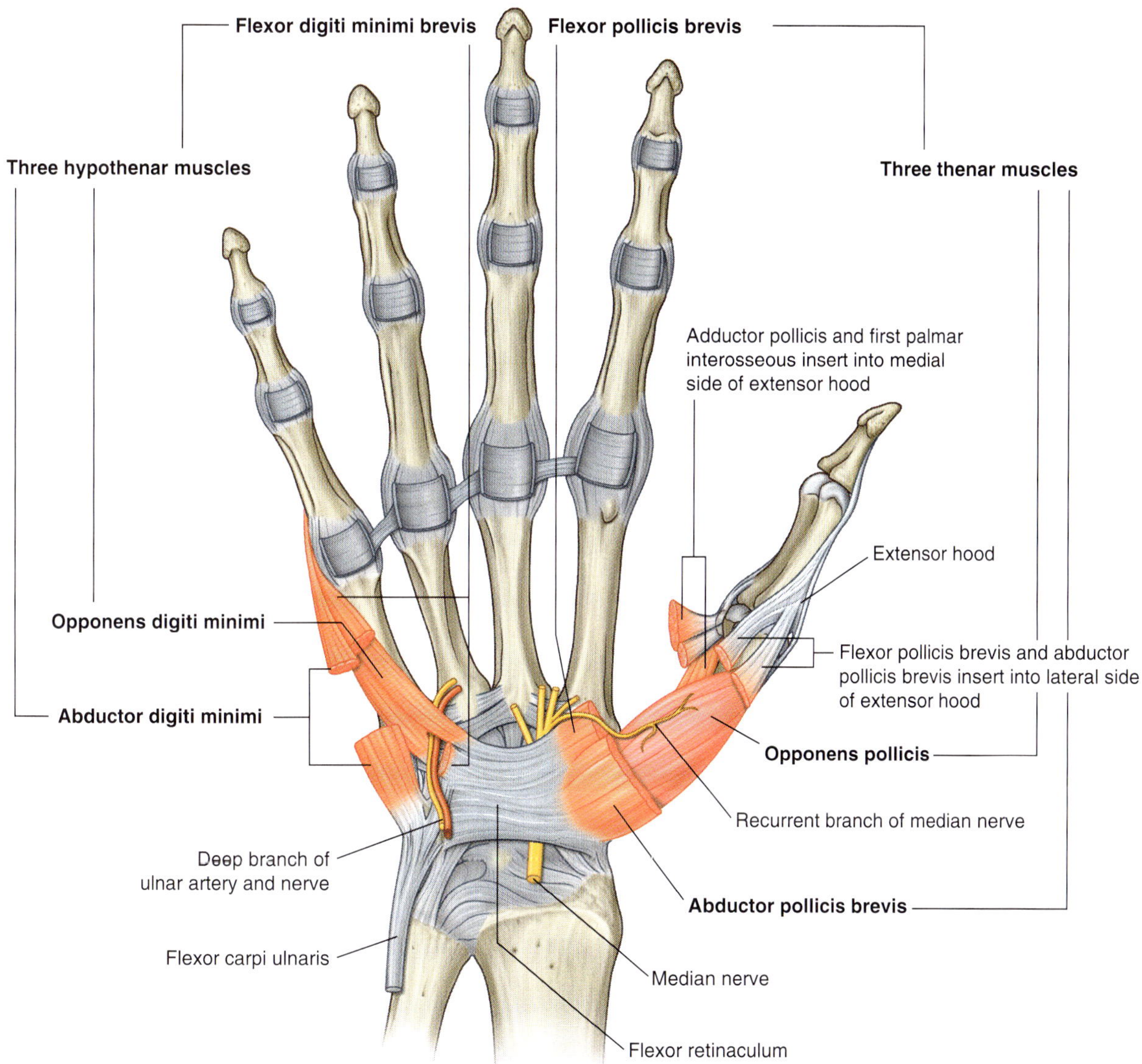

Fig. 2.103 Thenar and hypothenar muscles, right hand.

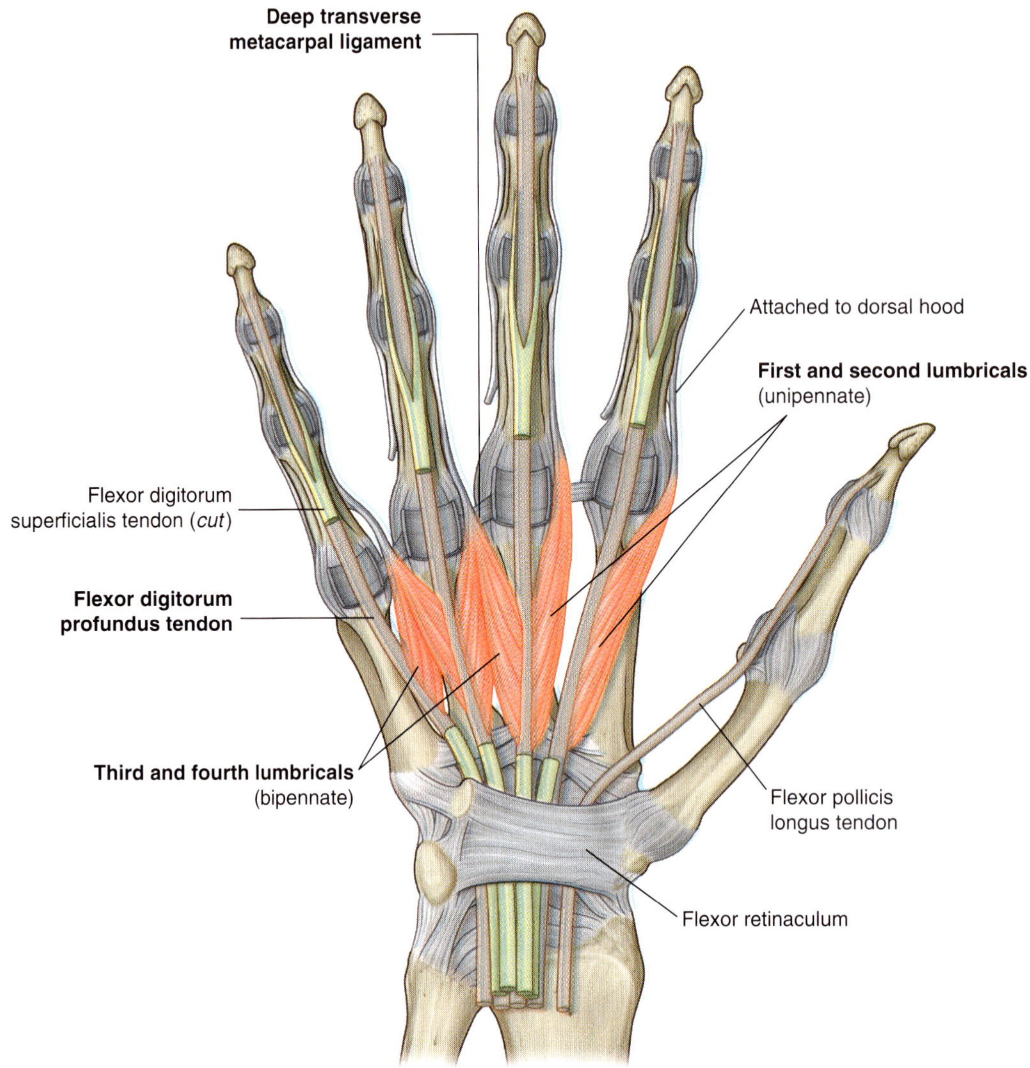

Fig. 2.104 Lumbrical muscles, right hand.

proximal phalanx and into the extensor hood of its related digit.

The tendons of the dorsal interossei pass dorsal to the deep transverse metacarpal ligaments:

- The first dorsal interosseous muscle is the largest and inserts into the lateral side of the index finger.
- The second and third dorsal interossei insert into the lateral and medial sides, respectively, of the middle finger.
- The fourth dorsal interosseous muscle inserts into the medial side of the ring finger.

In addition to generating flexion and extension movements of the fingers through their attachments to the extensor hoods, the dorsal interossei are the major abductors of the index, middle, and ring fingers, at the metacarpophalangeal joints (Table 2.15).

The middle finger can abduct medially and laterally with respect to the long axis of the middle finger and consequently has a dorsal interosseous muscle on each side. The thumb and little finger have their own abductors in the thenar and hypothenar muscle groups, respectively, and therefore do not have dorsal interossei.

The radial artery passes between the two heads of the first dorsal interosseous muscle as it passes from the anatomical snuffbox on the posterolateral side of the wrist into the deep aspect of the palm.

Table 2.15 Intrinsic muscles of the hand

Muscle	Origin	Insertion	Innervation	Function
Palmaris brevis	Palmar aponeurosis and flexor retinaculum	Dermis of skin on the medial margin of the hand	Superficial branch of the ulnar nerve (C8, **T1**)	Improves grip
Dorsal interossei (four muscles)	Adjacent sides of metacarpals	Extensor hood and base of proximal phalanges of index, middle, and ring fingers	Deep branch of ulnar nerve (C8, **T1**)	Abduction of index, middle, and ring fingers at the metacarpophalangeal joints
Palmar interossei (three or four muscles)	Sides of metacarpals	Extensor hoods of the thumb, index, ring, and little fingers and the proximal phalanx of thumb	Deep branch of ulnar nerve (C8, **T1**)	Adduction of the thumb, index, ring, and little fingers at the metacarpophalangeal joints
Adductor pollicis	Transverse head—metacarpal III; oblique head—capitate and bases of metacarpals II and III	Base of proximal phalanx and extensor hood of thumb	Deep branch of ulnar nerve (C8, **T1**)	Adducts thumb
Lumbricals (four muscles)	Tendons of flexor digitorum profundus	Extensor hoods of index, ring, middle, and little fingers	Medial two by the deep branch of the ulnar nerve; lateral two by digital branches of the median nerve	Flex metacarpophalangeal joints while extending interphalangeal joints
THENAR MUSCLES				
Opponens pollicis	Tubercle of trapezium and flexor retinaculum	Lateral margin and adjacent palmar surface of metacarpal I	Recurrent branch of median nerve (C8, **T1**)	Medially rotates thumb
Abductor pollicis brevis	Tubercles of scaphoid and trapezium and adjacent flexor retinaculum	Proximal phalanx and extensor hood of thumb	Recurrent branch of median nerve (C8, **T1**)	Abducts thumb at metacarpophalangeal joint
Flexor pollicis brevis	Tubercle of the trapezium and flexor retinaculum	Proximal phalanx of the thumb	Recurrent branch of median nerve (C8, **T1**)	Flexes thumb at metacarpophalangeal joint
HYPOTHENAR MUSCLES				
Opponens digiti minimi	Hook of hamate and flexor retinaculum	Medial aspect of metacarpal V	Deep branch of ulnar nerve (C8, **T1**)	Laterally rotates metacarpal V
Abductor digiti minimi	Pisiform, the pisohamate ligament, and tendon of flexor carpi ulnaris	Proximal phalanx of little finger	Deep branch of ulnar nerve (C8, **T1**)	Abducts little finger at metacarpophalangeal joint
Flexor digiti minimi brevis	Hook of the hamate and flexor retinaculum	Proximal phalanx of little finger	Deep branch of ulnar nerve (C8, **T1**)	Flexes little finger at metacarpophalangeal joint

Note: Spinal segments indicated in bold are the major segments innervating the muscle.

Palmar interossei

The three (or four) **palmar interossei** are anterior to the dorsal interossei, and are unipennate muscles originating from the metacarpals of the digits with which each is associated (Fig. 2.101).

The first palmar interosseous muscle is rudimentary and often considered part of either the adductor pollicis or the flexor pollicis brevis. When present, it originates from the medial side of the palmar surface of metacarpal I and inserts into both the base of the proximal phalanx of the thumb and the extensor hood. A sesamoid bone often occurs in the tendon attached to the base of the phalanx.

The second palmar interosseous muscle originates from the medial surface of metacarpal II and inserts into the medial side of the extensor hood of the index finger.

The third and fourth palmar interossei originate from the lateral surfaces of metacarpals IV and V and insert into the lateral sides of the respective extensor hoods.

Like the tendons of the dorsal interossei, the tendons of the palmar interossei pass dorsal to the deep transverse metacarpal ligaments.

The palmar interossei adduct the thumb, index, ring, and little fingers with respect to a long axis through the middle finger. The movements occur at the metacarpophalangeal joints. Because the muscles insert into the extensor hoods, they also produce complex flexion and extension movements of the digits (Table 2.15).

Adductor pollicis

The **adductor pollicis** is a large triangular muscle anterior to the plane of the interossei that crosses the palm (Fig. 2.102). It originates as two heads:

- A **transverse head**, from the anterior aspect of the shaft of metacarpal III
- An **oblique head**, from the capitate and adjacent bases of metacarpals II and III

The two heads converge laterally to form a tendon, which often contains a sesamoid bone that inserts into both the medial side of the base of the proximal phalanx of the thumb and the extensor hood.

The radial artery passes anteriorly and medially between the two heads of the muscle to enter the deep plane of the palm and form the deep palmar arch.

The adductor pollicis is a powerful adductor of the thumb and opposes the thumb to the rest of the digits in gripping (Table 2.15).

Thenar muscles

The three thenar muscles (the opponens pollicis, flexor pollicis brevis, and abductor pollicis brevis muscles) are associated with opposition of the thumb to the fingers and with delicate movements of the thumb (Fig. 2.103) and are responsible for the prominent swelling (**thenar eminence**) on the lateral side of the palm at the base of the thumb.

The thenar muscles are innervated by the recurrent branch of the median nerve.

Opponens pollicis

The **opponens pollicis** muscle is the largest of the thenar muscles and lies deep to the other two (Fig. 2.103). Originating from the tubercle of the trapezium and the adjacent flexor retinaculum, it inserts along the entire length of the lateral margin and adjacent lateral palmar surface of metacarpal I.

The opponens pollicis rotates and flexes metacarpal I on the trapezium, so bringing the pad of the thumb into a position facing the pads of the fingers (Table 2.15).

Abductor pollicis brevis

The **abductor pollicis brevis** muscle overlies the opponens pollicis and is proximal to the flexor pollicis brevis muscle (Fig. 2.103). It originates from the tubercles of the scaphoid and trapezium and from the adjacent flexor retinaculum, and inserts into the lateral side of the base of the proximal phalanx of the thumb and into the extensor hood.

The abductor pollicis brevis abducts the thumb, principally at the metacarpophalangeal joint. Its action is most apparent when the thumb is maximally abducted and the proximal phalanx is moved out of line with the long axis of the metacarpal bone (Table 2.15).

Flexor pollicis brevis

The **flexor pollicis brevis** muscle is distal to the abductor pollicis brevis (Fig. 2.103). It originates mainly from the tubercle of the trapezium and adjacent flexor retinaculum, but it may also have deeper attachments to other carpal bones and associated ligaments. It inserts into the lateral side of the base of the proximal phalanx of the thumb. The tendon often contains a sesamoid bone.

The flexor pollicis brevis flexes the metacarpophalangeal joint of the thumb (Table 2.15).

Hypothenar muscles

The hypothenar muscles (the opponens digiti minimi, abductor digiti minimi, and flexor digiti minimi brevis) contribute to the swelling (**hypothenar eminence**) on the medial side of the palm at the base of the little finger (Fig. 2.103). The hypothenar muscles are similar to the thenar muscles in name and in organization.

Unlike the thenar muscles, the hypothenar muscles are innervated by the deep branch of the ulnar nerve and not by the recurrent branch of the median nerve.

Opponens digiti minimi

The **opponens digiti minimi** muscle lies deep to the other two hypothenar muscles (Fig. 2.103). It originates from the hook of the hamate and from the adjacent flexor retinaculum and it inserts into the medial margin and palmar surface of metacarpal V. Its base is penetrated by the deep branches of the ulnar nerve and ulnar artery.

The opponens digiti minimi rotates metacarpal V toward the palm; however, because of the simple shape of the carpometacarpal joint and the presence of a deep transverse metacarpal ligament, which attaches the head of metacarpal V to that of the ring finger, the movement is much less dramatic than that of the thumb (Table 2.15).

Abductor digiti minimi

The **abductor digiti minimi** muscle overlies the opponens digiti minimi (Fig. 2.103). It originates from the pisiform bone, the pisohamate ligament, and the tendon of the flexor carpi ulnaris, and inserts into the medial side of the base of the proximal phalanx of the little finger and into the extensor hood.

The abductor digiti minimi is the principal abductor of the little finger (Table 2.15).

Flexor digiti minimi brevis

The **flexor digiti minimi** brevis muscle is lateral to the abductor digiti minimi (Fig. 2.103). It originates from the hook of the hamate bone and the adjacent flexor retinaculum and inserts with the abductor digiti minimi muscle into the medial side of the base of the proximal phalanx of the little finger.

The flexor digiti minimi brevis flexes the metacarpophalangeal joint.

Lumbrical muscles

There are four lumbrical (worm-like) muscles, each of which is associated with one of the fingers. The muscles originate from the tendons of the flexor digitorum profundus in the palm:

- The medial two lumbricals are bipennate and originate from the flexor digitorum profundus tendons associated with the middle and ring fingers and the ring and little fingers, respectively.
- The lateral two lumbricals are unipennate muscles, originating from the flexor digitorum profundus tendons associated with the index and middle fingers, respectively.

The lumbricals pass dorsally around the lateral side of each finger, and insert into the extensor hood (Fig. 2.104). The tendons of the muscles are anterior to the deep transverse metacarpal ligaments.

The lumbricals are unique because they link flexor tendons with extensor tendons. Through their insertion into the extensor hoods, they participate in flexing the metacarpophalangeal joints and extending the interphalangeal joints.

The medial two lumbricals are innervated by the deep branch of the ulnar nerve; the lateral two lumbricals are innervated by digital branches of the median nerve (Table 2.15).

Arteries and veins

The blood supply to the hand is by the radial and ulnar arteries, which form two interconnected vascular arches (superficial and deep) in the palm (Fig. 2.105). Vessels to the digits, muscles, and joints originate from the two arches and the parent arteries:

- The radial artery contributes substantially to the supply of the thumb and the lateral side of the index finger.
- The remaining digits and the medial side of the index finger are supplied mainly by the ulnar artery.

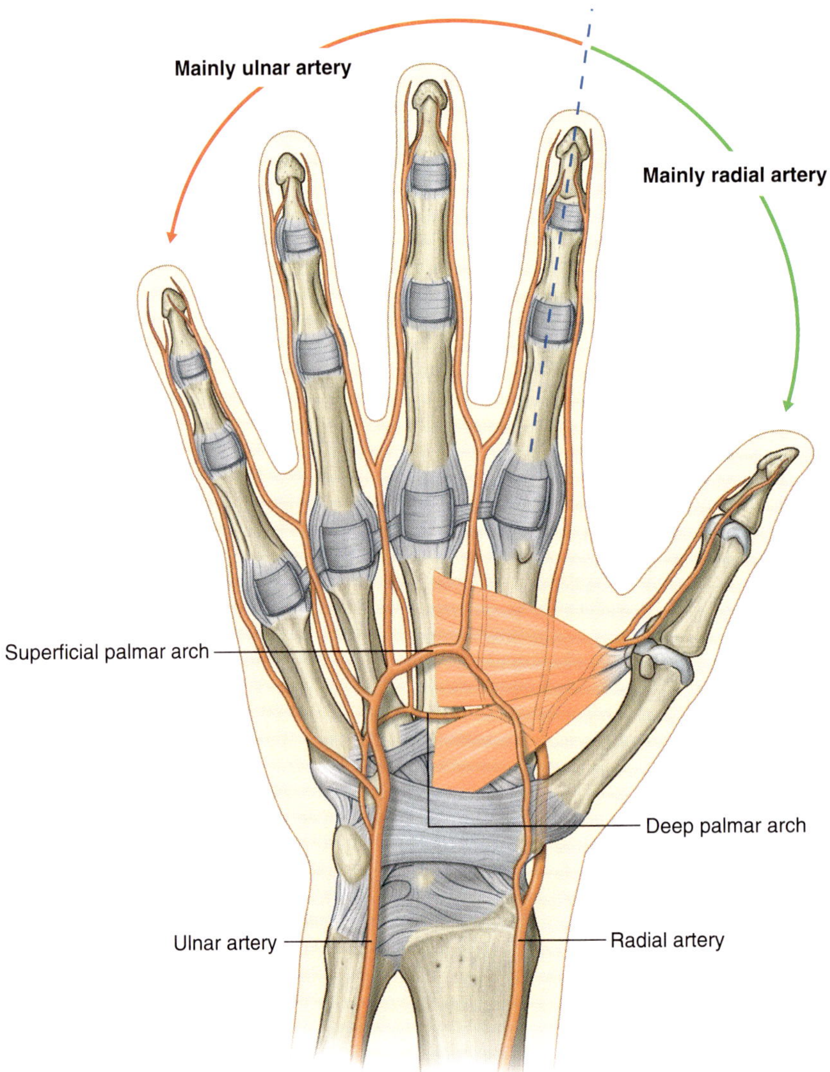

Fig. 2.105 Arterial supply of the right hand.

Ulnar artery and superficial palmar arch

The **ulnar artery** and ulnar nerve enter the hand on the medial side of the wrist (Fig. 2.106). The vessel lies between the palmaris brevis and the flexor retinaculum and is lateral to the ulnar nerve and the pisiform bone. Distally, the ulnar artery is medial to the hook of the hamate bone and then swings laterally across the palm, forming the **superficial palmar arch**, which is superficial to the long flexor tendons of the digits and just deep to the palmar aponeurosis. On the lateral side of the palm, the arch communicates with a palmar branch of the radial artery.

One branch of the ulnar artery in the hand is the **deep palmar branch** (Figs. 2.105 and 2.106), which arises from the medial aspect of the ulnar artery, just distal to the pisiform, and penetrates the origin of the hypothenar muscles. It curves medially around the hook of the hamate to access the deep plane of the palm and to anastomose with the deep palmar arch derived from the radial artery.

Branches from the superficial palmar arch include:

- A palmar digital artery to the medial side of the little finger.
- Three large, **common palmar digital arteries**, which ultimately provide the principal blood supply to the lateral side of the little finger, both sides of the ring and middle fingers, and the medial side of the index finger (Fig. 2.106); they are joined by palmar metacarpal arteries from the deep palmar arch before bifurcating into the **proper palmar digital arteries**, which enter the fingers.

Radial artery and deep palmar arch

The **radial artery** curves around the lateral side of the wrist and passes over the floor of the anatomical snuffbox and into the deep plane of the palm by penetrating anteriorly through the back of the hand (Figs. 2.105 and 2.107). It passes between the two heads of the first dorsal interosseous muscle and then between the two heads of the adductor pollicis to access the deep plane of the palm and form the deep palmar arch.

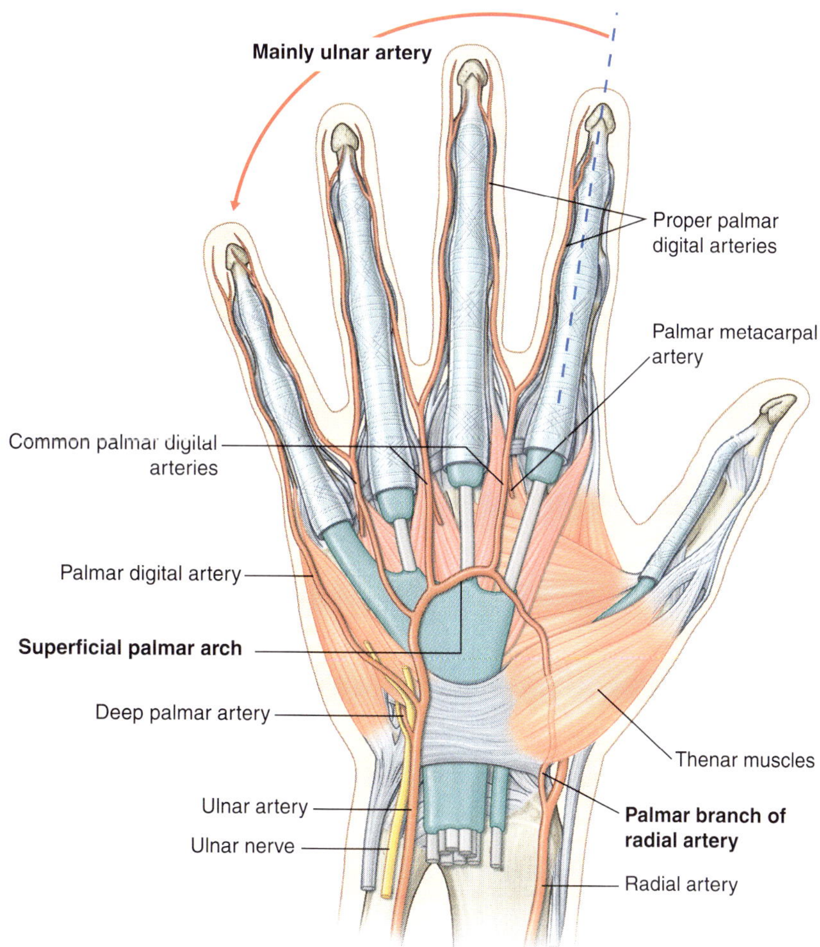

Fig. 2.106 Superficial palmar arch, right hand.

The **deep palmar arch** passes medially through the palm between the metacarpal bones and the long flexor tendons of the digits. On the medial side of the palm, it communicates with the deep palmar branch of the ulnar artery (Figs. 2.105 and 2.107).

Before penetrating the back of the hand, the radial artery gives rise to two vessels:

- A **dorsal carpal branch**, which passes medially as the **dorsal carpal arch**, across the wrist and gives rise to **three dorsal metacarpal arteries**, which subsequently divide to become small dorsal digital arteries, which enter the fingers
- The **first dorsal metacarpal artery**, which supplies adjacent sides of the index finger and thumb

Two vessels, the **princeps pollicis artery** and the **radialis indicis artery**, arise from the radial artery in the plane between the first dorsal interosseous and adductor pollicis. The princeps pollicis artery is the major blood supply to the thumb, and the radialis indicis artery supplies the lateral side of the index finger.

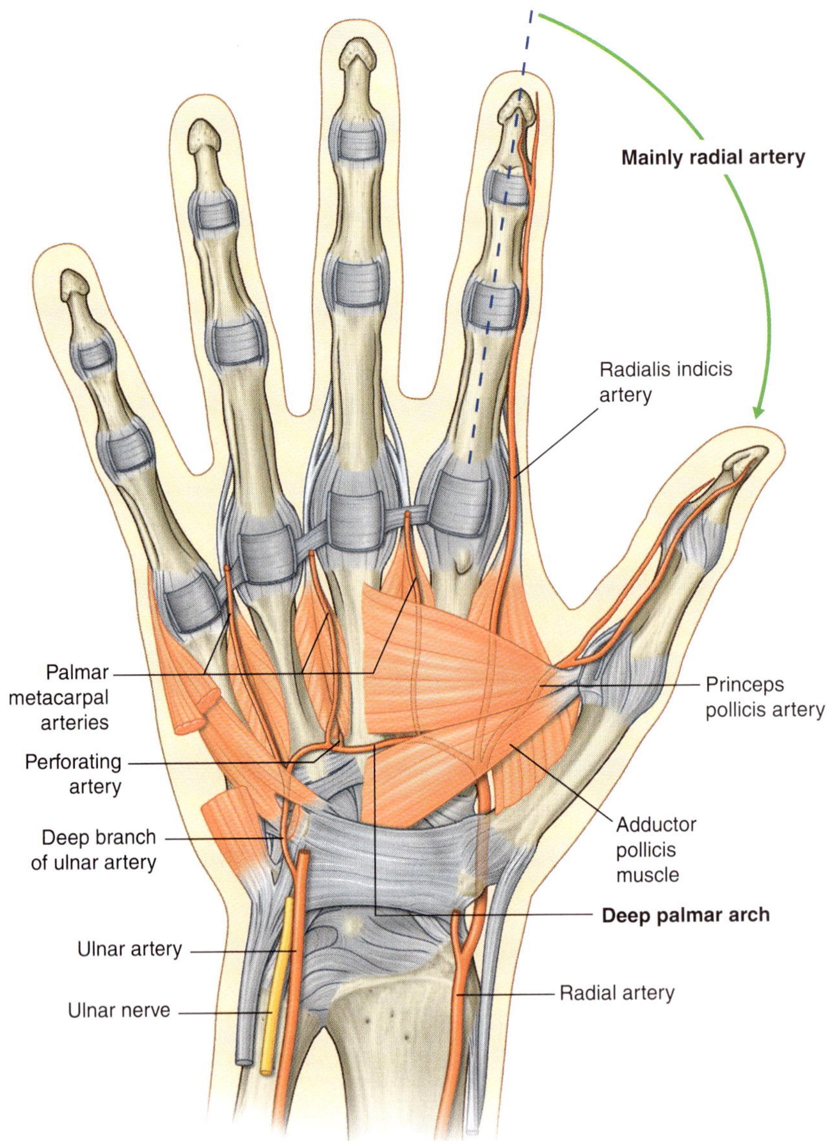

Fig. 2.107 Deep palmar arch, right hand.

The deep palmar arch gives rise to:

- Three **palmar metacarpal arteries**, which join the common palmar digital arteries from the superficial palmar arch
- Three **perforating branches**, which pass posteriorly between the heads of origin of the dorsal interossei to anastomose with the dorsal metacarpal arteries from the dorsal carpal arch

Early clinical exposure

Allen's test

To test for adequate anastomoses between the radial and ulnar arteries, compress both the radial and ulnar arteries at the wrist, then release pressure from one or the other, and determine the filling pattern of the hand. If there is little connection between the deep and superficial palmar arteries, only the thumb and lateral side of the index finger will fill with blood (become red) when pressure on the radial artery alone is released.

Veins

As generally found in the upper limb, the hand contains interconnected networks of deep and superficial veins. The deep veins follow the arteries; the superficial veins drain into a dorsal venous network on the back of the hand over the metacarpal bones (Fig. 2.108).

The cephalic vein originates from the lateral side of the dorsal venous network and passes over the anatomical snuffbox into the forearm.

The basilic vein originates from the medial side of the dorsal venous network and passes into the dorsomedial aspect of the forearm.

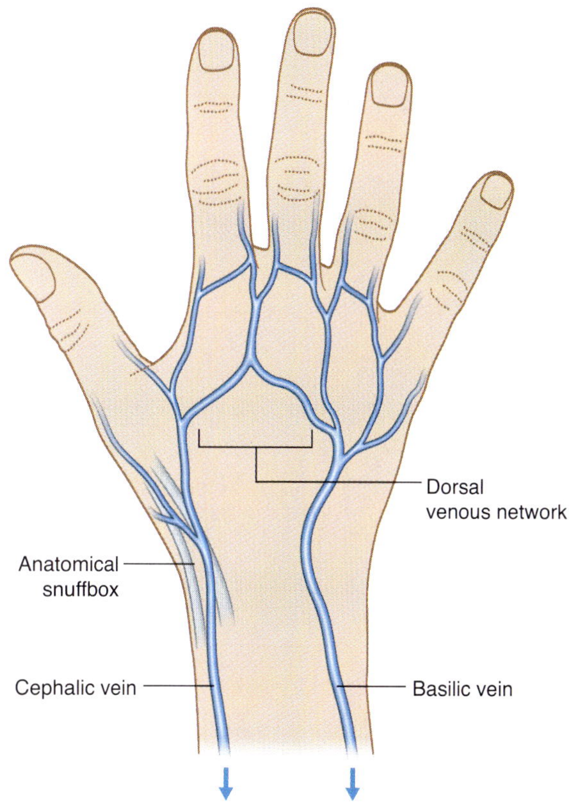

Fig. 2.108 Dorsal venous arch of the right hand.

Early clinical exposure

Venipuncture

In many patients, venous access is necessary for obtaining blood for laboratory testing and administering fluid and intravenous drugs. The ideal sites for venous access are typically in the cubital fossa and in the cephalic vein adjacent to the anatomical snuffbox. The veins are simply distended by use of a tourniquet. A tourniquet should be applied enough to allow the veins to become prominent. For straightforward blood tests the antecubital vein is usually the preferred site, and although it may not always be visible, it is easily palpated. The cephalic vein is generally the preferred site for a short-term intravenous cannula.

Nerves

The hand is supplied by the ulnar, median, and radial nerves (Fig. 2.109–2.111A). All three nerves contribute to cutaneous or general sensory innervation. The ulnar nerve innervates all intrinsic muscles of the hand except for the three thenar muscles and the two lateral lumbricals, which are innervated by the median nerve. The radial nerve only innervates skin on the dorsolateral side of the hand.

Ulnar nerve

The ulnar nerve enters the hand lateral to the pisiform and posteromedially to the ulnar artery (Fig. 2.109). Immediately distal to the pisiform, it divides into a deep branch, which is mainly motor, and a superficial branch, which is mainly sensory.

The deep branch of the ulnar nerve passes with the deep branch of the ulnar artery (Fig. 2.109). It penetrates and supplies the hypothenar muscles to reach the deep aspect of the palm, arches laterally across the palm, deep to the long flexors of the digits, and supplies the interossei, the adductor pollicis, and the two medial lumbricals. In addition, the deep branch of the ulnar nerve contributes small articular branches to the wrist joint.

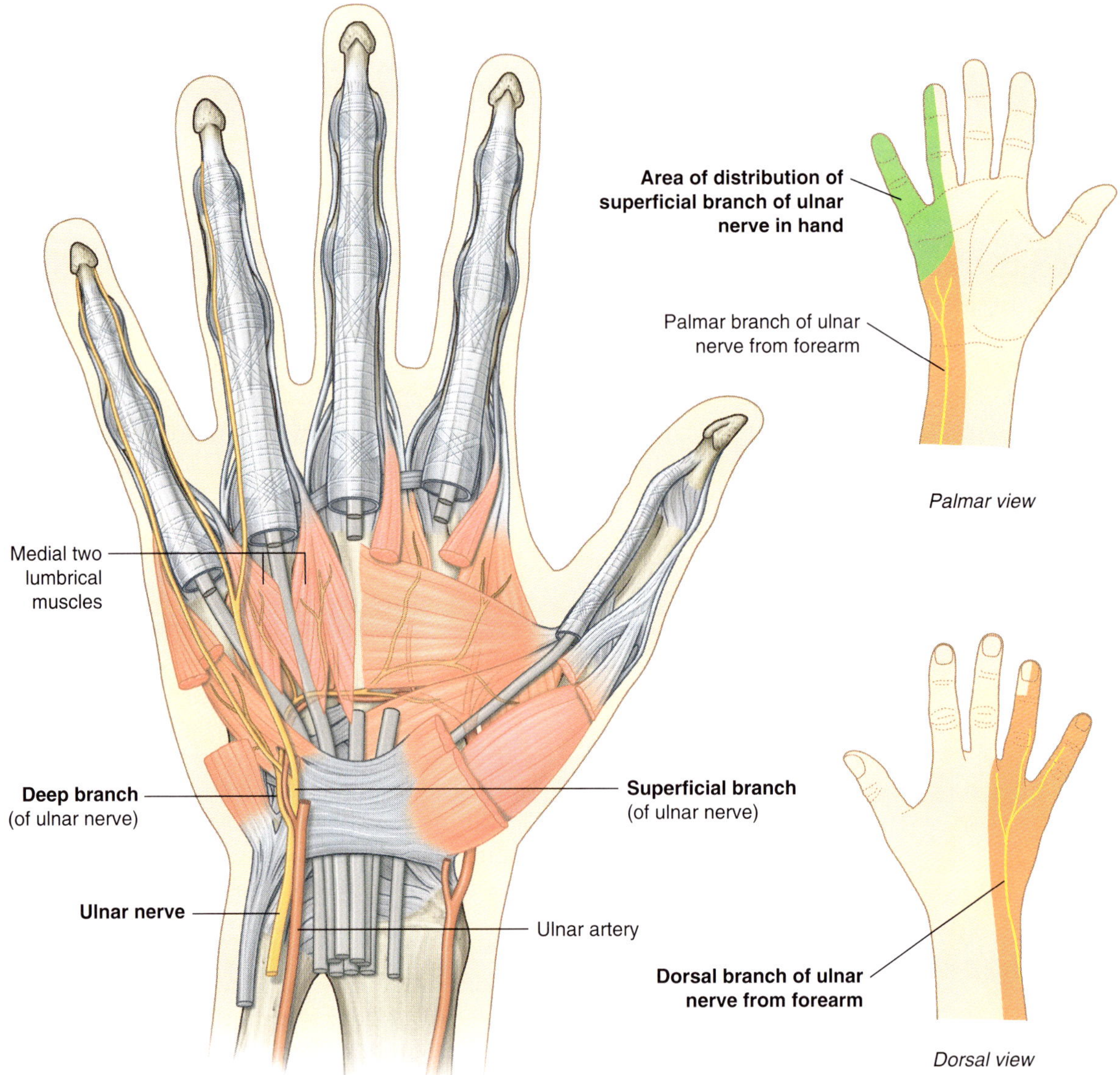

Fig. 2.109 Ulnar nerve in the right hand.

As the **deep branch** of the ulnar nerve passes across the palm, it lies in a fibro-osseous tunnel (Guyon's canal) between the hook of the hamate and the flexor tendons. Occasionally, small outpouchings of synovial membrane (ganglia) from the joints of the carpus compress the nerve within this canal, producing sensory and motor symptoms.

The superficial branch of the ulnar nerve innervates the palmaris brevis muscle and continues across the palm to supply skin on the palmar surface of the little finger and the medial half of the ring finger (Fig. 2.109).

Early clinical exposure

Ulnar nerve injury

The ulnar nerve is most commonly injured at two sites: the elbow and the wrist.

- At the elbow, the nerve lies posterior to the medial epicondyle.
- At the wrist, the ulnar nerve passes superficial to the flexor retinaculum and lies lateral to the pisiform bone.

Ulnar nerve lesions are characterized by "clawing" of the hand, in which the metacarpophalangeal joints of the fingers are hyperextended and the interphalangeal joints are flexed because the function of most of the intrinsic muscles of the hand is lost (Fig. 2.110).

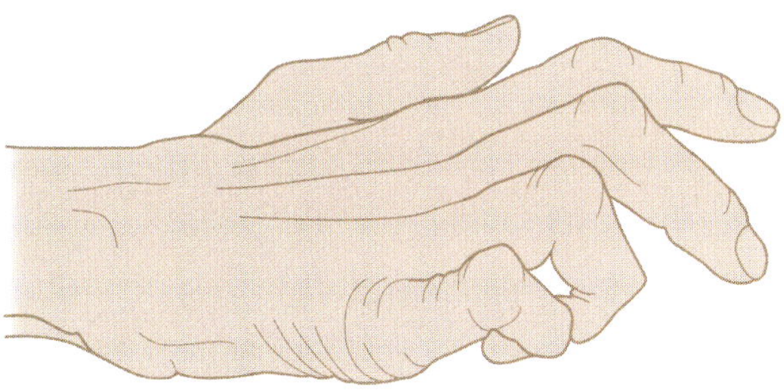

Fig. 2.110 Typical appearance of a "clawed hand" due to a lesion of the ulnar nerve.

Clawing is most pronounced in the medial fingers because the function of all intrinsic muscles of these digits is lost while in the lateral two digits, the lumbricals are innervated by the median nerve. Function of the adductor pollicis muscle is also lost.

In lesions of the ulnar nerve at the elbow, function of the flexor carpi ulnaris muscle and flexor digitorum profundus to the medial two digits is lost as well. Clawing of the hand, particularly of the little and ring fingers, is worse with lesions of the ulnar nerve at the wrist than at the elbow because interruption of the nerve at the elbow paralyzes the ulnar half of the flexor digitorum profundus, which leads to lack of flexion at the distal interphalangeal joints in these fingers.

Ulnar nerve lesions at the elbow and wrist result in impaired sensory innervation on the palmar aspect of the medial one and one-half digits.

Damage to the ulnar nerve at the wrist or at a site proximal to the wrist can be distinguished by evaluating the status of function of the **dorsal branch** (cutaneous) of the ulnar nerve, which originates in distal regions of the forearm. This branch innervates skin over the dorsal surface of the hand on the medial side.

Median nerve

The median nerve is the most important sensory nerve in the hand because it innervates skin on the thumb, index and middle fingers, and lateral side of the ring finger (Fig. 2.111A). The nervous system, using touch, gathers information about the environment from this area, particularly from the skin on the thumb and index finger. In addition, sensory information from the lateral three and one-half digits enables the fingers to be positioned with the appropriate amount of force when using precision grip.

The median nerve also innervates the thenar muscles that are responsible for opposition of the thumb to the other digits.

The median nerve enters the hand by passing through the carpal tunnel and divides into a recurrent branch and palmar digital branches (Fig. 2.111A).

The **recurrent branch** of the median nerve innervates the three thenar muscles. Originating from the lateral side of the median nerve near the distal margin of the flexor retinaculum, it curves around the margin

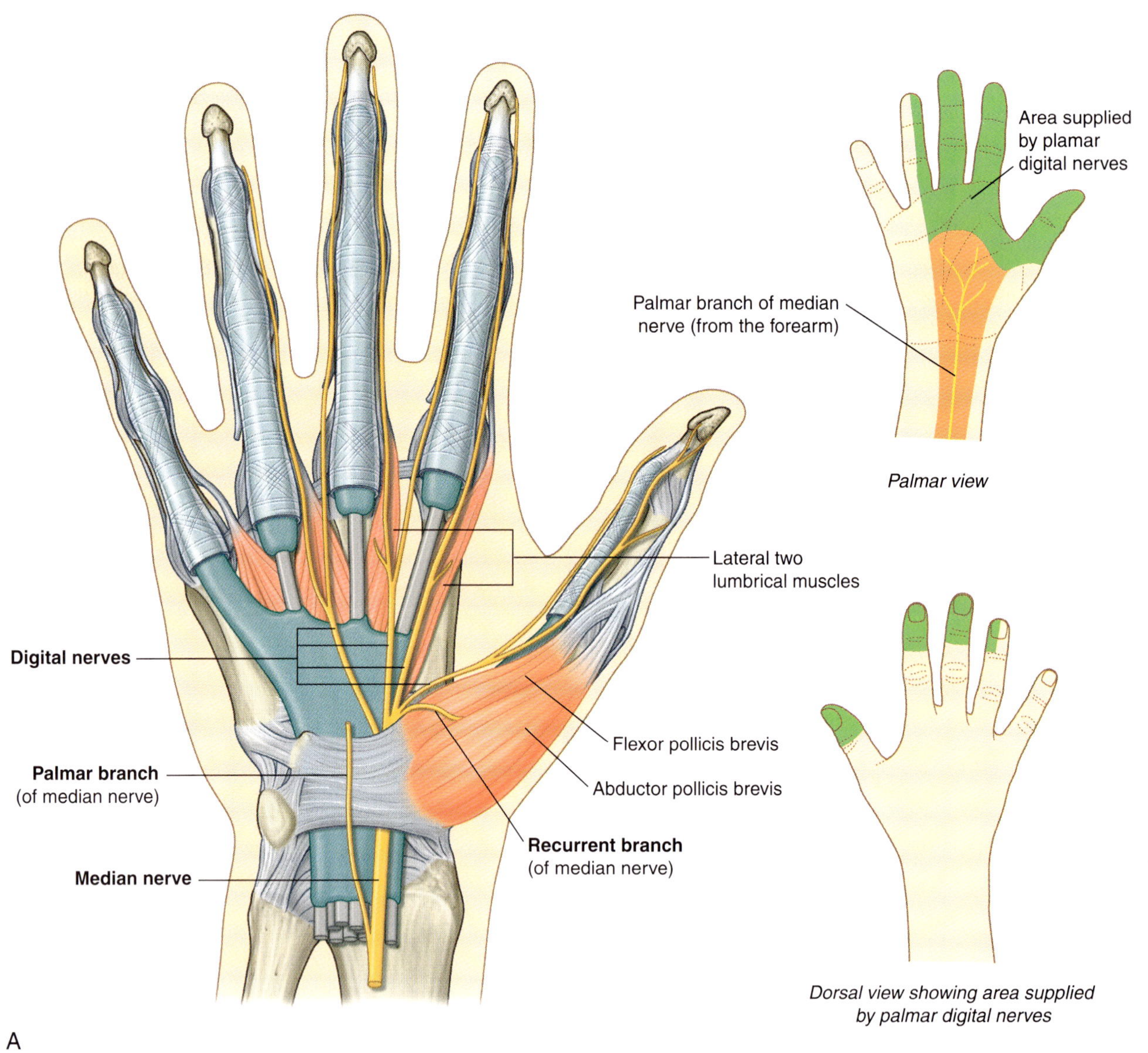

Fig. 2.111 (A) Median nerve in the hand.

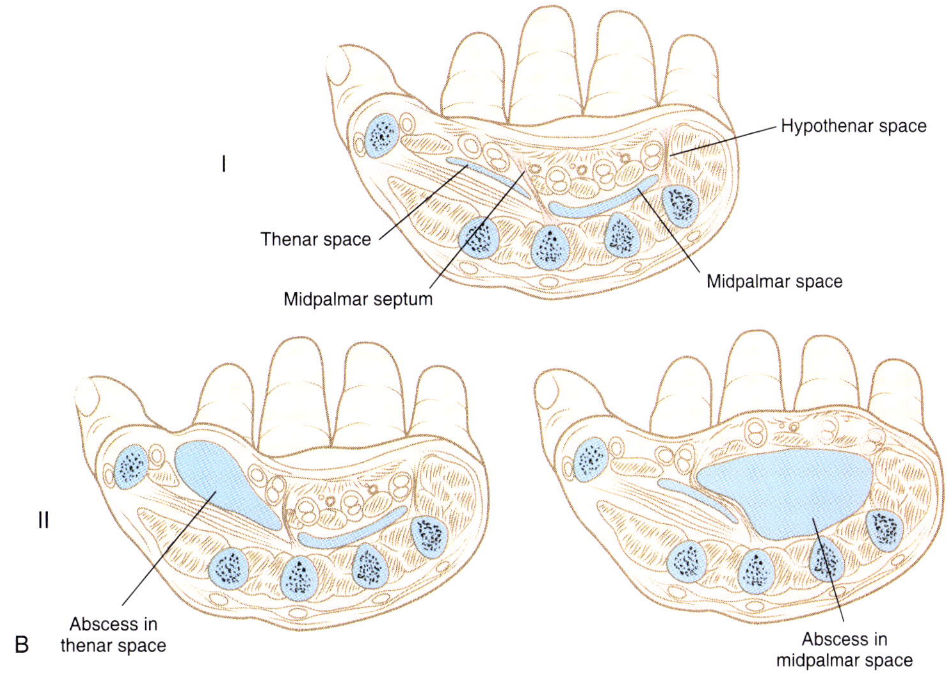

Fig. 2.111, cont'd (B) Fascial spaces of the palm. Deep palmar spaces. **(I)** Potential spaces of the mid palm. **(II)** Abscess in the thenar space. **(III)** Abscess in the midpalmar space. *Source:* David P. Green, Scott W. Wolfe, Robert N. Hotchkiss, Scott H. Kozin, William C. Pederson. Green's Operative Hand Surgery, Acute Infections. Churchill Livingstone, 2010:41–84.

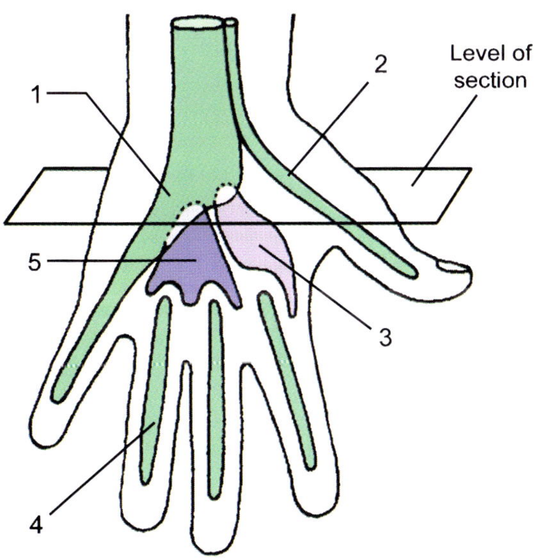

LD Fig. 2.111B.1 Synovial sheaths of the hand.

Question

2.111B.1 Name the structures indicated by the labels.

Answer

2.111B.1 The structures indicated by the labels are

1. Ulnar bursa
2. Radial bursa
3. Thenar space
4. Digital synovial sheath of the fourth digit
5. Midpalmar space

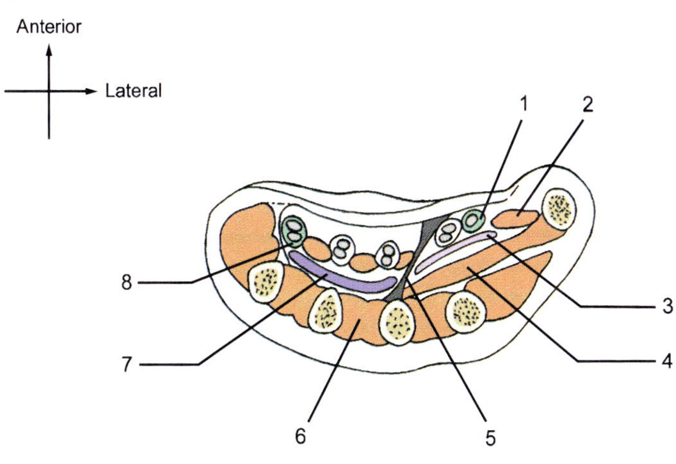

LD Fig. 2.111B.2 Palmar spaces.

Question

2.111B.2 Name the structures indicated by the labels.

Answer

2.111B.2 The structures indicated by the labels are

1. Radial bursa
2. Thenar eminence
3. Thenar space
4. Adductor pollicis
5. Midpalmar septum
6. Interosseous muscles
7. Thenar space
8. Ulnar bursa

of the retinaculum and passes proximally over the flexor pollicis brevis muscle. The recurrent branch then passes between the flexor pollicis brevis and abductor pollicis brevis to end in the opponens pollicis.

The **palmar digital nerves** cross the palm deep to the palmar aponeurosis and the superficial palmar arch and enter the digits. They innervate skin on the palmar surfaces of the lateral three and one-half digits and cutaneous regions over the dorsal aspects of the distal phalanges (nail beds) of the same digits. In addition to skin, the digital nerves supply the lateral two lumbrical muscles.

Superficial branch of the radial nerve

The only part of the radial nerve that enters the hand is the superficial branch (Fig. 2.112). It enters the hand by passing over the anatomical snuffbox on the dorsolateral side of the wrist. Terminal branches of the nerve can be palpated or "rolled" against the tendon of the extensor pollicis longus as they cross the anatomical snuffbox.

The superficial branch of the radial nerve innervates skin over the dorsolateral aspect of the palm and the dorsal aspects of the lateral three and one-half digits distally to approximately the terminal interphalangeal joints.

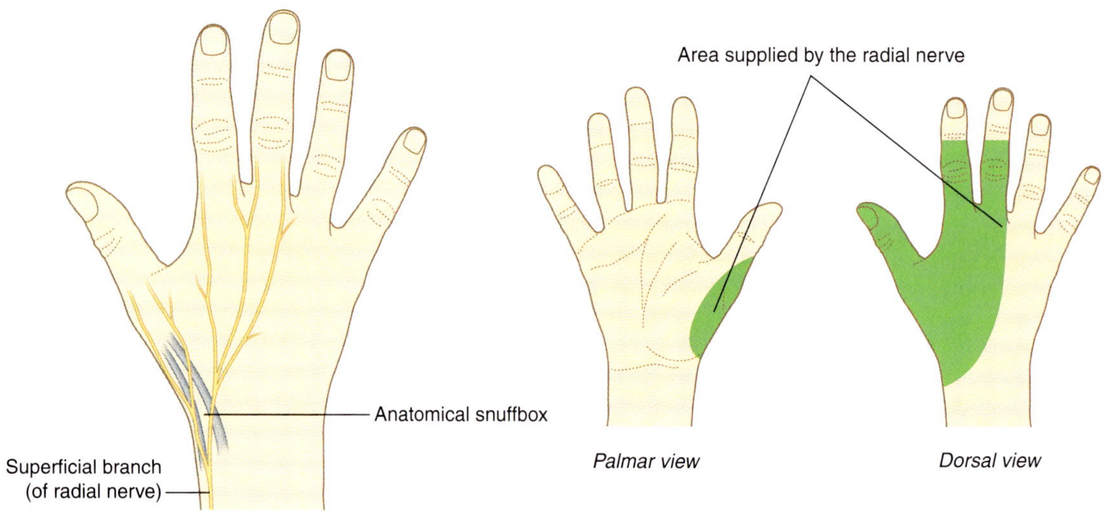

Fig. 2.112 Radial nerve in the hand.

Early clinical exposure

Radial nerve injury

Around the elbow joint, the radial nerve divides into its two terminal branches—the superficial branch and the deep branch.

The most common radial nerve injury is damage to the nerve in the radial groove of the humerus, which produces a global paralysis of the muscles of the posterior compartment, resulting in **wrist drop**. Radial nerve damage can result from fracture of the shaft of the humerus as the radial nerve spirals around in the radial groove. The typical injury produces reduction of sensation in the cutaneous distribution, predominantly over the posterior aspect of the hand. Severing the posterior interosseous nerve (continuation of deep branch of radial nerve) may paralyze the muscles of the posterior compartment of the forearm, but the nerve supply is variable. Typically, the patient may not be able to extend the fingers.

The distal branches of the superficial branch of the radial nerve can be readily palpated as "cords" passing over the tendon of the extensor pollicis longus in the anatomical snuffbox. Damage to these branches is of little consequence because they supply only a small area of skin.

Fascial spaces of the palm

The fascial spaces of the hand are potential spaces filled with connective tissue, limited by fibrous septa, and present on the dorsal and palmar aspects of the hand.

On the palmar aspect, there are the thenar space, midpalmar space, pulp space, and forearm space of Parona.

On the dorsal aspect, there are the dorsal subcutaneous space and dorsal subaponeurotic space.

The palmar fascial spaces are limited by fibrous septae extending from the palmar aponeurosis to the first metacarpal on the radial side and the fifth metacarpal on the ulnar side (Fig. 2.111B).

The thenar space is triangular in shape and located deep to the outer half of the hollow of the palm. The boundaries of the space are: anteriorly, the flexor tendons of index finger with the first and second lumbricals; posteriorly, the transverse head of adductor pollicis; laterally, the tendon of flexor pollicis longus with its synovial sheath; and, medially, the septum separating the thenar and midpalmar spaces

The midpalmar space is also triangular in shape and is located deep to the inner half of the hollow of the hand. The boundaries of the space are: anteriorly, the flexors of the little, ring, and middle fingers with their synovial sheaths and the third and fourth lumbricals; posteriorly, the dense fascia covering the interossei and metacarpals; laterally, the septum separating it from the thenar space; and, medially, the hypothenar muscles. Proximally, this space is continuous with the forearm space of Parona (Fig. 2.111B).

Forearm space of Parona: This is a potential fascial space in the distal part of forearm bounded anteriorly by the flexor digitorum profundus and posteriorly by the pronator quadratus muscle. This space extends distally to the wrist and proximally it is continuous with the forearm intermuscular space.

Early clinical exposure

Palmar space infection

Thenar and midpalmar space infection can occur following a penetrating injury to the hand. Thenar space infection can be drained by an incision between the thumb and index finger. In midpalmar space infection, the concavity of the palm is lost and this space is drained through a palmar incision along one of the lumbrical canals to avoid the neurovascular bundle.

Surface anatomy

Upper limb surface anatomy

Tendons, muscles, and bony landmarks in the upper limb are used to locate major arteries, veins, and nerves. Asking patients to maneuver their upper limbs in specific ways is essential for performing neurological examinations.

- Tendons are used to test reflexes associated with specific spinal cord segments.
- Vessels are used clinically as points of entry into the vascular system (for collecting blood and administering pharmaceuticals and nutrients), and for taking blood pressure and pulses.
- Nerves can become entrapped or be damaged in regions where they are related to bone or pass through confined spaces.

Bony landmarks and muscles of the posterior scapular region

The medial border, inferior angle, and part of the lateral border of the scapula can be palpated on a patient, as can the spine and acromion. The superior border and angle of the scapula are deep to soft tissue and are not readily palpable. The supraspinatus and infraspinatus muscles can be palpated above and below the spine, respectively (Fig. 2.113).

The trapezius muscle is responsible for the smooth contour of the lateral side of the neck and over the superior aspect of the shoulder.

The deltoid muscles form the muscular eminence inferior to the acromion and around the glenohumeral joint. The axillary nerve passes posteriorly around the surgical neck of the humerus deep to the deltoid muscle.

The latissimus dorsi muscle forms much of the muscle mass underlying the posterior axillary skin fold extending obliquely upward from the trunk to the arm. The teres major muscle passes from the inferior angle of the scapula to the upper humerus and contributes to this posterior axillary skin fold laterally.

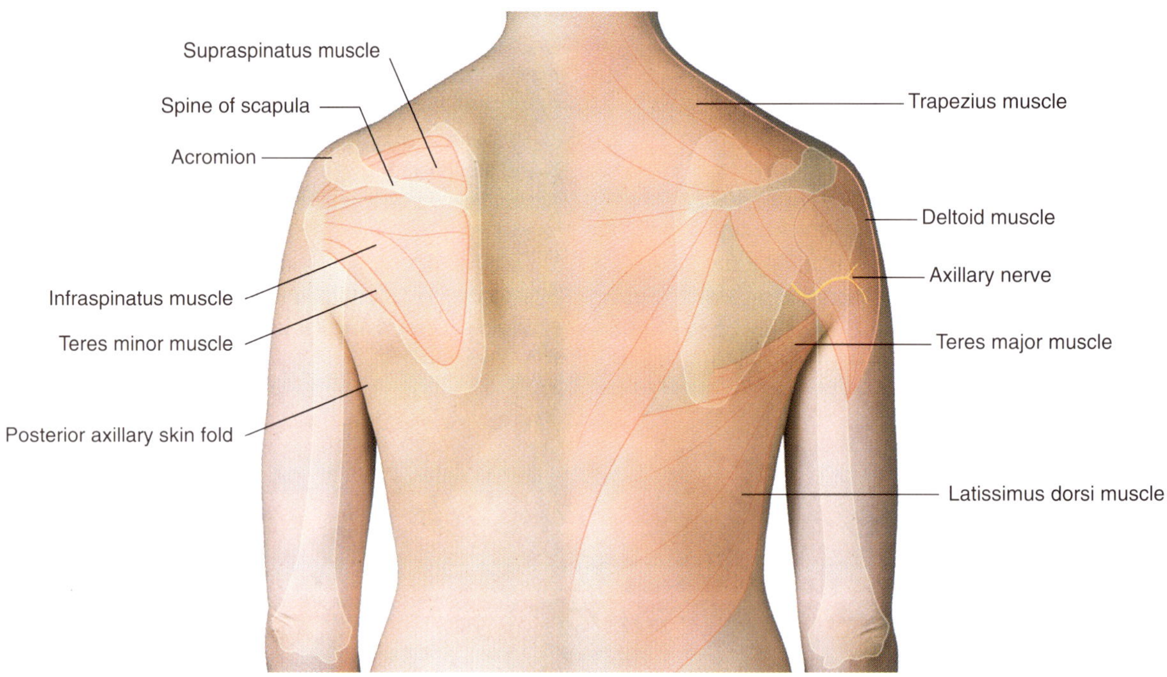

Fig. 2.113 Bony landmarks and muscles of the posterior scapular region. Posterior view of shoulder and back.

Visualizing the axilla and locating contents and related structures

The axillary inlet and outlet and walls of the axilla can be established using skin folds and palpable bony landmarks (Fig. 2.114).

- The anterior margin of the axillary inlet is the clavicle, which can be palpated along its entire length. The lateral limit of the axillary inlet is approximated by the tip of the coracoid process, which is palpable immediately below the lateral third of the clavicle and deep to the medial margin of the deltoid muscle.
- The inferior margin of the anterior axillary wall is the anterior axillary skin fold, which overlies the lower margin of the pectoralis major muscle.
- The inferior margin of the posterior axillary wall is the posterior axillary skin fold, which overlies the margins of the teres major muscle laterally and latissimus dorsi muscle medially.
- The medial wall of the axilla is the upper part of the serratus anterior muscle overlying the thoracic wall. The

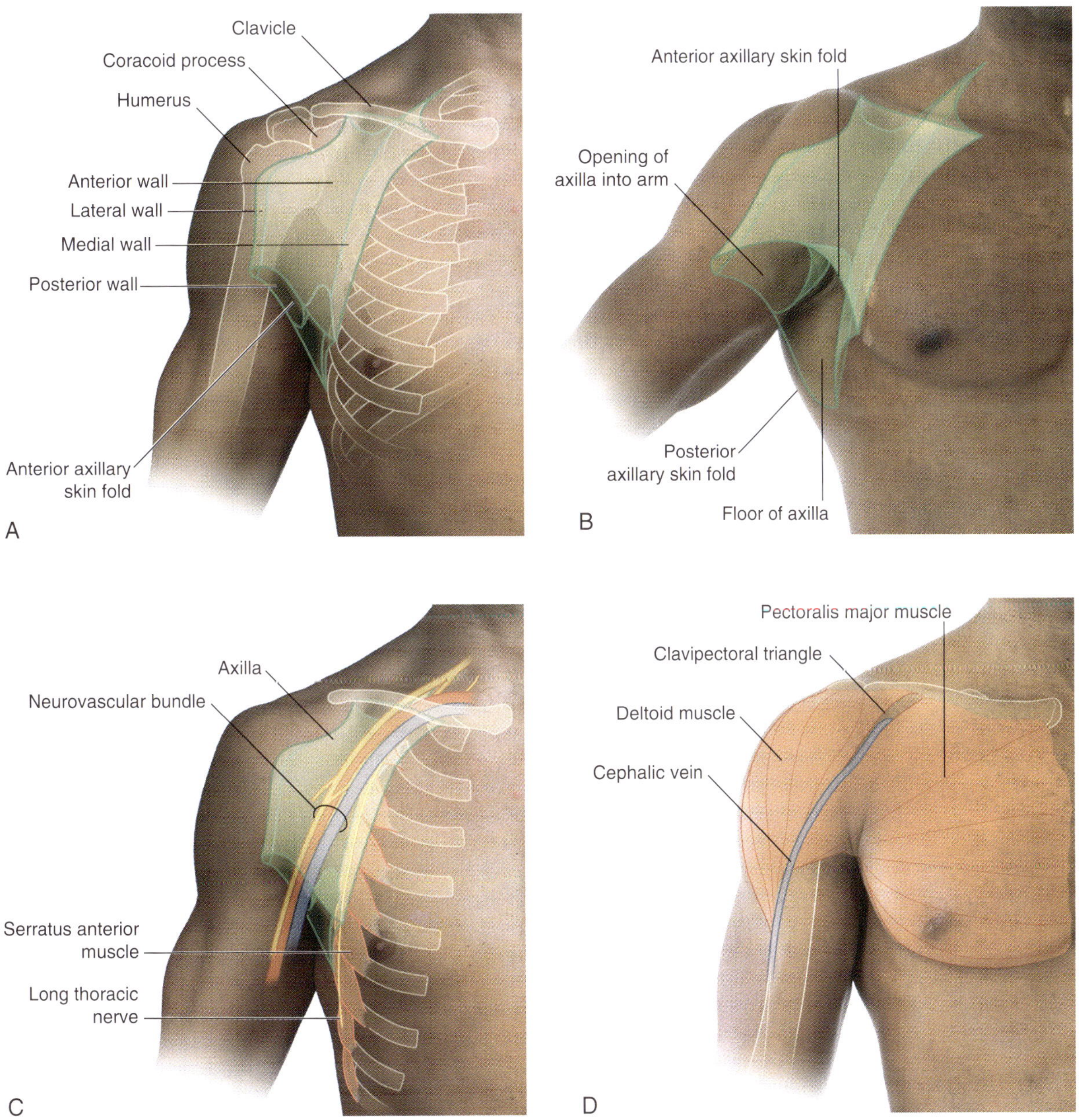

Fig. 2.114 Visualizing the axilla and locating its contents and related structures. **(A)** Anterior shoulder showing folds and walls of the axilla. **(B)** Anterior shoulder showing outlet and floor of the axilla. **(C)** Anterior view showing the axillary neurovascular bundle and long thoracic nerve. **(D)** Anterior view of the shoulder showing the clavipectoral triangle with the cephalic vein.

long thoracic nerve passes vertically out of the axilla and down the lateral surface of the serratus anterior muscle in a position just anterior to the posterior axillary skin fold.

- The lateral boundary of the axilla is the humerus.
- The floor of the axilla is the dome of skin between the posterior and anterior axillary skin folds.

Major vessels, nerves, and lymphatics travel between the upper limb and the trunk by passing through the axilla.

The axillary artery, axillary vein, and components of the brachial plexus pass through the axilla and into the arm by traveling lateral to the dome of skin that forms the floor. This neurovascular bundle can be palpated by placing a hand into this dome of skin and pressing laterally against the humerus.

The cephalic vein travels in superficial fascia in the cleft between the deltoid muscle and the pectoralis major muscle and penetrates deep fascia in the clavipectoral triangle to join with the axillary vein.

Locating the brachial artery in the arm

The brachial artery is on the medial side of the arm in the cleft between the biceps brachii and triceps brachii muscles (Fig. 2.115). The median nerve courses with the brachial artery, whereas the ulnar nerve deviates posteriorly from the vessel in distal regions.

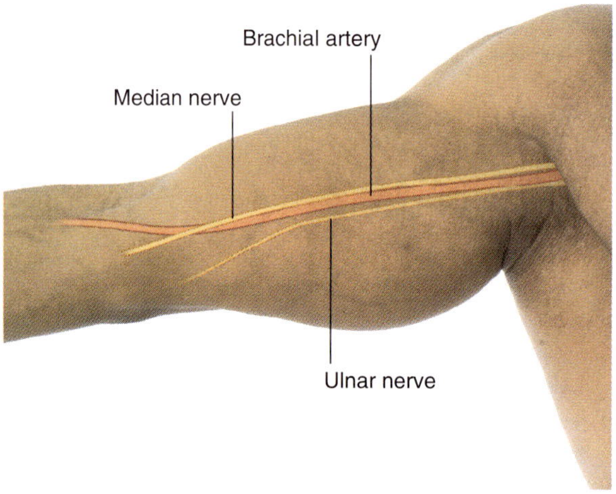

Fig. 2.115 Locating the brachial artery in the right arm (medial view of arm with brachial artery, median nerve, and ulnar nerve).

The triceps brachii tendon and position of the radial nerve

The triceps brachii muscle forms the soft tissue mass posterior to the humerus, and the tendon inserts onto the olecranon of the ulna, which is readily palpable and forms the bony protuberance at the "tip" of the elbow (Fig. 2.116).

The brachioradialis muscle is also visible as a muscular bulge on the lateral aspect of the arm. It is particularly prominent when the forearm is half pronated, flexed at the elbow against resistance, and viewed anteriorly.

The radial nerve in the distal arm emerges from behind the humerus to lie deep to the brachioradialis muscle.

Cubital fossa (anterior view)

The cubital fossa lies anterior to the elbow joint and contains the biceps brachii tendon, the brachial artery, and the median nerve (Fig. 2.117).

The base of the cubital fossa is an imaginary line between the readily palpable medial and lateral epicondyles of the humerus. The lateral and medial borders are formed by the brachioradialis and pronator teres muscles, respectively. The margin of the brachioradialis can be found by asking a subject to flex the semipronated forearm against resistance. The margin of the pronator teres can be estimated by an oblique line extending between the medial epicondyle and the midpoint along the length of the lateral surface of the forearm. The approximate apex of the cubital fossa is where this line meets the margin of the brachioradialis muscle.

Contents of the cubital fossa, from lateral to medial, are the tendon of the biceps brachii, the brachial artery, and the median nerve. The tendon of the biceps brachii is easily palpable. Often the cephalic, basilic, and median cubital veins are visible in the subcutaneous fascia overlying the cubital fossa.

The ulnar nerve passes behind the medial epicondyle of the humerus and can be "rolled" here against the bone.

The radial nerve travels into the forearm deep to the margin of the brachioradialis muscle anterior to the elbow joint.

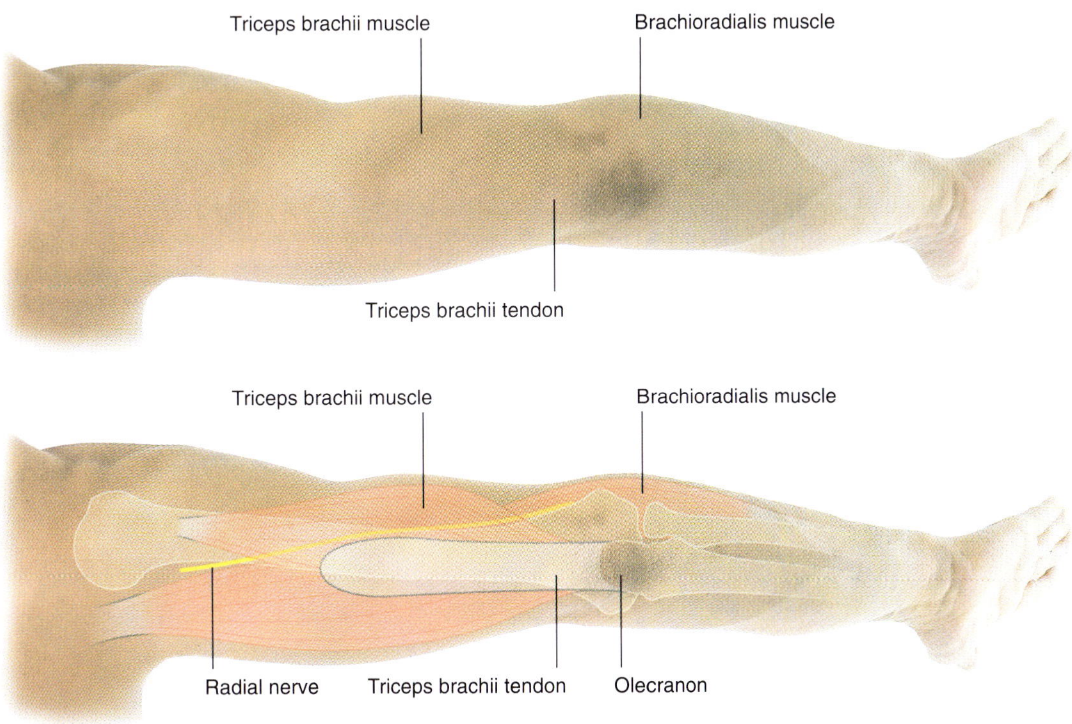

Fig. 2.116 Triceps brachii tendon and position of the radial nerve (posterior view of right arm).

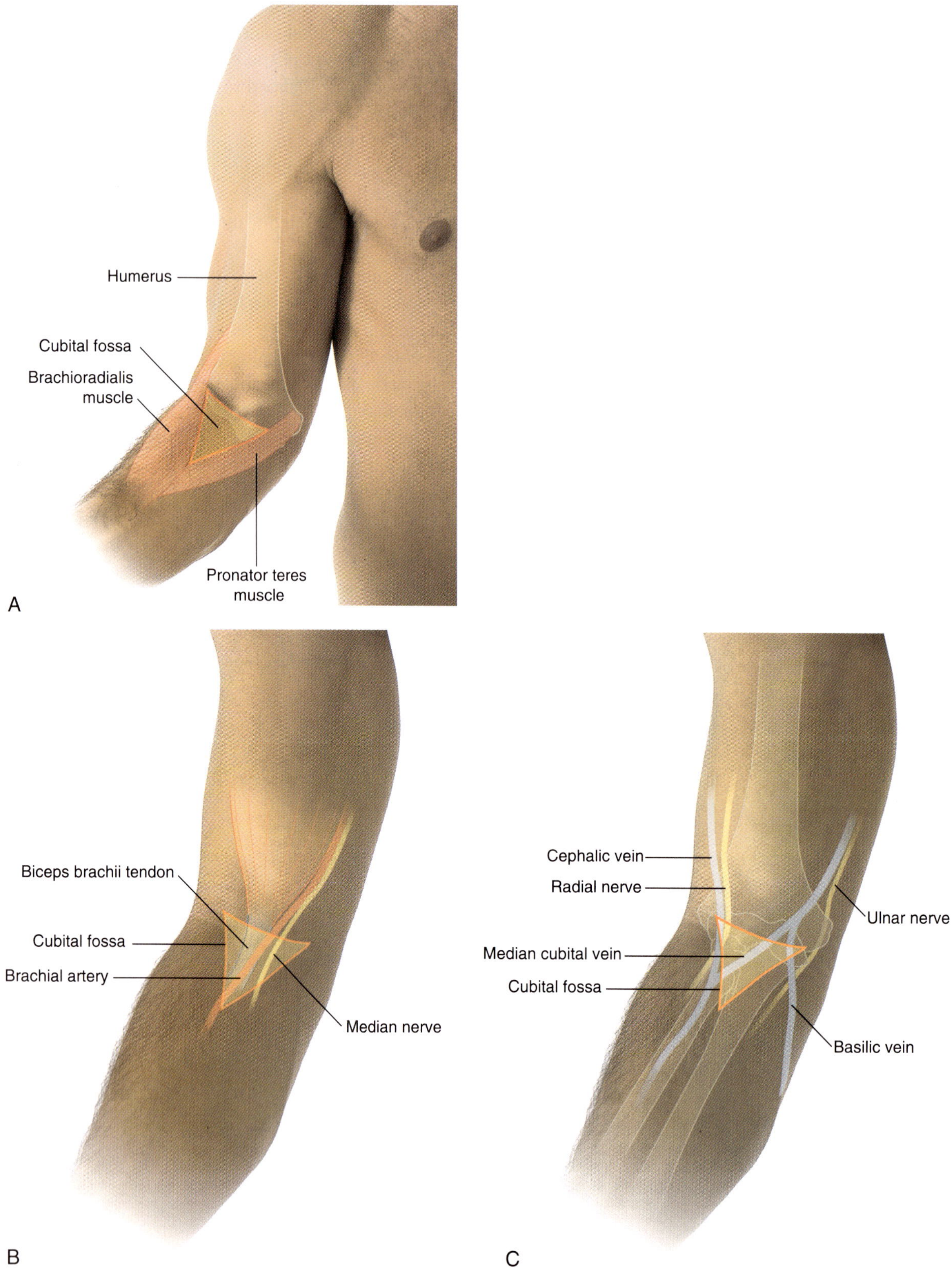

Fig. 2.117 Cubital fossa (anterior view, right arm). **(A)** Anterior view. **(B)** Boundaries and contents. **(C)** Showing radial and ulnar nerves, and veins.

Identifying tendons and locating major vessels and nerves in the distal forearm

Tendons that pass from the forearm into the hand are readily visible in the distal forearm and can be used as landmarks to locate major vessels and nerves.

In the anterior aspect of the distal forearm, the tendons of the flexor carpi radialis, flexor carpi ulnaris, and palmaris longus muscles can be easily located either by palpating or by asking a patient to flex the wrist against resistance.

- The tendon of flexor carpi radialis is located approximately at the junction between the lateral and middle thirds of an imaginary line drawn transversely across the distal forearm. The radial artery is immediately lateral to this tendon and this site is used for taking a radial pulse (Fig. 2.118A).
- The tendon of the flexor carpi ulnaris is easily palpated along the medial margin of the forearm and inserts on the pisiform, which can also be palpated by following the tendon to the base of the hypothenar eminence of the hand. The ulnar artery and ulnar nerve travel through the distal forearm and into the hand under the lateral lip of the flexor carpi ulnaris tendon and lateral to the pisiform.
- The palmaris longus tendon may be absent, but when present, lies medial to the flexor carpi radialis tendon and is particularly prominent when the wrist is flexed

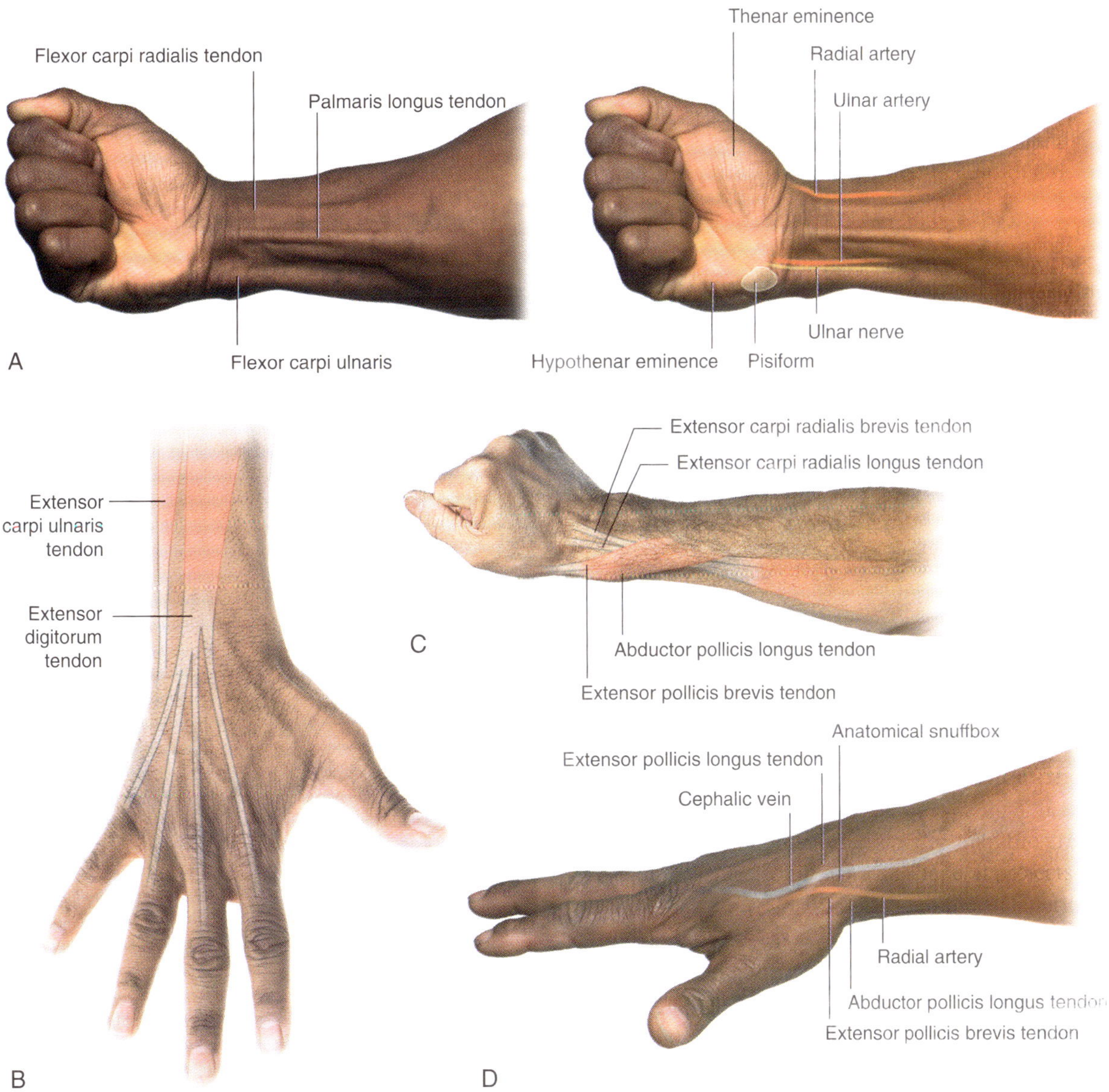

Fig. 2.118 Identifying tendons and locating major vessels and nerves in the distal right forearm. **(A)** Anterior distal forearm and wrist. **(B)** Posterior distal forearm and wrist. **(C)** Lateral view of posterior wrist and forearm. **(D)** Anatomical snuffbox.

against resistance. The median nerve is also medial to the flexor carpi radialis tendon and lies under the palmaris longus tendon.

- The long tendons of the digits of the hand are deep to the median nerve and between the long flexors of the wrist. Their position can be visualized by rapidly and repeatedly flexing and extending the fingers from medial to lateral.
- In the posterior distal forearm and wrist, the tendons of the extensor digitorum (Fig. 2.118B) are in the midline and radiate into the index, middle, ring, and little fingers from the wrist.
- The distal ends of the tendons of the extensor carpi radialis longus and brevis muscles are on the lateral side of the wrist (Fig. 2.118C) and can be accentuated by making a tight fist and extending the wrist against resistance.
- The tendon of the extensor carpi ulnaris can be felt on the far medial side of the wrist between the distal end of the ulna and the wrist.
- Hyperextension and abduction of the thumb reveals the anatomical snuffbox (Fig. 2.118D). The medial margin of this triangular area is the tendon of the extensor pollicis longus, which swings around the dorsal tubercle of the radius and then travels into the thumb. The lateral margin is formed by the tendons of the extensor pollicis brevis and abductor pollicis longus. The radial artery passes through the anatomical snuffbox when traveling laterally around the wrist to reach the back of the hand and penetrate the base of the first dorsal interosseous muscle to access the deep aspect of the palm of the hand. The pulse of the radial artery can be felt in the floor of the anatomical snuffbox in the relaxed wrist. The cephalic vein crosses the roof of the anatomical snuffbox, and cutaneous branches of the radial nerve can be felt by moving a finger back and forth along the tendon of the extensor pollicis longus muscle.

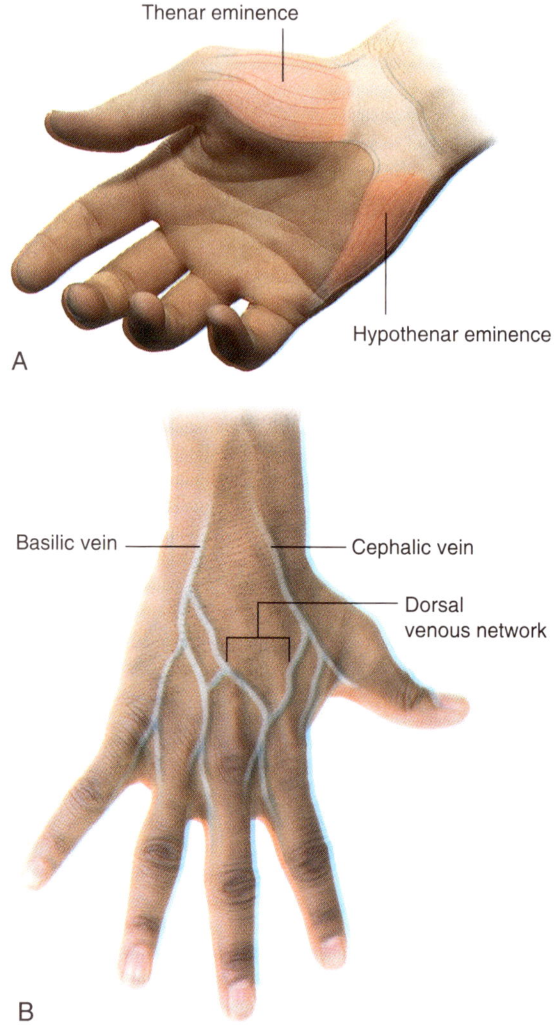

Fig. 2.119 Normal appearances of the right hand. **(A)** Palmar view with the thenar and hypothenar eminences and finger arcade. **(B)** Dorsal view with dorsal venous network.

Normal appearance of the hand

In the resting position, the palm and digits of the hand have a characteristic appearance. The fingers form a flexed arcade, with the little finger flexed the most and the index finger flexed the least (Fig. 2.119A). The pad of the thumb is positioned at a 90° angle to the pads of the fingers.

A thenar eminence occurs at the base of the thumb and is formed by the underlying thenar muscles. A similar hypothenar eminence occurs along the medial margin of the palm at the base of the little finger. The appearance of the thenar and hypothenar eminences and the positions of the fingers change when the ulnar and median nerves are compromised.

Major superficial veins of the upper limb begin in the hand from a dorsal venous network (Fig. 2.119B), which overlies the metacarpals. The basilic vein originates from the medial side of the network and the cephalic vein originates from the lateral side.

Position of the flexor retinaculum and the recurrent branch of the median nerve

The proximal margin of the flexor retinaculum can be determined using two bony landmarks:

- The pisiform bone is readily palpable at the distal end of the flexor carpi ulnaris tendon.
- The tubercle of the scaphoid can be palpated at the distal end of the flexor carpi radialis tendon as it enters the wrist (Fig. 2.120).

An imaginary line between these two points marks the proximal margin of the flexor retinaculum. The distal margin of the flexor retinaculum is approximately deep to the point where the anterior margin of the thenar eminence meets the hypothenar eminence near the base of the palm.

The recurrent branch of the median nerve lies deep to the skin and deep fascia overlying the anterior margin of the thenar eminence near the midline of the palm.

Motor function of the median and ulnar nerves in the hand

The ability to flex the metacarpophalangeal joints while at the same time extending the interphalangeal joints of the fingers is entirely dependent on the intrinsic muscles of the hand (Fig. 2.121A). These muscles are mainly innervated by the deep branch of the ulnar nerve, which carries fibers from spinal cord level (C8)T1.

Adducting the fingers to grasp an object placed between them is caused by the palmar interossei muscles, which are innervated by the deep branch of the ulnar nerve carrying fibers from spinal cord level (C8)T1.

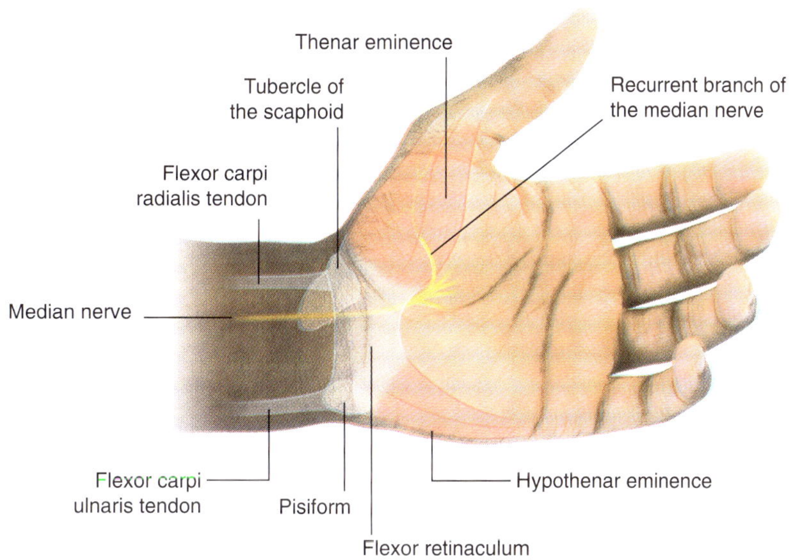

Fig. 2.120 Anterior left hand to show the position of the flexor retinaculum and recurrent branch of the median nerve.

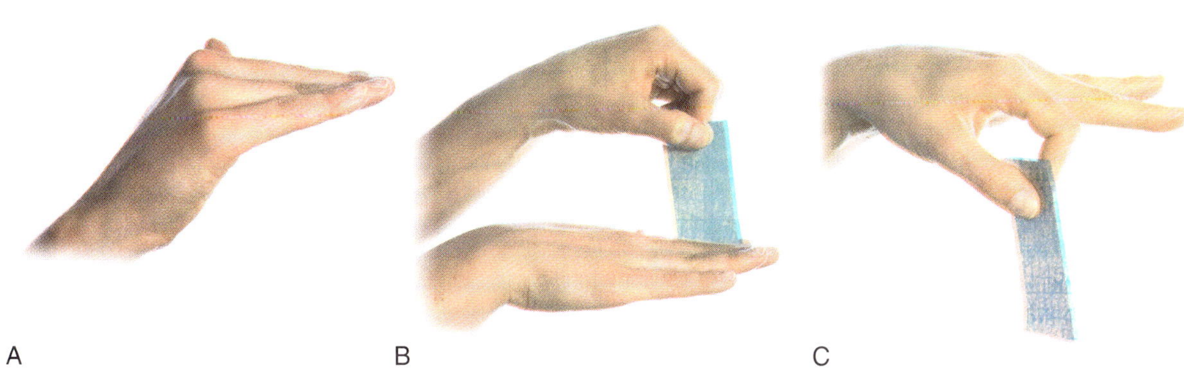

Fig. 2.121 Motor function of the ulnar and median nerves in the hand. **(A)** Flexing the metacarpophalangeal joints and extending the interphalangeal joints: the "ta-ta" position. **(B)** Grasping an object between the fingers. **(C)** Grasping an object between the pad of the thumb and pad of the index finger.

The ability to grasp an object between the pad of the thumb and the pad of one of the fingers depends on normal functioning of the thenar muscles, which are innervated by the recurrent branch of the median nerve carrying fibers from spinal cord level C8(T1).

Visualizing the positions of the superficial and deep palmar arches

The positions of the superficial and deep palmar arches in the hand can be visualized using bony landmarks, muscle eminences, and skin creases (Fig. 2.122).

- The superficial palmar arch begins as a continuation of the ulnar artery, which lies lateral to the pisiform bone at the wrist. The arch curves laterally across the palm anterior to the long flexor tendons in the hand. The arch reaches as high as the proximal transverse skin crease of the palm and terminates laterally by joining a vessel of variable size, which crosses the thenar eminence from the radial artery in the distal forearm.
- The deep palmar arch originates on the lateral side of the palm deep to the long flexor tendons and between the proximal ends of metacarpals I and II. It arches medially across the palm and terminates by joining the deep branch of the ulnar artery, which passes through the base of the hypothenar muscles and between the pisiform and hook of the hamate. The deep palmar arch is more proximal in the hand than the superficial palmar arch and lies approximately one-half of the distance between the distal wrist crease and the proximal transverse skin crease of the palm.

Pulse points

Peripheral pulses can be felt at six locations in the upper limb (Fig. 2.123).

- Axillary pulse: axillary artery in the axilla lateral to the apex of the dome of skin covering the floor of the axilla.
- Brachial pulse in midarm: brachial artery on the medial side of the arm in the cleft between the biceps brachii and triceps brachii muscles. This is the position where a blood pressure cuff is placed.
- Brachial pulse in the cubital fossa: brachial artery medial to the tendon of the biceps brachii muscle. This is the position where a stethoscope is placed to hear the pulse of the vessel when taking a blood pressure reading.
- Radial pulse in the distal forearm: radial artery immediately lateral to the tendon of the flexor carpi radialis muscle. This is the most common site for "taking a pulse."
- Ulnar pulse in the distal forearm: ulnar artery immediately under the lateral margin of the flexor carpi ulnaris tendon and proximal to the pisiform.
- Radial pulse in the anatomical snuffbox: radial artery as it crosses the lateral side of the wrist between the tendon of the extensor pollicis longus muscle and the tendons of the extensor pollicis brevis and abductor pollicis longus muscles.

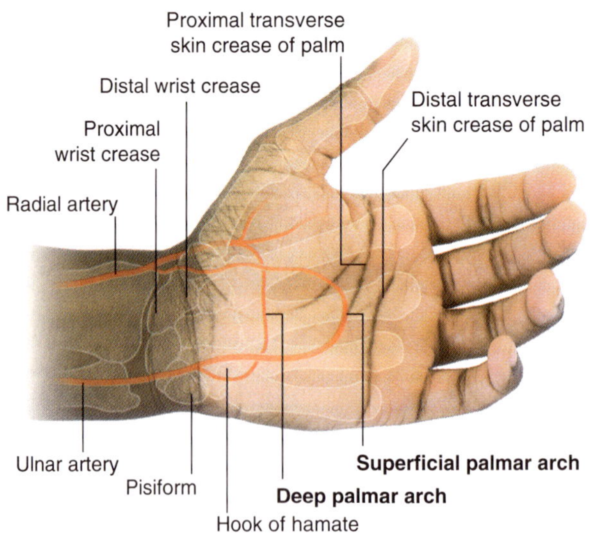

Fig. 2.122 Visualizing the positions of the superficial and deep palmar arches, left hand. The proximal transverse skin crease of the palm and distal wrist crease are labeled and the superficial and deep palmar arches shown in overlay. This also shows the position of the pisiform and the hook of the hamate.

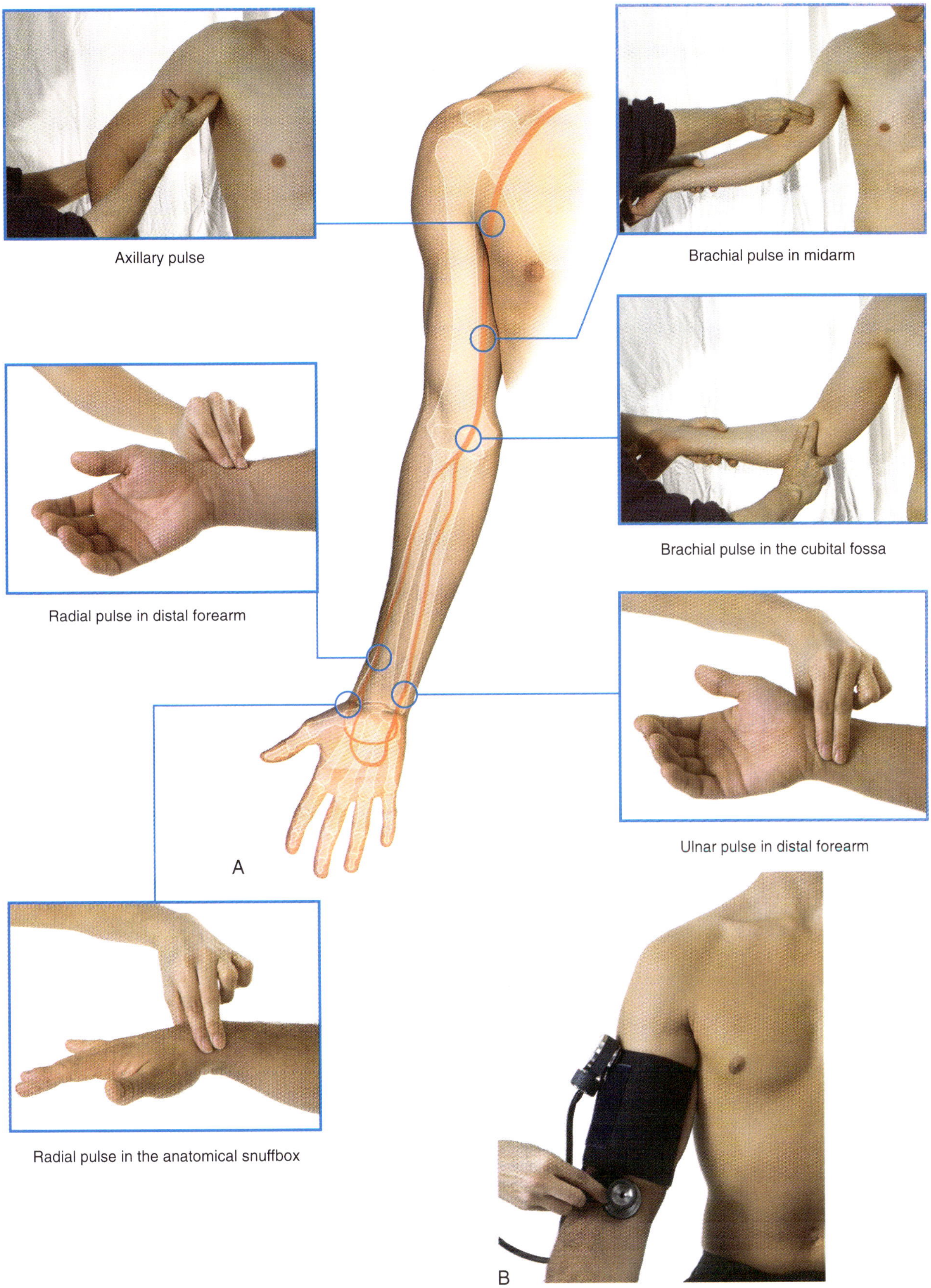

Fig. 2.123 Where to take peripheral artery pulses in the upper limb. **(A)** Pulse points. **(B)** Placement of blood pressure cuff and stethoscope.

Clinical cases

Case 1

SHOULDER PROBLEM AFTER FALLING ON AN OUTSTRETCHED HAND

A 45-year-old man came to his physician complaining of pain and weakness in his right shoulder. The pain began after a fall on his outstretched hand approximately 6 months earlier. The patient recalled having some minor shoulder tenderness but no other specific symptoms. He was otherwise fit and well.

On examination of the shoulder, there was marked wasting of the muscles in the supraspinous and infraspinous fossae. The patient found initiation of abduction difficult and there was a weakness of lateral rotation of the humerus.

The wasted muscles were the supraspinatus and infraspinatus. The cause of the muscle wasting was disuse.

Muscle atrophy (wasting) occurs through a variety of disorders. Disuse atrophy is one of the most common causes. Examples of disuse atrophy include the loss of muscle bulk after fracture immobilization in a plaster cast. The opposite effect can also be demonstrated—when muscles are overused, they become bulkier (hypertrophy).

The supraspinatus and infraspinatus muscles are supplied by the suprascapular nerve (C5, C6), which originates from the superior trunk of the brachial plexus. Given that only these muscles were involved, it is highly likely that the muscle atrophy is caused by denervation. Denervation may result from a direct nerve transection, nerve compression, or a pharmacological effect on the nerve.

The typical site for compression of the suprascapular nerve is the suprascapular notch (foramen) on the superior margin of the scapula.

The patient's apparently minor injury damaged the fibrocartilaginous glenoid labrum, which allowed a cyst to form and pass along the superior border of the scapula to the suprascapular notch (foramen), where the cyst compressed the suprascapular nerve.

Surgical excision of the damaged glenoid labrum and removal of the cyst improved the patient's symptoms.

Case 2

BRACHIAL PLEXUS NERVE BLOCK

A surgeon wished to carry out a complex procedure on a patient's wrist, and asked the anesthesiologist whether the whole arm could be numbed while the patient was awake. Within 20 minutes, the anesthesiologist had carried out the procedure after injecting 10 mL of local anesthetic into the axilla. The surgeon went ahead with the operation and the patient did not feel a thing.

The anesthetic was injected into the axillary sheath.

It would be almost impossible to anesthetize the wrist in the forearm because local anesthetic would have to be placed accurately around the ulnar, median, and radial nerves. Furthermore, all of the cutaneous branches of the forearm would also have to be anesthetized individually, which would take a considerable amount of time and probably produce subtotal anesthesia.

The nerves of the upper limb originate from the brachial plexus, which surrounds the axillary artery within the axilla. Importantly, the axillary artery, axillary vein, and brachial plexus lie within the sleeve-like covering of fascia termed the axillary sheath. By injecting the anesthetic into the space enclosed by the axillary sheath, all of the nerves of the brachial plexus were paralyzed.

It is possible with a patient's arm abducted and externally rotated (palm behind the head) to easily palpate the axillary artery and therefore locate the position of the axillary sheath. Once the axillary artery has been identified, a small needle can be placed beside the vessel and local anesthetic can be injected on both sides of it. The local anesthetic tracks along the axillary sheath in this region. The brachial plexus surrounding the axillary artery is therefore completely anesthetized and an effective local anesthetic "block" is achieved.

"Could there be any complications?" asks the patient.

Potential complications are a direct needle spike of the branches of the brachial plexus, damage to the axillary artery, and inadvertent arterial injection of the local anesthetic. Fortunately, these are rare in skilled hands.

Case 3

COMPLICATION OF A FRACTURED FIRST RIB

A 25-year-old woman was involved in a motor vehicle accident and thrown from her motorcycle. When she was admitted to the emergency room, she was unconscious. A series of tests and investigations were performed, one of which included chest radiography. The attending physician noted a complex fracture of the first rib on the left.

Many important structures that supply the upper limb pass over rib I.

It is important to test the nerves that supply the arm and hand, although this is extremely difficult to do in an unconscious patient. However, some muscle reflexes can be determined using a tendon hammer. Also, it may be possible to test for pain reflexes in patients with altered consciousness levels. Palpation of the axillary artery, brachial artery, radial artery, and ulnar artery pulses is necessary because a fracture of the first rib can sever and denude the subclavian artery, which passes over it.

A chest drain was immediately inserted because the lung had collapsed. The fractured first rib had damaged the visceral and parietal pleurae, allowing air from a torn lung to escape into the pleural cavity. The lung collapsed, and the pleural cavity filled with air, which impaired lung function.

A tube was inserted between the ribs, and the air was sucked out to reinflate the lung.

The first rib is a deep structure at the base of the neck. It is not uncommon for ribs to be broken after minor injuries, including sports injuries. However, rib I, which lies at the base of the neck, is surrounded by muscles and soft tissues that provide it with considerable protection. Therefore, a patient with a fracture of the first rib has undoubtedly been subjected to a considerable force, which usually occurs in a deceleration injury. Other injuries should always be sought and the patient should be managed with a high level of concern for deep neck and mediastinal injuries.

Case 4

MEDIAN NERVE COMPRESSION

A 35-year-old woman comes to her physician complaining of tingling and numbness in the fingertips of the first, second, and third digits (thumb, index, and middle fingers). The symptoms were provoked by arm extension. Local anesthesia was also present around the base of the thenar eminence.

The problem was diagnosed as median nerve compression.

The median nerve is formed from the lateral and medial cords of the brachial plexus anterior to the axillary artery and passes into the arm anterior to the brachial artery. At the level of the elbow joint, it sits medial to the brachial artery, both of which are medial to the tendon of the biceps. In the forearm, the nerve courses through the anterior compartment and passes deep to the flexor retinaculum. It innervates most of the muscles of the forearm, the thenar muscles, the two lateral lumbricals, and the skin over the palmar surface of the lateral three and one-half digits and over the lateral side of the palm and the middle of the wrist.

In this patient, the median nerve initially was believed to be trapped below the flexor retinaculum (carpal tunnel syndrome).

Carpal tunnel syndrome is a common problem in young to middle-aged patients. Typically the nerve becomes compressed within the carpal tunnel. This syndrome may be associated with a number of medical conditions, such as thyroid disease and pregnancy. Occasionally a small ganglion or a tumor situated within the carpal tunnel can also compress the nerve. Other possibilities include tenosynovitis in patients with rheumatoid arthritis.

Nerve conduction studies were performed to confirm the clinical findings. Nerve conduction studies are a series of tests that send small electrical impulses along the length of a variety of nerves in order to measure the speed at which the nerve conducts these pulses. The speed of the nerve pulse can be measured and is referred to as the latency. In our patient, it was noted that the nerve had normal latency to the elbow joint; however, below the elbow joint, there was increased latency.

The nerve conduction studies indicated that the compression site was at the elbow joint.

The clinical findings are not consistent with carpal tunnel syndrome. The clinician should have been alerted to this problem given that the patient experienced numbness over the thenar eminence of the hand. This clue indicates an understanding of the anatomy. Compression of the nerve within the carpal tunnel does not produce this numbness, because the small cutaneous branch that supplies this region is proximal to the flexor retinaculum.

The nerve compromise was caused by the ligament of Struthers, which is an embryological remnant of the coracobrachialis muscle. It is an extremely rare finding. Occasionally it may ossify and cross the nerve, artery, and vein to produce compression in arm extension. Although this is very rare and unusual, it illustrates the complex course of the median nerve.

Case 5

TORN SUPRASPINATUS TENDON

A 70-year-old woman came to an orthopedic surgeon with right shoulder pain and failure to initiate abduction of the shoulder. Further examination revealed loss of muscle bulk in the supraspinous fossa. The supraspinatus muscle was damaged.

Abduction of the humerus at the glenohumeral joint is initiated by the supraspinatus muscle. After the shoulder has been abducted to 10–15°, the deltoid muscle continues the movement. The patient was able to abduct her arm by lowering and tilting the glenohumeral joint inferiorly to enable the deltoid to obtain its mechanical advantage.

The loss of muscle bulk in the supraspinous fossa suggested muscle atrophy.

Muscle atrophy occurs when a muscle is not used. The orthopedic surgeon thought that there was a tear of the supraspinatus tendon beneath the acromion. If this was so, the muscle would atrophy.

The diagnosis was confirmed by ultrasound scan.

The patient was seated on a stool and her right shoulder was uncovered. The patient's hand was placed over her right buttock, a position that acts to externally rotate and extend the shoulder, exposing the supraspinatus tendon for ultrasound scan examination. The ultrasound revealed a completely torn tendon with fluid in the subacromial subdeltoid bursa (Fig. 2.124). The patient underwent a surgical repair and made a good recovery.

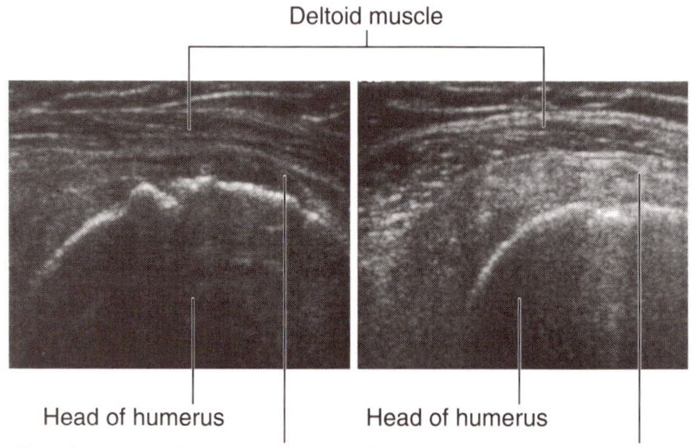

Fig. 2.124 Ultrasound showing a completely torn supraspinatus tendon with fluid in the subacromial subdeltoid bursa.

Case 6

HOW TO EXAMINE THE HAND

A resident was asked to carry out a clinical assessment of a patient's hand. He examined the following:

Musculoskeletal system

The musculoskeletal system includes the bones, joints, muscles, and tendons. The resident looked for abnormalities and muscle wasting. Knowing which areas are wasted identifies the nerve that supplies them. She palpated the individual bones and palpated the scaphoid with the wrist in ulnar deviation. She examined the movement of joints because they may be restricted by joint disease or inability of muscular contraction.

Circulation

Palpation of both radial and ulnar pulses is necessary. The resident looked for capillary return to assess how well the hand was perfused.

Examination of the nerves

The three main nerves to the hand should be tested.

Median nerve

The median nerve innervates the skin on the palmar aspect of the lateral three and one-half digits, the dorsal aspect of the distal phalanx, half of the middle phalanges of the same fingers, and a variable amount on the radial side of the palm of the hand. Median nerve damage results in wasting of the thenar eminence, absence of abduction of the thumb, and absence of opposition of the thumb.

Ulnar nerve

The ulnar nerve innervates the skin of the anterior and posterior surfaces of the little finger and the ulnar side of the ring finger, the skin over the hypothenar eminence, and a similar strip of skin posteriorly. Sometimes the ulnar nerve innervates all the skin of the ring finger and the ulnar side of the middle finger.

An ulnar nerve palsy results in wasting of the hypothenar eminence, absent flexion of the distal interphalangeal joints of the little and ring fingers, and absent abduction and adduction of the fingers. Adduction of the thumb also is affected.

Case 6 *(continued)*

Radial nerve

The radial nerve innervates a small area of skin over the lateral aspect of metacarpal I and the back of the first web space.

The radial nerve also produces extension of the wrist and extension of the metacarpophalangeal and interphalangeal joints and of the digits.

A very simple examination would include tests for the median nerve by opposition of the thumb, for the ulnar nerve by abduction and adduction of the digits, and for the radial nerve by extension of the wrist and fingers and feeling on the back of the first web space.

Case 7

SHOULDER JOINT PROBLEM

A 35-year-old baseball pitcher came to the clinic with a history of a recurrent dislocation of the shoulder (Fig. 2.125). An MRI scan was performed to assess the shoulder joint prior to any treatment.

The MRI demonstrates the anatomical structures in multiple planes, allowing the physician to obtain an overview of the shoulder and to assess any intra-articular or extra-articular structures that may have been damaged and require surgical repair.

The MRI demonstrated a divot in the posterosuperior aspect of the humeral head and a small fragment of bone and glenoid labrum that had become separated in the anteroinferior aspect of the glenoid cavity.

Shoulder dislocation is not an uncommon problem and may occur as a "once-off" or with repetitive injury may be recurrent. Recurrent dislocations may be bilateral and symmetrical (a memory aid is "torn loose or born loose").

The MRI findings are typical for an anteroinferior dislocation, which is the most common type; moreover, the MRI demonstrates the injuries that occur within the joint at the time of dislocation. These injuries include the abutment of the posterosuperior aspect of the humeral head on the anteroinferior aspect of the glenoid cavity. This type of injury, when recurrent, may avulse a small fragment of the glenoid labrum, and in some cases this may attach to a small fragment of bone (the Bankart lesion). When the shoulder is relocated, the integrity of the capsular attachment anteroinferiorly has been disrupted, potentially making the shoulder somewhat prone to further dislocation.

An arthroscopic repair was performed.

Arthroscopy of the shoulder is an established method for assessing the shoulder joint. Portals of entry are anterior and posterior and small holes in the capsule are made percutaneously. The shoulder joint is filled with saline, which distends it, allowing the arthroscope to move around the joint and inspect the joint surfaces, including the labrum. The labrum and its bony fragment were reattached and sutured using anchor sutures (somewhat similar to staples). The anterior aspect of the capsule was also tightened.

The patient made an uneventful recovery.

After the procedure, the arm was held in internal rotation and remained adducted. Gentle exercise and physiotherapy were performed and the patient returned to playing baseball.

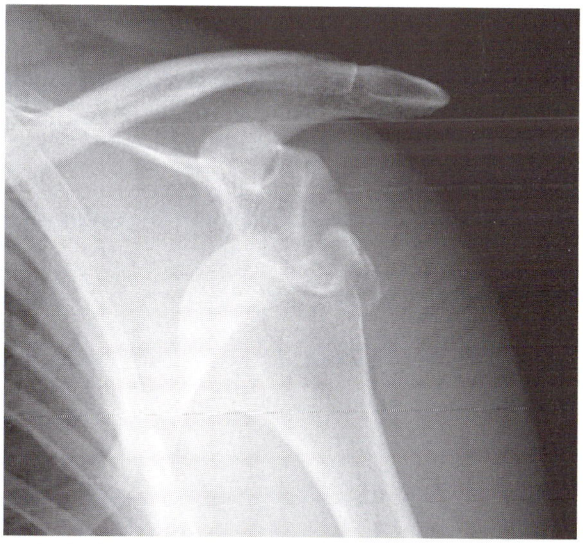

Fig. 2.125 The radiograph, anteroposterior view, demonstrates an anteroinferior dislocation of the humeral head at the glenohumeral joint.

Case 8

WINGED SCAPULA

A 57-year-old woman underwent a right mastectomy for a breast cancer. The surgical note reported that all of the breast tissue had been removed, including the axillary process. In addition, the surgeon had dissected all lymph nodes within the axilla with their surrounding fat. The patient made an uneventful recovery.

At the first follow-up appointment, the patient's husband told the surgeon that she had now developed a bony "spike" on her back. The surgeon was intrigued and asked the patient to reveal this spike. At examination, the spike was the inferior angle of the scapula, which appeared to be sticking out posteriorly ("winged"). Raising the arms accentuated this structure.

The medial border of the scapula was accentuated and it was noted that there was some loss of bulk of the serratus anterior muscle, which attaches to the tip of the scapula.

The nerve to this muscle was damaged.

During the surgery on the axilla, the long thoracic nerve was damaged as it passed down the lateral thoracic wall on the external surface of the serratus anterior, just deep to the skin and subcutaneous fascia.

Because the nerve was transected, it is unlikely that the patient will improve, but she was happy that she had an adequate explanation for the spike.

Case 9

IMMOBILIZING THE EXTENSOR DIGITORUM MUSCLE

After a hard day's studying, two medical students decided to meet for coffee. The senior student told the fresher that he would bet him Rs 50 that he could not lift a matchbook with a finger. The fresher placed Rs 50 on the table and the bet was on.

The senior medical student told the fresher to make a fist and place it in a palm-downward position, so that the middle phalanges of the fingers were in direct contact with the bar counter. He was then told to extend his middle finger so that it stuck forward while maintaining the middle phalanges of the index finger, the ring finger, and the little finger on the bar surface.

A matchbook was placed on top of the fresher's middle fingernail and he was told to flip it. He couldn't. He lost the Rs 50.

Extension of the index, middle, ring, and little fingers is performed by the extensor digitorum muscle.

Placing the fist in a palm-down position on the table and pressing the middle phalanges onto the table effectively immobilizes the action of the extensor digitorum. The fresher was therefore unable to elevate his middle finger (which was sticking out). It is important to remember that if this same procedure is carried out leaving either the index or the little finger free to move, they do move upwards. This is because these two digits are extended not only by the extensor digitorum muscle but also by the extensor indicis muscle (index finger) and extensor digiti minimi muscle (little finger).

3

Lower Limb

ADDITIONAL LEARNING RESOURCES for Chapter 3, Lower Limb, on MedEnact (www.MedEnact.com):

- Multiple-Choice Questions
- Short Questions—these are questions requiring short responses
- Medical Clinical Case Studies
  Femoral hernia
  Deep venous thrombosis

FREE Online Anatomy Self-Study Course

- Anatomy modules 26 through 31

Competency: The first-year medical students should be able to apply their knowledge of the course, relations, and distribution of the major arteries and nerves of the lower limb and the actions of the muscles at various joints and explain the anatomical basis of common clinical conditions and procedures.

Conceptual overview

SET INDUCTION—CASE SCENARIO 1: SUPERIOR GLUTEAL NERVE INJURY

A 33-year-old man who had been involved in a street fight walked into the emergency department. His pelvis dropped on the unsupported side when his leg swung forward. He was diagnosed to have weakness of the abductor muscles of the hip on the stance side. The possibility of damage to the superior gluteal nerve was considered.

It is necessary to know the anatomy of the hip joint before one can manage a patient with muscle weakness in the lower limb.

<table>
<tr><td rowspan="2">REMEMBER
[Recall Facts]</td><td colspan="3">OUTLINE 1. CONCEPTUAL OVERVIEW AND INTRODUCTION—LEARNING OBJECTIVES
[By the end of this section the student should be able to:]</td><td rowspan="2" colspan="2">EVALUATE
[Explain Concepts]</td></tr>
<tr><td colspan="3">DEMONSTRATE AND ANALYZE RELATIONSHIPS
[Identify structures in a Prosected Specimen or Figure]</td></tr>
<tr><td rowspan="7">1. Describe the subdivisions of the lower limb
2. Describe briefly the bones and joints of the lower limb
3. Describe some of the determinants of gait
4. List the structures that pass between the pelvic bone and the inguinal ligament
5. List the structures that pass between the pelvis and the lower limb via the greater sciatic foramen
6. List the structures that pass between the perineum and the lower limb via the lesser sciatic foramen
7. List the structures that pass through the obturator canal
8. Describe briefly the nerves, vessels, and lymphatics of the lower limb
9. Describe the regions of the skin of the lower limb innervated by peripheral nerves
10. Name the structure separating the superficial and deep groups of veins</td><td>Level I</td><td>Level II</td><td>Level III</td><td rowspan="2" colspan="2">■ Movements at the hip joint and the muscles causing them
■ Passage of structures into and out of the gluteal region
■ Line of gravity in relation to the joints of the lower limb</td></tr>
<tr><td rowspan="6">■ Great saphenous vein
■ Small saphenous vein
■ Landmarks on the bony pelvis and proximal part of the femur
■ Lumbar plexus
■ Sacral plexus
■ Common fibular nerve
■ Tibial nerve
■ Piriformis
■ Femoral artery and vein
■ Femoral sheath
■ Femoral canal</td><td rowspan="6">■ Obturator canal
■ Superior and inferior gluteal nerves and vessels
■ Saphenous opening
■ Adductor canal</td><td rowspan="6">■ Superficial inguinal lymph nodes
■ Cutaneous nerves in the lower limb</td></tr>
<tr><td colspan="2">EARLY CLINICAL EXPOSURE
[Apply Anatomical Knowledge]</td></tr>
<tr><td>Surgical Anatomy/ Pathology/ Trauma</td><td>Imaging/ Surface Anatomy</td></tr>
<tr><td>■ Trauma to the common fibular nerve at the neck of the fibula
■ Pelvic fractures</td><td>■ List the autonomous zones in the dermatomes of the lower limb
■ Vascular access to the femoral artery and vein</td></tr>
<tr><td colspan="2">PROBLEM SOLVING/ CLINICAL CASES
[Interpret]</td></tr>
<tr><td colspan="2">■ Testing of myotomes using joint movements and reflexes
■ Testing of somatic sensory and motor functions using tendon reflexes</td></tr>
</table>

Lower Limb

GENERAL INTRODUCTION

The lower limb articulates with the axial skeleton by a sacroiliac joint and by strong ligaments, which link the hip bone to the sacrum. It is separated from the abdomen, back, and perineum by a continuous line (Fig. 3.1). This line:

- Connects the pubic tubercle to the anterior superior iliac spine (position of the inguinal ligament) and then continues along the iliac crest to the posterior superior iliac spine—to separate the lower limb from the anterior and lateral abdominal walls.
- Passes from the posterior superior iliac spine and along the dorsolateral surface of the sacrum to the coccyx—to separate the lower limb from the muscles of the back.
- Joins the medial margin of the sacrotuberous ligament, the ischial tuberosity, the ischiopubic ramus, and the pubic symphysis—to separate the lower limb from the perineum.

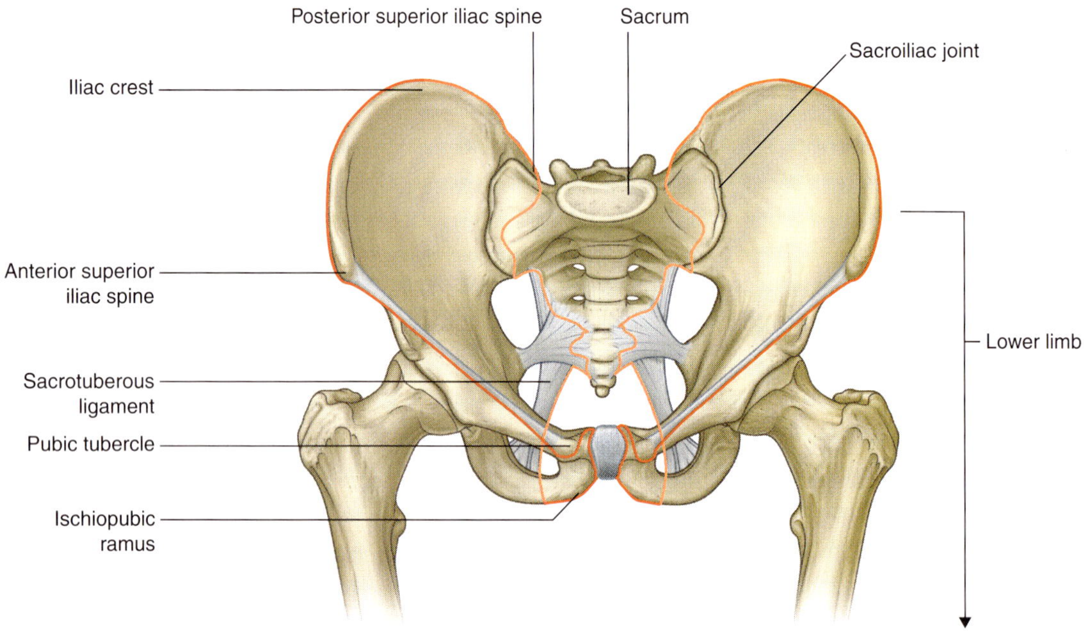

Fig. 3.1 Upper margin of the lower limb.

The lower limb is divided into the gluteal region, thigh, leg, and foot on the basis of major joints, component bones, and superficial landmarks (Fig. 3.2):

- The **gluteal region** is posterolateral and between the iliac crest and the fold of skin (gluteal fold) that defines the lower limit of the buttocks.
- Anteriorly, the **thigh** is between the inguinal ligament and the knee joint—the hip joint is just inferior to the middle third of the inguinal ligament, and the posterior thigh is between the gluteal fold and the knee.
- The **leg** is between the knee and ankle joint.
- The **foot** is distal to the ankle joint.

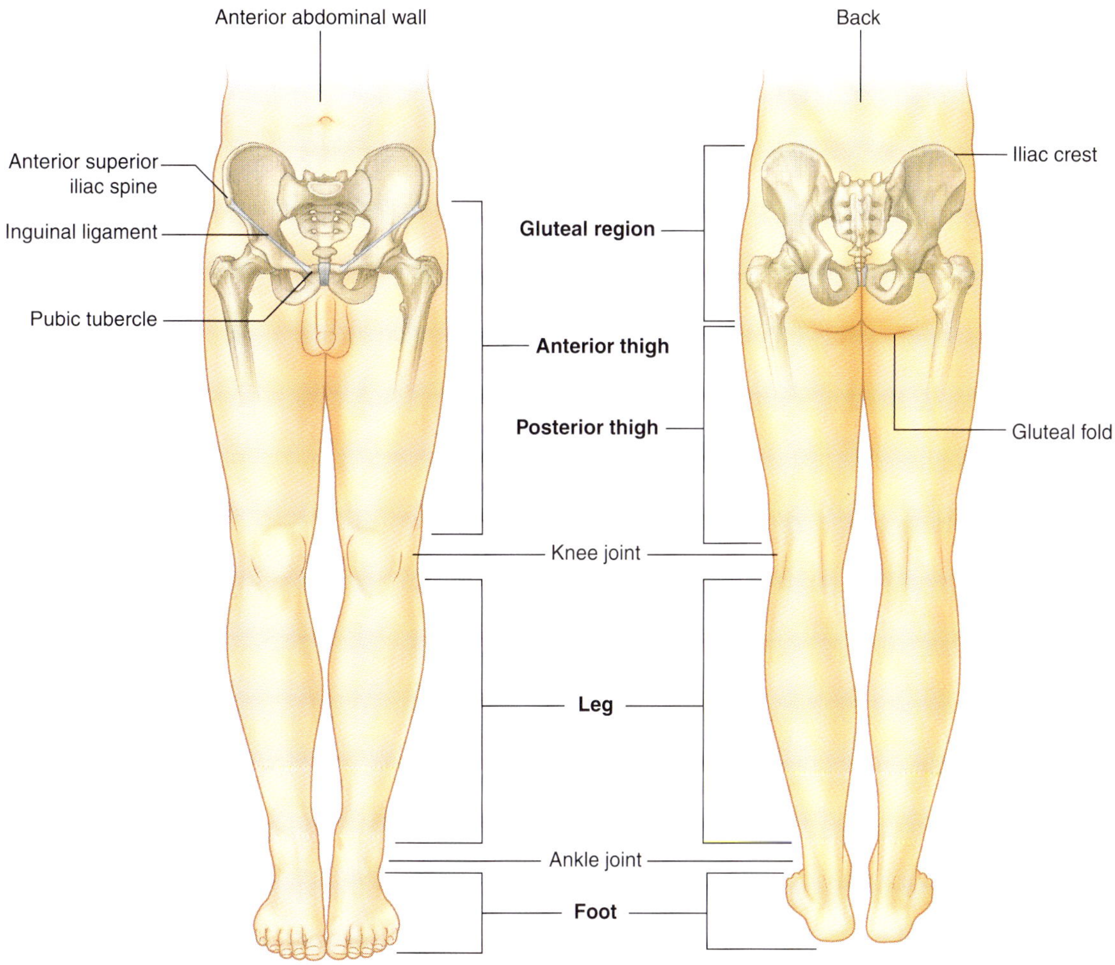

Fig. 3.2 Regions of the lower limb.

The femoral triangle, popliteal fossa, and posteromedial side of the ankle are important areas of transition. At these areas, blood vessels and nerves pass between subdivisions of the lower limb and generally change their names (Fig. 3.3). For example, the femoral triangle is the area containing the beginning of the femoral artery and the termination of the femoral vein and nerve.

The **femoral triangle** is a pyramid-shaped depression formed by muscles in the proximal regions of the thigh and by the inguinal ligament, which forms the base of the triangle. The major blood supply and one of the nerves of the limb (femoral nerve) enter into the thigh from the abdomen by passing deep to the inguinal ligament and into the femoral triangle.

The **popliteal fossa** is posterior to the knee joint and is a diamond-shaped region formed by muscles of the thigh and leg. Major vessels and nerves pass between the thigh and leg through the popliteal fossa.

Most nerves, vessels, and flexor tendons that pass between the leg and foot pass through a series of canals (collectively termed the **tarsal tunnel**) on the posteromedial side of the ankle. The canals are formed by adjacent bones and a flexor retinaculum, which holds the tendons in position.

FUNCTION

Support the body weight

A major function of the lower limb is to support the weight of the body with minimal expenditure of energy. When standing erect, the center of gravity is anterior to the edge of the S2 vertebra in the pelvis (Fig. 3.4). The vertical line through the center of gravity is slightly posterior to the hip joints, anterior to the knee and ankle joints, and directly over the almost circular support base formed by the feet on the ground and holds the knee and hip joints in extension.

The organization of ligaments at the hip and knee joints, together with the shape of the articular surfaces, particularly at the knee, facilitates "locking" of these joints into position when standing, thereby reducing the muscular energy required to maintain a standing position.

Locomotion

A second major function of the lower limbs is to move the body. This involves the integration of movements at all joints in the lower limb to position the foot on the ground and to move the body over the foot.

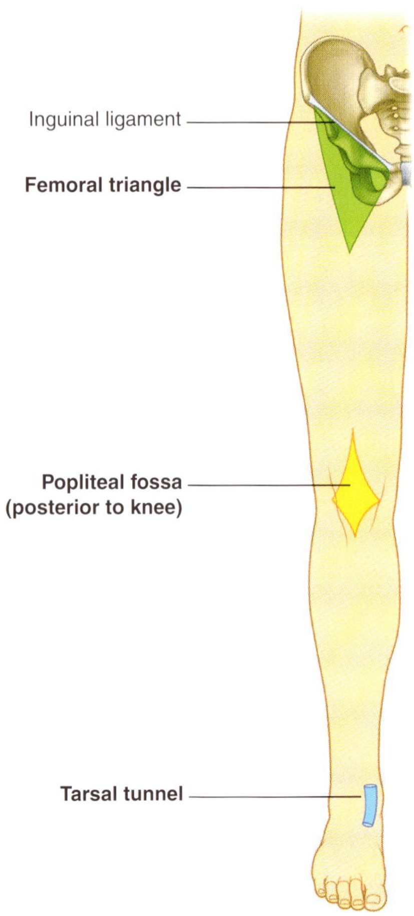

Fig. 3.3 Areas of transition.

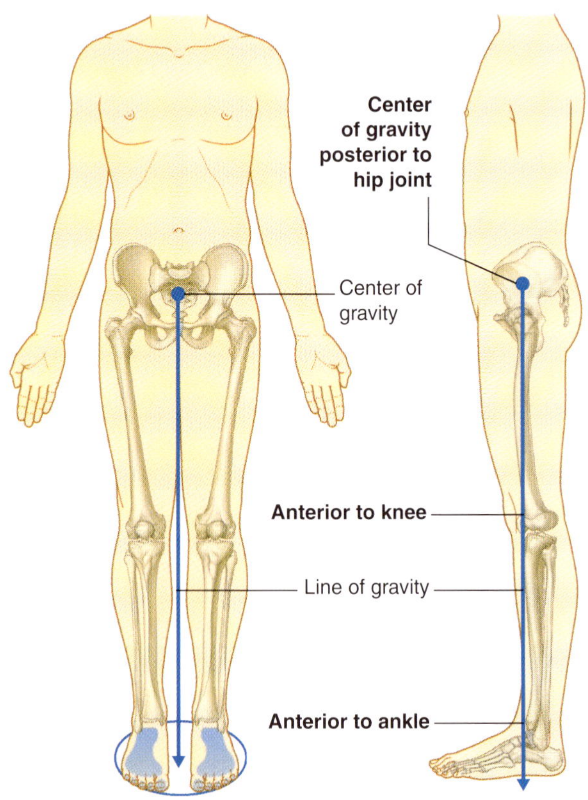

Fig. 3.4 Center and line of gravity.

Movements at the hip joint are: (a) flexion, extension, (b) abduction, adduction, (c) medial and lateral rotation, and (d) circumduction (Fig. 3.5 and 3.29). Flexion is in the sagittal plane around a transverse axis, abduction is in the coronal plane around an anteroposterior axis, and rotation occurs around a vertical axis.

The knee and ankle joints are primarily hinge joints. Movements at the knee are mainly flexion and extension (Fig. 3.6A). Movements at the ankle are dorsiflexion (movement of the dorsal side of the foot toward the leg) and plantar flexion (Fig. 3.6B).

During walking, many anatomical features of the lower limbs contribute to minimizing fluctuations in the body's center of gravity and thereby reduce the amount of energy needed to maintain locomotion and produce a smooth,

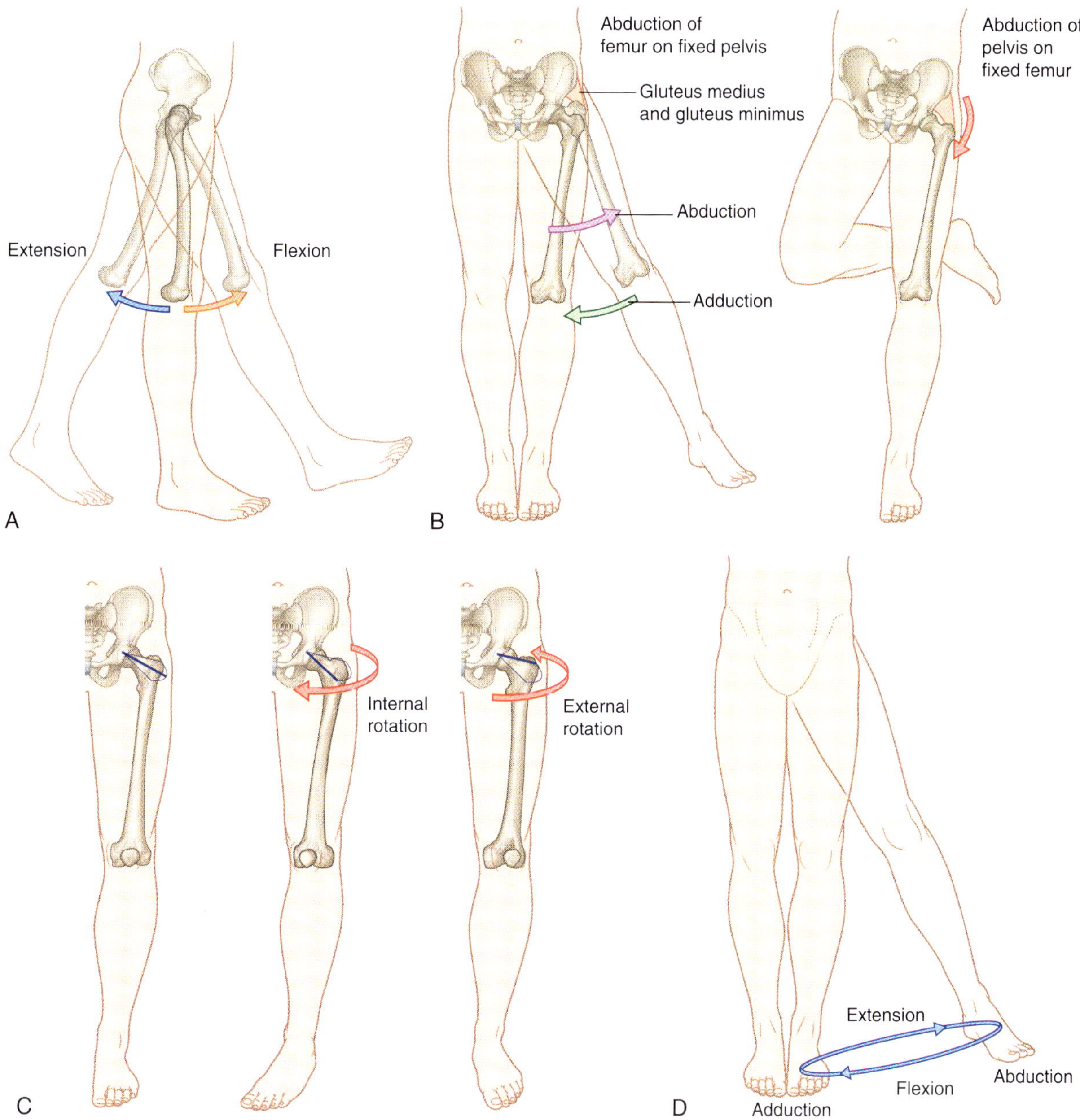

Fig. 3.5 Movements of the hip joint. **(A)** Flexion and extension. **(B)** Abduction and adduction. **(C)** External and internal rotation. **(D)** Circumduction.

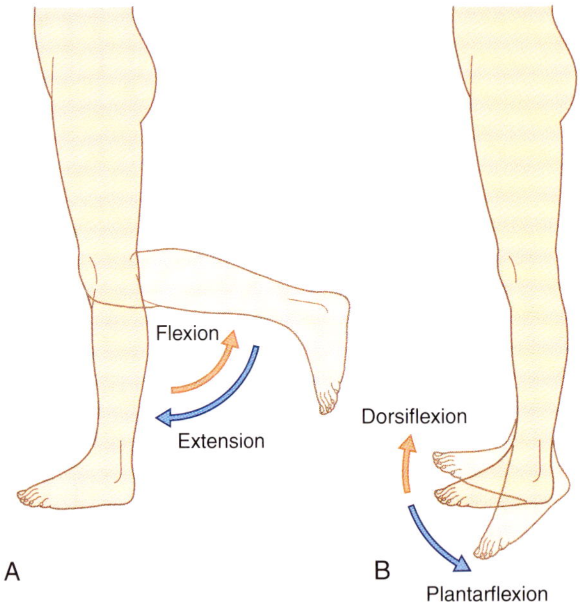

Fig. 3.6 Movements of the knee and ankle. **(A)** Knee flexion and extension. **(B)** Ankle dorsiflexion and plantar flexion.

efficient gait (Fig. 3.7). They include: (a) pelvic rotation in the transverse plane, (b) flexion of the knees, (c) pelvic tilt in the coronal plane, and (d) movement of the knees toward the midline, and complex interactions between the hip, knee, and ankle. As a result, during walking, the body's center of gravity normally fluctuates only 5 cm in both vertical and lateral directions.

COMPONENT PARTS

Bones and joints

The bones of the gluteal region and the thigh are the **pelvic bone** and the **femur** (Fig. 3.8). The large ball and socket joint between these two bones is the hip joint.

The femur is the bone of the thigh. At its distal end, its major weight-bearing articulation is with the **tibia**, but it also articulates anteriorly with the **patella** (knee cap). The patella is the largest sesamoid bone in the body and is embedded in the quadriceps femoris tendon.

The joint between the femur and tibia is the principal articulation of the knee joint, but the joint between the patella and femur shares the same articular cavity. Although the main movements at the knee are flexion and extension, the knee joint also allows the femur to rotate externally on the tibia. This rotation contributes to "locking" of the knee when fully extended, particularly when standing.

The leg contains two bones:

- The tibia is medial in position, is larger than the laterally positioned **fibula**, and is the weight-bearing bone.
- The fibula does not take part in the knee joint and forms only the most lateral part of the ankle joint—proximally, it forms a small synovial joint (superior tibiofibular joint) with the inferolateral surface of the head of the tibia.

The tibia and fibula are linked along their lengths by an interosseous membrane, and at their distal ends by a fibrous inferior tibiofibular joint, and little movement occurs between them. The distal surfaces of the tibia and fibula together form a deep recess. The ankle joint is formed by this recess and part of one of the tarsal bones of the foot (talus), which projects into the recess. The ankle is most stable when dorsiflexed.

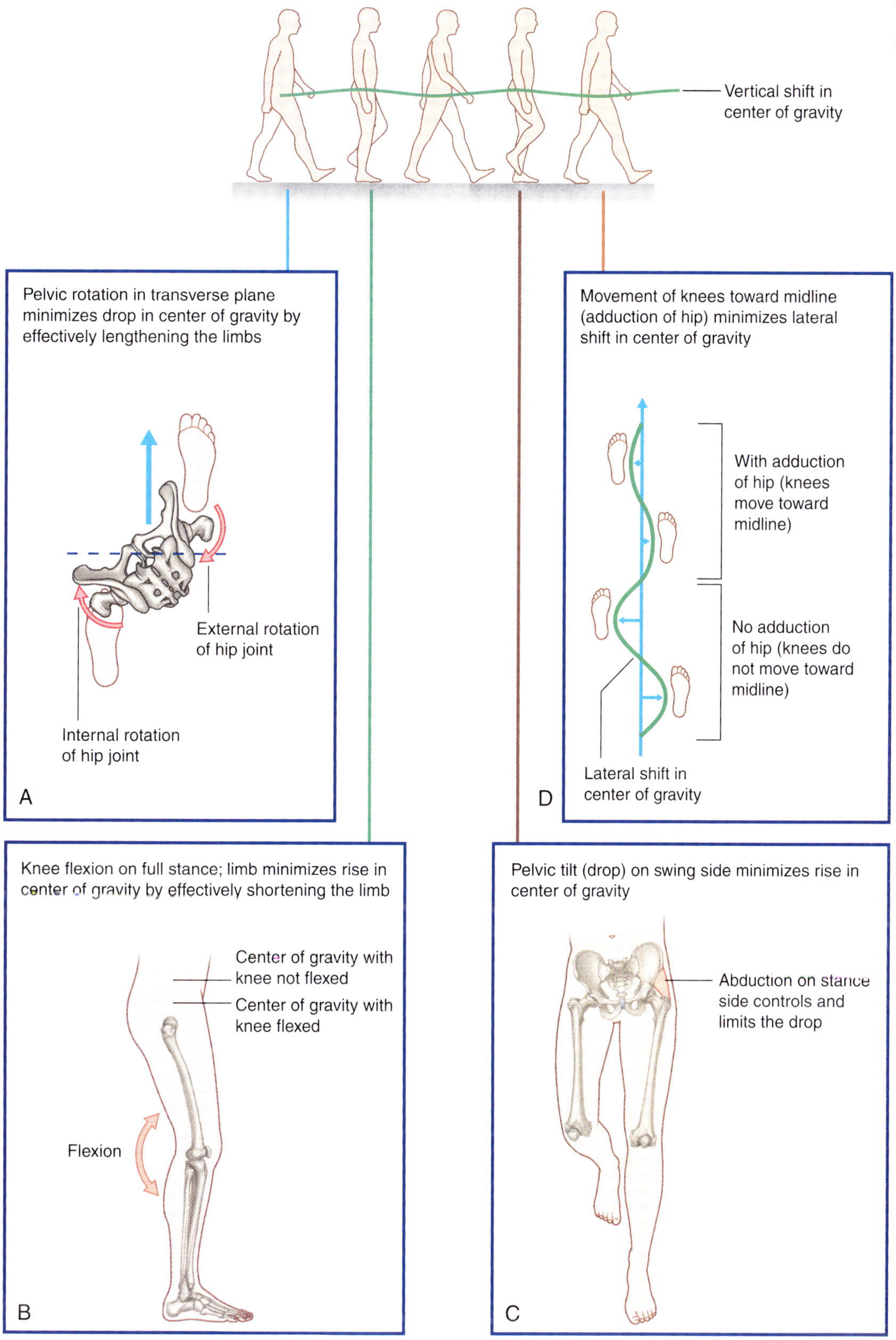

Fig. 3.7 Some of the determinants of gait. **(A)** Rotation of the hip joint. **(B)** Flexion of the knee joint, **(C)** Abduction of the hip joint on the stance side. **(D)** Adduction of the hip joint.

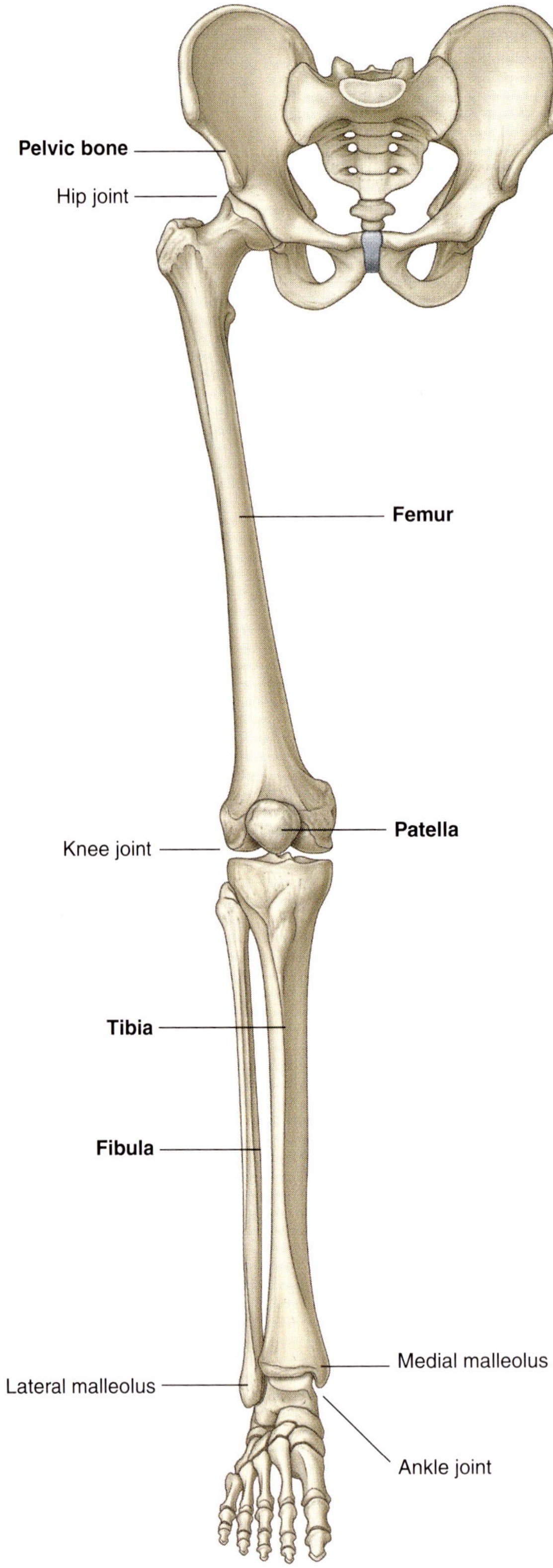

Fig. 3.8 Bones and joints of the lower limb.

The bones of the foot consist of the **tarsal bones**, the **metatarsals**, and the **phalanges** (Fig. 3.9). There are seven tarsal bones, which are organized in two rows with an intermediate bone between the two rows on the medial side. Inversion and eversion of the foot, or turning the sole of the foot inward and outward, respectively, occur at joints between the tarsal bones, such as the subtarsal joint.

The tarsal bones articulate with the metatarsals at tarsometatarsal joints, which allow only limited sliding movements.

Independent movements of the metatarsals are restricted by deep transverse metatarsal ligaments, which effectively link together the distal heads of the bones at the metatarsophalangeal joints. There is a metatarsal for each of the five digits, and each digit has three phalanges except for the great toe (digit I), which has only two.

The metatarsophalangeal joints allow flexion, extension, abduction, and adduction of the digits, but the range of movement is more restricted than in the hand.

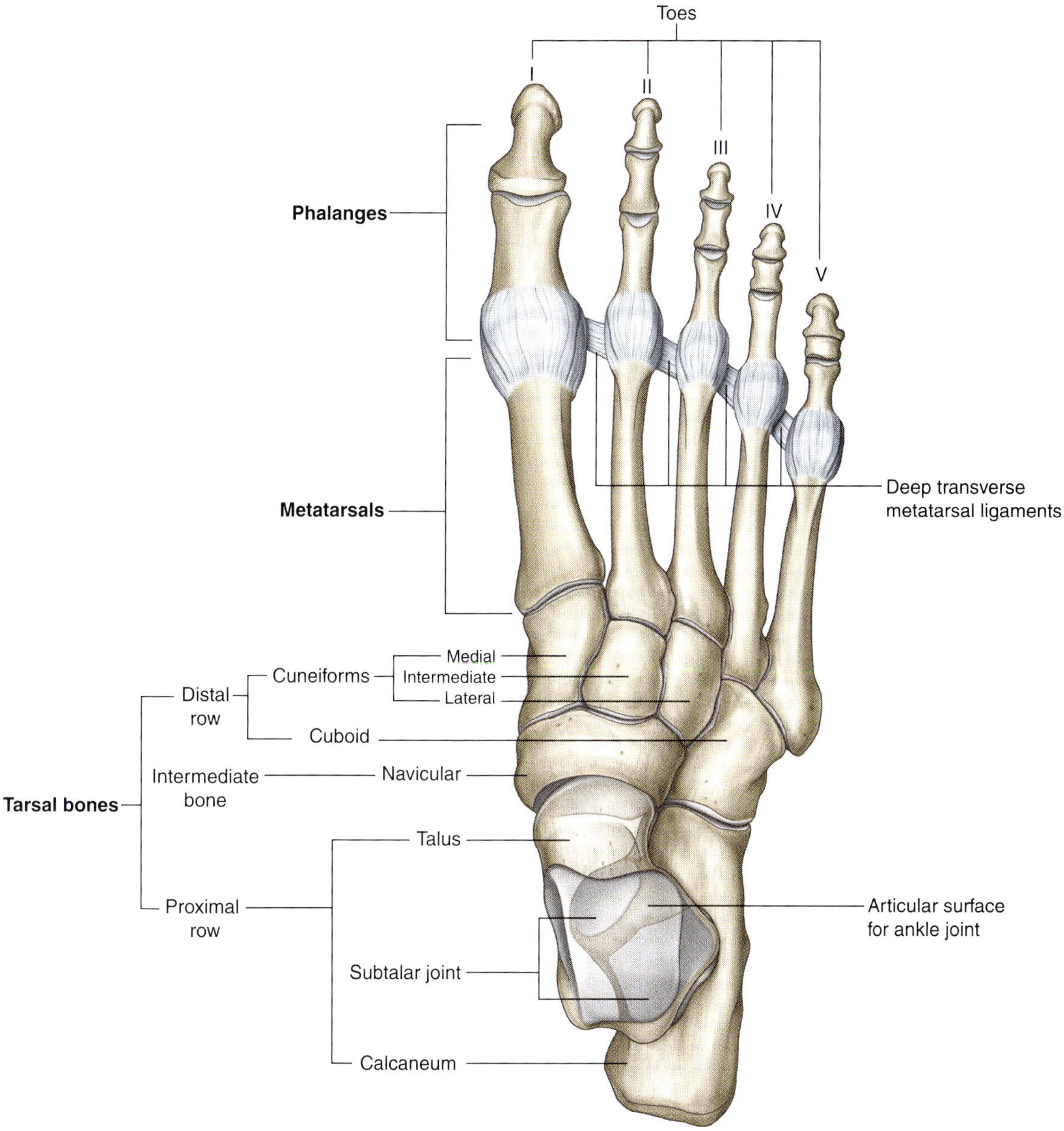

Fig. 3.9 Bones of the foot. The talus is shown as if transparent.

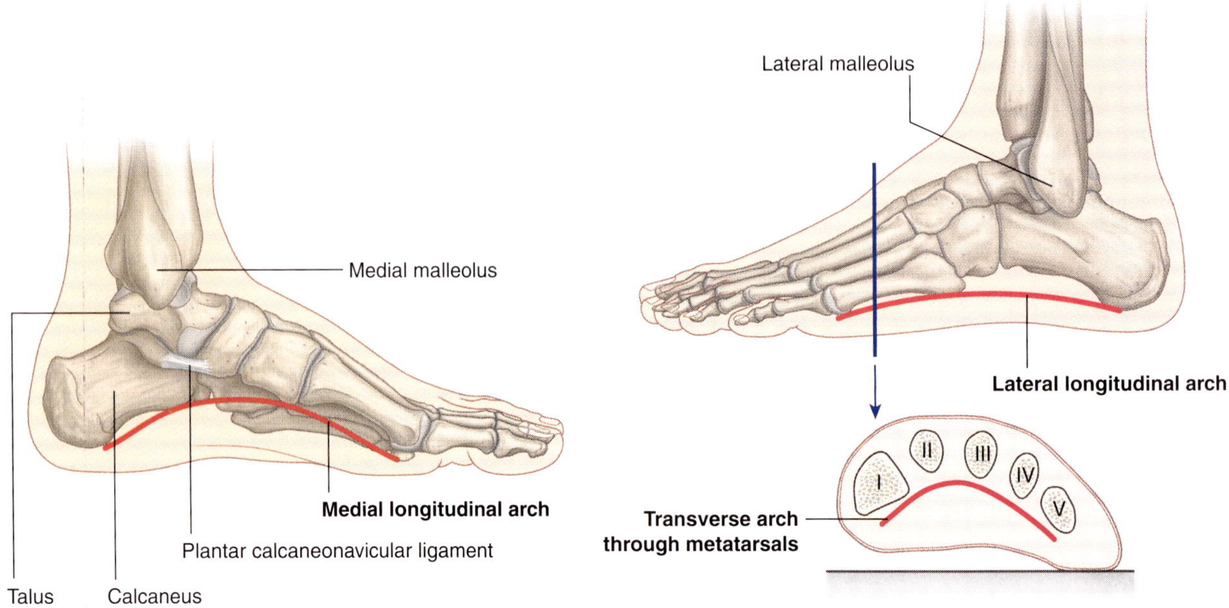

Fig. 3.10 Longitudinal and transverse arches of the foot.

The interphalangeal joints are hinge joints and allow flexion and extension.

The bones of the foot are not organized in a single plane so that they lie flat on the ground. Rather, the metatarsals and tarsals form **longitudinal and transverse arches** (Fig. 3.10). The longitudinal arch is highest on the medial side of the foot. The arches are flexible in nature and are supported by muscles and ligaments. They absorb and transmit forces during walking and standing.

Muscles

Muscles of the gluteal region consist predominantly of extensors, abductors, and rotators of the hip joint (Fig. 3.11). In addition to moving the thigh on a fixed pelvis, these muscles also control the movement of the pelvis relative to the limb bearing the body's weight (weight-bearing or stance limb) while the other limb swings forward (swing limb) during walking.

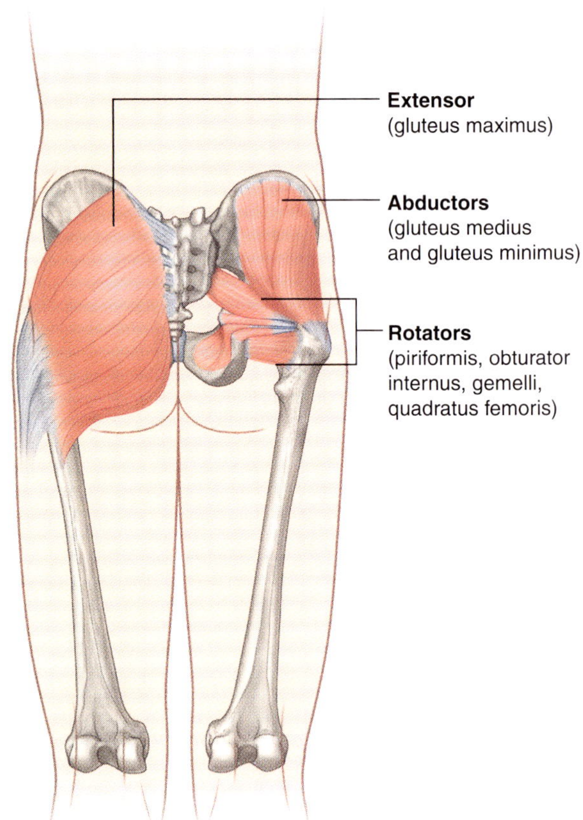

Fig. 3.11 Muscles of the gluteal region.

Major flexor muscles of the hip (iliopsoas—psoas major and iliacus) do not originate in the gluteal region or the thigh. Instead, they are attached to the posterior abdominal wall and descend through the gap between the inguinal ligament and pelvic bone to attach to the proximal end of the femur (Fig. 3.12).

Muscles in the thigh and leg are separated into three compartments by layers of fascia, bones, and ligaments (Fig. 3.13).

In the thigh, there are **medial** (adductor), **anterior** (extensor), and **posterior** (flexor) compartments:

- Most muscles in the medial compartment act mainly on the hip joint.
- The large muscles (hamstrings) in the posterior compartment act on the hip (extension) and knee (flexion) because they attach to both the pelvis and bones of the leg.
- Muscles in the anterior compartment (quadriceps femoris) predominantly extend the knee.
- Muscles in the leg are divided into **lateral** (fibular), **anterior**, and **posterior** compartments:
  - Muscles in the lateral compartment predominantly evert the foot.
  - Muscles in the anterior compartment dorsiflex the foot and extend the digits.
  - Muscles in the posterior compartment plantarflex the foot and flex the digits; some of the muscles can also flex the knee because they attach superiorly to the femur.

Specific muscles in each of the three compartments in the leg also provide dynamic support for the arches of the foot.

Muscles found entirely in the foot (intrinsic muscles) modify the forces produced by tendons entering the toes from the leg and provide dynamic support for the longitudinal arches of the foot when walking, particularly when levering the body forward on the stance limb just before toe-off.

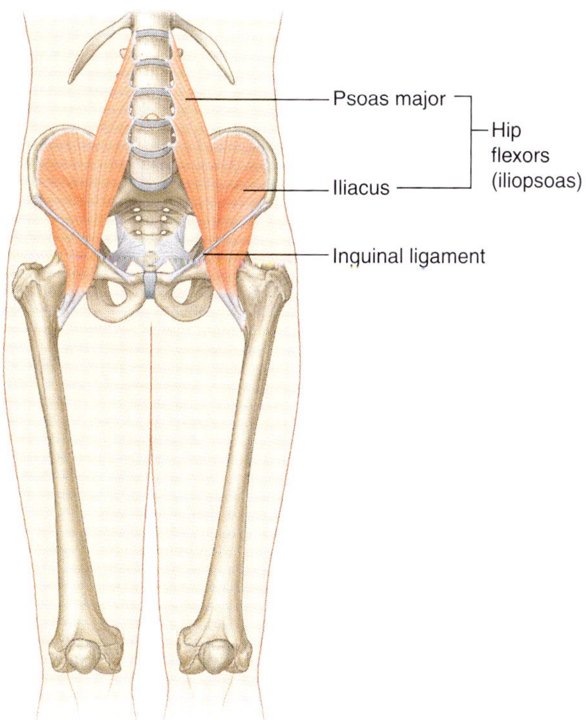

Fig. 3.12 Major flexors of the hip.

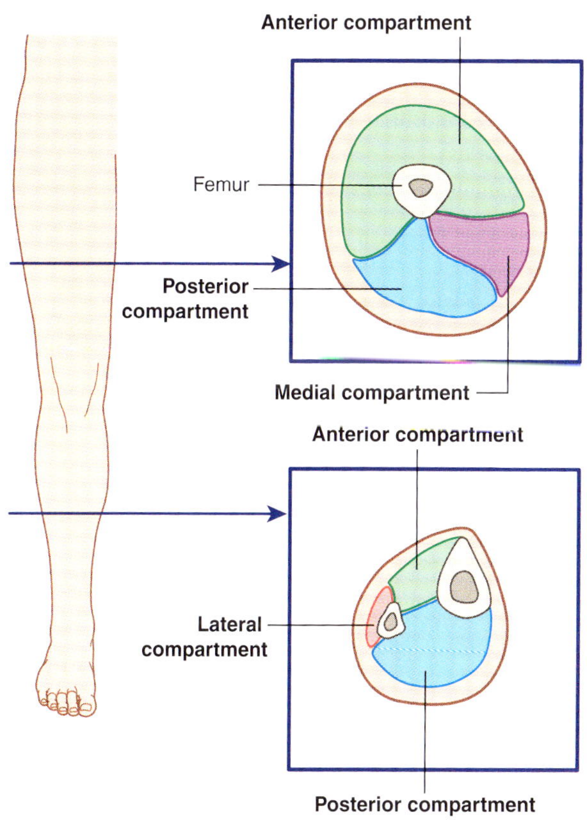

Fig. 3.13 Muscle compartments in the thigh and leg.

RELATIONSHIP TO OTHER REGIONS

Unlike in the upper limb where most structures pass between the neck and limb through a single axillary inlet, in the lower limb, there are four major entry and exit points between the lower limb and the abdomen, pelvis, and perineum (Fig. 3.14 and 4.12). These are

- The gap between the inguinal ligament and pelvic bone
- The greater sciatic foramen
- The obturator canal (at the top of the obturator foramen)
- The lesser sciatic foramen

Abdomen

The lower limb communicates directly with the abdomen through a gap between the pelvic bone and the inguinal ligament (Fig. 3.14 and 4.12). Structures passing though this gap include:

- Muscles—psoas major, iliacus, and pectineus
- Nerves—femoral and femoral branch of the genitofemoral nerves, and the lateral cutaneous nerve of the thigh
- Vessels—femoral artery and vein
- Lymphatics

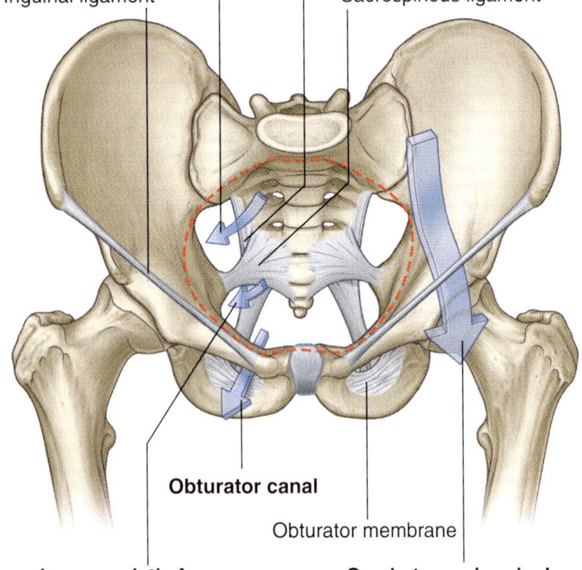

Fig. 3.14 Apertures of communication between the lower limb and other regions.

This gap between the pelvic bone and the inguinal ligament is a weak area in the abdominal wall and often associated with abnormal protrusion of the abdominal cavity and contents into the thigh (femoral hernia). This type of hernia usually occurs where the lymphatic vessels pass through the gap medially (the femoral canal) (see Fig. 3.42).

Pelvis

Structures within the pelvis communicate with the lower limb through two major apertures (Fig. 3.14 and 5.31).

Posteriorly, structures communicate with the gluteal region through the greater sciatic foramen and include:

- A muscle—piriformis
- Nerves—sciatic, superior and inferior gluteal, and pudendal nerves
- Vessels—superior and inferior gluteal arteries and veins, and the internal pudendal artery

The sciatic nerve is the largest peripheral nerve of the body and is the major nerve of the lower limb.

Anteriorly, the obturator nerve and vessels pass between the pelvis and thigh through the obturator canal. This canal is formed between bone at the top of the obturator foramen and the obturator membrane, which closes most of the foramen during life.

Perineum

Structures pass between the perineum and gluteal region through the lesser sciatic foramen (Fig. 3.14 and 5.31). The most important with respect to the lower limb is the tendon of the obturator internus muscle.

The artery and nerve of the perineum (the internal pudendal artery and pudendal nerve) pass out of the pelvis through the greater sciatic foramen into the gluteal region and then immediately pass around the ischial spine and sacrospinous ligament and through the lesser sciatic foramen to enter the perineum.

KEY POINTS

Innervation is by lumbar and sacral spinal nerves

Somatic motor and general sensory innervation of the lower limb is by peripheral nerves emanating from the lumbar and sacral plexuses on the posterior abdominal and pelvic walls. These plexuses are formed by the anterior rami of L1 to L3 and most of L4 (lumbar plexus, see Fig. 4.160) and L4 to S3 (sacral plexus, Fig. 4.160).

Nerves originating from the lumbar and sacral plexuses and entering the lower limb carry fibers from spinal cord levels L1 to S3 (Fig. 3.15). Nerves from lower sacral segments innervate the perineum. Terminal nerves exit the abdomen and pelvis through a number of apertures and foramina and enter the limb. As a consequence of this innervation, lumbar and upper sacral nerves are tested clinically by examining the lower limb. In addition, clinical signs (such as pain, pins-and-needles sensations, paresthesia, and fascicular muscle twitching) resulting from any disorder affecting these spinal nerves (e.g., herniated intervertebral disc in the lumbar region) appear in the lower limb (see Fig. 7.30).

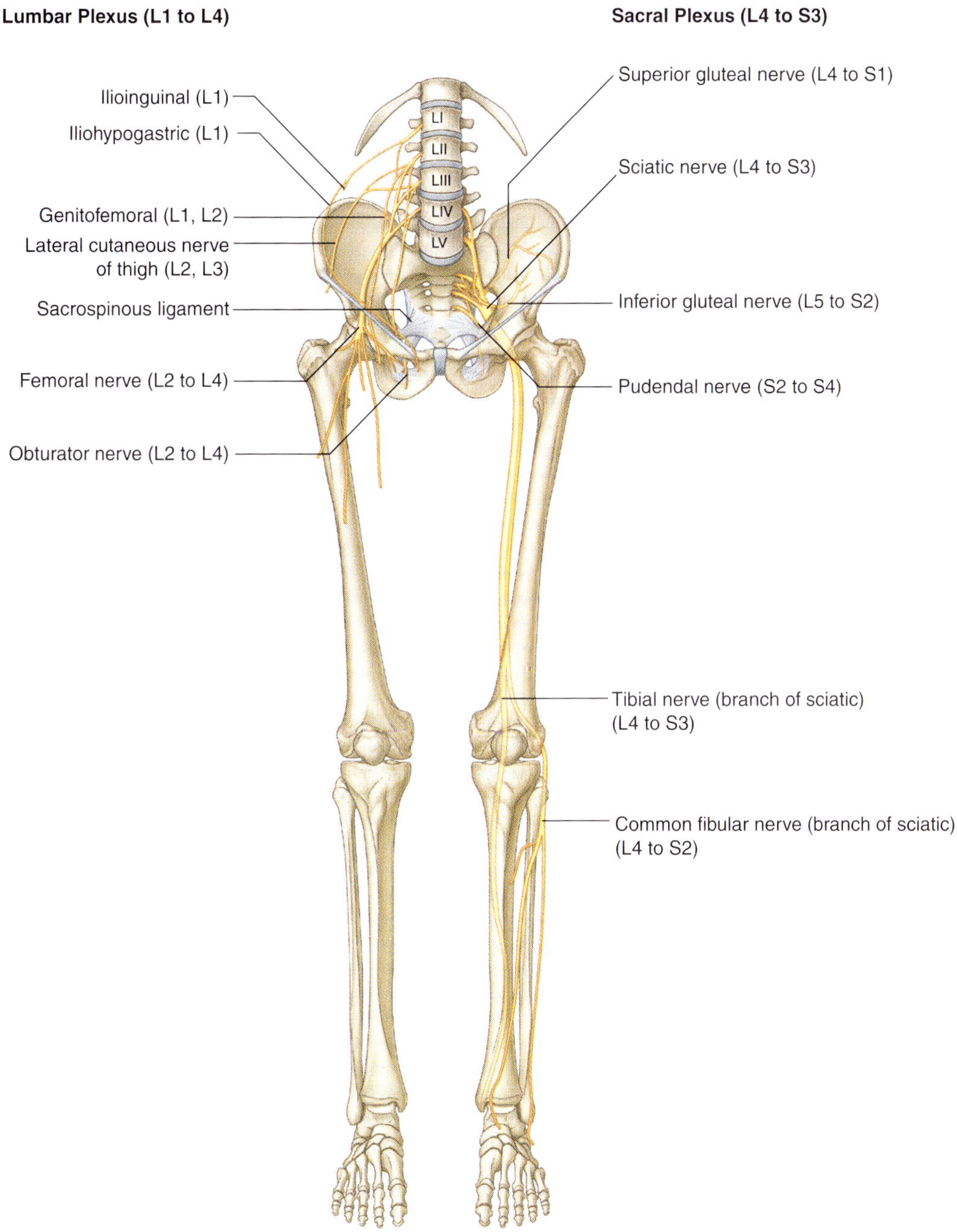

Fig. 3.15 Innervation of the lower limb.

Dermatomes in the lower limb are shown in Fig. 3.16. The arrangement can be explained by the development of the lower limb. Initially there is a preaxial border with the proximal dermatomes and a postaxial border with the distal dermatomes. Medial rotation of the lower limb occurs around a longitudinal axis passing through digit II. This results in the numerical sequence of the dermatomes which are seen to descend downwards and medially anteriorly (so the skin over the tibia is supplied by L4). Digit II is supplied by L5, and in the posterior view the numerical sequence ascends upwards and laterally:

- Over the inguinal ligament—L1
- Lateral side of the thigh—L2
- Lower medial side of the thigh—L3
- Medial side of the great toe (digit I)—L4
- Medial side of digit II—L5
- Little toe (digit V)—S1
- Back of the thigh—S2
- Skin over the gluteal fold—S3

The dermatomes of S4 and S5 are tested in the perineum.

Selected joint movements are used to test myotomes (Fig. 3.17). For example:

- Flexion of the hip is controlled primarily by L1 and L2.
- Extension of the knee is controlled mainly by L3 and L4.
- Dorsiflexion of the foot is controlled mainly by L4 and L5.
- Knee flexion is controlled mainly by L5 to S2.
- Plantar flexion of the foot is controlled predominantly by S1 and S2.
- Adduction of the digits is controlled by S2 and S3.

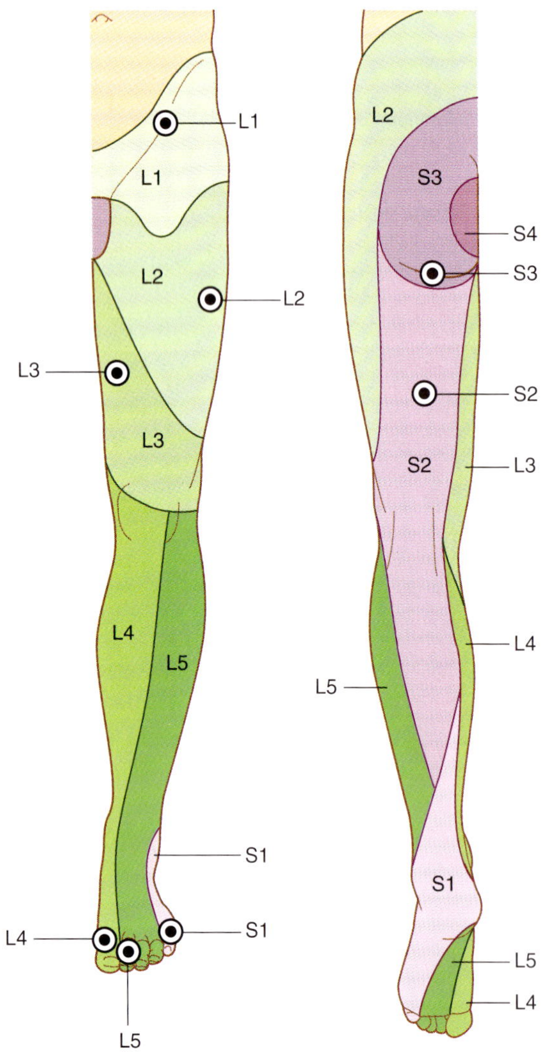

Fig. 3.16 Dermatomes of the lower limb. Dots indicate autonomous zones (i.e., with minimal overlap).

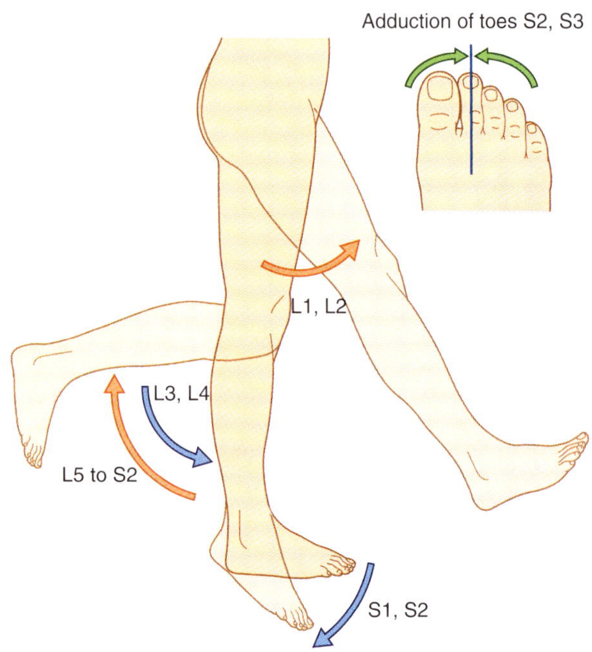

Fig. 3.17 Movements generated by myotomes.

In an unconscious patient, both somatic sensory and somatic motor functions of spinal cord levels can be tested using tendon reflexes:

- A tap on the patellar ligament at the knee tests predominantly L3 and L4.
- A tendon tap on the calcaneal tendon posterior to the ankle (tendon of gastrocnemius and soleus) tests S1 and S2.

Each of the major muscle groups or compartments in the lower limb is innervated primarily by one or more of the major nerves that originate from the lumbar and sacral plexuses (Fig. 3.18):

- Large muscles in the gluteal region are innervated by the superior and inferior gluteal nerves.

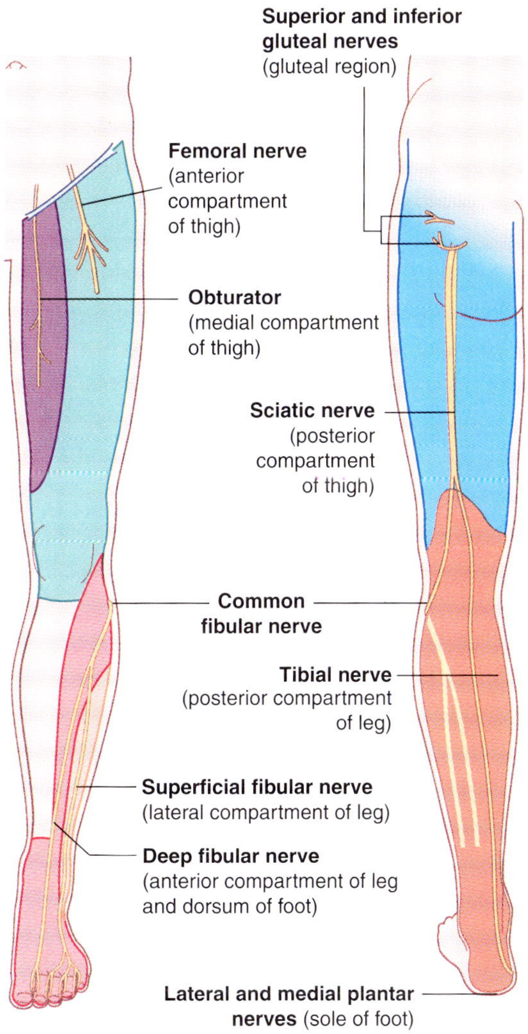

Fig. 3.18 Major nerves of the lower limb (colors indicate regions of motor innervation).

- Most muscles in the anterior compartment of the thigh are innervated by the femoral nerve (except the tensor fasciae latae, which are innervated by the superior gluteal nerve).
- Most muscles in the medial compartment are innervated mainly by the obturator nerve (except the pectineus, which is innervated by the femoral nerve, and part of the adductor magnus, which is innervated by the tibial division of the sciatic nerve).
- Most muscles in the posterior compartment of the thigh and the leg and in the sole of the foot are innervated by the tibial part of the sciatic nerve (except the short head of the biceps femoris in the posterior thigh, which is innervated by the common fibular division of the sciatic nerve).
- The anterior and lateral compartments of the leg and muscles associated with the dorsal surface of the foot are innervated by the common fibular part of the sciatic nerve.

In addition to innervating major muscle groups, each of the major peripheral nerves originating from the lumbar and sacral plexuses carries general sensory information from patches of skin (Fig. 3.19). Sensation from these areas can be used to test for peripheral nerve lesions:

- The femoral nerve innervates skin on the anterior thigh, medial side of the leg, and medial side of the ankle.
- The obturator nerve innervates the medial side of the thigh.
- The tibial nerve innervates the lateral side of the ankle and foot.
- The common fibular nerve innervates the lateral side of the leg and the dorsum of the foot.

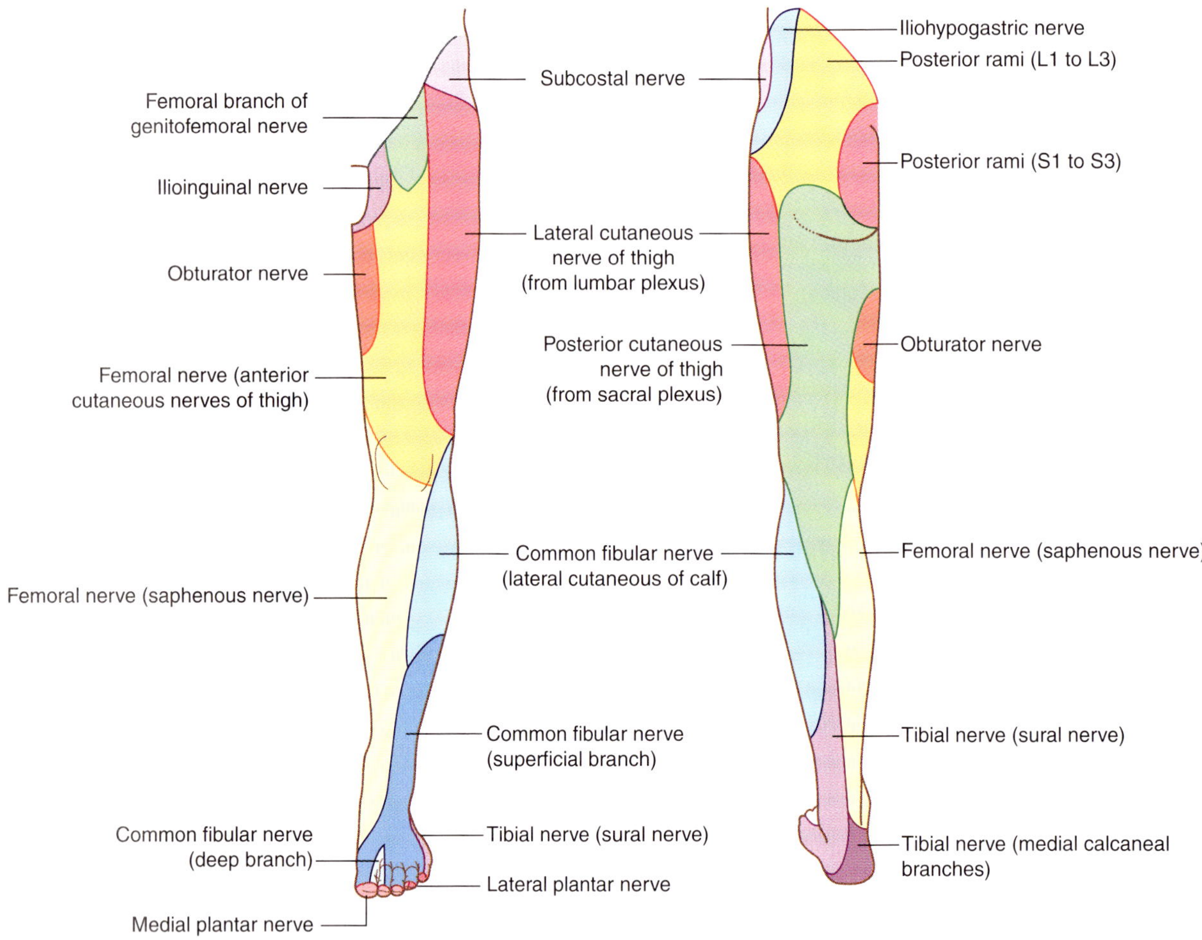

Fig. 3.19 Regions of skin innervated by peripheral nerves.

Nerves related to bone

The common fibular branch of the sciatic nerve curves laterally around the neck of the fibula when passing from the popliteal fossa into the leg (Fig. 3.20). The nerve can be rolled against bone just distal to the attachment of biceps femoris to the head of the fibula. In this location, the nerve can be damaged by impact injuries, fractures to the bone, or leg casts that are placed too high.

Superficial veins

Large veins embedded in the subcutaneous (superficial) fascia of the lower limb (Fig. 3.21) often become distended (varicose). These vessels can also be used for vascular transplantation.

The most important superficial veins are the great and small saphenous veins, which originate from the medial and lateral sides, respectively, of a dorsal venous arch in the foot.

- The great saphenous vein passes up the medial side of the leg, knee, and thigh to pass through an opening in deep fascia covering the femoral triangle and join with the femoral vein.
- The small saphenous vein passes behind the distal end of the fibula (lateral malleolus) and up the back of the leg to penetrate deep fascia and join the popliteal vein posterior to the knee.

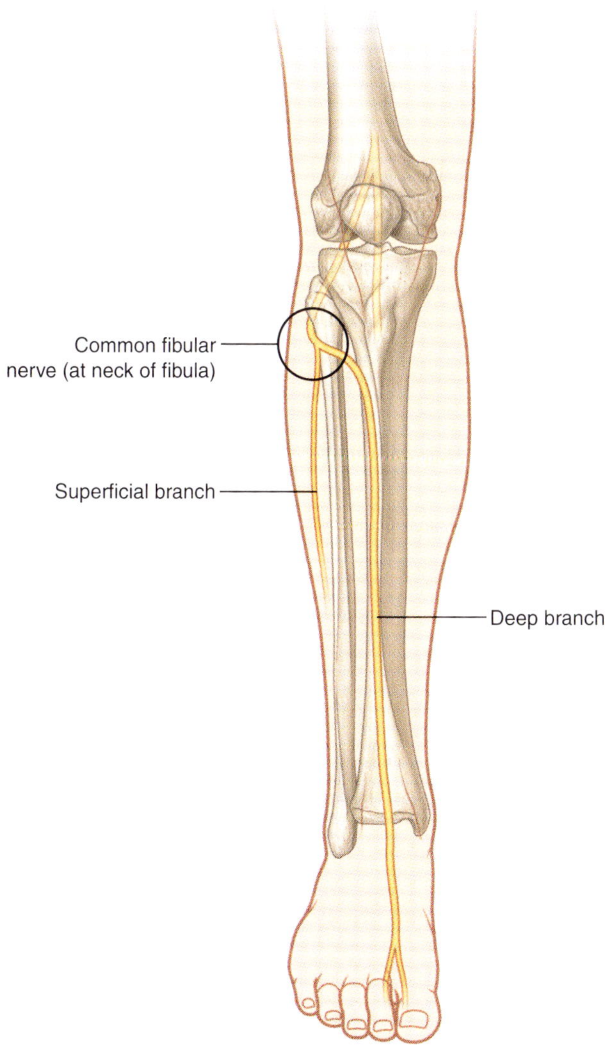

Fig. 3.20 Nerves related to bone.

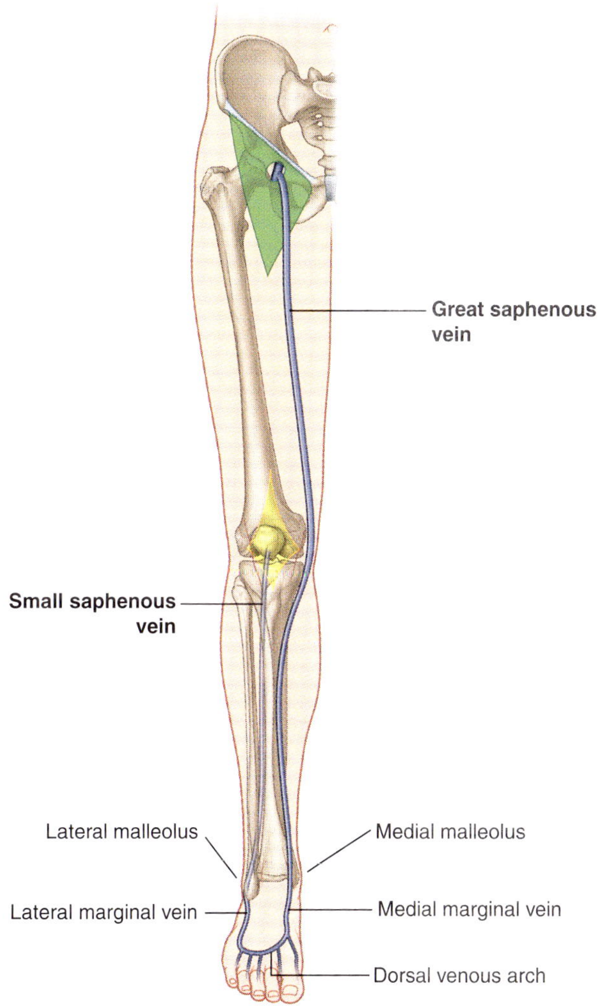

Fig. 3.21 Superficial veins.

Regional anatomy

Bony pelvis

The external surfaces of the pelvic bones, sacrum, and coccyx are predominantly the regions of the pelvis associated with the lower limb, although some muscles do originate from the deep or internal surfaces of these bones and from the surfaces of the lumbar vertebrae, above (Fig. 3.22).

Each pelvic bone is formed by three bones (ilium, ischium, and pubis), which fuse during childhood. The **ilium** is superior and the **pubis** and **ischium** are anteroinferior and posteroinferior, respectively.

The ilium articulates with the sacrum. The pelvic bone is further anchored to the end of the vertebral column (sacrum and coccyx) by the sacrotuberous and sacrospinous ligaments, which attach to a tuberosity and spine on the ischium.

The outer surface of the ilium and the adjacent surfaces of the sacrum, coccyx, and sacrotuberous ligament are associated with the gluteal region of the lower limb and provide extensive muscle attachment. The ischial tuberosity provides attachment for many of the muscles in the posterior compartment of the thigh, and the ischiopubic ramus and body of the pubis are associated mainly with muscles in the medial compartment of the thigh. The head of the femur articulates with the acetabulum on the lateral surface of the pelvic bone.

Ilium

The upper fan-shaped part of the ilium is associated on its inner side with the abdomen and on its outer side with the lower limb. The top of this region is the **iliac crest**, which ends anteriorly as the **anterior superior iliac spine** and posteriorly as the **posterior superior iliac spine**. A prominent lateral expansion of the crest just posterior to

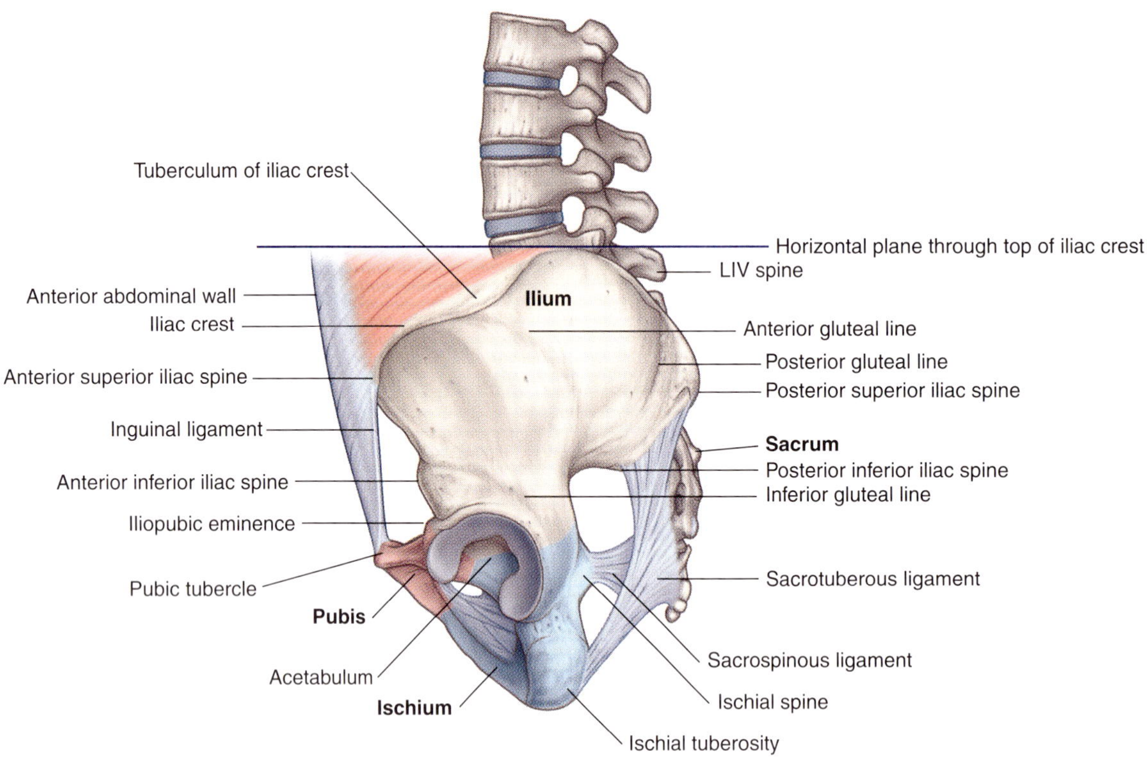

Fig. 3.22 External surface of the bony pelvis. Lateral view.

the anterior superior iliac spine is the **tubercle of the iliac crest**.

The anterior inferior iliac spine is on the anterior margin of the ilium, and below this, where the ilium fuses with the pubis, is a raised area of bone (the **iliopubic eminence**).

The gluteal surface of the ilium faces posterolaterally and lies below the iliac crest. It is marked by three curved lines (inferior, anterior, and posterior gluteal lines), which divide the surface into four regions:

- The **inferior gluteal line** originates just superior to the anterior inferior iliac spine and curves inferiorly across the bone to end near the posterior margin of the acetabulum—the rectus femoris muscle attaches to the anterior inferior iliac spine and to a roughened patch of bone between the superior margin of the acetabulum and the inferior gluteal line.
- The **anterior gluteal line** originates from the lateral margin of the iliac crest between the anterior superior iliac spine and the tuberculum of the iliac crest, and arches inferiorly across the ilium to disappear just superior to the upper margin of the greater sciatic foramen—the gluteus minimus muscle originates from between the inferior and anterior gluteal lines.
- The **posterior gluteal line** descends almost vertically from the iliac crest to a position near the posterior inferior iliac spine—the gluteus medius muscle attaches to bone between the anterior and posterior gluteal lines, and the gluteus maximus muscle attaches posterior to the posterior gluteal line.

Ischial tuberosity

The **ischial tuberosity** is posteroinferior to the acetabulum and is associated mainly with the hamstring muscles of the posterior thigh (Fig. 3.23). It is divided into upper and lower areas by a transverse line.

The upper area of the ischial tuberosity is oriented vertically and is further subdivided into two parts by an oblique line, which descends, from medial to lateral, across the surface:

- The more medial part of the upper area is for the attachment of the combined origin of the semitendinosus muscle and the long head of the biceps femoris muscle.
- The lateral part is for the attachment of the semimembranosus muscle.

The lower area of the ischial tuberosity is oriented horizontally and is divided into medial and lateral regions by a ridge of bone:

- The lateral region provides attachment for part of the adductor magnus muscle.
- The medial part faces inferiorly and is covered by connective tissue and by a bursa.

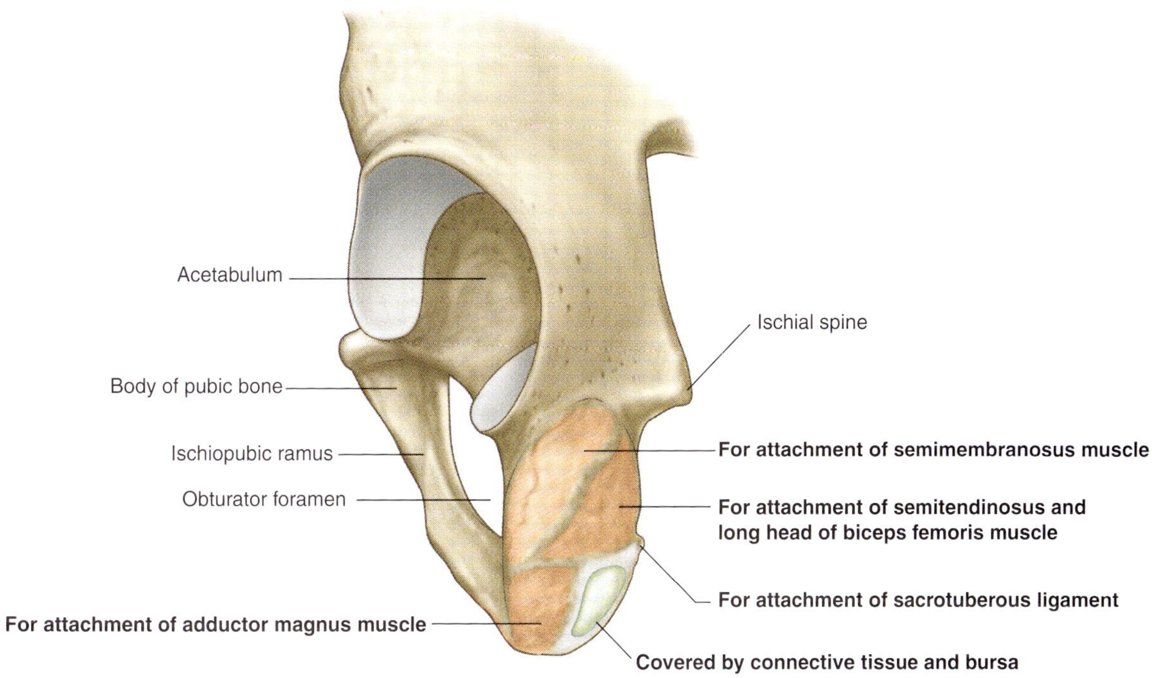

Fig. 3.23 Ischial tuberosity. Posterolateral view.

When sitting, this medial part supports the body weight.

The sacrotuberous ligament is attached to a sharp ridge on the medial margin of the ischial tuberosity.

Ischiopubic ramus and pubic bone

The external surfaces of the ischiopubic ramus anterior to the ischial tuberosity and the body of the pubis provide attachment for muscles of the medial compartment of the thigh (Fig. 3.23). These muscles include the adductor longus, adductor brevis, adductor magnus, pectineus, and gracilis (see Fig. 3.60).

Acetabulum

The large cup-shaped **acetabulum** for articulation with the head of the femur is on the lateral surface of the pelvic bone in the region where the ilium, pubis, and ischium fuse (Fig. 3.24).

The margin of the acetabulum is marked inferiorly by a prominent notch (**acetabular notch**).

The wall of the acetabulum consists of nonarticular and articular parts:

- The nonarticular part is rough and forms a shallow circular depression (the **acetabular fossa**) in central and inferior parts of the acetabular floor—the acetabular notch is continuous with the acetabular fossa.
- The articular surface is broad and surrounds the anterior, superior, and posterior margins of the acetabular fossa.

The smooth crescent-shaped articular surface (the **lunate surface**) is broadest superiorly where most of the body's weight is transmitted through the pelvis to the femur. The lunate surface is deficient inferiorly at the acetabular notch (see Fig. 3.30).

The acetabular fossa provides attachment for the ligament of the head of the femur, whereas blood vessels and nerves pass through the acetabular notch.

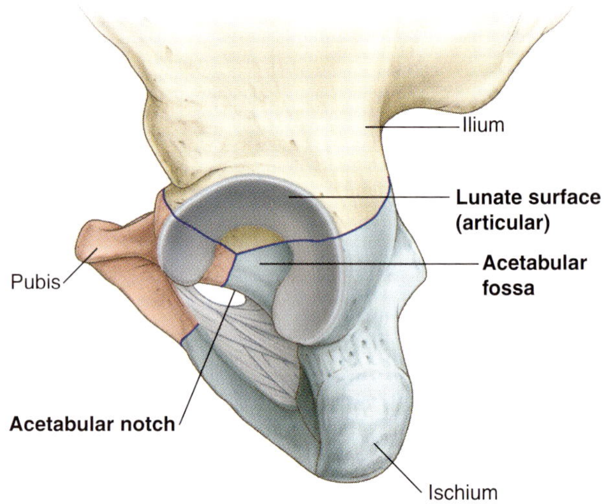

Fig. 3.24 Acetabulum.

Early clinical exposure

Pelvic fractures

The pelvic bones, sacrum, and associated joints form a bony ring surrounding the pelvic cavity. Soft tissue and visceral organ damage must be suspected when the pelvis is fractured. Patients with multiple injuries and evidence of chest, abdominal, and lower limb trauma should also be investigated for pelvic trauma.

Pelvic fractures can be associated with appreciable blood loss (concealed exsanguination) and blood transfusion is often required. In addition, this bleeding tends to form a significant pelvic hematoma, which can compress nerves, press on organs, and inhibit pelvic visceral function (Fig. 3.25).

There are many ways of classifying pelvic fractures, which enable the surgeon to determine the appropriate treatment and the patient's prognosis. Pelvic fractures are generally of four types:

- Type 1 injuries occur without disruption of the bony pelvic ring (e.g., a fracture of the iliac crest). These types of injuries are unlikely to represent significant trauma, though in the case of a fracture of the iliac crest, blood loss needs to be assessed.
- Type 2 injuries occur with a single break in the bony pelvic ring. An example of this would be a single fracture with diastasis (separation) of the symphysis pubis. Again, these injuries are relatively benign in nature, but it may be appropriate to assess for blood loss.

Early clinical exposure—cont'd

- Type 3 injuries occur with double breaks in the bony pelvic ring. These include bilateral fractures of the pubic rami, which may produce urethral damage.
- Type 4 injuries occur at and around the acetabulum.

Other types of pelvic ring injuries include fractures of the pubic rami and disruption of the sacroiliac joint with or without dislocation. This may involve significant visceral pelvic trauma and hemorrhage.

Other general pelvic injuries include stress fractures and insufficiency fractures, as seen in athletes and elderly patients with osteoporosis, respectively.

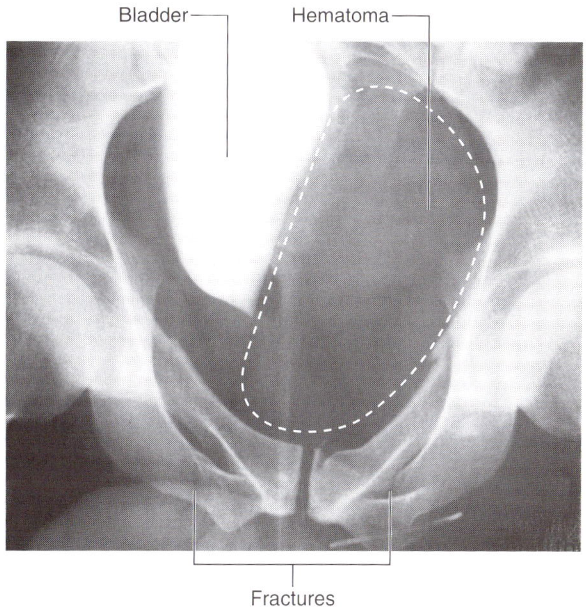

Fig. 3.25 Multiple fractures of the pelvis. Radiograph with contrast in the bladder. A large accumulation of blood is deforming the bladder.

Proximal femur

The femur is the bone of the thigh and the longest bone in the body. Its proximal end is characterized by a head and neck, and two large projections (the greater and lesser trochanters) on the upper part of the shaft (Fig. 3.26).

The **head** of the femur is spherical and articulates with the acetabulum of the pelvic bone. It is characterized by a nonarticular pit (**fovea**) on its medial surface for the attachment of the ligament of the head.

The **neck** of the femur is a cylindrical strut of bone that connects the head to the shaft of the femur. It projects superomedially from the shaft at an angle of approximately 125°, and projects slightly forward. The orientation of the neck relative to the shaft increases the range of movement of the hip joint.

The upper part of the **shaft** of the femur bears a greater and lesser trochanter, which are attachment sites for muscles that move the hip joint.

Greater and lesser trochanters

The **greater trochanter** extends superiorly from the shaft of the femur just lateral to the region where the shaft joins the neck of the femur (Fig. 3.26). It continues posteriorly where its medial surface is deeply grooved to form the **trochanteric fossa**. This fossa bears a distinct oval depression for attachment of the obturator externus muscle (see Fig. 3.61).

The greater trochanter has an elongate ridge on its anterolateral surface for attachment of the gluteus minimus and a similar ridge more posteriorly on its lateral surface for attachment of the gluteus medius. Between these two points, the greater trochanter is palpable.

On the medial side of the superior aspect of the greater trochanter and just above the trochanteric fossa is a small impression for attachment of the obturator internus and its associated gemelli muscles, and immediately above and behind this feature is an impression on the margin of the trochanter for attachment of the piriformis muscle.

The **lesser trochanter** is smaller than the greater trochanter and has a blunt conical shape. It projects posteromedially from the shaft of the femur just inferior to the junction with the neck (Fig. 3.26). It is the attachment site for the combined tendons of psoas major and iliacus muscles (see Fig. 3.57).

Extending between the two trochanters and separating the shaft from the neck of the femur are the intertrochanteric line and intertrochanteric crest.

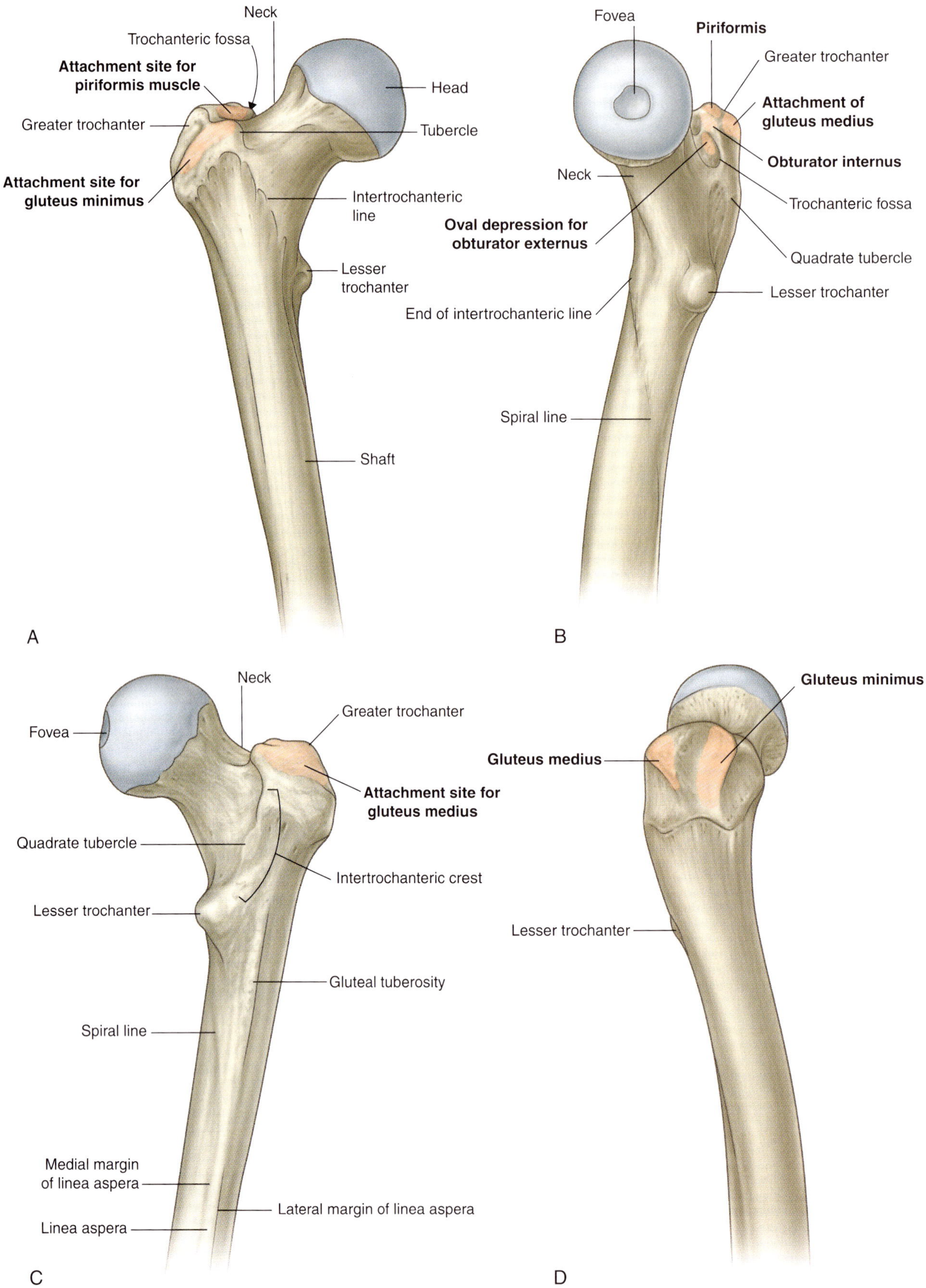

Fig. 3.26 Proximal end of the femur (*right*). **(A)** Anterior view. **(B)** Medial view. **(C)** Posterior view. **(D)** Lateral view.

Intertrochanteric line

The **intertrochanteric line** is a ridge of bone on the anterior surface of the upper margin of the shaft that descends medially from a tubercle on the anterior surface of the base of the greater trochanter to a position just anterior to the base of the lesser trochanter (Fig. 3.26). It is continuous with the **spiral line**, which curves medially below the lesser trochanter and around the shaft of the femur to merge with the medial margin of the **linea aspera** on the posterior aspect of the femur.

Intertrochanteric crest

The **intertrochanteric crest** is on the posterior surface of the femur and descends medially across the bone from the posterior margin of the greater trochanter to the base of the lesser trochanter (Fig. 3.26). It is a broad smooth ridge of bone with a prominent tubercle (the **quadrate tubercle**) on its upper half, which provides attachment for the quadratus femoris muscle.

Shaft of the femur

The shaft of the femur descends from lateral to medial in the coronal plane at an angle of 7° from the vertical axis (Fig. 3.27). The distal end of the femur is therefore closer to the midline than the upper end of the shaft.

The middle third of the shaft of the femur is triangular in shape with smooth lateral and medial margins between anterior, lateral (posterolateral), and medial (posteromedial) surfaces. The posterior margin is broad and forms a prominent raised crest (the linea aspera).

The linea aspera is a major site of muscle attachment in the thigh. In the proximal third of the femur, the medial and lateral margins of the linea aspera diverge and continue superiorly as the spiral line and gluteal tuberosity, respectively (Fig. 3.27):

- The spiral line curves anteriorly under the lesser trochanter and joins the intertrochanteric line.
- The gluteal tuberosity is a broad linear roughening that curves laterally to the base of the greater trochanter.
- The pectineal line extends vertically from the lesser trochanter.

The gluteus maximus muscle is attached to the gluteal tuberosity.

The triangular area enclosed by the spiral line, the gluteal tuberosity, and the intertrochanteric crest is the posterior surface of the proximal end of the femur.

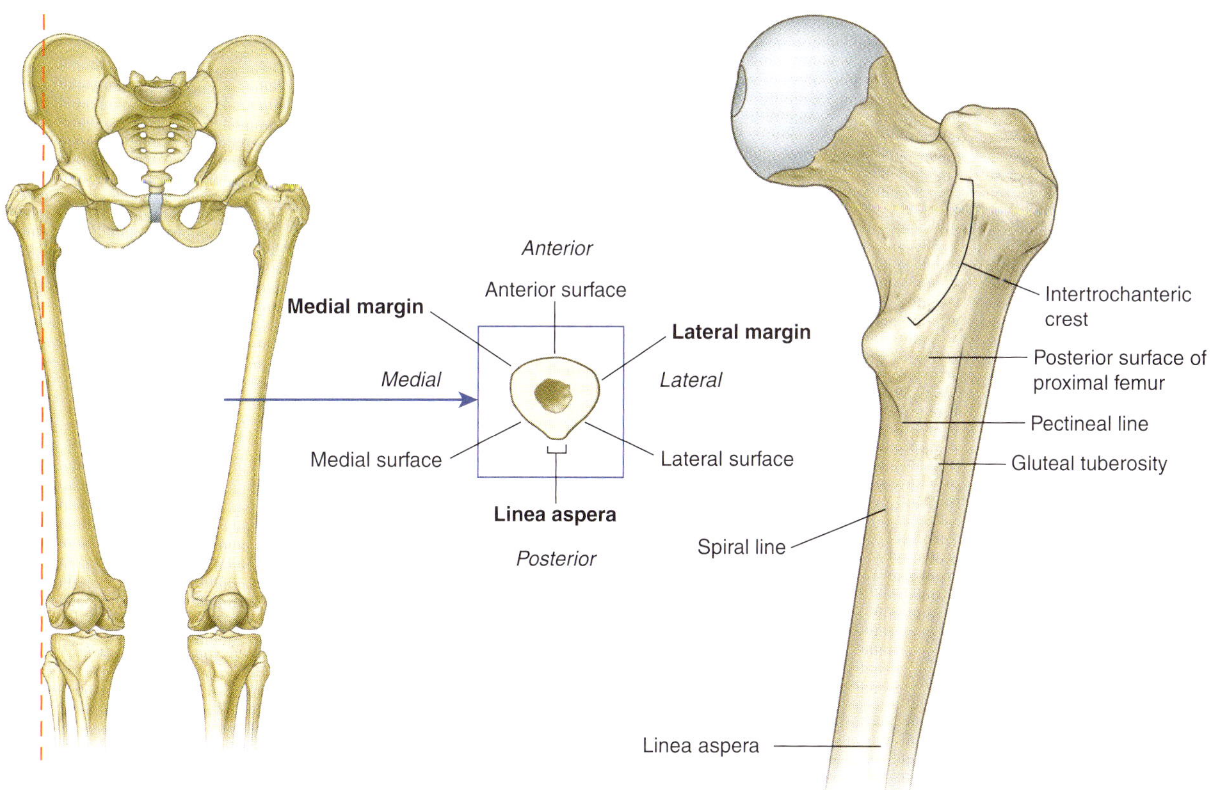

Fig. 3.27 Shaft of the femur. On the right is a posterior view of proximal shaft of right femur.

The neck–shaft angle (Mikulicz angle) is the angle between the long axis of the femoral shaft and the axis of femoral neck (125–140°). It appears that the femoral neck is rotated anteriorly (anteverted) and it is thought to be due to medial rotation of the limb bud in early intrauterine life. The femoral angle of anteversion (or angle of femoral torsion) is the angle subtended between the femoral neck and the line extending to the posterior borders of the femoral condyles in the axial plane (10–15°).

Early clinical exposure

Femoral neck fractures

Femoral neck fractures (Fig. 3.28A) can be diagnosed by noting the presence of a discontinuity or irregularity in Shenton's line. This is an imaginary line drawn along the inferior edge of the neck of the femur and the inferior edge of the superior ramus of the pubis in an X-ray of the hip joint. Such fractures can interrupt the blood supply to the femoral head. The blood supply to the head and neck is primarily from an arterial ring formed around the base of the femoral neck (see Fig. 3.33). From here, vessels course along the neck, penetrate the capsule, and supply the femoral head. The blood supply to the femoral head and femoral neck is further enhanced by the artery of the ligamentum teres, which is generally small and variable. Femoral neck fractures may disrupt associated vessels and lead to necrosis of the femoral head. A fracture of the neck of femur can be diagnosed by drawing Bryant's triangle or the iliofemoral triangle on both sides. A horizontal line is drawn passing through the anterior superior iliac spine. A vertical line is drawn from the tip of the greater trochanter to the horizontal line. The third line is drawn between the anterior superior iliac spine and the tip of the greater trochanter. The triangles of the two sides are compared.

The third line mentioned can be drawn up to the ischial tuberosity (Nelaton's line). The tip of the greater trochanter lies above this line if the upper end of the femur is displaced upwards in fracture of the femur.

Femoral neck fractures can be divided into three categories depending on the location of the fracture line: subcapital (fracture line passes across the femoral head–neck junction), transcervical (fracture line passes through the midportion of the femoral neck), and basicervical (fracture line passes across the base of the neck). Subcapital fractures have the highest risk of developing necrosis of the femoral head, and basicervical fractures have the lowest risk. Elderly patients with osteoporosis tend to have transverse subcapital fractures following low-energy trauma such as a fall from a standing height. Conversely, younger patients usually sustain more vertical fractures of the distal femoral neck (basicervical) after high-energy trauma such as a fall from a great height or due to axial load applied to an abducted knee, such as during a motor vehicle accident.

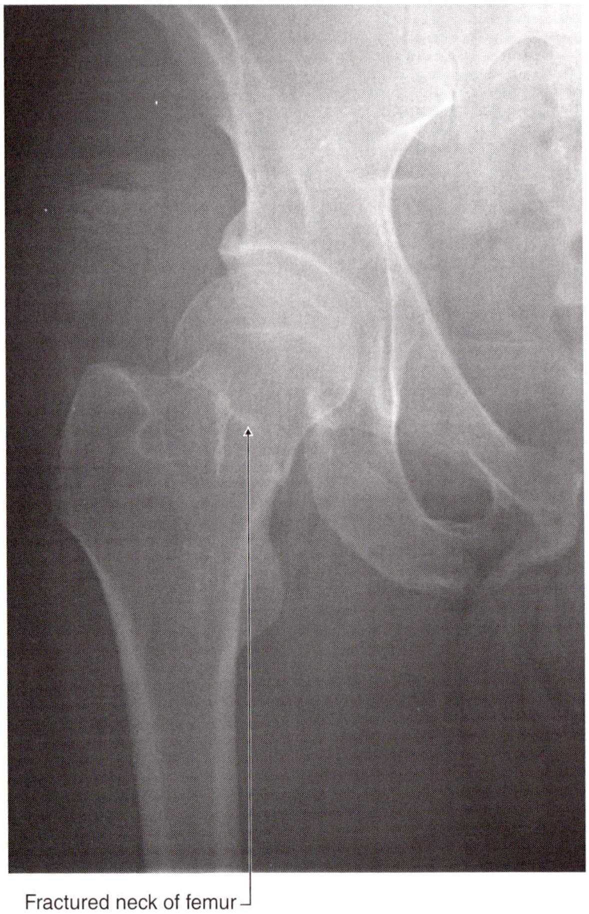

Fig. 3.28A Radiograph of the pelvis, anteroposterior view, demonstrating a fracture of the neck of the femur.

Early clinical exposure

Intertrochanteric fractures

In these fractures, the break usually runs from the greater trochanter through to the lesser trochanter and does not involve the femoral neck. Intertrochanteric fractures preserve the femoral neck blood supply and do not render the femoral head ischemic. They are most commonly seen in the elderly and result from low-energy impact (Fig. 3.28B).

Sometimes isolated fractures of the greater or the lesser trochanter can occur. An isolated fracture of the lesser trochanter in adults is most commonly pathological (due to an underlying pathology) and due to an underlying malignant deposit.

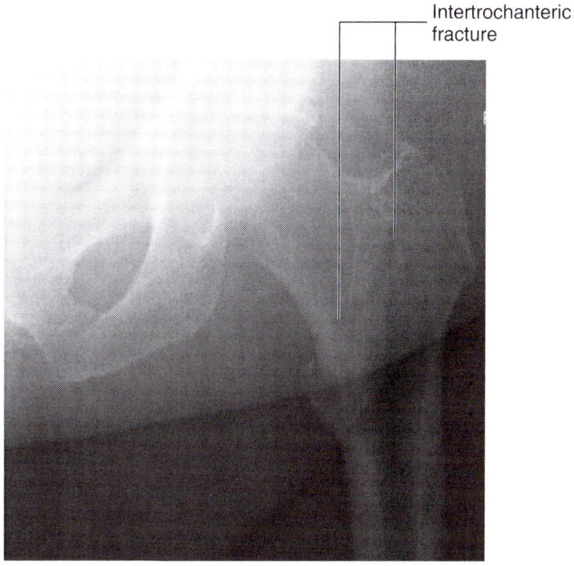

Fig. 3.28B Anteroposterior radiograph showing an intertrochanteric fracture of proximal end of femur.

Early clinical exposure

Femoral shaft fractures

An appreciable amount of energy is needed to fracture the femoral shaft. This type of injury is therefore accompanied by damage to the surrounding soft tissues, which include the muscle compartments and the structures they contain.

Hip joint

The hip joint is a synovial articulation between the head of the femur and the acetabulum of the pelvic bone (Fig. 3.29A). The joint is a multiaxial ball and socket joint designed for stability and weight-bearing at the expense of mobility. Movements at the joint include flexion, extension, abduction, adduction, medial and lateral rotation, and circumduction (Fig. 3.5).

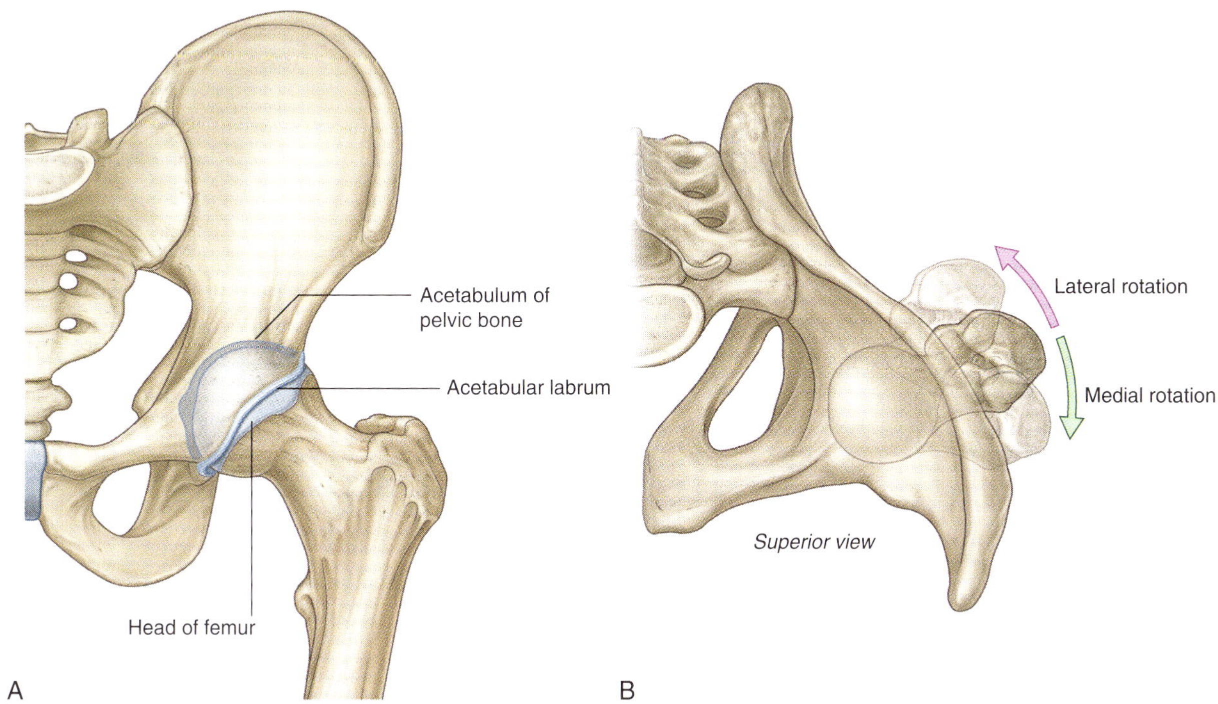

Fig. 3.29 Hip joint. **(A)** Articular surfaces: anterior view. **(B)** Movement of the neck of the femur during medial and lateral rotation: superior view.

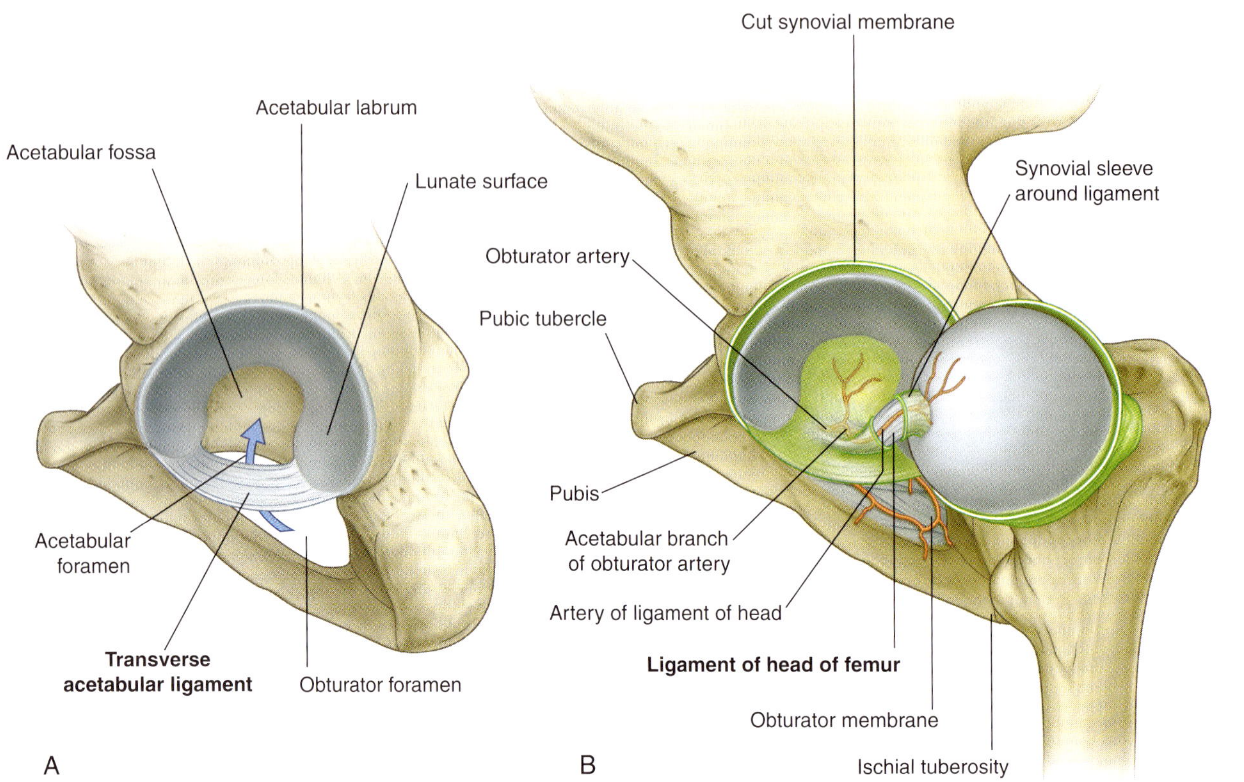

Fig. 3.30 Hip joint. **(A)** Transverse acetabular ligament. **(B)** Ligament of the head of the femur. The head of the femur has been laterally rotated out of the acetabulum to show the ligament.

When considering the effects of muscle action on the hip joint, the long neck of the femur and the angulation of the neck on the shaft of the femur must be borne in mind. For example, medial and lateral rotation of the femur involves muscles that move the greater trochanter forward and backward, respectively, relative to the acetabulum (Fig. 3.29B). The axis of rotation is an imaginary vertical line that passes through the femoral head.

The articular surfaces of the hip joint are

- The spherical head of the femur
- The lunate surface of the acetabulum of the pelvic bone

The acetabulum almost entirely encompasses the hemispherical head of the femur and contributes substantially to joint stability. The nonarticular acetabular fossa contains loose connective tissue. The lunate surface is covered by hyaline cartilage and is broadest superiorly.

Except for the fovea, the head of the femur is also covered by hyaline cartilage.

The rim of the acetabulum is raised slightly by a fibrocartilaginous collar (the acetabular labrum). Inferiorly, the labrum bridges across the acetabular notch as the **transverse acetabular ligament** and converts the notch into a foramen (Fig. 3.30A).

The **ligament of the head of the femur** is a flat band of delicate connective tissue that attaches at one end to the fovea on the head of the femur and at the other end to the acetabular fossa, transverse acetabular ligament, and margins of the acetabular notch (Fig. 3.30B). It carries a small branch of the obturator artery, which contributes to the blood supply of the head of the femur.

The synovial membrane attaches to the margins of the articular surfaces of the femur and acetabulum, forms a tubular covering around the ligament of the head of the femur, and lines the fibrous membrane of the joint (Fig. 3.30B and 3.31). From its attachment to the margin of the head of the femur, the synovial membrane covers the neck of the femur before reflecting onto the fibrous membrane (Fig. 3.31).

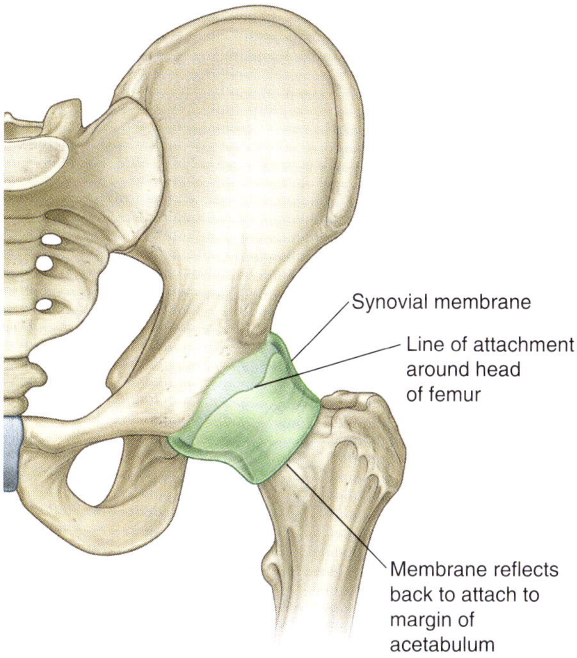

Fig. 3.31 Synovial membrane of the hip joint.

The fibrous membrane that encloses the hip joint is strong and generally thick. Medially, it is attached to the margin of the acetabulum, the transverse acetabular ligament, and the adjacent margin of the obturator foramen (Fig. 3.32A). Laterally, it is attached to the intertrochanteric line on the anterior aspect of the femur and to the neck of the femur just proximal to the intertrochanteric crest on the posterior surface.

Ligaments

Three ligaments reinforce the external surface of the fibrous membrane and stabilize the joint: the iliofemoral, pubofemoral, and ischiofemoral ligaments.

- The **iliofemoral ligament or Bigelow's ligament** is anterior to the hip joint and is triangular shaped (Fig. 3.32B). Its apex is attached to the ilium between the anterior inferior iliac spine and the margin of the acetabulum and its base is attached along the intertrochanteric line of the femur. Parts of the ligament attached to the upper and lower parts of the intertrochanteric line are thicker than the part attached to the central part of the line. This results in the ligament having a Y appearance.
- The **pubofemoral ligament** is anteroinferior to the hip joint (Fig. 3.32B). It is also triangular in shape, with its base attached medially to the iliopubic eminence, adjacent bone, and obturator membrane. Laterally, it blends with the fibrous membrane and with the deep surface of the iliofemoral ligament.
- The **ischiofemoral ligament** reinforces the posterior aspect of the fibrous membrane (Fig. 3.32C). It is attached medially to the ischium, just posteroinferior to the acetabulum, and laterally to the greater trochanter deep to the iliofemoral ligament.

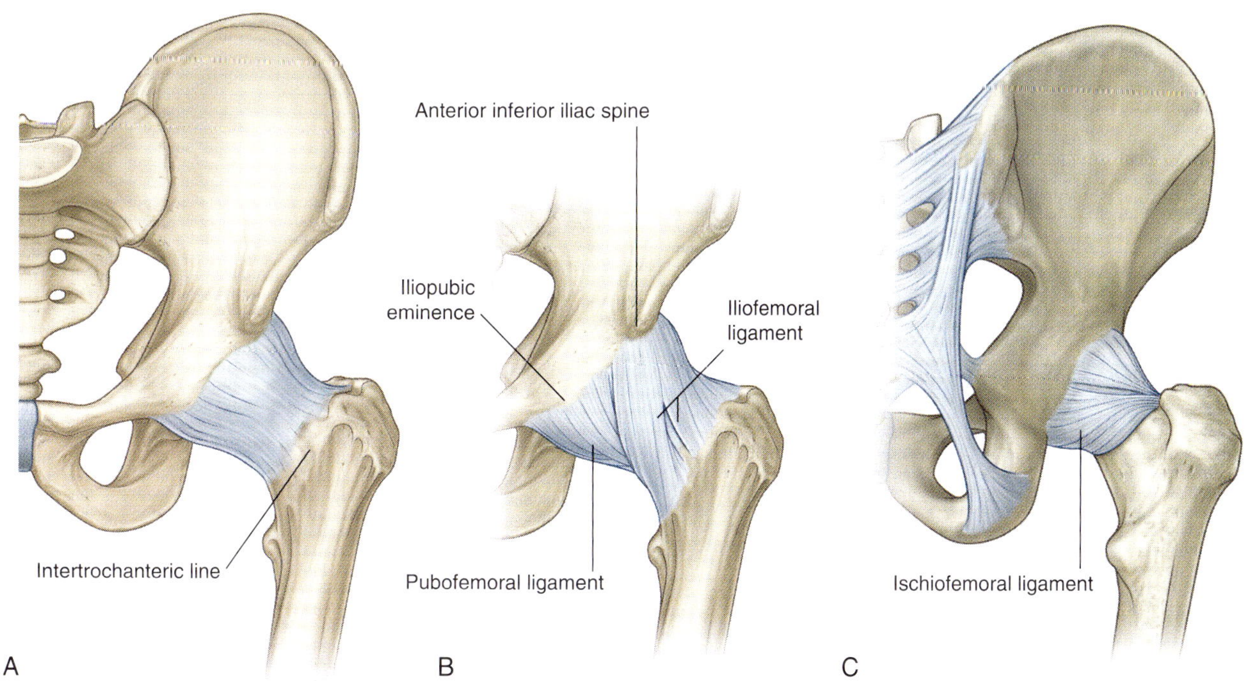

Fig. 3.32 Fibrous membrane and ligaments of the hip joint. **(A)** Fibrous membrane of the joint capsule: anterior view. **(B)** Iliofemoral and pubofemoral ligaments: anterior view. **(C)** Ischiofemoral ligament: posterior view.

The fibers of all three ligaments are oriented in a spiral fashion around the hip joint so that they become taut when the joint is extended. This stabilizes the joint and reduces the amount of muscle energy required to maintain a standing position.

Vascular supply to the hip joint is predominantly through branches of the obturator artery, medial and lateral circumflex femoral arteries, superior and inferior gluteal arteries, and the first perforating branch of the deep artery of the thigh. The articular branches of these vessels form a network around the joint (Fig. 3.33).

The hip joint is innervated by articular branches from the femoral, obturator, and superior gluteal nerves, and the nerve to the quadratus femoris.

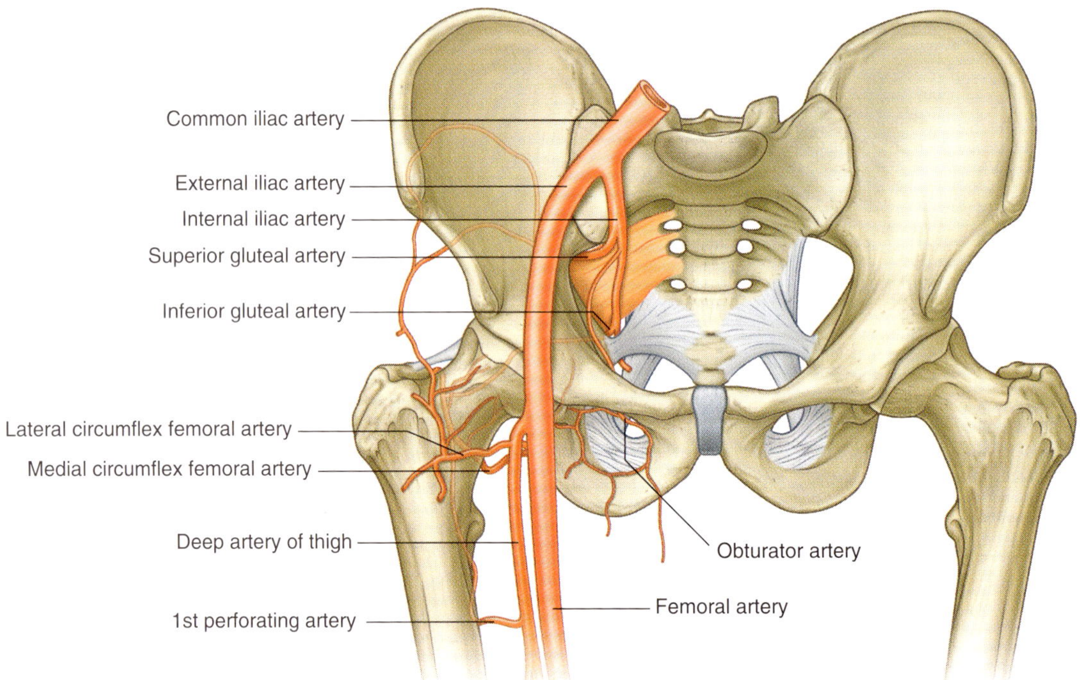

Fig. 3.33 Blood supply of the hip joint.

Gateways to the lower limb

There are four major routes by which structures pass from the abdomen and pelvis into and out of the lower limb. These are the obturator canal, the greater sciatic foramen, the lesser sciatic foramen, and the gap between the inguinal ligament and the anterosuperior margin of the pelvis (Fig. 3.34).

Obturator canal

The **obturator canal** is an almost vertically oriented passageway at the anterosuperior edge of the obturator foramen (Fig. 3.34). It is bordered:

- Above by a groove (**obturator groove**) on the inferior surface of the superior ramus of the pubic bone.
- Below by the upper margin of the obturator membrane, which fills most of the obturator foramen, and by muscles (obturator internus and externus) attached to the inner and outer surfaces of the obturator membrane and surrounding bone.

The obturator canal connects the abdominopelvic region with the medial compartment of the thigh. The obturator nerve and vessels pass through the canal.

Greater sciatic foramen

The **greater sciatic foramen** is formed on the posterolateral pelvic wall and is the major route for structures to pass between the pelvis and the gluteal region of the lower limb (Fig. 3.34). The margins of the foramen are formed by:

- The greater sciatic notch
- Parts of the upper borders of the sacrospinous and sacrotuberous ligaments
- The lateral border of the sacrum

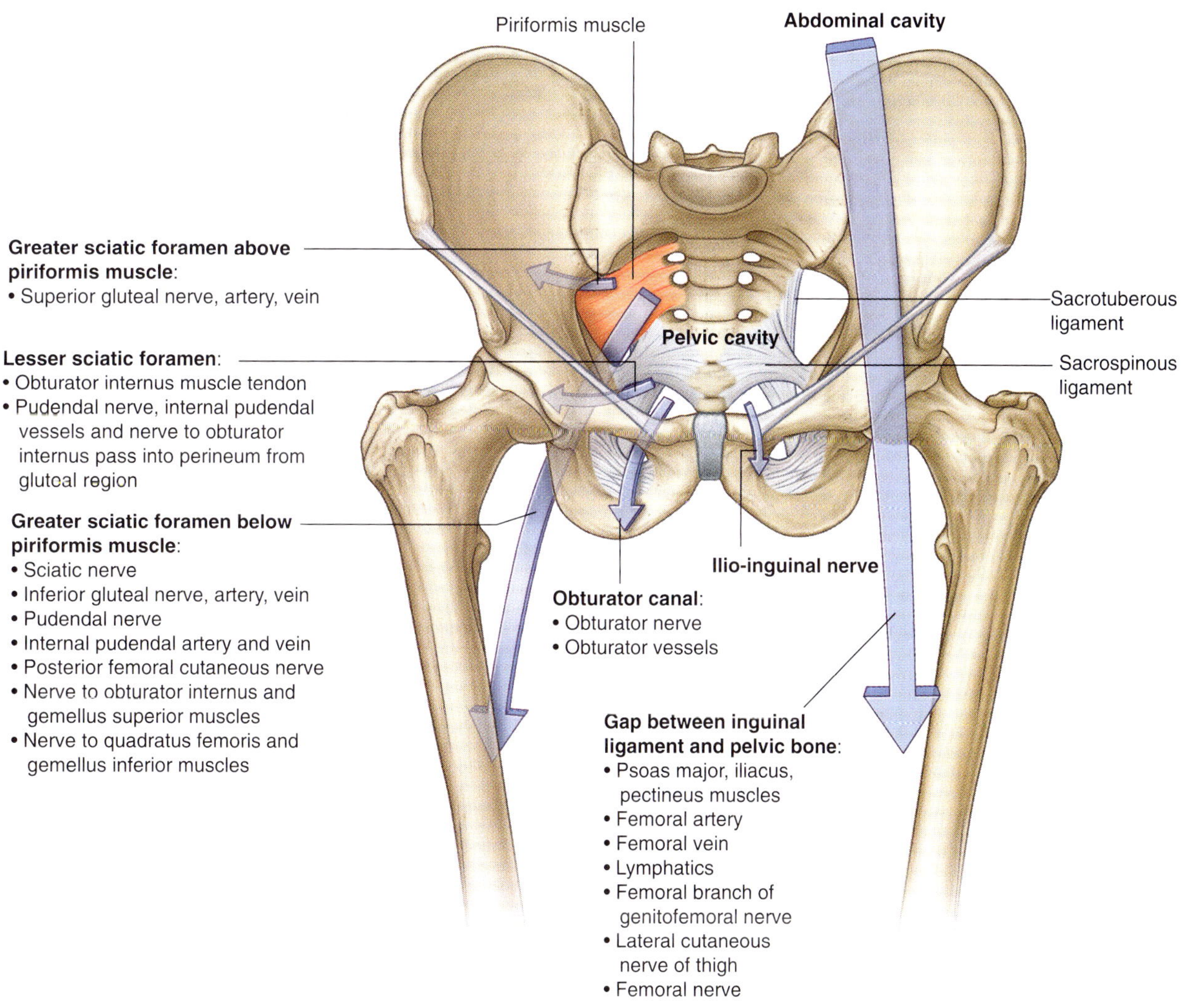

Fig. 3.34 Gateways to the lower limb.

The piriformis muscle passes out of the pelvis into the gluteal region through the greater sciatic foramen and separates the foramen into two parts, a part above the muscle and a part below:

- The superior gluteal nerve and vessels pass through the greater sciatic foramen above the piriformis.
- The sciatic nerve, inferior gluteal nerve and vessels, pudendal nerve and internal pudendal vessels, posterior cutaneous nerve of the thigh, nerve to the obturator internus and gemellus superior, and nerve to the quadratus femoris and gemellus inferior pass through the greater sciatic foramen below the muscle.

Lesser sciatic foramen

The **lesser sciatic foramen** is inferior to the greater sciatic foramen on the posterolateral pelvic wall (Fig. 3.34). It is also inferior to the lateral attachment of the pelvic floor (levator ani and coccygeus muscles) to the pelvic wall and therefore connects the gluteal region with the perineum:

- The tendon of the obturator internus passes from the lateral pelvic wall through the lesser sciatic foramen into the gluteal region to insert on the femur (see Fig. 3.47).
- The pudendal nerve and internal pudendal vessels, which first exit the pelvis by passing through the greater sciatic foramen below the piriformis muscle, enter the perineum below the pelvic floor by passing around the sacrospinous ligament and ischial spine and medially through the lesser sciatic foramen.

Gap between the inguinal ligament and pelvic bone

The large crescent-shaped gap between the inguinal ligament above and the anterosuperior margin of the pelvic bone below is the major route of communication between the abdomen and the anteromedial aspect of the thigh (Fig. 3.34). The psoas major, iliacus, and pectineus muscles pass through this gap to insert onto the femur. The major blood vessels (femoral artery and vein) and lymphatics of the lower limb also pass through it, as does the femoral nerve, to enter the femoral triangle of the thigh (see Fig. 3.42).

Nerves

Nerves that enter the lower limb from the abdomen and pelvis are terminal branches of the lumbosacral plexus on the posterior wall of the abdomen and the posterolateral walls of the pelvis (Fig. 3.35 and Table 3.1).

The **lumbar plexus** is formed by the anterior rami of spinal nerves L1 to L3 and part of L4 (see Chapter 4, p. 571). The rest of the anterior ramus of L4 and the anterior ramus of L5 combine to form the **lumbosacral trunk**, which enters the pelvic cavity and joins with the anterior rami of S1 to S3 to form the **sacral plexus** (see Chapter 5, p. 667).

Major nerves that originate from the lumbar and sacral plexuses and leave the abdomen and pelvis to enter the lower limb include the femoral nerve, obturator nerve, sciatic nerve, superior gluteal nerve, and inferior gluteal nerve. Other nerves that also originate from the plexus and enter the lower limb to supply skin or muscle include the lateral cutaneous nerve of the thigh, nerve to the obturator internus, nerve to the quadratus femoris, posterior cutaneous nerve of the thigh, perforating cutaneous nerve, and branches of the ilioinguinal and genitofemoral nerves.

Femoral nerve

The **femoral nerve** carries contributions from the anterior rami of L2 to L4 and leaves the abdomen by passing through the gap between the inguinal ligament and superior margin of the pelvis to enter the femoral triangle on the anteromedial aspect of the thigh (Fig. 3.35 and Table 3.1). In the femoral triangle, it is lateral to the femoral artery. The femoral nerve:

- Innervates all muscles in the anterior compartment of the thigh.
- In the abdomen, gives rise to branches that innervate the iliacus and pectineus muscles.
- Innervates skin over the anterior aspect of the thigh, the anteromedial side of the knee, the medial side of the leg, and the medial side of the foot (see Fig. 3.18 and 3.19).

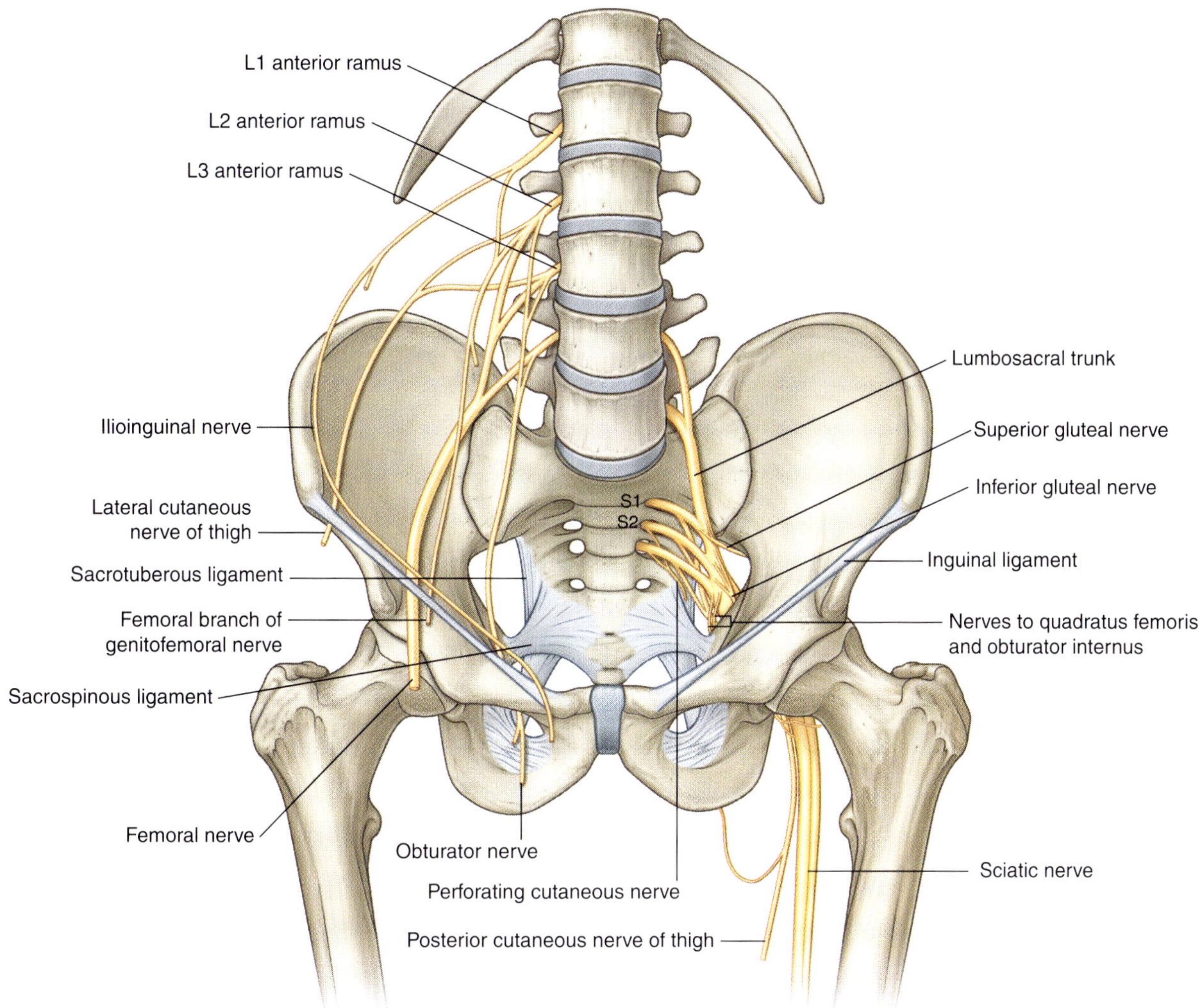

Fig. 3.35 Branches of the lumbar and sacral plexus.

Table 3.1 Branches of the lumbar and sacral plexus associated with the lower limb

Branch	Spinal segments	Function: motor	Function: sensory (cutaneous)
Ilioinguinal	L1	No motor function in lower limb, but innervates muscles of the abdominal wall	Skin over anteromedial part of upper thigh and adjacent skin of perineum
Genitofemoral	L1, L2	No motor function in lower limb, but genital branch innervates cremaster muscle in the wall of the spermatic cord in men	Femoral branch innervates skin on anterior central part of upper thigh; the genital branch innervates skin in anterior part of perineum (anterior scrotum in men, and mons pubis and anterior labia majora in women)
Femoral	L2 to L4	All muscles in the anterior compartment of thigh; in the abdomen, also gives rise to branches that supply iliacus and pectineus	Skin over the anterior thigh, anteromedial knee, medial side of the leg, and the medial side of the foot
Obturator	L2 to L4	All muscles in the medial compartment of thigh (except pectineus and the part of adductor magnus attached to the ischium); also innervates obturator externus	Skin over upper medial aspect of thigh

Continued

Table 3.1 Branches of the lumbar and sacral plexus associated with the lower limb—cont'd

Branch	Spinal segments	Function: motor	Function: sensory (cutaneous)
Sciatic	L4 to S3	All muscles in the posterior compartment of thigh and the part of adductor magnus attached to the ischium; all muscles in the leg and foot	Skin over lateral side of leg and foot, and over the sole and dorsal surface of foot
Superior gluteal	L4 to S1	Muscles of the gluteal region (gluteus medius, gluteus minimus, tensor fasciae latae)	
Inferior gluteal	L5 to S2	Muscle of the gluteal region (gluteus maximus)	
Lateral cutaneous nerve of thigh	L2, L3		Parietal peritoneum in iliac fossa; skin over anterolateral thigh
Posterior cutaneous nerve of thigh	S1 to S3		Skin over gluteal fold and upper medial aspect of thigh and adjacent perineum, posterior aspect of thigh, and upper posterior leg
Nerve to quadratus femoris	L4 to S1	Muscles of gluteal region (quadratus femoris and gemellus inferior)	
Nerve to obturator internus	L5 to S2	Muscles of gluteal region (obturator internus and gemellus superior)	
Perforating cutaneous nerve	S2, S3		Skin over medial aspect of gluteal fold

Obturator nerve

The **obturator nerve**, like the femoral nerve, originates from L2 to L4. It descends along the posterior abdominal wall, passes through the pelvic cavity, and enters the thigh by passing through the obturator canal (Fig. 3.35 and Table 3.1). The obturator nerve innervates:

- All muscles in the medial compartment of the thigh, except the part of the adductor magnus muscle that originates from the ischium and the pectineus muscle, which are innervated by the sciatic and the femoral nerves, respectively.
- The obturator externus muscle.
- Skin on the medial side of the upper thigh (see Fig. 3.18 and 3.19).

Sciatic nerve

The **sciatic nerve** is the largest nerve of the body and carries contributions from L4 to S3. It leaves the pelvis through the greater sciatic foramen inferior to the piriformis muscle, enters and passes through the gluteal region (Fig. 3.35 and Table 3.1), and then enters the posterior compartment of the thigh where it divides into its two major branches:

- The common fibular nerve
- The tibial nerve

Posterior divisions of L4 to S2 are carried in the common fibular part of the nerve and the anterior divisions of L4 to S3 are carried in the tibial part.

The sciatic nerve innervates:

- All muscles in the posterior compartment of the thigh.
- The part of the adductor magnus originating from the ischium.
- All muscles in the leg and foot.
- Skin on the lateral side of the leg and the lateral side and sole of the foot (see Fig. 3.18 and 3.19).

Gluteal nerves

The gluteal nerves are major motor nerves of the gluteal region.

The **superior gluteal nerve** (Fig. 3.35 and Table 3.1) carries contributions from the anterior rami of L4 to S1, leaves the pelvis through the greater sciatic foramen above the piriformis muscle, and innervates:

- The gluteus medius and minimus muscles
- The tensor fasciae latae muscle

The **inferior gluteal nerve** (Fig. 3.35 and Table 3.1) is formed by contributions from L5 to S2, leaves the pelvis through the greater sciatic foramen inferior to the piriformis muscle, and enters the gluteal region to supply the gluteus maximus.

Ilioinguinal and genitofemoral nerves

Terminal sensory branches of the ilioinguinal nerve (L1) and the genitofemoral nerve (L1, L2) descend into the upper thigh from the lumbar plexus.

The **ilioinguinal nerve** originates from the superior part of the lumbar plexus, descends around the abdominal wall in the plane between the transversus abdominis and internal oblique muscles, and then passes through the inguinal canal to leave the abdominal wall through the superficial inguinal ring (Fig. 3.35 and Table 3.1). Its terminal branches innervate skin on the medial side of the upper thigh and adjacent parts of the perineum.

The **genitofemoral nerve** passes anteroinferiorly through the psoas major muscle on the posterior abdominal wall and descends on the anterior surface of the psoas major (Fig. 3.35 and Table 3.1). Its femoral branch passes into the thigh by crossing under the inguinal ligament where it is lateral to the femoral artery. It passes superficially to innervate skin over the upper central part of the anterior thigh (see Fig. 4.161).

Lateral cutaneous nerve of thigh

The **lateral cutaneous nerve of the thigh** originates from L2 and L3. It leaves the abdomen either by passing through the gap between the inguinal ligament and the pelvic bone just medial to the anterior superior iliac spine or by passing directly through the inguinal ligament (Fig. 3.35 and Table 3.1). It supplies skin on the lateral side of the thigh (Fig. 3.19).

Nerve to quadratus femoris and nerve to obturator internus

The **nerve to the quadratus femoris** (L4 to S1) and the **nerve to the obturator internus** (L5 to S2) are small motor nerves that originate from the sacral plexus. Both nerves pass through the greater sciatic foramen inferior to the piriformis muscle and enter the gluteal region (Fig. 3.35 and Table 3.1):

- The nerve to the obturator internus supplies the gemellus superior muscle in the gluteal region and then loops around the ischial spine and enters the perineum through the lesser sciatic foramen to penetrate the perineal surface of the obturator internus muscle.
- The nerve to the quadratus femoris supplies the gemellus inferior and quadratus femoris muscles.

Posterior cutaneous nerve of thigh

The **posterior cutaneous nerve of the thigh** is formed by contributions from S1 to S3 and leaves the pelvic cavity through the greater sciatic foramen inferior to the piriformis muscle (Fig. 3.35 and Table 3.1). It passes vertically through the gluteal region deep to the gluteus maximus and enters the posterior thigh and innervates:

- A longitudinal band of skin over the posterior aspect of the thigh that continues into the upper leg.
- Skin over the gluteal fold, over the upper medial part of the thigh, and in the adjacent regions of the perineum.

Perforating cutaneous nerve

The **perforating cutaneous nerve** is a small sensory nerve formed by contributions from S2 and S3. It leaves the pelvic cavity by penetrating directly through the sacrotuberous ligament (Fig. 3.35 and Table 3.1) and passes inferiorly around the lower border of the gluteus maximus where it overlaps with the posterior cutaneous nerve of the thigh in innervating skin over the medial aspect of the gluteal fold.

Arteries

Femoral artery

The major artery supplying the lower limb is the **femoral artery** (Fig. 3.36), which is the continuation of the external iliac artery in the abdomen. The external iliac artery becomes the femoral artery as the vessel passes under the inguinal ligament to enter the femoral triangle in the anterior aspect of the thigh. Branches supply most of the thigh and all of the leg and foot.

Superior and inferior gluteal arteries and the obturator artery

Other vessels supplying parts of the lower limb include the superior and inferior gluteal arteries and the obturator artery (Fig. 3.36).

The **superior and inferior gluteal arteries** originate in the pelvic cavity as branches of the internal iliac artery (see Chapter 5, p. 677) and supply the gluteal region. The superior gluteal artery leaves the pelvis through the greater sciatic foramen above the piriformis muscle, and the inferior gluteal artery leaves through the same foramen but below the piriformis muscle.

The **obturator artery** is also a branch of the internal iliac artery in the pelvic cavity (see Chapter 5, p. 677) and passes through the obturator canal to enter and supply the medial compartment of the thigh.

Branches of the femoral, inferior gluteal, superior gluteal, and obturator arteries, together with branches from the internal pudendal artery of the perineum, interconnect to form an anastomotic network in the upper thigh and gluteal region. The presence of these anastomotic channels may provide collateral circulation when one of the vessels is interrupted.

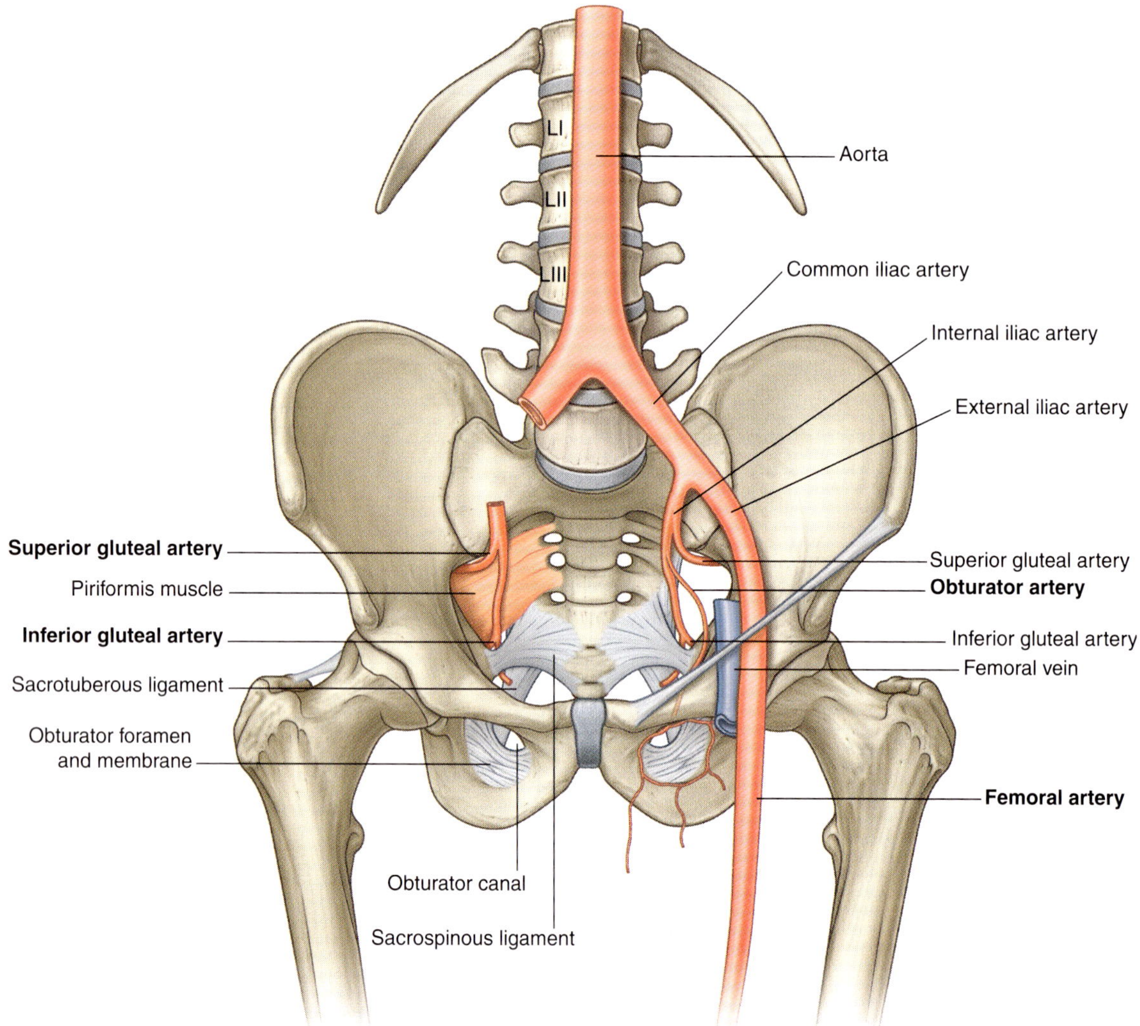

Fig. 3.36 Arteries of the lower limb.

Veins

Veins draining the lower limb form superficial and deep groups.

The **deep veins** generally follow the arteries (femoral, superior gluteal, inferior gluteal, and obturator). The major deep vein draining the limb is the **femoral vein** (Fig. 3.37). It becomes the external iliac vein when it passes deep to the inguinal ligament to enter the abdomen.

The **superficial veins** are in the subcutaneous connective tissue and are interconnected with and ultimately drain into the deep veins. The superficial veins form two major channels—the great saphenous vein and the small saphenous vein. Both veins originate from a dorsal venous arch in the foot:

- The **great saphenous vein** originates from the medial side of the dorsal venous arch where it joins the medial marginal vein. It ascends upward anterior to the medial malleolus, along the medial side of the leg, then a hand-breadth behind the patella, and then along the medial aspect of thigh to connect with the femoral vein just inferior to the inguinal ligament.

  Tributaries of the great saphaneous vein include:

1. Formative tributaries: the dorsal venous arch and the medial marginal vein
2. Tributaries in the leg: the anterior leg vein and posterior arch vein
3. Tributaries in the thigh: one or more anterolateral and posteromedial veins
4. Tributaries that it receives immediately before it pierces the saphenous opening: the superficial epigastric, superficial circumflex iliac, and superficial external pu dendal veins

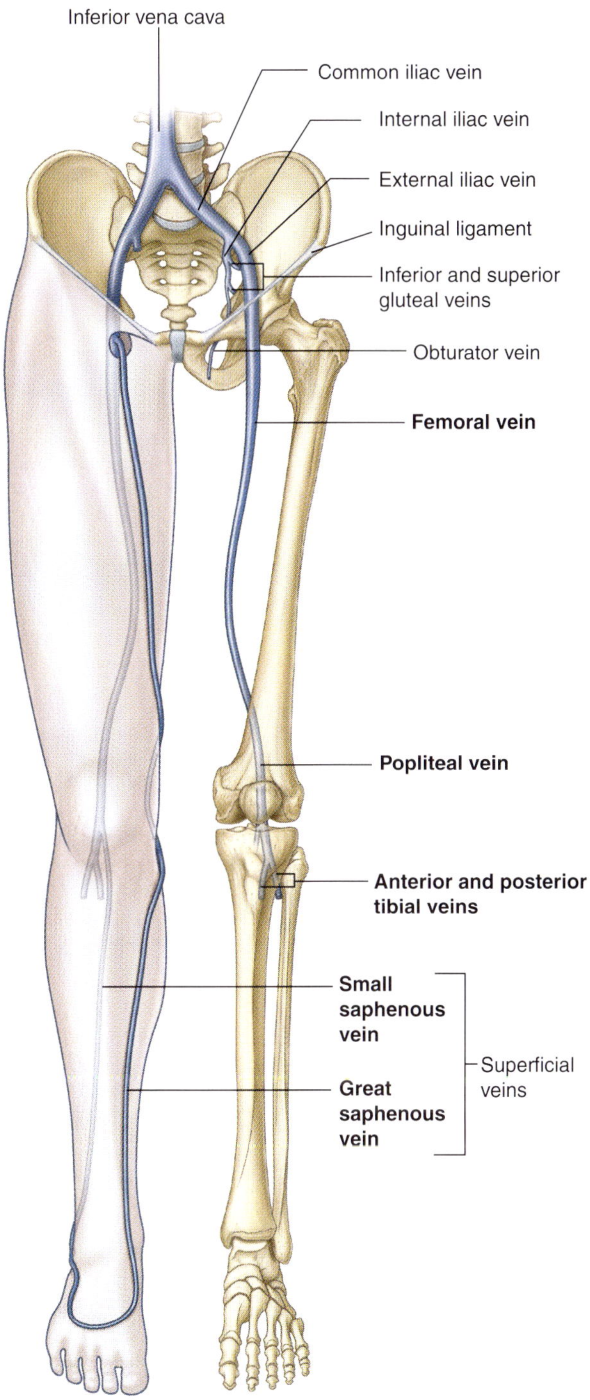

Fig. 3.37 Veins of the lower limb.

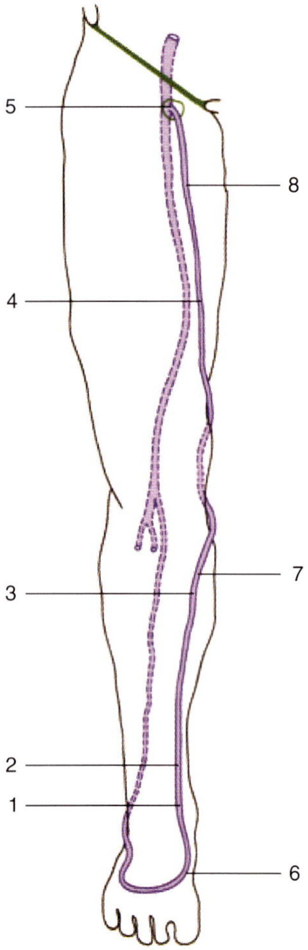

LD Fig. 3.37.1 Veins of the lower limb.

Questions

3.37.1A How are the veins of the lower limb classified, and what is the basis of this classification?

3.37.1B Mention the locations and names of the tributaries of the great saphenous vein labeled 6, 7, 8, and 5.

3.37.1C List the perforators present in the lower limb at the locations labeled 1–5, and mention any mnemonic for these.

3.37.1D In addition to these direct perforators which connect the superficial and deep veins, is there any other way in which the superficial veins drain into the deep veins?

3.37.1E Name the deep veins of the lower limb.

Answers

3.37.1A These veins are classified as superficial veins and deep veins. These veins are named in relation to the deep fascia.

3.37.1B The locations and names of the labeled tributaries of the great saphenous vein are

6. At the origin—the medial marginal vein and the dorsal venous arch
7. In the leg—anterior vein of leg; and just below the knee—the posterior arch vein
8. In the thigh—anterolateral and posteromedial veins
5. Before piercing the cribriform fascia—superficial circumflex iliac vein, superficial epigastric vein, and the superficial external pudendal vein; and after piercing the cribriform fascia—the deep external pudendal vein

3.37.1C The perforators present in the lower limb at the locations labeled 1–5 are

1. Ankle perforator
2. Lower leg perforator
3. Below-knee perforator
4. Mid-thigh perforator
5. Sapheno-femoral perforator

A mnemonic for some of these perforators is "CBD," which is an abbreviation for common bile duct, and also can stand for the Cockett's, Boyd's, and Dodd's perforators.

3.37.1D There is an indirect pathway where the superficial veins drain into the muscular veins which drain into the deep veins.

3.37.1E The deep veins of the lower limb are the:

Medial and lateral plantar veins

Venae comitantes of the dorsalis pedis, anterior tibial and posterior tibial arteries

Popliteal and femoral veins

Blood flow is from the superficial system to the deep veins through perforating or perforator veins. These have valves. The perforator veins include:

1. A midthigh perforator, or Hunter's canal perforator (Dodd's perforator)
2. A below-knee perforator, or gastrocnemius perforator (Boyd's perforator)
3. A lower leg perforator (Cockett's perforator)
4. An ankle perforator (May's or Kuster's perforator)

- The **small saphenous vein** originates from the lateral side of the dorsal venous arch, ascends up the posterior surface of the leg, and then penetrates deep fascia to join the popliteal vein posterior to the knee; proximal to the knee, the popliteal vein becomes the femoral vein.

Early clinical exposure

Varicose veins

The normal flow of blood in the lower limbs is from the skin and subcutaneous tissues to the superficial veins, which drain via perforating veins to the deep veins, which in turn drain into the iliac veins and inferior vena cava.

The normal flow of blood in the venous system depends on the presence of competent valves, which prevent reflux. Venous return is supplemented with contraction of the muscles in the lower limb, which pump the blood toward the heart. When venous valves become incompetent, they tend to place extra pressure on more distal valves, which may also become incompetent. This condition produces dilated tortuous superficial veins (varicose veins) in the distribution of the great (long) and small (short) saphenous venous systems.

Varicose veins occur more commonly in women than in men, and symptoms are often aggravated by pregnancy. Some individuals have a genetic predisposition to developing varicose veins. Valves may also be destroyed when a deep vein thrombosis occurs if the clot incorporates the valve into its interstices; during the process of healing and recanalization, the valve is destroyed, rendering it incompetent.

Typical sites for valvular incompetence include the junction between the great (long) saphenous vein and the femoral vein, perforating veins in the midthigh, and the junction between the small (short) saphenous vein and the popliteal vein.

Varicose veins may be unsightly, and soft tissue changes may occur with chronic venous incompetence. As the venous pressure rises, increased venular and capillary pressure damages the cells, and blood and blood products extrude into the soft tissue. This may produce a brown pigmentation in the skin, and venous eczema may develop. Furthermore, if the pressure remains high, the skin may break down and ulcerate, and many weeks of hospitalization may be needed for this to heal.

Treatments for varicose veins include tying off the valve, "stripping" (removing) the great (long) and small (short) saphenous systems, and in some cases valvular reconstruction.

Early clinical exposure

Deep vein thrombosis

Thrombosis may occur in the deep veins of the lower limb and within the pelvic veins. Its etiology was eloquently described by Virchow, who described the classic triad (venous stasis, injury to the vessel wall, and hypercoagulable states) that precipitates thrombosis.

In some patients, a deep vein thrombosis (DVT) in the calf veins may propagate into the femoral veins. This clot may break off and pass through the heart to enter the pulmonary circulation, resulting in occlusion of the pulmonary artery, cardiopulmonary arrest, and death.

A significant number of patients undergoing surgery are likely to develop a DVT, so most surgical patients are given specific prophylactic treatment to prevent thrombosis. A typical DVT prophylactic regimen includes anticoagulant injections and graduated stockings (to prevent deep venous stasis and facilitate emptying of the deep veins).

Although physicians aim to prevent the formation of DVT, it is not always possible to detect it because there may be no clinical signs. Calf muscle tenderness, postoperative pyrexia, and limb swelling can be helpful clues. The diagnosis is made by duplex Doppler sonography or ascending venography.

If DVT is confirmed, intravenous and oral anticoagulation are started to prevent extension of the thrombus.

Lymphatics

Most lymphatic vessels in the lower limb drain into superficial and deep inguinal nodes located in the fascia just inferior to the inguinal ligament (Fig. 3.38).

Superficial inguinal nodes

The **superficial inguinal nodes**, approximately 10 in number, are in the superficial fascia and parallel the course of the inguinal ligament in the upper thigh as the superolateral and superomedial groups. Medially, they extend inferiorly along the terminal part of the great saphenous vein as the inferior group.

The superolateral group receives lymph from the gluteal region, and lower abdominal wall below the umbilicus. The superomedial group receives lymph from the external genitalia excluding the testis, perineum, lower part of anal canal and vagina, and uterine lymphatics that accompany the round ligament. The inferior group receives lymph from the superficial regions of the lower limb. They drain, via vessels that accompany the femoral vessels, into **external iliac nodes** associated with the external iliac artery in the abdomen.

Deep inguinal nodes

The **deep inguinal nodes**, up to three in number, are medial to the femoral vein (Fig. 3.38).

The deep inguinal nodes receive lymph from deep lymphatics associated with the femoral vessels and from the glans penis (or clitoris) in the perineum. They interconnect with the superficial inguinal nodes and drain into the

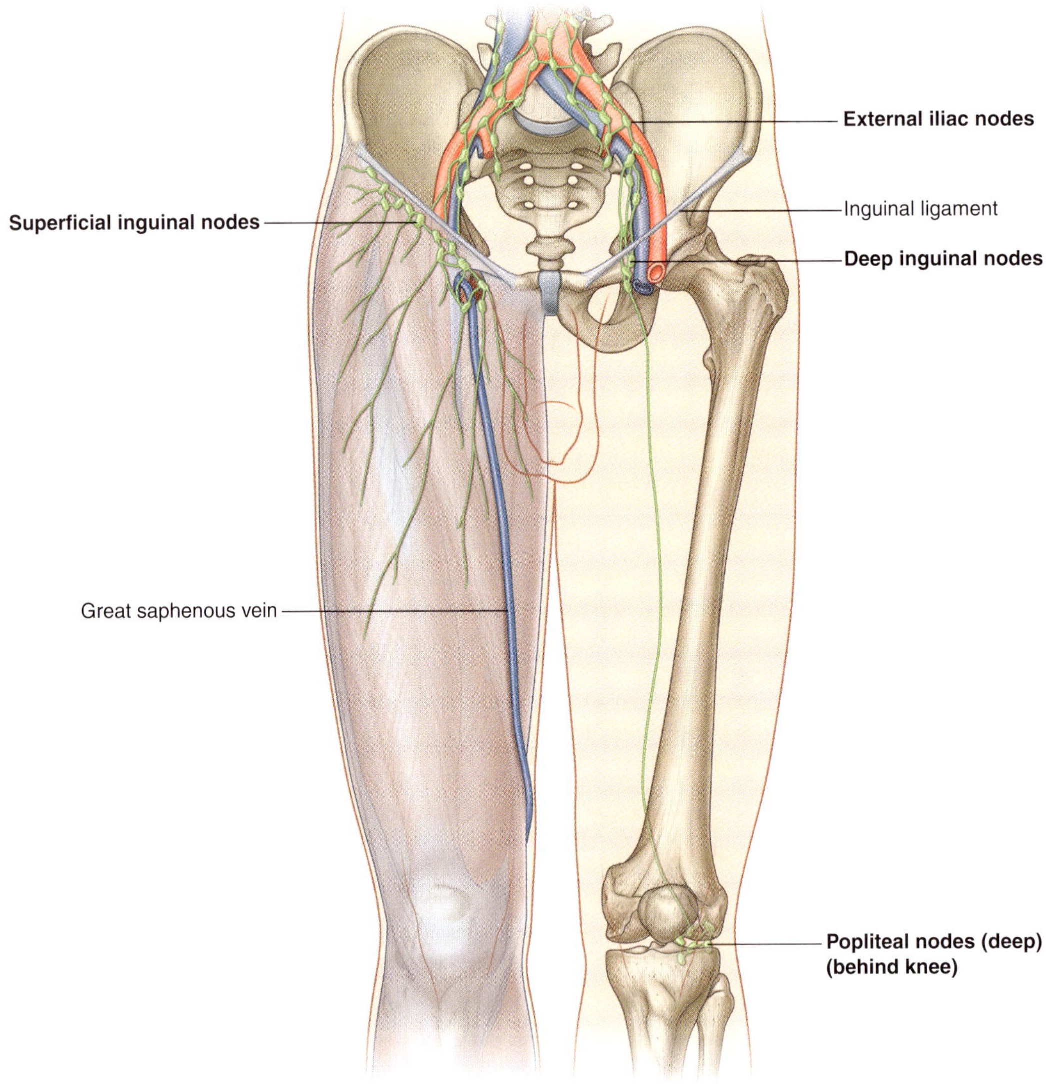

Fig. 3.38 Lymphatic drainage of the lower limb.

external iliac nodes via vessels that pass along the medial side of the femoral vein as it passes deep to the inguinal ligament. The space through which the lymphatic vessels pass under the inguinal ligament is the femoral canal.

Popliteal nodes

In addition to the inguinal nodes, there is a small collection of deep nodes posterior to the knee close to the popliteal vessels (Fig. 3.38). These **popliteal nodes** receive lymph from superficial vessels, which accompany the small saphenous vein, and from deep areas of the leg and foot. They ultimately drain into the deep and superficial inguinal nodes.

Deep fascia and the saphenous opening

Fascia lata

The outer layer of deep fascia in the lower limb forms a thick "stocking-like" membrane, which covers the limb and lies beneath the superficial fascia (Fig. 3.39A). This deep fascia is particularly thick in the thigh and gluteal region and is termed the **fascia lata**.

The fascia lata is anchored superiorly to bone and soft tissues along a line of attachment that defines the upper margin of the lower limb. Beginning anteriorly and circling laterally around the limb, this line of attachment includes the inguinal ligament, iliac crest, sacrum, coccyx, sacrotuberous ligament, inferior ramus of the pubic bone, body of the pubic bone, and superior ramus of the pubic bone.

Inferiorly, the fascia lata is continuous with the deep fascia of the leg.

Iliotibial tract

The fascia lata is thickened laterally into a longitudinal band (the **iliotibial tract**), which descends along the lateral margin of the limb from the tubercle of the iliac crest to a bony attachment just below the knee onto a tubercle on the lateral part of the upper end of the tibia (Gerdy's tubercle) (Fig. 3.39B).

The superior aspect of the fascia lata in the gluteal region splits anteriorly to enclose the tensor fasciae latae muscle and posteriorly to enclose the gluteus maximus muscle:

- The tensor fasciae latae muscle is partially enclosed by and inserts into the superior and anterior aspects of the iliotibial tract.
- Most of the gluteus maximus muscle inserts into the posterior aspect of the iliotibial tract.

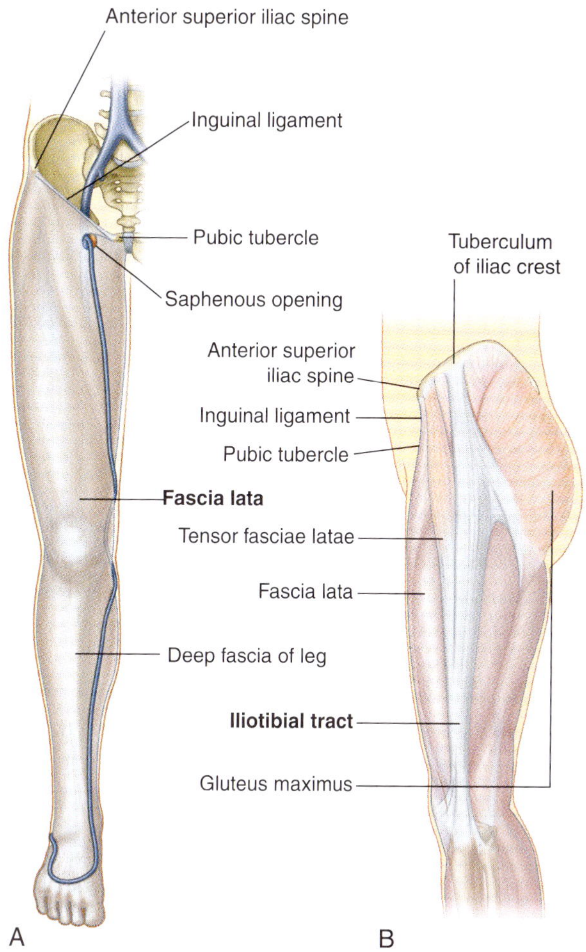

Fig. 3.39 Fascia lata. Right lower limb. **(A)** Anterior view. **(B)** Lateral view.

The tensor fasciae latae and gluteus maximus muscles, working through their attachments to the iliotibial tract, hold the leg in extension once other muscles have extended the leg at the knee joint. The iliotibial tract and its two associated muscles also stabilize the hip joint by preventing lateral displacement of the proximal end of the femur away from the acetabulum.

Saphenous opening

The fascia lata has one prominent aperture on the anterior aspect of the thigh just inferior to the medial end of the inguinal ligament (the **saphenous opening**), which allows the great saphenous vein to pass from superficial fascia through the deep fascia to connect with the femoral vein (Fig. 3.40).

The margin of the saphenous opening is called the saphenous ring. It is formed by the free medial edge of the fascia lata as it descends from the inguinal ligament and spirals around the lateral side of the great saphenous vein and medially under the femoral vein to attach to the pectineal line (pecten pubis) of the pelvic bone.

Femoral triangle

The femoral triangle is a wedge-shaped depression formed by muscles in the upper thigh at the junction between the anterior abdominal wall and the lower limb (Fig. 3.41):

- The base of the triangle is the inguinal ligament.
- The medial border is the medial margin of the adductor longus muscle in the medial compartment of the thigh.
- The lateral margin is the medial margin of the sartorius muscle in the anterior compartment of the thigh.
- The floor of the triangle is formed medially by the pectineus and adductor longus muscles in the medial compartment of the thigh and laterally by the iliopsoas muscle descending from the abdomen.
- The apex of the femoral triangle points inferiorly and is continuous with a fascial canal (**adductor canal**), which descends medially down the thigh and posteriorly through an aperture in the lower end of the adductor magnus muscle to open into the popliteal fossa behind the knee.

The femoral nerve, artery, and vein and lymphatics pass between the abdomen and lower limb deep to the inguinal

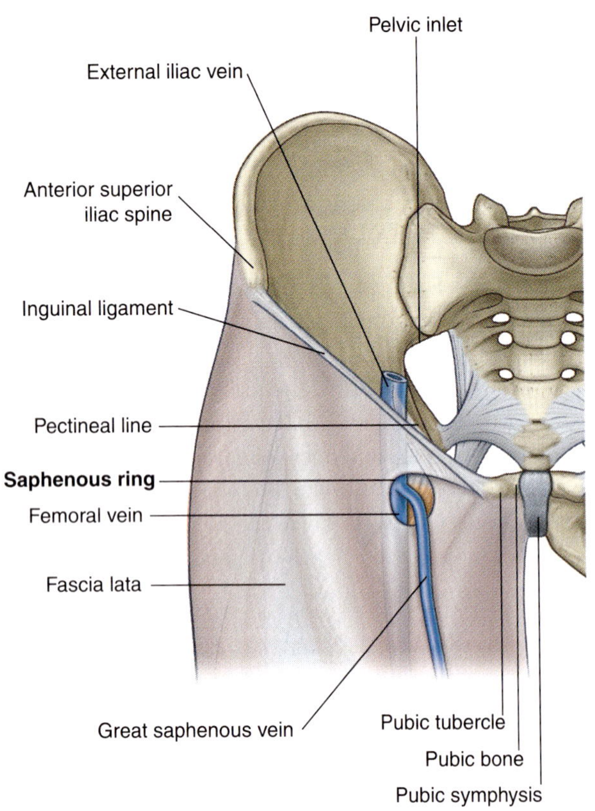

Fig. 3.40 Saphenous ring. Anterior view.

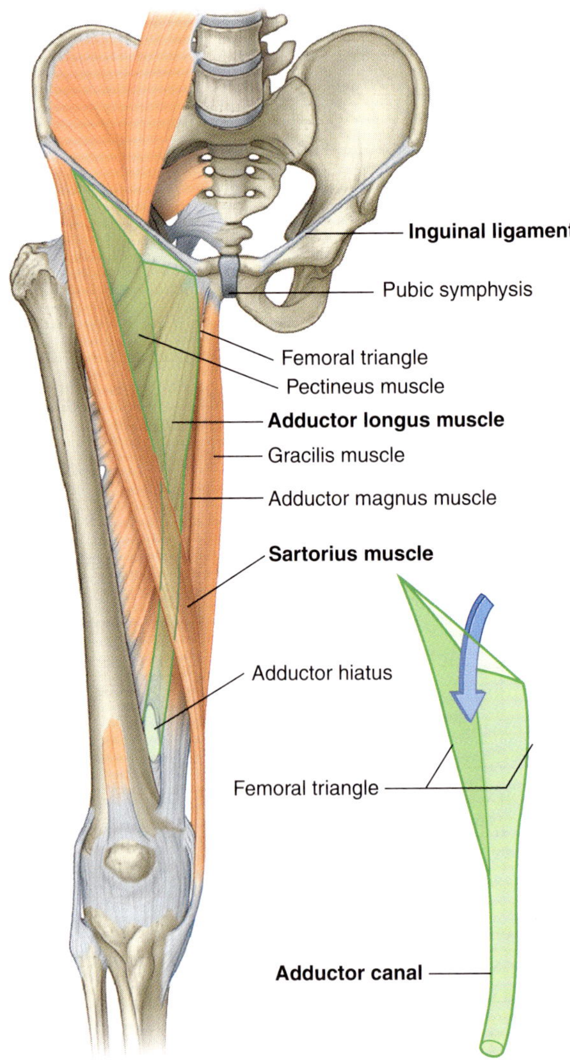

Fig. 3.41 Boundaries of the femoral triangle.

ligament and in the femoral triangle (Fig. 3.42). The femoral artery and vein pass inferiorly through the adductor canal and become the popliteal vessels behind the knee where they meet and are distributed with branches of the sciatic nerve, which descends through the posterior thigh from the gluteal region.

From lateral to medial, major structures in the femoral triangle are the femoral nerve, the femoral artery, the femoral vein, and lymphatic vessels. The femoral artery can be palpated in the femoral triangle just inferior to the inguinal ligament and midway between the anterior superior iliac spine and the pubic symphysis.

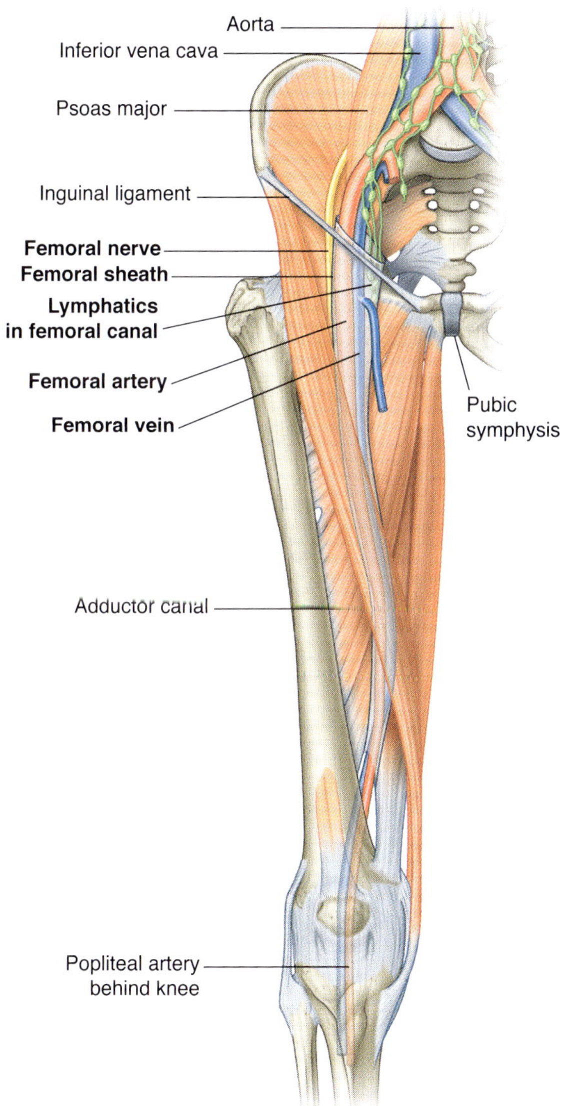

Fig. 3.42 Contents of the femoral triangle.

Femoral sheath

In the femoral triangle, the femoral artery and vein and the associated lymphatic vessels are surrounded by a funnel-shaped sleeve of fascia (the **femoral sheath**). The sheath is continuous superiorly with the transversalis fascia and iliac fascia of the abdomen and merges inferiorly with connective tissue associated with the vessels. Each of the three structures surrounded by the sheath is contained within a separate fascial compartment within the sheath. The most medial compartment (the femoral canal) contains the lymphatic vessels and is conical in shape. The opening of this canal superiorly is potentially a weak point in the lower abdomen and is the site for femoral hernias. The femoral nerve is lateral to and not contained within the femoral sheath.

Early clinical exposure

Vascular access to the lower limb

Deep and inferior to the inguinal ligament are the femoral artery and femoral vein. The femoral artery is palpable as it passes anterior to the femoral head and may be easily demonstrated using ultrasound. If arterial or venous access is needed rapidly, a physician can use the femoral approach to these vessels.

Many radiological procedures involve catheterization of the femoral artery or the femoral vein to obtain access to the contralateral lower limb, the ipsilateral lower limb, the vessels of the thorax and abdomen, and the cerebral vessels.

Cardiologists also use the femoral artery to place catheters in vessels around the arch of the aorta and into the coronary arteries to perform coronary angiography and angioplasty.

Access to the femoral vein permits catheters to be maneuvered into the renal veins, the gonadal veins, the right atrium, and the right side of the heart, including the pulmonary artery and distal vessels of the pulmonary tree. Access to the superior vena cava and the great veins of the neck is also possible.

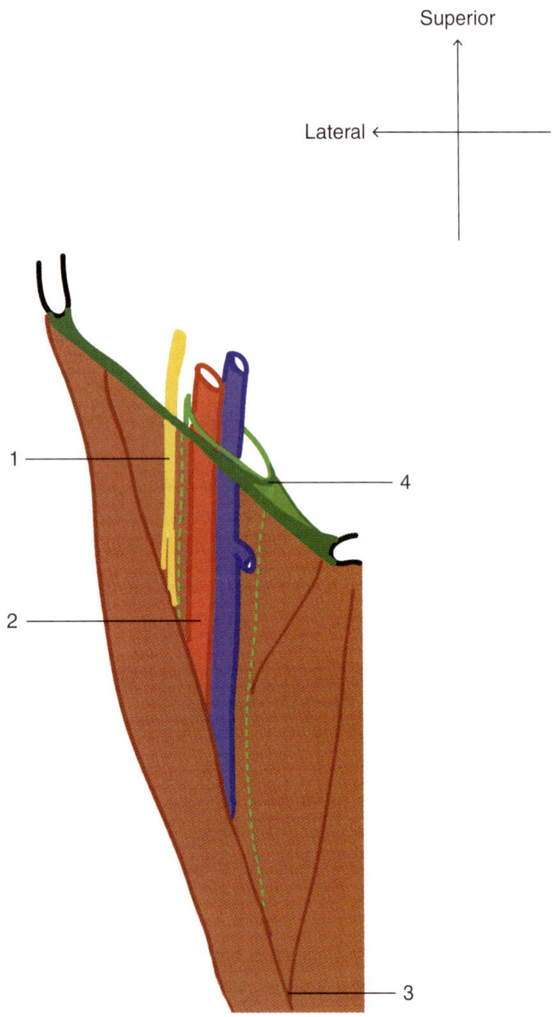

LD Fig. 3.42.1 Boundaries and contents of the femoral triangle.

Questions

3.42.1A Name the structures indicated by the labels.

3.42.1B Describe the part of the femoral triangle located at label 3?

3.42.1C List the boundaries of the femoral triangle.

3.42.1D List the main contents of the femoral triangle in a classified manner.

3.42.1E Mention any mnemonic for some of the main contents of the femoral triangle and highlight the clinical importance of the position of the femoral artery.

3.42.1F What is the clinical importance of the structure labeled 4?

3.42.1G Explain why the femoral nerve is located outside the femoral sheath, whereas the femoral vessels are inside the femoral sheath.

3.42.1H What does the dotted line on the right side indicate?

Answers

3.42.1A The structures indicated by the labels are

1. Femoral nerve
2. Femoral artery
3. Apex of the femoral triangle
4. Lacunar ligament

3.42.1B The apex of the femoral triangle where the medial borders of the sartorius and adductor longus meet.

3.42.1C The boundaries of the femoral triangle are the medial border of the adductor longus medially, the medial border of the sartorius laterally, and the inguinal ligament superiorly. The floor is formed by the adductor longus, pectineus, iliacus, and psoas. The roof is formed by the fascia lata.

3.42.1D The main contents of the femoral triangle are the:

Femoral vessels with their branches and tributaries—the main vessels of the lower limb

Femoral nerve and its terminal branches—located in the groove between the psoas and iliacus

Femoral canal, which is the medial compartment of the femoral sheath and contains the deep inguinal lymph nodes

3.42.1E A mnemonic is "VAN," which stands for the following structures from medial to lateral: the femoral vein, femoral artery, and femoral nerve. The artery is in the middle and is also at the midinguinal point (midway between the anterior superior iliac spine and the pubic symphysis) where it can be compressed.

3.42.1F The lacunar ligament is the boundary of the femoral ring which can be cut or incised to release a strangulated femoral hernia. Care must be taken to look for and to avoid cutting the aberrant obturator artery which may be lying medial to it. This abnormal artery is part of an anastomosis between the external iliac and internal iliac arteries called corona mortis.

3.42.1G The femoral sheath is formed as a downward prolongation of the fascia transversalis and fascia iliaca. As the femoral nerve lies posterior to the fascia iliaca, it lies outside the femoral sheath. The femoral vessels are continuations of the external iliac vessels, which are located between these layers of fascia.

3.42.1H The dotted line on the right side indicates the continuity of the contents of the femoral triangle and the contents of the adductor canal.

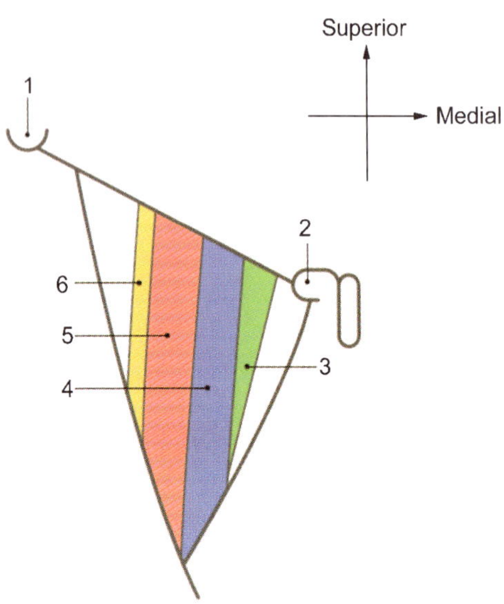

LD Fig. 3.42.2 Contents of the femoral triangle.

Question

3.42.2 Name the structures indicated by the labels.

Answer

3.42.2

1. Anterior superior iliac spine
2. Pubic tubercle
3. Femoral canal
4. Femoral vein
5. Femoral artery
6. Femoral nerve

GLUTEAL REGION

SET INDUCTION—CASE SCENARIO 2: SCIATICA

A 35-year-old woman presented to the outpatient department with pain in the buttock which radiated down the back of the lower limb. A diagnosis of sciatica was made. The possibility of compression of the sciatic nerve by the piriformis was considered.

It is necessary to know the anatomy of the gluteal region before one can manage a patient with sciatica.

<table>
<tr><th rowspan="2">REMEMBER
[Recall Facts]</th><th colspan="3">OUTLINE 2. GLUTEAL REGION—LEARNING OBJECTIVES
[By the end of this section the student should be able to:]</th><th colspan="2" rowspan="2">EVALUATE
[Explain Concepts]</th></tr>
<tr><th colspan="3">DEMONSTRATE AND ANALYZE RELATIONSHIPS
[Identify structures in a Prosected Specimen or Figure]</th></tr>
<tr><td rowspan="6">1. Mention the extent of the gluteal region
2. Describe in detail the hip joint
3. List the muscles of the gluteal region and mention their origin, insertion, action, and nerve supply
4. Name one strong flexor and extensor of the hip joint
5. Describe the boundaries of the greater sciatic foramen and list the structures passing through it
6. Describe the boundaries of the lesser sciatic foramen and list the structures passing through it
7. Describe briefly the course of the sciatic nerve in the gluteal region
8. Describe the relations of the piriformis</td><td>Level I</td><td>Level II</td><td>Level III</td><td colspan="2">■ Movements at the hip joint and the muscles causing them
■ Passage of structures into and out of the gluteal region</td></tr>
<tr><td rowspan="5">■ Bony markings on the hip bone
■ Gluteus maximus
■ Gluteus medius
■ Gluteus minimus
■ Tensor fasciae latae
■ Piriformis
■ Obturator internus
■ Quadratus femoris
■ Sciatic nerve
■ Pudendal nerve</td><td rowspan="5">■ Gemelli
■ Superior and inferior gluteal nerves and vessels
■ Nerve to obturator internus</td><td rowspan="5">■ Nerve supply of quadratus femoris
■ Posterior cutaneous nerve of the thigh</td><td colspan="2">EARLY CLINICAL EXPOSURE
[Apply Anatomical Knowledge]</td></tr>
<tr><td>Surgical Anatomy/ Pathology/ Trauma</td><td>Imaging/ Surface Anatomy</td></tr>
<tr><td>■ Intramuscular injections
■ Fracture of neck of femur
■ Dislocation of the hip joint</td><td>■ Radiograph of the normal and dislocated hip joint
■ Radiograph of fracture of neck of the femur
■ Course of the sciatic nerve</td></tr>
<tr><td colspan="2">PROBLEM SOLVING/ CLINICAL CASES
[Interpret]</td></tr>
<tr><td colspan="2">■ Trendelenburg's sign
■ Position of the lower limb in a patient with fracture of the neck of femur</td></tr>
</table>

The gluteal region lies posterolateral to the bony pelvis and proximal end of the femur (Fig. 3.43). Muscles in the region mainly abduct, extend, and laterally rotate the femur relative to the pelvic bone.

The gluteal region communicates anteromedially with the pelvic cavity and perineum through the greater sciatic foramen and lesser sciatic foramen, respectively. Inferiorly, it is continuous with the posterior thigh.

The sciatic nerve enters the lower limb from the pelvic cavity by passing through the greater sciatic foramen and descending through the gluteal region into the posterior thigh and then into the leg and foot (Fig. 3.15).

The pudendal nerve and internal pudendal vessels pass between the pelvic cavity and perineum by passing first through the greater sciatic foramen to enter the gluteal region and then immediately passing through the lesser sciatic foramen to enter the perineum. The nerve to the obturator internus and gemellus superior follows a similar course. Other nerves and vessels that pass through the greater sciatic foramen from the pelvic cavity supply structures in the gluteal region itself (see Fig. 3.47).

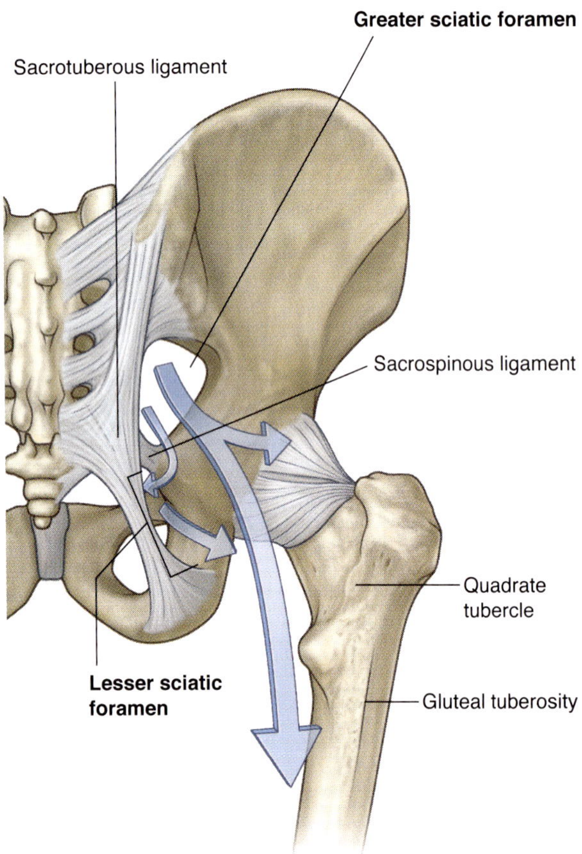

Fig. 3.43 Gluteal region. Posterior view.

Muscles

Muscles of the gluteal region (Table 3.2) are composed mainly of two groups:

- A deep group of small muscles, which are mainly lateral rotators of the femur at the hip joint and include the piriformis, obturator internus, gemellus superior, gemellus inferior, and quadratus femoris.
- A more superficial group of larger muscles, which mainly abduct and extend the hip and include the gluteus minimus, gluteus medius, and gluteus maximus; an additional muscle in this group, the tensor fasciae latae, stabilizes the knee in extension by acting on a specialized longitudinal band of deep fascia (the iliotibial tract) that passes down the lateral side of the thigh to attach to the proximal end of the tibia in the leg.

Many of the important nerves in the gluteal region are in the plane between the superficial and deep groups of muscles.

Table 3.2 Muscles of the gluteal region

Muscle	**Origin**	**Insertion**	**Innervation**	**Function**
Piriformis	Anterior surface of sacrum between anterior sacral foramina	Medial side of superior border of greater trochanter of femur	Branches from S1 and **S2**	Laterally rotates the extended femur at hip joint; abducts flexed femur at hip joint
Obturator internus	Anterolateral wall of true pelvis; deep surface of obturator membrane and surrounding bone	Medial side of greater trochanter of femur	Nerve to obturator internus (L5, **S1**)	Laterally rotates the extended femur at hip joint; abducts flexed femur at hip joint
Gemellus superior	External surface of ischial spine	Along length of superior surface of the obturator internus tendon and into the medial side of greater trochanter of femur with obturator internus tendon	Nerve to obturator internus (L5, **S1**)	Laterally rotates the extended femur at hip joint; abducts flexed femur at hip joint
Gemellus inferior	Upper aspect of ischial tuberosity	Along length of inferior surface of the obturator internus tendon and into the medial side of greater trochanter of femur with obturator internus tendon	Nerve to quadratus femoris (**L5, S1**)	Laterally rotates the extended femur at hip joint; abducts flexed femur at hip joint
Quadratus femoris	Lateral aspect of the ischium just anterior to the ischial tuberosity	Quadrate tubercle on the intertrochanteric crest of the proximal femur	Nerve to quadratus femoris (**L5, S1**)	Laterally rotates femur at hip joint
Gluteus minimus	External surface of ilium between inferior and anterior gluteal lines	Linear facet on the anterolateral aspect of the greater trochanter	Superior gluteal nerve (**L4, L5**, S1)	Abducts femur at hip joint; holds pelvis secure over stance leg and prevents pelvic drop on the opposite swing side during walking; medially rotates thigh
Gluteus medius	External surface of ilium between anterior and posterior gluteal lines	Elongate facet on the lateral surface of the greater trochanter	Superior gluteal nerve (**L4, L5**, S1)	Abducts femur at hip joint; holds pelvis secure over stance leg and prevents pelvic drop on the opposite swing side during walking; medially rotates thigh
Gluteus maximus	Fascia covering gluteus medius, external surface of ilium behind posterior gluteal line, fascia of erector spinae, dorsal surface of lower sacrum, lateral margin of coccyx, external surface of sacrotuberous ligament	Posterior aspect of iliotibial tract of fascia lata and gluteal tuberosity of proximal femur	Inferior gluteal nerve (**L5, S1**, S2)	Powerful extensor of flexed femur at hip joint; stabilizer of hip joint and knee joint in extension; laterally rotates and abducts thigh
Tensor fasciae latae	Lateral aspect of crest of ilium between anterior superior iliac spine and tubercle of the crest	Iliotibial tract of fascia lata	Superior gluteal nerve (**L4, L5**, S1)	Stabilizes the knee in extension

Note: Spinal segments in bold are the major segments innervating the muscle.

Deep group

Piriformis

The **piriformis** muscle is the most superior of the deep group of muscles (Fig. 3.44) and is a muscle of the pelvic wall and of the gluteal region. It originates from between the anterior sacral foramina on the anterolateral surface of the sacrum and passes laterally and inferiorly through the greater sciatic foramen.

In the gluteal region, the piriformis passes posterior to the hip joint and attaches to a facet on the upper margin of the greater trochanter of the femur.

The piriformis externally rotates and abducts the femur at the hip joint and is innervated in the pelvic cavity by the nerve to the piriformis, which originates as branches from S1 and S2 of the sacral plexus (see Chapter 5, p. 672).

In addition to its action on the hip joint, the piriformis is an important landmark because it divides the greater sciatic foramen into two regions, one above and one below the piriformis. Vessels and nerves pass between the pelvis and gluteal region by passing through the greater sciatic foramen either above or below the piriformis.

Obturator internus

The **obturator internus** muscle, like the piriformis muscle, is a muscle of the pelvic wall and of the gluteal region (Fig. 3.44). It is a flat fan-shaped muscle originating from the medial surface of the obturator membrane and adjacent bone of the obturator foramen (see Chapter 5, p. 627). Because the pelvic floor attaches to a thickened band of fascia across the medial surface of the obturator internus, the obturator internus forms:

- The anterolateral wall of the pelvic cavity above the pelvic floor
- The lateral wall of the ischioanal fossa in the perineum below the pelvic floor

The muscle fibers of the obturator internus converge to form a tendon, which bends 90° around the ischium between the ischial spine and ischial tuberosity and passes through the lesser sciatic foramen to enter the gluteal region. The tendon then passes posteroinferior to the hip joint and attaches to the medial surface of the superior

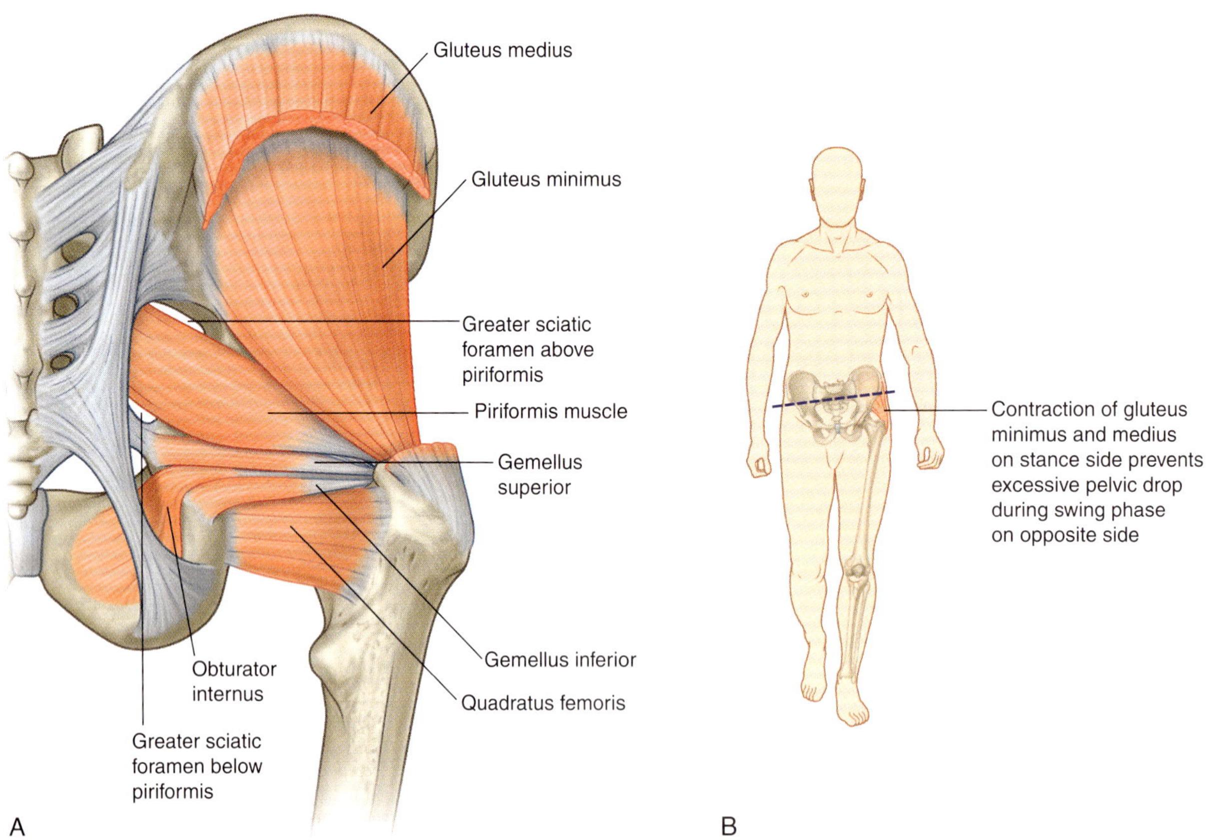

Fig. 3.44 Deep muscles in the gluteal region. **(A)** Posterior view. **(B)** Function.

margin of the greater trochanter of the femur just inferior to the attachment of the piriformis muscle.

The obturator internus laterally rotates and abducts the femur at the hip joint and is innervated by the nerve to the obturator internus (L5, S1, S2).

Gemellus superior and inferior

The gemellus superior and inferior (*gemelli* is Latin for "twins") are a pair of triangular muscles associated with the upper and lower margins of the obturator internus tendon (Fig. 3.44):

- The base of the **gemellus superior** originates from the gluteal surface of the ischial spine.
- The base of the **gemellus inferior** originates from the upper gluteal and pelvic surfaces of the ischial tuberosity.

Fibers of the gemellus muscles attach along the length of the obturator internus tendon, and the apices of the two muscles insert with the tendon of the obturator internus on the greater trochanter of the femur.

The gemellus superior is innervated by the nerve to the obturator internus, and the gemellus inferior is innervated by the nerve to the quadratus femoris. The gemellus muscles act with the obturator internus muscle to laterally rotate and abduct the femur at the hip joint.

Quadratus femoris

The **quadratus femoris** muscle is the most inferior of the deep group of muscles in the gluteal region (Fig. 3.44). It is a flat, rectangular muscle below the obturator internus muscle and its associated gemellus muscles.

The quadratus femoris is attached at one end to a linear roughening on the lateral aspect of the ischium just anterior to the ischial tuberosity and at the other end to the quadrate tubercle on the intertrochanteric crest of the proximal femur.

The quadratus femoris laterally rotates the femur at the hip joint and is innervated by the nerve to the quadratus femoris (L4, L5, S1).

Superficial group

Gluteus minimus and medius

The gluteus minimus and medius muscles are two muscles of the more superficial group in the gluteal region (Fig. 3.44).

The **gluteus minimus** is a fan-shaped muscle that originates from the external surface of the expanded upper part of the ilium, between the inferior gluteal line and the anterior gluteal line. The muscle fibers converge inferiorly and laterally to form a tendon, which inserts into a broad linear facet on the anterolateral aspect of the greater trochanter.

The **gluteus medius** overlies the gluteus minimus and is also fan shaped. It has a broad origin from the external surface of the ilium between the anterior gluteal line and posterior gluteal line and inserts on an elongate facet on the lateral surface of the greater trochanter.

The gluteus medius and minimus muscles abduct the lower limb at the hip joint and reduce pelvic drop over the opposite swing limb during walking by securing the position of the pelvis on the stance limb (Fig. 3.44B). Both muscles are innervated by the superior gluteal nerve.

The action of each muscle of the hip joint can be determined by considering the line of force of the muscle in relation to the three axes of the joint (Fig. 3.5 and 3.29B). For example, the line of force of the gluteus maximus is vertically upwards passing behind the transverse axis and so it causes extension. The line of force of the psoas is vertically upwards passing in front of this axis and so it causes flexion. The line of force of each of the six short lateral rotators and the gluteus maximus is directed medially and passes posterior to the vertical axis. Hence, these muscles cause lateral rotation of the hip joint. The line of force of the abductors passes above the anteroposterior axis and the line of force of the adductors passes below this axis.

Early clinical exposure

Trendelenburg's sign

Trendelenburg's sign occurs in people with weak or paralyzed abductor muscles (gluteus medius and gluteus minimus) of the hip. The sign is demonstrated by asking the patient to stand on one limb. When the patient stands on the affected limb, the pelvis severely drops over the swing limb.

Positive signs are typically found in patients with damage to the superior gluteal nerve. Damage to this nerve may occur with associated pelvic fractures, with space-occupying lesions within the pelvis extending into the greater sciatic foramen, and in some cases relating to hip surgery during which there has been disruption of and subsequent atrophy of the insertion of the gluteus medius and gluteus minimus tendons on the greater trochanter.

In patients with a positive Trendelenburg's sign, gait also is abnormal. Typically during the stance phase of the affected limb, the weakened abductor muscles allow the pelvis to tilt inferiorly over the swing limb. The patient compensates for the pelvic drop by lurching the trunk to the affected side to maintain the level of the pelvis throughout the gait cycle.

Gluteus maximus

The gluteus maximus is the largest muscle in the gluteal region and overlies most of the other gluteal muscles (Fig. 3.45).

The gluteus maximus is quadrangular in shape and has a broad origin extending from a roughened area of the ilium behind the posterior gluteal line and along the dorsal surface of the lower sacrum and the lateral surface of the coccyx to the external surface of the sacrotuberous ligament. It is also attached to fascia overlying the gluteus medius muscle and, between the ilium and sacrum, to fascia covering the erector spinae muscle, and is often described as being enclosed within two layers of the fascia lata, which covers the thigh and gluteal region.

Laterally, the upper and superficial lower parts of the gluteus maximus insert into the posterior aspect of a tendinous thickening of the fascia lata (the iliotibial tract), which passes over the lateral surface of the greater trochanter and descends down the thigh and into the upper leg. Deep distal parts of the muscle attach to the elongate gluteal tuberosity of the proximal femur.

The gluteus maximus mainly extends the flexed thigh at the hip joint. Through its insertion into the iliotibial tract, it also stabilizes the knee and hip joints. It is innervated by the inferior gluteal nerve.

Tensor fasciae latae

The tensor fasciae latae muscle is the most anterior of the superficial group of muscles in the gluteal region and overlies the gluteus minimus and the anterior part of the gluteus medius (Fig. 3.46).

The tensor fasciae latae originates from the outer margin of the iliac crest from the anterior superior iliac spine to approximately the tubercle of the iliac crest. The muscle

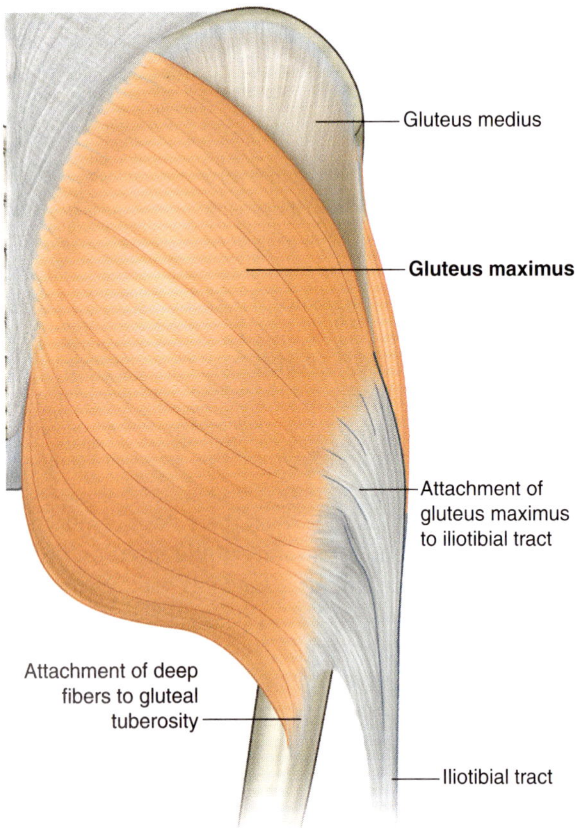

Fig. 3.45 Gluteus maximus muscle. Posterior view.

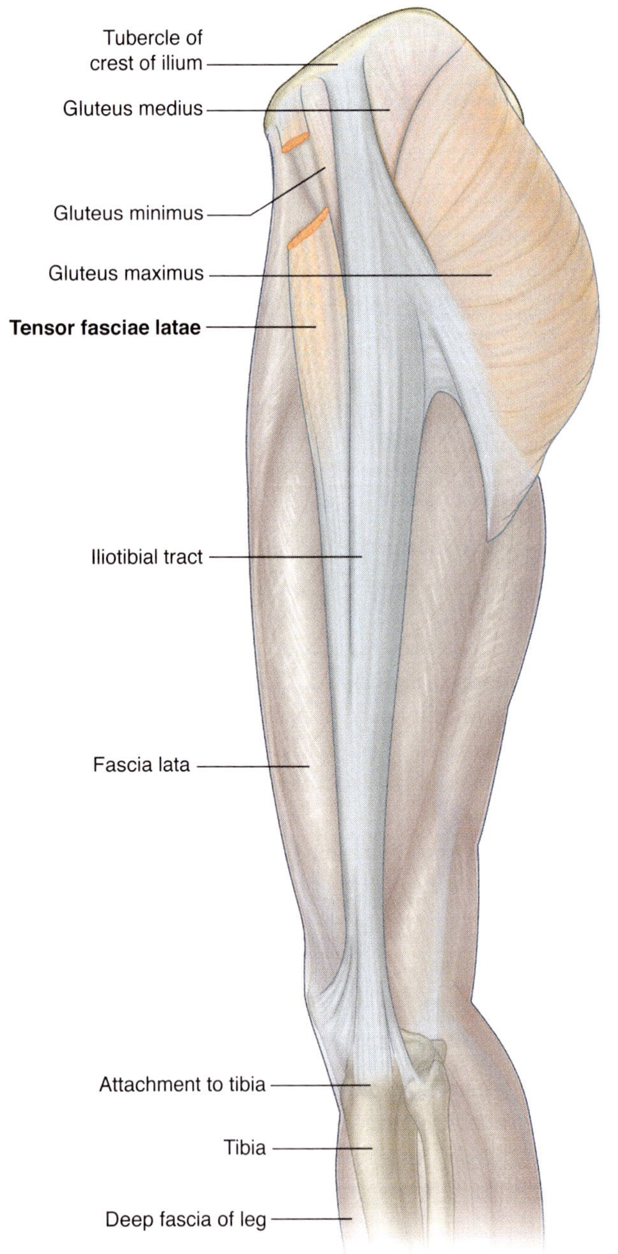

Fig. 3.46 Tensor fasciae latae. Left gluteal region, lateral view.

fibers descend to insert into the anterior aspect of the iliotibial tract of deep fascia, which runs down the lateral side of the thigh and attaches to the upper tibia. Like the gluteus maximus muscle, the tensor fasciae latae is enclosed within a compartment of the fascia lata.

The tensor fasciae latae stabilizes the knee in extension and, working with the gluteus maximus muscle on the iliotibial tract lateral to the greater trochanter, stabilizes the hip joint by holding the head of the femur in the acetabulum (Fig. 3.46). It is innervated by the superior gluteal nerve (L4, L5, S1).

Nerves

Seven nerves enter the gluteal region from the pelvis through the greater sciatic foramen (Fig. 3.47): the superior gluteal nerve, sciatic nerve, nerve to the quadratus femoris, nerve to the obturator internus, posterior cutaneous nerve of the thigh, pudendal nerve, and inferior gluteal nerve.

An additional nerve, the perforating cutaneous nerve, enters the gluteal region by passing directly through the sacrotuberous ligament.

Some of these nerves, such as the sciatic and pudendal nerves, pass through the gluteal region en route to other areas. Nerves such as the superior and inferior gluteal nerves innervate structures in the gluteal region. Many of the nerves in the gluteal region are in the plane between the superficial and deep groups of muscles.

Superior gluteal nerve

Of all the nerves that pass through the greater sciatic foramen, the superior gluteal nerve is the only one that passes above the piriformis muscle (Fig. 3.47). After entering the gluteal region, the nerve loops up over the inferior margin of the gluteus minimus and travels anteriorly and laterally in the plane between the gluteus minimus and medius muscles.

The superior gluteal nerve supplies branches to the gluteus minimus and medius muscles and terminates by innervating the tensor fasciae latae muscle.

Sciatic nerve

The sciatic nerve enters the gluteal region through the greater sciatic foramen inferior to the piriformis muscle (Fig. 3.47). It descends in the plane between the superficial

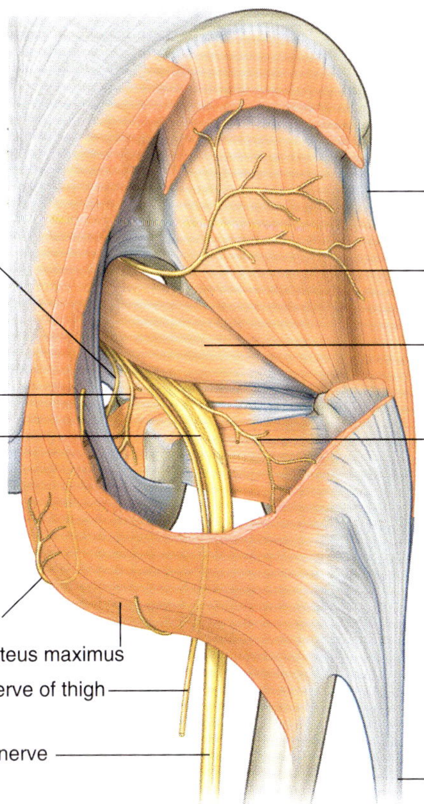

Fig. 3.47 Nerves of the gluteal region. Posterior view.

and deep groups of gluteal region muscles, crossing the posterior surfaces of first the obturator internus and associated gemellus muscles and then the quadratus femoris muscle. It lies just deep to the gluteus maximus at the midpoint between the ischial tuberosity and the greater trochanter. At the lower margin of the quadratus femoris muscle, the sciatic nerve enters the posterior thigh.

The sciatic nerve is the largest nerve in the body and innervates all muscles in the posterior compartment of the thigh that flex the knee and all muscles that move the ankle and foot. It also innervates a large area of skin in the lower limb (Fig. 3.18).

Nerve to quadratus femoris

The nerve to the quadratus femoris enters the gluteal region through the greater sciatic foramen inferior to the piriformis muscle and deep to the sciatic nerve (Fig. 3.47). Unlike other nerves in the gluteal region, the nerve to the quadratus femoris lies anterior to the plane of the deep muscles.

The nerve to the quadratus femoris descends along the ischium deep to the tendon of the obturator internus muscle and associated gemellus muscles to penetrate and innervate the quadratus femoris. It supplies a small branch to the gemellus inferior.

Nerve to obturator internus

The nerve to the obturator internus enters the gluteal region through the greater sciatic foramen inferior to the piriformis muscle and between the posterior cutaneous nerve of the thigh and the pudendal nerve (Fig. 3.47). It supplies a small branch to the gemellus superior and then passes over the ischial spine and through the lesser sciatic foramen to innervate the obturator internus muscle from the medial surface of the muscle in the perineum.

Posterior cutaneous nerve of the thigh

The posterior cutaneous nerve of the thigh enters the gluteal region through the greater sciatic foramen inferior to the piriformis muscle and immediately medial to the sciatic nerve (Fig. 3.47). It descends through the gluteal region just deep to the gluteus maximus and enters the posterior thigh.

The posterior cutaneous nerve of the thigh has a number of gluteal branches, which loop around the lower margin of the gluteus maximus muscle to innervate skin over the gluteal fold. A small perineal branch passes medially to contribute to the innervation of the skin of the scrotum or labia majora in the perineum. The main trunk of the posterior cutaneous nerve of the thigh passes inferiorly, giving rise to branches that innervate the skin on the posterior thigh and leg.

Pudendal nerve

The pudendal nerve enters the gluteal region through the greater sciatic foramen inferior to the piriformis muscle and medial to the sciatic nerve (Fig. 3.47). It passes over the sacrospinous ligament and immediately passes through the lesser sciatic foramen to enter the perineum. The course of the pudendal nerve in the gluteal region is short and the nerve is often hidden by the overlying upper margin of the sacrotuberous ligament.

The pudendal nerve is the major somatic nerve of the perineum and has no branches in the gluteal region.

Inferior gluteal nerve

The inferior gluteal nerve enters the gluteal region through the greater sciatic foramen inferior to the piriformis muscle and along the posterior surface of the sciatic nerve (Fig. 3.47). It penetrates and supplies the gluteus maximus muscle.

Perforating cutaneous nerve

The perforating cutaneous nerve is the only nerve in the gluteal region that does not enter the area through the greater sciatic foramen. It is a small nerve that leaves the sacral plexus in the pelvic cavity by piercing the sacrotuberous ligament. It then loops around the lower border of the gluteus maximus to supply the skin over the medial aspect of the gluteus maximus (Fig. 3.47).

Early clinical exposure

Intramuscular injections

From time to time it is necessary to administer drugs intramuscularly, that is, by direct injection into muscles. This procedure must be carried out without injuring neurovascular structures. A typical site for an intramuscular injection is the gluteal region. The sciatic nerve passes through this region and needs to be avoided. The safest place to inject is the upper outer quadrant of either gluteal region.

The gluteal region can be divided into quadrants by two imaginary lines positioned using palpable bony landmarks (Fig. 3.48). One line descends vertically from the highest point of the iliac crest. Another line is horizontal and passes through the first line midway between the highest point of the iliac crest and the horizontal plane through the ischial tuberosity.

It is important to remember that the gluteal region extends as far forward as the anterior superior iliac spine. The sciatic nerve curves through the upper lateral corner of the lower medial quadrant and descends along the medial margin of the lower lateral quadrant.

Occasionally, the sciatic nerve bifurcates into its tibial and common fibular branches in the pelvis, in which case the common fibular nerve passes into the gluteal region through, or even above, the piriformis muscle.

The superior gluteal nerve and vessels normally enter the gluteal region above the piriformis and pass superiorly and forward.

The anterior corner of the upper lateral quadrant is normally used for injections to avoid injuring any part of the sciatic nerve or other nerves and vessels in the gluteal region. A needle placed in this region enters the gluteus medius anterosuperior to the margin of the gluteus maximus.

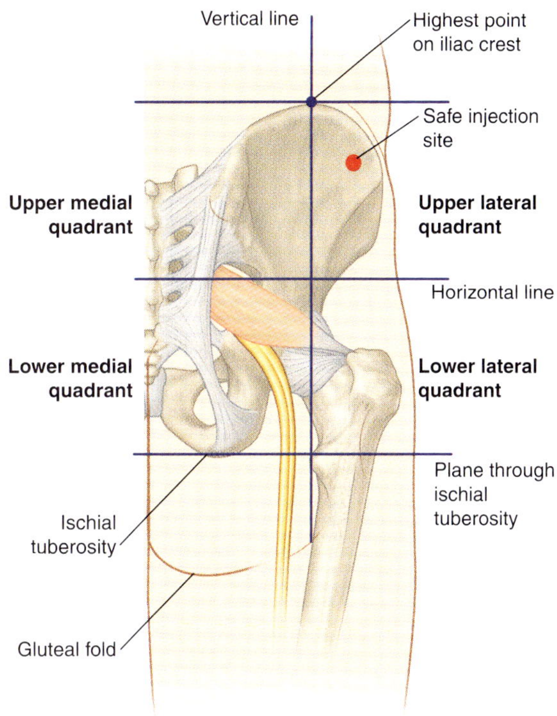

Fig. 3.48 Site for intramuscular injections in the gluteal region.

Arteries

Two arteries enter the gluteal region from the pelvic cavity through the greater sciatic foramen, the inferior gluteal artery and the superior gluteal artery (Fig. 3.49). They supply structures in the gluteal region and posterior thigh and have important collateral anastomoses with branches of the femoral artery.

Inferior gluteal artery

The inferior gluteal artery originates from the anterior trunk of the internal iliac artery in the pelvic cavity. It leaves the pelvic cavity with the inferior gluteal nerve through the greater sciatic foramen inferior to the piriformis muscle (Fig. 3.49).

The inferior gluteal artery supplies adjacent muscles and descends through the gluteal region and into the posterior thigh where it supplies adjacent structures and anastomoses with perforating branches of the femoral artery. It also supplies a branch to the sciatic nerve (companion artery of the sciatic nerve).

Superior gluteal artery

The superior gluteal artery originates from the posterior trunk of the internal iliac artery in the pelvic cavity. It leaves the pelvic cavity with the superior gluteal nerve through the greater sciatic foramen above the piriformis muscle (Fig. 3.49). In the gluteal region, it divides into a superficial branch and a deep branch:

- The superficial branch passes onto the deep surface of the gluteus maximus muscle.
- The deep branch passes between the gluteus medius and minimus muscles.

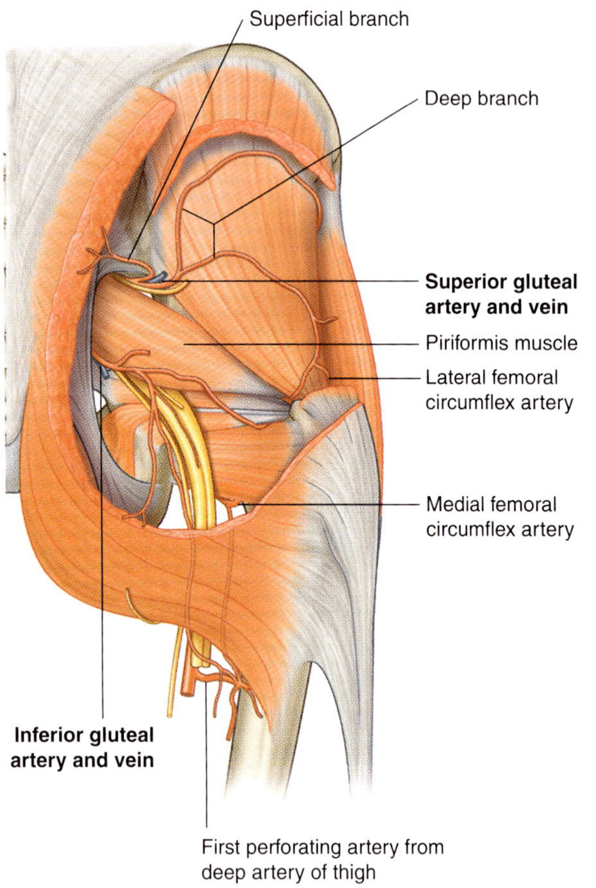

Fig. 3.49 Arteries of the gluteal region.

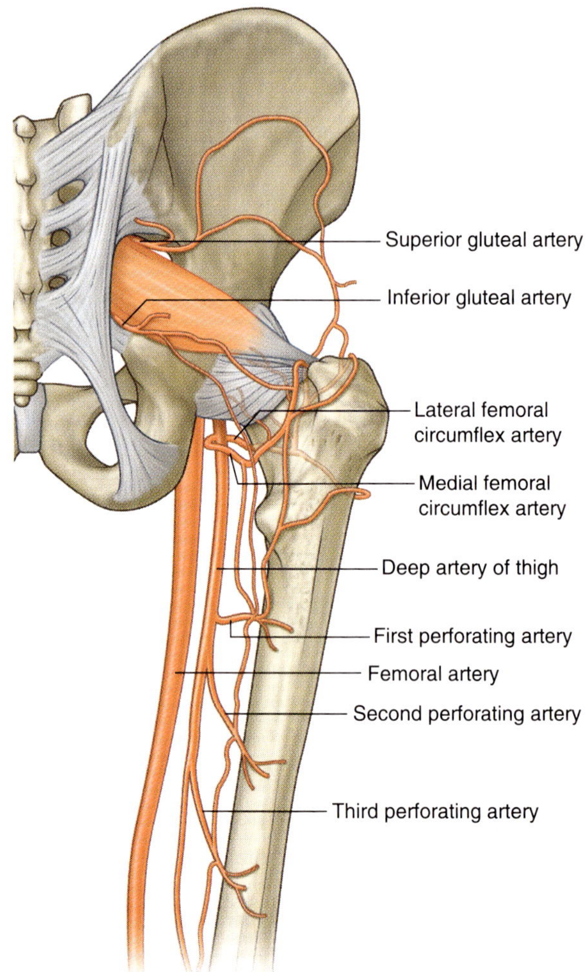

Fig. 3.50 Anastomoses between gluteal arteries and vessels originating from the femoral artery in the thigh. Posterior view.

In addition to adjacent muscles, the superior gluteal artery contributes to the supply of the hip joint. Branches of the artery also anastomose with the lateral and medial femoral circumflex arteries from the deep femoral artery in the thigh, and with the inferior gluteal artery (Fig. 3.50).

Veins

Inferior and superior gluteal veins follow the inferior and superior gluteal arteries into the pelvis where they join the pelvic plexus of veins. Peripherally, the veins anastomose with superficial gluteal veins, which ultimately drain anteriorly into the femoral vein.

Lymphatics

Deep lymphatic vessels of the gluteal region accompany the blood vessels into the pelvic cavity and connect with internal iliac nodes.

Superficial lymphatics drain into the superficial inguinal nodes on the anterior aspect of the thigh.

THIGH

SET INDUCTION—CASE SCENARIO 3: FEMORAL HERNIA

A 25-year-old woman presented to the outpatient department with complaints of pain and swelling in the left groin. On examination, a swelling was found which was present just below the center of the inguinal ligament. The swelling became bigger when the patient coughed. A diagnosis of femoral hernia was made and a plan was made to reduce the hernia by incising the lacunar ligament to widen the femoral ring.

It is important to know the anatomy of the femoral triangle to successfully reduce a femoral hernia.

REMEMBER [Recall Facts]	**OUTLINE 3. THIGH—LEARNING OBJECTIVES [By the end of this section the student should be able to:] DEMONSTRATE AND ANALYZE RELATIONSHIPS [Identify structures in a Prosected Specimen or Figure]**		
	Level I	**Level II**	**Level III**
1. Mention the areas drained by the superficial and deep inguinal lymph nodes 2. Describe in detail the great saphenous vein 3. Describe in detail the knee joint 4. List the names of the compartments of the thigh and mention the nerve that supplies the muscles in each one 5. List the muscles of the thigh and mention their origin, insertion, action, and nerve supply 6. Name the flexors and extensors of the knee joint 7. Describe the boundaries and contents of the femoral triangle 8. Describe the boundaries and contents of the adductor canal 9. Describe the boundaries and contents of the popliteal fossa 10. Describe the course and relations of the femoral artery and nerve 11. Describe the course and relations of the sciatic nerve 12. Describe the arterial anastomoses in the thigh and around the knee	■ Bony markings on the femur ■ Inguinal ligament ■ Femoral triangle and its contents ■ Adductor canal and its contents ■ Popliteal fossa and its contents ■ Muscles of the anterior compartment ■ Muscles of the medial compartment ■ Muscles of the posterior compartment ■ Nerves and vessels in the compartments of the thigh ■ Ligaments of the knee joint	■ Insertion of semimembranosus ■ Iliotibial tract ■ Nerve to obturator internus	■ Psoas minor ■ Hybrid muscles ■ Obturator artery ■ Articularis genu

EVALUATE [Explain Concepts]
■ Movements at the knee joint and the muscles causing them ■ Fascia lata and its importance in varicose veins

EARLY CLINICAL EXPOSURE [Apply Anatomical Knowledge]	
Surgical Anatomy/ Pathology/ Trauma	**Imaging/ Surface Anatomy**
■ Intramuscular injections ■ Fracture of the femur ■ Tear of the anterior cruciate ligament ■ Varicose veins	■ Radiograph of the normal knee joint ■ MRI of the knee joint ■ Course of the popliteal artery

PROBLEM SOLVING/ CLINICAL CASES [Interpret]
■ Trendelenburg's sign ■ Parts of the knee joint most susceptible to injury

The thigh is the region of the lower limb that is approximately between the hip and knee joints (Fig. 3.51):

- Anteriorly, it is separated from the abdominal wall by the inguinal ligament.
- Posteriorly, it is separated from the gluteal region by the gluteal fold superficially, and by the inferior margins of the gluteus maximus and quadratus femoris on deeper planes.

Structures enter and leave the top of the thigh by three routes:

- Posteriorly, the thigh is continuous with the gluteal region and the major structure passing between the two regions is the sciatic nerve.
- Anteriorly, the thigh communicates with the abdominal cavity through the aperture between the inguinal ligament and pelvic bone, and major structures passing through this aperture are the iliopsoas and pectineus muscles; the femoral nerve, artery, and vein; and lymphatic vessels.
- Medially, structures (including the obturator nerve and associated vessels) pass between the thigh and pelvic cavity through the obturator canal.

The thigh is divided into three compartments by intermuscular septa between the posterior aspect of the femur and the fascia lata (the thick layer of deep fascia that completely surrounds or invests the thigh; Fig. 3.51C):

- The **anterior compartment of the thigh** contains muscles that mainly extend the leg at the knee joint.

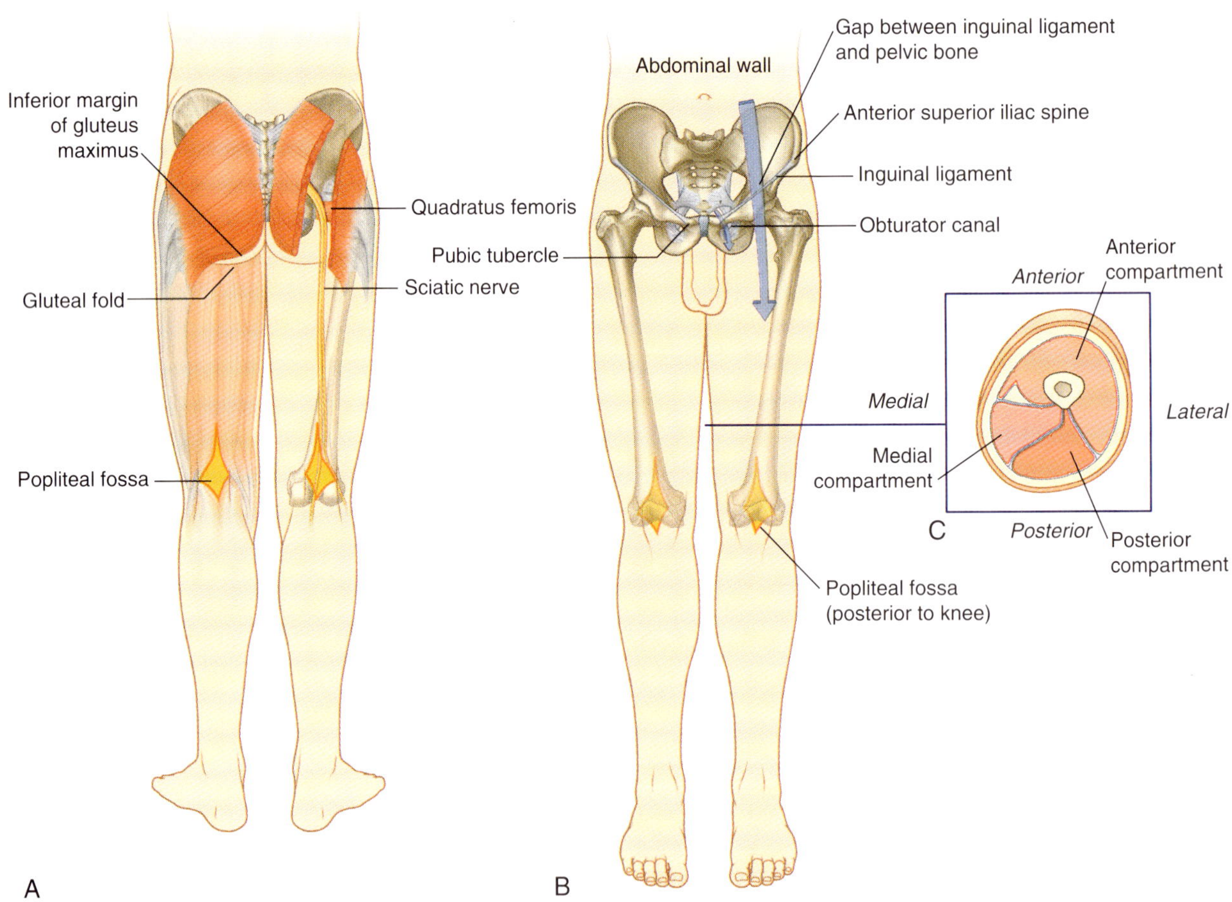

Fig. 3.51 Thigh. **(A)** Posterior view. **(B)** Anterior view. **(C)** Cross-section through the midthigh.

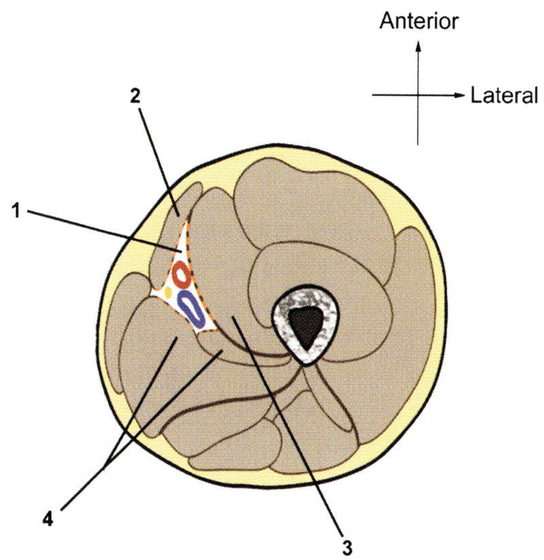

LD Fig. 3.51C.1 Adductor canal.

Questions

3.51C.1A What is the extent of the space labeled 1?

3.51C.1B Name the structures labelled 2, 3 and 4 and mention which boundary of this space that each one of these structures form.

3.51C.1C List the contents of this space.

Answers

3.51C.1A The adductor canal extends from the apex of the femoral triangle to the adductor hiatus.

3.51C.1B The labelled structures and the boundary of the adductor canal that each of them form are:

2. Sartorius, antero-medial wall
3. Vastus medialis, antero-lateral wall
4. Adductor longus and adductor magnus, posterior wall

3.51C.1C The contents of the adductor canal are the femoral vessels, saphenous nerve, nerve to vastus medialis, and the descending genicular artery.

- The **posterior compartment of the thigh** contains muscles that mainly flex the leg at the knee joint and extend the thigh at the hip joint.
- The **medial compartment of the thigh** consists of muscles that mainly adduct the thigh at the hip joint.

The sciatic nerve innervates muscles in the posterior compartment of the thigh, the femoral nerve innervates muscles in the anterior compartment of the thigh, and the obturator nerve innervates most muscles in the medial compartment of the thigh.

The major artery, vein, and lymphatic channels enter the thigh anterior to the pelvic bone and pass through the femoral triangle inferior to the inguinal ligament. Vessels and nerves passing between the thigh and leg pass through the popliteal fossa posterior to the knee joint.

Bones

The skeletal support for the thigh is the femur. Most of the large muscles in the thigh insert into the proximal ends of the two bones of the leg (tibia and fibula) and flex and extend the leg at the knee joint. The distal end of the femur provides origin for the gastrocnemius muscle, which is predominantly in the posterior compartment of the leg and plantarflexes the foot.

Shaft and distal end of femur

The shaft of the femur is bowed forward and has an oblique course from the neck of the femur to the distal end (Fig. 3.52). As a consequence of this oblique orientation, the knee is close to the midline under the body's center of gravity.

The middle part of the shaft of the femur is triangular in cross-section (Fig. 3.52D). In the middle part of the shaft, the femur has smooth medial (posteromedial), lateral (posterolateral), and anterior surfaces and medial, lateral, and posterior borders. The medial and lateral borders are rounded, whereas the posterior border forms a broad roughened crest—the **linea aspera**.

In proximal and distal regions of the femur, the linea aspera widens to form an additional posterior surface. At the distal end of the femur, this posterior surface forms the floor of the popliteal fossa, and its margins form the **medial** and **lateral supracondylar lines**. The medial supracondylar line terminates at a prominent tubercle (the **adductor tubercle**) on the superior aspect of the **medial condyle** of the distal end. Just lateral to the lower end of

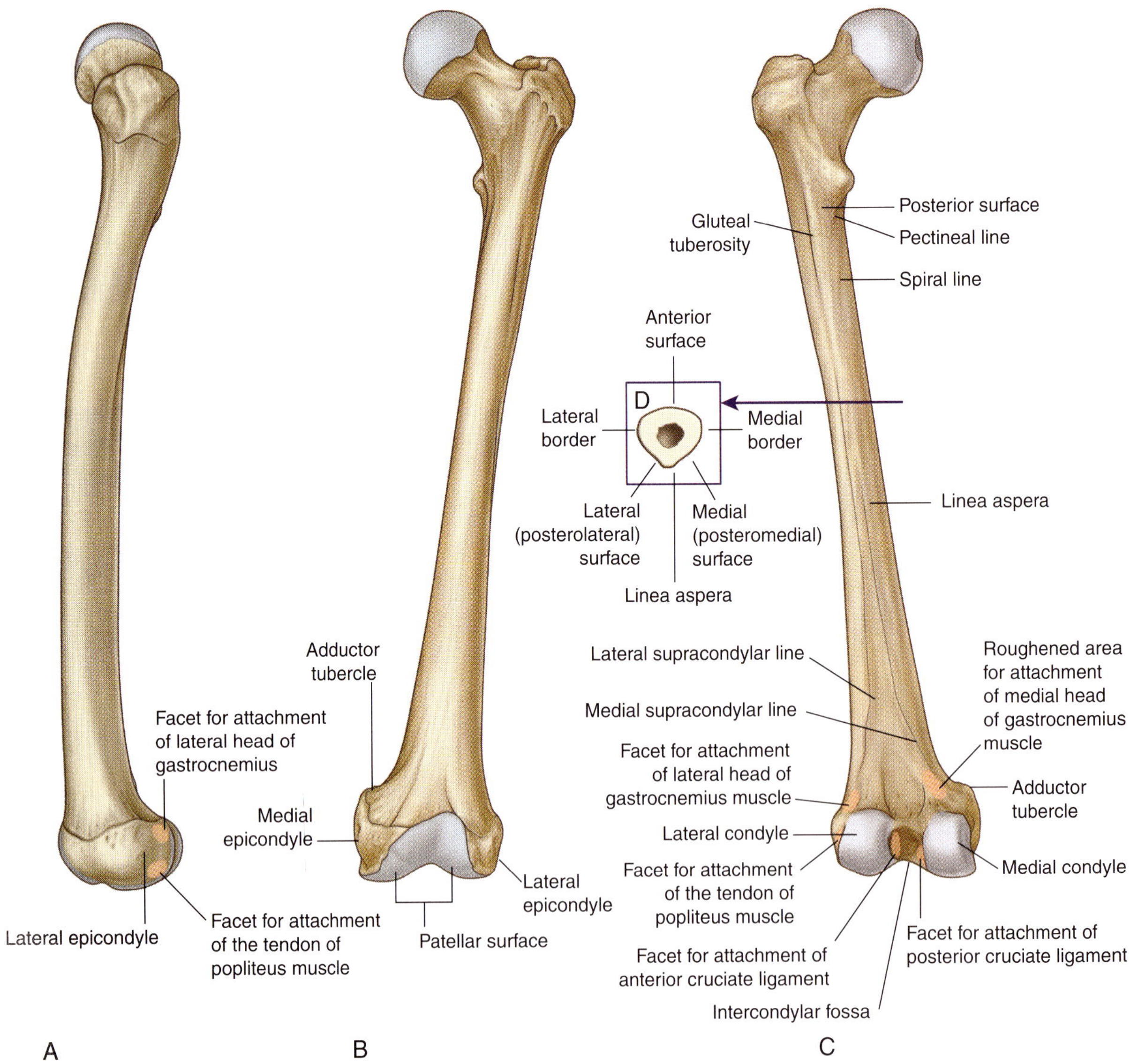

Fig. 3.52 Shaft and distal end of femur. **(A)** Lateral view. **(B)** Anterior view. **(C)** Posterior view. **(D)** Cross-section through shaft of femur.

the medial supracondylar line is an elongate roughened area of bone for the proximal attachment of the medial head of the gastrocnemius muscle (Fig. 3.52).

The distal end of the femur is characterized by two large condyles, which articulate with the proximal head of the tibia. The condyles are separated posteriorly by an **intercondylar fossa** and are joined anteriorly where they articulate with the patella.

The surfaces of the condyles that articulate with the tibia are rounded posteriorly and become flatter inferiorly. On each condyle, a shallow oblique groove separates the surface that articulates with the tibia from the more anterior surface that articulates with the patella. The surfaces of the medial and lateral condyles that articulate with the patella form a V-shaped trench, which faces anteriorly. The lateral surface of the trench is larger and steeper than the medial surface.

The walls of the intercondylar fossa bear two facets for the superior attachment of the cruciate ligaments, which stabilize the knee joint (Fig. 3.52):

- The wall formed by the lateral surface of the medial condyle has a large oval facet, which covers most of the inferior half of the wall, for attachment of the proximal end of the **posterior cruciate ligament** (see Fig. 3.69).
- The wall formed by the medial surface of the lateral condyle has a posterosuperior smaller oval facet for attachment of the proximal end of the **anterior cruciate ligament**.

Epicondyles, for the attachment of collateral ligaments of the knee joint, are bony elevations on the nonarticular outer surfaces of the condyles (Fig. 3.52). Two facets separated by a groove are just posterior to the **lateral epicondyle**:

- The upper facet is for attachment of the lateral head of the gastrocnemius muscle.
- The inferior facet is for attachment of the popliteus muscle.

The tendon of the popliteus muscle lies in the groove separating the two facets (Fig. 3.69).

The **medial epicondyle** is a rounded eminence on the medial surface of the medial condyle. Just posterosuperior to the medial epicondyle is the adductor tubercle.

Patella

The patella (knee cap) is the largest sesamoid bone (a bone formed within the tendon of a muscle) in the body. It is formed within the tendon of the quadriceps femoris muscle as it crosses anterior to the knee joint to insert on the tibia.

The patella is triangular:

- Its apex is pointed inferiorly for attachment to the patellar ligament, which connects the patella to the tibia (Fig. 3.53).
- Its base is broad and thick for the attachment of the quadriceps femoris muscle from above.
- Its posterior surface articulates with the femur and has medial and lateral facets, which slope away from a raised smooth ridge—the lateral facet is larger than the medial facet for articulation with the larger corresponding surface on the lateral condyle of the femur.

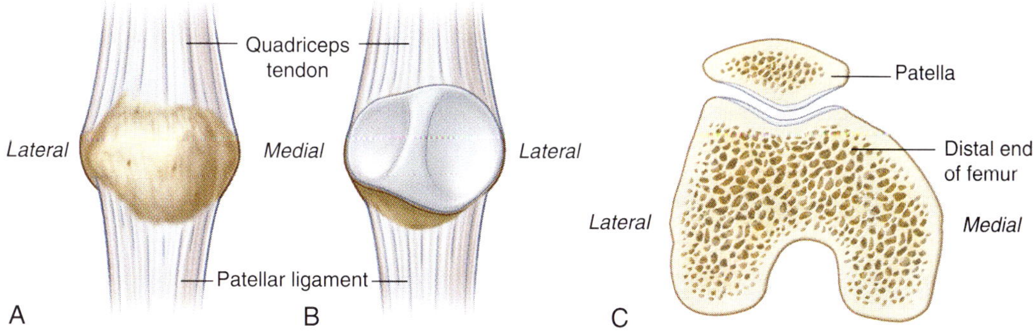

Fig. 3.53 Patella. **(A)** Anterior view. **(B)** Posterior view. **(C)** Superior view.

Proximal end of tibia

The tibia is the medial and larger of the two bones in the leg, and is the only one that articulates with the femur at the knee joint.

The proximal end of the tibia is expanded in the transverse plane for weight-bearing and consists of a **medial condyle** and a **lateral condyle**, both of which are flattened in the horizontal plane and overhang the shaft (Fig. 3.54).

The superior surfaces of the medial and lateral condyles are articular and separated by an intercondylar region, which contains sites of attachment for strong ligaments (cruciate ligaments) and interarticular cartilages (menisci) of the knee joint.

The articular surfaces of the medial and lateral condyles and the intercondylar region together form a "tibial plateau," which articulates with and is anchored to the distal end of the femur. Inferior to the condyles on the proximal part of the shaft is a large **tibial tuberosity** and roughenings for muscle and ligament attachments.

Tibial condyles and intercondylar areas

The tibial condyles are thick horizontal discs of bone attached to the top of the tibial shaft (Fig. 3.54).

The medial condyle is larger than the lateral condyle and is better supported over the shaft of the tibia. Its superior surface is oval for articulation with the medial condyle of the femur. The articular surface extends laterally onto the side of the raised **medial intercondylar tubercle**.

The superior surface of the lateral condyle is circular and articulates above with the lateral condyle of the femur. The medial edge of this surface extends onto the side of the **lateral intercondylar tubercle**.

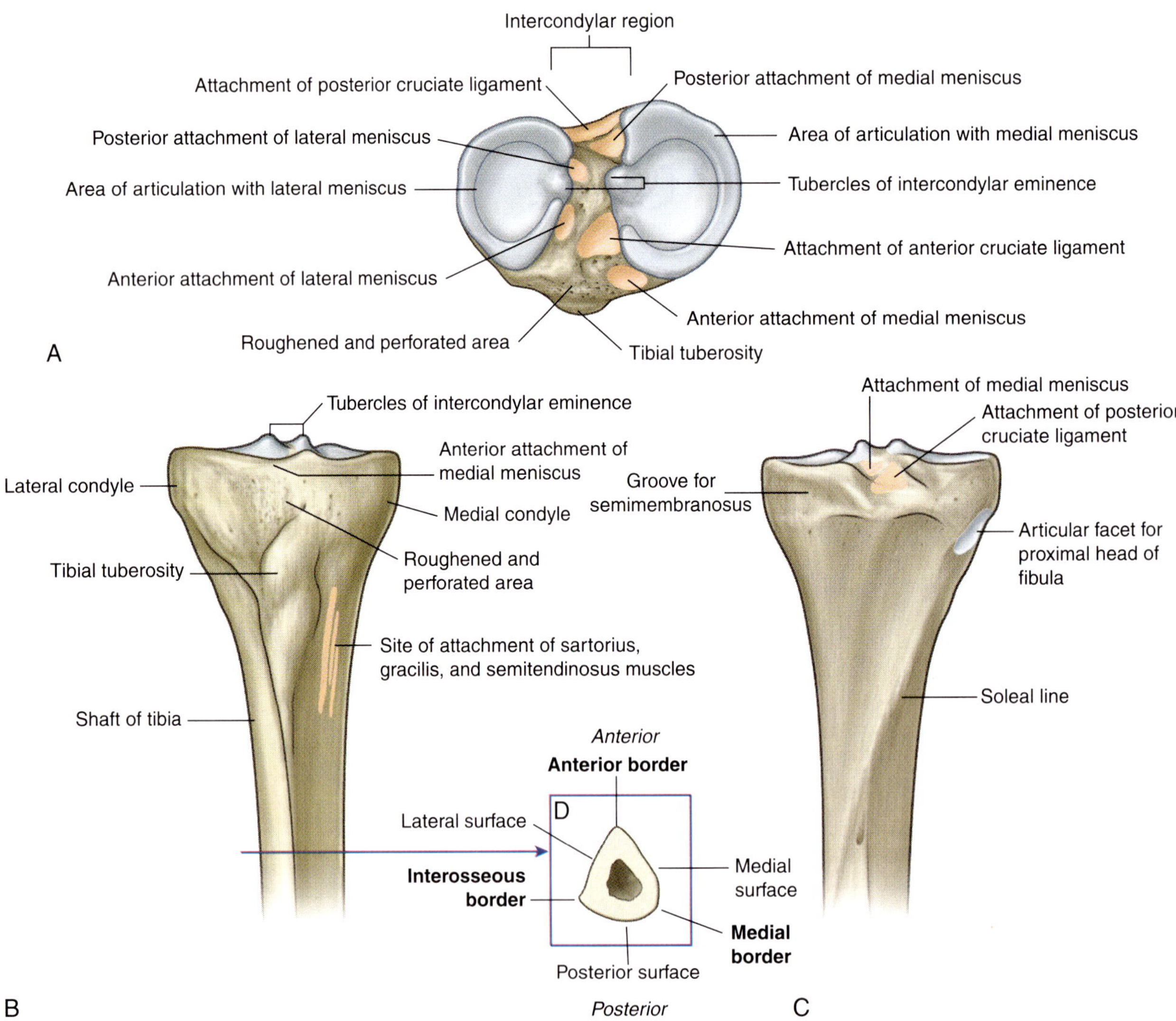

Fig. 3.54 Proximal end of the tibia. **(A)** Superior view, tibial plateau. **(B)** Anterior view. **(C)** Posterior view. **(D)** Cross-section through the shaft of tibia.

The superior articular surfaces of both the lateral and medial condyles are concave, particularly centrally. The outer margins of the surfaces are flatter and are the regions in contact with the interarticular discs (menisci) of fibrocartilage in the knee joint.

The nonarticular posterior surface of the medial condyle bears a distinct horizontal groove for part of the attachment of the semimembranosus muscle, and the undersurface of the lateral condyle bears a distinct circular facet for articulation with the proximal head of the fibula.

The intercondylar region of the tibial plateau lies between the articular surfaces of the medial and lateral condyles (Fig. 3.54). It is narrow centrally where it is raised to form the **intercondylar eminence**, the sides of which are elevated further to form medial and lateral intercondylar tubercles.

The intercondylar region bears six distinct facets for the attachment of menisci and cruciate ligaments. The anterior intercondylar area widens anteriorly and bears three facets:

- The most anterior facet is for attachment of the anterior end (horn) of the medial meniscus.
- Immediately posterior to the most anterior facet is a facet for the attachment of the anterior cruciate ligament.
- A small facet for the attachment of the anterior end (horn) of the lateral meniscus is just lateral to the site of attachment of the anterior cruciate ligament.

The posterior intercondylar area also bears three attachment facets:

- The most anterior is for attachment of the posterior horn of the lateral meniscus.
- Posteromedial to the most anterior facet is the site of attachment for the posterior horn of the medial meniscus.
- Behind the site of attachment for the posterior horn of the medial meniscus is a large facet for the attachment of the posterior cruciate ligament.

In other words, the attachments of the medial menisci are beyond, or external to, those of the lateral menisci; the attachment of the anterior cruciate ligament is posterior to the anterior horn of the medial meniscus, and the attachment of the posterior cruciate ligament is most posterior.

In addition to these six sites of attachment for menisci and cruciate ligaments, a large anterolateral region of the anterior intercondylar area is roughened and perforated by numerous small nutrient foramina for blood vessels. This region is continuous with a similar surface on the front of the tibia above the tuberosity and lies against infrapatellar connective tissue.

Tibial tuberosity

The **tibial tuberosity** is a palpable inverted triangular area on the anterior aspect of the tibia below the site of junction between the two condyles (Fig. 3.54). It is the site of attachment for the **patellar ligament**, which is a continuation of the quadriceps femoris tendon below the patella.

Shaft of tibia

The shaft of the tibia is triangular in cross-section and has three surfaces (posterior, medial, and lateral) and three borders (anterior, interosseous, and medial) (Fig. 3.54D):

- The **anterior border** is sharp and descends from the tibial tuberosity where it is continuous superiorly with a ridge that passes along the lateral margin of the tuberosity and onto the lateral condyle.
- The **interosseous border** is a subtle vertical ridge that descends along the lateral aspect of the tibia from the region of bone anterior and inferior to the articular facet for the head of the fibula.
- The medial border is indistinct superiorly where it begins at the anterior end of the groove on the posterior surface of the medial tibial condyle, but is sharp in midshaft.

The large **medial surface** of the shaft of the tibia, between the anterior and medial borders, is smooth and subcutaneous, and is palpable along almost its entire extent. Medial and somewhat inferior to the tibial tuberosity, this medial surface bears a subtle, slightly roughened elongate elevation. This elevation is the site of the combined attachment of three muscles (sartorius, gracilis, and semitendinosus), which descend from the thigh.

The **posterior surface** of the shaft of the tibia, between the interosseous and medial borders, is widest superiorly where it is crossed by a roughened oblique line (the **soleal line**).

The **lateral surface**, between the anterior and interosseous borders, is smooth and unremarkable.

Proximal end of fibula

The fibula is the lateral bone of the leg and does not take part in formation of the knee joint or in weight-bearing. It is much smaller than the tibia and has a small proximal head, a narrow neck, and a delicate shaft, which ends as the lateral malleolus at the ankle.

The **head** of the fibula is a globe-shaped expansion at the proximal end of the fibula (Fig. 3.55). A circular facet on the superomedial surface is for articulation above with a similar facet on the inferior aspect of the lateral condyle of the tibia. Just posterolateral to this facet, the bone projects superiorly as a blunt apex (styloid process).

The lateral surface of the head of the fibula bears a large impression for the attachment of the biceps femoris muscle. A depression near the upper margin of this impression is for attachment of the fibular collateral ligament of the knee joint.

The **neck** of the fibula separates the expanded head from the **shaft**. The common fibular nerve lies against the posterolateral aspect of the neck.

Like the tibia, the shaft of the fibula has three borders (anterior, posterior, and interosseous) and three surfaces (lateral, posterior, and medial), which lie between the borders (Fig. 3.55):

- The **anterior border** is sharp in the middle of the shaft and begins superiorly from the anterior aspect of the head.
- The **posterior border** is rounded and descends from the region of the styloid process of the head.
- The **interosseous border** is medial in position.

The three surfaces of the fibula are associated with the three muscular compartments (lateral, posterior, and anterior) of the leg.

A useful way to determine the side to which a fibula belongs is to determine with which hand it is possible to perform the following—to hold the lower end of the fibula like a pen with the index finger and thumb such that the thumb is placed in the malleolar fossa and does not cover the triangular articular surface of the fibula.

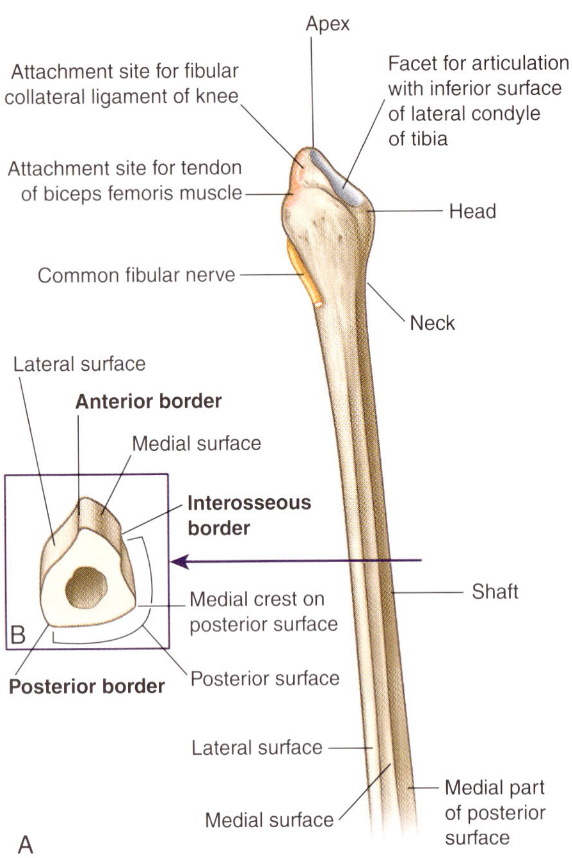

Fig. 3.55 Proximal end of the fibula. **(A)** Anterior view. **(B)** Cross-section through the shaft of fibula.

Muscles

Muscles of the thigh are arranged in three compartments separated by intermuscular septa (Fig. 3.56).

The **anterior compartment of the thigh** contains the sartorius and the four large quadriceps femoris muscles (rectus femoris, vastus lateralis, vastus medialis, and vastus intermedius). All are innervated by the femoral nerve. In addition, the terminal ends of the psoas major and iliacus muscles pass into the upper part of the anterior compartment from sites of origin on the posterior abdominal wall. These muscles are innervated by branches directly from the anterior rami of L1 to L3 (psoas major) or from the femoral nerve (iliacus) as it passes down the abdominal wall.

The **medial compartment of the thigh** contains six muscles (gracilis, pectineus, adductor longus, adductor brevis, adductor magnus, and obturator externus). All except the pectineus, which is innervated by the femoral nerve, and part of the adductor magnus, which is innervated by the sciatic nerve, are innervated by the obturator nerve.

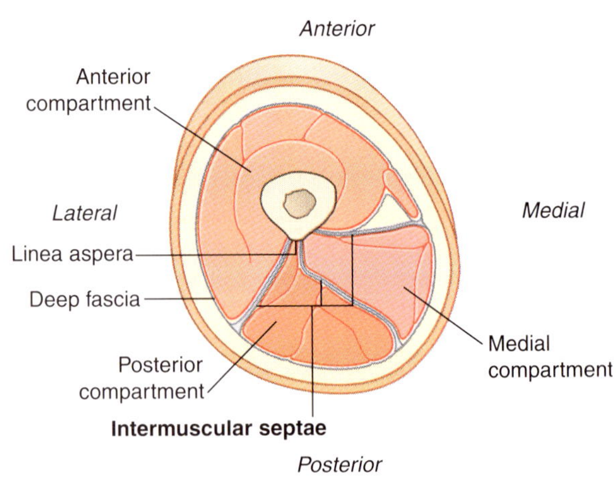

Fig. 3.56 Transverse section through the midthigh.

The **posterior compartment of the thigh** contains three large muscles termed the "hamstrings." All are innervated by the sciatic nerve (Flowchart 3.1).

Early clinical exposure

Compartment syndrome

Compartment syndrome occurs when there is swelling within a fascial enclosed muscle compartment in the limbs. Typical causes include limb trauma, intracompartment hemorrhage, and limb compression. As pressure within the compartment elevates, capillary blood flow and tissue perfusion is compromised, which can ultimately lead to neuromuscular damage if not treated.

Anterior compartment

Muscles in the anterior compartment (Table 3.3) act on the hip and knee joints:

- The psoas major and iliacus act on the hip joint.
- The sartorius and rectus femoris act on both the hip and knee joints.
- The vastus muscles act on the knee joint

This compartment is also called the extensor compartment because most of the muscles in this compartment act to extend the knee joint.

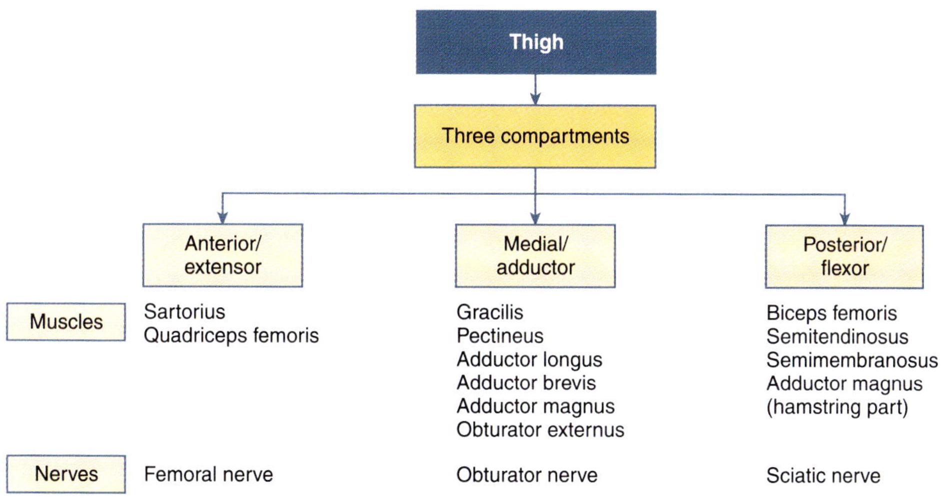

Flowchart 3.1 Compartments of thigh and their nerve supply.

Table 3.3 Muscles of the anterior compartment of thigh

Muscle	Origin	Insertion	Innervation	Function
Psoas major (Fig. 3.57)	Posterior abdominal wall (lumbar transverse processes, intervertebral discs, and adjacent bodies from TXII to LV and tendinous arches between these points)	Lesser trochanter of femur	Anterior rami (**L1, L2**, L3)	Flexes the thigh at the hip joint
Iliacus (Fig. 3.57)	Posterior abdominal wall (iliac fossa)	Lesser trochanter of femur	Femoral nerve (**L2**, L3)	Flexes the thigh at the hip joint
Vastus medialis (Fig. 3.26 and 3.58)	Femur—medial part of intertrochanteric line, pectineal line, medial lip of the linea aspera, medial supracondylar line	Quadriceps femoris tendon and medial border of patella	Femoral nerve (L2, **L3, L4**)	Extends the leg at the knee joint
Vastus intermedius	Femur—upper two-thirds of anterior and lateral surfaces	Quadriceps femoris tendon, lateral margin of patella, and lateral condyle of tibia	Femoral nerve (L2, **L3, L4**)	Extends the leg at the knee joint
Vastus lateralis	Femur—lateral part of intertrochanteric line, margin of greater trochanter, lateral margin of gluteal tuberosity, lateral lip of the linea aspera	Quadriceps femoris tendon and lateral margin of patella	Femoral nerve (L2, **L3, L4**)	Extends the leg at the knee joint
Rectus femoris	Straight head originates from the anterior inferior iliac spine; reflected head originates from the ilium just superior to the acetabulum	Quadriceps femoris tendon	Femoral nerve (L2, **L3, L4**)	Extends the leg at the knee joint and flexes the thigh at the hip joint
Sartorius	Anterior superior iliac spine	Medial surface of tibia just inferomedial to tibial tuberosity	Femoral nerve (**L2, L3**)	Flexes the leg at the knee joint and flexes the thigh at the hip joint

Note: Spinal segments in bold are the major segments innervating the muscle.

Iliopsoas—psoas major and iliacus

The **psoas major** and **iliacus** muscles originate on the posterior abdominal wall and descend into the upper part of the anterior compartment of the thigh through the lateral half of the gap between the inguinal ligament and the pelvic bone (Fig. 3.57).

Although the iliacus and psoas major originate as separate muscles in the abdomen, both insert by a common tendon onto the lesser trochanter of the femur and together are usually referred to as the **iliopsoas** muscle.

The iliopsoas is a powerful flexor of the thigh at the hip joint and can also contribute to lateral rotation of the thigh. The psoas major is innervated by branches from the anterior rami of L1 to L3 and the iliacus is innervated by branches from the femoral nerve in the abdomen.

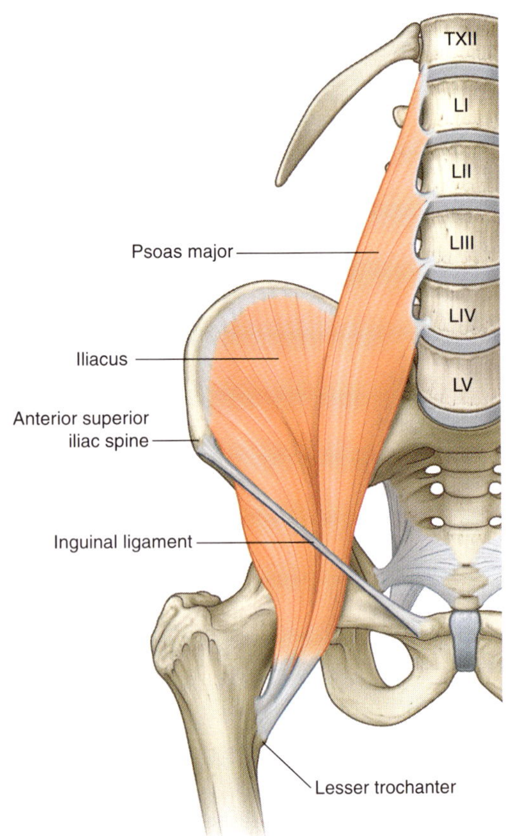

Fig. 3.57 Psoas major and iliacus muscles.

Quadriceps femoris—vastus medialis, intermedius, and lateralis and rectus femoris

The large **quadriceps femoris** muscle consists of four heads. These are the three vastus muscles (vastus medialis, vastus intermedius, and vastus lateralis) and the rectus femoris muscle (Fig. 3.58).

The quadriceps femoris muscle mainly extends the leg at the knee joint, but the rectus femoris component also assists flexion of the thigh at the hip joint. Because the vastus muscles insert into the margins of the patella as well as into the quadriceps femoris tendon, they stabilize the position of the patella during knee joint movement.

The quadriceps femoris is innervated by the femoral nerve with contributions mainly from spinal segments L3 and L4. A tap with a tendon hammer on the patellar ligament therefore tests reflex activity mainly at spinal cord levels L3 and L4.

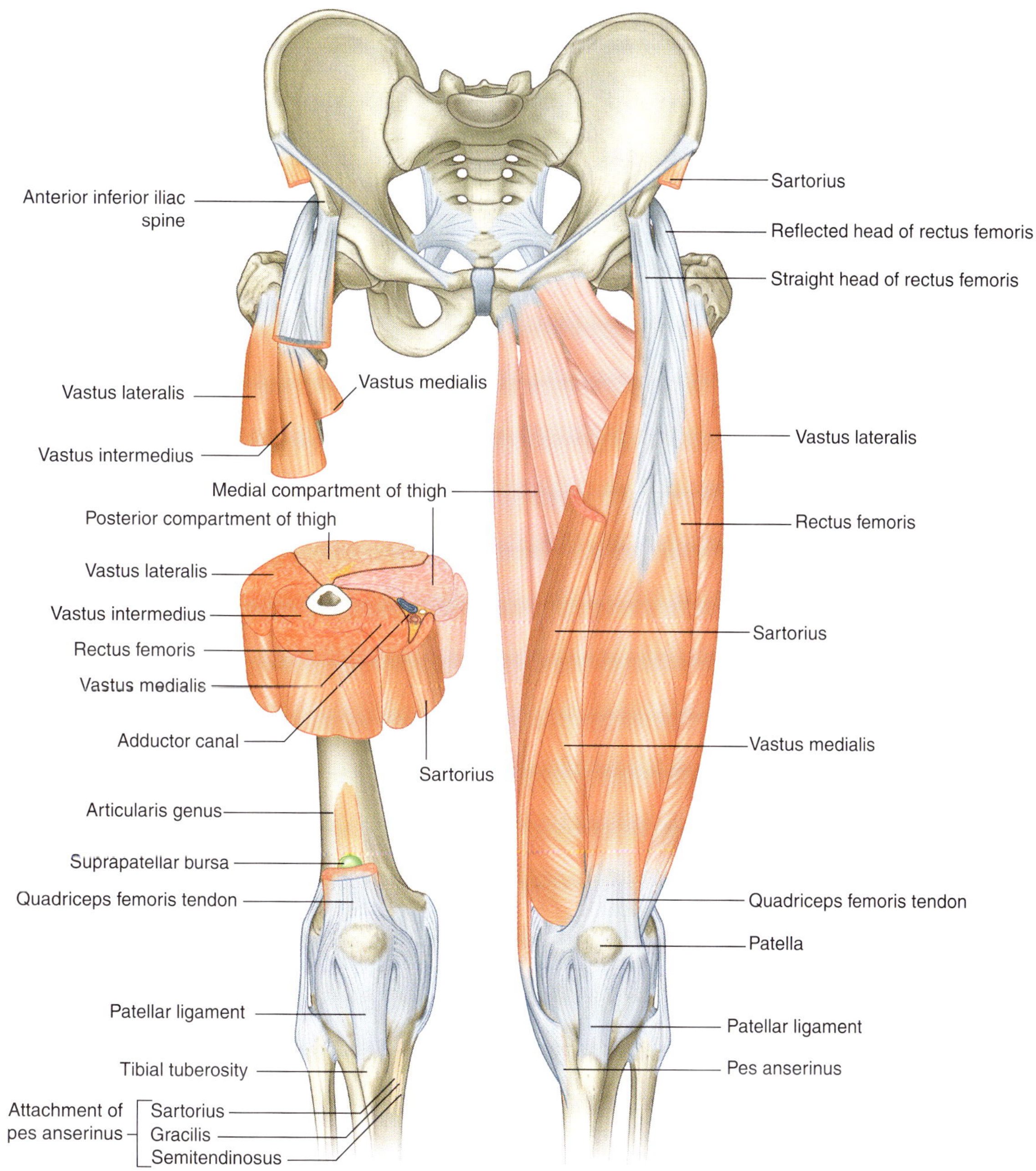

Fig. 3.58 Muscles of the anterior compartment of thigh.

Vastus muscles

The vastus muscles originate from the femur, whereas the rectus femoris muscle originates from the pelvic bone. All attach first to the patella by the quadriceps femoris tendon and then to the tibial tuberosity by the **patellar ligament**.

The **vastus medialis** originates from a continuous line of attachment on the femur, which begins anteromedially on the intertrochanteric line and continues posteroinferiorly along the pectineal line and then descends along the medial lip of the linea aspera and onto the medial supracondylar line (Fig. 3.26). The fibers converge onto the medial aspect of the quadriceps femoris tendon and the medial border of the patella (Fig. 3.58).

The **vastus intermedius** originates mainly from the upper two-thirds of the anterior and lateral surfaces of the femur and the adjacent intermuscular septum (Fig. 3.58). It merges into the deep aspect of the quadriceps femoris tendon and also attaches to the lateral margin of the patella and lateral condyle of the tibia.

A tiny muscle (**articularis genus**) originates from the femur just inferior to the origin of the vastus intermedius and inserts into the suprapatellar bursa associated with the knee joint (Fig. 3.58). This articular muscle, which is often part of the vastus intermedius muscle, pulls the bursa away from the knee joint during extension.

The **vastus lateralis** is the largest of the vastus muscles (Fig. 3.58). It originates from a continuous line of attachment, which begins anterolaterally from the superior part of the intertrochanteric line of the femur and then circles laterally around the bone to attach to the lateral margin of the gluteal tuberosity and continues down the upper part of the lateral lip of the linea aspera. Muscle fibers converge mainly onto the quadriceps femoris tendon and the lateral margin of the patella.

Rectus femoris

Unlike the vastus muscles, which cross only the knee joint, the **rectus femoris** muscle crosses both the hip and the knee joints (Fig. 3.58).

The rectus femoris has two tendinous heads of origin from the pelvic bone:

- One from the anterior inferior iliac spine (**straight head**)
- The other from a roughened area of the ilium immediately superior to the acetabulum (**reflected head**) (Fig. 3.58)

The two heads of the rectus femoris unite to form an elongate muscle belly, which lies anterior to the vastus intermedius muscle and between the vastus lateralis and vastus medialis muscles, to which it is attached on either side. At the distal end, the rectus femoris muscle converges on the quadriceps femoris tendon and inserts on the base of the patella.

Patellar ligament

The patellar ligament is functionally the continuation of the quadriceps femoris tendon below the patella and is attached above to the apex and margins of the patella and below to the tibial tuberosity (Fig. 3.58). The more superficial fibers of the quadriceps femoris tendon and the patellar ligament are continuous over the anterior surface of the patella, and lateral and medial fibers are continuous with the ligament on the sides of the margins of the patella.

Sartorius

The **sartorius** muscle is the most superficial muscle in the anterior compartment of the thigh and is a long strap-like muscle that descends obliquely through the thigh from the anterior superior iliac spine to the medial surface of the proximal shaft of the tibia (Fig. 3.58). Its flat aponeurotic insertion into the tibia is immediately anterior to the insertion of the gracilis and semitendinosus muscles.

The sartorius, gracilis, and semitendinosus muscles attach to the tibia in a three-pronged pattern on the tibia, so their combined tendons of insertion are often termed the **pes anserinus** (Latin for "goose foot").

In the upper one-third of the thigh, the medial margin of the sartorius forms the lateral margin of the femoral triangle.

In the middle one-third of the thigh, the sartorius forms the anterior wall of the adductor canal.

The sartorius muscle assists in flexing the leg at the knee joint and the thigh at the hip joint. It also abducts the thigh and rotates it laterally, as when resting the foot on the opposite knee when sitting. This is the leg folding position, or "palthi posture."

The sartorius is innervated by the femoral nerve.

Medial compartment

There are six muscles in the medial compartment of the thigh (Table 3.4): gracilis, pectineus, adductor longus, adductor brevis, adductor magnus, and obturator externus (Fig. 3.59). Collectively, all these muscles except the obturator externus mainly adduct the thigh at the hip joint; the adductor muscles may also medially rotate the thigh. Obturator externus is a lateral rotator of the thigh at the hip joint.

Gracilis

The **gracilis** is the most superficial of the muscles in the medial compartment of thigh and descends almost vertically down the medial side of the thigh (Fig. 3.59). It is attached above to the outer surface of the ischiopubic ramus of the pelvic bone and below to the medial surface of the proximal shaft of the tibia, where it lies sandwiched between the tendon of sartorius in front and the tendon of the semitendinosus behind.

Table 3.4 Muscles of the medial compartment of thigh

Muscle	Origin	Insertion	Innervation	Function
Gracilis (Fig. 3.59)	A line on the external surfaces of the body of the pubis, the inferior pubic ramus, and the ramus of the ischium	Medial surface of proximal shaft of tibia	Obturator nerve (**L2**, L3)	Adducts thigh at hip joint and flexes leg at knee joint
Pectineus	Pectineal line (pecten pubis) and adjacent bone of pelvis	Oblique line extending from base of lesser trochanter to linea aspera on posterior surface of proximal femur	Femoral nerve (**L2**, L3)	Adducts and flexes thigh at hip joint
Adductor longus	External surface of body of pubis (triangular depression inferior to pubic crest and lateral to pubic symphysis)	Linea aspera on middle one-third of shaft of femur	Obturator nerve (anterior division) (**L2, L3**, L4)	Adducts and medially rotates thigh at hip joint
Adductor brevis	External surface of body of pubis and inferior pubic ramus	Posterior surface of proximal femur and upper one-third of linea aspera	Obturator nerve (**L2, L3**)	Adducts and medially rotates thigh at hip joint
Adductor magnus	Adductor part—ischiopubic ramus	Posterior surface of proximal femur, linea aspera, medial supracondylar line	Obturator nerve (**L2, L3**, L4)	Adducts and medially rotates thigh at hip joint
	Hamstring part—ischial tuberosity	Adductor tubercle and medial supracondylar line	Sciatic nerve (tibial division) (**L2, L3**, L4)	Extends thigh at hip joint
Obturator externus	External surface of obturator membrane and adjacent bone	Trochanteric fossa	Obturator nerve (posterior division) (L3, **L4**)	Laterally rotates thigh at hip joint

Note: Spinal segments in bold are the major segments innervating the muscle.

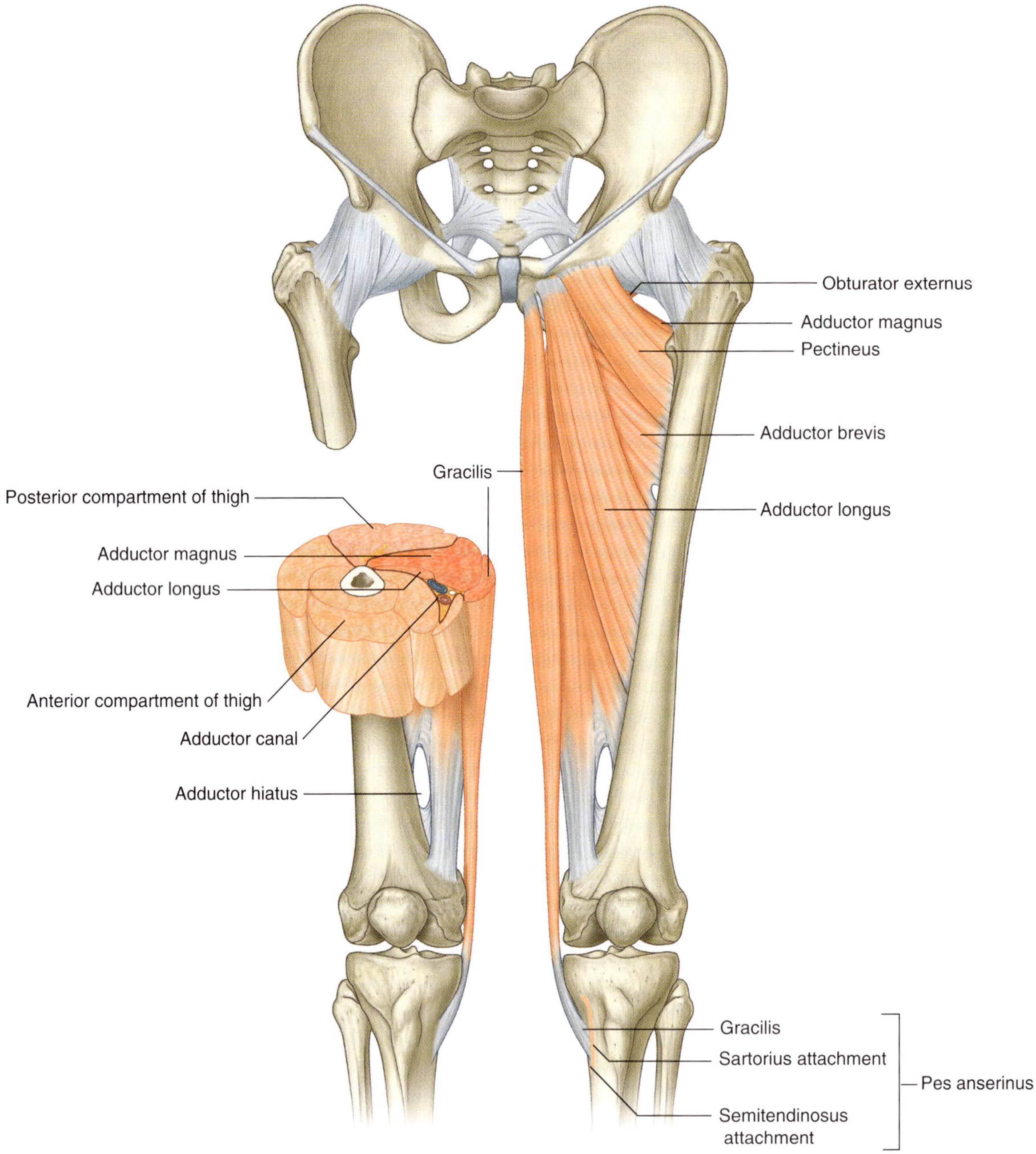

Fig. 3.59 Muscles of the medial compartment of thigh. Anterior view.

Pectineus

The **pectineus** is a flat quadrangular muscle (Fig. 3.60). It is attached above to the pectineal line of the pelvic bone and adjacent bone, and descends laterally to attach to an oblique line extending from the base of the lesser trochanter to the linea aspera on the posterior surface of the proximal femur.

From its origin on the pelvic bone, the pectineus passes into the thigh below the inguinal ligament and forms part of the floor of the medial half of the femoral triangle (Fig. 3.41).

The pectineus adducts and flexes the thigh at the hip joint and is innervated by the femoral nerve.

Adductor longus

The **adductor longus** is a flat fan-shaped muscle that originates from a small, rough, triangular area on the external surface of the body of the pubis just inferior to the pubic crest and lateral to the pubic symphysis (Fig. 3.60). It expands as it descends posterolaterally to insert via an aponeurosis into the middle third of the linea aspera.

The adductor longus contributes to the floor of the femoral triangle, and its medial margin forms the medial border of the femoral triangle. The muscle also forms the proximal posterior wall of the adductor canal.

The adductor longus adducts and medially rotates the thigh at the hip joint and is innervated by the anterior division of the obturator nerve.

Adductor brevis

The **adductor brevis** lies posterior to the pectineus and adductor longus. It is a triangular muscle attached at its apex to the body of the pubis and inferior pubic ramus just superior to the origin of the gracilis muscle (Fig. 3.60). The

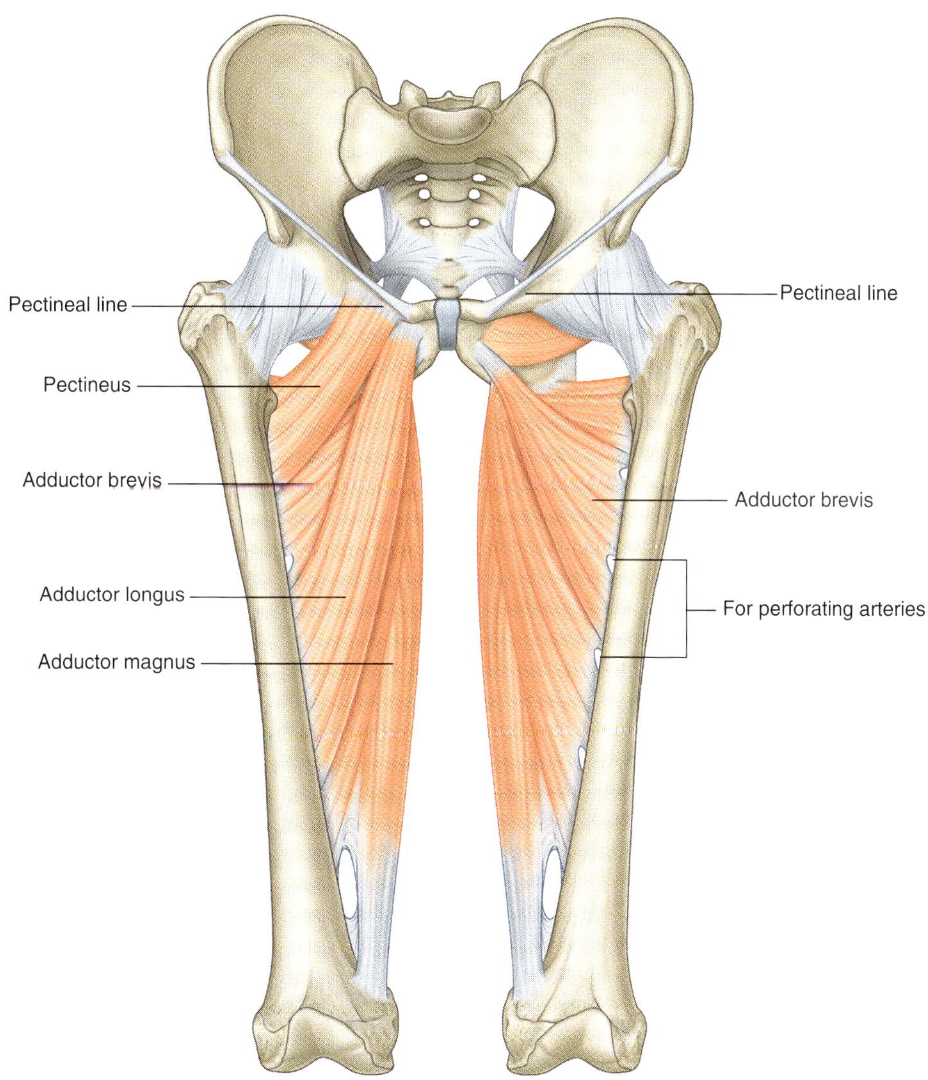

Fig. 3.60 Pectineus, adductor longus, and adductor brevis muscles. Anterior view.

muscle is attached into the upper aspect of the linea aspera by its expanded base via an aponeurosis to a vertical line extending from lateral to the insertion of the pectineus lateral to the attachment of the adductor longus.

The adductor brevis adducts and medially rotates the thigh at the hip joint and is innervated by the obturator nerve.

Adductor magnus

The **adductor magnus** is the largest and deepest of the muscles in the medial compartment of the thigh (Fig. 3.61). The muscle forms the distal posterior wall of the adductor canal. Like the adductor longus and brevis muscles, the adductor magnus is a triangular or fan-shaped muscle anchored by its apex to the pelvis and attached by its expanded base to the femur.

On the pelvis, the adductor magnus is attached along a line that extends from the inferior pubic ramus, above the attachments of the adductor longus and brevis muscles, and along the ramus of the ischium to the ischial tuberosity. The part of the muscle that originates from the ischiopubic ramus expands laterally and inferiorly to insert on the femur along a vertical line of attachment that extends from just inferior to the quadrate tubercle and medial to the gluteal tuberosity, along the linea aspera and onto the medial supracondylar line. This lateral part of the muscle is often termed the "adductor part" of the adductor magnus.

The medial part of the adductor magnus, often called the "hamstring part," originates from the ischial tuberosity of the pelvic bone and descends almost vertically along the thigh to insert via a rounded tendon into the adductor tubercle on the medial condyle of the femur. It also inserts via an aponeurosis up onto the medial supracondylar line. A large circular gap inferiorly between the hamstring and adductor parts of the muscle is the **adductor hiatus** (Fig. 3.61), which allows the femoral artery and associated veins to pass between the adductor canal on the anteromedial aspect of the thigh and the popliteal fossa posterior to the knee.

The adductor magnus adducts and medially rotates the thigh at the hip joint. The adductor part of the muscle is innervated by the obturator nerve and the hamstring part is innervated by the sciatic nerve (tibial division).

Obturator externus

The **obturator externus** is a flat fan-shaped muscle. Its expansive body is attached to the external aspect of the obturator membrane and adjacent bone (Fig. 3.61). The muscle fibers converge posterolaterally to form a tendon, which passes posterior to the hip joint and neck of the femur to insert on an oval depression on the trochanteric fossa.

The obturator externus externally rotates the thigh at the hip joint and is innervated by the posterior division of the obturator nerve.

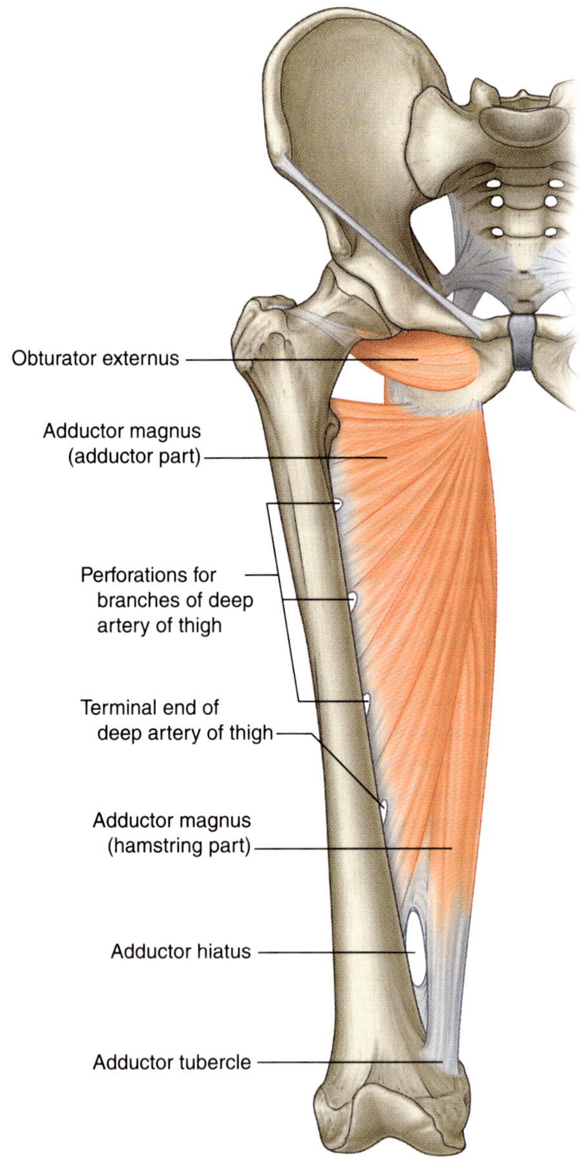

Fig. 3.61 Adductor magnus and obturator externus muscles. Anterior view. The neck of the femur is shown as if transparent.

Posterior compartment

There are three long muscles in the posterior compartment of the thigh: biceps femoris, semitendinosus, and semimembranosus (Table 3.5)—and they are collectively known as the **hamstrings** (Fig. 3.62). All except the short head of the biceps femoris cross both the hip and knee joints. As a group, the hamstrings flex the leg at the knee joint and extend the thigh at the hip joint. They are also rotators at both joints.

Biceps femoris

The **biceps femoris** muscle is lateral in the posterior compartment of the thigh and has two heads (Fig. 3.62):

- The **long head** originates with the semitendinosus muscle from the inferomedial part of the upper area of the ischial tuberosity.
- The **short head** arises from the lateral lip of the linea aspera on the shaft of the femur.

The muscle belly of the long head crosses the posterior thigh obliquely from medial to lateral and is joined by the short head distally. Together, fibers from the two heads form a tendon, which is palpable on the lateral side of the distal thigh. The main part of the tendon inserts into the lateral surface of the head of the fibula. Extensions from the tendon blend with the fibular collateral ligament and with ligaments associated with the lateral side of the knee joint.

The biceps femoris flexes the leg at the knee joint. The long head also extends and laterally rotates the hip. When the knee is partly flexed, the biceps femoris can laterally rotate the leg at the knee joint.

The long head is innervated by the sciatic nerve (tibial division) and the short head is innervated by the sciatic nerve (common fibular division).

Table 3.5 Muscles of the posterior compartment of thigh

Muscle	Origin	Insertion	Innervation	Function
Biceps femoris (Fig. 3.62 and 3.63)	Long head—inferomedial part of the upper area of the ischial tuberosity; short head—lateral lip of linea aspera	Head of fibula	Sciatic nerve (L5, **S1**, S2)	Flexes and laterally rotates leg at knee joint; extends and laterally rotates thigh at hip joint
Semitendinosus	Inferomedial part of the upper area of the ischial tuberosity	Medial surface of proximal tibia	Sciatic nerve (L5, **S1**, S2)	Flexes and medially rotates leg at knee joint; extends and medially rotates thigh at hip joint, and leg at knee joint
Semimembranosus (Fig. 3.54)	Superolateral impression on the ischial tuberosity	Groove and adjacent bone on medial and posterior surface of medial tibial condyle	Sciatic nerve (L5, **S1**, S2)	Flexes leg at knee joint and extends thigh at hip joint; medially rotates thigh at hip joint and leg at knee joint

Note: Spinal segments in bold are the major segments innervating the muscle.

Semitendinosus

The **semitendinosus** muscle is medial to the biceps femoris muscle in the posterior compartment of the thigh (Fig. 3.62). It originates with the long head of the biceps femoris muscle from the inferomedial part of the upper area of the ischial tuberosity. The spindle-shaped muscle belly ends in the lower half of the thigh and forms a long cord-like tendon, which lies on the semimembranosus muscle and descends to the knee. The tendon curves around the medial condyle of the tibia and inserts into the medial surface of the tibia just posterior to the tendons of the gracilis and sartorius muscles as part of the pes anserinus (Fig. 3.58).

The semitendinosus flexes the leg at the knee joint and extends the thigh at the hip joint. Working with the semimembranosus, it also medially rotates the thigh at the hip joint and medially rotates the leg at the knee joint.

The semitendinosus muscle is innervated by the sciatic nerve (tibial division).

Semimembranosus

The **semimembranosus** muscle lies deep to the semitendinosus muscle in the posterior compartment of the thigh

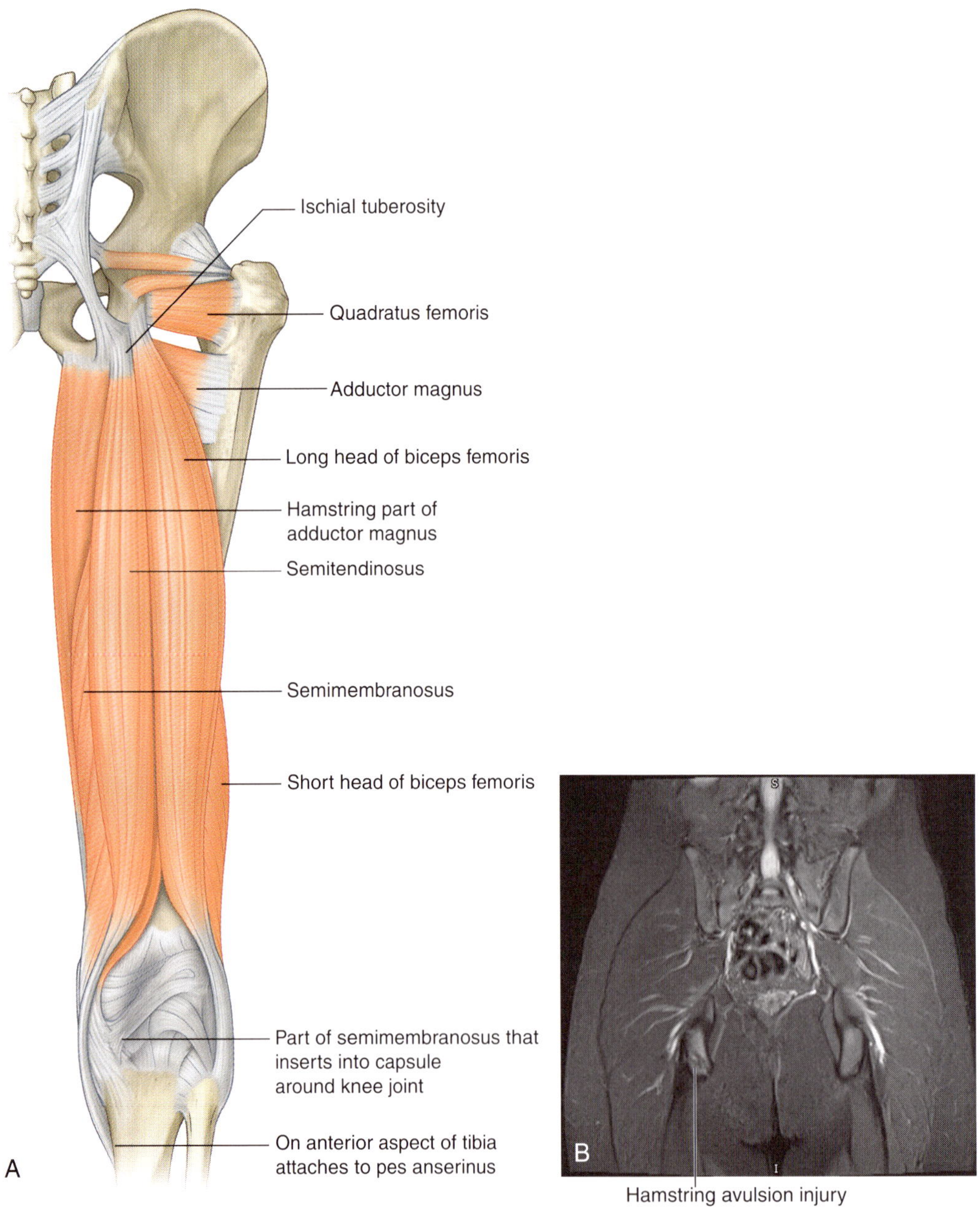

Fig. 3.62 (A) Muscles of the posterior compartment of thigh. Posterior view. **(B)** Coronal MRI of the posterior pelvis and thigh showing a hamstring avulsion injury.

(Fig. 3.62). It is attached above to the superolateral impression on the ischial tuberosity and below mainly to the groove and adjacent bone on the medial and posterior surfaces of the medial tibial condyle (Fig. 3.54). Expansions from the tendon also insert into and contribute to the formation of the oblique popliteal ligament and fascia around the knee joint (see Fig. 3.73).

The semimembranosus flexes the leg at the knee joint and extends the thigh at the hip joint. Working with the semitendinosus muscle, it medially rotates the thigh at the hip joint and the leg at the knee joint.

The semimembranosus muscle is innervated by the sciatic nerve (tibial division).

Early clinical exposure

Muscle injuries to the lower limb

Muscle injuries may occur as a result of direct trauma or as part of an overuse syndrome.

Muscle injuries may occur as a minor muscle tear, which may be demonstrated as a focal area of fluid within the muscle. With increasingly severe injuries, further muscle fibers are torn and this may eventually result in a complete muscle tear. The usual muscles in the thigh that tear include the hamstring muscles. Tears in the muscles below the knee typically occur within the soleus muscle, though other muscles may be affected.

Hamstring muscle injury

Injury to the hamstring muscles is a common source of pain in athletes, particularly in those competing in sports requiring a high degree of power and speed (such as sprinting, track and field, football) where the hamstring muscles are very susceptible to injury from excessive stretching.

The injury can range from a mild muscle strain to a complete tear of a muscle or a tendon. It usually occurs during sudden accelerations and decelerations or rapid change in direction. In adults, the most commonly injured is the muscle–tendon junction, which is a wide transition zone between the muscle and the tendon. An avulsion of the ischial tuberosity with proximal hamstring origin attachment is common in the adolescent population, particularly during sudden hip flexion because the ischial apophysis is the weakest element of the proximal hamstring unit in this age group. Both ultrasound and MRI can be used to assess the hamstring injury with the MRI providing not only the information about the extent of the injury but also some indication about the prognosis (future risk of retear, loss of function, etc.).

Arteries

Three arteries enter the thigh: the femoral artery, the obturator artery, and the inferior gluteal artery. Of these, the femoral artery is the largest and supplies most of the lower limb. The three arteries contribute to an anastomotic network of vessels around the hip joint.

Femoral artery

The femoral artery is the continuation of the external iliac artery and begins as the external iliac artery passes deep to the inguinal ligament to enter the femoral triangle on the anterior aspect of the upper thigh (Fig. 3.63). The femoral artery is palpable in the femoral triangle just inferior to the

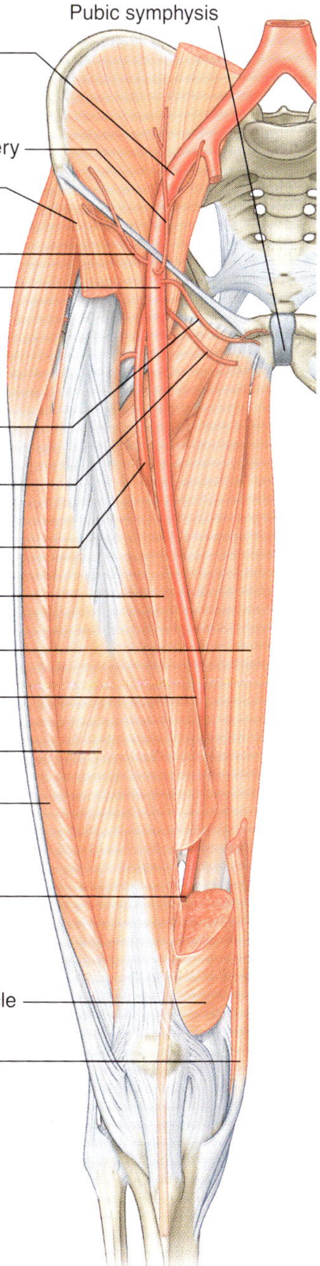

Fig. 3.63 Femoral artery.

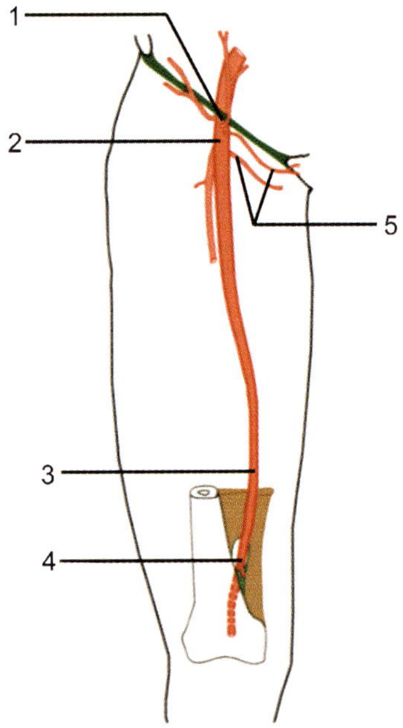

LD Fig. 3.63.1 Femoral artery.
Questions
3.63.1A Identify the labeled structures and mention the location of each label.
3.63.1B Name the branches of the femoral artery.

Answers
3.63.1A The labeled structures and their location are the
1. Beginning of the femoral artery as a continuation of the external iliac artery deep to the inguinal ligament at the midinguinal point
2. Femoral artery in the femoral triangle
3. Femoral artery in the adductor canal
4. Termination of the femoral artery as it passes through the adductor hiatus to form the popliteal artery

3.63.1B The branches of the femoral artery are the superficial circumflex iliac artery, superficial epigastric artery, superficial external pudendal artery, deep external pudendal artery, profunda femoris artery (which passes laterally and downwards), muscular branches, and the descending genicular artery (which passes medially and downwards).

inguinal ligament midway between the anterior superior iliac spine and the pubic symphysis.

The femoral artery passes vertically through the femoral triangle and then continues down the thigh in the adductor canal. It leaves the canal by passing through the adductor hiatus in the adductor magnus muscle and becomes the popliteal artery behind the knee.

A cluster of four small branches—**superficial epigastric artery**, **superficial circumflex iliac artery**, **superficial external pudendal artery**, and **deep external pudendal artery**—originate from the femoral artery in the femoral triangle and supply cutaneous regions of the upper thigh, lower abdomen, and perineum.

Deep artery of thigh

The largest branch of the femoral artery in the thigh is the **deep artery of the thigh** (profunda femoris artery), which originates from the lateral side of the femoral artery in the femoral triangle and is the major source of blood supply to the thigh (Fig. 3.63). The deep artery of the thigh:

- Immediately passes posteriorly between the pectineus and adductor longus muscles and then between the adductor longus and adductor brevis muscles.
- Then travels inferiorly between the adductor longus and adductor magnus, eventually penetrating through the adductor magnus to connect with branches of the popliteal artery behind the knee.

The deep artery of the thigh has lateral and medial circumflex femoral branches and three perforating branches.

Lateral circumflex femoral artery

- The **lateral circumflex femoral artery** normally originates proximally from the lateral side of the deep artery of the thigh, but may arise directly from the femoral artery (Fig. 3.64). It passes deep to the sartorius and rectus femoris and divides into three terminal branches:
- The **ascending branch** ascends laterally deep to the tensor fasciae latae muscle and connects with a branch of the medial circumflex femoral artery to form a channel, which circles the neck of the femur and supplies the neck and head of the femur.
- The **descending branch** descends deep to the rectus femoris, penetrates the vastus lateralis muscle, and connects with a branch of the popliteal artery near the knee.
- The **transverse branch** passes laterally to pierce the vastus lateralis and then circles around the proximal shaft of the femur to anastomose with branches from the medial femoral circumflex artery, the inferior gluteal artery, and the first perforating artery to form the cruciate anastomosis around the hip.

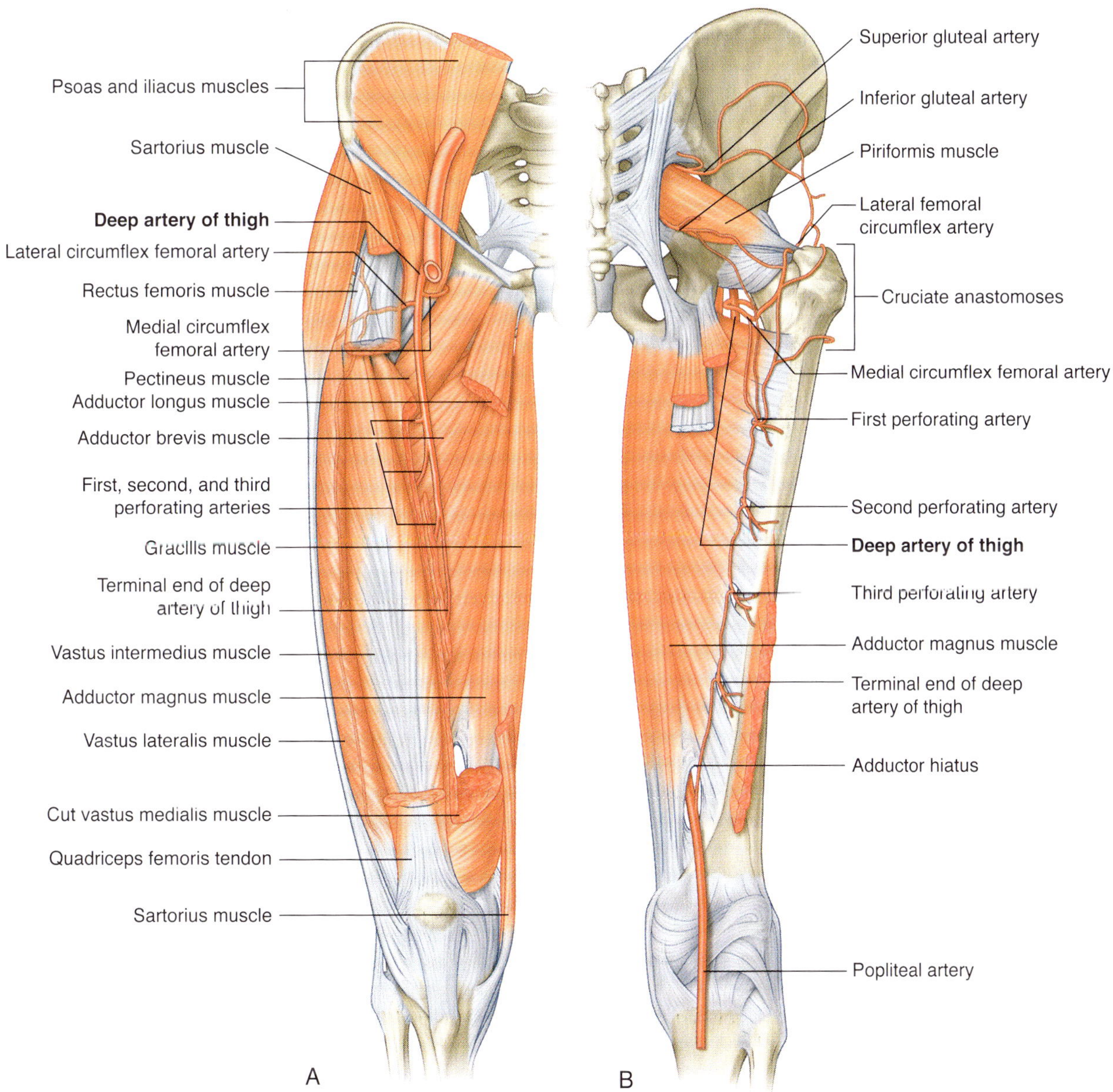

Fig. 3.64 Deep artery of thigh. **(A)** Anterior view. **(B)** Posterior view.

Medial circumflex femoral artery

The **medial circumflex femoral artery** normally originates proximally from the posteromedial aspect of the deep artery of the thigh, but may originate from the femoral artery (Fig. 3.64). It passes medially around the shaft of the femur, first between the pectineus and iliopsoas and then between the obturator externus and adductor brevis muscles. Near the margin of the adductor brevis, the vessel gives off a small branch, which enters the hip joint through the acetabular notch and anastomoses with the acetabular branch of the obturator artery.

The main trunk of the medial circumflex femoral artery passes over the superior margin of the adductor magnus and divides into two major branches deep to the quadratus femoris muscle:

- One branch ascends to the trochanteric fossa and connects with branches of the gluteal and lateral circumflex femoral arteries (trochanteric anastomosis).
- The other branch passes laterally to participate with branches from the lateral circumflex femoral artery, the inferior gluteal artery, and the first perforating artery in forming an anastomotic network of vessels around the hip (cruciate anastomosis).

Perforating arteries

The three **perforating arteries** branch from the deep artery of the thigh (Fig. 3.64) as it descends anterior to the adductor brevis muscle—the first originates above the muscle, the second originates anterior to the muscle, and the third originates below the muscle. All three penetrate through the adductor magnus near its attachment to the linea aspera to enter and supply the posterior compartment of the thigh. Here, the vessels have ascending and descending branches, which interconnect to form a longitudinal channel, which participates above in forming an anastomotic network of vessels around the hip and inferiorly anastomoses with branches of the popliteal artery behind the knee.

Obturator artery

The **obturator artery** originates as a branch of the internal iliac artery in the pelvic cavity and enters the medial compartment of the thigh through the obturator canal (Fig. 3.65). As it passes through the canal, it bifurcates into an **anterior branch** and a **posterior branch**, which together form a channel that circles the margin of the obturator membrane and lies within the attachment of the obturator externus muscle.

Vessels arising from the anterior and posterior branches supply adjacent muscles and anastomose with the inferior gluteal and medial circumflex femoral arteries. In addition, an acetabular vessel originates from the posterior branch, enters the hip joint through the acetabular notch, and contributes to the supply of the head of the femur.

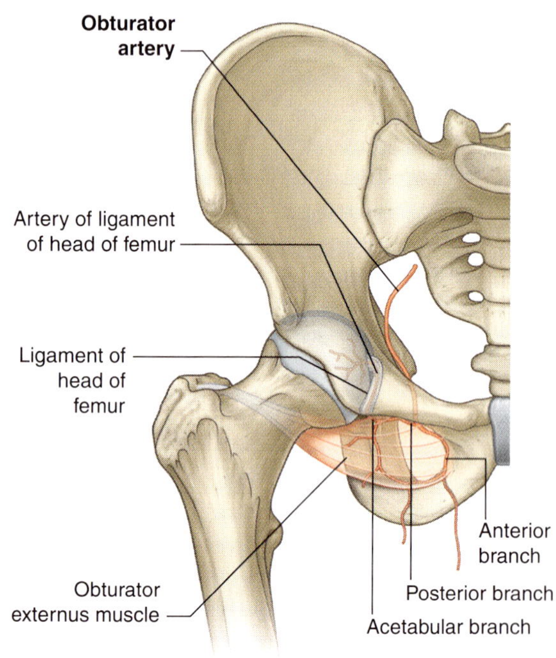

Fig. 3.65 Obturator artery.

Early clinical exposure

Peripheral vascular disease

Peripheral vascular disease is often characterized by reduced blood flow to the legs. This disorder may be caused by stenoses (narrowing) and/or occlusions (blockages) in the lower aorta and the iliac, femoral, tibial, and fibular vessels. Patients typically have chronic leg ischemia and "acute on chronic" leg ischemia.

Chronic leg ischemia

Chronic leg ischemia is a disorder in which vessels have undergone atheromatous change, and often there is significant luminal narrowing (usually over 50%). Most patients with peripheral arterial disease have widespread arterial disease (including cardiovascular and cerebrovascular disease), which may be clinically asymptomatic. Some of these patients develop such severe ischemia that the viability of the limb is threatened (**critical limb ischemia**).

The commonest symptom of chronic leg ischemia is **intermittent claudication**. Patients typically have a history of pain that develops in the calf muscles (usually associated with occlusions or narrowing in the femoral artery) or the buttocks (usually associated with occlusion or narrowing in the aortoiliac segments). The pain experienced in these muscles is often cramp-like and occurs with walking. The patient rests and is able to continue walking up to the same distance until the pain recurs and stops walking as before.

Acute on chronic ischemia

In some patients with chronic limb ischemia, an acute event blocks the vessels or reduces the blood supply to such a degree that the viability of the limb is threatened.

Occasionally a leg may become acutely ischemic with no evidence of underlying atheromatous disease. In these instances, a blood clot is likely to have embolized from the heart. Patients with mitral valve disease and atrial fibrillation are prone to embolic disease.

Critical limb ischemia

Critical limb ischemia occurs when the blood supply to the limb is so poor that the viability of the limb is severely threatened, and in this case many patients develop gangrene, ulceration, and severe rest pain in the foot. These patients require urgent treatment, which may be in the form of surgical reconstruction, radiological angioplasty, or even amputation.

Veins

Veins in the thigh consist of superficial and deep veins. Deep veins generally follow the arteries and have similar names. Superficial veins are in the superficial fascia, interconnect with deep veins, and do not generally accompany arteries. The largest of the superficial veins in the thigh is the great saphenous vein.

Great saphenous vein

The great saphenous vein originates from a venous arch on the dorsal aspect of the foot and ascends along the medial side of the lower limb to the proximal anterior part of the thigh (see p. 269). Here it pierces the deep fascia by passing through the saphenous opening to connect with the femoral vein in the femoral triangle (see p. 269).

Nerves

There are three major nerves in the thigh, each associated with one of the three compartments. The femoral nerve is associated with the anterior compartment of the thigh, the obturator nerve is associated with the medial compartment of the thigh, and the sciatic nerve is associated with the posterior compartment of the thigh.

Femoral nerve

The femoral nerve originates from the lumbar plexus (spinal cord segments L2–L4) on the posterior abdominal wall and enters the femoral triangle of the thigh by passing deep to the inguinal ligament (Fig. 3.66). In the femoral triangle, the femoral nerve lies on the lateral side of the femoral artery and is outside the femoral sheath, which surrounds the vessels.

Before entering the thigh, the femoral nerve supplies branches to the iliacus and pectineus muscles.

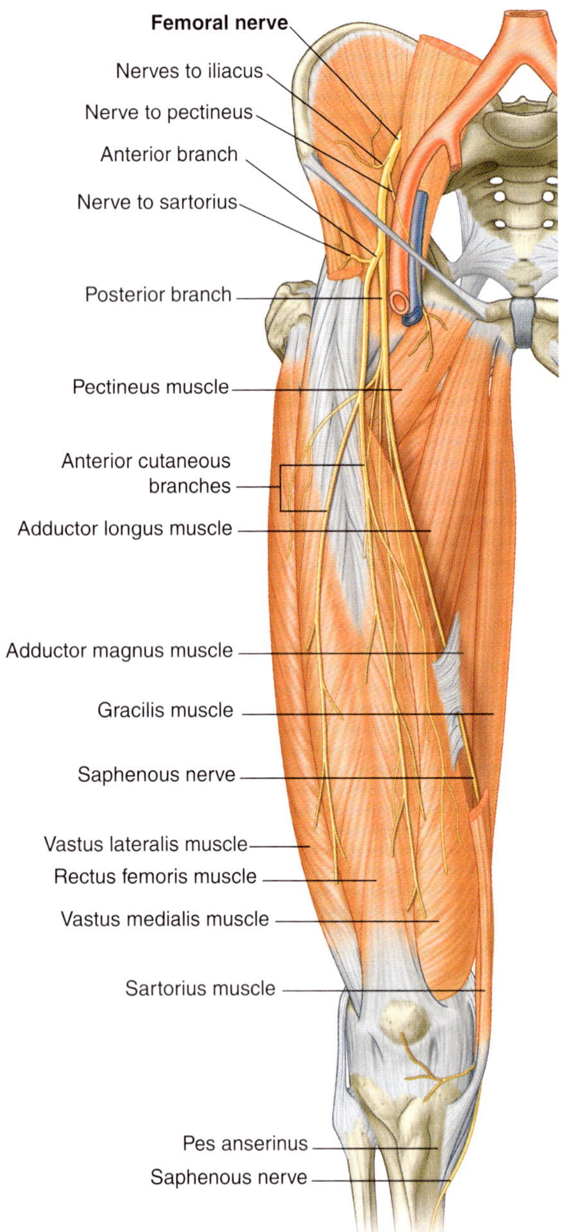

Fig. 3.66 Femoral nerve.

Immediately after passing deep to the inguinal ligament, the femoral nerve divides into anterior and posterior branches, which supply muscles of the anterior compartment of the thigh and skin on the anterior and medial aspects of the thigh and on the medial sides of the leg and foot.

Branches of the femoral nerve (Fig. 3.66) include:

- Anterior cutaneous branches, which penetrate deep fascia to supply skin on the front of the thigh and knee
- Numerous motor nerves, which supply the quadriceps femoris muscles (rectus femoris, vastus lateralis, vastus intermedius, and vastus medialis muscles) and the sartorius muscle
- One long cutaneous nerve, the saphenous nerve, which supplies skin as far distally as the medial side of the foot

The **saphenous nerve** accompanies the femoral artery through the adductor canal, but does not pass through the adductor hiatus with the femoral artery. Rather, the saphenous nerve penetrates directly through connective tissues near the end of the canal to appear between the sartorius and gracilis muscles on the medial side of the knee. Here the saphenous nerve penetrates deep fascia and continues down the medial side of the leg to the foot, and supplies skin on the medial side of the knee, leg, and foot (Flowchart 3.2).

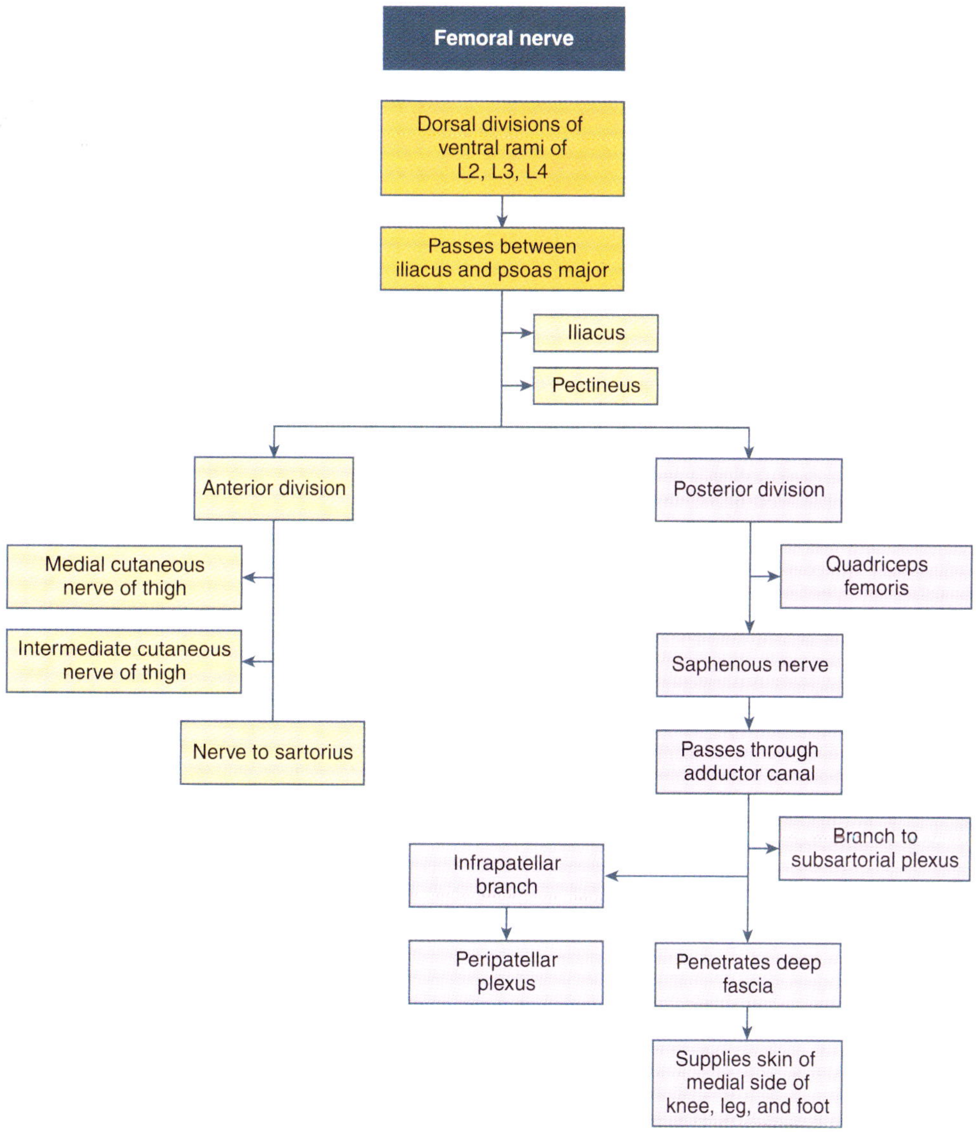

Flowchart 3.2 Course and distribution of femoral nerve.

Obturator nerve

The obturator nerve is a branch of the lumbar plexus (spinal cord segments L2–L4) on the posterior abdominal wall. It descends in the psoas muscle, and then passes out of the medial margin of the psoas muscle to enter the pelvis (Fig. 3.67). The obturator nerve continues along the lateral pelvic wall and then enters the medial compartment of the thigh by passing through the obturator canal. It supplies most of the adductor muscles and skin on the medial aspect of the thigh. As the obturator nerve enters the thigh, it divides into two branches, an anterior branch and a posterior branch, which are separated by the adductor brevis muscle:

- The **posterior branch** descends behind the adductor brevis muscle and on the anterior surface of the adductor magnus muscle, and supplies the obturator externus and adductor brevis muscles and the part of the adductor magnus that attaches to the linea aspera.
- The **anterior branch** descends on the anterior surface of the adductor brevis muscle and is behind the pectineus and adductor longus muscles—it supplies branches to the adductor longus, gracilis, and adductor brevis muscles, and often contributes to the supply of the pectineus muscle, and cutaneous branches innervate the skin on the medial side of the thigh (Flowchart 3.3).

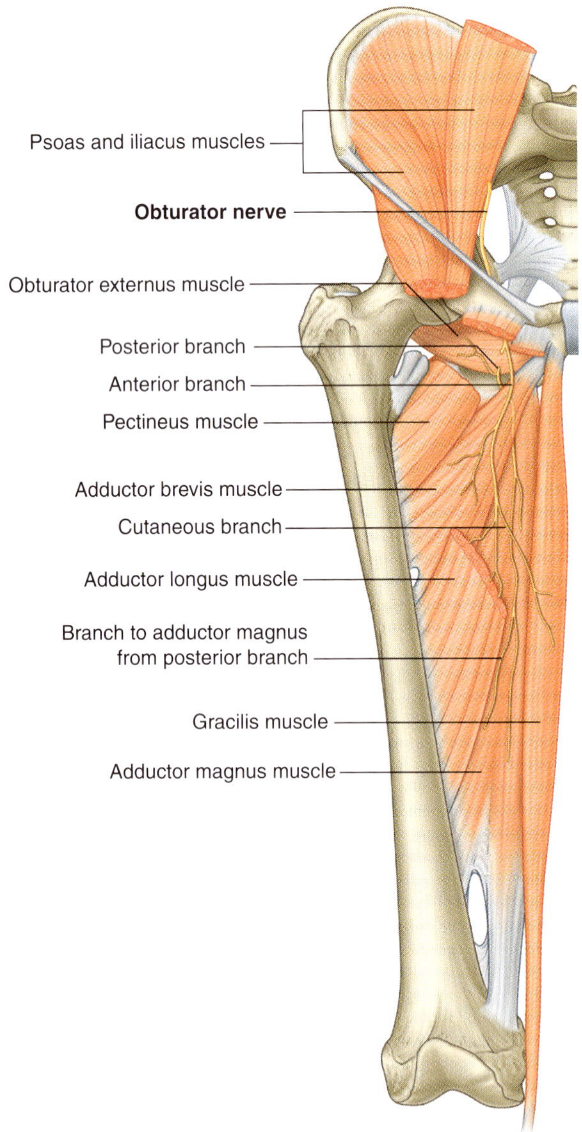

Fig. 3.67 Obturator nerve.

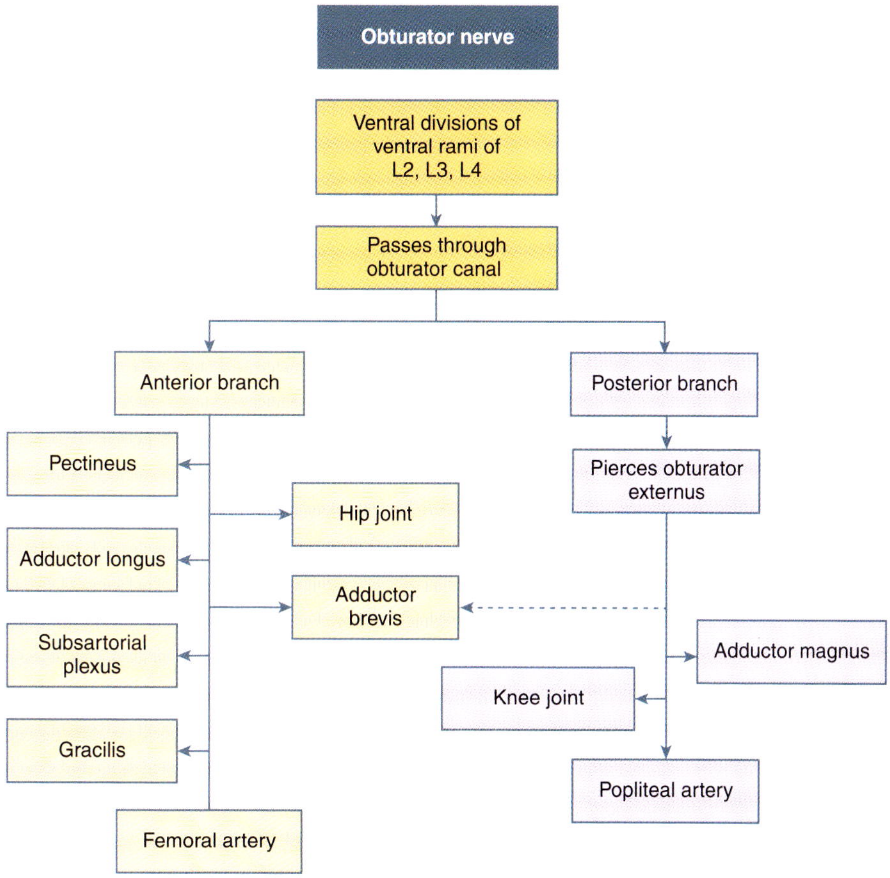

Flowchart 3.3 Course and distribution of obturator nerve.

Sciatic nerve

The sciatic nerve is a branch of the sacral plexus (spinal cord segments L4–S3) and descends into the posterior compartment of the thigh from the gluteal region (Fig. 3.68). It innervates all muscles in the posterior compartment of the thigh and then its branches continue into the leg and foot.

In the posterior compartment of the thigh, the sciatic nerve lies on the adductor magnus muscle and is crossed by the long head of the biceps femoris muscle.

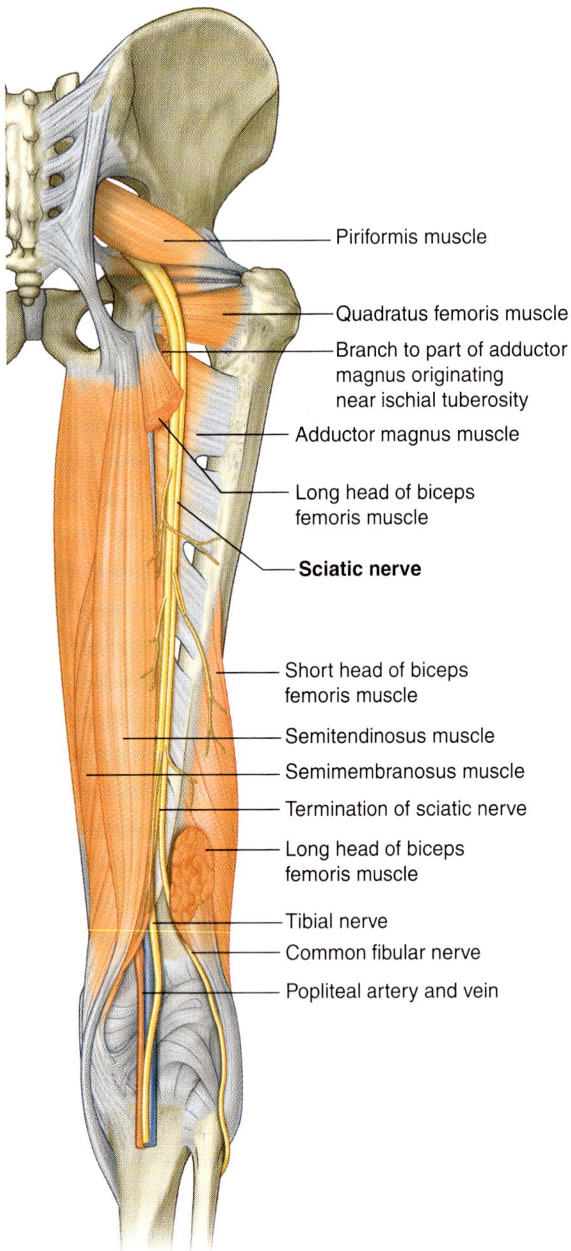

Fig. 3.68 Sciatic nerve.

In the middle third of the thigh, and sometimes within the pelvis, the sciatic nerve divides into its two terminal branches: the **tibial nerve** and the **common fibular nerve**. These nerves travel vertically down the thigh and enter the popliteal fossa posterior to the knee. Here, they meet the popliteal artery and vein (Flowchart 3.4).

Tibial nerve

The tibial part of the sciatic nerve, either before or after its separation from the common fibular nerve, supplies branches to all muscles in the posterior compartment of the thigh (long head of biceps femoris, semimembranosus, semitendinosus) except the short head of the biceps femoris, which is innervated by the common fibular part (Fig. 3.68).

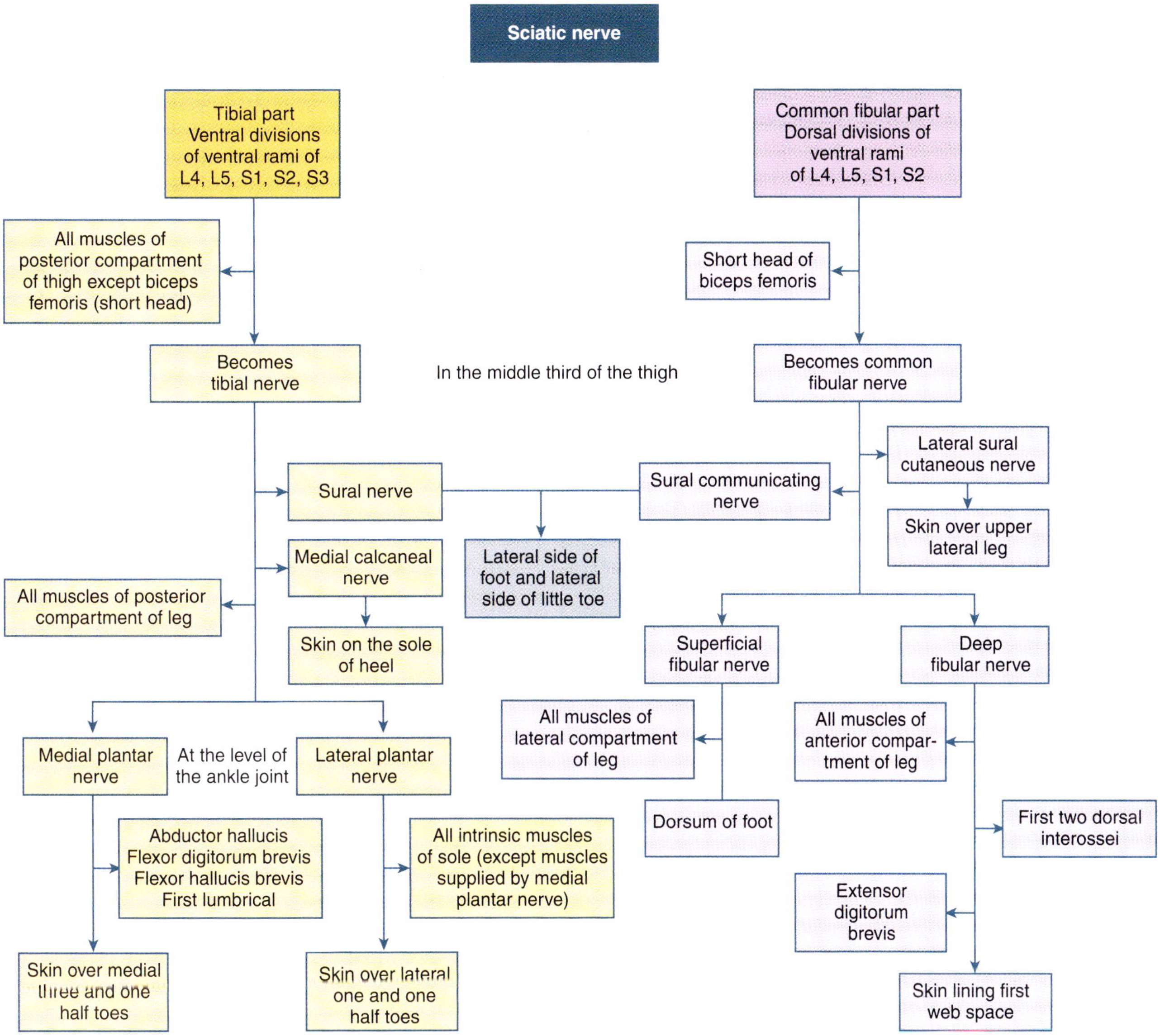

Flowchart 3.4 Course and distribution of sciatic nerve.

The **tibial nerve** descends through the popliteal fossa, enters the posterior compartment of the leg, and its terminal branches continue into the sole of the foot.

The tibial nerve innervates:

- All muscles in the posterior compartment of the leg.
- All intrinsic muscles in the sole of the foot including the first two dorsal interossei muscles, which also may receive innervation from the deep fibular nerve.
- Skin on the posterolateral side of the lower half of the leg and lateral side of the ankle, foot, and little toe, and skin on the sole of the foot and toes (Fig. 3.19).

Common fibular nerve

The common fibular part of the sciatic nerve innervates the short head of the biceps femoris in the posterior compartment of the thigh and then its terminal branches continue into the lateral and anterior compartments of the leg and onto the foot (Fig. 3.68).

The common fibular nerve innervates:

- All muscles in the anterior and lateral compartments of the leg.
- One muscle (extensor digitorum brevis) on the dorsal aspect of the foot.
- The first two dorsal interossei muscles in the sole of the foot.
- Skin over the lateral aspect of the leg, and ankle, and over the dorsal aspect of the foot and toes (Fig. 3.19).

Knee joint

The knee joint is the largest synovial joint in the body. It is a condylar joint and consists of:

- The articulation between the femur and tibia, which is weight-bearing.
- The articulation between the patella and the femur, which allows the pull of the quadriceps femoris muscle to be directed anteriorly over the knee to the tibia without tendon wear (Fig. 3.69).

Two fibrocartilaginous menisci, one on each side, between the femoral condyles and tibia accommodate changes in the shape of the articular surfaces during joint movements.

The detailed movements of the knee joint are complex, but basically the joint is a modified hinge joint that allows mainly flexion and extension. Like all hinge joints, the knee joint is reinforced by collateral ligaments, one on each side of the joint. In addition, two very strong ligaments (the cruciate ligaments) interconnect the adjacent ends of the femur and tibia and maintain their opposed positions during movement.

Because the knee joint is involved in weight-bearing, it has an efficient "locking" mechanism to reduce the amount of muscle energy required to keep the joint extended when standing.

Articular surfaces

The articular surfaces of the bones that contribute to the knee joint are covered by hyaline cartilage. The major surfaces involved include:

- The two femoral condyles
- The adjacent surfaces of the superior aspect of the tibial condyles

The surfaces of the femoral condyles that articulate with the tibia in flexion of the knee are curved or round, whereas the surfaces that articulate in full extension are flat (Fig. 3.70).

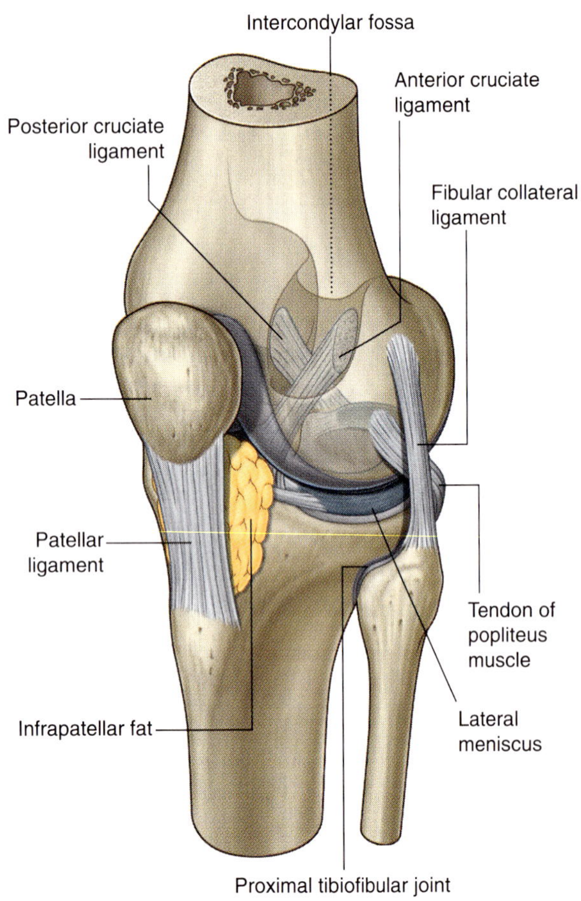

Fig. 3.69 Knee joint. Joint capsule is not shown.

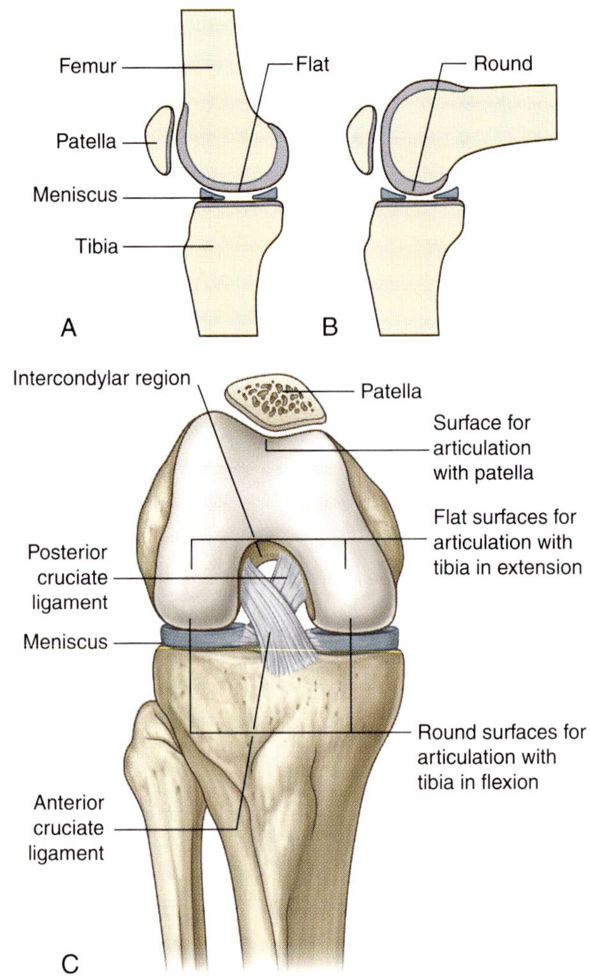

Fig. 3.70 Articular surfaces of the knee joint. **(A)** Extended. **(B)** Flexed. **(C)** Anterior view (flexed).

The articular surfaces between the femur and patella are the V-shaped trench on the anterior surface of the distal end of the femur where the two condyles join and the adjacent surfaces on the posterior aspect of the patella. The joint surfaces are all enclosed within a single articular cavity, as are the intra-articular menisci between the femoral and tibial condyles.

Menisci

There are two menisci, which are fibrocartilaginous C-shaped cartilages, in the knee joint, one medial (**medial meniscus**) and the other lateral (**lateral meniscus**) (Fig. 3.71). Both are attached at each end to facets in the intercondylar region of the tibial plateau.

The medial meniscus is attached around its margin to the capsule of the joint and to the tibial collateral ligament, whereas the lateral meniscus is unattached to the capsule. Therefore, the lateral meniscus is more mobile than the medial meniscus.

The menisci are interconnected anteriorly by a transverse ligament of the knee. The lateral meniscus is also connected to the tendon of the popliteus muscle, which passes superolaterally between this meniscus and the capsule to attach to the femur.

The menisci improve congruency between the femoral and tibial condyles during joint movements where the surfaces of the femoral condyles articulating with the tibial plateau change from small curved surfaces in flexion to large flat surfaces in extension.

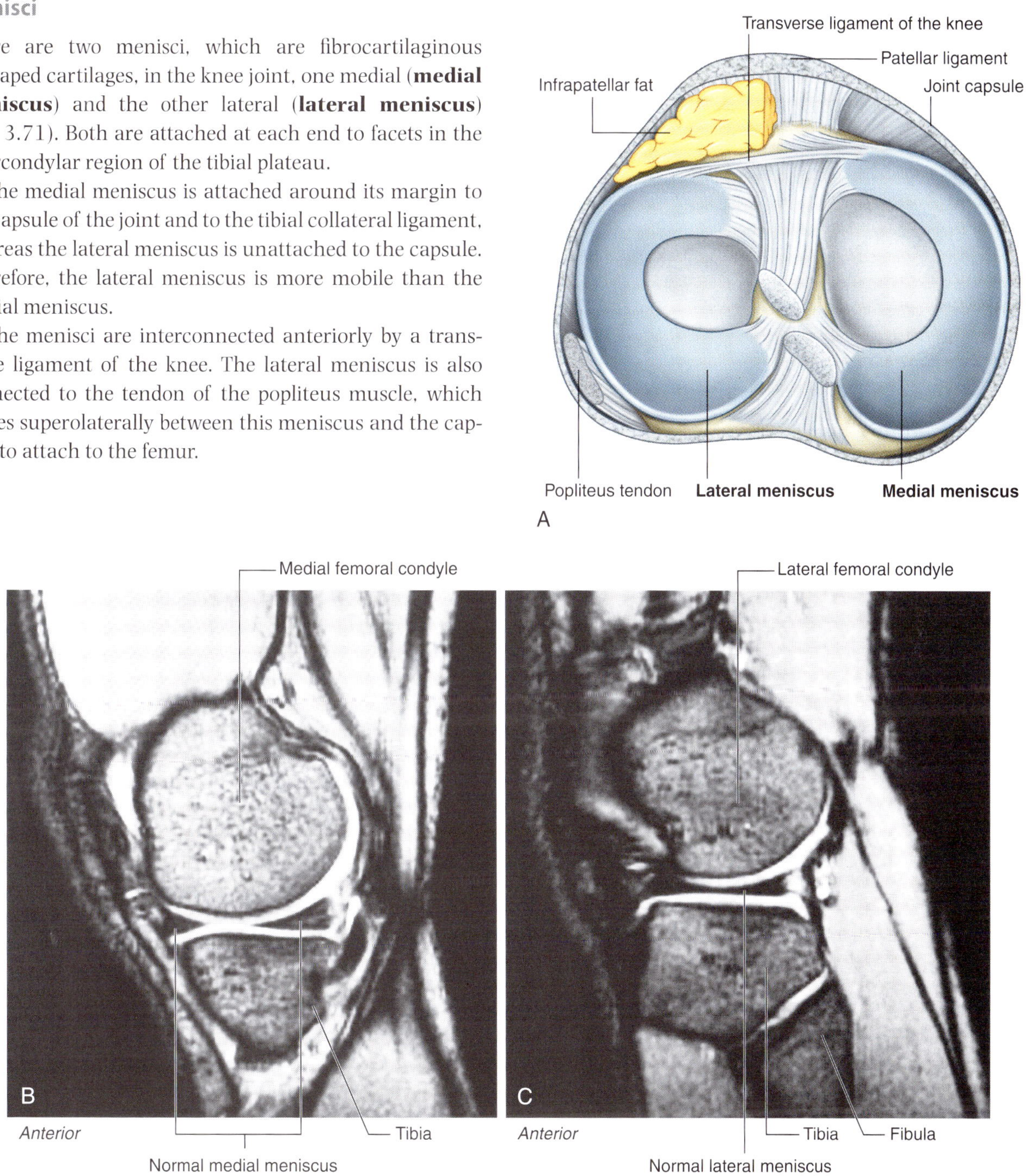

Fig. 3.71 Menisci of the knee joint. **(A)** Superior view. Menisci of the knee joint. **(B)** Normal knee joint showing the medial meniscus. **(C)** Normal knee joint showing the lateral meniscus.

Continued

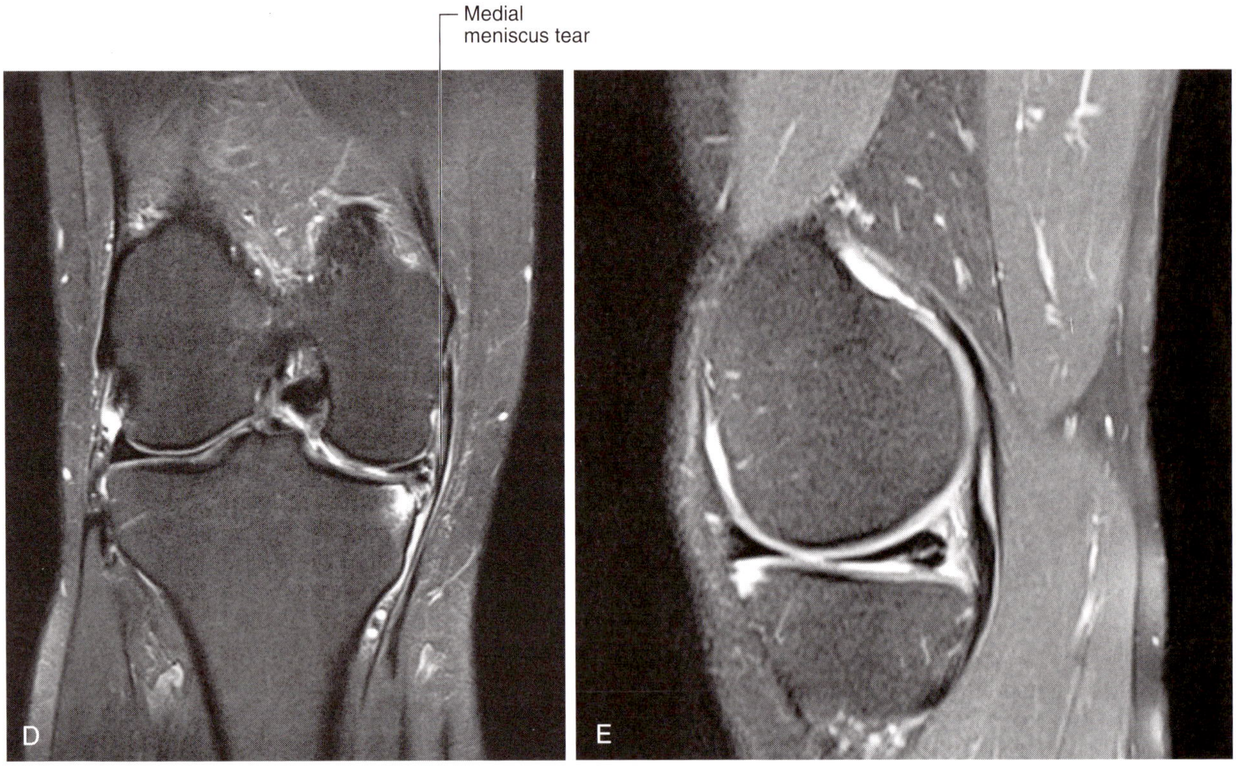

Fig. 3.71, cont'd (D) Sagittal MRI of a knee joint showing tear of the medial meniscus. **(E)** Coronal MRI of a knee showing a truncated lateral meniscus after partial meniscectomy to treat a tear.

Early clinical exposure

Meniscal injuries

Menisci can get torn during forceful rotation or twisting of the knee, but significant trauma is not always necessary for a tear to occur. There are various patterns of meniscal tearing depending on the cleavage plane such as vertical tears (perpendicular to the tibial plateau), horizontal tears (parallel to the long axis of the meniscus and perpendicular to the tibial plateau), or bucket handle tears (longitudinal tear where the torn portion of the meniscus forms a handle-shaped fragment which gets displaced into the intercondylar notch).

The patient usually complains of pain localized to the medial or lateral side of the knee, knee locking or clicking, sensation of knee giving way, and swelling, which can be intermittent and usually delayed.

MRI is the modality of choice to assess meniscal tears and detect other associated injuries, such as ligamentous tears and articular cartilage damage (Fig. 3.71E). Arthroscopy is usually performed to repair a tear, debride the damaged meniscal material, or rarely remove the entire torn meniscus (Fig. 3.71E).

Synovial membrane

The synovial membrane of the knee joint attaches to the margins of the articular surfaces and to the superior and inferior outer margins of the menisci (Fig. 3.72A). The two cruciate ligaments, which attach in the intercondylar region of the tibia below and the intercondylar fossa of the femur above, are outside the articular cavity, but enclosed within the fibrous membrane of the knee joint.

Posteriorly, the synovial membrane reflects off the fibrous membrane of the joint capsule on either side of the posterior cruciate ligament and loops forward around both ligaments, thereby excluding them from the synovial-lined articular cavity. The joint cavity contains only synovial fluid.

Anteriorly, the synovial membrane is separated from the patellar ligament by an **infrapatellar fat pad**. On each side of the pad, the synovial membrane forms a fringed margin (an **alar fold**), which projects into the articular cavity. In addition, the synovial membrane covering the upper part of the infrapatellar fat pad is raised into a sharp midline fold directed posteriorly (the **infrapatellar synovial fold**), which attaches to the margin of the intercondylar fossa of the femur.

The synovial membrane of the knee joint forms pouches in two locations to provide low-friction surfaces for the movement of tendons associated with the joint:

- The smallest of these expansions is the **subpopliteal recess** (Fig. 3.72A), which extends posterolaterally from the articular cavity and lies between the lateral meniscus and the tendon of the popliteus muscle, which passes through the joint capsule.
- The second expansion is the **suprapatellar bursa** (Fig. 3.72B), a large bursa that is a continuation of the articular cavity superiorly between the distal end of the shaft of the femur and the quadriceps femoris muscle and tendon—the apex of this bursa is attached to the small articularis genus muscle, which pulls the bursa away from the joint during extension of the knee.

Other bursae associated with the knee but not normally communicating with the articular cavity include the subcutaneous prepatellar bursa, deep and subcutaneous infrapatellar bursae, and numerous other bursae associated with tendons and ligaments around the joint (Fig. 3.72B).

The prepatellar bursa is subcutaneous and anterior to the patella. The deep and subcutaneous infrapatellar bursae are on the deep and subcutaneous sides of the patellar ligament, respectively.

Fibrous membrane

The fibrous membrane or fibrous capsule of the knee joint is extensive and is partly formed and reinforced by extensions from tendons of the surrounding muscles (Fig. 3.73). In general, the fibrous membrane encloses the articular cavity and the intercondylar region:

- On the medial side of the knee joint, the fibrous membrane blends with the tibial collateral ligament and is attached on its internal surface to the medial meniscus.
- Laterally, the external surface of the fibrous membrane is separated by a space from the fibular collateral ligament and the internal surface of the fibrous membrane is not attached to the lateral meniscus.
- Anteriorly, the fibrous membrane is attached to the margins of the patella where it is reinforced with tendinous expansions from the vastus lateralis and vastus medialis muscles. The fibrous membrane also merges above with the quadriceps femoris tendon and below with the patellar ligament.

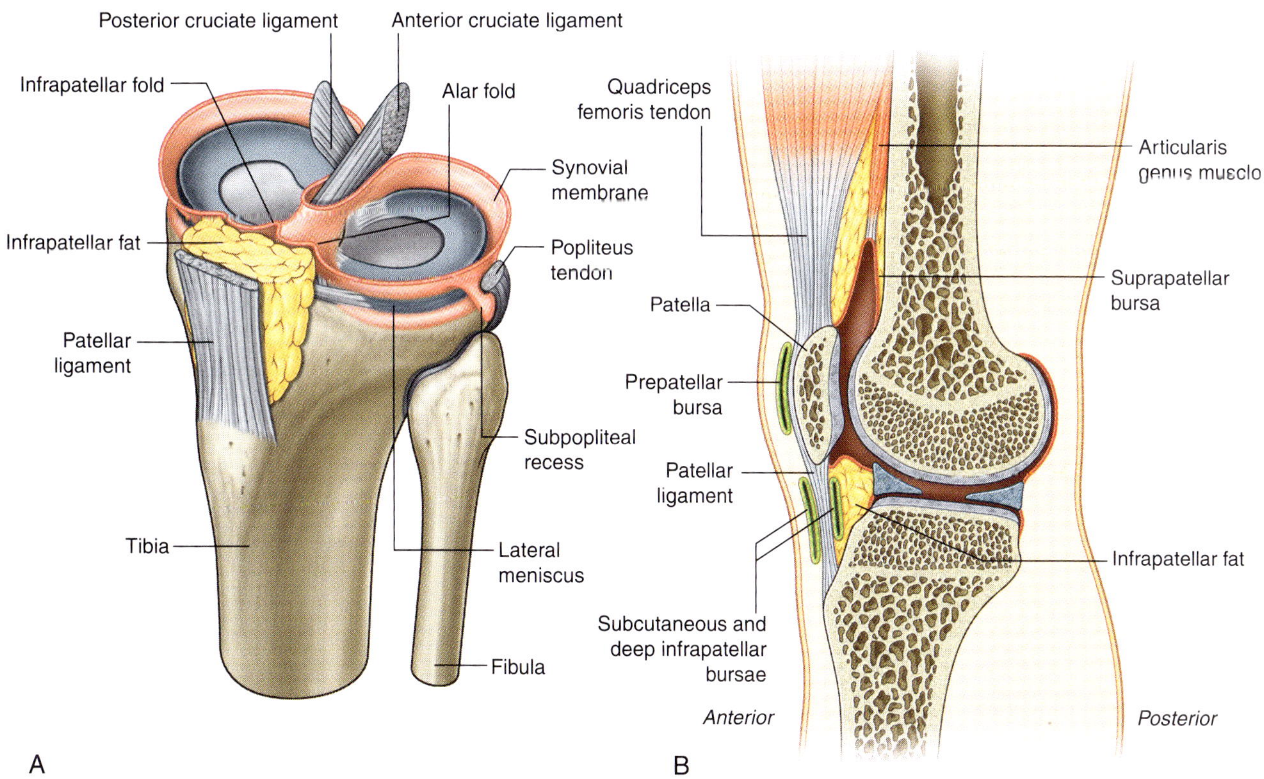

Fig. 3.72 Synovial membrane of the knee joint and associated bursae. **(A)** Superolateral view; patella and femur not shown. **(B)** Paramedial sagittal section through the knee.

The fibrous membrane is reinforced anterolaterally by a fibrous extension from the iliotibial tract and posteromedially by an extension from the tendon of the semimembranosus (the **oblique popliteal ligament**), which reflects superolaterally across the back of the fibrous membrane.

The upper end of the popliteus muscle passes through an aperture in the posterolateral aspect of the fibrous membrane of the knee and is enclosed by the fibrous membrane as its synovial-lined tendon travels around the joint to insert on the lateral aspect of the lateral femoral condyle. The tendons of this muscle along with the menisci and cruciate ligaments are intracapsular and extrasynovial.

Ligaments

The major ligaments associated with the knee joint are the patellar ligament, the tibial (medial) and fibular (lateral) collateral ligaments, and the anterior and posterior cruciate ligaments.

Patellar ligament

The **patellar ligament** is basically the continuation of the quadriceps femoris tendon inferior to the patella (Fig. 3.73). It is attached to the margins and apex of the patella superiorly and to the tibial tuberosity inferiorly.

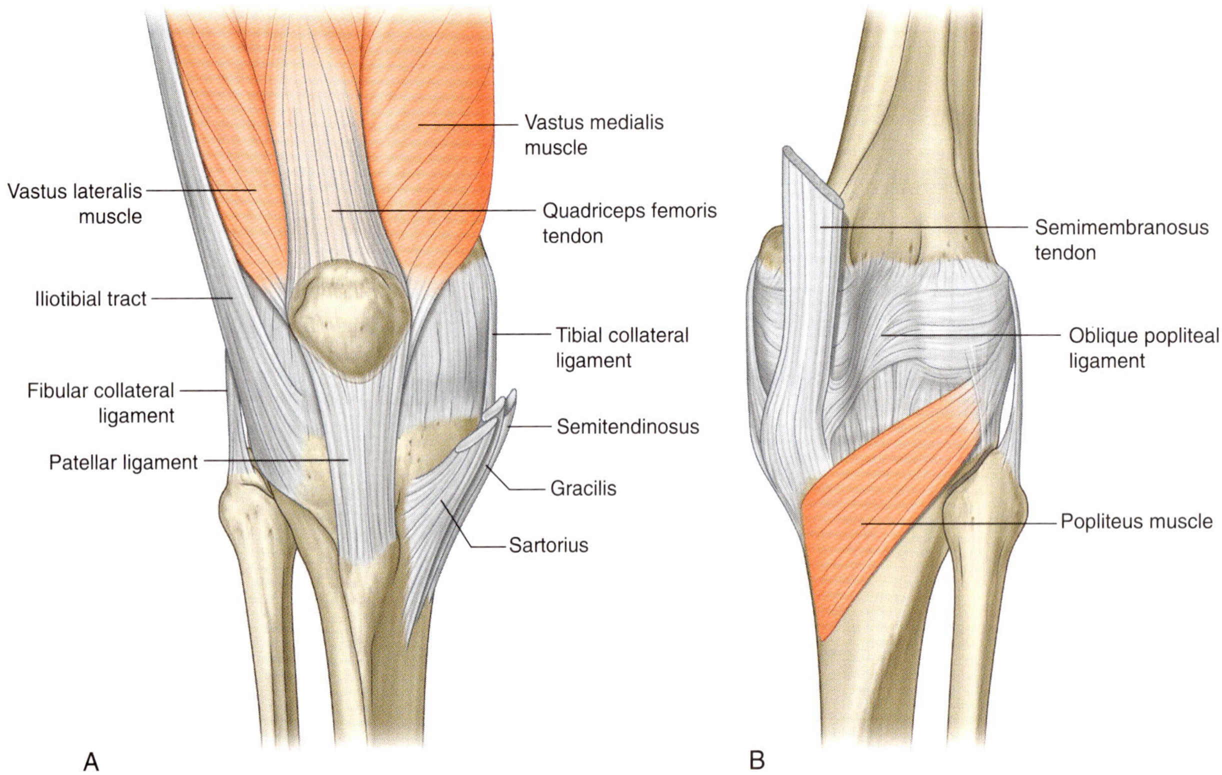

Fig. 3.73 Fibrous membrane of the knee joint capsule. **(A)** Anterior view. **(B)** Posterior view.

Collateral ligaments

The collateral ligaments, one on each side of the joint, stabilize the hinge-like motion of the knee (Fig. 3.74).

The cord-like **fibular collateral ligament** is attached superiorly to the lateral femoral epicondyle just above the groove for the popliteus tendon. Inferiorly, it is attached to a depression on the lateral surface of the fibular head. It is separated from the fibrous membrane by a bursa.

The broad and flat **tibial collateral ligament** is attached by much of its deep surface to the underlying fibrous membrane. It is anchored superiorly to the medial femoral epicondyle just inferior to the adductor tubercle and descends anteriorly to attach to the medial margin of the medial condyle and medial surface of the tibia above and behind the attachment of the sartorius, gracilis, and semitendinosus tendons.

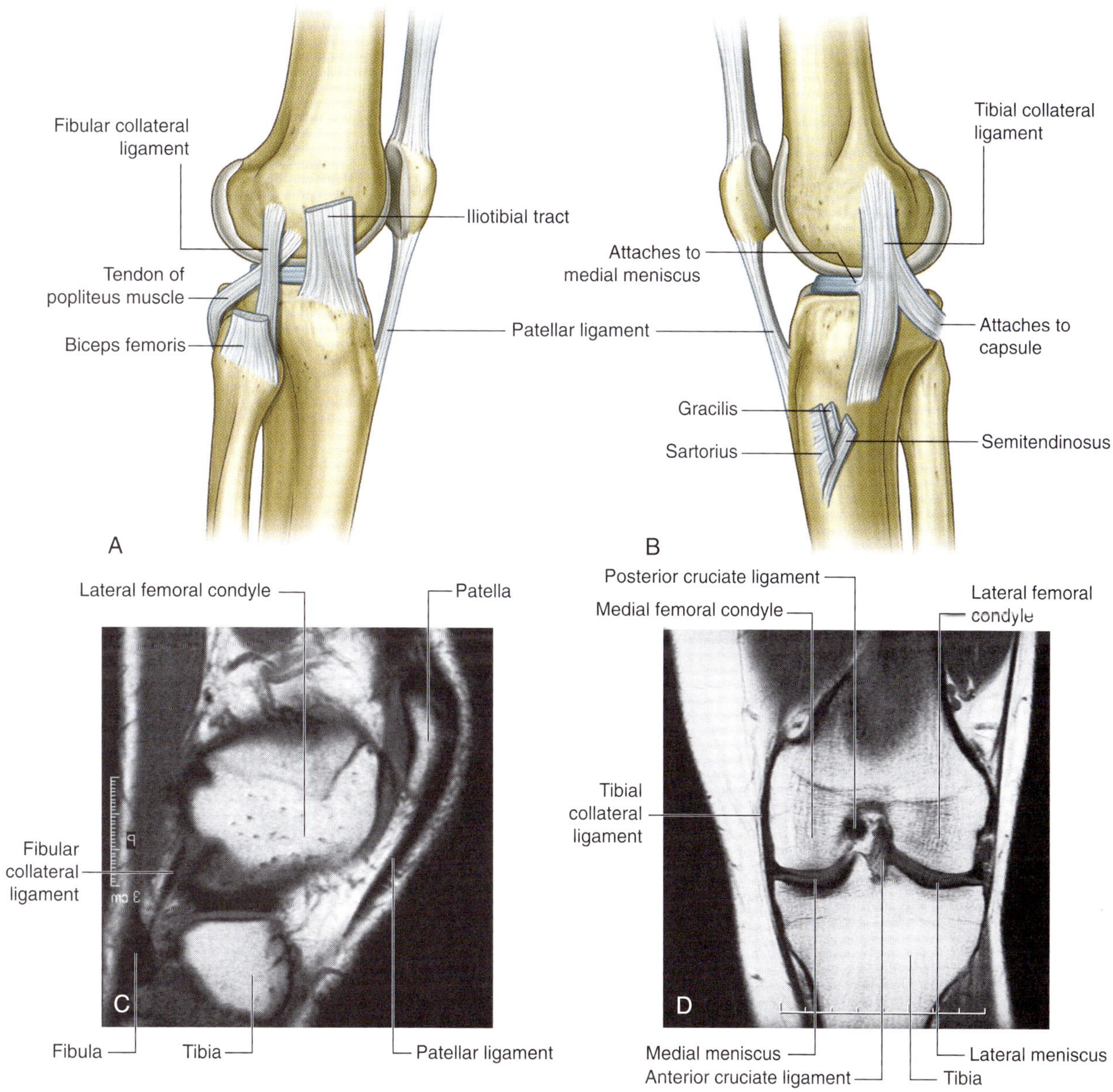

Fig. 3.74 Collateral ligaments of the knee joint. **(A)** Lateral view. **(B)** Medial view. **(C)** Normal knee joint showing the patellar ligament and the fibular collateral ligament. T1-weighted magnetic resonance image in the sagittal plane. **(D)** Normal knee joint showing the tibial collateral ligament, the medial and lateral menisci, and the anterior and posterior cruciate ligaments. T1-weighted magnetic resonance image in the coronal plane.

Cruciate ligaments

The two cruciate ligaments are in the intercondylar region of the knee and interconnect the femur and tibia (Fig. 3.74D and 3.75). They are termed "cruciate" (Latin for "shaped like a cross") because they cross each other in the sagittal plane between their femoral and tibial attachments:

- The **anterior cruciate ligament** attaches to a facet on the anterior part of the intercondylar area of the tibia and ascends posteriorly to attach to a facet at the back of the lateral wall of the intercondylar fossa of the femur.
- The **posterior cruciate ligament** attaches to the posterior aspect of the intercondylar area of the tibia and ascends anteriorly to attach to the medial wall of the intercondylar fossa of the femur.

The anterior cruciate ligament crosses lateral to the posterior cruciate ligament as they pass through the intercondylar region.

The anterior cruciate ligament prevents anterior displacement of the tibia relative to the femur and the posterior cruciate ligament restricts posterior displacement (Fig. 3.75).

Locking mechanism

When standing, the knee joint is locked into position, thereby reducing the amount of muscle work needed to maintain the standing position (Fig. 3.76).

One component of the locking mechanism is a change in the shape and size of the femoral surfaces that articulate with the tibia:

- In flexion, the surfaces are the curved and rounded areas on the posterior aspects of the femoral condyles.
- As the knee is extended, the surfaces move to the broad and flat areas on the inferior aspects of the femoral condyles.

Consequently, the joint surfaces become larger and more stable in extension.

Another component of the locking mechanism is medial rotation of the femur on the tibia during extension. Medial rotation and full extension tightens all the associated ligaments.

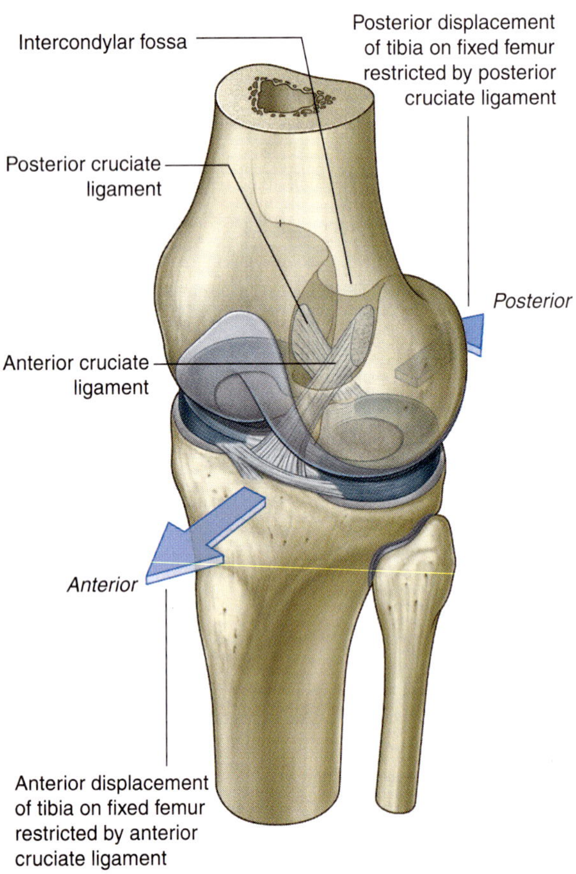

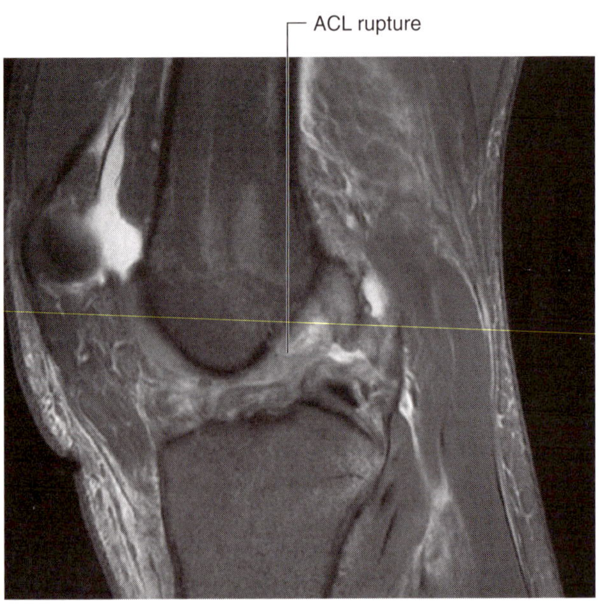

Fig. 3.75 **(A)** Cruciate ligaments of the knee joint. Superolateral view. **(B)** Sagittal MRI of knee joint showing rupture of the anterior cruciate ligament.

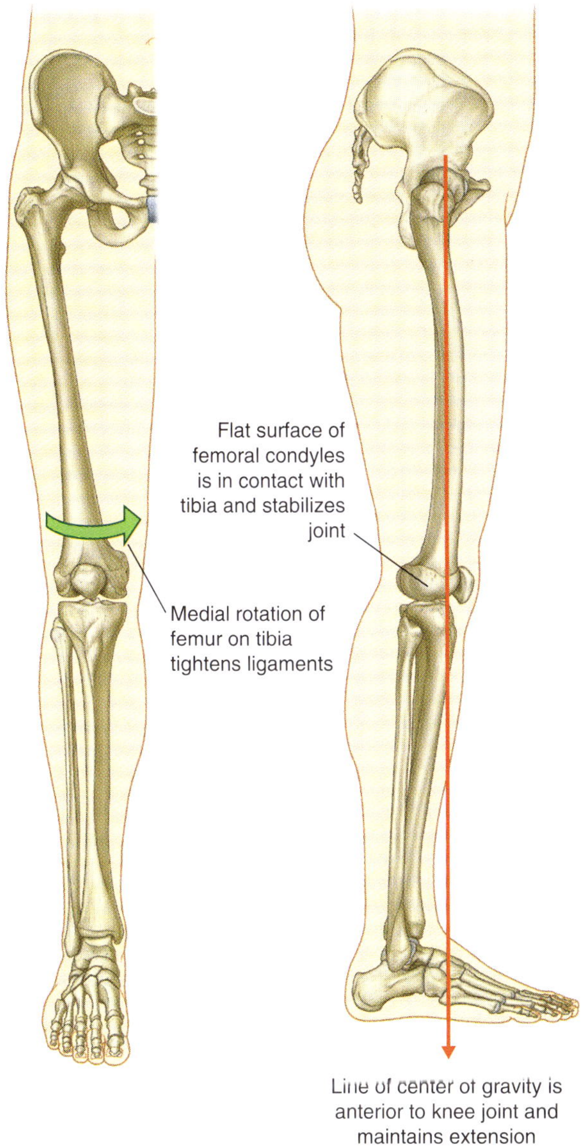

Fig. 3.76 Knee "locking" mechanism.

Another feature that keeps the knee extended when standing is that the body's center of gravity is positioned along a vertical line that passes anterior to the knee joint.

The popliteus muscle unlocks the knee by initiating lateral rotation of the femur on the tibia.

Vascular supply and innervation

Vascular supply to the knee joint is predominantly through descending and genicular branches from the femoral, popliteal, and lateral circumflex femoral arteries in the thigh and the circumflex fibular artery and recurrent branches from the anterior tibial artery in the leg. These vessels form an anastomotic network around the joint (Fig. 3.77).

The knee joint is innervated by branches from the obturator, femoral, tibial, and common fibular nerves.

The Q angle of the knee is the angle formed by a line drawn from the anterior superior iliac spine to the center of the patella and a second line drawn from the center of the patella to the tibial tubercle. An increased Q angle is a risk factor for patellar subluxation.

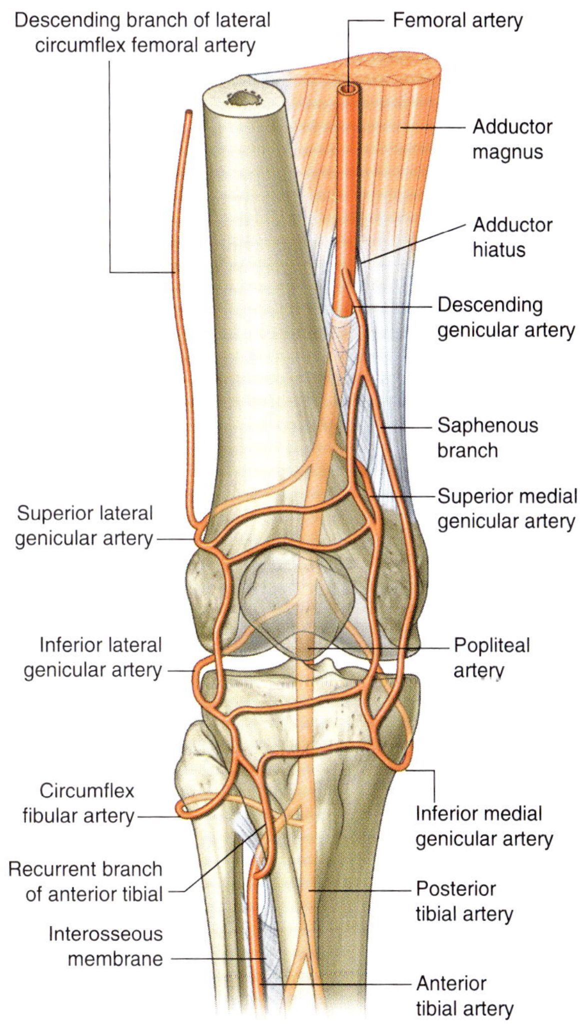

Fig. 3.77 Anastomoses of arteries around the knee. Anterior view.

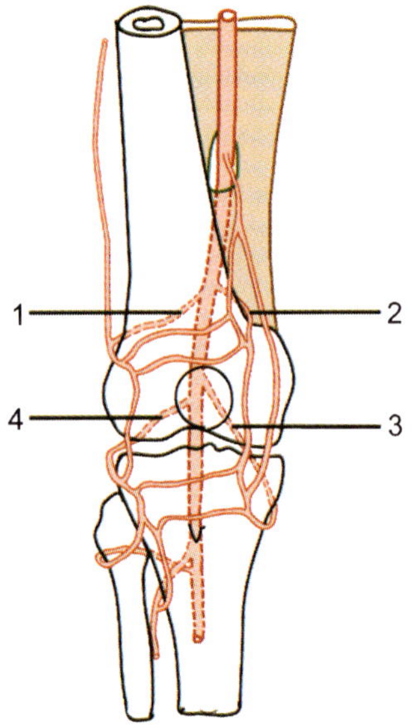

LD Fig. 3.77.1 Anastomosis around the knee.
Questions
3.77.1A Name the labeled structures.
3.77.1B What are these arteries branches of?
3.77.1C Name the other arteries involved in this anastomosis, and what are they branches of?

Answers
3.77.1A The labeled structures are
1. Superior lateral genicular artery
2. Superior medial genicular artery
3. Inferior medial genicular artery
4. Inferior lateral genicular artery

3.77.1B These arteries are branches of the popliteal artery.
3.77.1C The other arteries involved in this anastomosis and what each of them is a branch of are:
Descending genicular artery-branch of the lateral circumflex artery
Descending genicular artery-branch of the femoral artery
Middle genicular artery-branch of the popliteal artery
Recurrent genicular artery-branch of the anterior tibial artery
Circumflex fibular artery-branch of the posterior tibial artery

Early clinical exposure

Collateral ligament injuries

The collateral ligaments are responsible for stabilizing the knee joint, controlling its sideway movements, and protecting the knee from excessive motion.

Injury to the fibular collateral ligament occurs when excessive outward force is applied to the medial side of the knee (varus force), and is less common than an injury to the tibial collateral ligament that is damaged when excessive force is applied inward to the lateral side of the joint (valgus force). Injuries to the tibial collateral ligament can be part of a so-called "unhappy triad" that also involves tears of the medial meniscus and the anterior cruciate ligament (ACL).

The spectrum of injuries to collateral ligaments of the knee ranges from minor sprains where the ligaments are slightly stretched, but still able to stabilize the knee joint, to full thickness tears where all fibers are torn and the ligaments lose their stabilizing function.

Cruciate ligament injuries

The ACL is most frequently injured during noncontact activities when there is a sudden change in the direction of movement (cutting or pivoting). Contact sports may also result in ACL injury due to sudden twisting, hyperextension, and valgus force related to direct collision. The injury usually affects the midportion of the ligament and manifests itself as a complete or partial discontinuity of the fibers or abnormal orientation and contour of the ligament. With an acute ACL tear, a sudden click or pop can be heard and the knee becomes rapidly swollen. Several tests are used to clinically assess the injury, and the diagnosis is usually confirmed by MRI. A full thickness ACL tear causes instability of the knee joint. The treatment depends on the desired level of activity of the patient. In those with high activity levels, surgical reconstruction of the ligament is required. Those with low activity levels may opt for knee bracing and physiotherapy; however, in the long term, the internal damage to the knee leads to the development of early osteoarthritis.

A tear to the posterior cruciate ligament (PCL) requires significant force, so it rarely occurs in isolation. It usually occurs during hyperextension of the knee or as a result of a direct blow to a bent knee such as when striking the knee against the dashboard in a motor vehicle accident. Typically, the injury presents as posterior displacement of the tibia on physical examination (the so-called tibial sag sign). Patients complain of knee pain and swelling, inability to bear weight, and instability. The diagnosis is confirmed on MRI. The management, as in ACL injury, depends on the degree of the injury (sprain, partial thickness, full thickness) and the level of desired activity.

Any soft tissue injury at and around the knee joint may involve the neurovascular bundle, and assessment of neurovascular structures is critical in the management of patients with injury to the soft tissues.

Early clinical exposure

Degenerative joint disease/osteoarthritis

Degenerative joint disease occurs in many joints in the body. Articular degeneration may result from an abnormal force across the joint with a normal cartilage or a normal force with abnormal cartilage.

Typically degenerative joint disease occurs in synovial joints and the process is called **osteoarthritis**. In the joints where osteoarthritis occurs, the cartilage and bony tissues are usually involved, with limited change within the synovial membrane. The typical findings include reduction in the joint space, eburnation (joint sclerosis), osteophytosis (small bony outgrowths), and bony cyst formation. As the disease progresses, the joint may become malaligned, its movement may become severely limited, and there may be significant pain.

The commonest sites for osteoarthritis include the small joints of the hands and wrist, and in the lower limb, the hip and knee are typically affected, though the tarsometatarsal and metatarsophalangeal articulations may undergo similar change.

The etiology of degenerative joint disease is unclear, but there are some associations, including genetic predisposition, increasing age (males tend to be affected younger than females), overuse or underuse of joints, and nutritional and metabolic abnormalities. Further factors include joint trauma and preexisting articular disease or deformity.

The histological findings of osteoarthritis consist of degenerative changes within the cartilage and the subchondral bone. Further articular damage worsens these changes, which promote further abnormal stresses upon the joint. As the disease progresses, the typical finding is pain, which is usually worse on rising from bed and at the end of a day's activity. Commonly it is aggravated by the extremes of movement or unaccustomed exertion. Stiffness and limitation of movement may ensue.

Treatment in the first instance includes alteration of lifestyle to prevent pain and simple analgesia. As symptoms progress, a joint replacement may be necessary, but although joint replacement appears to be the panacea for degenerative joint disease, it is not without risks and complications, which include infection and failure in the short and long term.

Early clinical exposure

Examination of the knee joint

It is important to establish the nature of the patient's complaint before any examination. The history should include information about the complaint, the signs and symptoms, and the patient's lifestyle (level of activity). This history may give a significant clue to the type of injury and the likely findings on clinical examination, for example, if the patient was kicked just below the medial aspect of the knee, a valgus deformity (the bone distal to the joint is directed outward) injury to the tibial collateral ligament might be suspected.

The examination should include assessment in the erect position, while walking, and on the couch. The affected side must be compared with the unaffected side.

There are many tests and techniques for examining the knee joint, including the following.

Tests for anterior instability

- Lachman's test—the patient lies on the couch. The examiner places one hand around the distal femur and the other around the proximal tibia and then elevates the knee, producing 20° of flexion. The patient's heel rests on the couch. The examiner's thumb must be on the tibial tuberosity. The hand on the tibia applies a brisk anteriorly directed force. If the movement of the tibia on the femur comes to a sudden stop, it is a firm end point. If it does not come to a sudden stop, the end point is described as soft and is associated with a tear of the anterior cruciate ligament.
- Anterior drawer test—a positive anterior drawer test is when the upper end of a patient's tibia can be pulled anteriorly on the femur. The patient lies supine on the couch. The knee is flexed to 90° and the heel and sole of the foot are placed on the couch. The examiner sits gently on the patient's foot, which has been placed in a neutral position. The index fingers are used to check that the hamstrings are relaxed while the other fingers encircle the upper end of the tibia and pull the tibia. If the tibia moves forward, the anterior cruciate ligament is torn. Other peripheral structures, such as the medial meniscus or meniscotibial ligaments, must also be damaged to elicit this sign.

Tests for posterior instability

- Posterior drawer test—a positive posterior drawer test occurs when the proximal head of a patient's tibia can be pushed posteriorly on the femur. The patient is placed in a supine position and the knee is flexed to approximately 90° with the foot in the neutral position. The examiner sits gently on the patient's foot placing both thumbs on the tibial tuberosity and pushing the tibia backward. If the tibial plateau moves, the posterior cruciate ligament is torn.

Early clinical exposure—cont'd

Assessment of other structures of the knee

- Assessment of the tibial collateral ligament can be performed by placing a valgus stress on the knee.
- Assessment of lateral and posterolateral knee structures requires more complex clinical testing.

The knee will also be assessed for:

- Joint line tenderness
- Patellofemoral movement and instability
- Presence of an effusion
- Muscle injury
- Popliteal fossa masses

Further investigations

After the clinical examination has been carried out, further investigations usually include **plain radiography** and possibly **magnetic resonance imaging**, which allows the radiologist to assess the menisci, cruciate ligaments, collateral ligaments, bony and cartilaginous surfaces, and soft tissues.

Arthroscopy may be carried out and damage to any internal structures repaired or trimmed. An arthroscope is a small camera that is placed into the knee joint through the anterolateral or anteromedial aspect of the knee joint. The joint is filled with a saline solution and the telescope is manipulated around the knee joint to assess the cruciate ligaments, menisci, and cartilaginous surfaces (see Fig. 1.25B).

Early clinical exposure

Anterolateral ligament of the knee

A ligament associated at its origin with the fibular collateral ligament of the knee has been described. This ligament (anterolateral ligament of the knee) courses from the lateral femoral epicondyle to the anterolateral region of the proximal end of the tibia and may control internal rotation of the tibia (*J Anat* 2013;223:321–328).

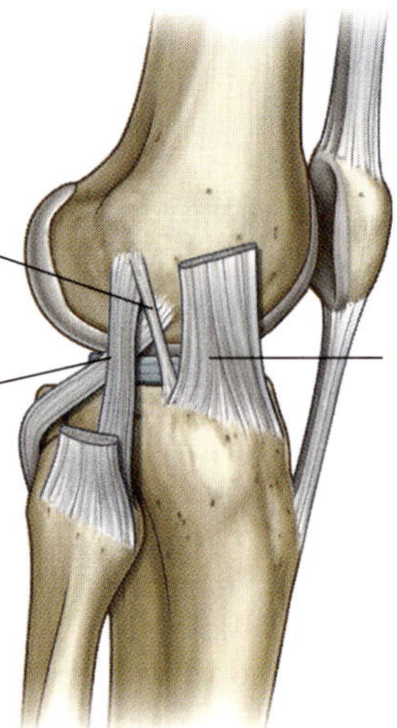

Tibiofibular joint

The small proximal tibiofibular joint is plane synovial in type and allows very little movement (Fig. 3.78). The opposing joint surfaces, on the undersurface of the lateral condyle of the tibia and on the superomedial surface of the head of the fibula, are flat and circular. The capsule is reinforced by anterior and posterior ligaments.

Popliteal fossa

The **popliteal fossa** is an important area of transition between the thigh and leg and is the major route by which structures pass from one region to the other.

The popliteal fossa is a diamond-shaped space behind the knee joint formed between muscles in the posterior compartments of the thigh and leg (Fig. 3.79A):

- The margins of the upper part of the diamond are formed medially by the distal ends of the semitendinosus and semimembranosus muscles and laterally by the distal end of the biceps femoris muscle.

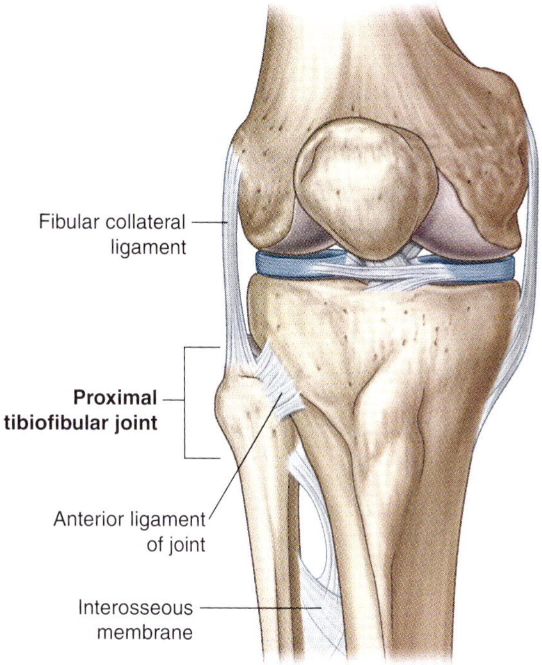

Fig. 3.78 Proximal tibiofibular joint.

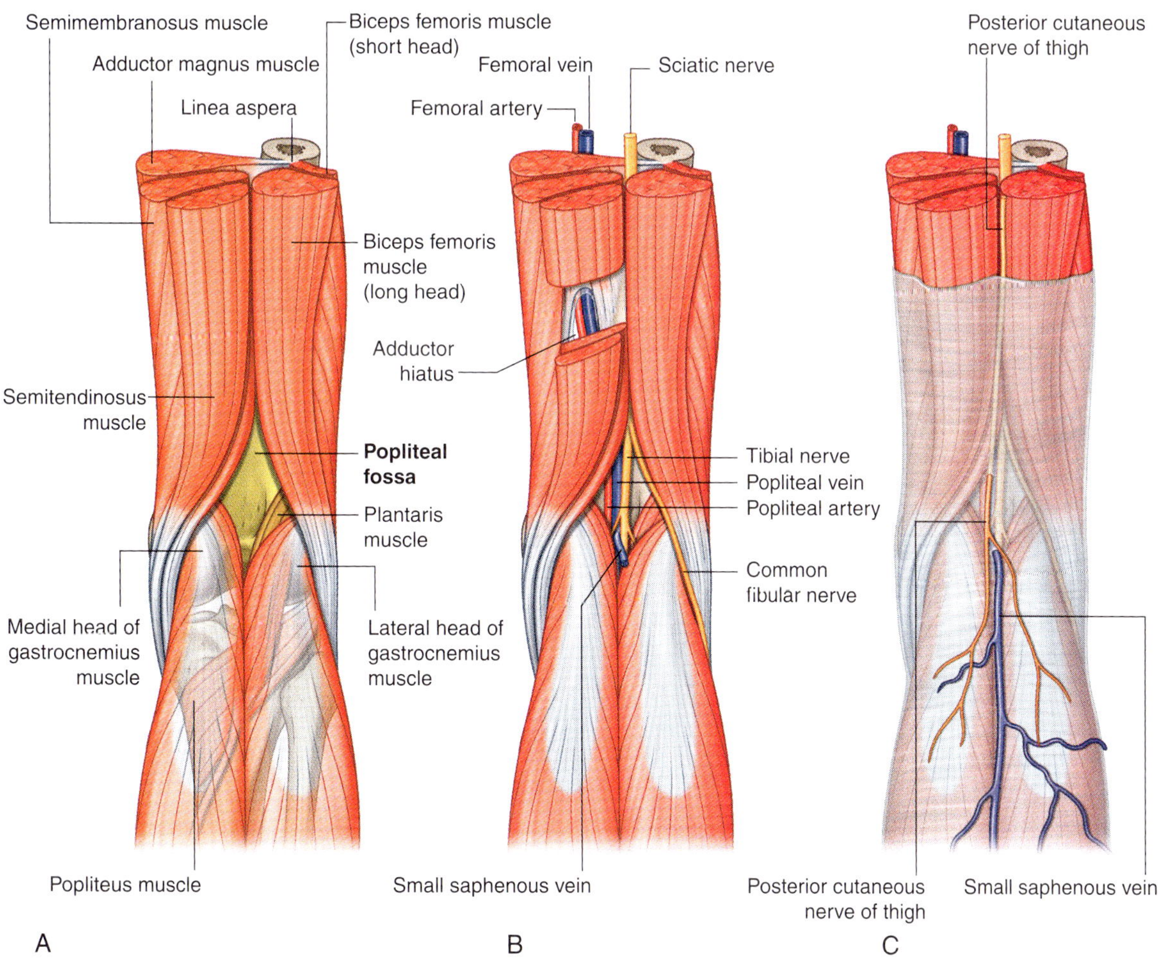

Fig. 3.79 Popliteal fossa. **(A)** Boundaries. **(B)** Nerves and vessels. **(C)** Superficial structures.

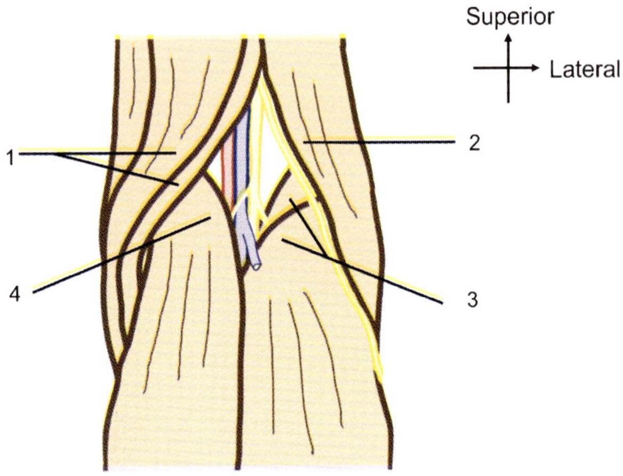

LD Fig. 3.79.1 Popliteal fossa.

Questions

3.79.1A Name the labeled structures and name the boundary of the popliteal fossa that each of them forms.

3.79.1B List the contents of this fossa in order.

3.79.1C Name one muscle that is seen in the floor of this fossa.

Answers

3.79.1A The labelled structures and the boundary of the popliteal fossa that each one of them forms is:

1. Semitendinosus and semimembranosus, superomedial boundary
2. Biceps femoris, superolateral boundary
3. Medial head of gastrocnemius, inferomedial boundary
4. Lateral head of gastrocnemius and plantaris, inferolateral boundary

3.79.1B The contents of the popliteal fossa in order from deep to superficial are: the popliteal artery, popliteal vein, and tibial nerve.

Other contents include the common fibular nerve, the posterior cutaneous nerve of the thigh, the small saphenous vein, the branches and tributaries of these structures, popliteal lymph nodes, and a variable amount of fat.

3.79.1C One muscle that is seen in the floor of this fossa is the popliteus.

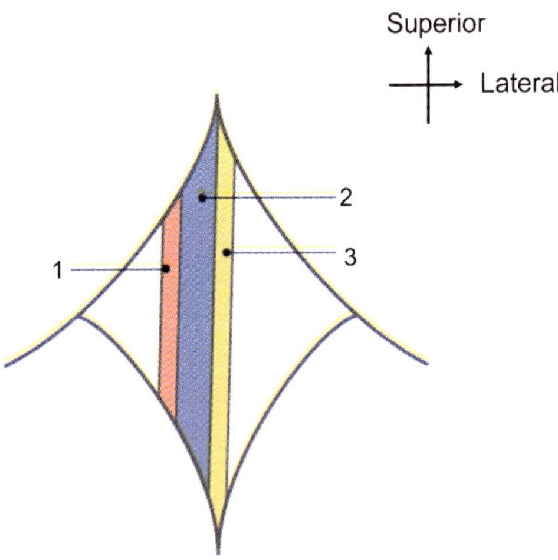

LD Fig. 3.79.2 Contents of the popliteal fossa.

Questions

3.79.2A Name the structures indicated by the labels.

3.79.2B What is the relation of these structures to each other?

Answers

3.79.2A The structures indicated by the labels are the:

1. Popliteal artery
2. Popliteal vein
3. Tibial nerve

3.79.2B These structures lie in order from medial to lateral and deep to superficial are the popliteal artery, popliteal vein, and tibial nerve.

- The margins of the smaller lower part of the space are formed medially by the medial head of the gastrocnemius muscle and laterally by the plantaris muscle and the lateral head of the gastrocnemius muscle.
- The floor of the fossa is formed by the capsule of the knee joint and adjacent surfaces of the femur and tibia, and, more inferiorly, by the popliteus muscle.
- The roof is formed by deep fascia, which is continuous above with the fascia lata of the thigh and below with deep fascia of the leg.

Contents

The major contents of the popliteal fossa are the popliteal artery, the popliteal vein, and the tibial and common fibular nerves (Fig. 3.79B).

Tibial and common fibular nerves

The tibial and common fibular nerves originate proximal to the popliteal fossa as the two major branches of the sciatic nerve. They are the most superficial of the neurovascular structures in the popliteal fossa and enter the region directly from above under the margin of the biceps femoris muscle:

- The tibial nerve descends vertically through the popliteal fossa and exits by passing deep to the margin of the plantaris muscle to enter the posterior compartment of the leg.
- The common fibular nerve exits by following the biceps femoris tendon over the lower lateral margin of the popliteal fossa. This nerve continues to the lateral side of the leg where it swings around the neck of the fibula and enters the lateral compartment of the leg.

Popliteal artery and vein

The popliteal artery is the continuation of the femoral artery in the anterior compartment of the thigh, and begins as the femoral artery passes posteriorly through the adductor hiatus in the adductor magnus muscle.

The popliteal artery appears in the popliteal fossa on the upper medial side under the margin of the semimembranosus muscle. It descends obliquely through the fossa with the tibial nerve and enters the posterior compartment of the leg where it ends just lateral to the midline of the leg by dividing into the anterior and posterior tibial arteries.

The popliteal artery is the deepest of the neurovascular structures in the popliteal fossa and is therefore difficult to palpate; however, a pulse can usually be detected by deep palpation near the midline.

In the popliteal fossa, the popliteal artery gives rise to branches, which supply adjacent muscles, and to a series of geniculate arteries, which contribute to vascular anastomoses around the knee.

The popliteal vein is superficial to and travels with the popliteal artery. It exits the popliteal fossa superiorly to become the femoral vein by passing through the adductor hiatus.

Roof of popliteal fossa

The roof of the popliteal fossa is covered by superficial fascia and skin (Fig. 3.79C). The most important structure in the superficial fascia is the small saphenous vein. This vessel ascends vertically in the superficial fascia on the back of the leg from the lateral side of the dorsal venous arch in the foot. It ascends to the back of the knee where it penetrates **deep fascia**, which forms the roof of the popliteal fossa, and joins with the popliteal vein.

One other structure that passes through the roof of the fossa is the posterior cutaneous nerve of the thigh, which descends through the thigh superficial to the hamstring muscles, passes through the roof of the popliteal fossa, and then continues inferiorly with the small saphenous vein to innervate skin on the upper half of the back of the leg.

LEG

SET INDUCTION—CASE SCENARIO 4: VARICOSE VEINS

A 64-year-old man presented to the outpatient department with swelling of the left foot and complaints of dilated and tortuous veins of the legs. A diagnosis of varicose veins was made, and a plan was made to surgically remove the dilated veins.

Knowledge of the anatomy of the veins of the leg is important to be able to manage a patient with varicose veins.

OUTLINE 4. LEG—LEARNING OBJECTIVES
[By the end of this section the student should be able to:]

REMEMBER [Recall Facts]	DEMONSTRATE AND ANALYZE RELATIONSHIPS [Identify structures in a Prosected Specimen or Figure]		
	Level I	**Level II**	**Level III**
1. Mention the areas drained by the popliteal lymph nodes 2. Describe in detail the small saphenous vein 3. Describe in detail the ankle joint 4. Describe briefly the superior and inferior tibiofibular joints 5. List the names of the compartments of the leg and mention the nerve that supplies the muscles in each one 6. List the muscles of the leg and mention their origin, insertion, action, and nerve supply 7. Name the dorsiflexors and plantarflexors of the ankle joint 8. Name the inverters and evertors of the subtalar and transverse tarsal joints 9. Describe the structures passing through the tarsal tunnel 10. Describe the course and relations of the deep and superficial fibular nerves 11. Describe the course and relations of the anterior and posterior tibial arteries 12. Describe the arterial anastomoses around the ankle joint	■ Bony markings on the tibia and fibula ■ Interosseous membrane ■ Tarsal tunnel and its contents ■ Muscles of the anterior compartment ■ Muscles of the lateral compartment ■ Muscles of the posterior compartment ■ Nerves and vessels in the leg ■ Retinacula around the ankle joint ■ Ligaments of the ankle joint	■ Insertion of semimembranosus ■ Iliotibial tract ■ Nerve to obturator internus	■ Psoas minor ■ Hybrid muscles ■ Articularis genu

EVALUATE [Explain Concepts]
■ Movements at the ankle and subtalar joints and the muscles causing them ■ Venous sinus in the soleus and its importance in varicose veins

EARLY CLINICAL EXPOSURE [Apply Anatomical Knowledge]	
Surgical Anatomy/ Pathology/ Trauma	**Imaging/ Surface Anatomy**
■ Intraosseous injections ■ Fracture of the femur ■ Tear of the ligaments of the ankle joint ■ Varicose veins	■ Radiograph of the normal ankle joint ■ Course of the tibial nerve

PROBLEM SOLVING/ CLINICAL CASES [Interpret]
■ Ankle sprain ■ Tear of the calcaneal tendon ■ Foot drop

The leg is the part of the lower limb between the knee joint and ankle joint (Fig. 3.80):

- Proximally, most major structures pass between the thigh and leg through or in relation to the **popliteal fossa** behind the knee.
- Distally, structures pass between the leg and foot mainly through the **tarsal tunnel** on the posteromedial side of the ankle, the exceptions being the anterior tibial artery and the ends of the deep and superficial fibular nerves, which enter the foot anterior to the ankle.

The bony framework of the leg consists of two bones, the tibia and fibula, arranged in parallel.

The **fibula** is much smaller than the tibia and is on the lateral side of the leg. It articulates superiorly with the inferior aspect of the lateral condyle of the proximal tibia, but does not take part in formation of the knee joint. The distal end of the fibula is firmly anchored to the tibia by a fibrous joint and forms the lateral malleolus of the ankle joint.

The **tibia** is the weight-bearing bone of the leg and is therefore much larger than the fibula. Above, it takes part in the formation of the knee joint and below it forms the medial malleolus and most of the bony surface for articulation of the leg with the foot at the ankle joint.

The leg is divided into anterior (extensor), posterior (flexor), and lateral (fibular) **compartments** by:

- An interosseous membrane, which links adjacent borders of the tibia and fibula along most of their length
- Two intermuscular septa, which pass between the fibula and deep fascia surrounding the limb
- Direct attachment of the deep fascia to the periosteum of the anterior and medial borders of the tibia (Fig. 3.80)

Muscles in the anterior compartment of the leg dorsiflex the ankle, extend the toes, and invert the foot. Muscles in the posterior compartment plantarflex the ankle, flex the toes, and invert the foot. Muscles in the lateral compartment evert the foot. Major nerves and vessels supply or pass through each compartment.

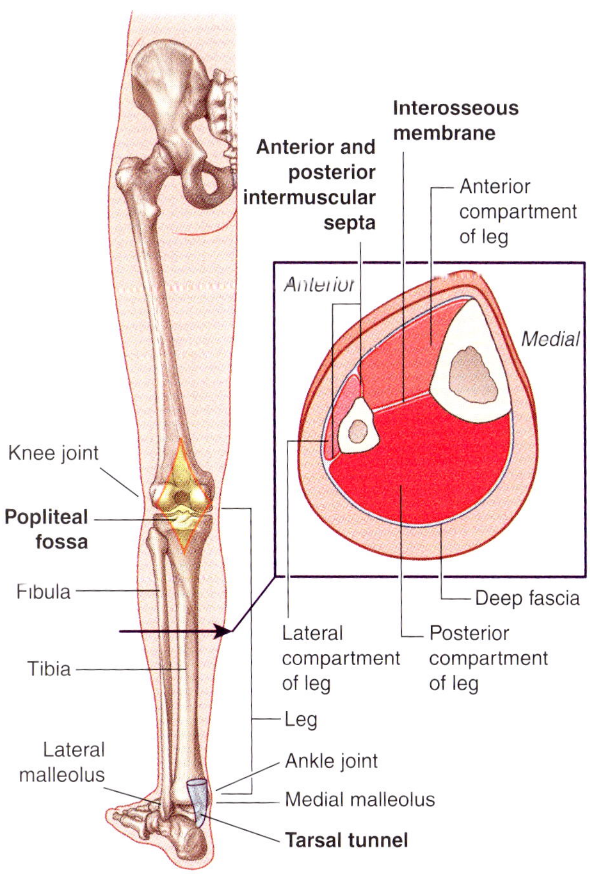

Fig. 3.80 Posterior view of leg; cross-section through the left leg (*inset*).

Bones

Shaft and distal end of tibia

The shaft of the tibia is triangular in cross-section and has anterior, interosseous, and medial borders and medial, lateral, and posterior surfaces (Fig. 3.81):

- The anterior and medial borders and the entire medial surface are subcutaneous and easily palpable.
- The interosseous border of the tibia is connected, by the interosseous membrane, along its length to the interosseous border of the fibula.
- The posterior surface is marked by an oblique line (the soleal line).

The soleal line descends across the bone from the lateral side to the medial side where it merges with the medial border. In addition, a vertical line descends down the upper part of the posterior surface from the midpoint of the soleal line. It disappears in the lower one-third of the tibia.

The shaft of the tibia expands at both the upper and lower ends to support the body's weight at the knee and ankle joints.

The distal end of the tibia is shaped like a rectangular box with a bony protuberance on the medial side (the **medial malleolus**; Fig. 3.81). The upper part of the box is continuous with the shaft of the tibia while the lower surface and the medial malleolus articulate with one of the tarsal bones (talus) to form a large part of the ankle joint.

The posterior surface of the box-like distal end of the tibia is marked by a vertical groove, which continues inferiorly and medially onto the posterior surface of the medial malleolus. The groove is for the tendon of the tibialis posterior muscle.

The lateral surface of the distal end of the tibia is occupied by a deep triangular notch (the **fibular notch**), to

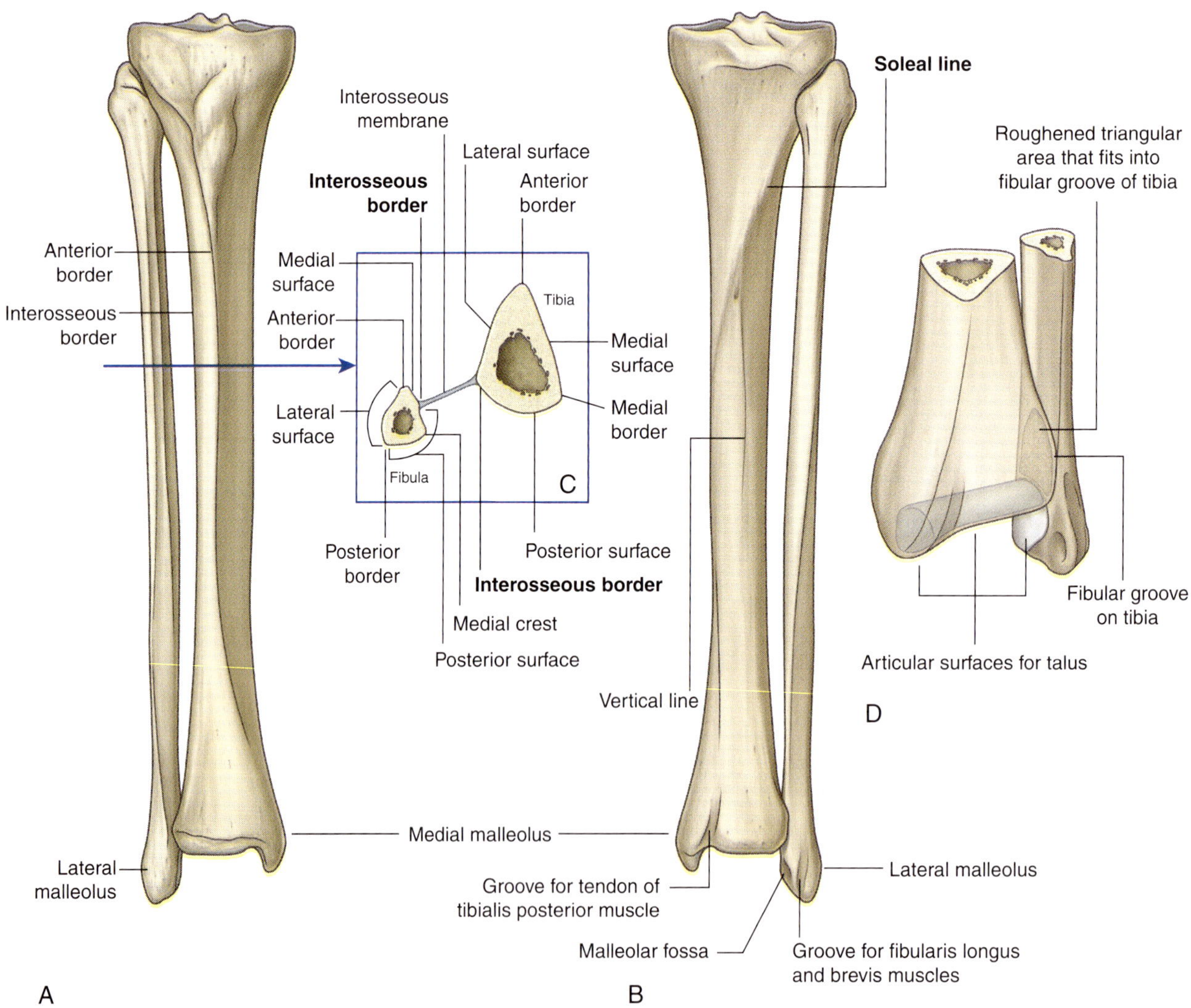

Fig. 3.81 Tibia and fibula. **(A)** Anterior view. **(B)** Posterior view. **(C)** Cross-section through shafts. **(D)** Posteromedial view of distal ends.

which the distal head of the fibula is anchored by a thickened part of the interosseous membrane.

Shaft and distal end of fibula

The fibula is not involved in weight-bearing. The fibular shaft is therefore much narrower than the shaft of the tibia. Also, and except for the ends, the fibula is enclosed by muscles.

Like the tibia, the shaft of the fibula is triangular in cross-section and has three borders and three surfaces for the attachment of muscles, intermuscular septa, and ligaments (Fig. 3.81). The interosseous border of the fibula faces and is attached to the interosseous border of the tibia by the interosseous membrane. Intermuscular septa attach to the anterior and posterior borders. Muscles attach to the three surfaces.

The narrow **medial surface** faces the anterior compartment of the leg, the **lateral surface** faces the lateral compartment of the leg, and the **posterior surface** faces the posterior compartment of the leg (Flowchart 3.5).

The posterior surface is marked by a vertical crest (**medial crest**), which divides the posterior surface into two parts, each attached to a different deep flexor muscle.

The distal end of the fibula expands to form the spade-shaped **lateral malleolus** (Fig. 3.81).

The medial surface of the lateral malleolus bears a triangular facet for articulation with the lateral surface of the talus, thereby forming the lateral part of the ankle joint. Just superior to this articular facet is a triangular area, which fits into the fibular notch on the distal end of the tibia. Here the tibia and fibula are joined together by the distal end of the interosseous membrane. Posteroinferior to the triangular facet for articulation with the talus is a pit or fossa (the **malleolar fossa**) for the attachment of the posterior talofibular ligament associated with the ankle joint.

The posterior surface of the lateral malleolus is marked by a shallow groove for the tendons of the fibularis longus and fibularis brevis muscles.

Joints

Interosseous membrane of leg

The interosseous membrane of the leg is a tough fibrous sheet of connective tissue that spans the distance between facing interosseous borders of the tibial and fibular shafts (Fig. 3.82). The collagen fibers descend obliquely from the interosseous border of the tibia to the interosseous border of the fibula, except superiorly where there is a ligamentous band, which ascends from the tibia to fibula.

There are two apertures in the interosseous membrane, one at the top and the other at the bottom, for vessels to pass between the anterior and posterior compartments of the leg.

The interosseous membrane not only links the tibia and fibula together but also provides an increased surface area for muscle attachment.

The distal ends of the fibula and tibia are held together by the inferior aspect of the interosseous membrane, which spans the narrow space between the fibular notch on the lateral surface of the distal end of the tibia and the

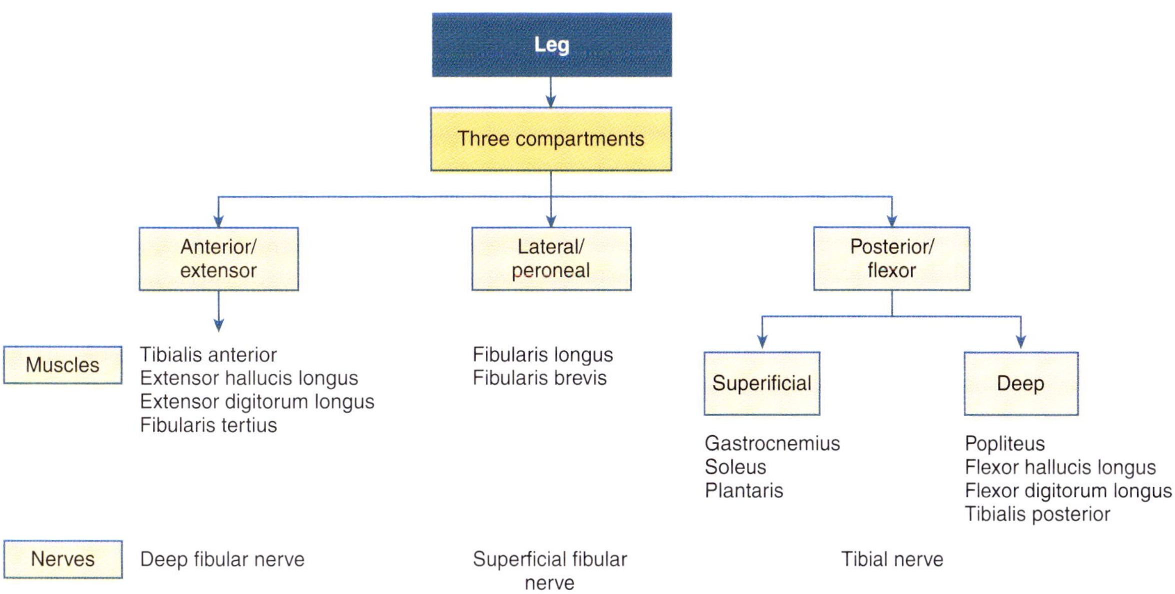

Flowchart 3.5 Compartments of the leg and their nerve supply.

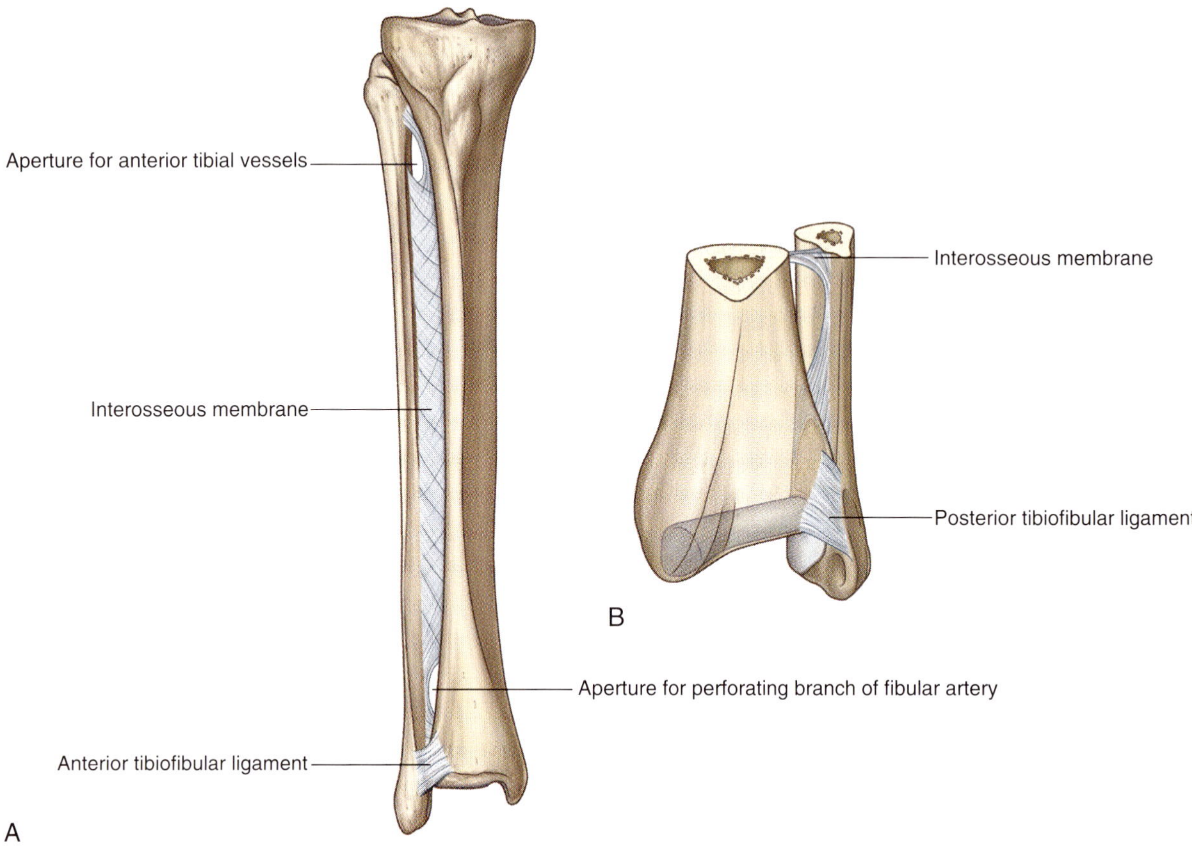

Fig. 3.82 Interosseous membrane. **(A)** Anterior view. **(B)** Posteromedial view.

corresponding surface on the distal end of the fibula. This expanded end of the interosseous membrane is reinforced by **anterior** and **posterior tibiofibular ligaments**. This firm linking together of the distal ends of the tibia and fibula is essential to produce the skeletal framework for articulation with the foot at the ankle joint.

Posterior compartment of leg

Muscles

Muscles in the posterior (flexor) compartment of the leg are organized into two groups, superficial and deep, separated by a layer of deep fascia. Generally, the muscles mainly plantarflex and invert the foot and flex the toes. All are innervated by the tibial nerve.

Superficial group

The superficial group of muscles in the posterior compartment of the leg comprises three muscles—the gastrocnemius, plantaris, and soleus (Table 3.6)—all of which insert onto the heel (calcaneus) of the foot and plantarflex the foot at the ankle joint (Fig. 3.83). As a unit, these muscles are large and powerful because they propel the body forward off the planted foot during walking and can elevate the body upward onto the toes when standing. Two of the muscles (gastrocnemius and plantaris) originate on the distal end of the femur and can also flex the knee.

Gastrocnemius

The **gastrocnemius** muscle is the most superficial of the muscles in the posterior compartment and is one of the largest muscles in the leg (Fig. 3.83). It originates from two heads, one lateral and one medial:

- The **medial head** is attached to an elongate roughening on the posterior aspect of the distal femur just behind the adductor tubercle and above the articular surface of the medial condyle.
- The **lateral head** originates from a distinct facet on the upper lateral surface of the lateral femoral condyle where it joins the lateral supracondylar line.

At the knee, the facing margins of the two heads of the gastrocnemius form the lateral and medial borders of the lower end of the popliteal fossa.

Table 3.6 Superficial group of muscles in the posterior compartment of leg

Muscle	Origin	Insertion	Innervation	Function
Gastrocnemius (Fig. 3.52 and 3.83)	Medial head—posterior surface of distal femur just superior to medial condyle; lateral head—upper posterolateral surface of lateral femoral condyle	Via calcaneal tendon, to posterior surface of calcaneus	Tibial nerve (**S1, S2**)	Plantarflexes foot and flexes knee
Plantaris (Fig. 3.73)	Inferior part of lateral supracondylar line of femur and oblique popliteal ligament of knee	Via calcaneal tendon, to posterior surface of calcaneus	Tibial nerve (**S1, S2**)	Plantarflexes foot and flexes knee
Soleus (Fig. 3.81)	Soleal line and medial border of tibia; posterior aspect of fibular head and adjacent surfaces of neck and proximal shaft; tendinous arch between tibial and fibular attachments	Via calcaneal tendon, to posterior surface of calcaneus	Tibial nerve (**S1, S2**)	Plantarflexes the foot

Note: Spinal segments in bold are the major segments innervating the muscle.

In the upper leg, the heads of the gastrocnemius combine to form a single elongate muscle belly, which forms much of the soft tissue bulge identified as the **calf**.

In the lower leg, the muscle fibers of the gastrocnemius converge with those of the deeper soleus muscle to form the **calcaneal tendon**, which attaches to the calcaneus (heel) of the foot.

The gastrocnemius plantarflexes the foot at the ankle joint and can also flex the leg at the knee joint. It is innervated by the tibial nerve.

Plantaris

The **plantaris** has a small muscle belly proximally and a long thin tendon, which descends through the leg and joins the calcaneal tendon (Fig. 3.83). The muscle takes origin superiorly from the lower part of the lateral supracondylar ridge of the femur and from the oblique popliteal ligament associated with the knee joint.

The short spindle-shaped muscle body of the plantaris descends medially, deep to the lateral head of the gastrocnemius, and forms a thin tendon, which passes between the gastrocnemius and soleus muscles and eventually fuses with the medial side of the calcaneal tendon near its attachment to the calcaneus.

The plantaris contributes to plantar flexion of the foot at the ankle joint and flexion of the leg at the knee joint, and is innervated by the tibial nerve.

Soleus

The **soleus** is a large flat muscle under the gastrocnemius muscle (Fig. 3.83). It is attached to the proximal ends of the fibula and tibia, and to a tendinous ligament, which spans the distance between the two heads of attachment to the fibula and tibia:

- On the proximal end of the fibula, the soleus originates from the posterior aspect of the head and adjacent surface of the neck and upper shaft of the fibula.
- On the tibia, the soleus originates from the soleal line and adjacent medial border (Fig. 3.81).
- The ligament, which spans the distance between the attachments to the tibia and fibula, arches over the popliteal vessels and tibial nerve as they pass from the popliteal fossa into the deep region of the posterior compartment of the leg.

In the lower leg, the soleus muscle narrows to join the calcaneal tendon that attaches to the calcaneus.

The soleus muscle, together with the gastrocnemius and plantaris, plantarflexes the foot at the ankle joint. It is innervated by the tibial nerve.

Early clinical exposure

Achilles tendon rupture

Rupture of the Achilles tendon is often related to sudden or direct trauma. This type of injury frequently occurs in a normal healthy tendon. In addition, there are certain conditions that may predispose the tendon to rupture. Among these conditions are tendinopathy (due to overuse or age-related degenerative changes) and previous Achilles tendon interventions such as injections of pharmaceuticals and the use of certain antibiotics (quinolone group). The diagnosis of Achilles tendon rupture is relatively straightforward. The patient typically complains of "being kicked" or "shot" behind the ankle, and clinical examination often reveals a gap in the tendon.

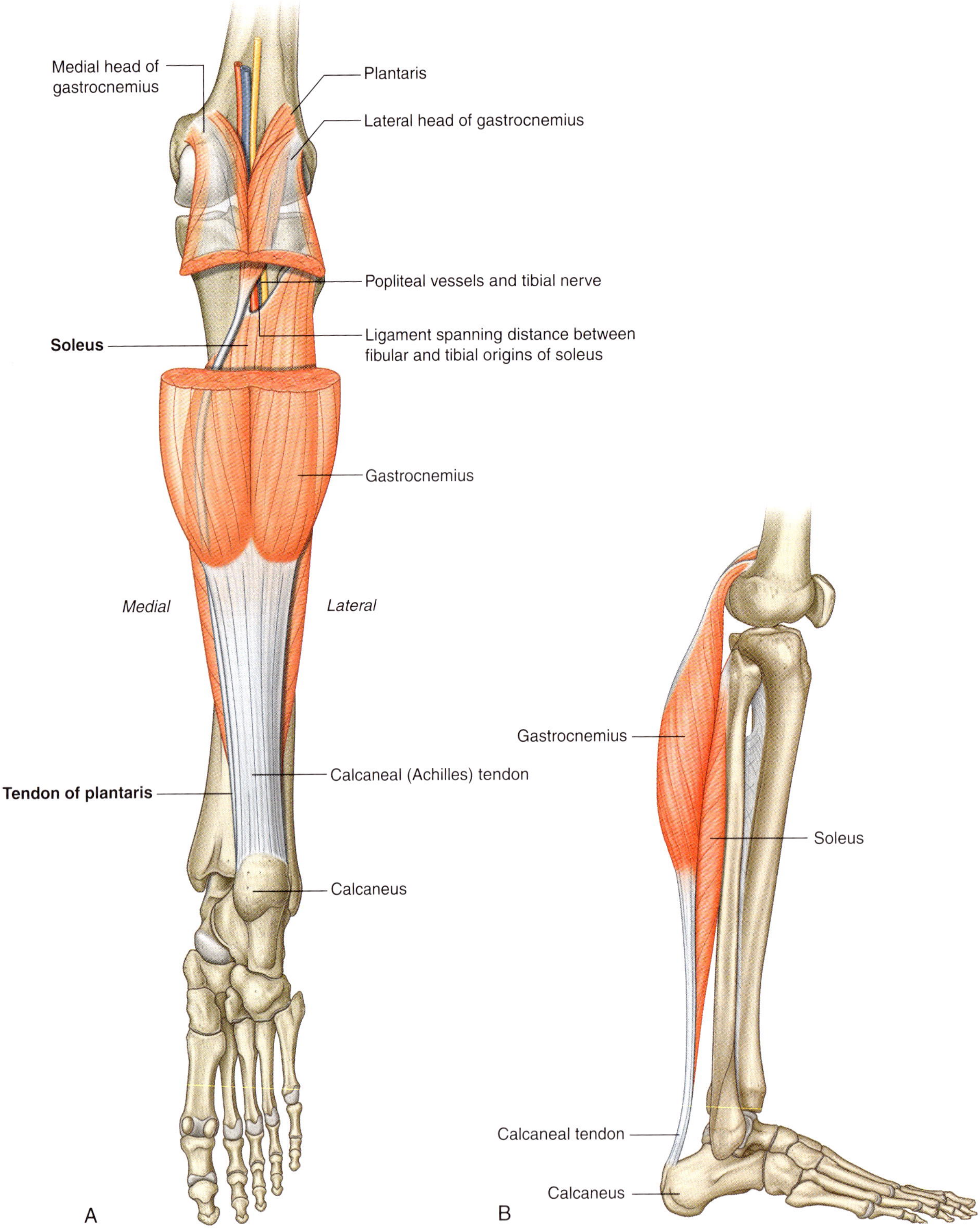

Fig. 3.83 Superficial group of muscles in the posterior compartment of leg. **(A)** Posterior view. **(B)** Lateral view.

Deep group

There are four muscles in the deep posterior compartment of the leg (Fig. 3.84)—the popliteus, flexor hallucis longus, flexor digitorum longus, and tibialis posterior (Table 3.7). The popliteus muscle acts on the knee, whereas the other three muscles act mainly on the foot.

Popliteus

The **popliteus** is the smallest and most superior of the deep muscles in the posterior compartment of the leg. It unlocks the extended knee at the initiation of flexion and stabilizes the knee by resisting lateral (external) rotation of the tibia on the femur. It is flat and triangular in shape and forms part of the floor of the popliteal fossa (Fig. 3.84). It is inserted into a broad triangular region above the soleal line on the posterior surface of the tibia.

The popliteus muscle ascends laterally across the lower aspect of the knee and forms a tendon, which penetrates the fibrous membrane of the joint capsule of the knee. The tendon ascends laterally around the joint where it passes between the lateral meniscus and the fibrous membrane and then into a groove on the inferolateral aspect of the lateral femoral condyle. The tendon attaches to a depression at the anterior end of the groove.

When initiating gait from a standing position, contraction of the popliteus laterally rotates the femur on the fixed tibia, unlocking the knee joint. The popliteus muscle is innervated by the tibial nerve.

Flexor hallucis longus

The flexor hallucis longus muscle originates on the lateral side of the posterior compartment of the leg and inserts into the plantar surface of the great toe on the medial side of the foot (Fig. 3.84). It arises mainly from the lower two-thirds of the posterior surface of the fibula and adjacent interosseous membrane.

The muscle fibers of the flexor hallucis longus converge inferiorly to form a large cord-like tendon, which passes behind the distal end of the tibia and then slips into a distinct groove on the posterior surface of the adjacent tarsal bone (talus) of the foot. The tendon curves anteriorly first under the talus and then under a shelf of bone (the sustentaculum tali), which projects medially from the calcaneus, and then continues anteriorly through the sole of the foot to insert on the inferior surface of the base of the distal phalanx of the great toe.

The flexor hallucis longus flexes the great toe. It is particularly active during the toe-off phase of walking when the body is propelled forward off the stance leg and the great toe is the last part of the foot to leave the ground. It can also contribute to plantar flexion of the foot at the ankle joint and is innervated by the tibial nerve.

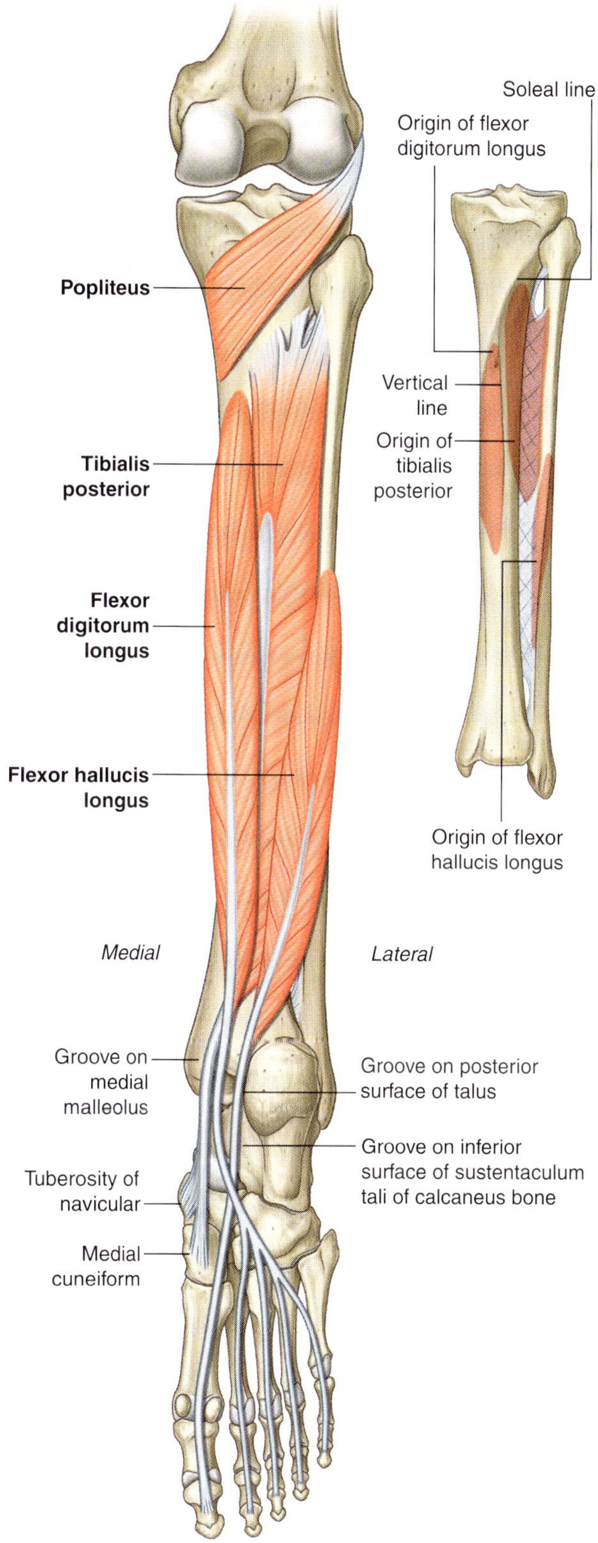

Fig. 3.84 Deep group of muscles in the posterior compartment of leg.

Table 3.7 Deep group of muscles in the posterior compartment of leg

Muscle	Origin	Insertion	Innervation	Function
Popliteus (Fig. 3.84)	Groove on inferolateral aspect of lateral femoral condyle	Posterior surface of proximal tibia	Tibial nerve (L4 to S1)	Stabilizes knee joint (resists lateral rotation of tibia on femur) Unlocks knee joint (laterally rotates femur on fixed tibia)
Flexor hallucis longus	Posterior surface of fibula and adjacent interosseous membrane	Plantar surface of distal phalanx of great toe	Tibial nerve (**S2**, S3)	Flexes great toe
Flexor digitorum longus	Medial side of posterior surface of the tibia	Plantar surfaces of bases of distal phalanges of the lateral four toes	Tibial nerve (**S2**, S3)	Flexes lateral four toes
Tibialis posterior	Posterior surfaces of interosseous membrane and adjacent regions of tibia and fibula	Mainly to tuberosity of navicular and adjacent region of medial cuneiform	Tibial nerve (L4, L5)	Inversion and plantar flexion of foot; support of medial arch of foot during walking

Note: Spinal segments in bold are the major segments innervating the muscle.

Flexor digitorum longus

The flexor digitorum longus muscle originates on the medial side of the posterior compartment of the leg and inserts into the lateral four digits of the foot (Fig. 3.84). It arises mainly from the medial side of the posterior surface of the tibia inferior to the soleal line.

The flexor digitorum longus descends in the leg and forms a tendon, which crosses posterior to the tendon of the tibialis posterior muscle near the ankle joint. The tendon continues inferiorly in a shallow groove behind the medial malleolus and then swings forward to enter the sole of the foot. It crosses inferior to the tendon of the flexor hallucis longus muscle to reach the medial side of the foot and then divides into four tendons, which insert on the plantar surfaces of the bases of the distal phalanges of digits II to V.

The flexor digitorum longus flexes the lateral four toes. It is involved with gripping the ground during walking and propelling the body forward off the toes at the end of the stance phase of gait. It is innervated by the tibial nerve.

Tibialis posterior

The tibialis posterior muscle originates from the interosseous membrane and the adjacent posterior surfaces of the tibia and fibula (Fig. 3.84). It lies between and is overlapped by the flexor digitorum longus and the flexor hallucis longus muscles.

Near the ankle, the tendon of the tibialis posterior is crossed superficially by the tendon of the flexor digitorum longus muscle and lies medial to this tendon in the groove on the posterior surface of the medial malleolus. The tendon curves forward under the medial malleolus and enters the medial side of the foot. It wraps around the medial margin of the foot to attach to the plantar surfaces of the medial tarsal bones, mainly to the tuberosity of the navicular and to the adjacent region of the medial cuneiform.

The tibialis posterior inverts and plantarflexes the foot, and supports the medial arch of the foot during walking. It is innervated by the tibial nerve.

Early clinical exposure

Neurological examination of the legs

Some of the commonest conditions that affect the legs are peripheral neuropathy (particularly associated with diabetes mellitus), lumbar nerve root lesions (associated with pathology of the intervertebral discs), fibular nerve palsy, and spastic paraparesis.

- Look for muscle wasting—loss of muscle mass may indicate loss of or reduced innervation.
- Test the power in muscle groups—hip flexion (L1, L2—iliopsoas—the patient lies supine and tries to raise the thigh with the knee extended, straight leg raise), knee flexion (L5 to S2—hamstrings—the patient tries to bend the knee against resistance, while the examiner applies force to the leg to hold the knee in extension), knee extension (L3, L4—quadriceps femoris—the patient attempts to keep the knee extended, while the examiner applies a force to the leg to flex the knee joint), ankle dorsiflexion (L4, L5—the patient pulls the foot upward, while the examiner applies a force to the dorsal aspect of the foot to plantarflex the ankle joint), and ankle plantar flexion (S1, S2—the patient pushes the foot down while the examiner applies a force to the plantar surface of the foot to dorsiflex the ankle joint).
- Examine knee and ankle reflexes—a tap with a tendon hammer on the patellar ligament (tendon) tests reflexes at the L3 to L4 spinal levels, and tapping the calcaneal tendon tests reflexes at the S1 to S2 spinal levels.
- Assess status of general sensory input to lumbar and upper sacral spinal cord levels—test light touch, pin prick, and vibration sense at dermatomes in the lower limb.

Arteries

Popliteal artery

The **popliteal artery** is the major blood supply to the leg and foot and enters the posterior compartment of the leg from the popliteal fossa behind the knee (Fig. 3.85).

The popliteal artery passes into the posterior compartment of the leg between the gastrocnemius and popliteus muscles. As it continues inferiorly, it passes under the tendinous arch formed between the fibular and tibial heads of the soleus muscle and enters the deep region of the posterior compartment of the leg where it immediately divides into the anterior tibial artery and the posterior tibial artery.

Two large sural arteries, one on each side, branch from the popliteal artery to supply the gastrocnemius, soleus, and plantaris muscles (Fig. 3.85). In addition, the popliteal artery gives rise to branches that contribute to a collateral network of vessels around the knee joint (see Fig. 3.77).

Anterior tibial artery

The **anterior tibial artery** passes forward through the aperture in the upper part of the interosseous membrane and enters and supplies the anterior compartment of the leg. It continues inferiorly onto the dorsal aspect of the foot.

Posterior tibial artery

The **posterior tibial artery** supplies the posterior and lateral compartments of the leg and continues into the sole of the foot (Fig. 3.85).

The posterior tibial artery descends through the deep region of the posterior compartment of the leg on the superficial surfaces of the tibialis posterior and flexor digitorum longus muscles. It passes through the tarsal tunnel behind the medial malleolus and into the sole of the foot.

In the leg, the posterior tibial artery supplies adjacent muscles and bone and has two major branches, the circumflex fibular artery and the fibular artery:

- The **circumflex fibular artery** passes laterally through the soleus muscle and around the neck of the fibula to connect with the anastomotic network of vessels surrounding the knee (Fig. 3.85; see also Fig. 3.77).
- The **fibular artery** parallels the course of the tibial artery, but descends along the lateral side of the posterior compartment adjacent to the medial crest on the posterior surface of the fibula, which separates the attachments of the tibialis posterior and flexor hallucis longus muscles.

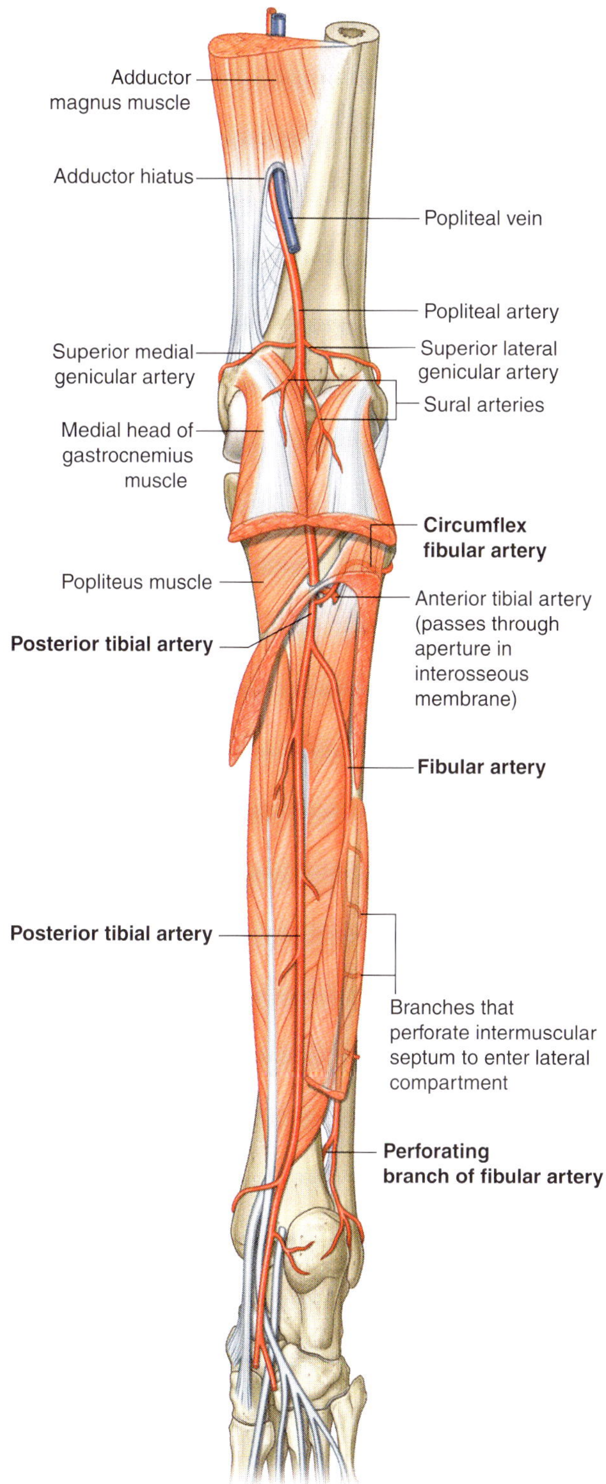

Fig. 3.85 Arteries in the posterior compartment of leg.

The fibular artery supplies adjacent muscles and bone in the posterior compartment of the leg and also has branches that pass laterally through the intermuscular septum to supply the fibularis muscles in the lateral compartment of the leg.

A **perforating branch** that originates from the fibular artery distally in the leg passes anteriorly through the inferior aperture in the interosseous membrane to anastomose with a branch of the anterior tibial artery.

The fibular artery passes behind the attachment between the distal ends of the tibia and fibula and terminates in a network of vessels over the lateral surface of the calcaneus.

Veins

Deep veins in the posterior compartment generally follow the arteries.

Nerves

Tibial nerve

The nerve associated with the posterior compartment of the leg is the tibial nerve (Fig. 3.86). It is a terminal branch of the sciatic nerve that descends into the posterior compartment from the popliteal fossa.

The tibial nerve passes under the tendinous arch formed between the fibular and tibial heads of the soleus muscle and passes vertically through the deep region of the posterior compartment of the leg on the surface of the tibialis posterior muscle with the posterior tibial vessels.

The tibial nerve leaves the posterior compartment of the leg at the ankle by passing through the tarsal tunnel behind the medial malleolus. It enters the foot to supply most of the intrinsic muscles and skin.

In the leg, the tibial nerve gives rise to:

- Branches that supply all the muscles in the posterior compartment of the leg
- Two cutaneous branches, the **sural nerve** and **medial calcaneal nerve**

Branches of the tibial nerve that innervate the superficial group of muscles of the posterior compartment and popliteus muscle of the deep group originate high in the leg between the two heads of the gastrocnemius muscle in the distal region of the popliteal fossa (Fig. 3.86). Branches innervate the gastrocnemius, plantaris, and soleus muscles, and pass more deeply into the popliteus muscle.

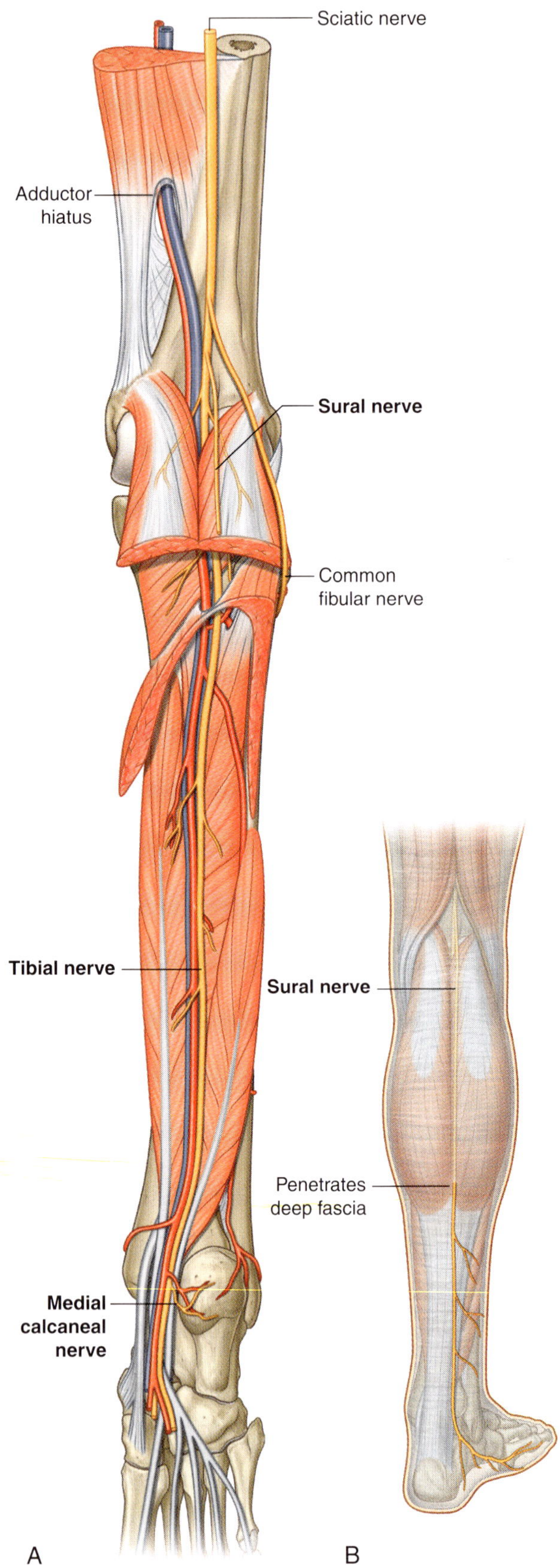

Fig. 3.86 Tibial nerve. **(A)** Posterior view. **(B)** Sural nerve.

Branches to the deep muscles of the posterior compartment originate from the tibial nerve deep to the soleus muscle in the upper half of the leg and innervate the tibialis posterior, flexor hallucis longus, and flexor digitorum longus muscles.

Sural nerve

The sural nerve originates high in the leg between the two heads of the gastrocnemius muscle (Fig. 3.86). It descends superficial to the belly of the gastrocnemius muscle and penetrates through the deep fascia approximately in the middle of the leg where it is joined by a sural communicating branch from the common fibular nerve (Fig. 3.88). It passes down the leg, below the lateral malleolus, and into the foot.

The sural nerve supplies skin on the lower posterolateral surface of the leg and the lateral side of the foot and little toe.

Medial calcaneal nerve

The medial calcaneal nerve is often multiple and originates from the tibial nerve low in the leg near the ankle and descends onto the medial side of the heel.

The medial calcaneal nerve innervates skin on the medial surface and sole of the heel (Fig. 3.86).

Lateral compartment of leg

Muscles

There are two muscles in the lateral compartment of the leg—the fibularis longus and fibularis brevis (Fig. 3.87 and Table 3.8). Both evert the foot (turn the sole outward) and are innervated by the superficial fibular nerve, which is a branch of the common fibular nerve.

Fibularis longus

The **fibularis longus** muscle arises in the lateral compartment of the leg, but its tendon crosses under the foot to attach to bones on the medial side (Fig. 3.87). It originates both from the upper two-thirds of the lateral surface of the fibula and from the anterior aspect of the fibular head and occasionally up onto the adjacent region of the lateral tibial condyle.

The common fibular nerve passes anteriorly around the fibular neck between the attachments of the fibularis longus to the fibular head and shaft.

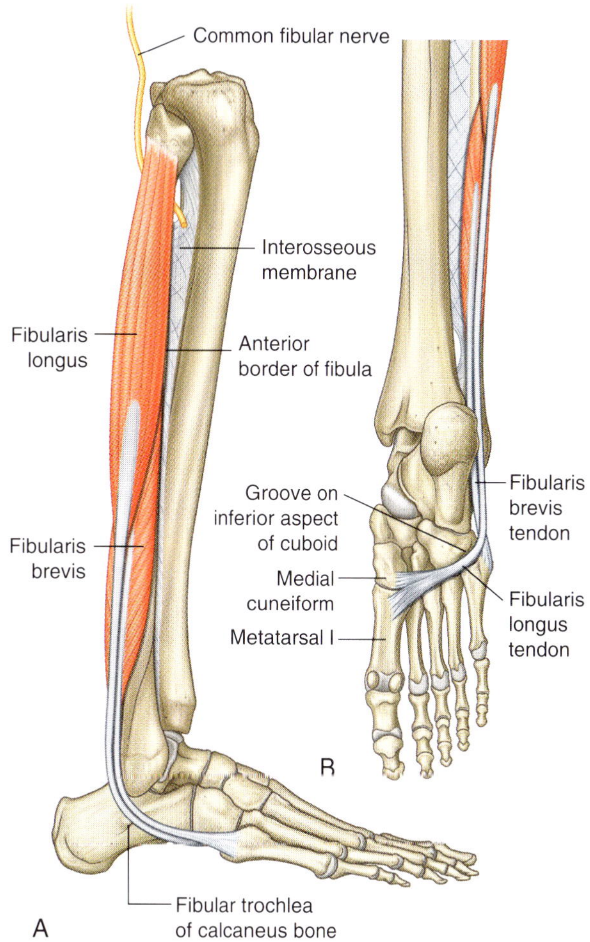

Fig. 3.87 Muscles in the lateral compartment of leg. **(A)** Lateral view. **(B)** Inferior view of the right foot, with the foot plantarflexed at the ankle.

Table 3.8 Muscles of the lateral compartment of leg

Muscle	Origin	Insertion	Innervation	Function
Fibularis longus	Upper two-thirds of lateral surface of fibula, head of fibula, and occasionally the lateral tibial condyle	Undersurface of lateral sides of distal end of medial cuneiform and base of metatarsal I	Superficial fibular nerve (**L5, S1**, S2)	Eversion and plantar flexion of foot; supports arches of foot
Fibularis brevis	Lower two-thirds of lateral surface of shaft of fibula	Lateral tubercle at base of metatarsal V	Superficial fibular nerve (**L5, S1**, S2)	Eversion of foot

Note: Spinal segments in bold are the major segments innervating the muscle.

Distally, the fibularis longus descends in the leg to form a tendon, which, in order:

- Passes posterior to the lateral malleolus in a shallow bony groove
- Swings forward to enter the lateral side of the foot
- Descends obliquely down the lateral side of the foot where it curves forward under a bony tubercle (fibular trochlea) of the calcaneus
- Enters a deep groove on the inferior surface of one of the other tarsal bones (the cuboid)
- Swings under the foot to cross the sole and attach to the inferior surfaces of the lateral sides of the distal end of the medial cuneiform and the base of metatarsal I

The fibularis longus everts and plantarflexes the foot. In addition, the fibularis longus, tibialis anterior, and tibialis posterior muscles, which all insert on the undersurfaces of bones on the medial side of the foot, together act as a stirrup to support the arches of the foot. The fibularis longus supports mainly the lateral and transverse arches.

The fibularis longus is innervated by the superficial fibular nerve.

Fibularis brevis

The fibularis brevis muscle is deep to the fibularis longus muscle in the leg and originates from the lower two-thirds of the lateral surface of the shaft of the fibula (Fig. 3.87).

The tendon of the fibularis brevis passes behind the lateral malleolus with the tendon of the fibularis longus muscle and then curves forward across the lateral surface of the calcaneus to attach to a tubercle on the lateral surface of the base of metatarsal V.

The fibularis brevis assists in eversion of the foot and is innervated by the superficial fibular nerve.

Arteries

No major artery passes vertically through the lateral compartment of the leg. It is supplied by branches (mainly from the fibular artery in the posterior compartment of the leg) that penetrate into the lateral compartment (Fig. 3.88).

Veins

Deep veins generally follow the arteries.

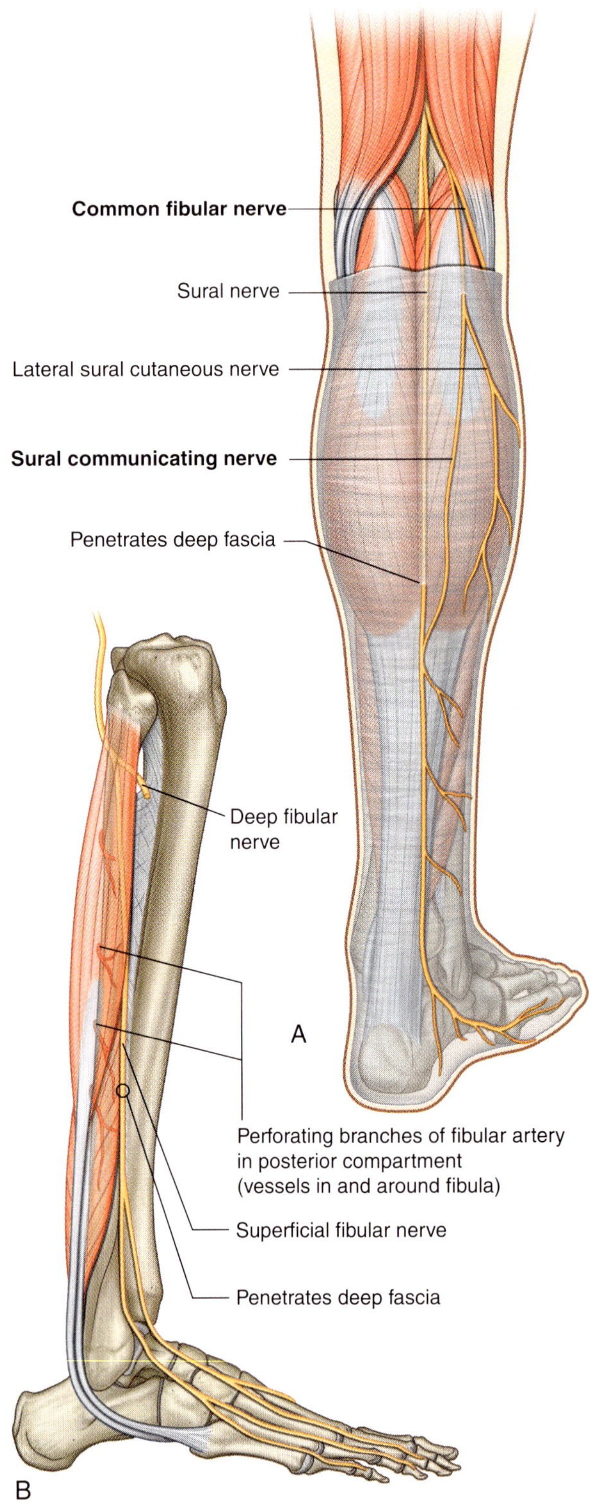

Fig. 3.88 Common fibular nerve, and nerves and arteries of the lateral compartment of leg. **(A)** Posterior view, right leg. **(B)** Lateral view, right leg.

Nerves

Superficial fibular nerve

The nerve associated with the lateral compartment of the leg is the **superficial fibular nerve**. This nerve originates as one of the two terminal branches of the common fibular nerve, which enters the lateral compartment of the leg from the popliteal fossa (Fig. 3.88B).

The common fibular nerve originates from the sciatic nerve in the posterior compartment of the thigh or in the popliteal fossa (Fig. 3.88A), and follows the medial margin of the biceps femoris tendon over the lateral head of the gastrocnemius muscle and toward the fibula. Here it gives origin to two cutaneous branches, which descend in the leg:

- The **sural communicating nerve**, which joins the sural branch of the tibial nerve and contributes to innervation of skin over the lower posterolateral side of the leg
- The **lateral sural cutaneous nerve**, which innervates skin over the upper lateral leg

The common fibular nerve continues around the neck of the fibula and enters the lateral compartment by passing between the attachments of the fibularis longus muscle to the head and shaft of the fibula. Here the common fibular nerve divides into its two terminal branches:

- The superficial fibular nerve
- The deep fibular nerve

The superficial fibular nerve descends in the lateral compartment deep to the fibularis longus and innervates the fibularis longus and fibularis brevis (Fig. 3.87B). It then penetrates deep fascia in the lower leg and enters the foot where it divides into medial and lateral branches, which supply dorsal areas of the foot and toes except for:

- The skin lining the web space between the great and second toes, which is supplied by the deep fibular nerve
- The lateral side of the little toe, which is supplied by the sural branch of the tibial nerve (see Fig. 3.122)

The deep fibular nerve passes anteromedially through the intermuscular septum into the anterior compartment of the leg, which it supplies.

Anterior compartment of leg

Muscles

There are four muscles in the anterior compartment of the leg—the tibialis anterior, extensor hallucis longus, extensor digitorum longus, and fibularis tertius (Fig. 3.89 and Table 3.9). Collectively they dorsiflex the foot at the ankle joint, extend the toes, and invert the foot. All are innervated by the deep fibular nerve, which is a branch of the common fibular nerve.

Tibialis anterior

The **tibialis anterior** muscle is the most anterior and medial of the muscles in the anterior compartment of the leg

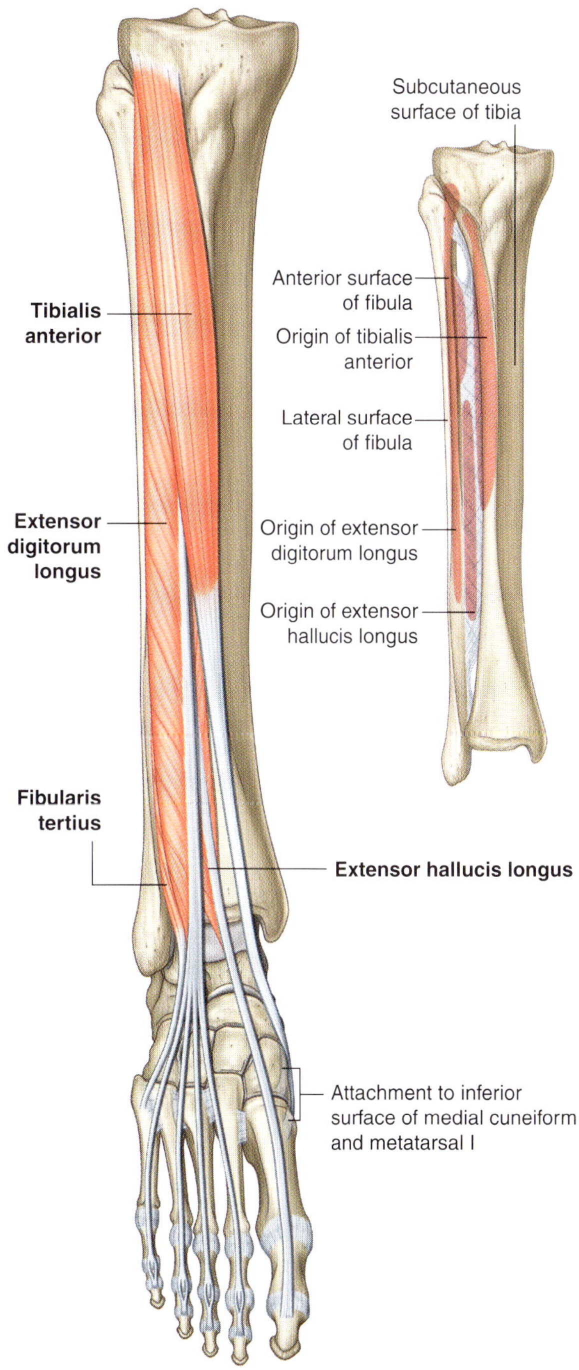

Fig. 3.89 Muscles of the anterior compartment of leg.

Table 3.9 Muscles of the anterior compartment of leg

Muscle	Origin	Insertion	Innervation	Function
Tibialis anterior	Lateral surface of tibia and adjacent interosseous membrane	Medial and inferior surfaces of medial cuneiform and adjacent surface on base of metatarsal I	Deep fibular nerve (**L4**, L5)	Dorsiflexion of foot at ankle joint; inversion of foot; dynamic support of medial arch of foot
Extensor hallucis longus	Middle one-half of medial surface of fibula and adjacent surface of interosseous membrane	Dorsal surface of base of distal phalanx of great toe	Deep fibular nerve (**L5, S1**)	Extension of great toe and dorsiflexion of foot
Extensor digitorum longus	Proximal one-half of medial surface of fibula and related surface of lateral tibial condyle	Via dorsal digital expansions into bases of distal and middle phalanges of lateral four toes	Deep fibular nerve (**L5, S1**)	Extension of lateral four toes and dorsiflexion of foot
Fibularis tertius	Distal part of medial surface of fibula	Dorsomedial surface of base of metatarsal V	Deep fibular nerve (**L5, S1**)	Dorsiflexion and eversion of foot

Note: Spinal segments in bold are the major segments innervating the muscle.

(Fig. 3.89). It originates mainly from the upper two-thirds of the lateral surface of the shaft of the tibia and adjacent surface of the interosseous membrane. It also originates from deep fascia.

The muscle fibers of the tibialis anterior converge in the lower one-third of the leg to form a tendon, which descends into the medial side of the foot, where it attaches to the medial and inferior surfaces of the medial cuneiform and adjacent parts of metatarsal I.

The tibialis anterior dorsiflexes the foot at the ankle joint and inverts the foot at the intertarsal joints. During walking, it provides dynamic support for the medial arch of the foot.

The tibialis anterior is innervated by the deep fibular nerve.

Extensor hallucis longus

The **extensor hallucis longus** muscle lies next to and is partly overlapped by the tibialis anterior muscle (Fig. 3.89). It originates from the middle one-half of the medial surface of the fibula and adjacent interosseous membrane.

The tendon of the extensor hallucis longus appears between the tendons of the tibialis anterior and extensor digitorum longus in the lower one-half of the leg and descends into the foot. It continues anteriorly on the medial side of the dorsal surface of the foot to near the end of the great toe where it inserts on the upper surface of the base of the distal phalanx.

The extensor hallucis longus extends the great toe. Because it crosses anterior to the ankle joint, it also dorsiflexes the foot at the ankle joint. Like all muscles in the anterior compartment of the leg, the extensor hallucis longus muscle is innervated by the deep fibular nerve.

Extensor digitorum longus

The **extensor digitorum longus** muscle is the most posterior and lateral of the muscles in the anterior compartment of the leg (Fig. 3.89). It originates mainly from the upper one-half of the medial surface of the fibula lateral to and above the origin of the extensor hallucis longus muscle, and extends superiorly onto the lateral condyle of the tibia. Like the tibialis anterior muscle, it also originates from deep fascia.

The extensor digitorum longus muscle descends to form a tendon, which continues into the dorsal aspect of the foot, where it divides into four tendons, which insert, via dorsal digital expansions, into the dorsal surfaces of the bases of the middle and distal phalanges of the lateral four toes.

The extensor digitorum longus extends the toes and dorsiflexes the foot at the ankle joint, and is innervated by the deep fibular nerve.

Fibularis tertius

The **fibularis tertius** muscle is normally considered part of the extensor digitorum longus (Fig. 3.89). The fibularis tertius originates from the medial surface of the fibula immediately below the origin of the extensor digitorum longus muscle and the two muscles are normally connected.

The tendon of the fibularis tertius descends into the foot with the tendon of the extensor digitorum longus. On the dorsal aspect of the foot, it deviates laterally to insert into the dorsomedial surface of the base of metatarsal V.

The fibularis tertius assists in dorsiflexion and possibly eversion of the foot, and is innervated by the deep fibular nerve.

Arteries

Anterior tibial artery

The artery associated with the anterior compartment of the leg is the **anterior tibial artery**, which originates from the popliteal artery in the posterior compartment of the leg and passes forward into the anterior compartment of the leg through an aperture in the interosseous membrane.

The anterior tibial artery descends through the anterior compartment on the interosseous membrane (Fig. 3.90). In the distal leg, it lies between the tendons of the tibialis anterior and extensor hallucis longus muscles. It leaves the leg by passing anterior to the ankle joint and continues onto the dorsal aspect of the foot as the dorsalis pedis artery.

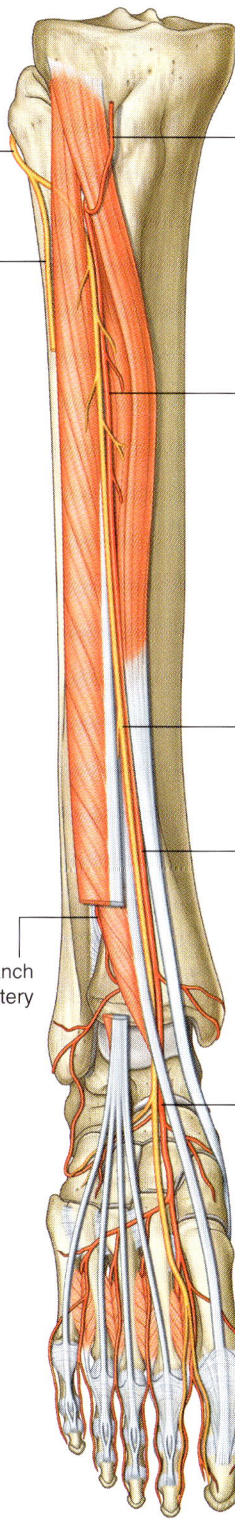

Fig. 3.90 Anterior tibial artery and deep fibular nerve.

In the proximal leg, the anterior tibial artery has a recurrent branch, which connects with the anastomotic network of vessels around the knee joint.

Along its course, the anterior tibial artery supplies numerous branches to adjacent muscles and is joined by the perforating branch of the fibular artery, which passes forward through the lower aspect of the interosseous membrane from the posterior compartment of the leg.

Distally, the anterior tibial artery gives rise to an **anterior medial malleolar artery** and an **anterior lateral malleolar artery**, which pass posteriorly around the distal ends of the tibia and fibula, respectively, and connect with vessels from the posterior tibial and fibular arteries to form an anastomotic network around the ankle.

Veins

Deep veins follow the arteries and have similar names.

Nerves

Deep fibular nerve

The nerve associated with the anterior compartment of the leg is the **deep fibular nerve** (Fig. 3.90). This nerve originates in the lateral compartment of the leg as one of the two divisions of the common fibular nerve.

The deep fibular nerve passes anteromedially through the intermuscular septum that separates the lateral from the anterior compartments of the leg and then passes deep to the extensor digitorum longus. It reaches the interosseous membrane where it meets and descends with the anterior tibial artery.

The deep fibular nerve:

- Innervates all muscles in the anterior compartment
- Then continues into the dorsal aspect of the foot where it innervates the extensor digitorum brevis, contributes to the innervation of the first two dorsal interossei muscles, and supplies the skin lining the adjacent sides of the great and second toes

Early clinical exposure

Foot drop

Foot drop is an inability to dorsiflex the foot. Patients with foot drop have a characteristic "steppage" gait. As the patient walks, the knee of the affected limb is elevated to an abnormal height during the swing phase to prevent the foot from dragging. At the end of the swing phase, the foot "slaps" the ground. Also, the unaffected limb often acquires a characteristic tiptoe pattern of gait during the stance phase. A typical cause of foot drop is damage to the common fibular nerve. Other causes include disc protrusion compressing the L5 nerve root, disorders of the sciatic nerve and the lumbar and sacral plexuses, and pathologies of the spinal cord and brain.

Common fibular nerve injury

The common fibular nerve is susceptible to injury as it passes around the lateral aspect of the neck of the fibula. It can be injured as a result of a direct trauma (blow or laceration), secondary to knee injury (knee dislocation), or as a consequence of a proximal fibular fracture. Sometimes damage to the nerve can be iatrogenic, that is, damaged during arthroscopy or knee surgery.

Symptoms of common fibular nerve injury are often observed in bed-bound patients, particularly in those with decreased levels of consciousness, due to prolonged external pressure to the knee leading to nerve compression and neuropathy. Similarly, application of a tight cast or a brace to the leg can compress the nerve, producing symptoms of fibular muscle palsy.

Apart from a foot drop, other symptoms of common fibular nerve injury include loss of sensation over the lateral aspect of the leg and dorsum of the foot, and wasting of fibular and anterior tibial muscles.

FOOT

SET INDUCTION—CASE SCENARIO 5: ANKLE SPRAIN

A 20-year-old girl was brought to the emergency department with a history of a fall while playing basketball. On examination, a swelling was found on the lateral side of the ankle joint. A diagnosis of a tear of the lateral ligament of the ankle joint was made.

Knowledge of the anatomy of the foot is needed to manage a patient with a sprain of the ankle joint.

<table>
<tr><th rowspan="2">REMEMBER
[Recall Facts]</th><th colspan="3">OUTLINE 5. FOOT—LEARNING OBJECTIVES
[By the end of this section the student should be able to:]</th><th colspan="2" rowspan="2">EVALUATE
[Explain Concepts]</th></tr>
<tr><th colspan="3">DEMONSTRATE AND ANALYZE RELATIONSHIPS
[Identify structures in a Prosected Specimen or Figure]</th></tr>
<tr><td rowspan="6">1. Mention the factors maintaining the arches of the foot
2. Describe in detail the talocalcaneonavicular joint
3. Describe long and short plantar ligaments
4. Describe briefly calcaneocuboid joint
5. Describe the contents of each of the layers of the sole of the foot
6. Describe the lateral and medial planar arteries and nerves
7. List the muscles of the foot and mention their origin, insertion, action, and nerve supply</td><td>Level I</td><td>Level II</td><td>Level III</td><td colspan="2" rowspan="2">■ Movements at the metatarsophalangeal and interphalangeal joints and the muscles causing them
■ Maintenance of the arches of the foot</td></tr>
<tr><td rowspan="5">■ Bony markings on the articulated foot
■ Plantar aponeurosis
■ Dorsal venous arch
■ Dorsalis pedis artery
■ Talocalcaneonavicular joint
■ Plantar calcaneonavicular ligament
■ Long and short plantar ligaments
■ Contents of the layers of the sole of the foot
■ Deep transverse metatarsal ligament</td><td rowspan="5">■ Interosseous talocalcaneal ligament
■ Bifurcate ligament</td><td rowspan="5">■ Plantar ligaments
■ Extensor hood</td></tr>
<tr><th colspan="2">EARLY CLINICAL EXPOSURE
[Apply Anatomical Knowledge]</th></tr>
<tr><th>Surgical Anatomy/ Pathology/ Trauma</th><th>Imaging/ Surface Anatomy</th></tr>
<tr><td>■ Fracture of the talus
■ Bunion
■ Hallux valgus</td><td>■ Radiograph of the normal foot
■ Plantar arterial arch</td></tr>
<tr><td colspan="2">PROBLEM SOLVING/ CLINICAL CASES
[Interpret]
■ Flat foot
■ Deep vein thrombosis</td></tr>
</table>

The foot is the region of the lower limb distal to the ankle joint. It is subdivided into the ankle, the metatarsus, and the digits.

There are five digits consisting of the medially positioned great toe (digit I) and four more laterally placed digits, ending laterally with the little toe (digit V) (Fig. 3.91).

The foot has a superior surface (**dorsum of foot**) and an inferior surface (**sole**; Fig. 3.91).

Abduction and adduction of the toes are defined with respect to the long axis of the second digit. Unlike in the hand, where the thumb is oriented 90° to the other fingers, the great toe is oriented in the same position as the other toes. The foot is the body's point of contact with the ground and provides a stable platform for upright stance. It also levers the body forward during walking.

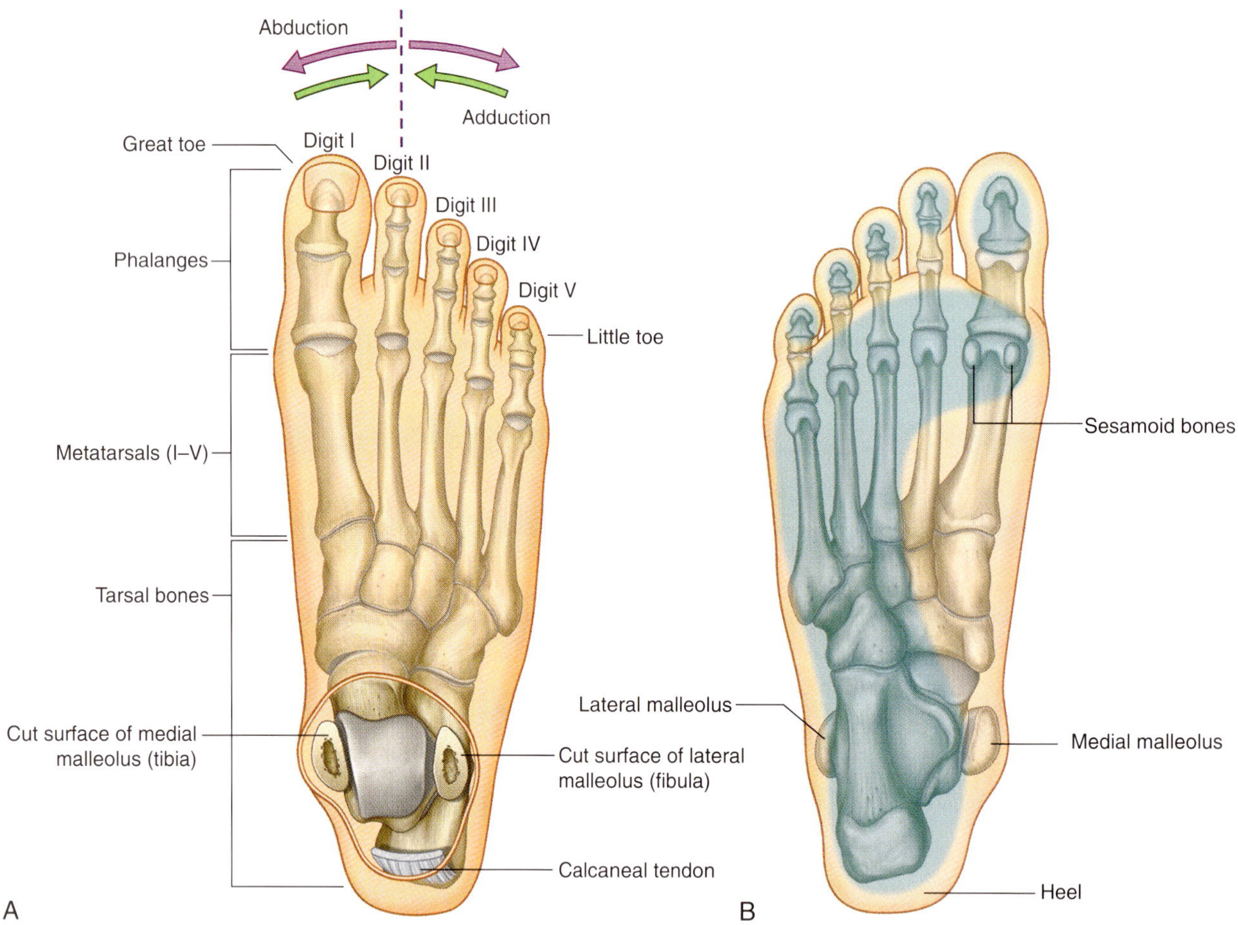

Fig. 3.91 Foot. **(A)** Dorsal aspect, right foot. **(B)** Plantar aspect, right foot, showing the surface in contact with the ground when standing.

Bones

There are three groups of bones in the foot (Fig. 3.92):

- The seven **tarsal bones**, which form the skeletal framework for the ankle.
- **Metatarsals (I to V)**, which are the bones of the metatarsus.
- The **phalanges**, which are the bones of the toes—each toe has three phalanges, except for the great toe, which has two.

Tarsal bones

The tarsal bones are arranged in a proximal group and a distal group with an intermediate bone between the two groups on the medial side of the foot (Fig. 3.92A).

Proximal group

The proximal group consists of two large bones, the talus (Latin for "ankle") and the calcaneus (Latin for "heel"):

- The **talus** is the most superior bone of the foot and sits on top of and is supported by the calcaneus (Fig. 3.92B)—it articulates above with the tibia and

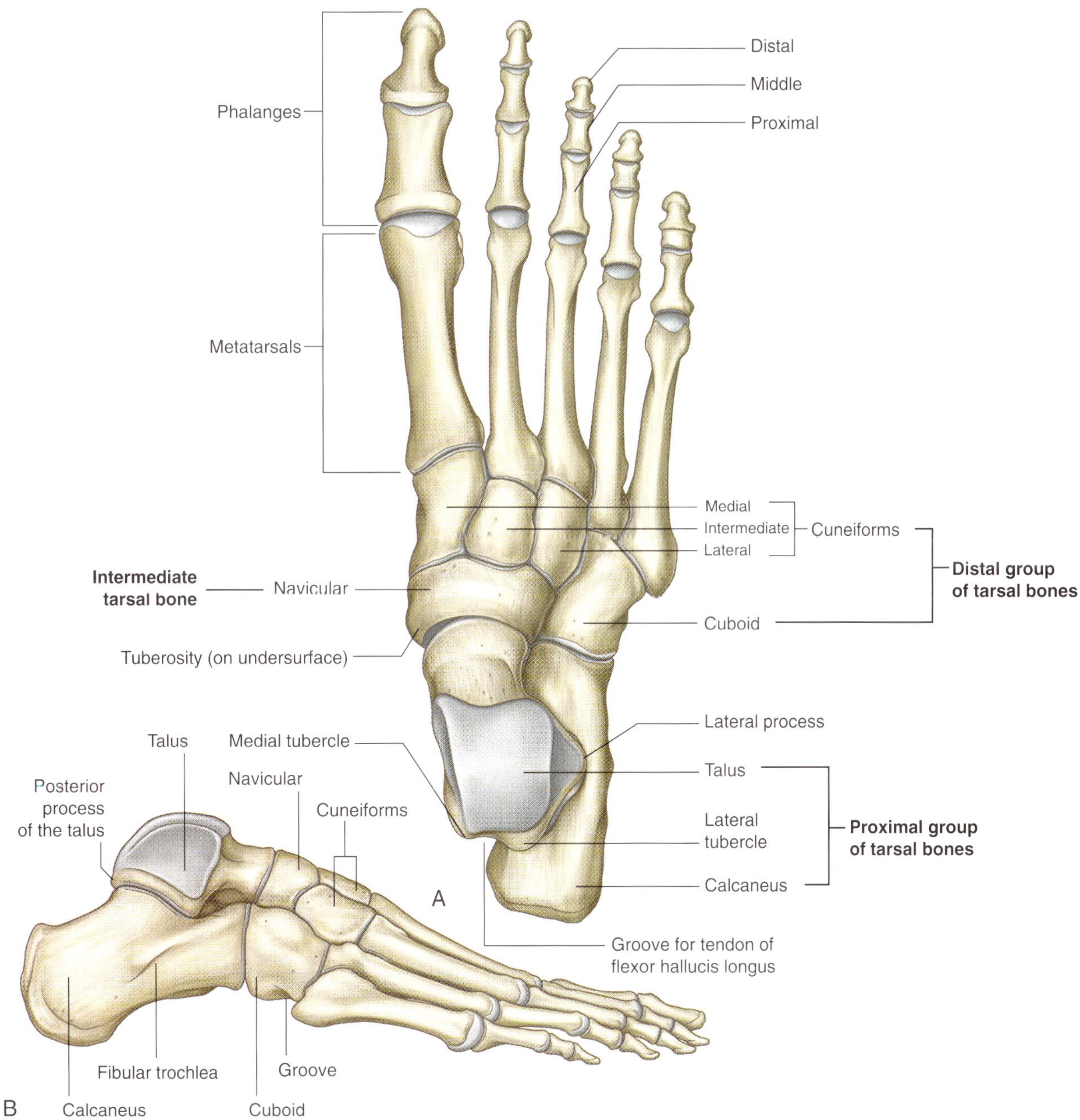

Fig. 3.92 Bones of the foot. **(A)** Dorsal view, right foot. **(B)** Lateral view, right foot.

fibula to form the ankle joint and also projects forward to articulate with the intermediate tarsal bone (navicular) on the medial side of the foot.
- The **calcaneus** is the largest of the tarsal bones—posteriorly it forms the bony framework of the heel and anteriorly it projects forward to articulate with one of the distal group of tarsal bones (cuboid) on the lateral side of the foot.

Talus

The talus, when viewed from the medial or lateral sides, is snail shaped (Fig. 3.93A and B). It has a rounded **head**, which is projected forward and medially at the end of a short broad **neck**, which is connected posteriorly to an expanded body.

Anteriorly, the head of the talus is dome-shaped for articulation with a corresponding circular depression on the posterior surface of the navicular bone. Inferiorly, this dome-shaped articular surface is continuous with an additional three articular facets separated by smooth ridges:

- The anterior and middle facets articulate with adjacent surfaces on the calcaneus bone.
- The other facet, medial to the facets for articulation with the calcaneus, articulates with a ligament—the plantar calcaneonavicular ligament (spring ligament)—which connects the calcaneus to the navicular under the head of the talus.

The neck of the talus is marked by a deep groove (the **sulcus tali**), which passes obliquely forward across the inferior surface from medial to lateral, and expands dramatically on the lateral side. Posterior to the sulcus tali is a large facet (posterior calcaneal surface) for articulation with the calcaneus at the subtalar joint (see Fig. 3.101).

The superior aspect of the body of the talus is elevated to fit into the socket formed by the distal ends of the tibia and fibula to form the ankle joint (see Fig. 3.97):

- The upper (trochlear) surface of this elevated region articulates with the inferior end of the tibia.
- The medial surface articulates with the medial malleolus of the tibia.
- The lateral surface articulates with the lateral malleolus of the fibula.

Because the lateral malleolus is larger and projects more inferiorly than the medial malleolus at the ankle joint, the corresponding lateral articular surface on the talus is larger and projects more inferiorly than the medial surface.

The lower part of the lateral surface of the body of the talus forms a bony projection (the **lateral process**). This is below the lower part of the facet for articulation with the fibula.

The inferior surface of the body of the talus has a large oval concave facet (the **posterior calcaneal articular facet**) for articulation with the calcaneus at the subtalar joint.

The posterior aspect of the body of the talus consists of a backward and medially facing projection (the **posterior process**). The posterior process is marked on its surface by a lateral tubercle and a medial tubercle, which bracket between them the **groove for the tendon of the flexor hallucis longus** as it passes from the leg into the foot.

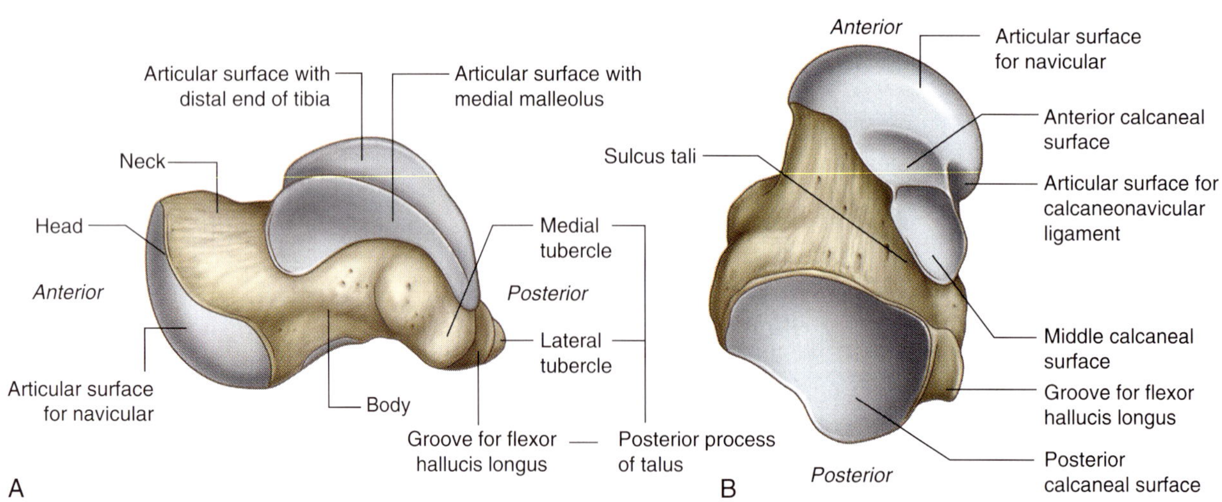

Fig. 3.93 Talus. **(A)** Medial view. **(B)** Inferior view.

Calcaneus

The calcaneus is inferior to and supports the talus. It is an elongate, irregular, box-shaped bone with its long axis generally oriented along the midline of the foot, but deviating lateral to the midline anteriorly (Fig. 3.94).

The calcaneus projects behind the ankle joint to form the skeletal framework of the heel. The posterior surface of this heel region is circular and divided into upper, middle, and lower parts. The calcaneal tendon (Achilles tendon) attaches to the middle part:

- The upper part is separated from the calcaneal tendon by a bursa.
- The lower part curves forward, is covered by subcutaneous tissue, is the weight-bearing region of the heel, and is continuous onto the plantar surface of the bone as the **calcaneal tuberosity**.

The calcaneal tuberosity projects forward on the plantar surface as a large medial process and a small lateral process separated from each other by a V-shaped notch (Fig. 3.94B). At the anterior end of the plantar surface is a tubercle (the **calcaneal tubercle**) for the posterior attachment of the short plantar ligament of the sole of the foot.

The lateral surface of the calcaneus has a smooth contour except for two slightly raised regions (Fig. 3.94C). One of these raised areas—the **fibular trochlea** (peroneal tubercle)—is anterior to the middle of the surface and often has two shallow grooves, which pass, one above the other, obliquely across its surface. The tendons of the fibularis brevis and longus muscles are bound to the trochlea as they pass over the lateral side of the calcaneus (Fig. 3.87).

Superior and posterior to the fibular trochlea is a second raised area or tubercle for attachment of the calcaneofibular part of the lateral collateral ligament of the ankle joint (see Fig. 3.99).

The medial surface of the calcaneus is concave and has one prominent feature associated with its upper margin (the **sustentaculum tali**; Fig. 3.94A), which is a shelf of bone projecting medially and supporting the more posterior part of the head of the talus.

The underside of the sustentaculum tali has a distinct groove running from posterior to anterior and along which the tendon of the flexor hallucis longus muscle travels into the sole of the foot.

The superior surface of the sustentaculum tali has a facet (**middle talar articular surface**) for articulation with the corresponding middle facet on the head of the talus.

Anterior and **posterior talar articular surfaces** are on the superior surface of the calcaneus itself (Fig. 3.94A):

- The anterior talar articular surface is small and articulates with the corresponding anterior facet on the head of the talus.

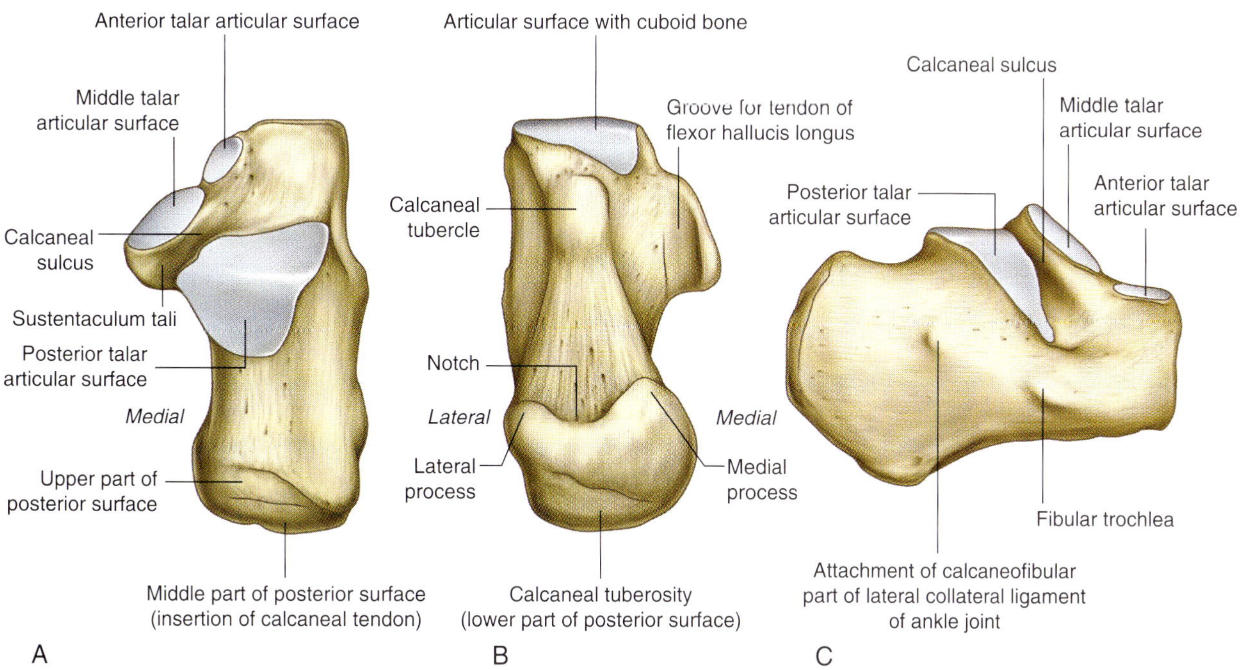

Fig. 3.94 Calcaneus. **(A)** Superior view. **(B)** Inferior view. **(C)** Lateral view.

- The posterior talar articular surface forms the subtalar joint. It is large and is approximately near the middle of the superior surface of the calcaneus.

Between the posterior talar articular surface and the other two articular surfaces, which articulate with the head of the talus, is a deep groove (the **calcaneal sulcus**; Fig. 3.94A and C).

The calcaneal sulcus on the superior surface of the calcaneus and the sulcus tali on the inferior surface of the talus together form the **tarsal sinus**, which is a large gap between the anterior ends of the calcaneus and talus that is visible when the skeleton of the foot is viewed from its lateral aspect (Fig. 3.95A and 3.101).

Intermediate tarsal bone

The intermediate tarsal bone on the medial side of the foot is the **navicular** (boat shaped) (Fig. 3.92). This bone articulates behind with the talus and articulates in front and on the lateral side with the distal group of tarsal bones (Fig. 3.84 and 3.98).

One distinctive feature of the navicular is a prominent rounded tuberosity for the attachment of the tibialis posterior tendon, which projects inferiorly on the medial side of the plantar surface of the bone.

Distal group

From lateral to medial, the distal group of tarsal bones consists of (Fig. 3.92):

- The **cuboid** (Greek for "cube"), which articulates posteriorly with the calcaneus, medially with the lateral cuneiform, and anteriorly with the bases of the lateral two metatarsals—the tendon of the fibularis longus muscle lies in a prominent groove on the anterior plantar surface, which passes obliquely forward across the bone from lateral to medial (see Fig. 3.92 and 3.103).
- Three **cuneiforms** (Latin for "wedge")—the **lateral**, **intermediate**, and **medial** cuneiform bones, in addition to articulating with each other, articulate posteriorly with the navicular bone and anteriorly with the bases of the medial three metatarsals.

Metatarsals

There are five metatarsals in the foot, numbered I to V from medial to lateral (Fig. 3.96). Metatarsal I, associated with the great toe, is shortest and thickest. The second is the longest.

Each metatarsal has a **head** at the distal end, an elongate **shaft** in the middle, and a proximal **base**.

The head of each metatarsal articulates with the proximal phalanx of a toe and the base articulates with one or more of the distal group of tarsal bones. The plantar surface of the head of metatarsal I also articulates with two sesamoid bones (Fig. 3.96).

The sides of the bases of metatarsals II to V also articulate with each other. The lateral side of the base of metatarsal V has a prominent **tuberosity**, which projects posteriorly and is the attachment site for the tendon of the fibularis brevis muscle.

Phalanges

The phalanges are the bones of the toes (Fig. 3.96). Each toe has three phalanges (**proximal**, **middle**, and **distal**), except for the great toe, which has only two (proximal and distal).

Each phalanx consists of a **base**, a **shaft**, and a distal **head**:

- The base of each proximal phalanx articulates with the head of the related metatarsal.
- The head of each distal phalanx is nonarticular and flattened into a crescent-shaped plantar tuberosity under the plantar pad at the end of the digit.

In each toe, the total length of the phalanges combined is much shorter than the length of the associated metatarsal.

Early clinical exposure

Talar beak

Occasionally there is a superior projection of the distal aspect of the talus, which is beak-shaped (Fig. 3.95B). It is often associated with the presence of a bony or fibrous joint between the talus and calcaneus.

Fracture of the talus

The talus is an unusual bone because it ossifies from a single primary ossification center, which initially appears in the neck. The posterior aspect of the talus appears to ossify last, normally after puberty. In up to 50% of people, there is a small accessory ossicle (the **os trigonum**) posterior to the lateral tubercle of the posterior process. Articular cartilage covers approximately 60% of the talar surface and there are no direct tendon or muscle attachments to the bone.

One of the problems with fractures of the talus is that the blood supply to the bone is vulnerable to damage. The main blood supply to the bone enters the talus through the **tarsal canal** from a branch of the posterior tibial artery. This vessel supplies most of the neck and the body of the talus.

Early clinical exposure—cont'd

Branches of the dorsalis pedis artery enter the superior aspect of the **talar neck** and supply the dorsal portion of the head and neck, and branches from the fibular artery supply a small portion of the lateral talus.

Fractures of the neck of the talus often interrupt the blood supply to the talus, so making the body and posterior aspect of the talus susceptible to osteonecrosis, which may in turn lead to premature osteoarthritis and require extensive surgery.

Midfoot fractures

Fractures of the midfoot are uncommon. They usually occur when heavy weights have been dropped onto the feet or when the feet have been run over by a vehicle. Plain radiographs are usually sufficient to demonstrate dislocations and fractures.

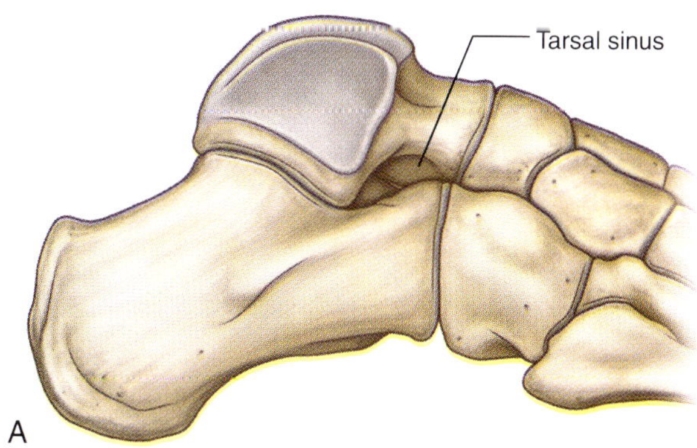

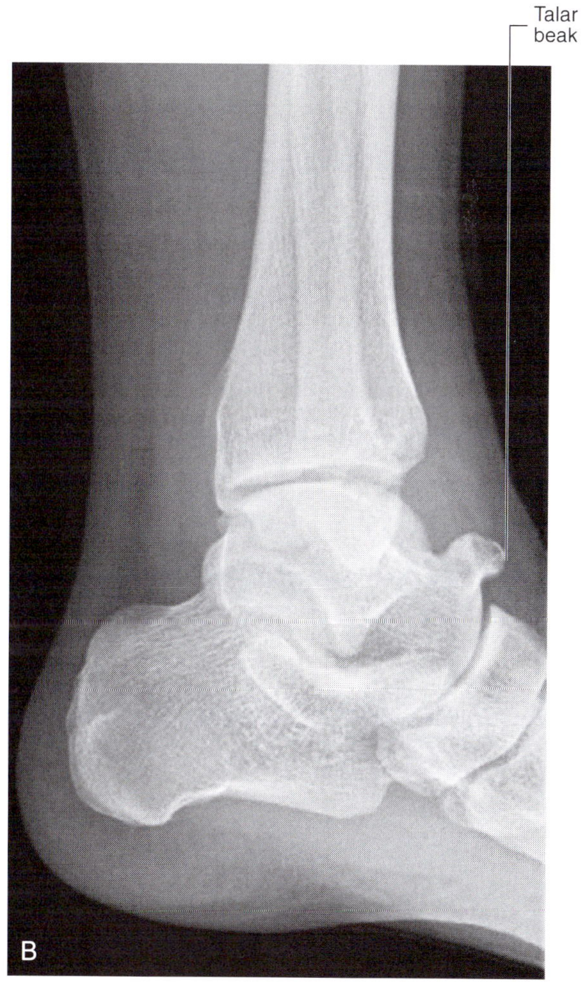

Fig. 3.95 **(A)** Tarsal sinus. Lateral view, right foot. **(B)** Radiograph of ankle showing talar beak.

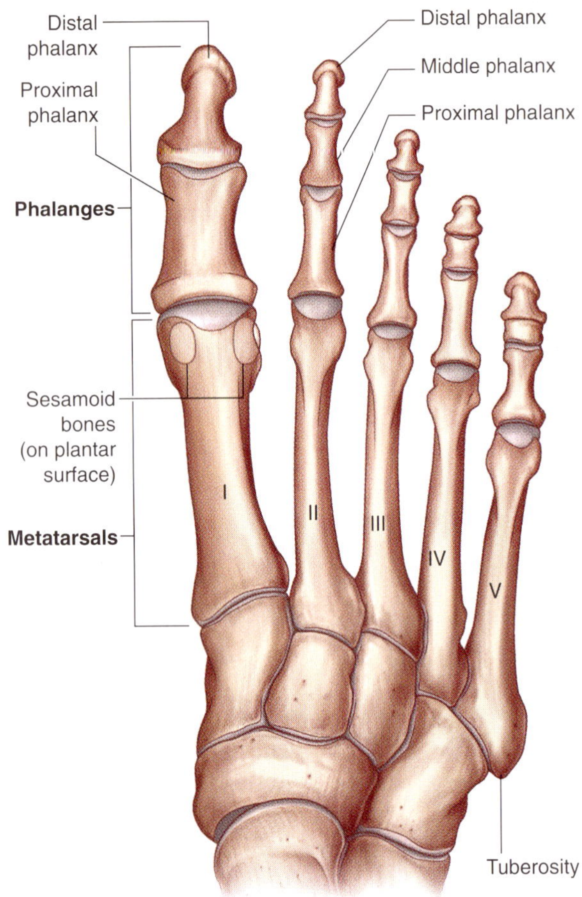

Fig. 3.96 Metatarsals and phalanges. Dorsal view. The head of the first metatarsal is shown as if transparent.

Joints

Ankle joint

The ankle joint is synovial hinge in type and involves the talus of the foot and the tibia and fibula of the leg (Fig. 3.97).

The ankle joint mainly allows hinge-like dorsiflexion and plantar flexion of the foot on the leg.

The distal end of the fibula is firmly anchored to the larger distal end of the tibia by strong ligaments. Together, the fibula and tibia create a deep bracket-shaped socket for the upper expanded part of the body of the talus:

- The roof of the socket is formed by the inferior surface of the distal end of the tibia.
- The medial side of the socket is formed by the medial malleolus of the tibia.
- The longer lateral side of the socket is formed by the lateral malleolus of the fibula.

The articular surfaces are covered by hyaline cartilage.

The articular part of the talus is shaped like a short half-cylinder tipped onto its flat side with one end facing lateral and the other end facing medial (Fig. 3.97B). The curved upper surface of the half-cylinder and the two ends are covered by hyaline cartilage and fit into the bracket-shaped socket formed by the distal ends of the tibia and fibula.

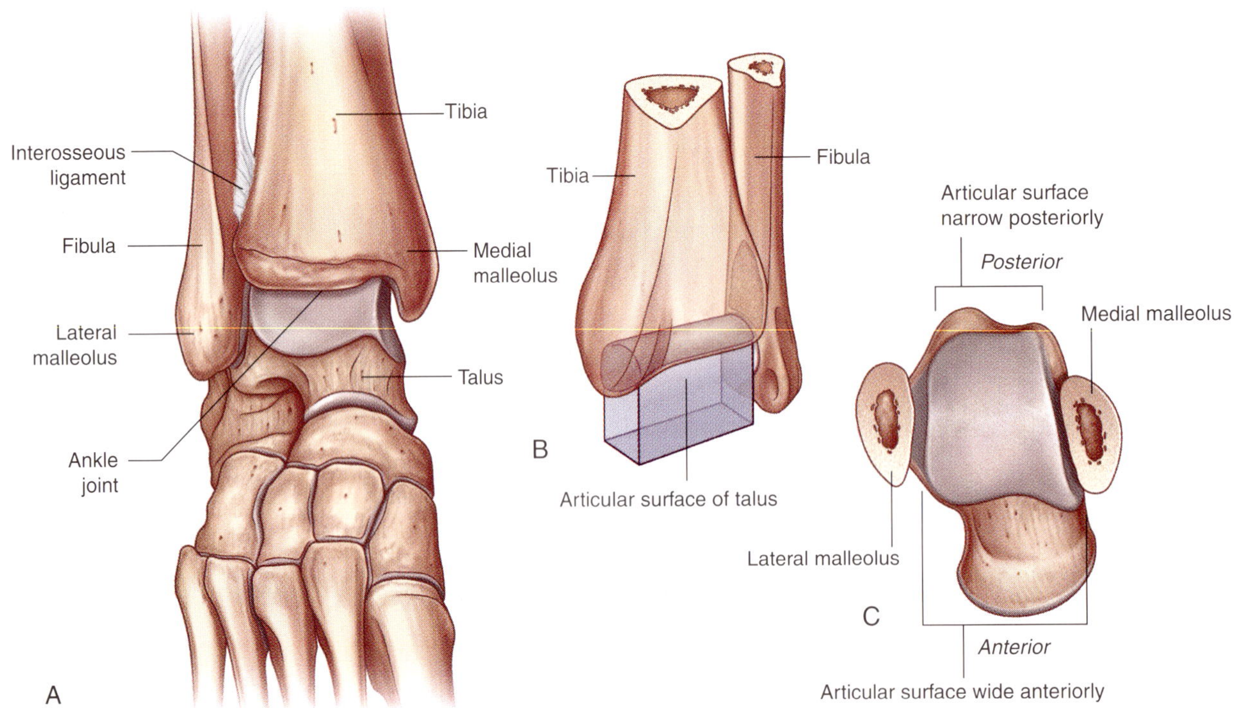

Fig. 3.97 Ankle joint. **(A)** Anterior view with foot plantarflexed. **(B)** Schematic of joint. **(C)** Superior view of the talus to show the shape of the articular surface.

When viewed from above, the articular surface of the talus is much wider anteriorly than it is posteriorly. As a result, the bone fits tighter into its socket when the foot is dorsiflexed and the wider surface of the talus moves into the ankle joint than when the foot is plantarflexed and the narrower part of the talus is in the joint. The joint is therefore most stable when the foot is dorsiflexed.

The articular cavity is enclosed by a synovial membrane, which attaches around the margins of the articular surfaces, and by a fibrous membrane, which covers the synovial membrane and is also attached to the adjacent bones.

The ankle joint is stabilized by **medial** (deltoid) and **lateral ligaments**.

Medial ligament (deltoid ligament)

The medial (deltoid) ligament is large, strong (Fig. 3.98), and triangular in shape. Its apex is attached above to the medial malleolus and its broad base is attached below to a line that extends from the tuberosity of the navicular bone in front to the medial tubercle of the talus behind.

The medial ligament is subdivided into four parts based on the inferior points of attachment:

- The part that attaches in front to the tuberosity of the navicular and the associated margin of the plantar calcaneonavicular ligament (spring ligament), which connects the navicular bone to the sustentaculum tali of the calcaneus bone behind, is the **tibionavicular part** of the medial ligament.
- The **tibiocalcaneal part**, which is more central, attaches to the sustentaculum tali of the calcaneus bone.
- The **posterior tibiotalar part** attaches to the medial side and medial tubercle of the talus.
- The fourth part (the **anterior tibiotalar part**) is deep to the tibionavicular and tibiocalcaneal parts of the medial ligament and attaches to the medial surface of the talus.

Lateral ligament

The lateral ligament of the ankle is composed of three separate ligaments, the anterior talofibular ligament, the posterior talofibular ligament, and the calcaneofibular ligament (Fig. 3.99):

- The **anterior talofibular ligament** is a short ligament, and attaches the anterior margin of the lateral malleolus to the adjacent region of the talus.
- The **posterior talofibular ligament** runs horizontally backward and medially from the malleolar fossa on the

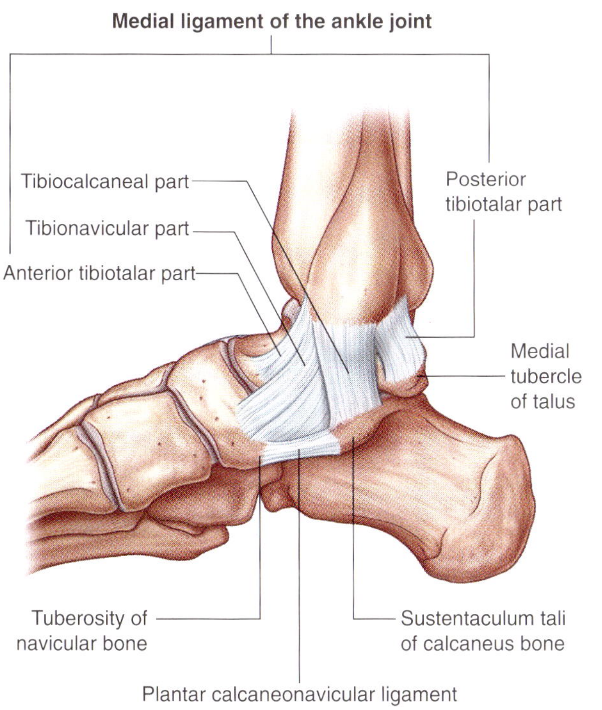

Fig. 3.98 Medial ligament of the ankle joint.

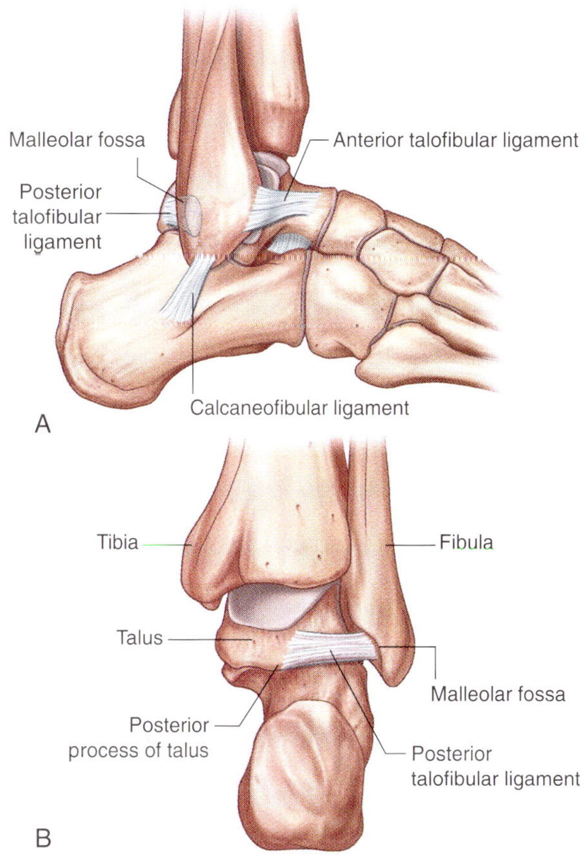

Fig. 3.99 Lateral ligament of the ankle joint. **(A)** Lateral view. **(B)** Posterior view.

medial side of the lateral malleolus to the posterior process of the talus.

- The **calcaneofibular ligament** is attached above to the malleolar fossa on the posteromedial side of the lateral malleolus and passes posteroinferiorly to attach below to a tubercle on the lateral surface of the calcaneus.

Intertarsal joints

The numerous synovial joints between the individual tarsal bones mainly invert, evert, supinate, and pronate the foot:

- Inversion and eversion is turning the whole sole of the foot inward and outward, respectively.
- Pronation is to move the front of the foot laterally relative to the back of the foot, and supination is the reverse movement.

Pronation and supination allow the foot to maintain normal contact with the ground when in different stances or when standing on irregular surfaces.

The major joints at which movements occur include the subtalar, talocalcaneonavicular, and calcaneocuboid joints (Fig. 3.100). The talocalcaneonavicular and calcaneocuboid joints together form what is often referred to as the **transverse tarsal joint**.

Intertarsal joints between the cuneiforms and between the cuneiforms and the navicular allow only limited movement.

The joint between the cuboid and navicular is normally fibrous.

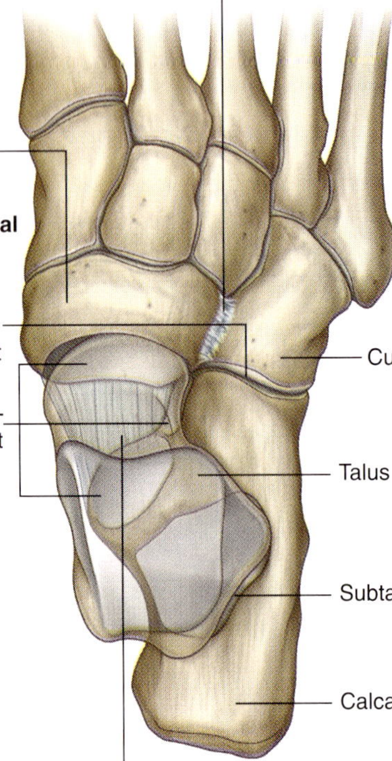

Fig. 3.100 Intertarsal joints. The talus is shown as it is transparent.

Early clinical exposure

Ankle fractures

An appreciation of ankle anatomy is essential to understand the wide variety of fractures that may occur at and around the ankle joint.

The ankle joint and related structures can be regarded as a fibro-osseous ring oriented in the coronal plane.

- The upper part of the ring is formed by the joint between the distal ends of the fibula and tibia and by the ankle joint itself.
- The sides of the ring are formed by the ligaments that connect the medial malleolus and lateral malleolus to the adjacent tarsal bones.
- The bottom of the ring is not part of the ankle joint, but consists of the subtalar joint and the associated ligaments.

Visualizing the ankle joint and surrounding structures as a fibro-osseous ring allows the physician to predict the type of damage likely to result from a particular type of injury. For example, an inversion injury may tear ligaments anchoring the lateral malleolus to the tarsal bones and fracture the medial malleolus.

The ring may be disrupted not only by damage to the bones (which produces fractures) but also by damage to the ligaments. Unlike bone fractures, damage to ligaments is unlikely to be appreciated on plain radiographs. When a fracture is noted on a plain radiograph, the physician must always be aware that there may also be appreciable ligamentous disruption.

Ottawa ankle rules

The Ottawa ankle rules were developed to assist clinicians in deciding whether patients with acute ankle injuries require investigation with radiographs in order to avoid unnecessary studies. Named after the hospital where they were developed, the rules are highly sensitive and have reduced the utilization of unwarranted ankle radiographs since their implementation.

Early clinical exposure—cont'd

An ankle X-ray series is required if there is ankle pain and any of the following:

- Bone tenderness along the distal 6 cm of the posterior tibia or tip of the medial malleolus
- Bone tenderness along the distal 6 cm of the posterior fibula or tip of the lateral malleolus
- Inability to bear weight for four steps both immediately after the injury and in the emergency department

A foot X-ray series is required if there is midfoot pain and any of the following:

- Bone tenderness at the base of the fifth metatarsal bone
- Bone tenderness at the navicular bone
- Inability to bear weight for four steps both immediately after the injury and in the emergency department

Subtalar joint

The **subtalar joint** is between:

- The large posterior calcaneal facet on the inferior surface of the talus
- The corresponding posterior talar facet on the superior surface of the calcaneus

The articular cavity is enclosed by synovial membrane, which is covered by a fibrous membrane.

The subtalar joint allows gliding and rotation, which are involved in inversion and eversion of the foot. **Lateral, medial, posterior**, and **interosseous talocalcaneal ligaments** stabilize the joint. The interosseous talocalcaneal ligament lies in the tarsal sinus (Fig. 3.101).

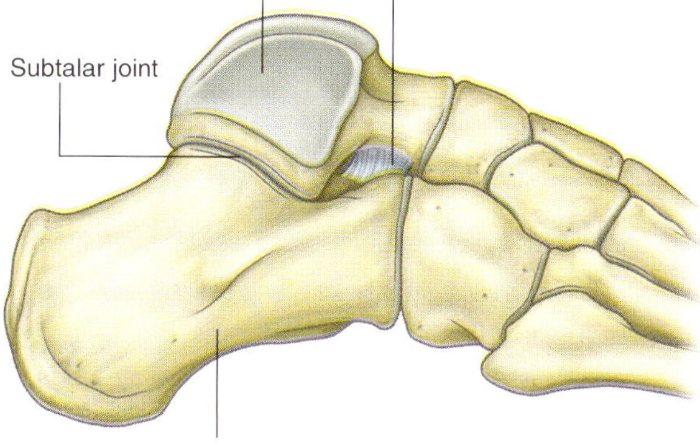

Fig. 3.101 Interosseous talocalcaneal ligament. Lateral view.

Talocalcaneonavicular joint

The **talocalcaneonavicular joint** is a complex joint in which the head of the talus articulates with the calcaneus and plantar calcaneonavicular ligament (spring ligament) below and the navicular in front (Fig. 3.102A).

The talocalcaneonavicular joint allows gliding and rotation movements, which together with similar movements of the subtalar joint are involved with inversion and eversion of the foot. It also participates in pronation and supination.

The parts of the talocalcaneonavicular joint between the talus and calcaneus are

- The anterior and middle calcaneal facets on the inferior surface of the talar head
- The corresponding anterior and middle talar facets on the superior surface and sustentaculum tali, respectively, of the calcaneus (Fig. 3.102B)

The part of the joint between the talus and the plantar calcaneonavicular ligament (spring ligament) is between the ligament and the medial facet on the inferior surface of the talar head (Fig. 3.93).

The joint between the navicular and talus is a ball ad socket joint. It is the largest part of the talocalcaneonavicular joint and is between the ovoid anterior end of the talar head and the corresponding concave posterior surface of the navicular.

Ligaments

The capsule of the talocalcaneonavicular joint, which is a synovial joint, is reinforced:

- Posteriorly by the interosseous talocalcaneal ligament
- Superiorly by the **talonavicular ligament**, which passes between the neck of the talus and adjacent regions of the navicular
- Inferiorly by the plantar calcaneonavicular ligament (spring ligament) (Fig. 3.102C and D)

The lateral part of the talocalcaneonavicular joint is reinforced by the calcaneonavicular part of the **bifurcate**

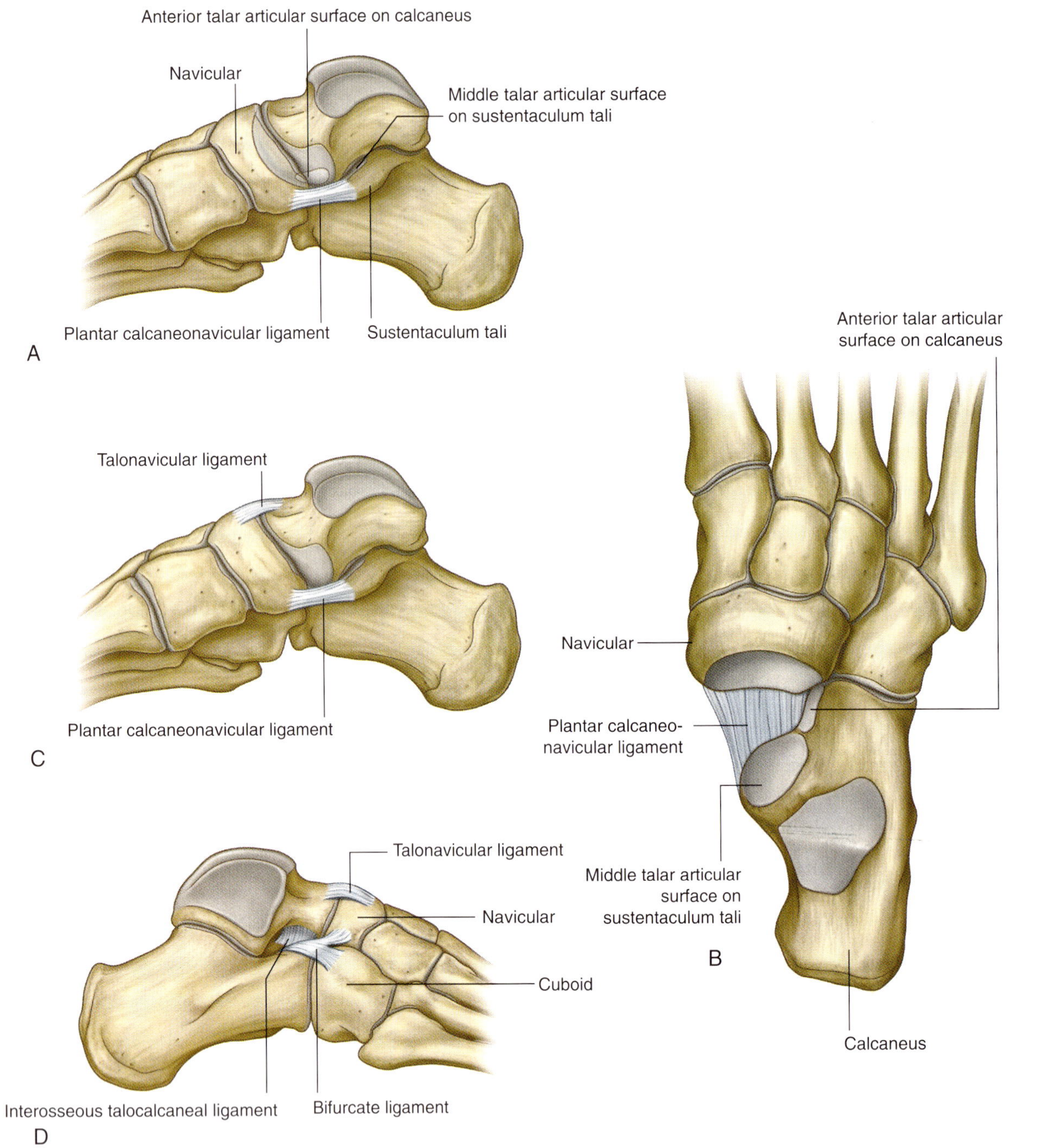

Fig. 3.102 Talocalcaneonavicular joint. **(A)** Medial view, right foot. **(B)** Superior view, right foot, talus removed. **(C)** Ligaments, medial view, right foot. **(D)** Ligaments, lateral view, right foot.

ligament, which is a Y-shaped ligament superior to the joint. The base of the bifurcate ligament is attached to the anterior aspect of the superior surface of the calcaneus and its arms are attached to:

- The dorsomedial surface of the cuboid (**calcaneocuboid ligament**)
- The dorsolateral part of the navicular (**calcaneonavicular ligament**)

The **plantar calcaneonavicular ligament** (spring ligament) is a broad thick ligament that spans the space between the sustentaculum tali behind and the navicular bone in front (Fig. 3.102B and C). It supports the head of the talus, takes part in the talocalcaneonavicular joint, and resists depression of the medial arch of the foot.

Calcaneocuboid joint

The **calcaneocuboid joint** is a synovial saddle joint between the facet on the anterior surface of the calcaneus and the corresponding facet on the posterior surface of the cuboid.

The calcaneocuboid joint allows sliding and rotating movements involved with inversion and eversion of the foot, and also contributes to pronation and supination of the forefoot on the hindfoot.

Ligaments

The calcaneocuboid joint is reinforced by the bifurcate ligament (see above) and by the long plantar ligament and the plantar calcaneocuboid ligament (short plantar ligament).

The **plantar calcaneocuboid ligament** (short plantar ligament) is short, wide, and very strong, and connects the calcaneal tubercle to the inferior surface of the cuboid (Fig. 3.103A). It not only supports the calcaneocuboid joint but also assists the long plantar ligament in resisting depression of the lateral arch of the foot.

The **long plantar ligament** is the longest ligament in the sole of the foot and lies inferior to the plantar calcaneocuboid ligament (Fig. 3.103B):

- Posteriorly, it attaches to the inferior surface of the calcaneus between the calcaneal tuberosity and the calcaneal tubercle.
- Anteriorly, it attaches to a broad ridge and a tubercle on the inferior surface of the cuboid bone behind the groove for the fibularis longus tendon.

More superficial fibers of the long plantar ligament extend to the bases of the metatarsal bones.

The long plantar ligament supports the calcaneocuboid joint and is the strongest ligament resisting depression of the lateral arch of the foot.

Tarsometatarsal joints

The **tarsometatarsal joints** between the metatarsal bones and adjacent tarsal bones are plane joints and allow limited sliding movements (Fig. 3.104).

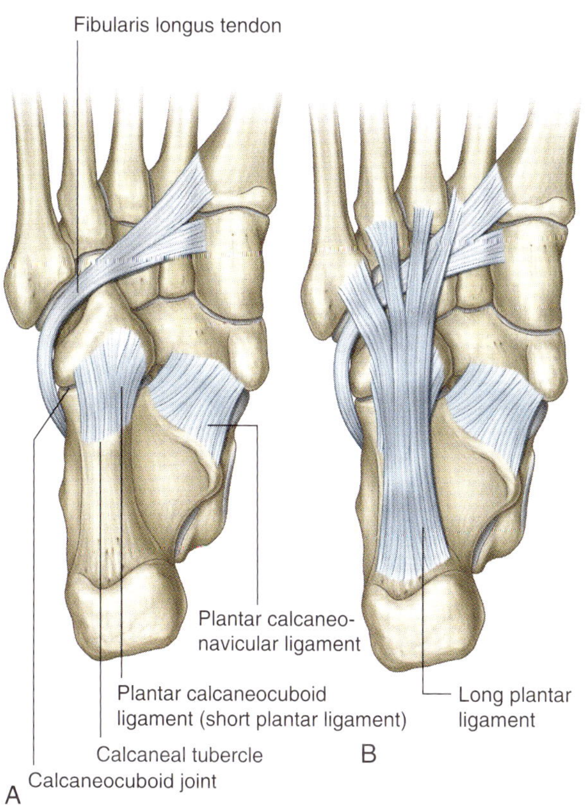

Fig. 3.103 Plantar ligaments. **(A)** Plantar calcaneocuboid ligament (short plantar ligament). **(B)** Long plantar ligament.

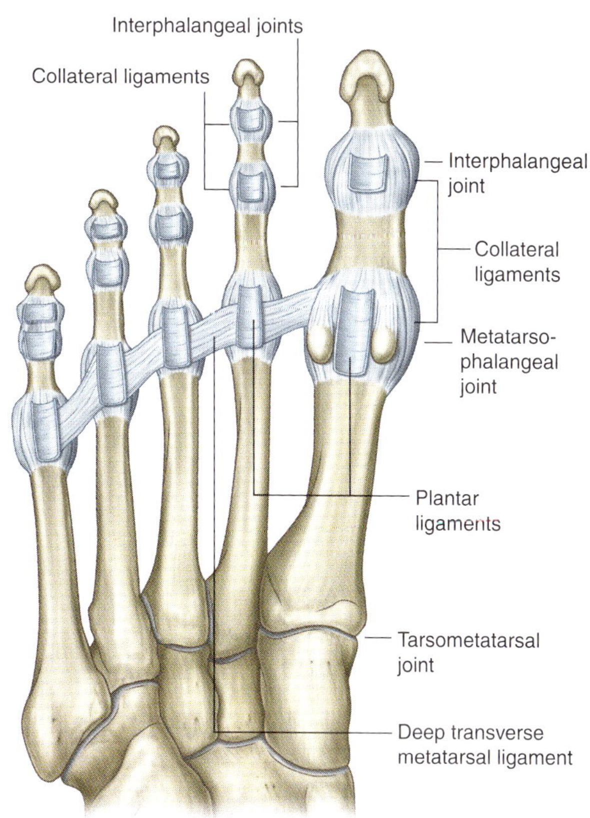

Fig. 3.104 Tarsometatarsal, metatarsophalangeal, and interphalangeal joints, and the deep transverse metatarsal ligaments.

The range of movement of the tarsometatarsal joint between the metatarsal of the great toe and the medial cuneiform is greater than that of the other tarsometatarsal joints and allows flexion, extension, and rotation. The tarsometatarsal joints, with the transverse tarsal joint, take part in pronation and supination of the foot.

Metatarsophalangeal joints

The metatarsophalangeal joints are ellipsoid synovial joints between the sphere-shaped heads of the metatarsals and the corresponding bases of the proximal phalanges of the digits.

The metatarsophalangeal joints allow extension and flexion, and limited abduction, adduction, and circumduction.

The joint capsules are reinforced by medial and lateral **collateral ligaments**, and by **plantar ligaments**, which have grooves on their plantar surfaces for the long tendons of the digits (Fig. 3.104).

Early clinical exposure

Bunions

A bunion occurs on the medial aspect of the first metatarsophalangeal joint. This is an extremely important area of the foot because it is crossed by tendons and ligaments, which transmit and distribute the body's weight during movement. It is postulated that abnormal stresses in this region of the joint may produce the bunion deformity.

Clinically, a bunion is a significant protuberance of bone that may include soft tissue around the medial aspect of the first metatarsophalangeal joint. As it progresses, the toe appears to move toward the smaller toes, producing crowding of the digits.

This deformity tends to occur among people who wear high-heeled or pointed shoes, but osteoporosis and a hereditary predisposition are also risk factors.

Typically the patient's symptoms are pain, swelling, and inflammation. The bunion tends to enlarge and may cause problems in wearing footwear.

Initial treatment is by adding padding to shoes, changing the type of footwear used, and taking anti-inflammatory drugs. Some patients may need surgery to correct the deformity and realign the toe.

Deep transverse metatarsal ligaments

Four **deep transverse metatarsal ligaments** link the heads of the metatarsals together and enable the metatarsals to act as a single unified structure (Fig. 3.104). The ligaments blend with the plantar ligaments of the adjacent metatarsophalangeal joints.

The metatarsal of the great toe is oriented in the same plane as the metatarsals of the other toes and is linked to the metatarsal of the second toe by a deep transverse metatarsal ligament. In addition, the joint between the metatarsal of the great toe and medial cuneiform has a limited range of motion. The great toe therefore has a very restricted independent function—unlike the thumb in the hand, where the metacarpal is oriented 90° to the metacarpals of the fingers, there is no deep transverse metacarpal ligament between the metacarpals of the thumb and index finger, and the saddle joint between the metacarpal and carpal bone allows a wide range of motion.

Interphalangeal joints

The interphalangeal joints are hinge joints that allow mainly flexion and extension. They are reinforced by medial and lateral **collateral ligaments** and by **plantar ligaments** (Fig. 3.104).

Tarsal tunnel, retinacula, and arrangement of major structures at the ankle

The tarsal tunnel is formed on the posteromedial side of the ankle by:

- A depression formed by the medial malleolus of the tibia, the medial and posterior surfaces of the talus, the medial surface of the calcaneus, and the inferior surface of the sustentaculum tali of the calcaneus.
- An overlying flexor retinaculum (Fig. 3.105).

Flexor retinaculum

The flexor retinaculum is a strap-like layer of connective tissue that spans the bony depression formed by the medial malleolus, the medial and posterior surfaces of the talus, the medial surface of the calcaneus, and the inferior surface of the sustentaculum tali (Fig. 3.105). It attaches above to the medial malleolus and below and behind to the inferomedial margin of the calcaneus.

The retinaculum is continuous above with the deep fascia of the leg and below with the deep fascia (plantar aponeurosis) of the foot.

Septa from the flexor retinaculum convert grooves on the bones into tubular connective tissue channels for the tendons of the flexor muscles as they pass into the sole of the foot from the posterior compartment of the leg (Fig. 3.105). Free movement of the tendons in the channels is facilitated by synovial sheaths, which surround the tendons.

Two compartments on the posterior surface of the medial malleolus are for the tendons of the tibialis posterior and flexor digitorum longus muscles. The tendon of the tibialis posterior is medial to the tendon of the flexor digitorum longus.

Immediately lateral to the tendons of the tibialis posterior and flexor digitorum longus, the posterior tibial artery with its associated veins and the tibial nerve pass through the tarsal tunnel into the sole of the foot. The pulse of the posterior tibial artery can be felt through the flexor retinaculum midway between the medial malleolus and the calcaneus.

Lateral to the tibial nerve is the compartment on the posterior surface of the talus and the undersurface of the sustentaculum tali for the tendon of the flexor hallucis longus muscle.

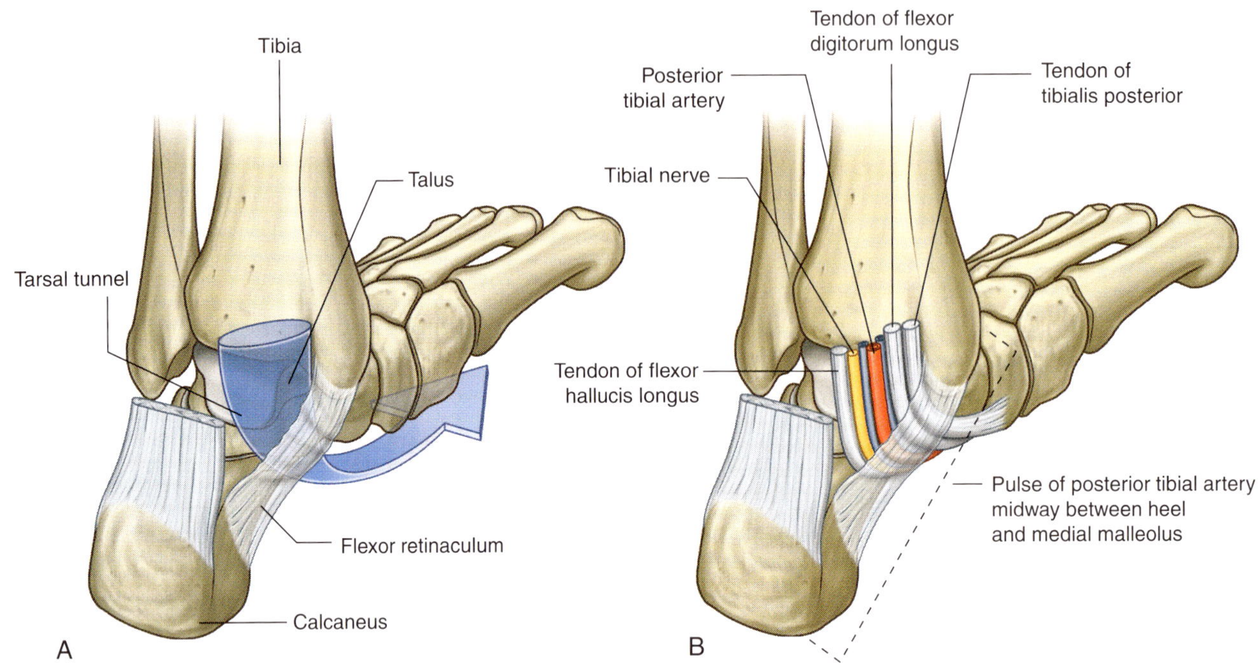

Fig. 3.105 Tarsal tunnel and flexor retinaculum. Posteromedial view. **(A)** Bones. **(B)** Tarsal tunnel and flexor retinaculum.

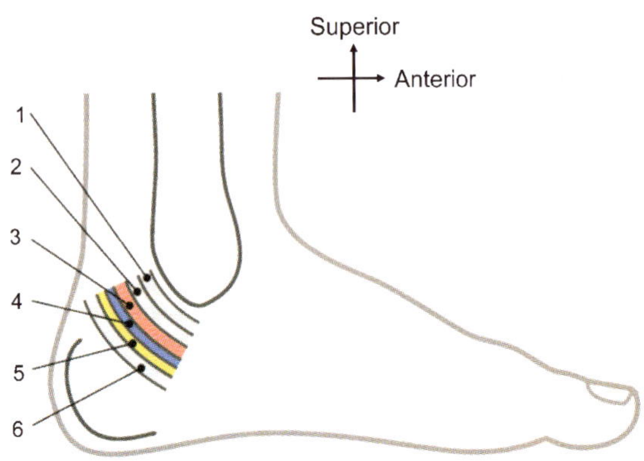

LD Fig. 105.1 Contents of the tarsal tunnel.

Question

105.1A Name the labeled structures in the tarsal tunnel in order from superior to inferior.

Answer

105.1A The labeled structures in the tarsal tunnel in order from superior to inferior are

1. Tibialis posterior
2. Flexor digitorum longus
3. Posterior tibial artery
4. Posterior tibial vein
5. Tibial nerve
6. Flexor hallucis longus

Extensor retinacula

Two extensor retinacula strap the tendons of the extensor muscles to the ankle region and prevent tendon bowing during dorsiflexion of the foot and extension of the toes (Fig. 3.106):

- The **superior extensor retinaculum** is a thickening of deep fascia in the distal leg just superior to the ankle joint and attached to the anterior borders of the fibula and tibia.
- The **inferior extensor retinaculum** is Y-shaped. It is attached by its base to the lateral side of the upper surface of the calcaneus, and crosses medially over the foot to attach by one of its arms to the medial malleolus. The other arm wraps medially around the foot and attaches to the medial side of the plantar aponeurosis.

The tendons of the extensor digitorum longus and fibularis tertius pass through a compartment on the lateral side of the proximal foot. Medial to these tendons, the dorsalis pedis artery (terminal branch of the anterior tibial artery), the tendon of the extensor hallucis longus muscle, and finally the tendon of the tibialis anterior muscle pass under the extensor retinacula.

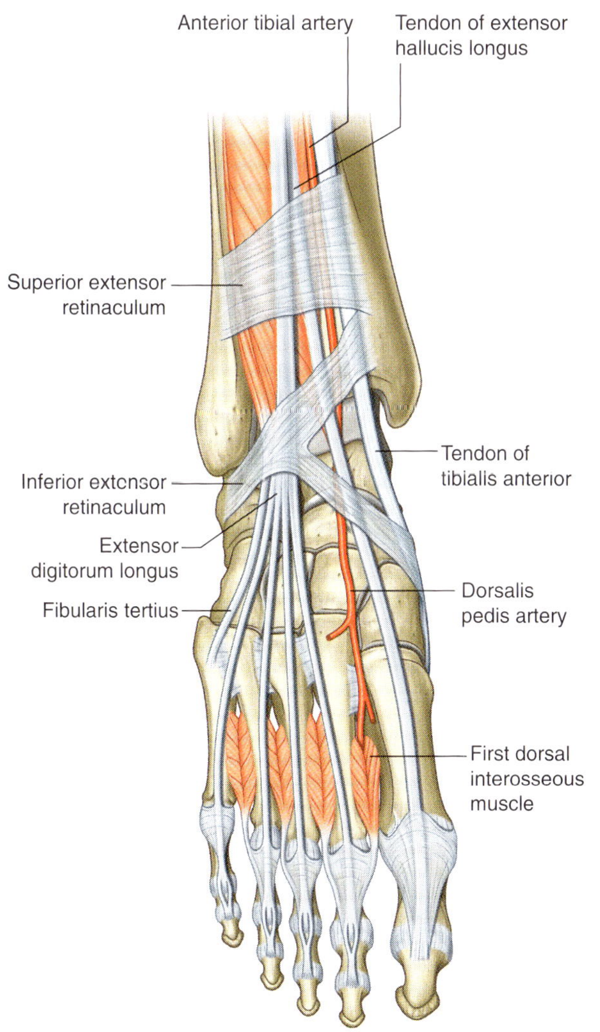

Fig. 3.106 Extensor retinacula.

Fibular retinacula

Fibular (peroneal) retinacula bind the tendons of the fibularis longus and fibularis brevis muscles to the lateral side of the foot (Fig. 3.107):

- **The superior fibular retinaculum** extends between the lateral malleolus and the calcaneus.
- **The inferior fibular retinaculum** attaches to the lateral surface of the calcaneus around the fibular trochlea and blends above with the fibers of the inferior extensor retinaculum.

At the fibular trochlea, a septum separates the compartment for the tendon of the fibularis brevis muscle above from that for the fibularis longus below.

Arches of the foot

The bones of the foot do not lie in a horizontal plane. Instead, they form longitudinal and transverse arches

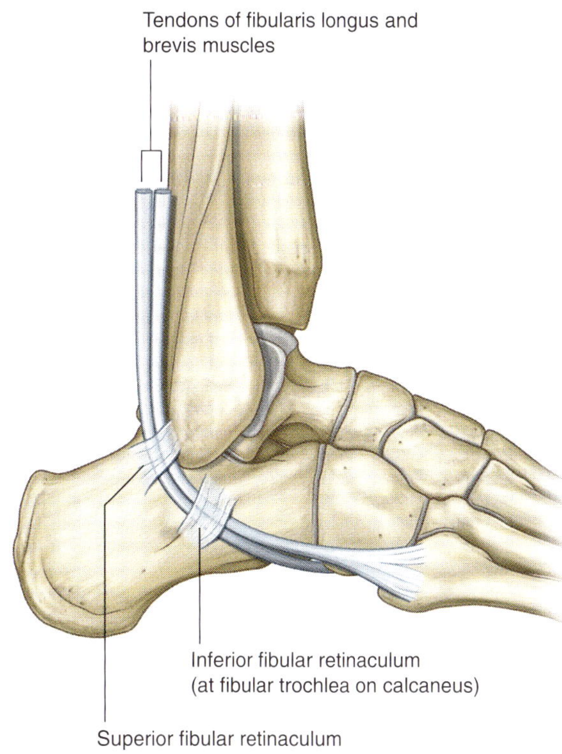

Fig. 3.107 Fibular retinacula. Lateral view, right foot.

relative to the ground (Fig. 3.108), which absorb and distribute downward forces from the body during standing and moving on different surfaces. It enables the foot to act as a segmented lever that is pliable for uneven surfaces. It protects the vessels and nerves within the arches.

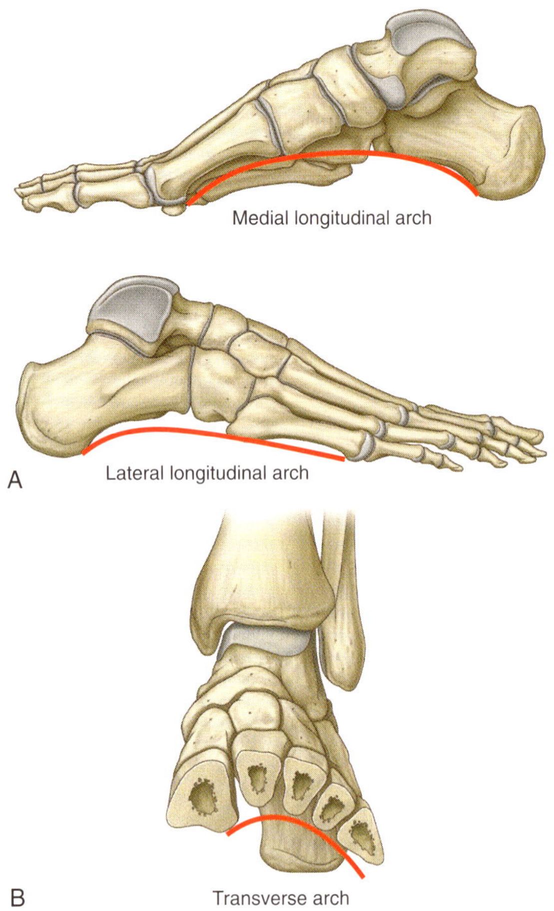

Fig. 3.108 Arches of the foot. **(A)** Longitudinal arches, right foot. **(B)** Transverse arch, left foot.

Longitudinal arch

The longitudinal arch of the foot is formed between the posterior end of the calcaneus and the heads of the metatarsals (Fig. 3.108A). It is highest on the medial side, where it forms the medial longitudinal arch (formed by the calcaneum, talus, navicular, cuneiforms, and medial three metatarsals), and lowest on the lateral side, where it forms the lateral longitudinal arch (formed by the calcaneum, cuboid, and lateral two metatarsals). Each arch has a keystone and anterior and posterior pillars of the arch. The summits or keystones of these arches are the talus and cuboid.

Transverse arch

The transverse arch of the foot is highest in a coronal plane that passes through the head of the talus and disappears near the heads of the metatarsals, where these bones are held together by the deep transverse metatarsal ligaments (Fig. 3.108B). The keystone is the intermediate cuneiform.

Mechanisms by which the muscles, ligaments, and the shapes of bones support the arches of the foot

The mechanisms which support the arches are indicated with inverted commas below:

- Muscles that provide dynamic support for the arches during walking include the tibialis anterior and posterior and the fibularis longus. The longitudinal arch is also maintained by the flexor digitorum longus and brevis, and the flexor hallucis longus. The transverse arch is maintained by the oblique head of the adductor hallucis. Muscles hold the ends of the arch together similar to a "bowstring." The tendons of tibialis anterior, tibialis posterior, peroneus longus, brevis, and tertius hold up the middle of the longitudinal arch like "slings" (Fig. 3.109B).

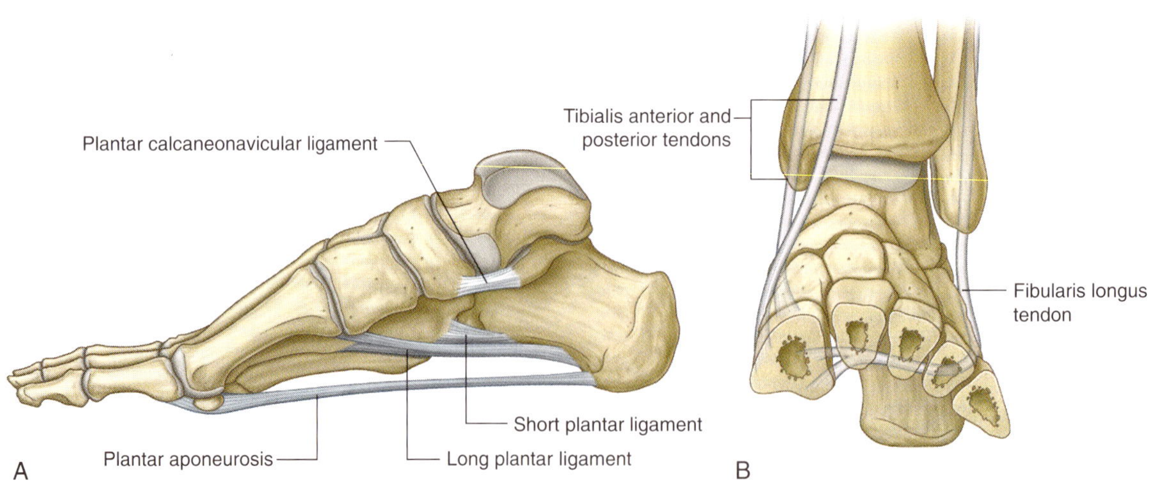

Fig. 3.109 Support for arches of the foot. **(A)** Ligaments. Medial view, right foot. **(B)** Cross-section through the foot to show tendons of muscles supporting the arches.

- Ligaments. These are the primary supports during standing. Ligaments that support the arches include the plantar calcaneonavicular (spring ligament), plantar calcaneocuboid (short plantar ligament), and long plantar ligaments, and the plantar aponeurosis (Fig. 3.109A). These ligaments hold the bones of the longitudinal arch together and are described as "intersegmental ties." The long planter ligament is the primary support of the lateral longitudinal arch. The intersegmental ties of the transverse arch include the deep transverse metatarsal ligament, transverse fibers of plantar aponeurosis, and transverse head of adductor hallucis.
- The superficial fibers of the deltoid ligament act as a "sling" to support the medial longitudinal arch.
- When the big toe is extended, the plantar aponeurosis is pulled distally and stretched, which accentuates the medial longitudinal arch.
- The ligaments and muscles which hold the ends of the arch together are called "tie-beams." For the longitudinal arch these include the plantar aponeurosis, flexor hallucis longus, flexor hallucis brevis, flexor digitorum longus, flexor digitorum brevis, abductor digiti minimi, and flexor digiti minimi brevis, and for the transverse arch these include the peroneus longus and tibialis posterior.
- Shape of the bones. The shape of the talus helps to maintain the medial longitudinal arch (Fig. 3.108). It is at the summit of the arch and functions as a "keystone." The cuneiforms and cuboid are wedge-shaped and maintain the transverse arch. The longitudinal arch has anterior and posterior pillars.
- Abnormalities of the arches of the foot include flatfoot (pes planus), a highly arched foot (pes cavus), and clubfoot (talipes equinovarus).

Plantar aponeurosis

The plantar aponeurosis is a thickening of deep fascia in the sole of the foot (Fig. 3.110A). It is firmly anchored to the medial process of the calcaneal tuberosity and extends forward as a thick band of longitudinally arranged connective tissue fibers. The fibers diverge as they pass anteriorly and form digital bands, which enter the toes and connect with bones, ligaments, and dermis of the skin.

Distal to the metatarsophalangeal joints, the digital bands of the plantar aponeurosis are interconnected by transverse fibers, which form **superficial transverse metatarsal ligaments**.

The plantar aponeurosis supports the longitudinal arch of the foot and protects deeper structures in the sole.

Early clinical exposure

Plantar fasciitis

The plantar aponeurosis is a flat band of connective tissue that supports the arch of the sole of the foot. It runs from the calcaneal tuberosity to the base of the toes. Overuse and increased strain on the plantar aponeurosis, such as excessive running and standing, and increased body weight, can lead to microtears and degeneration within the aponeurosis at the heel with disorganization of the collagen fibers. Patients typically present with mild to severe heel pain, which appears thickened on imaging (Fig. 3.110B). It is usually successfully treated with intense physiotherapy, but may require image-guided injection therapies. In severe cases, the diseased section of the fascia needs to be surgically removed.

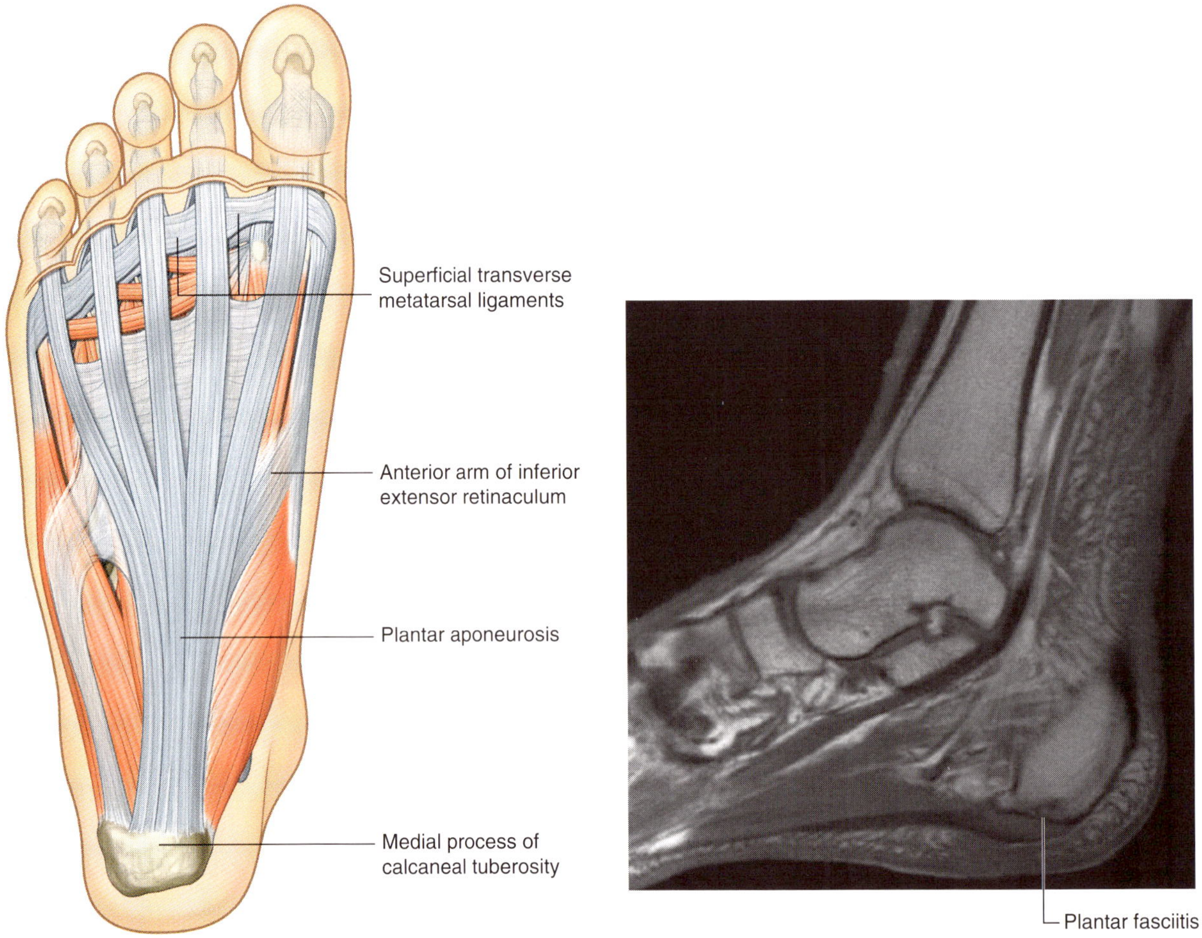

Fig. 3.110 (A) Plantar aponeurosis. **(B)** MRI of posterior foot in a patient with plantar fasciitis shows thickening of the plantar aponeurosis at the calcaneal insertion and a calcaneal spur.

Fibrous sheaths of toes

The tendons of the flexor digitorum longus, flexor digitorum brevis, and flexor hallucis longus muscles enter fibrous digital sheaths or tunnels on the plantar aspect of the digits (Fig. 3.111). These fibrous digital sheaths begin anterior to the metatarsophalangeal joints and extend to the distal phalanges. They are formed by fibrous arches and cruciate (cross-shaped) ligaments attached superiorly to the margins of the phalanges and to the plantar ligaments associated with the metatarsophalangeal and interphalangeal joints.

These fibrous tunnels hold the tendons to the bony plane and prevent tendon bowing when the toes are flexed. Within each tunnel, the tendons are surrounded by a synovial sheath.

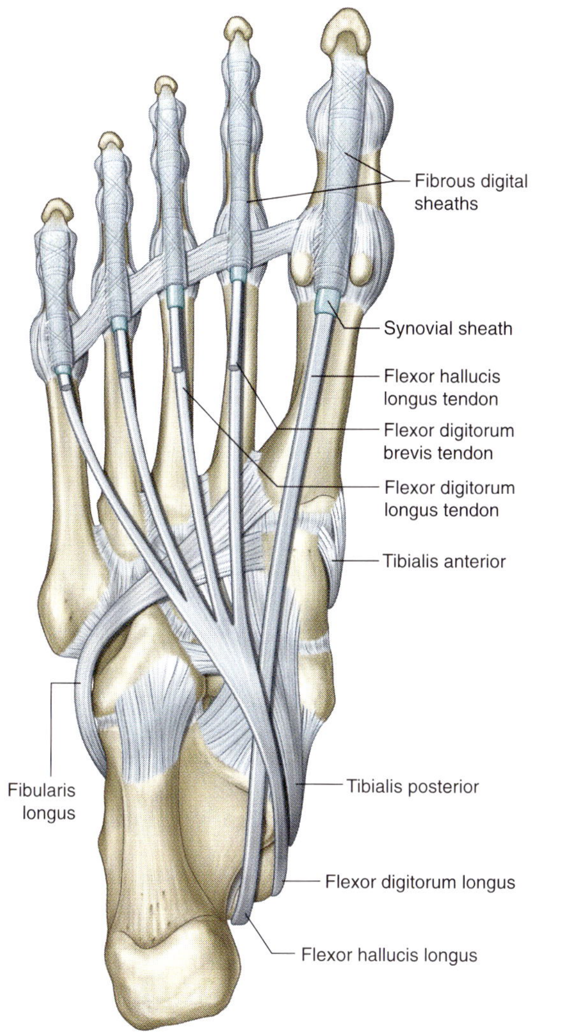

Fig. 3.111 Fibrous digital sheaths.

Extensor hoods

The tendons of the extensor digitorum longus, extensor digitorum brevis, and extensor hallucis longus pass into the dorsal aspect of the digits and expand over the proximal phalanges to form complex dorsal digital expansions ("extensor hoods") (Fig. 3.112).

Each extensor hood is triangular in shape with the apex attached to the distal phalanx, the central region attached to the middle (toes II to V) or proximal (toe I) phalanx. Each corner of the base is wrapped around the sides of the metatarsophalangeal joint and is attached mainly to the deep transverse metatarsal ligaments.

The lumbricals and interossei, which are intrinsic muscles of the foot, insert into the free margin of the hood on each side. The attachment of these muscles into the extensor hoods allows the forces from these muscles to be distributed over the toes to cause flexion of the metatarsophalangeal joints while at the same time extending the interphalangeal joints (Fig. 3.112). The function of these movements in the foot is uncertain, but they may prevent overextension of the metatarsophalangeal joints and flexion of the interphalangeal joints when the heel is elevated off the ground and the toes grip the ground during walking.

Intrinsic muscles

Intrinsic muscles of the foot originate and insert in the foot:

- The extensor digitorum brevis and extensor hallucis brevis on the dorsal aspect of the foot (Fig. 3.113).

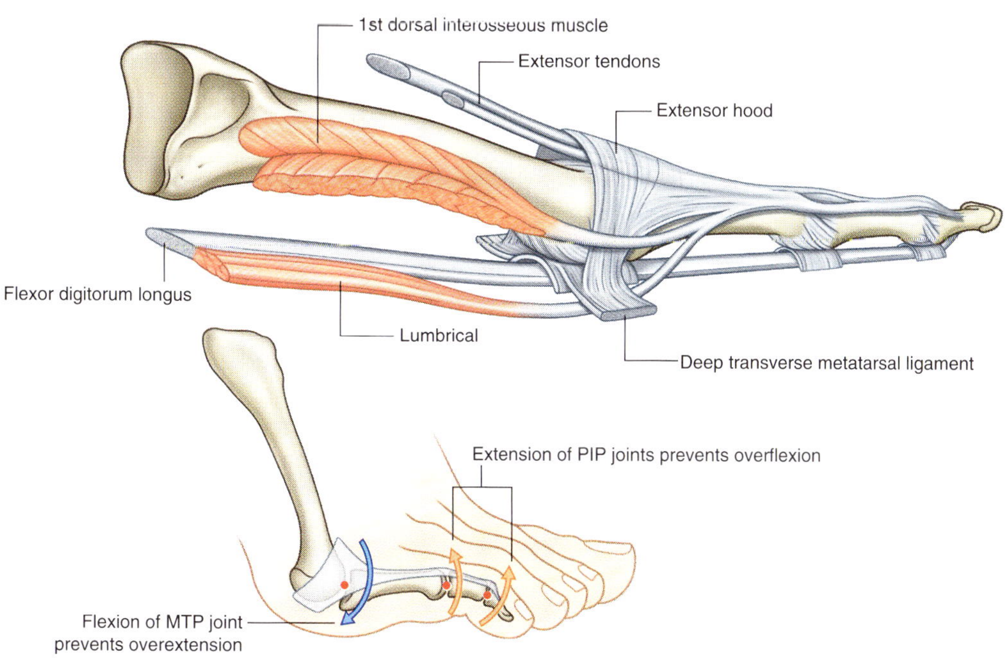

Fig. 3.112 Extensor hoods.

- All other intrinsic muscles—the dorsal and plantar interossei, flexor digiti minimi brevis, flexor hallucis brevis, flexor digitorum brevis, quadratus plantae (flexor accessorius), abductor digiti minimi, abductor hallucis, and lumbricals—are on the plantar side of the foot in the sole where they are organized into four layers.

Intrinsic muscles mainly modify the actions of the long tendons and generate fine movements of the toes.

All intrinsic muscles of the foot are innervated by the medial and lateral plantar branches of the tibial nerve except for the extensor digitorum brevis, which is innervated by the deep fibular nerve. The first two dorsal interossei also may receive part of their innervation from the deep fibular nerve.

On the dorsal aspect

Extensor digitorum brevis and extensor hallucis brevis

The **extensor digitorum brevis** is attached to a roughened area on the superolateral surface of the calcaneus lateral to the tarsal sinus (Fig. 3.113 and Table 3.10).

The flat muscle belly passes anteromedially over the foot, deep to the tendons of the extensor digitorum longus, and forms three tendons, which enter digits II, III, and IV. The tendons join the lateral sides of the tendons of the extensor digitorum longus. The extensor digitorum brevis extends the middle three toes through attachments to the long extensor tendons and extensor hoods. It is innervated by the deep fibular nerve.

The **extensor hallucis brevis** originates in continuity with the extensor digitorum brevis. Its tendon attaches to the base of the proximal phalanx of the great toes. The muscle extends the metatarsophalangeal joint of the great toe and is innervated by the deep fibular nerve.

In the sole

The muscles in the sole of the foot are organized into four layers. From superficial to deep, or plantar to dorsal, these layers are the first, second, third, and fourth layers.

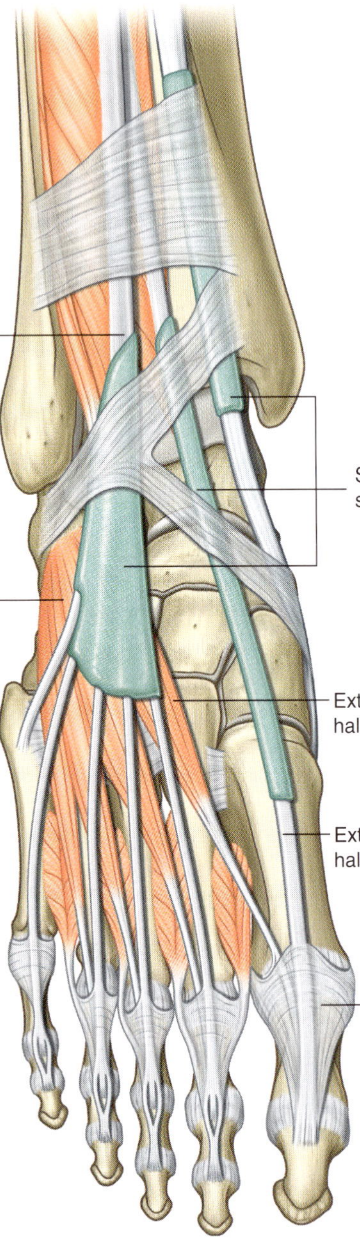

Fig. 3.113 Extensor digitorum brevis muscle.

Table 3.10 Muscles of the dorsal aspect of the foot

Muscle	Origin	Insertion	Innervation	Function
Extensor digitorum brevis	Superolateral surface of the calcaneus	Lateral sides of the tendons of extensor digitorum longus of toes II to IV	Deep fibular nerve (**S1, S2**)	Extension of metacarpal joints of toes II to IV
Extensor hallucis brevis	Superolateral surface of calcaneus	Base of proximal phalanx of great toe	Deep fibular nerve (**S1, S2**)	Extension of metatarsophalangeal joint of great toe

Note: Spinal segments in bold are the major segments innervating the muscle.

First layer

There are three components in the first layer of muscles, which is the most superficial of the four layers and is immediately deep to the plantar aponeurosis (Fig. 3.114 and Table 3.11). From medial to lateral, these muscles are the abductor hallucis, flexor digitorum brevis, and abductor digiti minimi.

Abductor hallucis

The **abductor hallucis** muscle forms the medial margin of the foot and contributes to a soft tissue bulge on the medial side of the sole (Fig. 3.114). It originates from the medial process of the calcaneal tuberosity and adjacent margins of the flexor retinaculum and plantar aponeurosis. It forms a tendon that inserts on the medial side of the base of the proximal phalanx of the great toe and on the medial sesamoid bone associated with the tendon of the flexor hallucis brevis muscle.

The abductor hallucis abducts and flexes the great toe at the metatarsophalangeal joint and is innervated by the medial plantar nerve.

Flexor digitorum brevis

The **flexor digitorum brevis** muscle lies immediately superior to the plantar aponeurosis and inferior to the tendons of the flexor digitorum longus in the sole of the foot (Fig. 3.114). The flat spindle-shaped muscle belly originates as a tendon from the medial process of the calcaneal tuberosity and from the adjacent plantar aponeurosis.

The muscle fibers of the flexor digitorum brevis diverge anteriorly to form four tendons, each of which enters one of the lateral four toes. Near the base of the proximal phalanx of the toe, each tendon splits to pass dorsally around each side of the tendon of the flexor digitorum longus and attaches to the margins of the middle phalanx.

The flexor digitorum brevis flexes the lateral four toes at the proximal interphalangeal joints and is innervated by the medial plantar nerve.

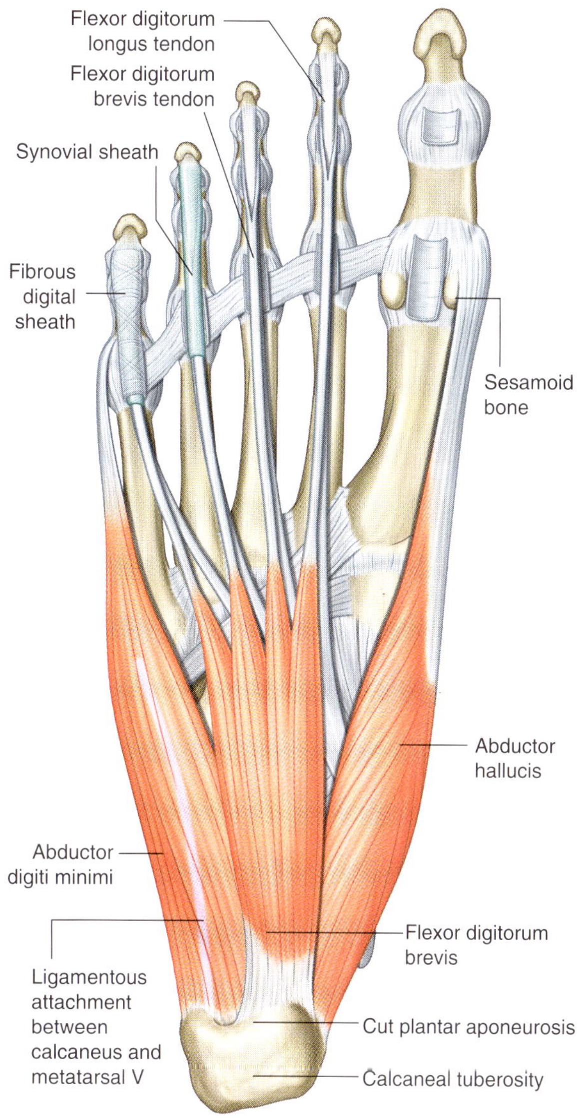

Fig. 3.114 First layer of muscles in the sole of the foot.

Table 3.11 First layer of muscles in the sole of the foot

Muscle	Origin	Insertion	Innervation	Function
Abductor hallucis	Medial process of calcaneal tuberosity	Medial side of base of proximal phalanx of great toe	Medial plantar nerve (**S1, S2, S3**)	Abducts and flexes great toe at metatarsophalangeal joint
Flexor digitorum brevis	Medial process of calcaneal tuberosity and plantar aponeurosis	Sides of plantar surface of middle phalanges of lateral four toes	Medial plantar nerve (**S1, S2, S3**)	Flexes lateral four toes at proximal interphalangeal joint
Abductor digiti minimi	Lateral and medial processes of calcaneal tuberosity, and band of connective tissue connecting calcaneus with base of metatarsal V	Lateral side of base of proximal phalanx of little toe	Lateral plantar nerve (**S1, S2, S3**)	Abducts little toe at the metatarsophalangeal joint

Note: Spinal segments in bold are the major segments innervating the muscle.

Abductor digiti minimi

The **abductor digiti minimi** muscle is on the lateral side of the foot and contributes to the large lateral plantar eminence on the sole (Fig. 3.114). It has a broad base of origin, mainly from the lateral and medial processes of the calcaneal tuberosity and from a fibrous band of connective tissue, which connects the calcaneus with the base of metatarsal V.

The abductor digiti minimi forms a tendon, which travels in a shallow groove on the plantar surface of the base of metatarsal V and continues forward to attach to the lateral side of the base of the proximal phalanx of the little toe.

The abductor digiti minimi abducts the little toe at the metatarsophalangeal joint and is innervated by the lateral plantar nerve.

Second layer

The second muscle layer in the sole of the foot is associated with the tendons of the flexor digitorum longus muscle, which pass through this layer, and consists of the quadratus plantae and four lumbrical muscles (Fig. 3.115 and Table 3.12). The tendons of flexor hallucis longus and flexor digitorum longus also pass though this layer.

Quadratus plantae

The **quadratus plantae** muscle is a flat quadrangular muscle with two heads of origin (Fig. 3.115):

- One of the heads originates from the medial surface of the calcaneus inferior to the sustentaculum tali.
- The other head originates from the inferior surface of the calcaneus anterior to the lateral process of the calcaneal tuberosity and the attachment of the long plantar ligament.

The quadratus plantae muscle inserts into the lateral side of the tendon of the flexor digitorum longus in the proximal half of the sole of the foot near where the tendon divides.

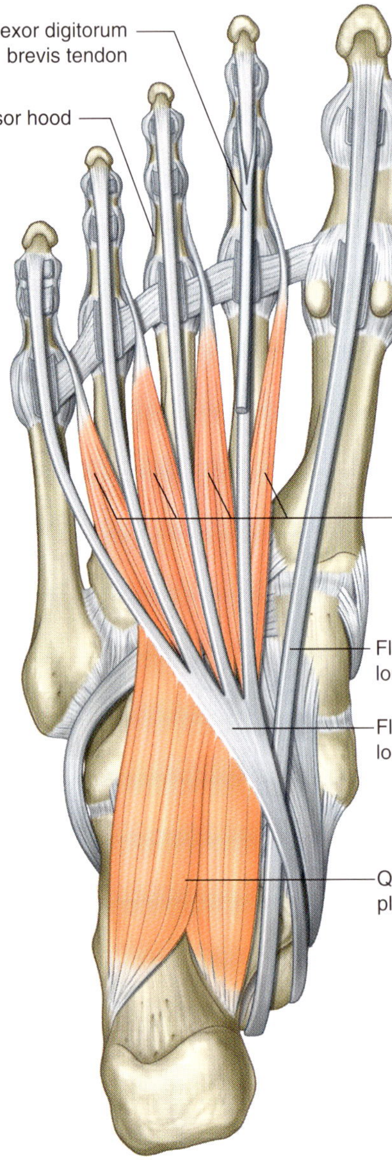

Fig. 3.115 Second layer of muscles in the sole of the foot.

Table 3.12 Second layer of muscles in the sole of the foot

Muscle	Origin	Insertion	Innervation	Function
Quadratus plantae	Medial surface of calcaneus and lateral process of calcaneal tuberosity	Lateral side of tendon of flexor digitorum longus in proximal sole of the foot	Lateral plantar nerve (**S1, S2, S3**)	Assists flexor digitorum longus tendon in flexing toes II to V
Lumbricals	First lumbrical—medial side of tendon of flexor digitorum longus associated with toe II; second, third, and fourth lumbricals—adjacent surfaces of adjacent tendons of flexor digitorum longus	Medial free margins of extensor hoods of toes II to V	First lumbrical—medial plantar nerve; second, third, and fourth lumbricals—lateral plantar nerve (**S2, S3**)	Flexion of metatarsophalangeal joint and extension of interphalangeal joints

Note: Spinal segments in bold are the major segments innervating the muscle.

The quadratus plantae assists the flexor digitorum longus tendon in flexing the toes and may also adjust the "line of pull" of this tendon as it enters the sole of the foot from the medial side. The muscle is innervated by the lateral plantar nerve.

Lumbricals

The lumbrical muscles are four worm-like muscles that originate from the tendons of the flexor digitorum longus and pass dorsally to insert into the free medial margins of the extensor hoods of the four lateral toes (Fig. 3.115).

The first lumbrical originates from the medial side of the tendon of the flexor digitorum longus that is associated with the second toe. The remaining three muscles are bipennate and originate from the sides of adjacent tendons.

The lumbrical muscles act through the extensor hoods to resist excessive extension of the metatarsophalangeal joints and flexion of the interphalangeal joints when the heel leaves the ground during walking.

The first lumbrical is innervated by the medial plantar nerve, while the other three are innervated by the lateral plantar nerve.

Third layer

There are three muscles in the third layer in the sole of the foot (Fig. 3.116 and Table 3.13):

- Two (the flexor hallucis brevis and adductor hallucis) are associated with the great toe.
- The third (the flexor digiti minimi brevis) is associated with the little toe.

Flexor hallucis brevis

The **flexor hallucis brevis** muscle has two tendinous heads of origin (Fig. 3.116):

- The **lateral head** originates from the plantar surface of the cuboid, behind the groove for the fibularis longus, and adjacent surface of the lateral cuneiform.

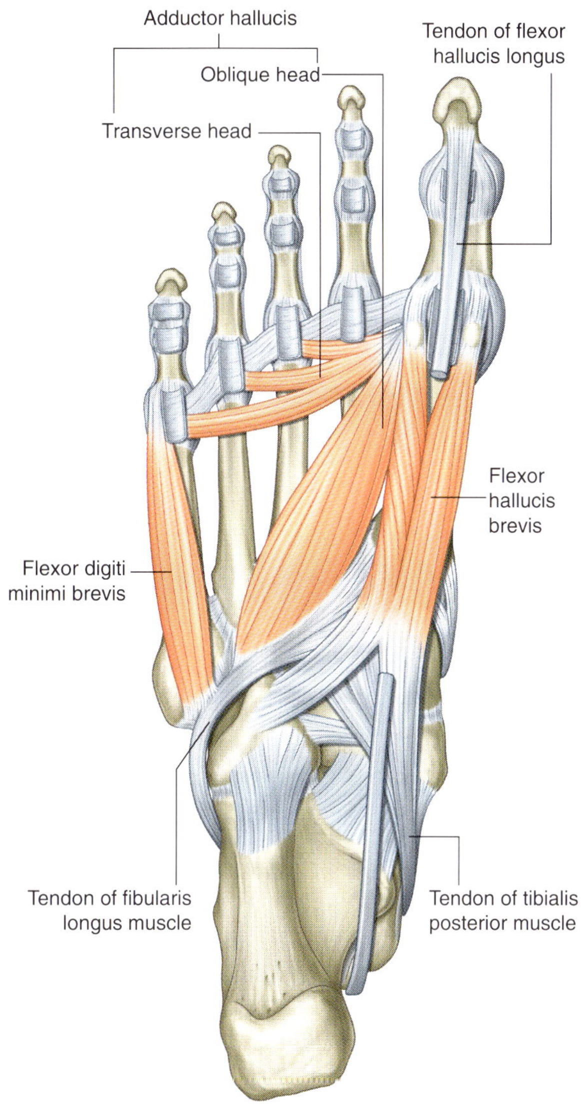

Fig. 3.116 Third layer of muscles in the sole of the foot.

Table 3.13 Third layer of muscles in the sole of the foot

Muscle	Origin	Insertion	Innervation	Function
Flexor hallucis brevis	Plantar surface of cuboid and lateral cuneiform; tendon of tibialis posterior	Lateral and medial sides of base of proximal phalanx of the great toe	Medial plantar nerve (**S1**, S2)	Flexes metatarsophalangeal joint of the great toe
Adductor hallucis	Transverse head—ligaments associated with metatarsophalangeal joints of lateral three toes; oblique head—bases of metatarsals II to IV and from sheath covering fibularis longus	Lateral side of base of proximal phalanx of great toe	Lateral plantar nerve (**S2, S3**)	Adducts great toe at metatarsophalangeal joint
Flexor digiti minimi brevis	Base of metatarsal V and related sheath of fibularis longus tendon	Lateral side of base of proximal phalanx of little toe	Lateral plantar nerve (**S2, S3**)	Flexes little toe at metatarsophalangeal joint

Note: Spinal segments in bold are the major segments innervating the muscle.

- The **medial head** originates from the tendon of the tibialis posterior muscle as it passes into the sole of the foot.

The medial and lateral heads unite and give rise to a muscle belly, which itself is separated into medial and lateral parts adjacent to the plantar surface of metatarsal I. Each part of the muscle gives rise to a tendon that inserts on either the lateral or medial side of the base of the proximal phalanx of the great toe.

A sesamoid bone occurs in each tendon of the flexor hallucis brevis as it crosses the plantar surface of the head of metatarsal I. The tendon of the flexor hallucis longus passes between the sesamoid bones.

The flexor hallucis brevis flexes the metatarsophalangeal joint of the great toe and is innervated by the medial plantar nerve.

Adductor hallucis

The **adductor hallucis** muscle originates by two muscular heads, transverse and oblique, which join near their ends to insert into the lateral side of the base of the proximal phalanx of the great toe (Fig. 3.116):

- The **transverse head** originates from the plantar ligaments associated with the metatarsophalangeal joints of the lateral three toes and from the associated deep transverse metatarsal ligaments—the muscle crosses the sole of the foot transversely from lateral to medial and joins the oblique head near the base of the great toe.
- The **oblique head** is larger than the transverse head and originates from the plantar surfaces of the bases of metatarsals II to IV and from the sheath covering the fibularis longus muscle—this head passes anteromedially through the sole of the foot and joins the transverse head.

The tendon of insertion of the adductor hallucis attaches to the lateral sesamoid bone associated with the tendon of the flexor hallucis brevis muscle in addition to attaching to the proximal phalanx.

The adductor hallucis adducts the great toe at the metatarsophalangeal joint and is innervated by the lateral plantar nerve.

Flexor digiti minimi brevis

The **flexor digiti minimi brevis** muscle originates from the plantar surface of the base of metatarsal V and adjacent sheath of the fibularis longus tendon (Fig. 3.116). It inserts on the lateral side of the base of the proximal phalanx of the little toe.

The flexor digiti minimi brevis flexes the little toe at the metatarsophalangeal joint and is innervated by the lateral plantar nerve.

Fourth layer

There are two muscle groups in the deepest muscle layer in the sole of the foot, the dorsal and plantar interossei (Fig. 3.117 and Table 3.14). The tendons of fibularis longus and tibialis posterior also pass through this layer.

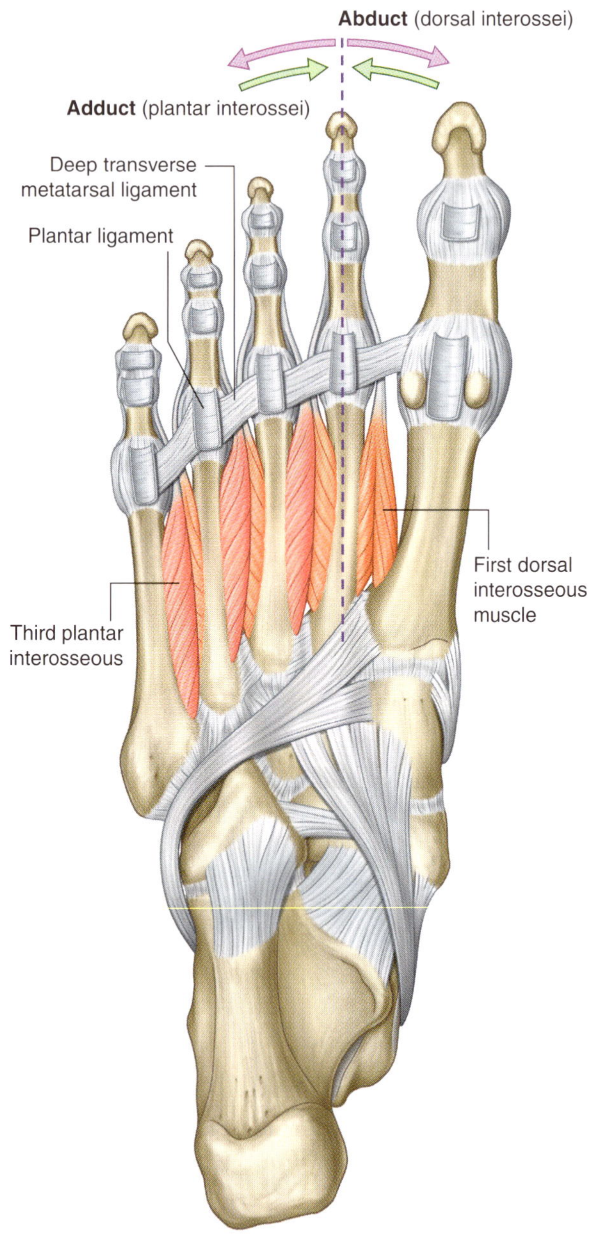

Fig. 3.117 Fourth layer of muscles in the sole of the foot.

Table 3.14 Fourth layer of muscles in the sole of the foot

Muscle	Origin	Insertion	Innervation	Function
Dorsal interossei	Sides of adjacent metatarsals	Extensor hoods and bases of proximal phalanges of toes II to IV	Lateral plantar nerve from tibial nerve; first and second dorsal interossei also innervated by deep fibular nerve (**S2, S3**)	Abduction of toes II to IV at metatarsophalangeal joints; resist extension of metatarsophalangeal joints and flexion of interphalangeal joints
Plantar interossei	Medial sides of metatarsals of toes III to V	Extensor hoods and bases of proximal phalanges of toes III to V	Lateral plantar nerve from tibial nerve (**S2, S3**)	Adduction of toes III to V at metatarsophalangeal joints; resist extension of the metatarsophalangeal joints and flexion of the interphalangeal joints

Note: Spinal segments in bold are the major segments innervating the muscle.

Dorsal interossei

The four **dorsal interossei** are the most superior muscles in the sole of the foot and abduct the second to fourth toes relative to the long axis through the second toe (Fig. 3.117). All four muscles are bipennate and originate from the sides of adjacent metatarsals.

The tendons of the dorsal interossei insert into the free margin of the extensor hoods and base of the proximal phalanges of the toes.

The second toe can be abducted to either side of its long axis, so it has two dorsal interossei associated with it, one on each side. The third and fourth toes have a dorsal interosseous muscle on their lateral sides only. The great and little toes have their own abductors (the abductor hallucis and abductor digiti minimi) in the first layer of muscles in the sole of the foot.

In addition to abduction, the dorsal interossei act through the extensor hoods to resist extension of the metatarsophalangeal joints and flexion of the interphalangeal joints.

The dorsal interossei are innervated by the lateral plantar nerve. The first and second dorsal interossei also receive branches on their superior surfaces from the deep fibular nerve.

Plantar interossei

The three plantar interossei adduct the third, fourth, and little toes toward the long axis through the second toe (Fig. 3.117).

Each plantar interosseous muscle originates from the medial side of its associated metatarsal and inserts into the medial free margin of the extensor hood and base of the proximal phalanx.

The great toe has its own adductor (the adductor hallucis) in the third layer of muscles in the sole of the foot and the second toe is adducted back to its longitudinal axis by using one of its dorsal interossei.

In addition to adduction, the plantar interossei act through the extensor hoods to resist extension of the metatarsophalangeal joints and flexion of the interphalangeal joints. All are innervated by the lateral plantar nerve.

Arteries

Blood supply to the foot is by branches of the posterior tibial and dorsalis pedis (dorsal artery of the foot) arteries.

The posterior tibial artery enters the sole and bifurcates into lateral and medial plantar arteries. The lateral plantar artery joins with the terminal end of the dorsalis pedis artery (the deep plantar artery) to form the deep plantar arch. Branches from this arch supply the toes.

The dorsalis pedis artery is the continuation of the anterior tibial artery, and passes onto the dorsal aspect of the foot and then inferiorly, as the deep plantar artery, between metatarsals I and II to enter the sole of the foot.

Posterior tibial artery and plantar arch

The posterior tibial artery enters the foot through the tarsal tunnel on the medial side of the ankle and posterior to the medial malleolus. Midway between the medial malleolus and the heel, the pulse of the posterior tibial artery is palpable because here the artery is covered only by a thin layer of retinaculum, by superficial connective tissue, and by skin. Near this location, the posterior tibial artery bifurcates into a small medial plantar artery and a much larger lateral plantar artery.

Lateral plantar artery

The **lateral plantar artery** passes anterolaterally into the sole of the foot, first deep to the proximal end of the abductor hallucis muscle and then between the quadratus plantae and flexor digitorum brevis muscles (Fig. 3.118). It reaches the base of metatarsal V where it lies in the groove between the flexor digitorum brevis and abductor digiti

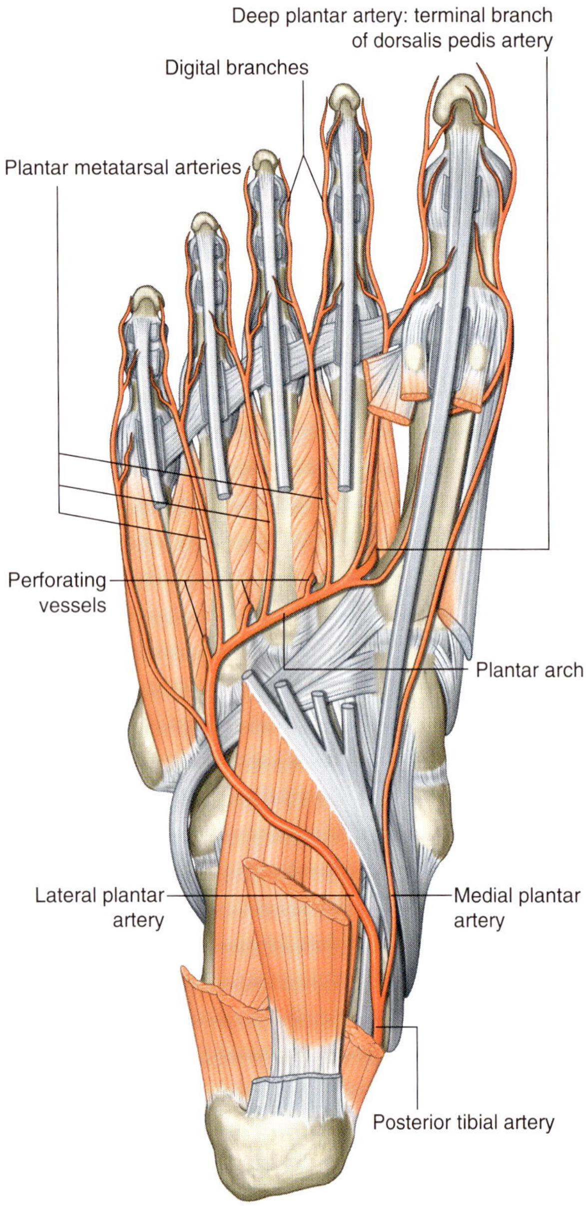

Fig. 3.118 Arteries in the sole of the foot.

minimi muscles. From here, the lateral plantar artery curves medially to form the **plantar arch**, which crosses the deep plane of the sole on the metatarsal bases and the interossei muscles.

Between the bases of metatarsals I and II, the plantar arch joins with the terminal branch (deep plantar artery) of the dorsalis pedis artery, which enters the sole from the dorsal side of the foot.

Major branches of the plantar arch include:

- A digital branch to the lateral side of the little toe
- Four plantar metatarsal arteries, which supply digital branches to adjacent sides of toes I to V and the medial side of the great toe
- Three perforating arteries, which pass between the bases of metatarsals II to V to anastomose with vessels on the dorsal aspect of the foot

Medial plantar artery

The **medial plantar artery** passes into the sole of the foot by passing deep to the proximal end of the abductor hallucis muscle (Fig. 3.118). It supplies a deep branch to adjacent muscles and then passes forward in the groove between the abductor hallucis and the flexor digitorum brevis muscles. It ends by joining the digital branch of the plantar arch, which supplies the medial side of the great toe.

Near the base of metatarsal I, the medial plantar artery gives rise to a superficial branch, which divides into three vessels that pass superficial to the flexor digitorum brevis muscle to join the plantar metatarsal arteries from the deep plantar arch.

Dorsalis pedis artery

The dorsalis pedis artery is the continuation of the anterior tibial artery and begins as the anterior tibial artery crosses the ankle joint (Fig. 3.119). It passes anteriorly over the dorsal aspect of the talus, navicular, and intermediate cuneiform bones, and then passes inferiorly, as the deep plantar artery, between the two heads of the first dorsal interosseous muscle to join the plantar arch in the sole of the foot. The pulse of the dorsalis pedis artery on the dorsal surface of the foot can be felt by gently palpating the vessel against the underlying tarsal bones between the tendons of the extensor hallucis longus and the extensor digitorum longus to the second toe (Fig. 3.106).

Branches of the dorsalis pedis artery include lateral and medial tarsal branches, an arcuate artery, and a first dorsal metatarsal artery:

- The **tarsal arteries** pass medially and laterally over the tarsal bones, supplying adjacent structures and anastomosing with a network of vessels formed around the ankle.
- The **arcuate artery** passes laterally over the dorsal aspect of the metatarsals near their bases and gives rise to three **dorsal metatarsal arteries**, which supply **dorsal digital arteries** to adjacent sides of digits II to V, and to a dorsal digital artery that supplies the lateral side of digit V.
- The **first dorsal metatarsal artery** (the last branch of the dorsalis pedis artery before the dorsalis pedis artery continues as the deep plantar artery into the sole of the foot) supplies dorsal digital branches to adjacent sides of the great and second toes, and medial side of the great toe.

The dorsal metatarsal arteries connect with perforating branches from the plantar arch and similar branches from the plantar metatarsal arteries.

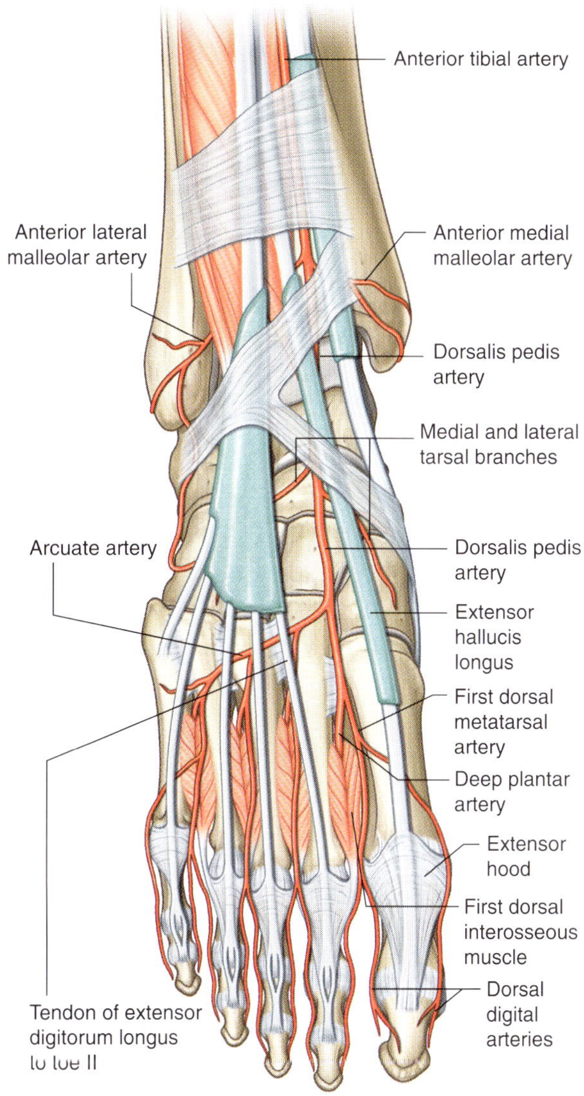

Fig. 3.119 Dorsalis pedis artery.

Veins

There are interconnected networks of deep and superficial veins in the foot. The deep veins follow the arteries. Superficial veins drain into a dorsal venous arch on the dorsal surface of the foot over the metatarsals (Fig. 3.120):

- The **great saphenous vein** originates from the medial side of the arch and passes anterior to the medial malleolus and onto the medial side of the leg.
- The **small saphenous vein** originates from the lateral side of the arch and passes posterior to the lateral malleolus and onto the back of the leg.

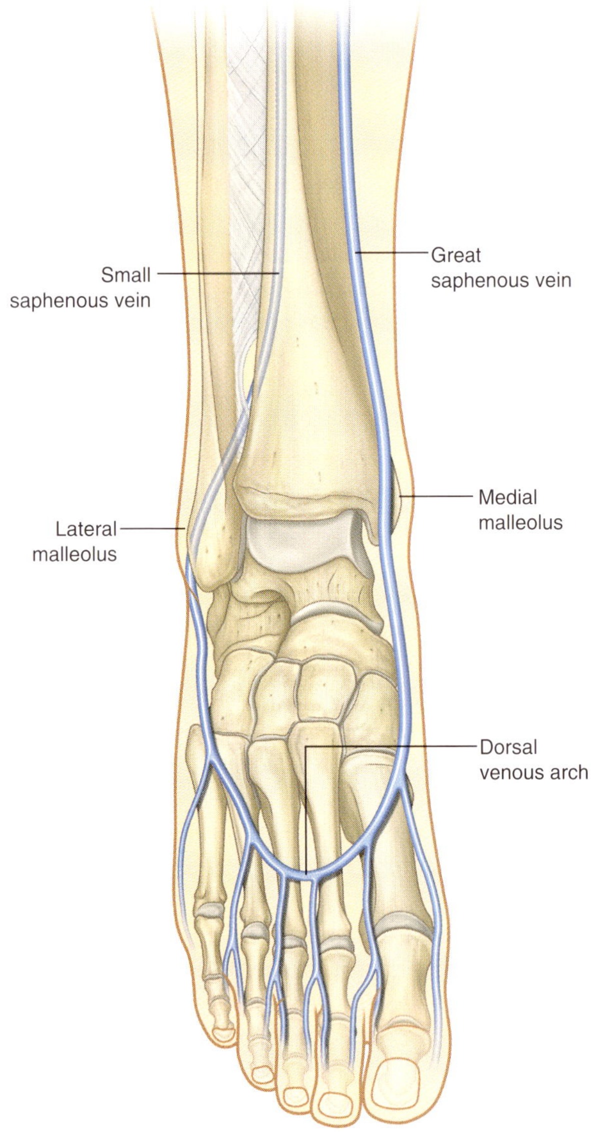

Fig. 3.120 Superficial veins of the foot. The tibia and fibula are shown as if transparent.

Nerves

The foot is supplied by the tibial, deep fibular, superficial fibular, sural, and saphenous nerves:

- All five nerves contribute to cutaneous or general sensory innervation.
- The tibial nerve innervates all intrinsic muscles of the foot except for the extensor digitorum brevis, which is innervated by the deep fibular nerve.
- The deep fibular nerve often also contributes to the innervation of the first and second dorsal interossei.

Tibial nerve

The **tibial nerve** enters the foot through the tarsal tunnel posterior to the medial malleolus (Fig. 3.86). In the tunnel, the nerve is lateral to the posterior tibial artery, and gives origin to **medial calcaneal branches**, which penetrate the flexor retinaculum to supply the heel. Midway between the medial malleolus and the heel, the tibial nerve bifurcates with the posterior tibial artery into:

- A large medial plantar nerve
- A smaller lateral plantar nerve (Fig. 3.121)

The medial and lateral plantar nerves lie together between their corresponding arteries.

Medial plantar nerve

The **medial plantar nerve** is the major sensory nerve in the sole of the foot (Fig. 3.121). It innervates skin on most of the anterior two-thirds of the sole and adjacent surfaces of the medial three and one-half toes, which includes the great toe. In addition to this large area of plantar skin, the nerve also innervates four intrinsic muscles—the abductor hallucis, flexor digitorum brevis, flexor hallucis brevis, and first lumbrical.

The medial plantar nerve passes into the sole of the foot deep to the abductor hallucis muscle and passes forward in the groove between the abductor hallucis and flexor digitorum brevis, supplying branches to both these muscles.

The medial plantar nerve supplies a digital branch (**proper plantar digital nerve**) to the medial side of the great toe and then divides into three nerves (**common plantar digital nerves**) on the plantar surface of the flexor digitorum brevis, which continue forward to supply proper plantar digital branches to adjacent surfaces of toes I to IV. The nerve to the first lumbrical originates from the first common plantar digital nerve.

Lateral plantar nerve

The **lateral plantar nerve** is an important motor nerve in the foot because it innervates all intrinsic muscles in the sole, except for the muscles supplied by the medial plantar nerve (the abductor hallucis, flexor digitorum brevis, flexor hallucis brevis, and first lumbrical) (Fig. 3.121). It also innervates a strip of skin on the lateral side of the anterior two-thirds of the sole and the adjacent plantar surfaces of the lateral one and one-half digits.

The lateral plantar nerve enters the sole of the foot by passing deep to the proximal attachment of the abductor hallucis muscle. It continues laterally and anteriorly across the sole between the flexor digitorum brevis and quadratus plantae muscles, supplying branches to both these muscles,

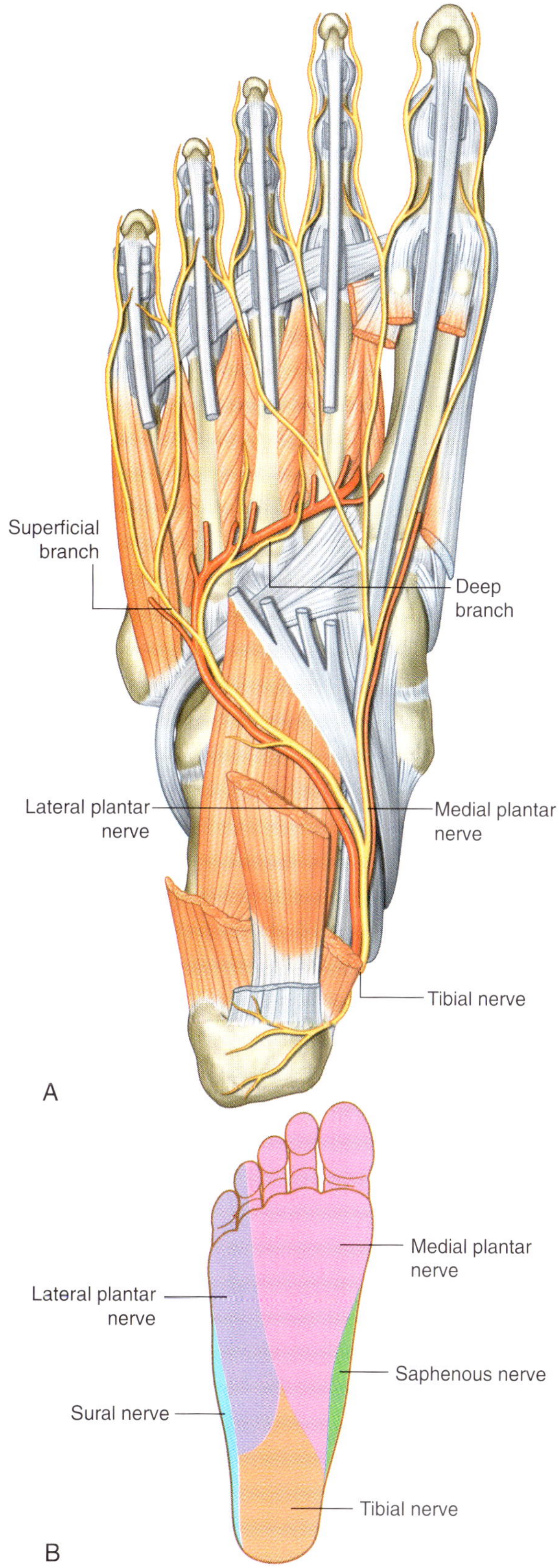

Fig. 3.121 Lateral and medial plantar nerves. **(A)** Sole of the right foot. **(B)** Cutaneous distribution.

and then divides near the head of metatarsal V into deep and superficial branches.

The **superficial branch** of the lateral plantar nerve gives rise to a **proper plantar digital nerve**, which supplies skin on the lateral side of the little toe, and to a **common plantar digital nerve**, which divides to supply proper plantar digital nerves to skin on the adjacent sides of toes IV and V.

The proper plantar digital nerve to the lateral side of the little toe also innervates the flexor digiti minimi brevis and the dorsal and plantar interossei muscles between metatarsals IV and V.

The **deep branch** of the lateral plantar nerve is motor and accompanies the lateral plantar artery deep to the long flexor tendons and the adductor hallucis muscle. It supplies branches to the second to fourth lumbrical muscles, the adductor hallucis muscle, and all interossei except those between metatarsals IV and V, which are innervated by the superficial branch.

Early clinical exposure

Morton's neuroma

A Morton's neuroma is an enlarged common plantar nerve, usually in the third interspace between the third and fourth toes. In this region of the foot, the lateral plantar nerve often unites with the medial plantar nerve. As the two nerves join, the resulting nerve is typically larger in diameter than those of the other toes. Also, it is in a relatively subcutaneous position, just above the fat pad of the foot close to the artery and the vein. Above the nerve is the deep transverse metatarsal ligament, which is a broad strong structure holding the metatarsals together. Typically, as the patient enters the "push-off" phase of walking, the interdigital nerve is sandwiched between the ground and the deep transverse metatarsal ligament. The forces tend to compress the common plantar nerve, which can be irritated, in which case there is usually some associated inflammatory change and thickening.

Typically, patients experience pain related to the third interspace, which may be sharp or dull and is usually worsened by wearing shoes and walking.

Treatment may include injection of anti-inflammatory drugs, or it may be necessary to surgically remove the lesion.

Deep fibular nerve

The **deep fibular nerve** innervates the extensor digitorum brevis, contributes to the innervation of the first two dorsal interossei muscles, and supplies general sensory branches to the skin on the adjacent dorsal sides of the first and second toes and on the web space between them (Fig. 3.122).

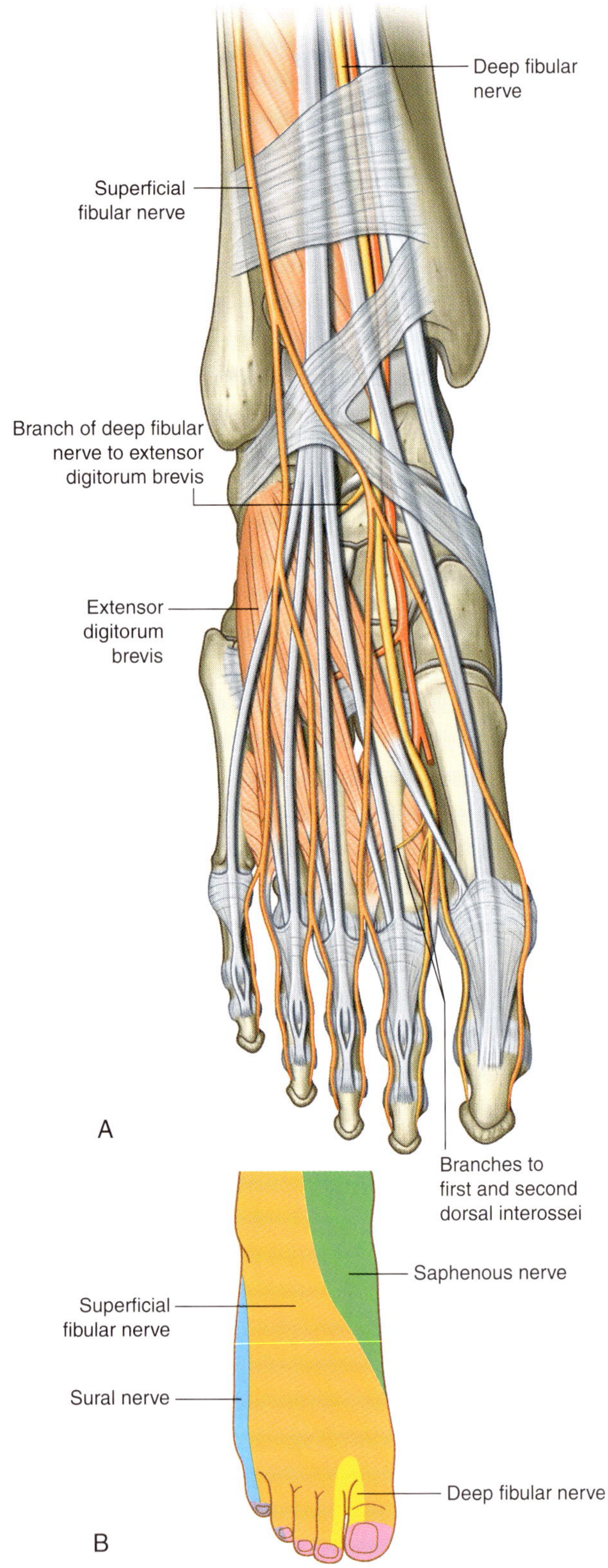

Fig. 3.122 **(A)** Terminal branches of superficial and deep fibular nerves in the foot. **(B)** Cutaneous distribution.

The deep fibular nerve enters the dorsal aspect of the foot on the lateral side of the dorsalis pedis artery, and is parallel with and lateral to the tendon of the extensor hallucis longus muscle. Just distal to the ankle joint, the nerve gives origin to a lateral branch, which innervates the extensor digitorum brevis from its deep surface.

The deep fibular nerve continues forward on the dorsal surface of the foot, penetrates deep fascia between metatarsals I and II near the metatarsophalangeal joints, and then divides into two **dorsal digital nerves**, which supply skin over adjacent surfaces of toes I and II down to the beginning of the nail beds.

Small motor branches, which contribute to the supply of the first two dorsal interossei muscles, originate from the deep fibular nerve before it penetrates deep fascia.

Superficial fibular nerve

The **superficial fibular nerve** is sensory to most skin on the dorsal aspect of the foot and toes except for skin on adjacent sides of toes I and II (which is innervated by the deep fibular nerve) and skin on the lateral side of the foot and little toe (which is innervated by the sural nerve; Fig. 3.122).

The superficial fibular nerve penetrates deep fascia on the anterolateral side of the lower leg and enters the dorsal aspect of the foot in superficial fascia. It gives rise to cutaneous branches and **dorsal digital nerves** along its course.

Sural nerve

The sural nerve is a cutaneous branch of the tibial nerve that originates high in the leg. It enters the foot in the superficial fascia posterior to the lateral malleolus close to the short saphenous vein. Terminal branches innervate skin on the lateral side of the foot and dorsolateral surface of the little toe (Fig. 3.122B).

Saphenous nerve

The saphenous nerve is a cutaneous branch of the femoral nerve that originates in the thigh. Terminal branches enter the foot in superficial fascia on the medial side of the ankle and supply skin on the medial side of the proximal foot (Fig. 3.122B).

Early clinical exposure

Clubfoot

Clubfoot is a congenital deformity in which babies are born with one or both feet pointing inward and downward. It is treated with gentle manipulation of the affected foot and with plaster casts to straighten the foot, which is usually followed by a minor surgical procedure where the calcaneal tendon is cut to release the foot into a better position.

Surface anatomy

LOWER LIMB SURFACE ANATOMY

Tendons, muscles, and bony landmarks in the lower limb are used to locate major arteries, veins, and nerves.

Because the vessels are large, they can be used as entry points to the vascular system. In addition, vessels in the lower limb are farthest from the heart and the most inferior in the body. Therefore, the nature of peripheral pulses in the lower limb can give important information about the status of the circulatory system in general.

Sensation and muscle action in the lower limb are tested to assess lumbar and sacral regions of the spinal cord.

Avoiding the sciatic nerve

The sciatic nerve innervates muscles in the posterior compartment of the thigh, muscles in the leg and foot, and an appreciable area of skin. It enters the lower limb in the gluteal region (Fig. 3.123) and passes inferiorly midway between two major palpable bony landmarks, the greater trochanter and the ischial tuberosity. The greater trochanter can be easily felt as a hard bony protuberance about one hand's width inferior to the midpoint of the iliac crest. The ischial tuberosity is palpable just above the gluteal fold.

The gluteal region can be divided into quadrants by two lines positioned using palpable bony landmarks:

- One line descends vertically from the highest point of the iliac crest.
- The other line passes horizontally through the first line midway between the highest point of the iliac crest and the horizontal plane through the ischial tuberosity.

The sciatic nerve curves through the upper lateral corner of the lower medial quadrant and descends along the lateral margin of the lower medial quadrant. Injections can be carried out in the anterior corner of the upper lateral quadrant to avoid injury to the sciatic nerve and major vessels in the region (Fig. 3.123B).

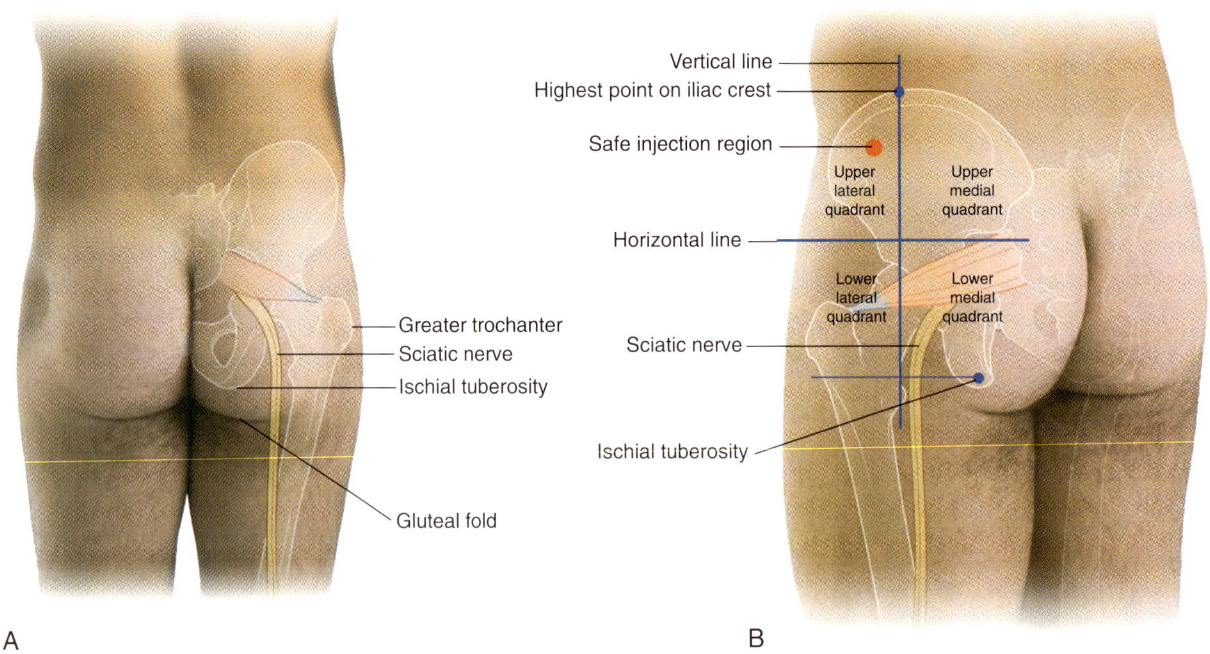

Fig. 3.123 Avoiding the sciatic nerve. **(A)** Posterior view of the gluteal region of a man with the position of the sciatic nerve indicated. **(B)** Posterolateral view of the left gluteal region with gluteal quadrants and the position of the sciatic nerve indicated.

Finding the femoral artery in the femoral triangle

The femoral artery passes into the femoral triangle (Fig. 3.124) of the lower limb from the abdomen.

The femoral triangle is the depression formed in the anterior thigh between the medial margin of the adductor longus muscle, the medial margin of the sartorius muscle, and the inguinal ligament.

The tendon of the adductor longus muscle can be palpated as a cord-like structure that attaches to bone immediately inferior to the pubic tubercle.

The sartorius muscle originates from the anterior superior iliac spine and crosses anteriorly over the thigh to attach to the medial aspect of the tibia below the knee joint.

The inguinal ligament attaches to the anterior superior iliac spine laterally and the pubic tubercle medially.

The femoral artery descends into the thigh from the abdomen by passing deep to the inguinal ligament and into the femoral triangle. In the femoral triangle, its pulse is easily felt just inferior to the inguinal ligament midway between the pubic symphysis and the anterior superior iliac spine. Medial to the artery is the femoral vein and medial to the vein is the femoral canal, which contains lymphatics and lies immediately lateral to the pubic tubercle. The femoral nerve lies lateral to the femoral artery.

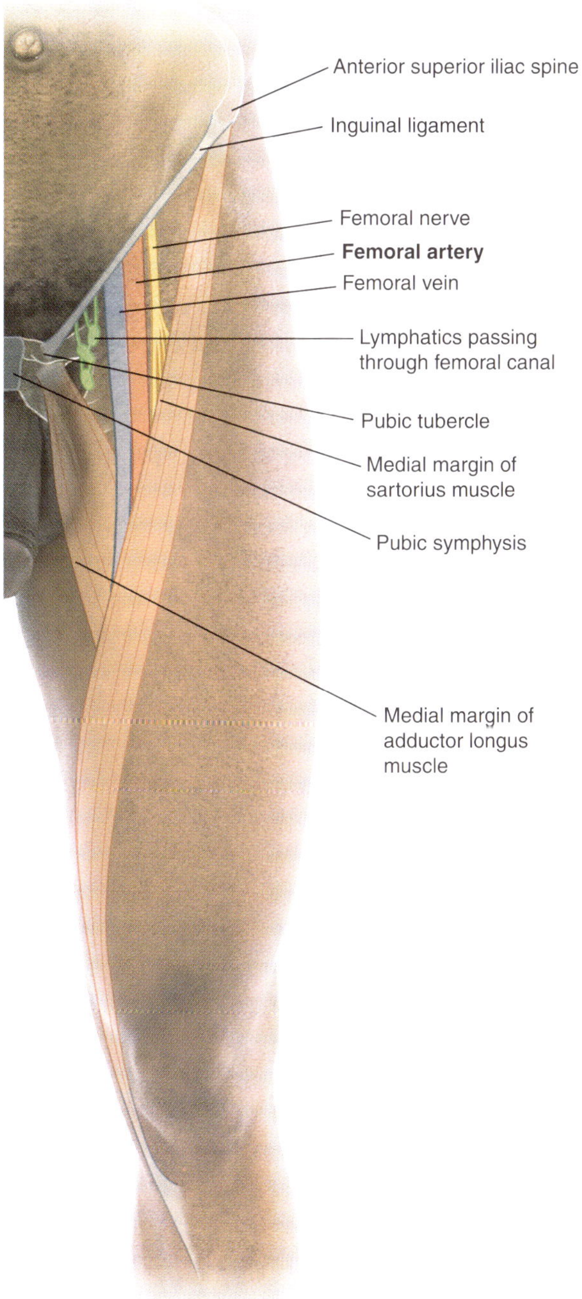

Fig. 3.124 Position of the femoral artery in the femoral triangle. Anterior thigh.

Identifying structures around the knee

The patella is a prominent palpable feature at the knee. The quadriceps femoris tendon attaches superiorly to it and the patellar ligament connects the inferior aspect of the patella to the tibial tuberosity (Fig. 3.125). The patellar ligament and the tibial tuberosity are easily palpable. A tap on the patellar ligament (tendon) tests reflex activity mainly at spinal cord levels L3 and L4.

The head of the fibula is palpable as a protuberance on the lateral surface of the knee just inferior to the lateral condyle of the tibia. It can also be located by following the tendon of the biceps femoris inferiorly.

The common fibular nerve passes around the lateral surface of the neck of the fibula just inferior to the head of the fibula and can often be felt as a cord-like structure in this position.

Another structure that can usually be located on the lateral side of the knee is the iliotibial tract. This flat tendinous structure, which attaches to the lateral tibial condyle, is most prominent when the knee is fully extended. In this position, the anterior edge of the tract raises a sharp vertical fold of skin posterior to the lateral edge of the patella.

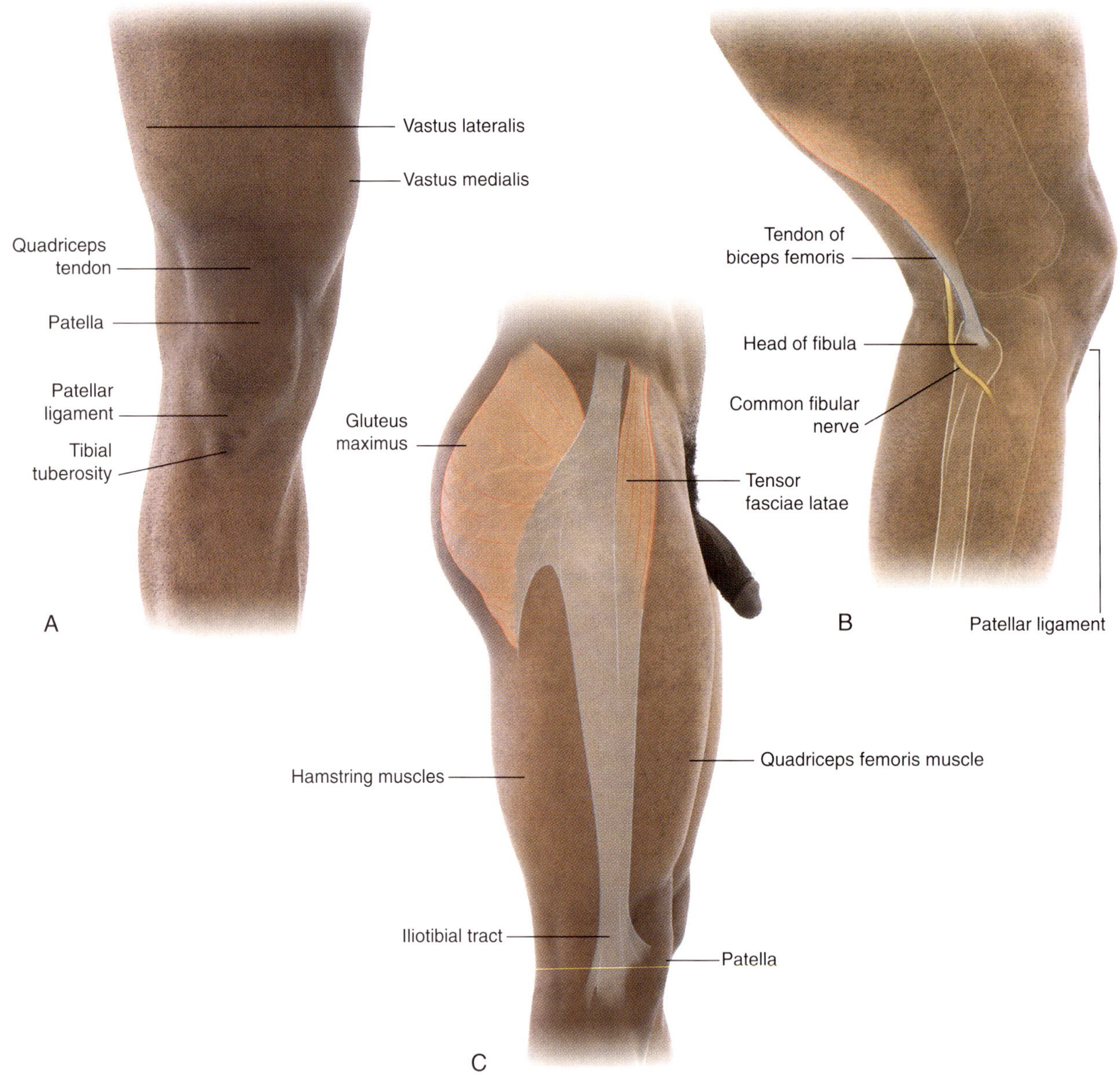

Fig. 3.125 Identifying structures around the knee. **(A)** Anterior view of the right knee. **(B)** Lateral view of the partially flexed right knee. **(C)** Lateral view of the extended right knee, thigh, and gluteal region.

Visualizing the contents of the popliteal fossa

The popliteal fossa is a diamond-shaped depression formed between the hamstrings and gastrocnemius muscle posterior to the knee. The inferior margins of the diamond are formed by the medial and lateral heads of the gastrocnemius muscle. The superior margins are formed laterally by the biceps femoris muscle and medially by the semimembranosus and semitendinosus muscles. The tendons of the biceps femoris muscle and the semitendinosus muscle are palpable and often visible.

The head of the fibula is palpable on the lateral side of the knee and can be used as a landmark for identifying the biceps femoris tendon and the common fibular nerve, which curves laterally out of the popliteal fossa and crosses the neck of the fibula just inferior to the head.

The popliteal fossa contains the popliteal artery, the popliteal vein, the tibial nerve, and the common fibular nerve (Fig. 3.126). The popliteal artery is the deepest of the structures in the fossa and descends through the region from the upper medial side. As a consequence of its position, the popliteal artery pulse is difficult to find, but usually can be detected on deep palpation just medial to the midline of the fossa.

The small saphenous vein penetrates deep fascia in the upper part of the posterior leg and joins the popliteal vein.

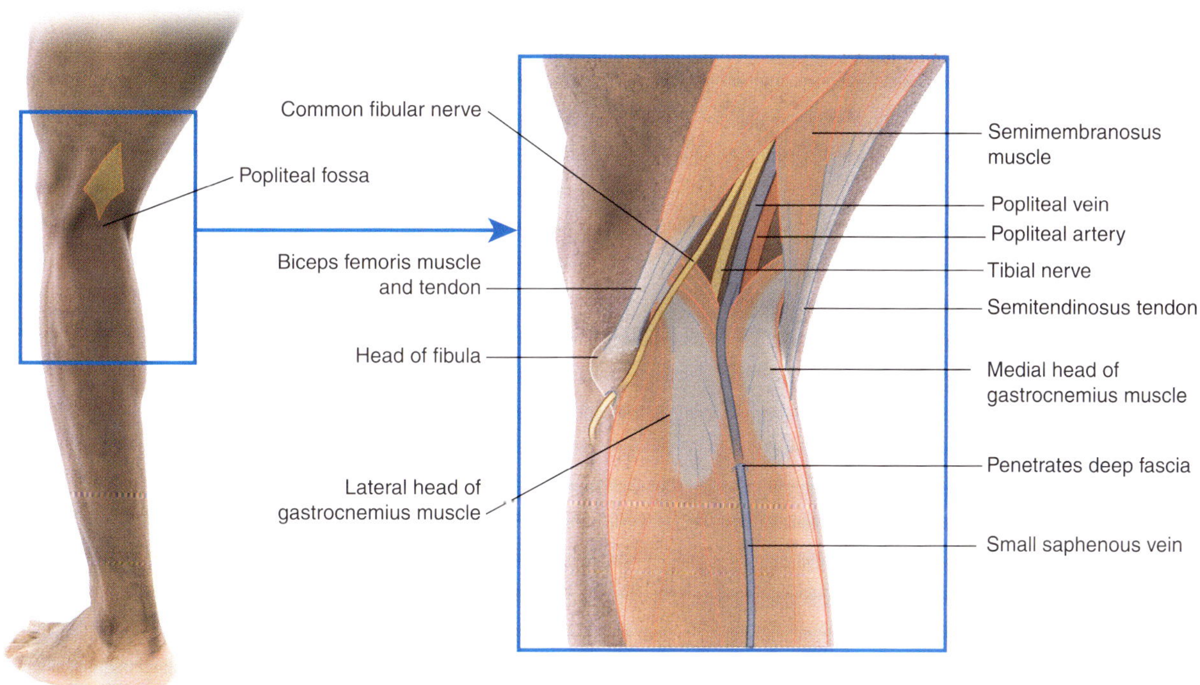

Fig. 3.126 Visualizing the contents of the popliteal fossa. Posterior view of the left knee.

Finding the tarsal tunnel—the gateway to the foot

The tarsal tunnel (Fig. 3.127) is formed on the medial side of the foot in the groove between the medial malleolus and the heel (calcaneal tuberosity) and by the overlying flexor retinaculum.

The posterior tibial artery and tibial nerve enter the foot through the tarsal tunnel. The tendons of the tibialis posterior, flexor digitorum longus, and flexor hallucis longus also pass through the tarsal tunnel in compartments formed by septa of the flexor retinaculum.

The order of structures passing through the tunnel from anteromedial to posterolateral are the tendon of the tibialis posterior, the tendon of the flexor digitorum longus, the posterior tibial artery and associated veins, the tibial nerve, and the tendon of the flexor hallucis longus ("Tom, Dick, and a very nervous Harry").

The tibial artery is palpable just posteroinferior to the medial malleolus on the anterior face of the visible groove between the heel and medial malleolus.

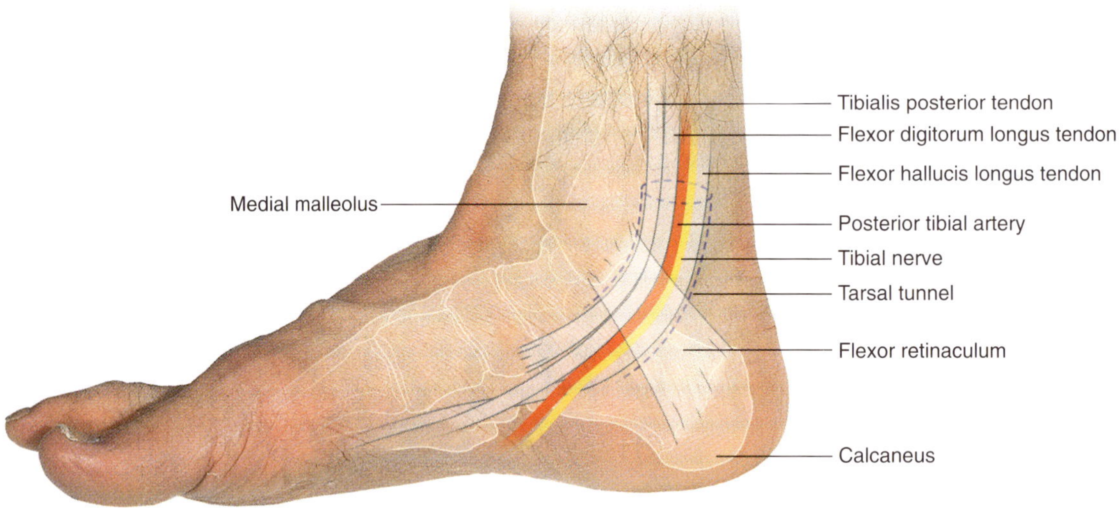

Fig. 3.127 Finding the tarsal tunnel—the gateway to the foot.

Identifying tendons around the ankle and in the foot

Numerous tendons can be identified around the ankle and in the foot (Fig. 3.128) and can be used as useful landmarks for locating vessels or testing spinal reflexes.

The tibialis anterior tendon is visible on the medial side of the ankle anterior to the medial malleolus.

The calcaneal tendon is the largest tendon entering the foot and is prominent on the posterior aspect of the foot as it descends from the leg to the heel. A tap with a tendon hammer on this tendon tests reflex activity of spinal cord levels S1 and S2.

When the foot is everted, the tendons of the fibularis longus and fibularis brevis raise a linear fold of skin, which descends from the lower leg to the posterior edge of the lateral malleolus.

The tendon of the fibularis brevis is often evident on the lateral surface of the foot descending obliquely to the base of metatarsal V. The tendons of the fibularis tertius, extensor

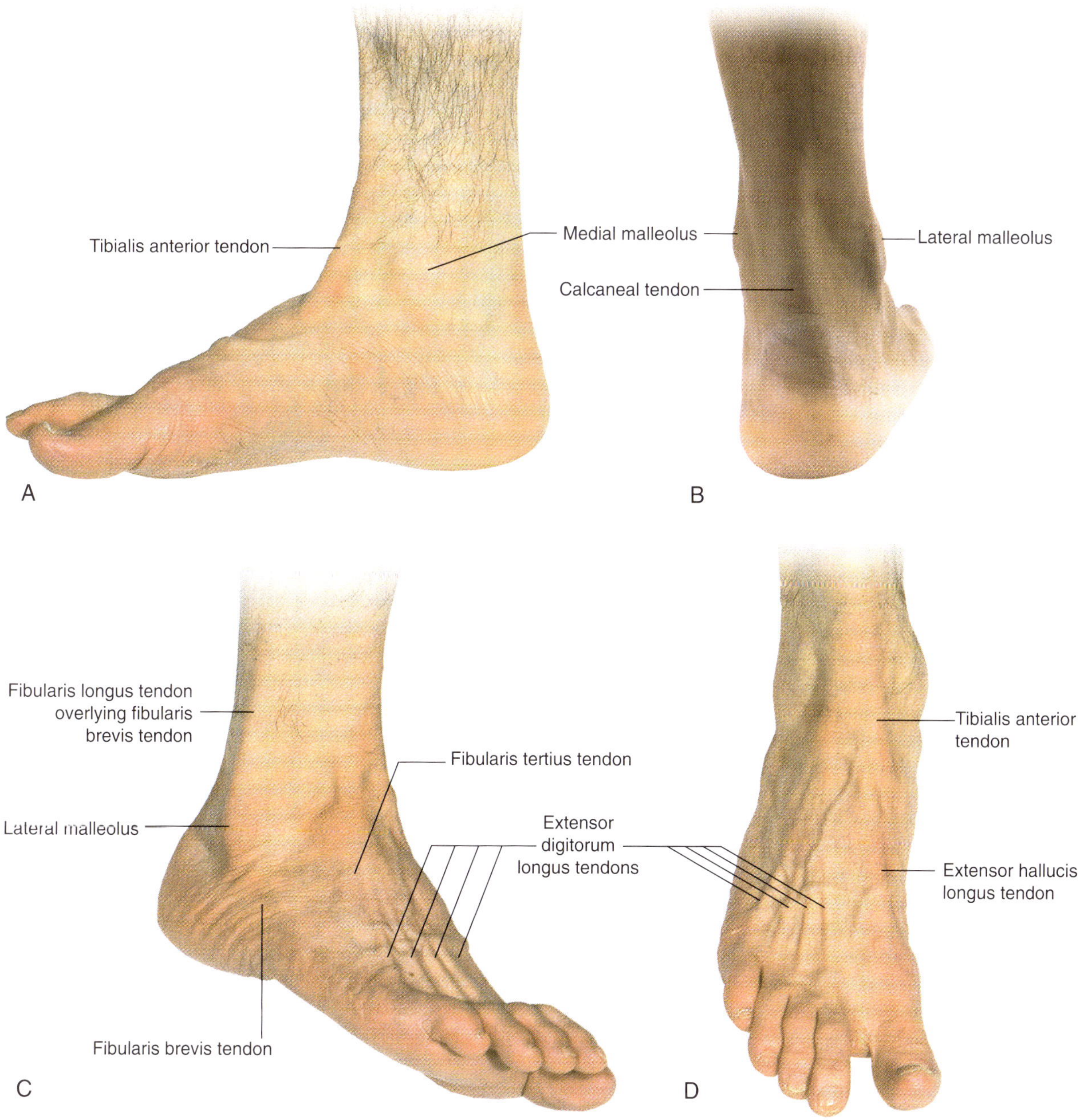

Fig. 3.128 Identifying tendons around the ankle and in the foot. **(A)** Medial side of the right foot. **(B)** Posterior aspect of the right foot. **(C)** Lateral side of the everted right foot. **(D)** Dorsal aspect of the right foot.

digitorum longus, and extensor hallucis longus are visible on the dorsal aspect of the foot from lateral to medial.

Finding the dorsalis pedis artery

The nature of the dorsalis pedis pulse (Fig. 3.129) is important for assessing peripheral circulation because the dorsalis pedis artery is the farthest palpable vessel from the heart. Also, it is the lowest palpable artery in the body when a person is standing.

The dorsalis pedis artery passes onto the dorsal aspect of the foot and anteriorly over the tarsal bones where it lies between and is parallel to the tendon of the extensor hallucis longus and the tendon of the extensor digitorum longus to the second toe. It is palpable in this position. The terminal branch of the dorsalis pedis artery passes into the plantar surface of the foot between the two heads of the first dorsal interosseous muscle.

Approximating the position of the plantar arterial arch

The blood supply of the foot is provided by branches of the posterior tibial and dorsalis pedis arteries.

The posterior tibial artery enters the plantar surface of the foot through the tarsal tunnel and divides into a lateral and a medial plantar artery.

The lateral plantar artery curves laterally across the posterior half of the sole and then curves medially as the plantar arch (Fig. 3.130) through the anterior sole. Between the bases of metatarsals I and II, the plantar arch joins the terminal branch (deep plantar artery) of the dorsalis pedis artery. Most of the foot is supplied by the plantar arch.

The medial plantar artery passes anteriorly through the sole, connects with branches of the plantar arch, and supplies the medial side of the great toe.

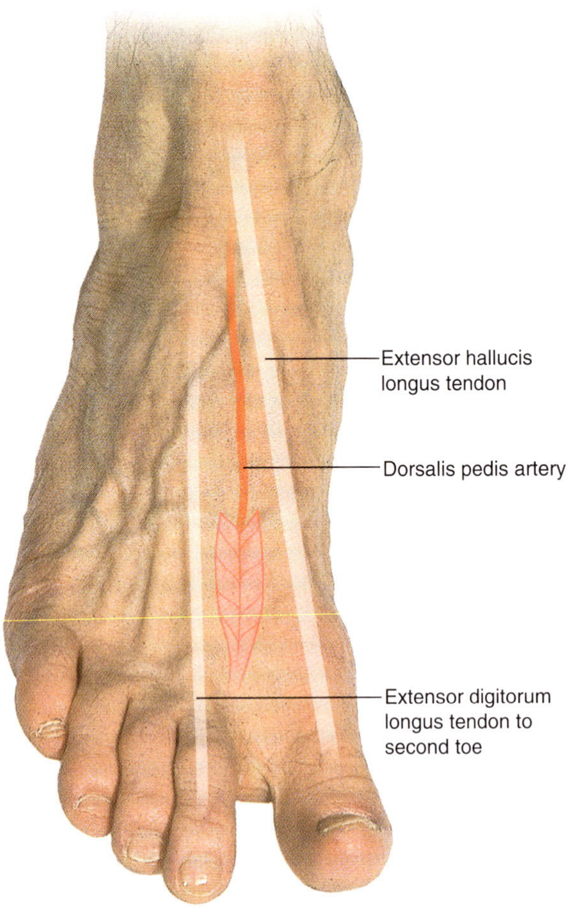

Fig. 3.129 Finding the dorsalis pedis artery.

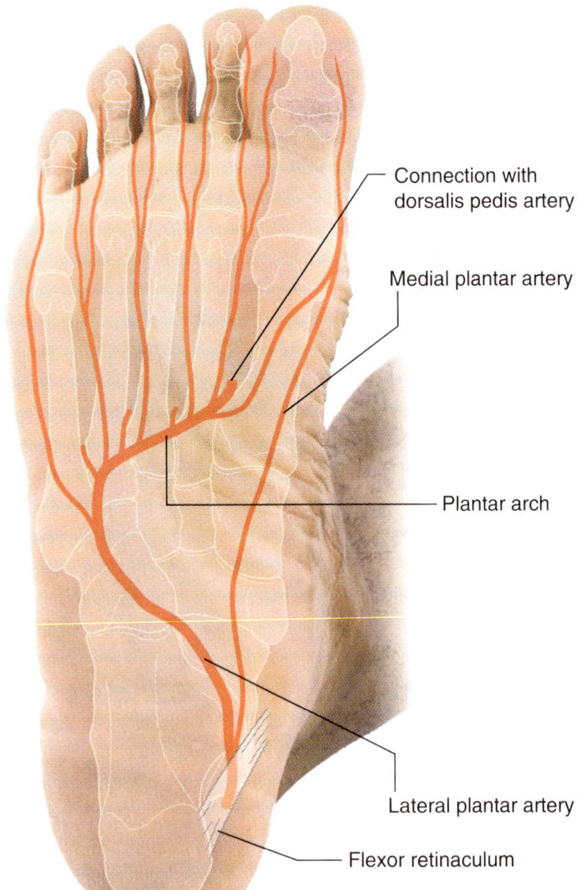

Fig. 3.130 Position of the plantar arch.

Major superficial veins

Superficial veins in the lower limb often become enlarged. Also, because the veins are long, they can be removed and used elsewhere in the body as vascular grafts.

Superficial veins (Fig. 3.131) in the lower limb begin as a dorsal venous arch in the foot. The medial side of the arch curves superiorly anterior to the medial malleolus and passes up the leg and thigh as the great saphenous vein. This vein passes through an aperture in the fascia lata (saphenous ring) to join with the femoral vein in the femoral triangle.

The lateral side of the dorsal venous arch in the foot passes posterior to the lateral malleolus and up the posterior surface of the leg as the small saphenous vein. This vessel pierces the deep fascia in the upper one-third of the leg and connects with the popliteal vein in the popliteal fossa posterior to the knee.

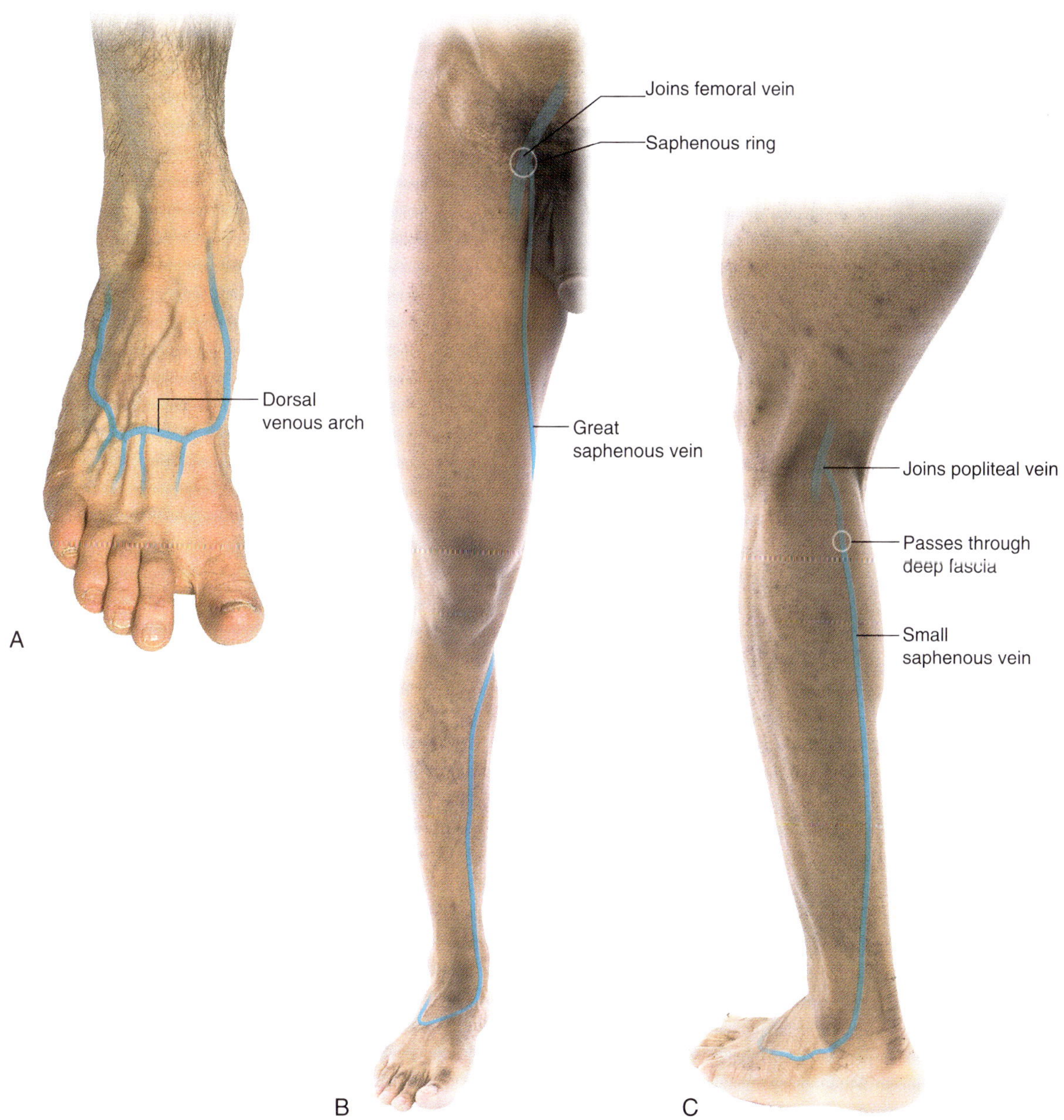

Fig. 3.131 Major superficial veins. **(A)** Dorsal aspect of the right foot. **(B)** Anterior view of right lower limb. **(C)** Posterior aspect of the left thigh, leg, and foot.

Pulse points

Peripheral pulses can be felt at four locations in the lower limb (Fig. 3.132):

- **Femoral pulse** in the femoral triangle—femoral artery inferior to the inguinal ligament and midway between the anterior superior iliac spine and the pubic symphysis (Fig. 3.124)
- **Popliteal pulse** in the popliteal fossa—popliteal artery deep in the popliteal fossa medial to the midline of the fossa (Fig. 3.126)
- **Posterior tibial pulse** in the tarsal tunnel—posterior tibial artery posteroinferior to the medial malleolus in the groove between the medial malleolus and the heel (calcaneal tuberosity, Fig. 3.127)
- **Dorsalis pedis pulse** on the dorsal aspect of the foot—dorsalis pedis artery as it passes distally over the tarsal bones between the tendon of the extensor hallucis longus and the tendon of the extensor digitorum longus to the second toe (Fig. 3.129)

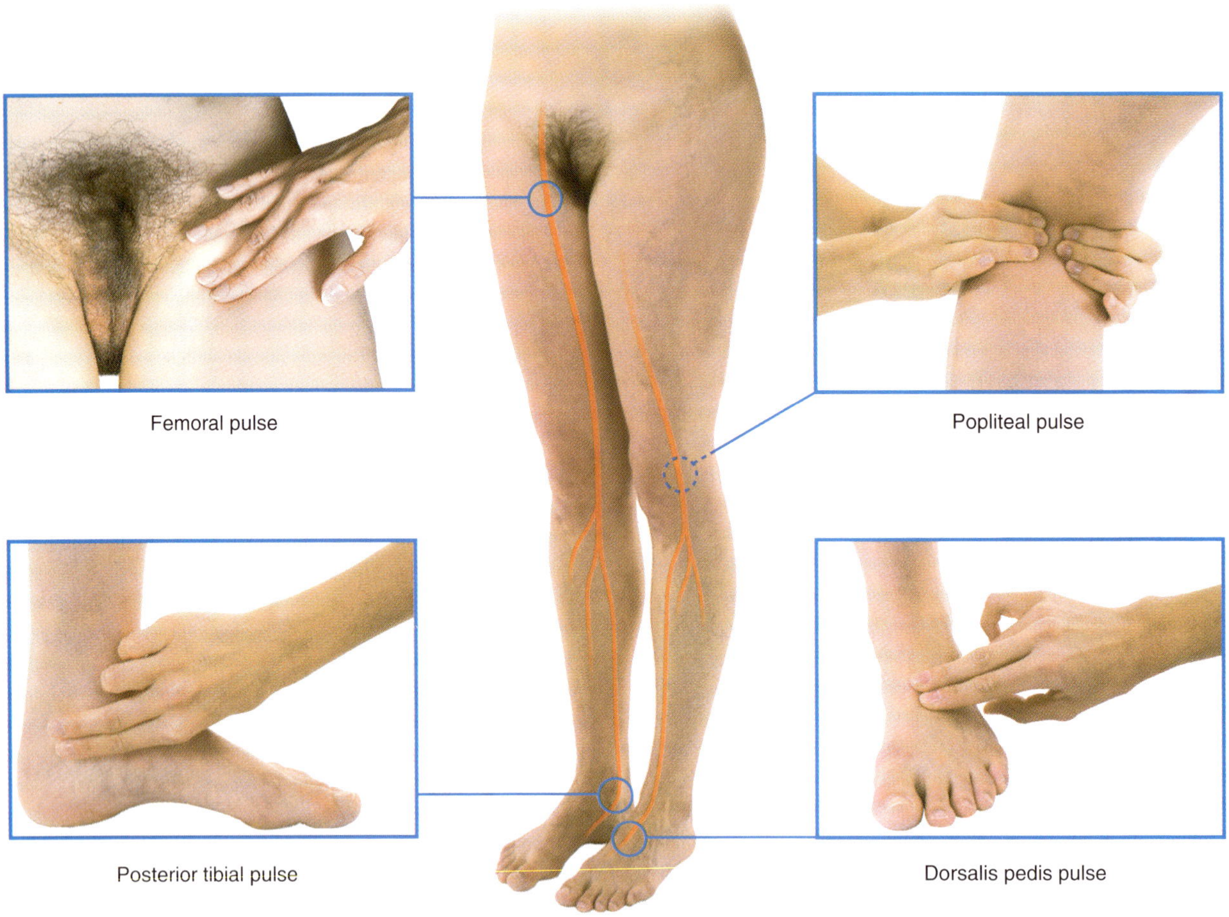

Fig. 3.132 Where to feel peripheral arterial pulses in the lower limb.

Clinical cases

Case 1

VARICOSE VEINS

A young woman came to a vascular surgeon with several large dilated tortuous veins in her right leg. The rest of her leg was otherwise normal.

A diagnosis of varicose veins was made and the surgeon needs to determine the site of valvular incompetence.

There are typical points where incompetent valves occur between the superficial and the deep veins. In these regions, the varicosities tend to become marked. The typical sites are

- At the saphenofemoral junction where the great saphenous vein joins the femoral vein—saphena varix
- In the midthigh where there is a perforating vein between the great saphenous vein and the femoral vein
- The three sites in the calf where perforators are present between the great saphenous vein and the deep veins of the calf are, 5, 10, and 15 cm above the medial malleolus
- At the junction of the small saphenous vein and the popliteal vein

The surgeon asked the patient to lie supine on the bed and elevated the leg. A tourniquet was placed around the upper thigh below the saphenofemoral junction and the patient was asked to stand up. No veins were demonstrated filling on the medial aspect of the thigh and lower limb.

The effect of the tourniquet is to compress the great saphenous vein while permitting blood to flow in the deep venous system of the femoral vein and the deep femoral vein.

Because there was no filling of the medial varicose veins below the level of the tourniquet, the surgeon assumed that the valve at the saphenofemoral junction was incompetent and would require surgical treatment.

However, during the tourniquet maneuver, the surgeon also noted some veins around the posterior and posterolateral aspect of the calf.

A similar technique was performed by application of a tourniquet just below the level of the knee joint while the leg was elevated. The patient stood up and no veins were demonstrated filling in the posterior and posterolateral aspect of the calf. These findings suggested to the surgeon that there was also incompetence of the valve for the small saphenous system where it drains into the popliteal vein.

Surgery was planned.

A small transverse incision was made below the level of the inguinal ligament where the great saphenous vein passes through the saphenous ring in the deep fascia. This can be easily palpated as a small circular defect in the fascia. The saphenofemoral junction was identified and the great saphenous vein was ligated, at its anastomosis with the femoral vein. The great saphenous vein was stripped using special surgical techniques and removed.

The patient was placed prone for the second part of the operation.

A small incision was made transversely at the level of the skin crease in the popliteal fossa. However, the surgeon had difficulty identifying the junction between the small saphenous vein and the popliteal vein. After considerable time, the surgeon located what he thought was the small saphenous vein and the structure was ligated and the wound closed.

The following day the patient was sent home, but returned to the clinic after 2 weeks complaining of difficulty in walking. On examination there was absence of dorsiflexion, a sensory disturbance over the lateral aspect of the leg and foot, and obvious wasting of the fibular muscles. As the

Continued

Case 1 *(continued)*

patient walked, the foot was dragged between steps. A clinical diagnosis of foot drop was made and a common fibular nerve injury was diagnosed. The injury occurred at the time of surgery.

Within the popliteal fossa are the popliteal artery, popliteal vein, tibial nerve, and common fibular nerve. The popliteal artery is the deepest structure. The popliteal vein is superficial to the artery and the tibial nerve is superficial to the vein (Fig. 3.133). Importantly, the sciatic nerve divides at the apex of the popliteal fossa. The tibial nerve continues into the popliteal fossa. The common fibular nerve passes laterally adjacent to the biceps femoris muscle to become superficial and wrap around the fibula neck.

It was concluded that the surgeon had accidentally ligated the common fibular nerve rather than the small saphenous vein, thus producing this patient's symptoms.

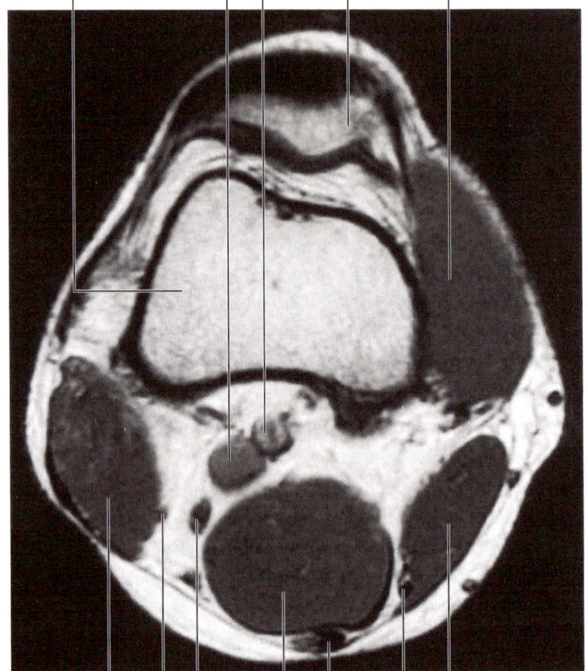

Fig. 3.133 Popliteal fossa showing position of the popliteal artery and vein and tibial nerve. T1-weighted magnetic resonance image in the axial plane.

Case 2

KNEE JOINT INJURY

A young man was enjoying a long weekend skiing at a European ski resort. While racing a friend, he caught the inner edge of his right ski. He lost his balance and fell. During his tumble, he heard an audible "click." After recovering from his fall, he developed tremendous pain in his right knee. He was unable to carry on skiing for that day, and by the time he returned to his hotel, his knee was significantly swollen. He went immediately to see an orthopedic surgeon.

The orthopedic surgeon carefully reviewed the mechanism of injury.

The man was skiing down the slope with both skis in parallel. The ankles were held rigid in the boots and the knees were slightly flexed. A momentary loss of concentration led to the skier catching the inner edge of his right ski. This effect was to force the boot and calf into external rotation. Furthermore, the knee was forced into a valgus position (bowed laterally away from the midline) and the skier tumbled. Both skis were detached from the boots as the bindings released them.

A series of structures within the knee joint were damaged sequentially.

Case 2 *(continued)*

As the knee went into external rotation and valgus, the anterior cruciate ligament became taut, acting as a fulcrum. The tibial collateral ligament was stressed and the lateral compartment of the knee compressed. As the force increased, the tibial collateral ligament was torn (Fig. 3.134A and B), as was the medial meniscus (Fig. 3.135C). Finally, the anterior cruciate ligament, which was taut, gave way (Fig. 3.135A and B).

The joint became swollen some hours afterward.

Disruption of the anterior cruciate ligament characteristically produces marked joint swelling. The ligament is extrasynovial and intracapsular and has a rich blood supply. As the ligament was torn, it ruptured into the joint. Blood from the tear irritates the synovial membrane and also enters the joint. These factors produce gradual swelling of the joint over the ensuing hours with significant fluid accumulation in the joint cavity.

The patient had a surgical reconstruction of the anterior cruciate ligament.

It is difficult to find a man-made substance that can act in the same way as the anterior cruciate ligament and demonstrate the same physical properties. Surgeons have devised ingenious ways of reconstructing the anterior cruciate ligament. Two of the commonest methods use the patellar ligament (tendon) and hamstrings to reconstruct the ligament.

The patient had further surgical procedures.

The tibial collateral ligament was explored and resutured. Using arthroscopic techniques, the tear in the medial meniscus was debrided to prevent further complications.

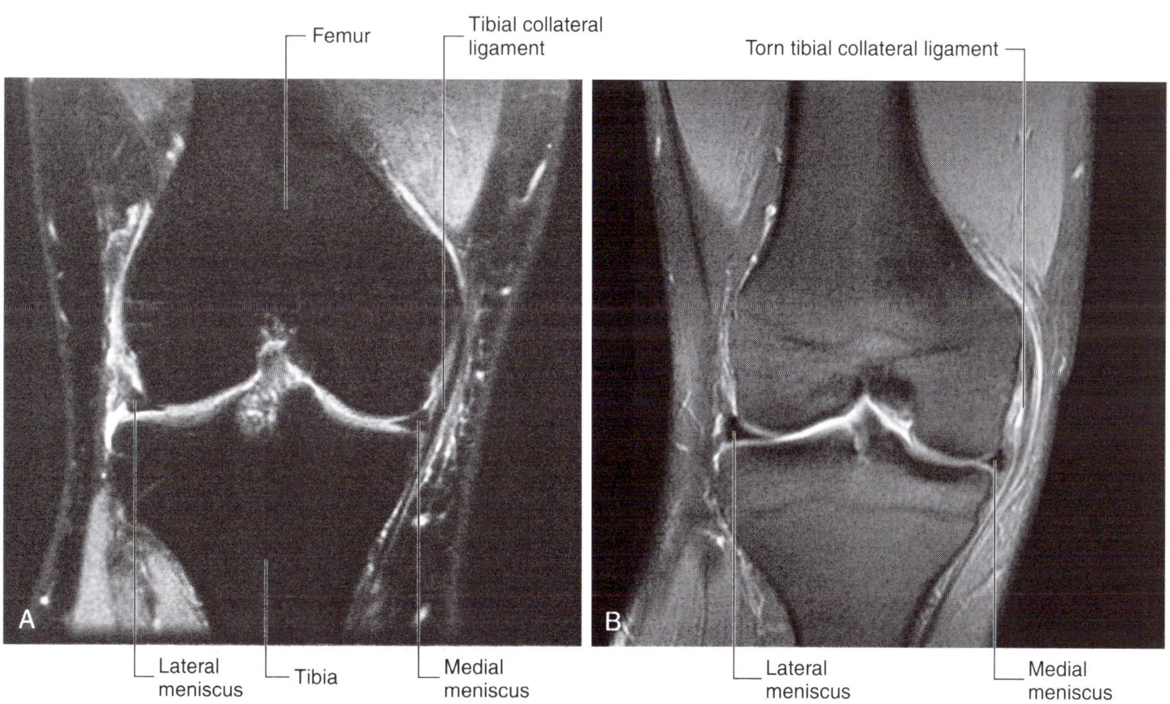

Fig. 3.134 (A) Normal knee joint showing the tibial collateral ligament and the medial and lateral menisci. Proton density (PD)-weighted magnetic resonance image in the coronal plane. **(B)** Knee joint showing a torn tibial collateral ligament. PD-weighted magnetic resonance image in the coronal plane.

Continued

Case 2 *(continued)*

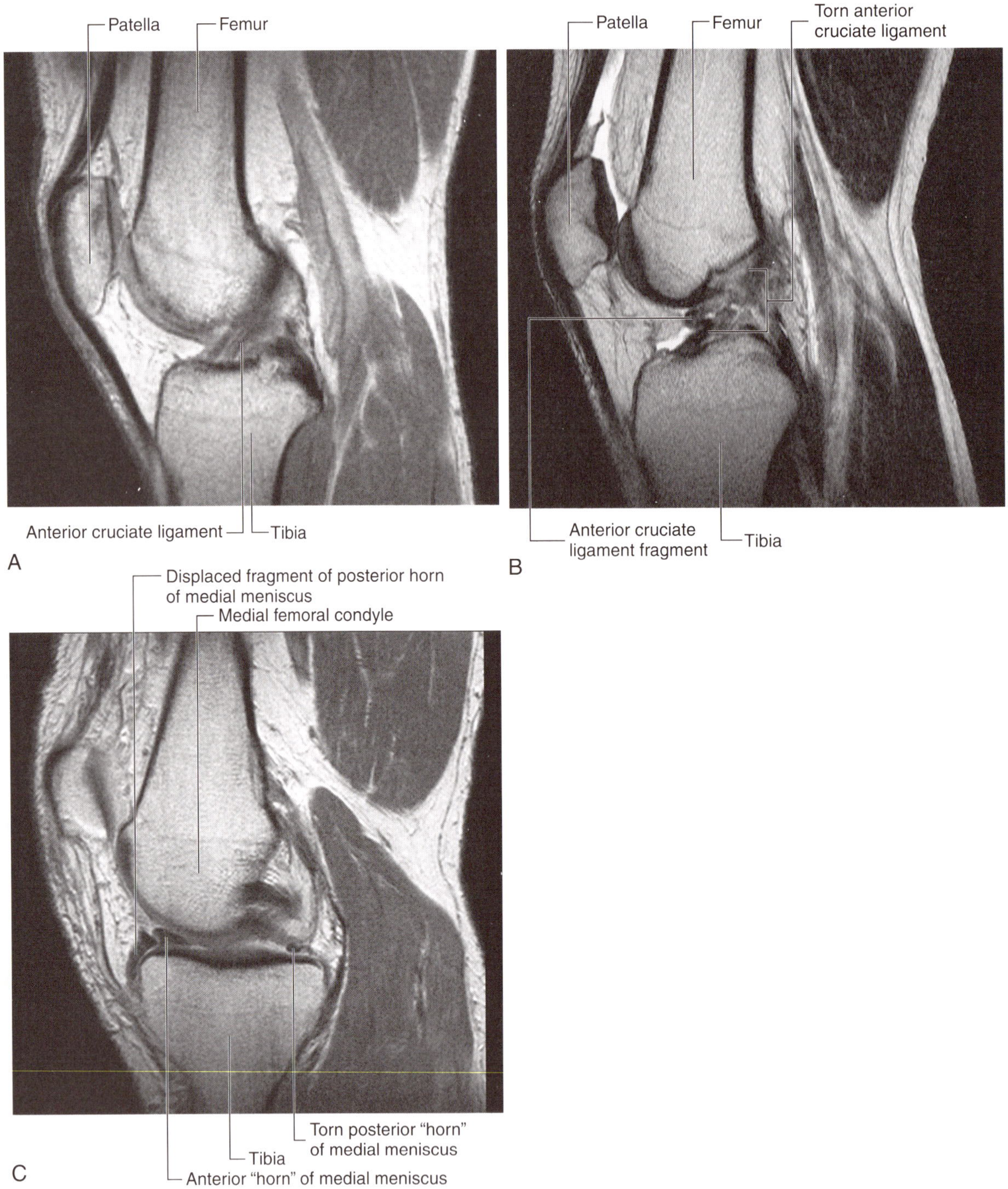

Fig. 3.135 (A) Knee joint showing an intact anterior cruciate ligament. T2-weighted magnetic resonance image in the sagittal plane. **(B)** Knee joint showing a torn anterior cruciate ligament. T2-weighted magnetic resonance image in the sagittal plane. **(C)** Knee joint showing a torn medial meniscus (the broken off portion of the posterior horn has moved into the anterior aspect of the joint giving the impression of a "double meniscus" in this location). Proton density-weighted magnetic resonance image in the sagittal plane.

Case 3

FRACTURE OF NECK OF FEMUR

A 72-year-old woman was admitted to the emergency room after falling at home. She complained of a severe pain in her right hip and had noticeable bruising on the right side of the face.

On admission it was noted that the patient's right lower limb was shorter than her left lower limb and the thigh was externally rotated.

An initial series of investigations was carried out, including a plain radiograph of the pelvis.

The plain radiograph of the pelvis demonstrated a displaced fracture through the right neck of the femur.

The apparent shortening and external rotation of the lower limb on clinical examination were accounted for by spasm of the muscles connecting the pelvis to the trochanters and proximal femur. Of the muscles that surround the hip joint, the largest group acting on the thigh is the adductor group (adductor longus, brevis, and magnus) and the psoas major. The psoas major inserts onto the lesser trochanter and its action is to internally rotate and flex the hip. The fulcrum of action of the psoas major is the femoral head in the acetabulum. However, when the femoral neck is detached, its overriding action pulls the femur proximally and into external rotation. The external rotation is exacerbated by the spasm in the adductor muscles.

Extensive medical testing was necessary before surgery. It is important to remember that elderly patients may have a number of coexisting diseases.

The patient then underwent a hemiarthroplasty. This is a surgical procedure in which the femoral head is removed from the acetabulum. The femoral neck is trimmed close to the trochanters and the medullary cavity of the femoral shaft is reamed. A metal hip prosthesis is inserted into the medullary cavity of the femur and the head of the prosthesis is placed into the acetabulum, in which it articulates.

The blood supply to the femoral head is from three sources—the artery within the ligament of the head of the femur, vessels in the medullary cavity, and vessels deep to the synovium running in the retinacula of the fibrous capsule of the hip joint. With increasing age, the medullary cavity undergoes fatty replacement of the normal red marrow, thus attenuating the medullary blood supply. The artery within the ligament of the head of the femur also becomes attenuated and this is often associated with atherosclerotic arterial disease.

Unfortunately for this patient, the sole blood supply to the head of the femur was via the vessels in the retinacula fibers, which were transected at the time of the fracture. If the patient had an intertrochanteric fracture instead, the vessels of the retinacula fibers would not have been damaged and a different approach to surgical fixation could be undertaken without the need for a hemiarthroplasty.

The patient had osteoporosis.

Osteoporosis is a common condition affecting older people, but is significantly more frequent in postmenopausal women. Many fractures of the femoral neck in elderly patients occur because the strength of the bone is significantly reduced when it is osteoporotic. Other common sites for osteoporotic fractures include the distal radius and the thoracic and lumbar vertebrae.

Case 4

DEEP VEIN THROMBOSIS

A 28-year-old woman was seen by her family practitioner for a routine pregnancy checkup at 36 weeks' gestational age. Neither the patient nor the family physician had any concerns about the pregnancy. However, the patient did complain of unilateral swelling of her left leg, which had gradually increased over the previous 2 days. Furthermore, the evening before her visit, she developed some sharp chest pain, which was exacerbated by taking deep breaths.

The family physician ordered a duplex ultrasound scan of the left leg venous system.

Ultrasound scanning of the vascular tree can demonstrate flow and occlusion of arteries and veins.

The probe was placed over the left femoral vein and no flow was demonstrated. Furthermore, the vein could not be compressed, and no alteration of flow with breathing could be demonstrated. Some flow was demonstrated in the deep femoral vein and in the great saphenous vein. No flow was demonstrated throughout the length of the left femoral vein, the popliteal vein, and the tibial veins.

The technician scanned the opposite side, where excellent flow was demonstrated within the right femoral venous system. In addition, when the calf was gently massaged, an augmentation to the flow was noted. It was possible to demonstrate alteration of flow with respiratory excursion and venous compression was satisfactory. A diagnosis of extensive left-sided deep vein thrombosis was made.

Certain patients are more prone to deep vein thrombosis.

Three major factors predispose a patient to thrombosis:

- Reduced or stagnant blood flow in the veins
- Injury to the vein wall
- Hypercoagulability of the blood

In this patient, compression of the left external iliac veins by the gravid uterus was the likely cause of stasis, which led to the deep vein thrombosis.

The chest pain was due to pulmonary emboli.

Small emboli were thrown off from the leading edge of the thrombus through the heart to lodge in the lungs. Small emboli cause typical pleuritic chest pain, which is exacerbated by breathing. In isolation, these small pulmonary emboli may affect respiratory function, but they may be the precursor to a large and potentially fatal pulmonary embolus (Fig. 3.136).

Anticoagulation was instituted and the patient had an uneventful delivery.

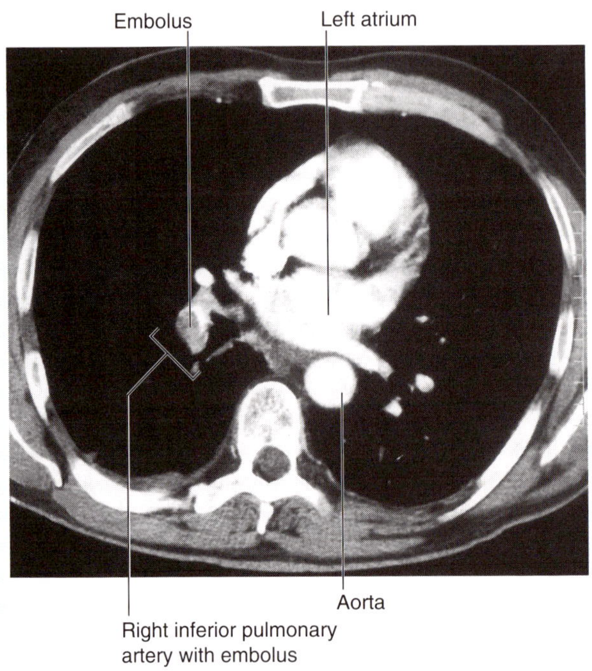

Fig. 3.136 Pulmonary embolus. Axial computed tomogram.

Case 5

RUPTURED CALCANEAL TENDON

A 45-year-old man had recently taken up squash. During a game he attempted a forehand shot and noticed severe sudden pain in his heel. He thought his opponent had hit him with his racket. When he turned, though, he realized his opponent was too far away to have hit him.

Within minutes there was marked swelling of the ankle. The patient was unable to plantarflex his foot and had to stop the game. Afterward, an appreciable subcutaneous hematoma developed in the ankle.

The diagnostic possibilities include a bone or soft tissue injury.

A bony injury was excluded because there was no bone tenderness.

The patient had a significant soft tissue injury. On examination he had significant swelling of the ankle with a subcutaneous hematoma. He was unable to stand on tiptoe on the right leg, and in the prone position a palpable defect was demonstrated within the calcaneal tendon.

A diagnosis of calcaneal tendon rupture was made.

This patient has a typical history of ruptured calcaneal tendon and the clinical findings support this. Magnetic resonance imaging was carried out and confirmed the diagnosis (Fig. 3.137).

The patient underwent an operative repair.

The tendon healed well, though the patient has not gone back to playing squash.

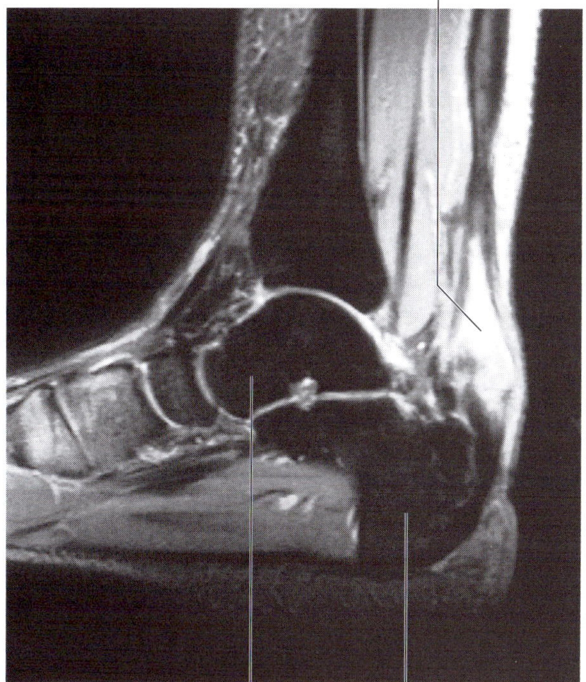

Fig. 3.137 Ankle showing a ruptured calcaneal tendon. T2-weighted magnetic resonance image in the sagittal plane.

Case 6

POPLITEAL ARTERY ANEURYSM

A 67-year-old man was noted to have a mass at the back of his knee. The mass measured approximately 4 cm in transverse diameter. The patient was otherwise fit and well and had no other history of note.

The mass was arising from one of the structures in the popliteal fossa.

Within the popliteal fossa, there is a neurovascular bundle that contains the tibial nerve, the popliteal artery, and the popliteal vein. There are also numerous small bursae associated with the posterior aspect of the knee joint and the muscles and tendons in this region. It is possible that this mass is arising from the posterior structures of the knee joint, which include synovial outpouchings, the menisci, and the muscles and tendons of this region.

The commonest masses demonstrated within the popliteal fossa are a popliteal cyst, a popliteal aneurysm, and an arterial adventitial cyst.

Further clinical examination revealed that this mass was pulsatile and demonstrated a bruit (an audible rumbling made by turbulent blood flow) on auscultation.

A diagnosis of popliteal artery aneurysm was made.

A popliteal artery aneurysm is an abnormal dilatation of the popliteal artery. It is unusual for it to be greater than 5 cm because symptoms usually develop before it reaches this size.

Unlike aneurysms elsewhere in the body, the natural history of popliteal aneurysms is to embolize, with the mural thrombus producing ischemia distal to the lesion, rather than rupture. It is mandatory to examine the rest of the arterial tree in patients with a popliteal aneurysm because aneurysms may be bilateral and there is an association with abdominal aortic aneurysms.

An ultrasound investigation was carried out.

Using real-time ultrasound the dimensions of the popliteal aneurysm were noted and the flow in the vessels was demonstrated. Furthermore, a popliteal cyst and adventitial cyst were completely excluded.

The patient underwent a surgical excision and graft interposition and has made an uneventful recovery.

Case 7

ANTERIOR TALOFIBULAR LIGAMENT TEAR

A young long-distance runner came to her physician with acute swelling around the lateral aspect of her ankle. This injury occurred directly after accidentally running into a pothole in the pavement.

A fractured ankle was suspected.

Plain anteroposterior and lateral radiographs of the ankle revealed no evidence of any bone injury to account for the patient's soft tissue swelling.

The patient was given a pair of crutches and analgesics and told to rest. A diagnosis of a simple sprain was made.

Over the ensuing weeks, the swelling and edema within the soft tissue of the ankle decreased and the patient began to run, but noted that the ankle kept "giving way." She went to an orthopedic surgeon for further assessment.

There was a positive anterior drawer test of the ankle joint.

At this stage it is important to review the mechanism of injury. Typically when running on a hard surface, the final phase of push-off involves supination of the foot. If the foot is caught in a pothole, this supinating maneuver continues and inversion occurs along with plantar flexion. This puts significant strain on the lateral ligament complex and, given the appropriate circumstances, disruption (in order) of the ligament structures occurs from anterior to posterior. First, the anterior talofibular ligament is disrupted, followed by the calcaneofibular ligament, and then the posterior talofibular ligament. As each of these ligaments is disrupted, the severity of the soft tissue injury is significantly enhanced and the chance of permanent ankle instability is increased.

On examination any positive anterior drawer test of the ankle (4–5 mm compared to the opposite side) suggests an injury to the anterior talofibular ligament.

The anterior talofibular ligament can be assessed by placing the foot in marked plantar flexion. If there is over 10° of difference between the affected foot and nonaffected foot, an anterior talofibular ligament disruption is suspected.

It is extremely rare for all three ligaments to be disrupted, and if so, there are usually other significant ankle injuries.

Magnetic resonance imaging (MRI) was carried out to assess ligament damage.

Case 7 *(continued)*

MRI is excellent for demonstrating the medial and lateral ligament complexes of the ankle as well as the soft tissues that support the bones of the posterior foot.

Unfortunately for this patient there was a tear of the anterior talofibular ligament (Fig. 3.138), which had to be repaired surgically.

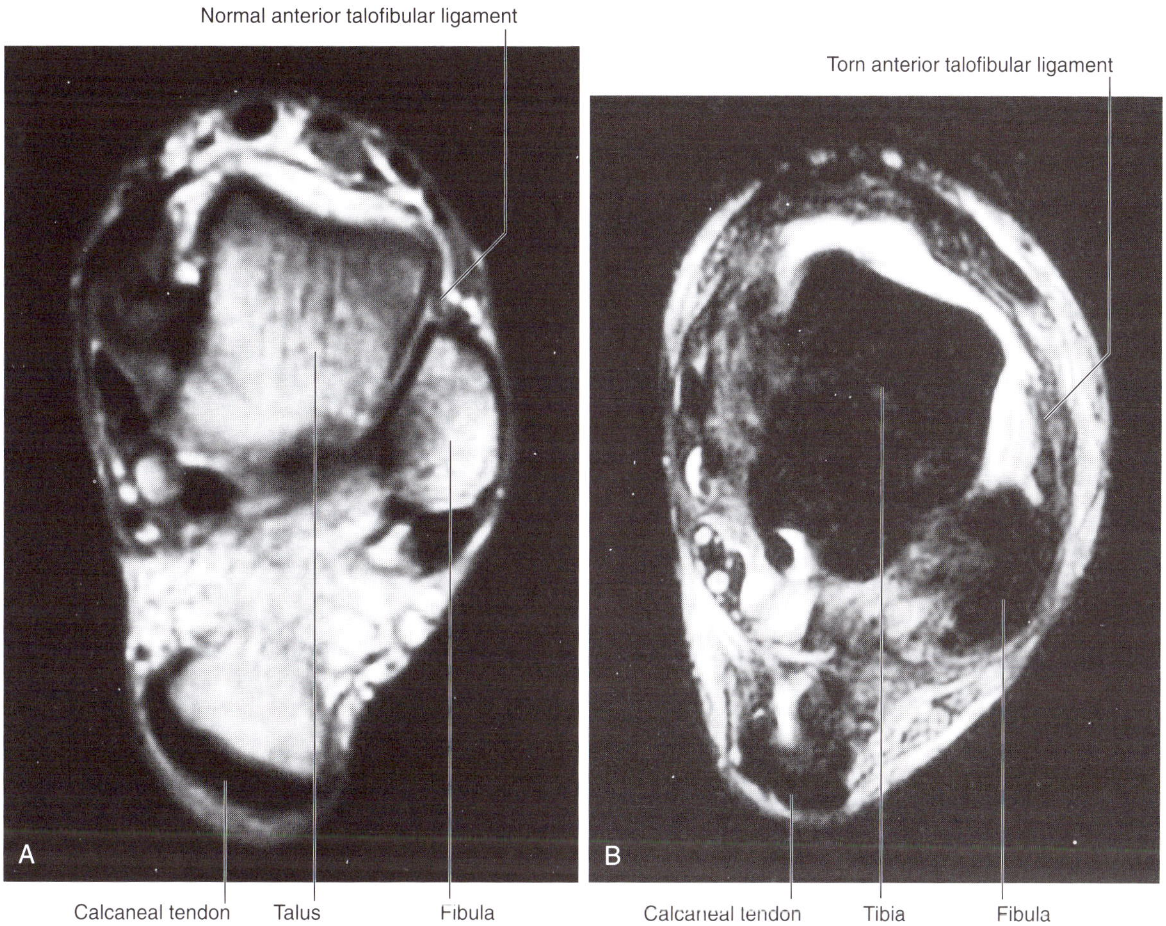

Fig. 3.138 (A) Normal ankle joint showing an intact anterior talofibular ligament. T1-weighted magnetic resonance image in the axial plane. **(B)** Ankle joint showing a torn anterior talofibular ligament. T2-weighted magnetic resonance image in the axial plane.

Case 8

OSTEOMYELITIS

A 45-year-old man with diabetes mellitus visited his nurse because he had an ulcer on his foot that was not healing despite daily dressings.

Diabetes can lead to vascular disease of large and medium arteries, narrowing the lumen and reducing blood supply to the extremities, thereby impairing healing. In addition, diabetes can also affect blood supply to nerves, which leads to peripheral neuropathy. Peripheral neuropathy results in reduced sensation, and therefore minor injuries can often go unnoticed.

This patient has developed an ulcer on his heel, which is a pressure point and likely to be under repeated strain. The nurse examined the ulcer and found that the ulcer was looking infected with pus at the base of the ulcer and asked for a specialist orthopedic opinion, who requested an X-ray and an MRI. Both the MRI and X-ray demonstrated infection invading into the calcaneus with destruction of the bone (Fig. 3.139A and B).

The patient required surgical washout with removal of the dead and infected bone (debridement) and was given long-term antibiotic treatment (Fig. 3.139C).

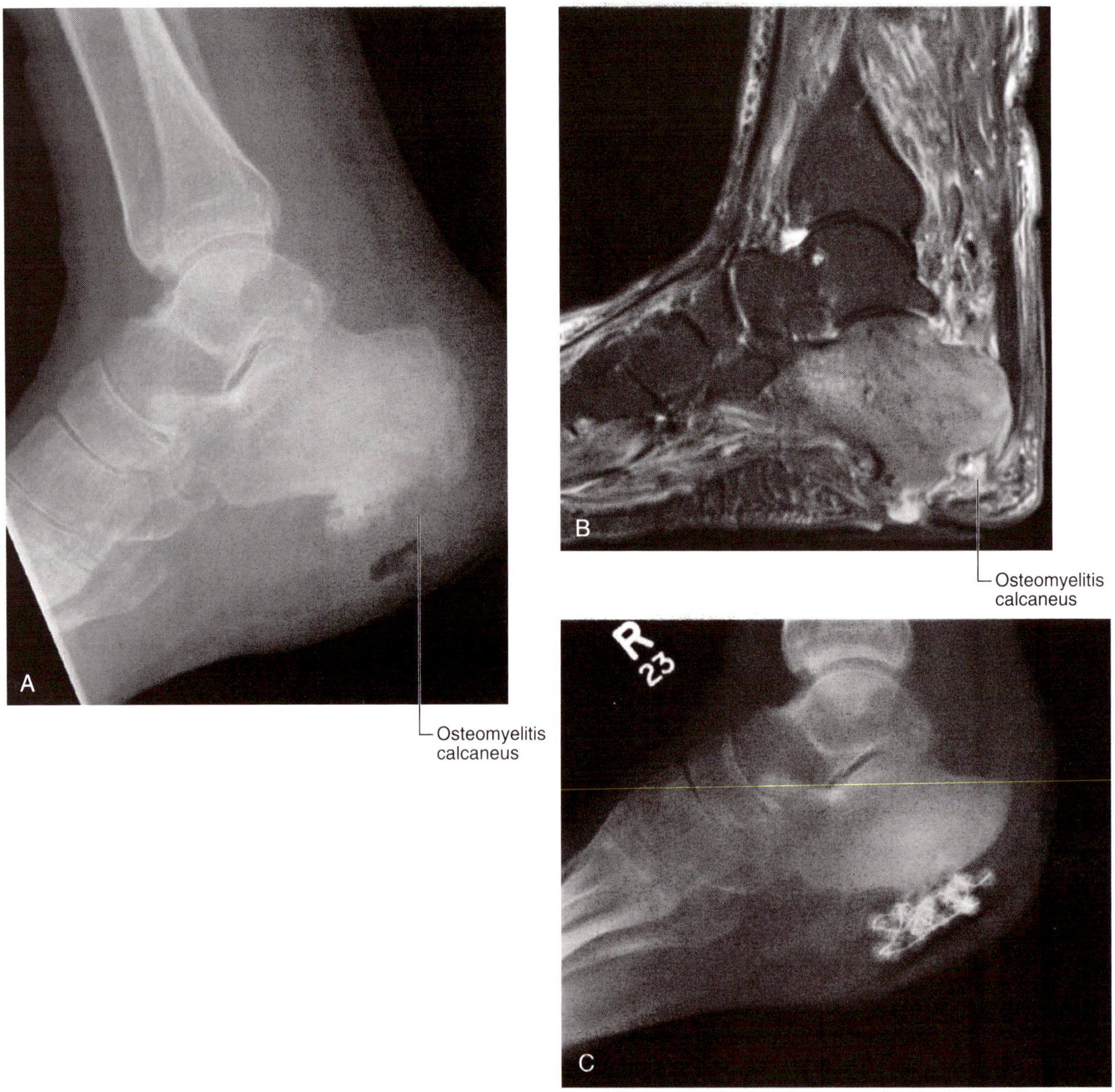

Fig. 3.139 Radiograph **(A)** and MRI **(B)** of soft tissue ulceration and erosion in the adjacent calcaneus. After debridement and placement of antibiotics beads in the wound, there is progressive healing **(C)**.

4

Abdomen

ADDITIONAL LEARNING RESOURCES for Chapter 4, Abdomen, on MedEnact (www.MedEnact.com):

- Multiple Choice Questions
- Short Questions—these are questions requiring short responses
- Medical Clinical Case Studies
  Aortoiliac occlusive disease
  Splenic rupture
  Intussusception
  Zollinger–Ellison syndrome
- MCQs

FREE Online Anatomy Self-Study Course

- Anatomy modules 10 through 17

Competency: The first-year medical students should be able to apply their knowledge of the anatomy of the abdominal walls and abdominal viscera to explain the anatomical basis of common clinical conditions and procedures.

Conceptual overview

SET INDUCTION—CASE SCENARIO 1: RECTUS SHEATH HEMATOMA

A 19-year-old male was brought to the emergency department with a history of abdominal pain of sudden origin, which had occurred while playing football. On examination, a localized tender swelling was found on the anterior abdominal wall. Anatomical knowledge of the rectus sheath is needed to make a diagnosis of rectus sheath hematoma.

<table>
<tr><th rowspan="2">REMEMBER
[Recall Facts]</th><th colspan="3">OUTLINE 1. CONCEPTUAL OVERVIEW, ANTERIOR ABDOMINAL WALL, AND RECTUS SHEATH—LEARNING OBJECTIVES
[By the end of this section the student should be able to:]</th><th rowspan="2" colspan="2">EVALUATE
[Explain Concepts]</th></tr>
<tr><th colspan="3">DEMONSTRATE AND ANALYZE RELATIONSHIPS
[Identify structures in a Prosected Specimen or Figure]</th></tr>
<tr><td rowspan="6">Conceptual overview
1. Describe the boundaries of the abdominal cavity
2. Classify the abdominal viscera
3. List the component parts of the walls of the abdominal cavity
4. Describe the types of peritoneum in relation to the dorsal mesentery in the fetus
5. Differentiate between intraperitoneal and retroperitoneal structures
6. Describe the development of the gut tube and the processes that qive rise to the mesenteries related to the gut tube
7. Describe the dermatomes of the anterior abdominal wall
8. Describe the processus vaginalis
9. List the arteries to the gut tube and the venous shunts from left to right
10. Describe briefly the hepatic portal vein and the portosystemic anastomosis
11. Describe the relationship of the abdominal cavity to neighboring regions
Anterior abdominal wall
1. Describe the fascia, muscles, vessels and nerves, and peritoneum of the anterior abdominal wall
2. Describe the topographic subdivisions of the anterior abdominal wall</td><td>Level I</td><td>Level II</td><td>Level III</td><td colspan="2">▪ Attachments, actions, modifications, and nerve supply of muscles of anterior abdominal wall
▪ Formation of rectus sheath at different levels
▪ Contents of rectus sheath
▪ Various planes and their levels</td></tr>
<tr><td rowspan="5">▪ Superficial fascia and its two layers:
  ▪ Fatty
  ▪ Membranous
▪ Superficial inguinal ring:
  ▪ Spermatic cord in male
  ▪ Round ligament of uterus in female
▪ External oblique muscle and aponeurosis
▪ Internal oblique muscle
▪ Transversus abdominis
▪ Anterior layer of rectus sheath
▪ Rectus abdominis muscle
▪ Pyramidalis muscle, if present
▪ Posterior layer of rectus sheath
▪ Superior and inferior epigastric vessels
▪ Arcuate line
▪ Linea alba
▪ Linea semilunaris</td><td rowspan="5">▪ Nerves with accompanying blood vessels:
  ▪ Lower intercostal nerves
  ▪ Subcostal nerve
  ▪ Iliohypogastric nerve
  ▪ Ilioinguinal nerve
▪ Intercostal nerves
▪ Subcostal nerve</td><td rowspan="5">▪ Anterior and lateral cutaneous nerves</td><th colspan="2">EARLY CLINICAL EXPOSURE
[Apply Anatomical knowledge]</th></tr>
<tr><th>Surgical Anatomy/ Pathology/ Trauma</th><th>Imaging/ Surface Anatomy</th></tr>
<tr><td>▪ Umbilical hernia and paraumbilical hernia
▪ Epigastric hernia
▪ Divarication of recti
▪ Paracentesis abdominis
▪ Caput medusae
▪ SVC blockage—lateral thoracic vein
▪ Anterior abdominal wall incisions</td><td>▪ Ultrasonography</td></tr>
<tr><th colspan="2">PROBLEM SOLVING/ CLINICAL CASES
[Interpret]</th></tr>
<tr><td colspan="2">▪ Formation of the rectus sheath at various levels</td></tr>
</table>

Abdomen

GENERAL DESCRIPTION

The abdomen is a roughly cylindrical chamber extending from the inferior margin of the thorax to the superior margin of the pelvis and the lower limb (Fig. 4.1A).

The **inferior thoracic aperture** forms the superior opening to the abdomen, and is closed by the diaphragm. Inferiorly, the deep aspect of the abdominal wall is continuous with the pelvic wall at the **pelvic inlet**. This is the junction of the abdominal cavity above and the pelvic cavity below (see Fig. 4.10). This is also the junction between the false pelvis above and the true pelvis below, when describing the bony pelvis. Superficially, the inferior limit of the abdominal wall is the superior margin of the lower limb.

The chamber enclosed by the abdominal wall contains a single large **peritoneal cavity**, which freely communicates with the pelvic cavity.

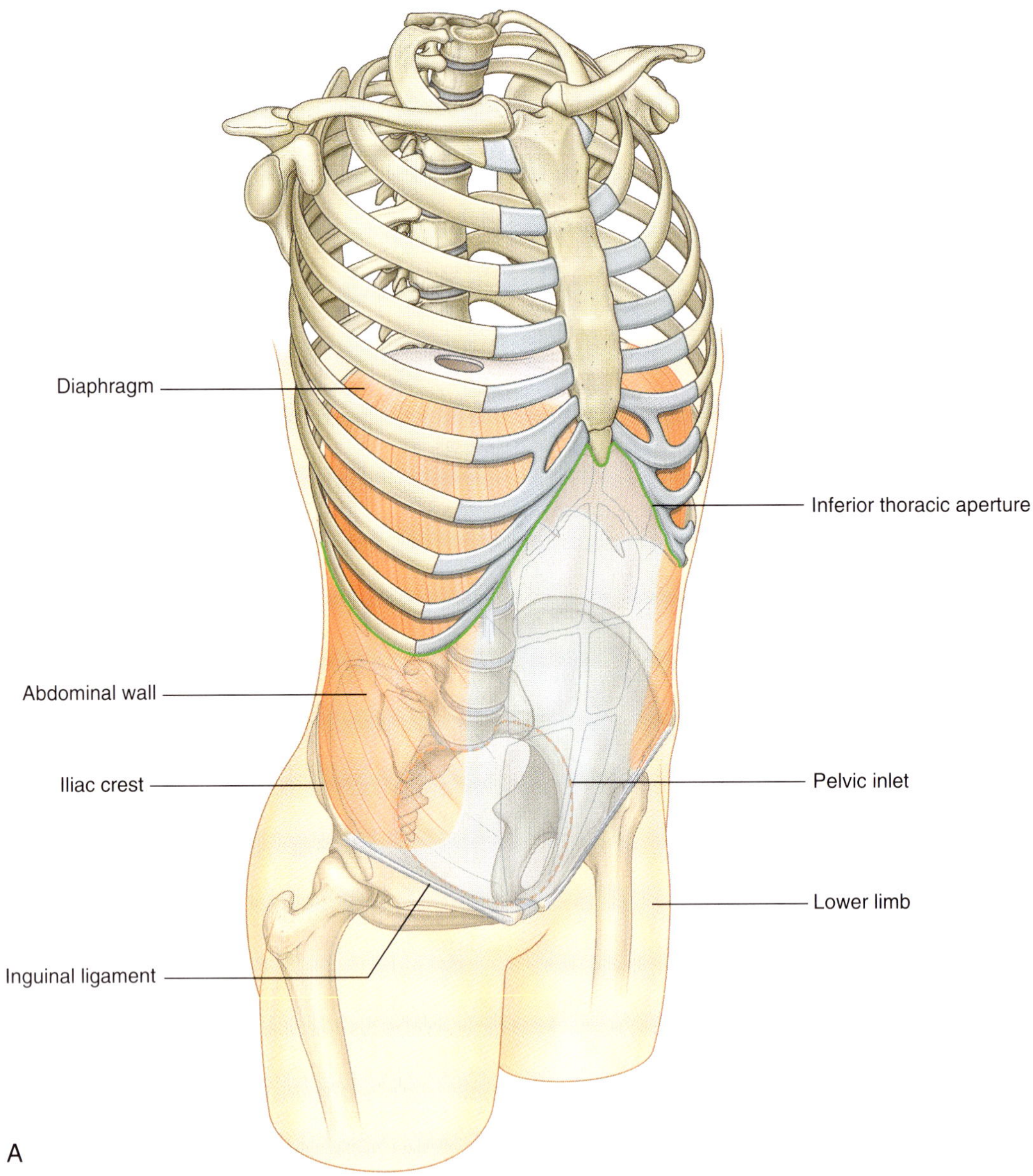

Fig. 4.1 Abdomen. **(A)** Boundaries.

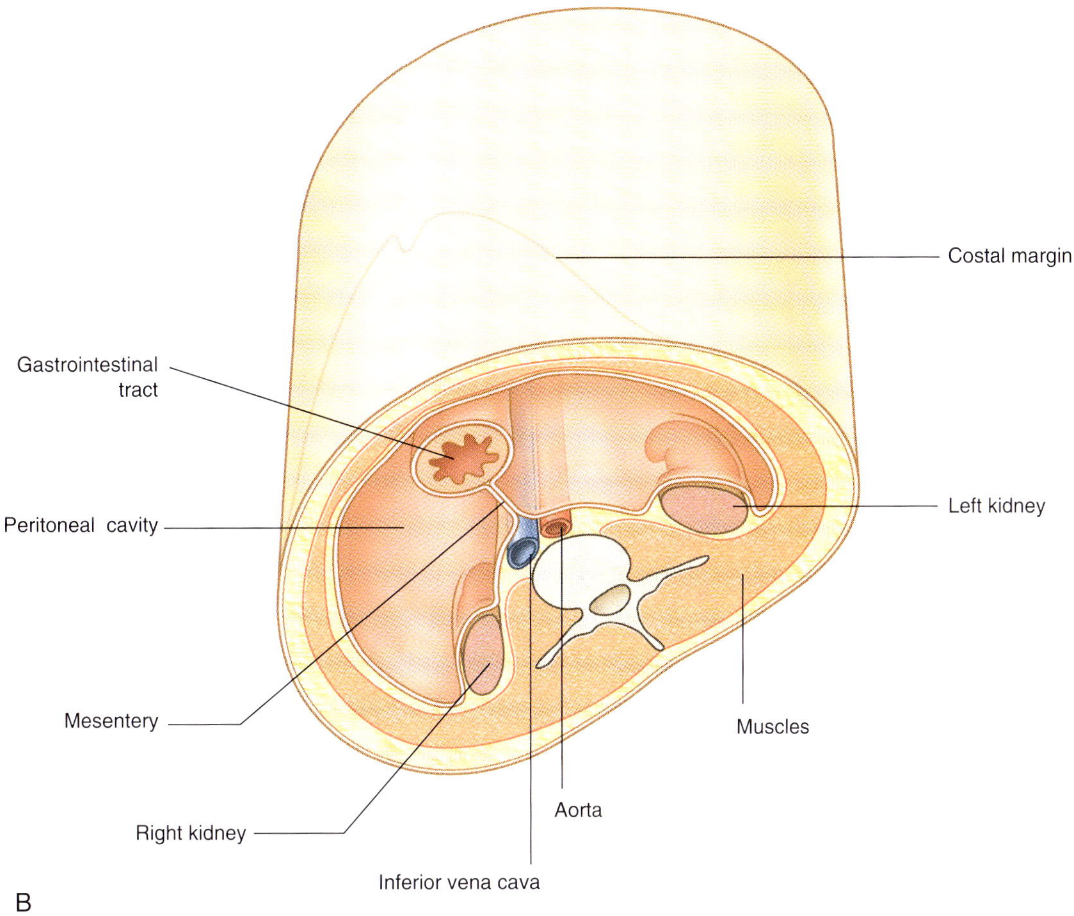

Fig. 4.1, cont'd (B) Arrangement of abdominal contents. Inferior view.

Abdominal viscera are either suspended in the peritoneal cavity by mesenteries (intraperitoneal) or positioned between the cavity and the musculoskeletal wall (retroperitoneal) (Fig. 4.1B; see also Fig. 4.6 and 4.52).

Abdominal viscera include:

- Major elements of the gastrointestinal system—the caudal end of the esophagus, stomach, small and large intestines, liver, pancreas, and gallbladder
- The spleen
- Components of the urinary system—kidneys and ureters
- The suprarenal glands
- Major neurovascular structures

FUNCTIONS

Houses and protects major viscera

The abdomen houses major elements of the gastrointestinal system (Fig. 4.2), the spleen, and parts of the urinary system.

Much of the liver, gallbladder, stomach, and spleen and parts of the colon are under the domes of the diaphragm, which project superiorly above the costal margin of the thoracic wall, and as a result these abdominal viscera are protected by the thoracic wall. The superior poles of the kidneys are deep to the lower ribs.

Viscera not under the domes of the diaphragm are supported and protected predominantly by the muscular walls of the abdomen.

Breathing

One of the most important roles of the abdominal wall is to assist in breathing:

- It relaxes during inspiration to accommodate expansion of the thoracic cavity and the inferior displacement of abdominal viscera during contraction of the diaphragm (Fig. 4.3).
- During expiration, it contracts to assist in elevating the domes of the diaphragm, thus reducing thoracic volume.

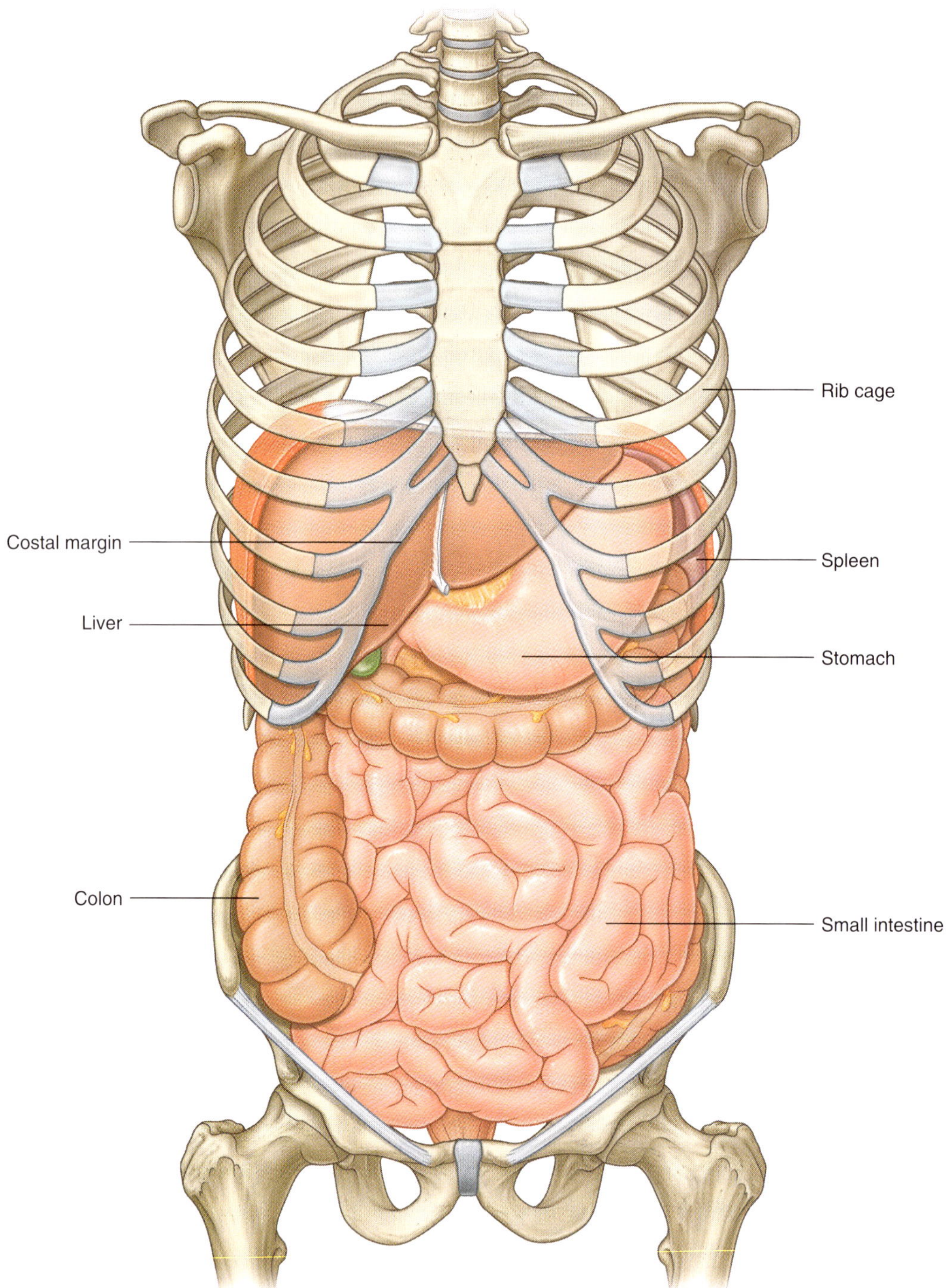

Fig. 4.2 The abdomen contains and protects the abdominal viscera.

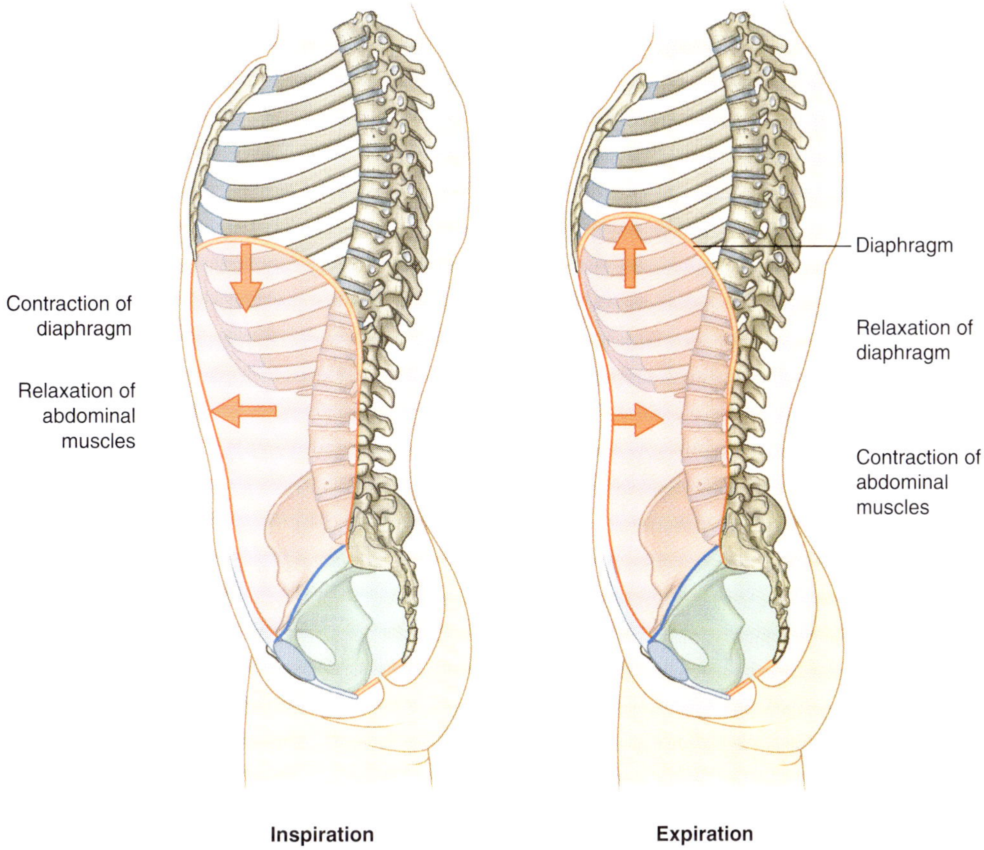

Fig. 4.3 The abdomen assists in breathing.

Material can be expelled from the airway by forced expiration using the abdominal muscles, as in coughing or sneezing.

Changes in intraabdominal pressure

Contraction of abdominal wall muscles can dramatically increase intraabdominal pressure when the diaphragm is in a fixed position (Fig. 4.4). Air is retained in the lungs by closing the glottis in the larynx in the neck. Increased intraabdominal pressure assists in emptying the contents of the bladder and rectum and in giving birth.

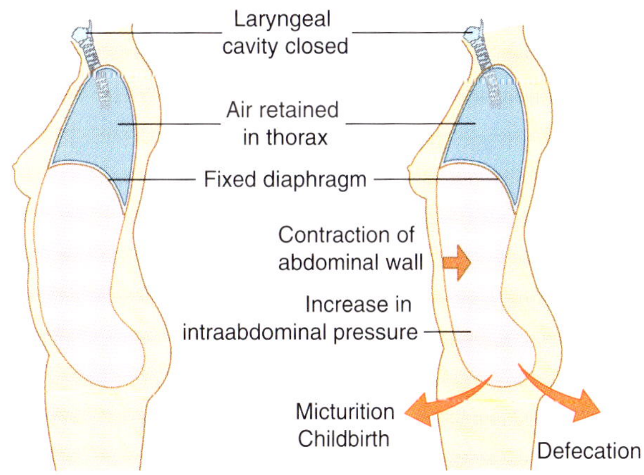

Fig. 4.4 Increasing intraabdominal pressure to assist in micturition, defecation, and childbirth.

COMPONENT PARTS

Wall

The abdominal wall consists partly of bone but mainly of muscle (Fig. 4.5). The skeletal elements of the wall (Fig. 4.5A) are

- The five lumbar vertebrae and their intervening intervertebral discs
- The superior expanded parts of the pelvic bones
- Bony components of the inferior thoracic wall, including the costal margin, rib XII, the anterior end of rib XI, and the xiphoid process

Muscles make up the rest of the abdominal wall (Fig. 4.5B):

- Lateral to the vertebral column, the diaphragm, quadratus lumborum, psoas major, and iliacus muscles reinforce the posterior aspect of the wall. The distal ends of the psoas major and iliacus muscles pass into the thigh and are major flexors of the hip joint.
- Lateral parts of the abdominal wall are predominantly formed by three layers of muscles, which are similar in orientation to the intercostal muscles of the thorax—transversus abdominis, internal oblique, and external oblique.

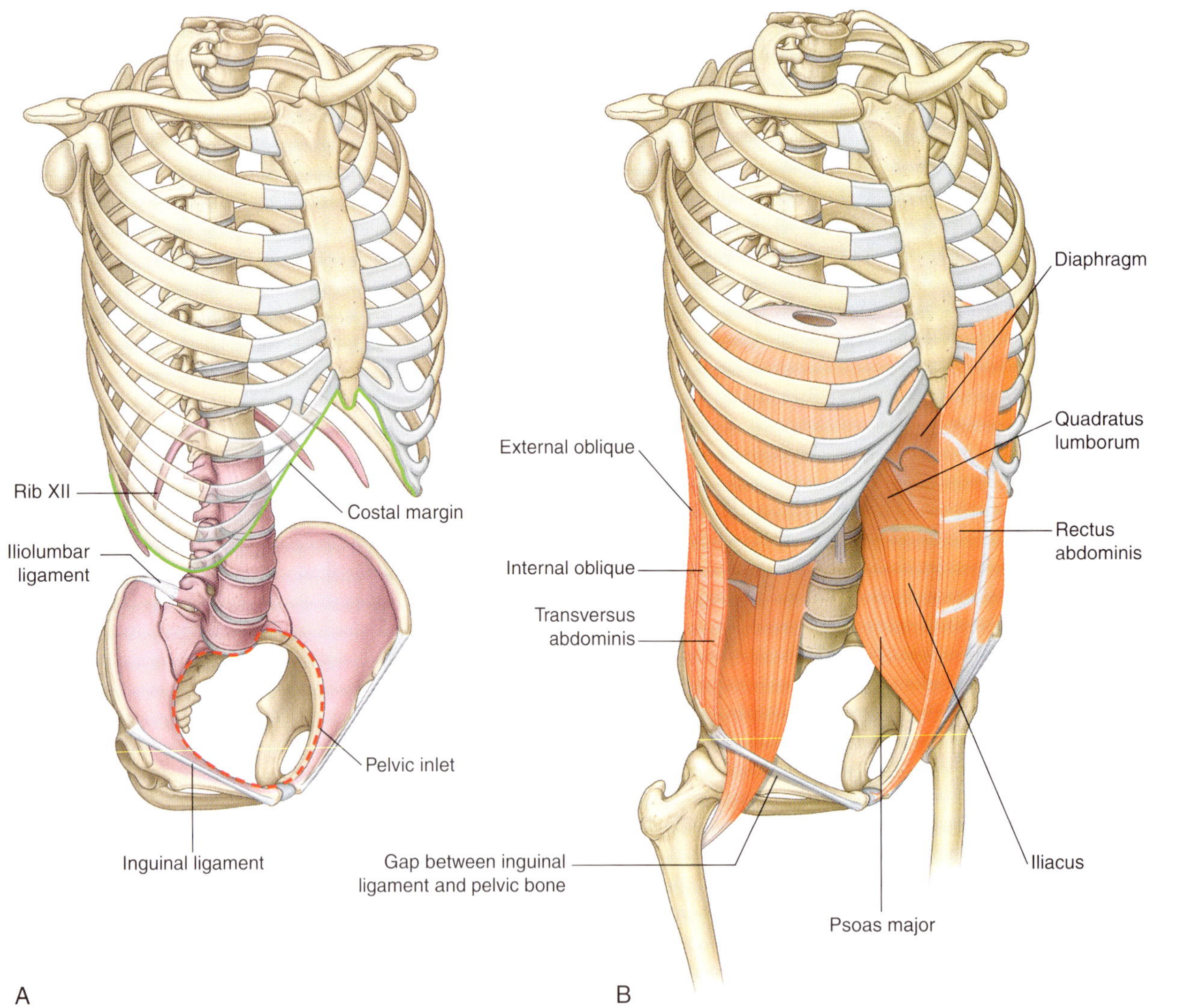

Fig. 4.5 Abdominal wall. **(A)** Skeletal elements. **(B)** Muscles.

- Anteriorly, a segmented muscle (the rectus abdominis) on each side spans the distance between the inferior thoracic wall and the pelvis.

Structural continuity between posterior, lateral, and anterior parts of the abdominal wall is provided by thick fascia posteriorly and by flat tendinous sheets (aponeuroses) derived from muscles of the lateral wall. A fascial layer of varying thickness separates the abdominal wall from the peritoneum, which lines the abdominal cavity. This fascia is named according to the structure to which it is related.

Abdominal cavity

The general organization of the abdominal cavity in the fetus is one in which a central gut tube (gastrointestinal system) is suspended from the posterior abdominal wall and partly from the anterior abdominal wall by thin sheets of tissue (**mesenteries**; Fig. 4.6):

- A ventral (anterior) mesentery for proximal regions of the gut tube
- A dorsal (posterior) mesentery along the entire length of the system

Different parts of these two mesenteries are named according to the organs they suspend or with which they are associated.

Major viscera, such as the kidneys, that are not suspended in the abdominal cavity by mesenteries are associated with the abdominal wall.

The abdominal cavity is lined by **peritoneum**, which consists of an epithelial-like single layer of cells (the **mesothelium**) together with a supportive layer of connective tissue. Peritoneum is similar to the pleura and serous pericardium in the thorax.

The peritoneum reflects off the abdominal wall to become a component of the mesenteries that suspend the viscera.

- **Parietal peritoneum** lines the abdominal wall.
- **Visceral peritoneum** covers suspended organs.

Normally, elements of the gastrointestinal tract and its derivatives completely fill the abdominal cavity, making the peritoneal cavity a potential space. Visceral peritoneum on organs and parietal peritoneum on the adjacent abdominal wall slide freely against one another due to the presence of a small quantity of peritoneal fluid, which is the only content of the peritoneal cavity.

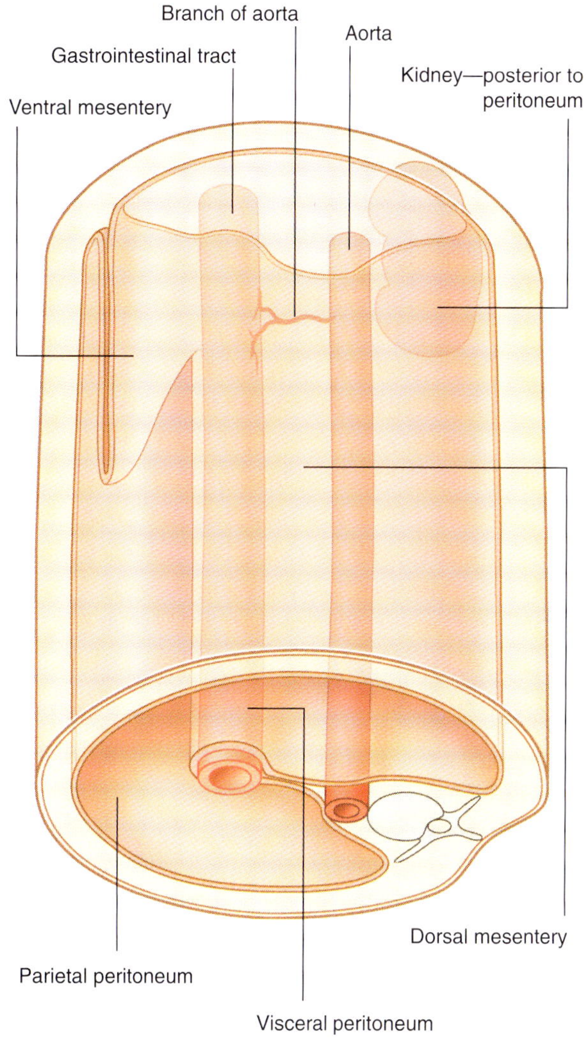

Fig. 4.6 The gut tube is suspended by mesenteries.

Abdominal viscera are either intraperitoneal or retroperitoneal:

- **Intraperitoneal** structures, such as elements of the gastrointestinal system, are suspended from the abdominal wall by mesenteries.
- Structures that are not suspended in the abdominal cavity by a mesentery and that lie between the parietal peritoneum and abdominal wall are **retroperitoneal** in position (see Fig. 4.52).

Retroperitoneal structures include the kidneys and ureters, which develop in the region between the peritoneum and the abdominal wall and remain in this position in the adult.

During development, some organs, such as parts of the small and large intestines, are suspended initially in the abdominal cavity by a mesentery, and later become retroperitoneal secondarily by fusing with the abdominal wall (Fig. 4.7).

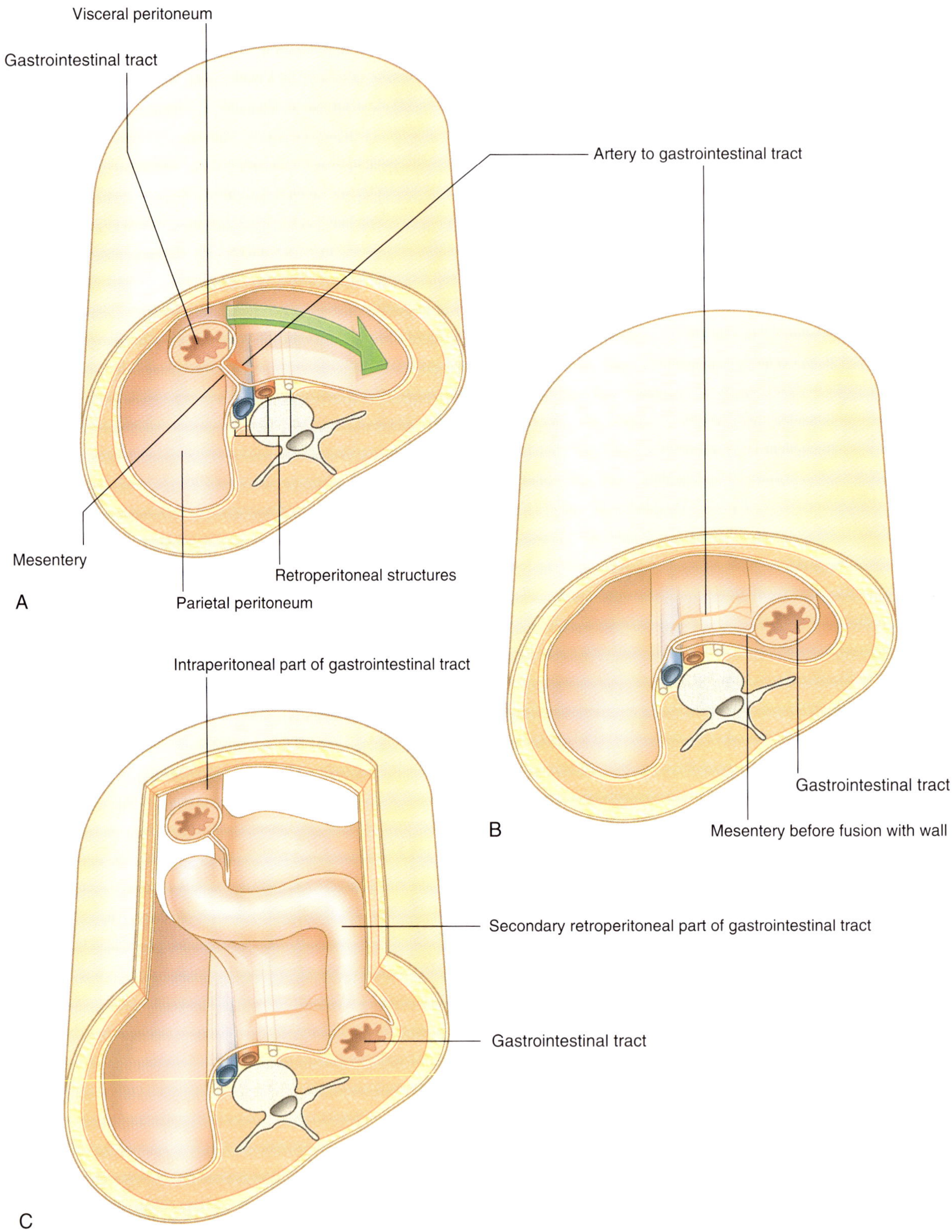

Fig. 4.7 A series showing the progression **(A–C)** from an intraperitoneal organ to a secondarily retroperitoneal organ.

Large vessels, nerves, and lymphatics are associated with the posterior abdominal wall along the median axis of the body in the region where, during development, the peritoneum reflects off the wall as the dorsal mesentery, which supports the developing gut tube. As a consequence, branches of the neurovascular structures that pass to parts of the gastrointestinal system are unpaired, are attached to the anterior aspects of their parent structures, and travel in mesenteries or pass retroperitoneally in areas where the mesenteries secondarily fuse to the abdominal wall.

Generally, vessels, nerves, and lymphatics to the abdominal wall and to organs that originate as retroperitoneal structures branch laterally from the central neurovascular structures and are usually paired, one on each side.

Inferior thoracic aperture

The superior aperture of the abdomen is the inferior thoracic aperture, which is closed by the diaphragm (see Fig. 6.4). The margin of the inferior thoracic aperture consists of vertebra TXII, rib XII, the anterior end of rib XI, the costal margin, and the xiphoid process of the sternum.

Diaphragm

The musculotendinous diaphragm separates the abdomen from the thorax.

The diaphragm attaches to the margin of the inferior thoracic aperture, but the attachment is complex posteriorly and extends into the lumbar area of the vertebral column (Fig. 4.8). On each side, a muscular extension (crus) firmly anchors the diaphragm to the anterolateral surface of the vertebral column as far down as vertebra LIII on the right and vertebra LII on the left.

Because the costal margin is not complete posteriorly, the diaphragm is anchored to arch-shaped (arcuate)

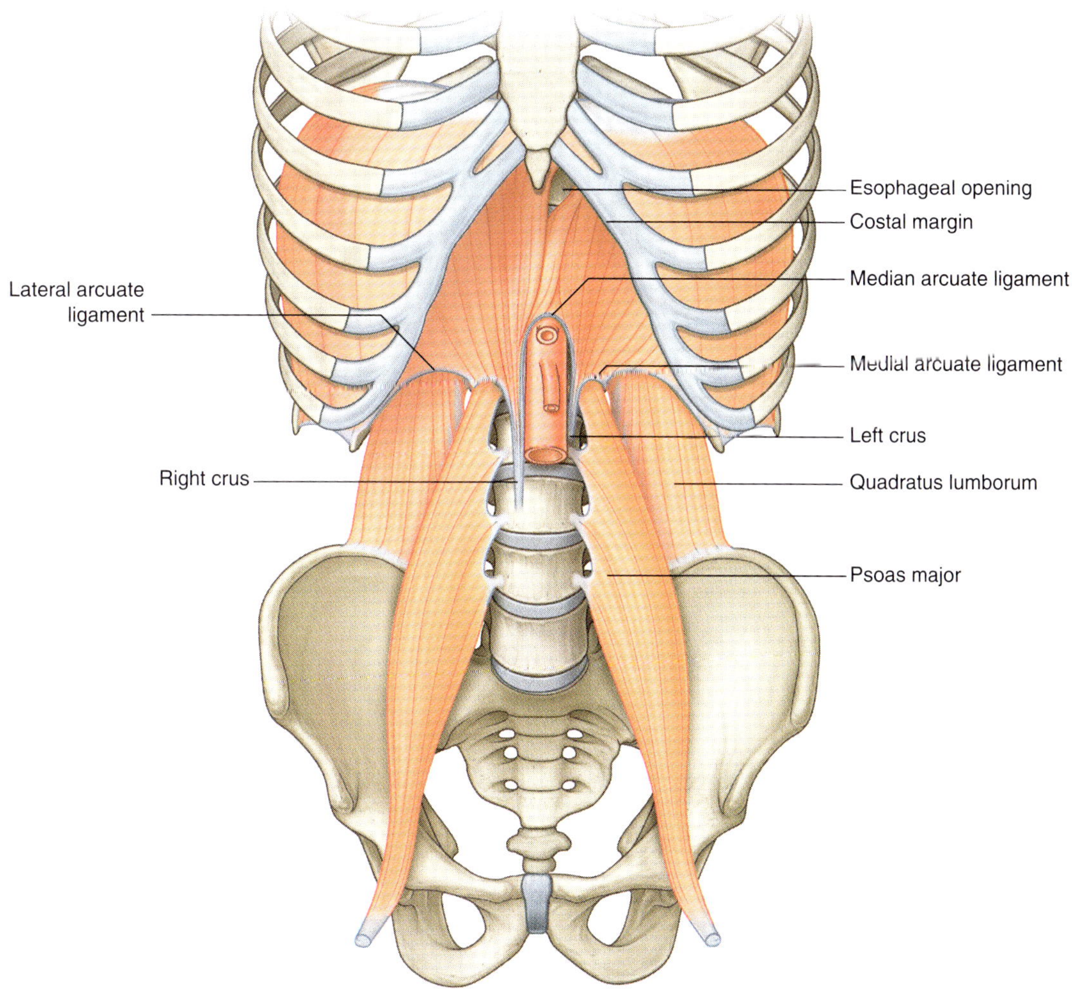

Fig. 4.8 Inferior thoracic aperture and the diaphragm.

ligaments, which span the distance between available bony points and the intervening soft tissues:

- **Medial** and **lateral arcuate ligaments** cross muscles of the posterior abdominal wall and attach to vertebrae, the transverse processes of vertebra LI and rib XII, respectively.
- A **median arcuate ligament** crosses the aorta and is continuous with the crus of the diaphragm on each side.

The posterior attachment of the diaphragm extends much farther inferiorly than the anterior attachment. Consequently, the diaphragm is an important component of the posterior abdominal wall, to which a number of viscera are related.

Pelvic inlet

The abdominal wall is continuous with the pelvic wall at the pelvic inlet, and the abdominal cavity is continuous with the pelvic cavity.

The circular margin of the pelvic inlet is formed entirely by bone:

- Posteriorly by the sacrum
- Anteriorly by the pubic symphysis
- Laterally, on each side, by a distinct bony rim on the pelvic bone (Fig. 4.9)

Because of the way in which the sacrum and attached pelvic bones are angled posteriorly on the vertebral column, the pelvic cavity is not oriented in the same vertical plane as the abdominal cavity. Instead, the pelvic cavity projects posteriorly, and the inlet opens anteriorly and somewhat superiorly (Fig. 4.10).

RELATIONSHIP TO OTHER REGIONS

Thorax

The abdomen is separated from the thorax by the diaphragm. Structures pass between the two regions through or posterior to the diaphragm (see Fig. 4.8).

Pelvis

The pelvic inlet opens directly into the abdomen and structures pass between the abdomen and pelvis through it.

The peritoneum lining the abdominal cavity is continuous with the peritoneum in the pelvis. Consequently, the

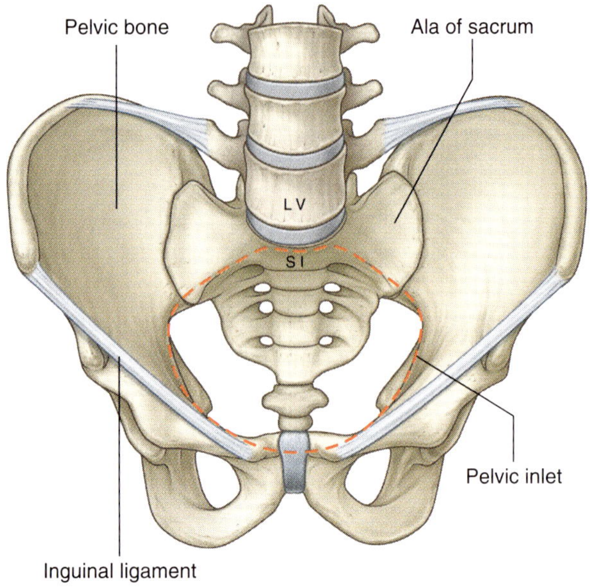

Fig. 4.9 Pelvic inlet.

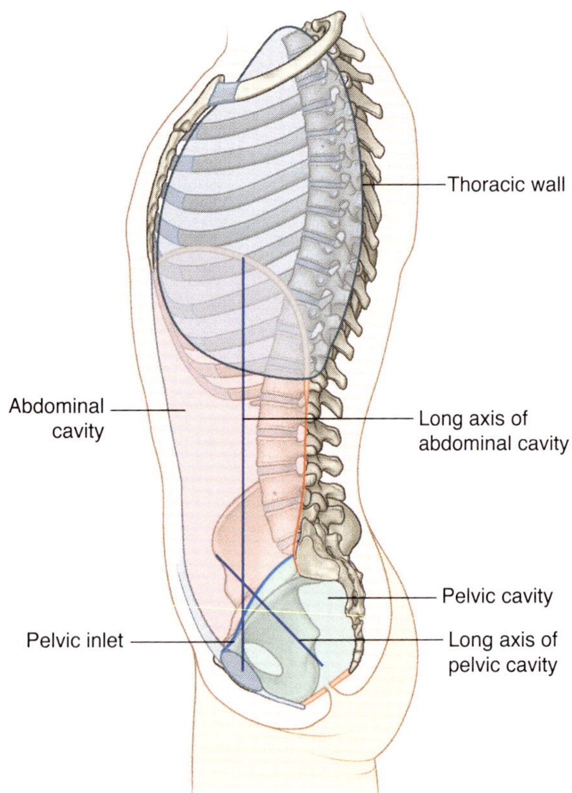

Fig. 4.10 Orientation of abdominal and pelvic cavities.

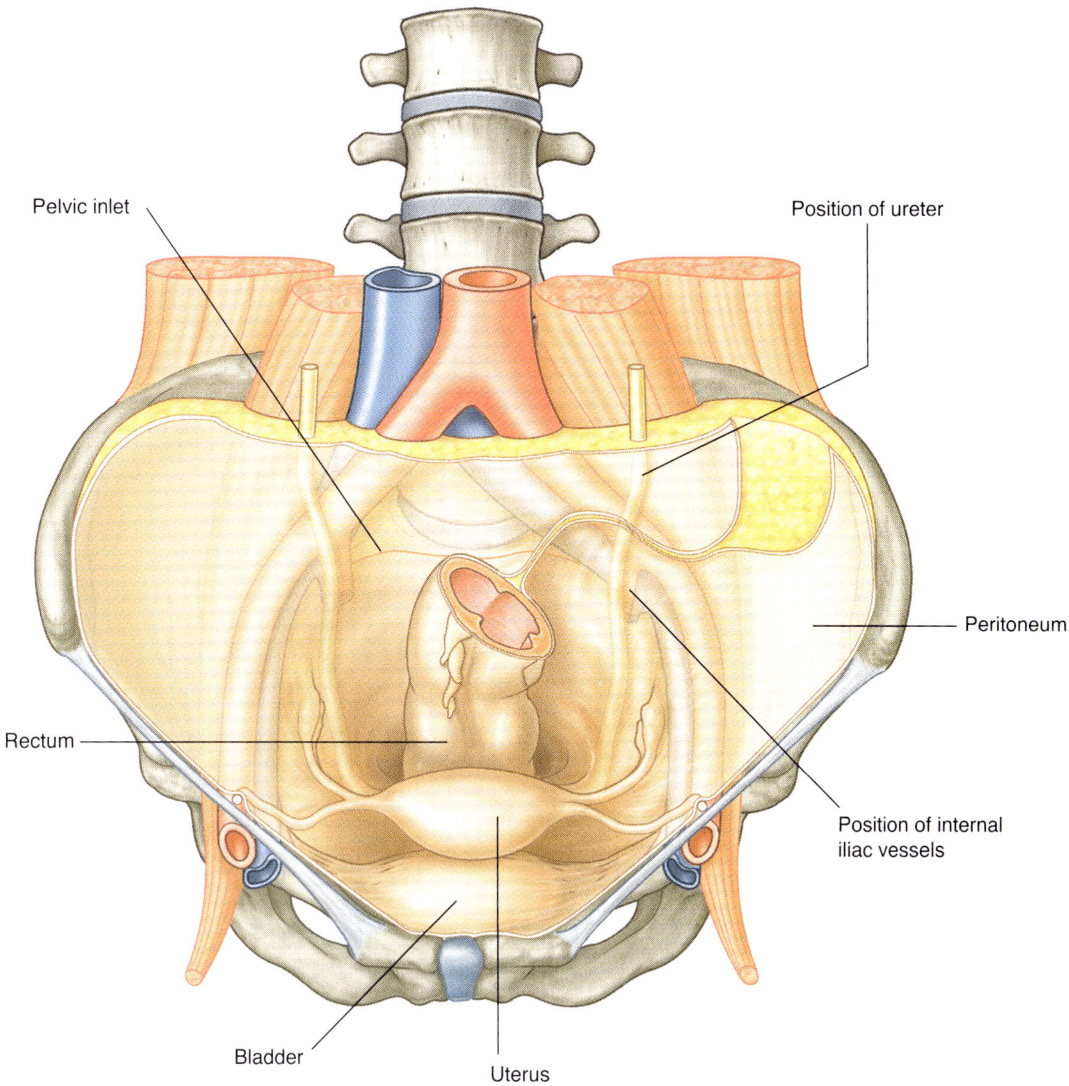

Fig. 4.11 The abdominal cavity is continuous with the pelvic cavity.

abdominal cavity is entirely continuous with the pelvic cavity (Fig. 4.11). Infections in one region can therefore freely spread into the other.

The bladder expands superiorly from the pelvic cavity into the abdominal cavity and, during pregnancy, the uterus expands freely superiorly out of the pelvic cavity into the abdominal cavity.

Lower limb

The abdomen communicates directly with the thigh through an aperture formed anteriorly between the inferior margin of the abdominal wall (marked by the inguinal ligament) and the pelvic bone (Fig. 4.12). Structures that pass through this aperture are

- The major artery and vein of the lower limb
- The femoral nerve, which innervates the quadriceps femoris muscle, which extends the knee joint
- Lymphatics
- The distal ends of psoas major and iliacus muscles, which flex the thigh at the hip joint

As vessels pass inferior to the inguinal ligament, their names change—the external iliac artery and vein of the abdomen become the femoral artery and vein of the thigh.

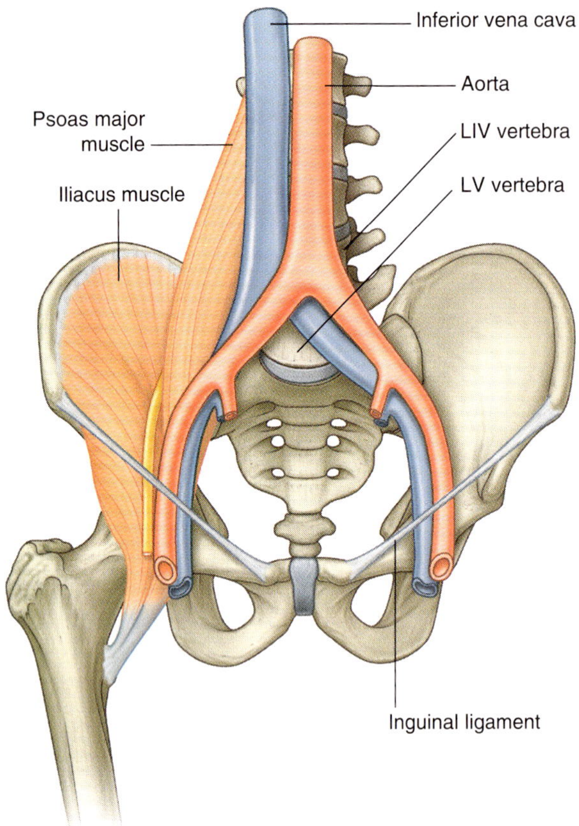

Fig. 4.12 Structures passing between the abdomen and thigh.

KEY FEATURES

Arrangement of abdominal viscera in the adult

A basic knowledge of the development of the gastrointestinal tract is needed to understand the arrangement of viscera and mesenteries in the abdomen (Fig. 4.13).

The gastrointestinal tract in the fetus is oriented longitudinally in the body cavity and is suspended from surrounding walls by a large dorsal mesentery and a much smaller ventral mesentery.

Superiorly, the dorsal and ventral mesenteries are anchored to the diaphragm.

The primitive gut tube consists of the foregut, the midgut, and the hindgut. Massive longitudinal growth of the gut tube, rotation of selected parts of the tube, and secondary fusion of some viscera and their associated mesenteries to the body wall participate in generating the adult arrangement of abdominal organs.

Development of the foregut

In abdominal regions, the **foregut** gives rise to the distal end of the esophagus, the stomach, and the proximal part of the duodenum. The foregut is the only part of the gut tube suspended from the wall by both the ventral and dorsal mesenteries.

A diverticulum from the anterior aspect of the foregut grows into the ventral mesentery, giving rise to the liver, gallbladder, and ventral part of the pancreas.

The dorsal part of the pancreas develops from an outgrowth of the foregut into the dorsal mesentery. The spleen develops in the dorsal mesentery in the region between the body wall and presumptive stomach.

In the foregut, the developing stomach rotates clockwise and the associated dorsal mesentery, containing the spleen, moves to the left and greatly expands. During this process, part of the mesentery becomes associated with, and secondarily fuses with, the left side of the body wall.

At the same time, the duodenum, together with its dorsal mesentery and an appreciable part of the pancreas, swings to the right and fuses to the body wall (Fig. 4.13).

Secondary fusion of the duodenum to the body wall, massive growth of the liver in the ventral mesentery, and fusion of the superior surface of the liver to the diaphragm restrict the opening to the space enclosed by the ballooned dorsal mesentery associated with the stomach. This restricted opening is the **omental foramen** (**epiploic foramen**).

The part of the abdominal cavity enclosed by the expanded dorsal mesentery, and posterior to the stomach, is the **omental bursa** (**lesser sac**). Access, through the omental foramen, to this space from the rest of the peritoneal cavity (**greater sac**) is inferior to the free edge of the ventral mesentery.

The part of the dorsal mesentery that initially forms part of the lesser sac greatly enlarges in an inferior direction, and the two opposing surfaces of the mesentery fuse to form an apron-like structure (the **greater omentum**). The greater omentum is suspended from the greater curvature of the stomach, lies over other viscera in the abdominal cavity, and is the first structure observed when the abdominal cavity is opened anteriorly (see Fig. 4.56).

Development of the midgut

The midgut develops into the distal part of the duodenum and the jejunum, ileum, cecum, appendix, ascending colon, and proximal two-thirds of the transverse colon. A small yolk sac projects anteriorly from the developing midgut into the umbilicus.

Rapid growth of the gastrointestinal system results in a loop of the midgut herniating out of the abdominal cavity and into the umbilical cord. As the body grows in size and the connection with the yolk sac is lost, the midgut returns to the abdominal cavity. While this process is occurring, the two limbs of the midgut loop rotate counterclockwise

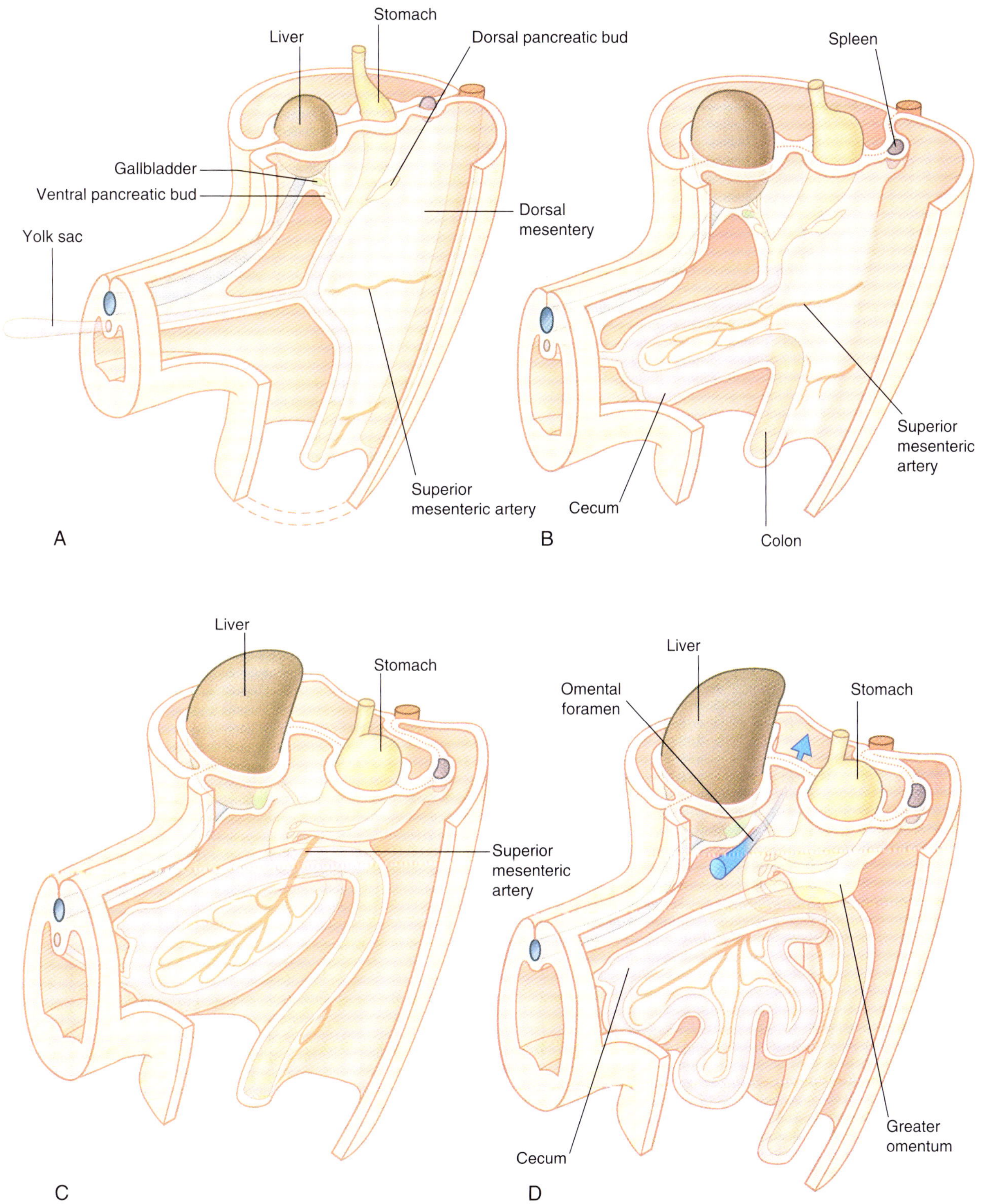

Fig. 4.13 A series **(A–H)** showing the development of the gut and mesenteries.

Continued

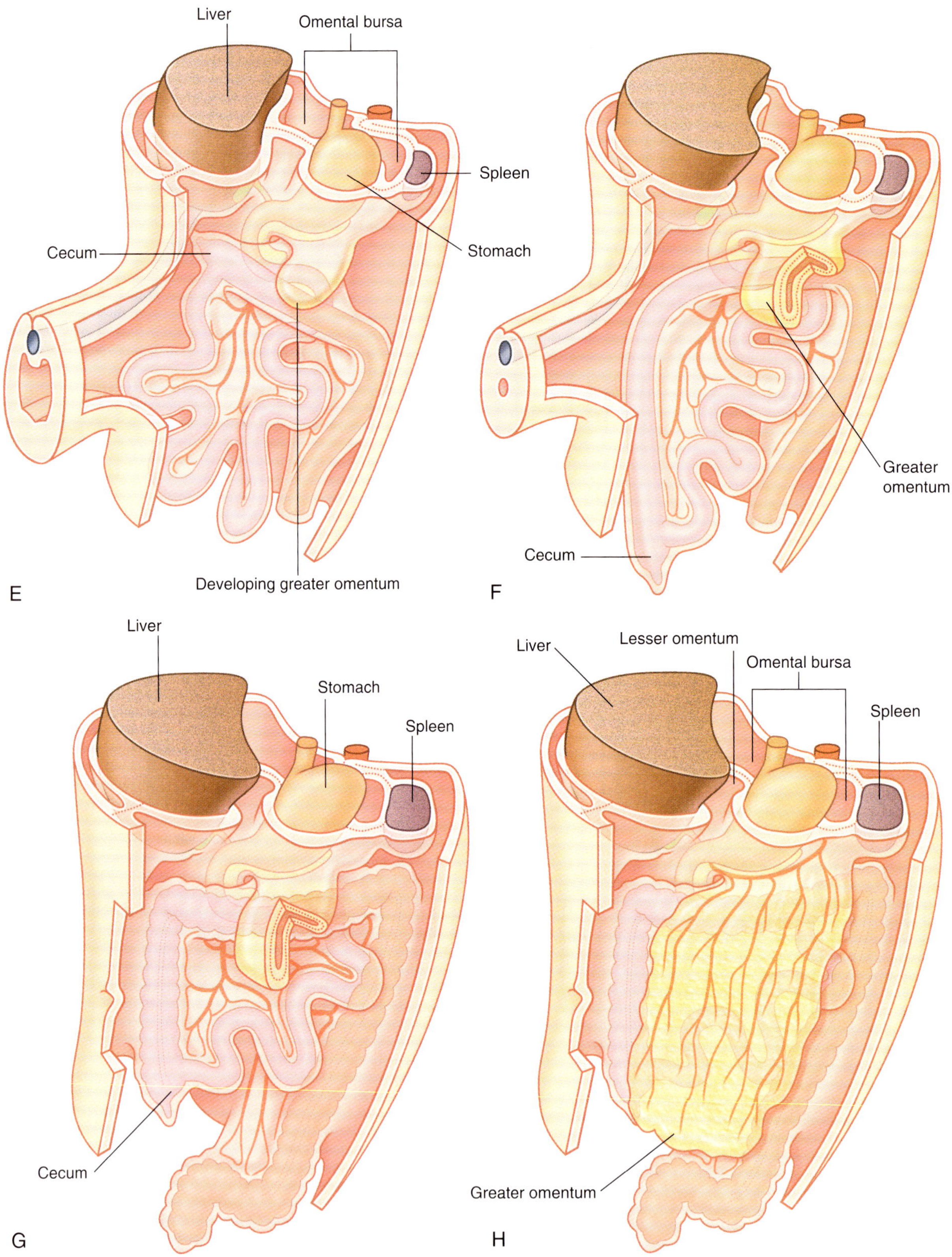

Fig. 4.13, cont'd

when viewed from front. This occurs around their combined central axis, and the part of the loop that becomes the cecum descends into the inferior right aspect of the cavity. The superior mesenteric artery, which supplies the midgut, is at the center of the axis of rotation.

The cecum remains intraperitoneal, the ascending colon fuses with the body wall becoming secondarily retroperitoneal, and the transverse colon remains suspended by its dorsal mesentery (transverse mesocolon). The greater omentum hangs over the transverse colon and the mesocolon and usually fuses with these structures.

Development of the hindgut

The distal one-third of the transverse colon, descending colon, sigmoid colon, and superior part of the rectum develop from the hindgut.

Proximal parts of the hindgut swing to the left and become the descending colon and sigmoid colon. The descending colon and its dorsal mesentery fuse to the body wall, while the sigmoid colon remains intraperitoneal. The sigmoid colon passes through the pelvic inlet and is continuous with the rectum at the level of vertebra SIII.

Skin and muscles of the anterior and lateral abdominal wall and thoracic intercostal nerves

The anterior rami of thoracic spinal nerves T7 to T12 follow the inferior slope of the lateral parts of the ribs and cross the costal margin to enter the abdominal wall (Fig. 4.14). Intercostal nerves T7 to T11 supply skin and muscle of the abdominal wall, as does the subcostal nerve T12. In addition, T5 and T6 supply upper parts of the external oblique muscle of the abdominal wall; T6 also supplies cutaneous innervation to skin over the xiphoid.

Skin and muscle in the inguinal and suprapubic regions of the abdominal wall are innervated by L1 and not by thoracic nerves.

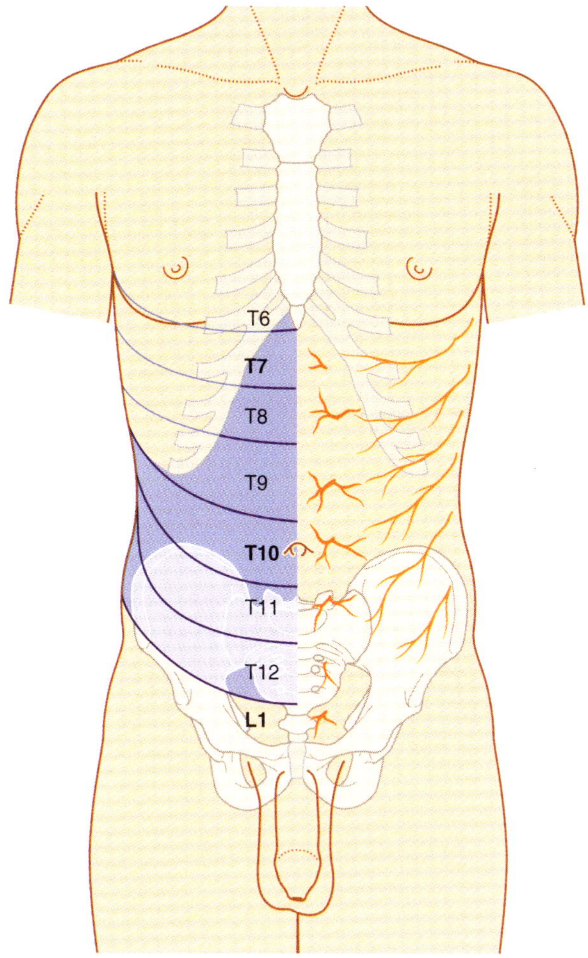

Fig. 4.14 Innervation of the anterior abdominal wall.

Dermatomes of the anterior abdominal wall are indicated in Fig. 4.14. In the midline, the dermatome of the skin over the infrasternal angle is T6 and that around the umbilicus is T10. L1 innervates skin in the inguinal and suprapubic regions.

Muscles of the abdominal wall are innervated segmentally in patterns that generally reflect the patterns of the overlying dermatomes.

The groin is a weak area in the anterior abdominal wall

During development, the gonads in both sexes descend from their sites of origin on the posterior abdominal wall into the pelvic cavity in women and the developing scrotum in men (Fig. 4.15).

Before descent, a cord of tissue (the **gubernaculum**) passes through the anterior abdominal wall and connects the inferior pole of each gonad with primordia of the scrotum in men and the labia majora in women (labioscrotal swellings).

A tubular extension (the **processus vaginalis**) of the peritoneal cavity and the accompanying muscular layers of the anterior abdominal wall project along the gubernaculum on each side into the labioscrotal swellings.

In men, the testis, together with its neurovascular structures and its efferent duct (the ductus deferens), descends into the scrotum along a path, initially defined by the gubernaculum, between the processus vaginalis and the accompanying coverings derived from the abdominal wall. All that remains of the gubernaculum is a connective tissue remnant that attaches the caudal pole of the testis to the scrotum.

The **inguinal canal** is the passage through the anterior abdominal wall created by the processus vaginalis. The **spermatic cord** is the tubular extension of the layers of the abdominal wall into the scrotum that contains all structures passing between the testis and the abdomen.

The distal sac-like terminal end of the spermatic cord on each side contains the testis, associated structures, and the now isolated part of the peritoneal cavity (the cavity of the tunica vaginalis).

In women, the gonads descend to a position just inside the pelvic cavity and never pass through the anterior abdominal wall. As a result, the only major structure passing through the inguinal canal is a derivative of the gubernaculum (the round ligament of the uterus).

In both men and women, the groin (inguinal region) is a weak area in the abdominal wall (see Fig. 4.15) and is the site of inguinal hernias.

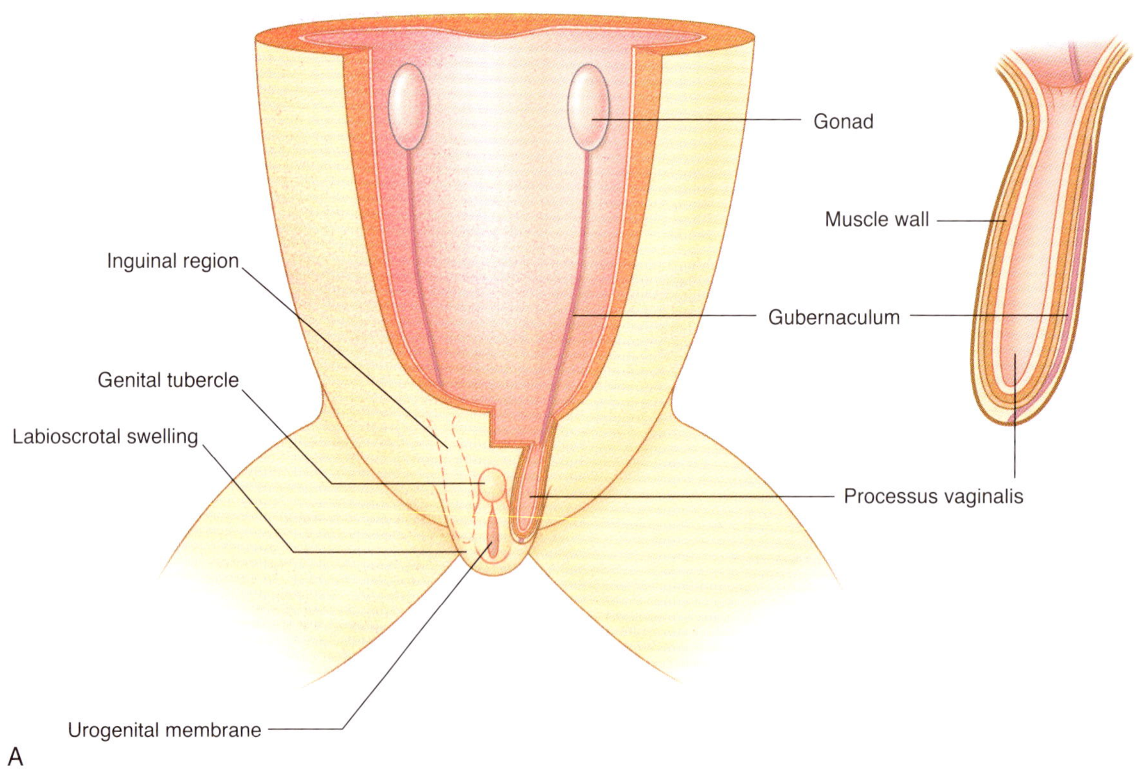

Fig. 4.15 Inguinal region. **(A)** During development.

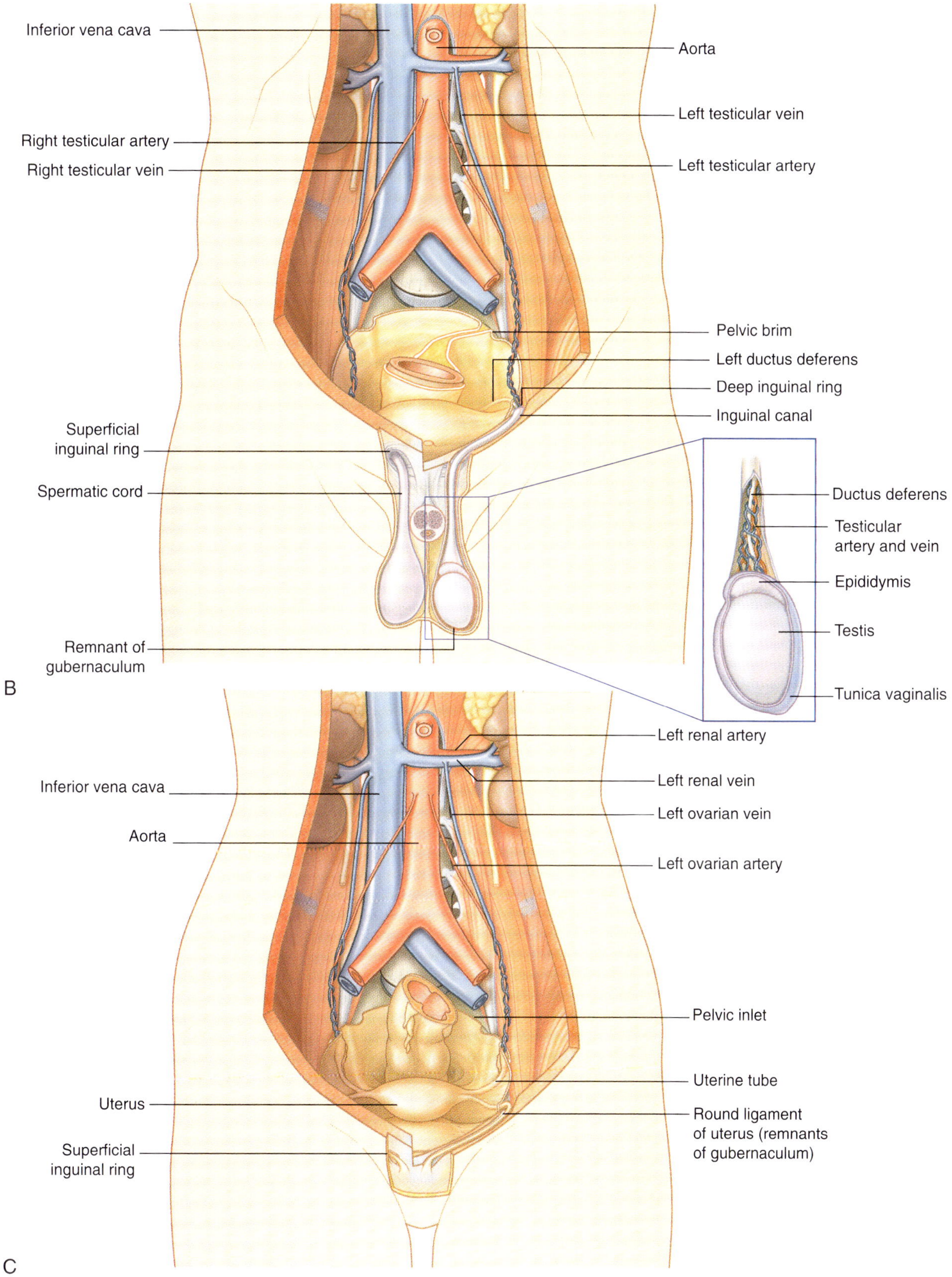

Fig. 4.15, cont'd (B) In men. **(C)** In women.

Vertebral level LI

The transpyloric plane is a horizontal plane that transects the body through the lower aspect of vertebra LI (Fig. 4.16). It:

- Is about midway between the jugular notch and the pubic symphysis, and crosses the costal margin on each side at the tip of the ninth costal cartilage.
- Crosses through the opening of the stomach into the duodenum (the pyloric orifice), which is just to the right of the body of LI; the duodenum then makes a characteristic C-shaped loop on the posterior abdominal wall and crosses the midline to open into the jejunum just to the left of the body of vertebra LII, whereas the head of the pancreas is bounded on the right side and above and below by the loop of the duodenum, and the body of the pancreas extends across the midline to the left.
- Crosses through the body of the pancreas.
- Approximately passes through the level of the hila of the kidneys; though because the left kidney is slightly higher than the right, the transpyloric plane crosses through the inferior aspect of the left hilum and the superior part of the right hilum.

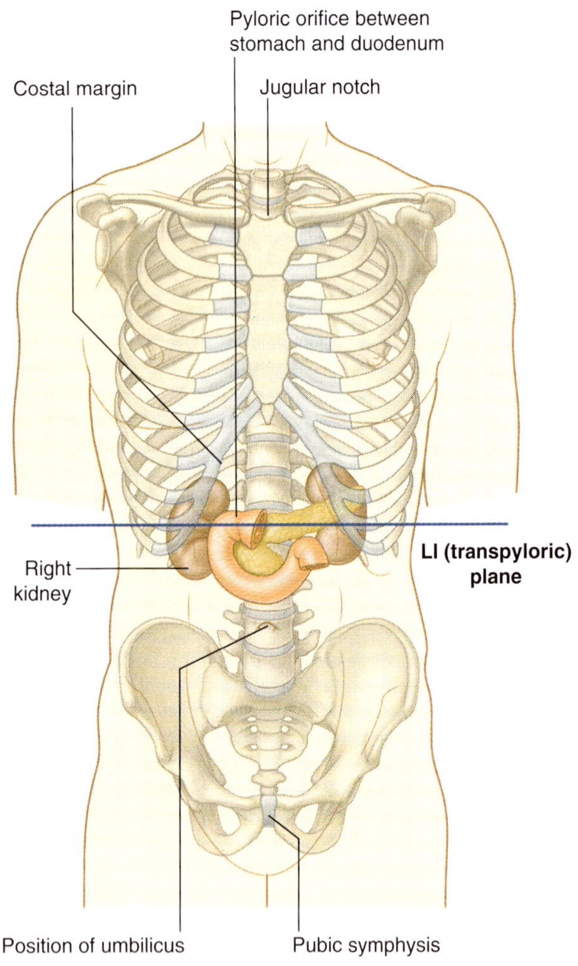

Fig. 4.16 Vertebral level LI.

The gastrointestinal system and its derivatives are supplied by three major arteries

Three large unpaired arteries branch from the anterior surface of the abdominal aorta to supply the abdominal part of the gastrointestinal tract and all of the structures (liver, pancreas, and gallbladder) to which this part of the gut gives rise during development (Fig. 4.17). These arteries pass through derivatives of the dorsal and ventral mesenteries to reach the target viscera. These vessels therefore also supply structures such as the spleen and lymph nodes that develop in the mesenteries. These three arteries are

- The **celiac artery**, which branches from the abdominal aorta at the upper border of vertebra LI and supplies the foregut (up to and including the point in the second part of the duodenum where the greater duodenal papilla opens).
- The **superior mesenteric artery**, which arises from the abdominal aorta at the lower border of vertebra LI and supplies the midgut (up to the right two-thirds of the transverse colon).
- The **inferior mesenteric artery**, which branches from the abdominal aorta at approximately vertebral level LIII and supplies the hindgut.

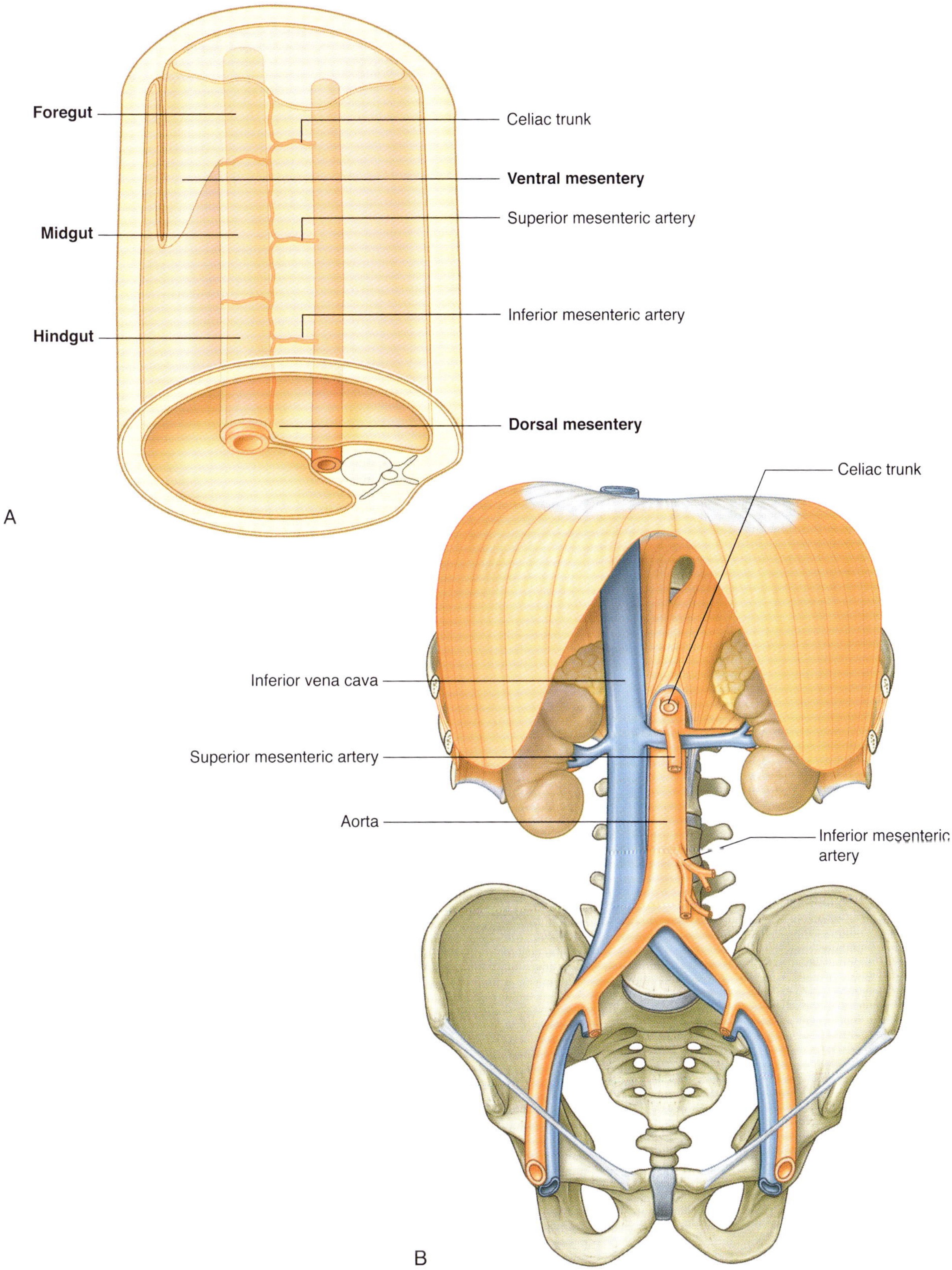

Fig. 4.17 Blood supply of the gut. **(A)** Relationship of vessels to the gut and mesenteries in the embryo. **(B)** Anterior view.

Venous shunts from left to right

All blood returning to the heart from regions of the body other than the lungs flows into the right atrium of the heart. The inferior vena cava is the major systemic vein in the abdomen and drains this region together with the pelvis, perineum, and both lower limbs (Fig. 4.18).

The inferior vena cava lies to the right of the vertebral column and penetrates the central tendon of the diaphragm at approximately vertebral level TVIII. A number of large vessels cross the midline to deliver blood from the left side of the body to the inferior vena cava.

- One of the most significant is the left renal vein, which drains the kidney, suprarenal gland, and gonad on the same side.
- Another is the left common iliac vein, which crosses the midline at approximately vertebral level LV to join with

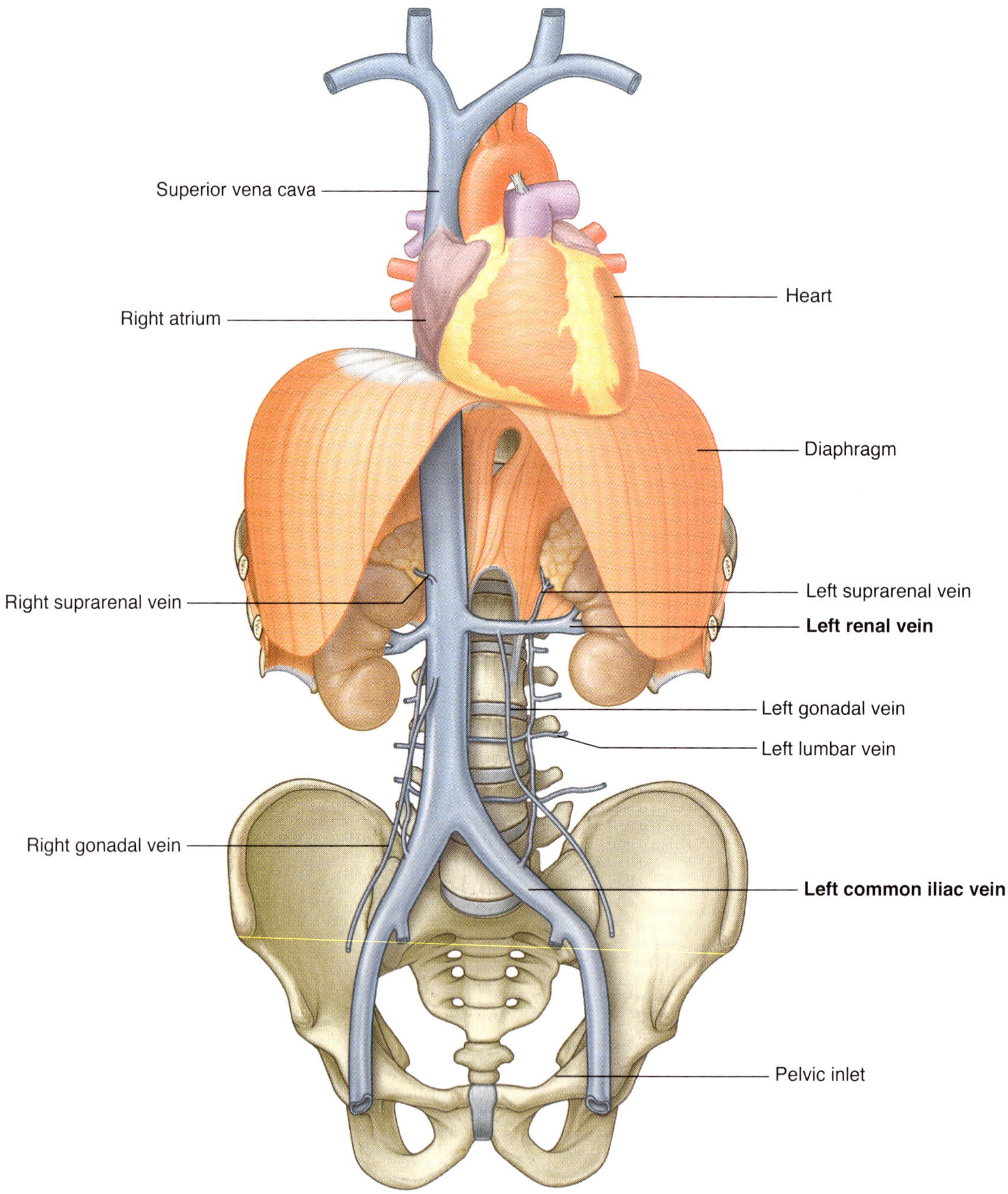

Fig. 4.18 Left-to-right venous shunts.

its partner on the right to form the inferior vena cava. These veins drain the lower limbs, the pelvis, the perineum, and parts of the abdominal wall.

- Other vessels crossing the midline include the left lumbar veins, which drain the back and posterior abdominal wall on the left side.

All venous drainage from the gastrointestinal system passes through the liver

The blood from the abdominal parts of the gastrointestinal system and the spleen passes through a second vascular capillary bed, in the liver, before ultimately returning to the heart (Fig. 4.19).

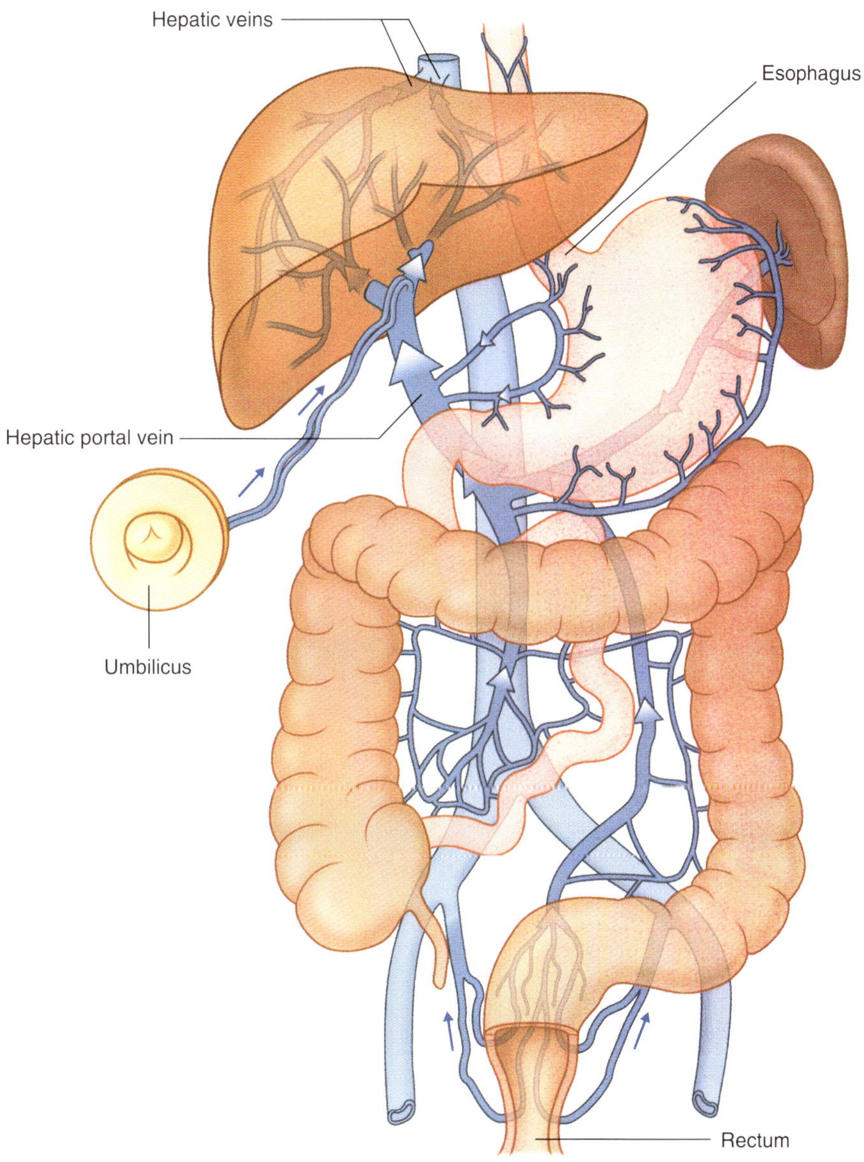

Fig. 4.19 Hepatic portal system.

Venous blood from the digestive tract, pancreas, gallbladder, and spleen enters the inferior surface of the liver through the large **hepatic portal vein**. This vein then ramifies like an artery to distribute blood to small endothelial-lined hepatic sinusoids, which form the vascular exchange network of the liver.

After passing through the sinusoids, the blood collects in a number of short **hepatic veins**, which drain into the inferior vena cava just before the inferior vena cava penetrates the diaphragm and enters the right atrium of the heart.

Normally, vascular beds drained by the hepatic portal system interconnect, through small veins, with beds drained by systemic vessels, which ultimately connect directly with either the superior or inferior vena cava.

Portacaval anastomoses

Among the clinically most important regions of overlap between the portal and caval systems are those at each end of the abdominal part of the gastrointestinal system:

- Around the inferior end of the esophagus
- Around the inferior part of the rectum

Small veins that accompany the obliterated umbilical vein (**round ligament of the liver**) establish another important portacaval anastomosis.

The round ligament of the liver connects the umbilicus of the anterior abdominal wall with the left branch of the portal vein as it enters the liver. The small veins that accompany this ligament form a connection between the portal system and paraumbilical regions of the abdominal wall, which drain into systemic veins.

Other regions where portal and caval systems interconnect include:

- Where the liver is in direct contact with the diaphragm (the bare area of the liver)
- Where the wall of the gastrointestinal tract is in direct contact with the posterior abdominal wall (retroperitoneal areas of the large and small intestine)
- The posterior surface of the pancreas (much of the pancreas is secondarily retroperitoneal)

Blockage of the hepatic portal vein or of vascular channels in the liver

Blockage of the hepatic portal vein or of vascular channels in the liver can affect the pattern of venous return from abdominal parts of the gastrointestinal system. Vessels that interconnect the portal and caval systems can become greatly enlarged and tortuous, allowing blood in tributaries of the portal system to bypass the liver, to enter the caval system, and thereby return to the heart. Portal hypertension can result in esophageal and rectal varices and in caput medusae in which systemic vessels that radiate from paraumbilical veins enlarge and become visible on the abdominal wall (see Fig. 4.122).

Abdominal viscera are supplied by a large prevertebral plexus

Innervation of the abdominal viscera is derived from a large prevertebral plexus associated mainly with the anterior and lateral surfaces of the aorta (Fig. 4.20). Branches are distributed to target tissues along vessels that originate from the abdominal aorta.

The prevertebral plexus contains sympathetic, parasympathetic, and visceral sensory components:

- Sympathetic components originate from spinal cord levels T5 to L2.
- Parasympathetic components are from the vagus nerve [X] and spinal cord levels S2 to S4.
- Visceral sensory fibers generally parallel the motor pathways.

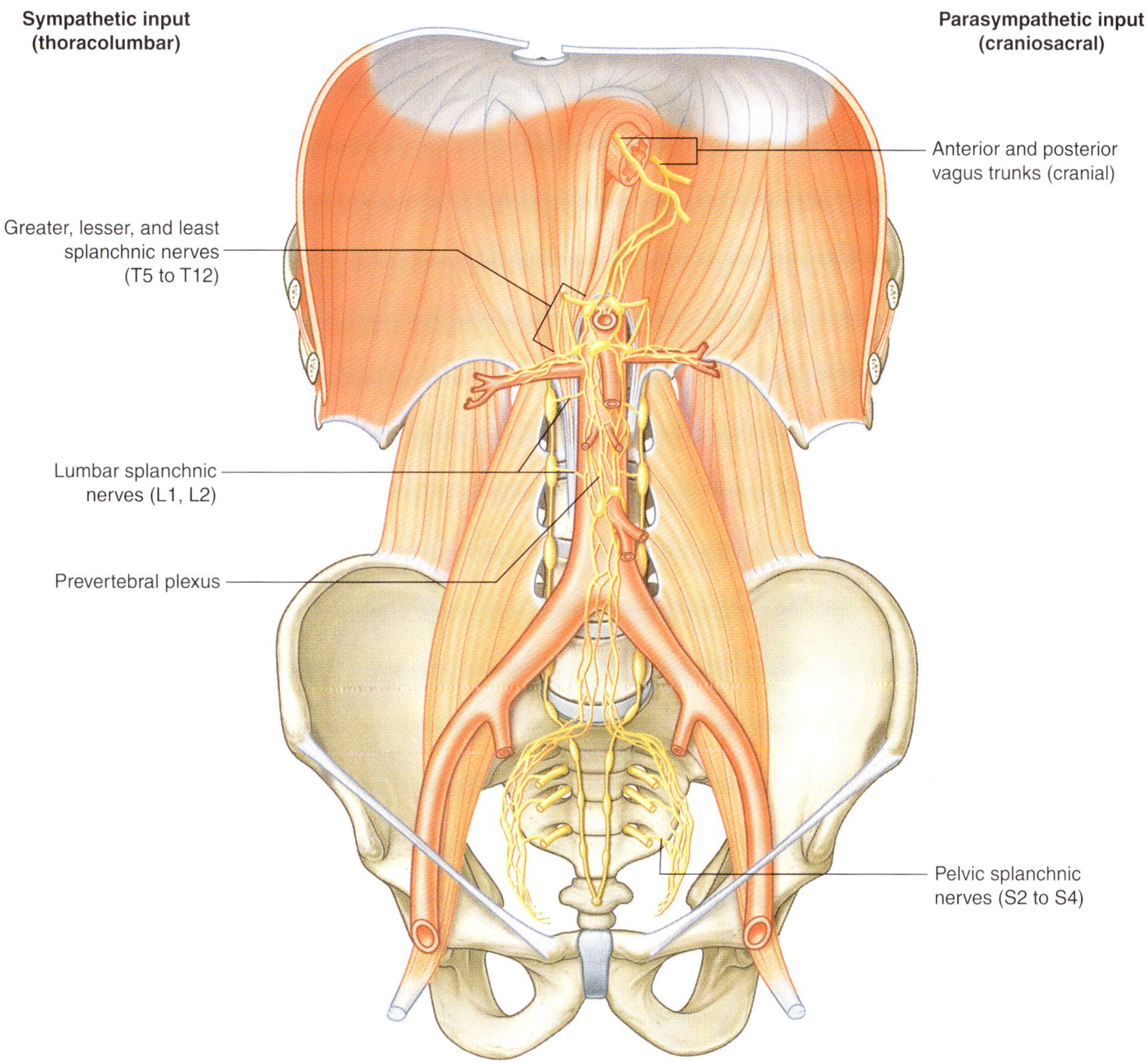

Fig. 4.20 Prevertebral plexus.

Regional anatomy

The abdomen is the part of the trunk inferior to the thorax (Fig. 4.21). Its musculomembranous walls surround a large cavity (the **abdominal cavity**), which is bounded superiorly by the diaphragm and inferiorly by the pelvic inlet.

The abdominal cavity may extend superiorly as high as the fourth intercostal space, and is continuous inferiorly with the pelvic cavity. It contains the **peritoneal cavity** and the abdominal viscera.

SURFACE TOPOGRAPHY

Topographical divisions of the abdomen are used to describe the location of abdominal organs and the pain associated with abdominal problems. The two schemes most often used are

- A four-quadrant pattern
- A nine-region pattern

Four-quadrant pattern

A horizontal transumbilical plane passing through the umbilicus and the intervertebral disc between vertebrae LIII and LIV and intersecting with the vertical median plane divides the abdomen into four quadrants—the right upper, left upper, right lower, and left lower quadrants (Fig. 4.22).

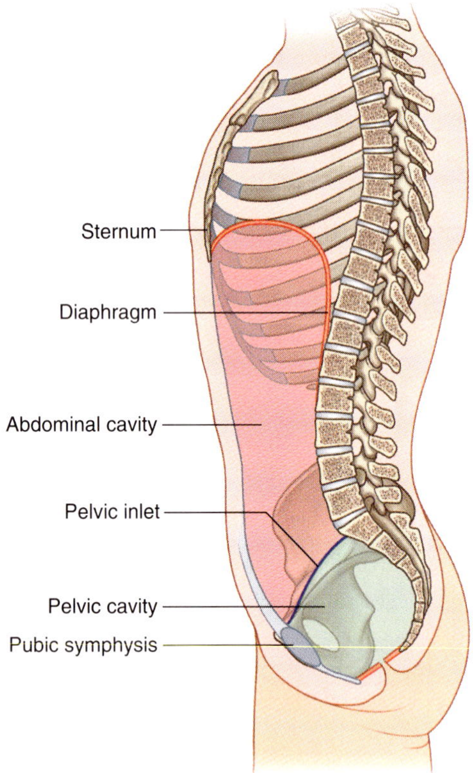

Fig. 4.21 Boundaries of the abdominal cavity.

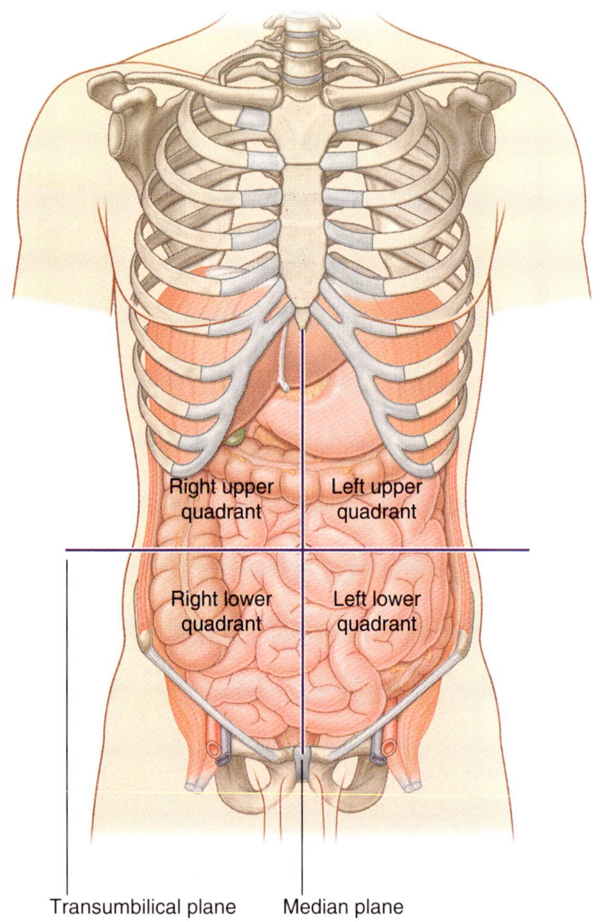

Fig. 4.22 Four-quadrant topographical pattern.

Nine-region pattern

The nine-region pattern is based on two horizontal and two vertical planes (Fig. 4.23).

- The superior horizontal plane (the **subcostal plane**) is immediately inferior to the costal margins, which places it at the lower border of the costal cartilage of rib X and passing posteriorly through the body of vertebra LIII. (Note, however, that sometimes the **transpyloric plane,** halfway between the jugular notch and the symphysis pubis or halfway between the umbilicus and the inferior end of the body of the sternum, passing posteriorly through the lower border of vertebra LI and intersecting with the costal margin at the anterior ends of the ninth costal cartilages, is used instead.)
- The inferior horizontal plane (the **intertubercular plane**) connects the tubercles of the iliac crests, which are palpable structures 5 cm posterior to the anterior superior iliac spines, and passes through the upper part of the body of vertebra LV.

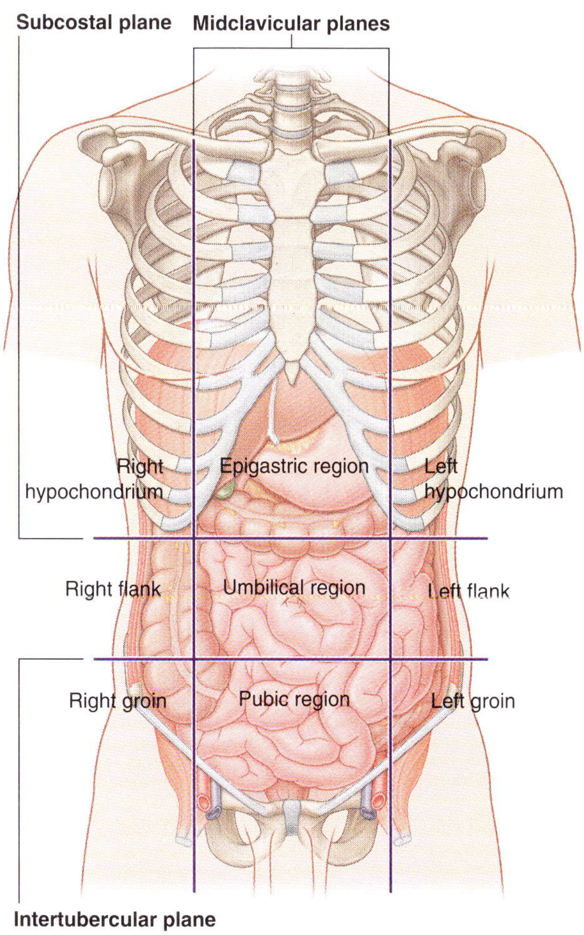

Fig. 4.23 Nine-region organizational pattern.

- The vertical planes pass from the midpoint of the clavicles inferiorly to a point midway between the anterior superior iliac spine and pubic symphysis at the midinguinal point.

These four planes establish the topographical divisions in the nine-region organization. The following designations are used for each region: superiorly the right hypochondrium, the epigastric region, and the left hypochondrium; inferiorly the right groin (right inguinal region or right iliac fossa), pubic region, and left groin; and in the middle the right flank (right lateral region), the umbilical region, and the left flank (see Fig. 4.23).

Early clinical exposure

Surgical incisions

Access to the abdomen and its contents is usually obtained through incisions in the anterior abdominal wall. Traditionally, incisions have been placed at and around the region of surgical interest. The size of these incisions was usually large to allow good access and optimal visualization of the abdominal cavity. As anesthesia has developed and muscle-relaxing drugs have become widely used, the abdominal incisions have become smaller.

Currently, the most commonly used large abdominal incision is a central craniocaudal incision from the xiphoid process to the symphysis pubis, which provides wide access to the whole of the abdominal contents and allows an exploratory procedure to be performed (laparotomy).

Cutting of nerves should be avoided wherever possible. To avoid the risk of denervation, muscles should be split in the direction of their fibers rather than transected, as in the gridiron incision (LD Fig. 4.23.1). However, the rectus muscle, may be transected because it has a segmental nerve supply. Muscles and abdominal organs should be retracted toward, and not away from their neurovascular supply, as in the right paramedian incision (LD Fig. 4.23.1), where the rectus abdominis is retracted laterally toward its nerve supply.

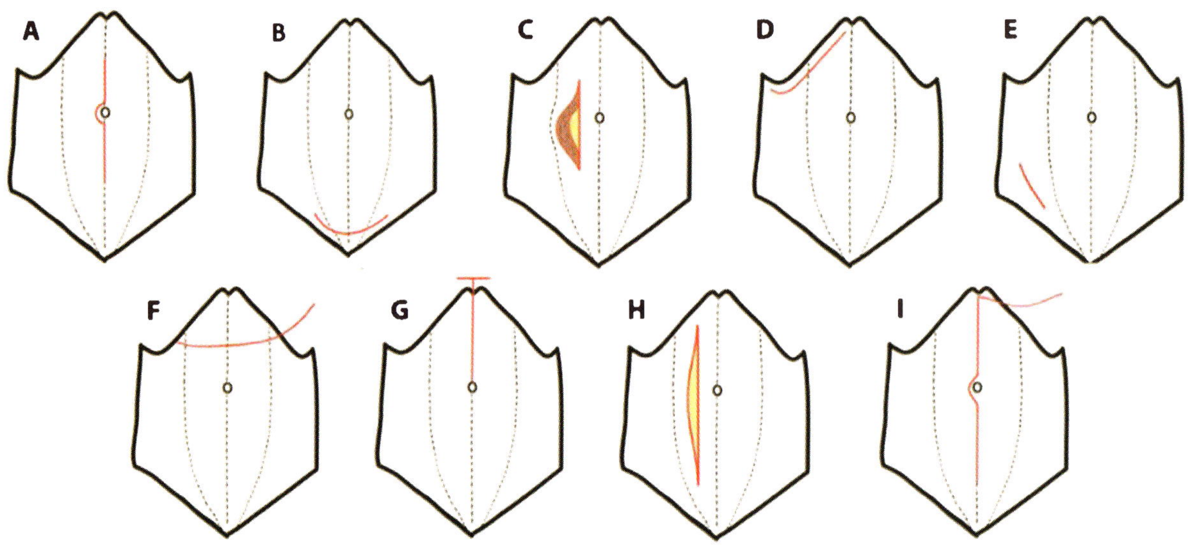

LD Fig. 4.23.1 Incisions of the anterior abdominal wall.
Question
LD Fig. 4.23.1 A Name the labelled incisions.

Answer
LD Fig. 4.23.1 A **(A)** Midline incision, **(B)** suprapubic incision, **(C)** right paramedian incision with muscle retraction, **(D)** subcostal incision, **(E)** Gridiron (McBurney) incision, **(F, G, I)** thoracoabdominal incisions, **(H)** paramedian (rectus) incision with muscle splitting.

Early clinical exposure

Laparoscopic surgery

Laparoscopic surgery, also known as minimally invasive or keyhole surgery, is performed by operating through a series of small incisions no more than 1–2 cm in length. As the incisions are much smaller than those used in traditional abdominal surgery, patients experience less postoperative pain and have shorter recovery times. There is also a favorable cosmetic outcome with smaller scars. Several surgical procedures such as appendicectomy, cholecystectomy, and hernia repair, as well as numerous orthopedic, urological, and gynecological procedures are now commonly performed laparoscopically.

During the operation, a camera known as a laparoscope is used to transmit live, magnified images of the surgical field to a monitor viewed by the surgeon. The camera is inserted into the abdominal cavity through a small incision, called a port site, usually at the umbilicus. In order to create enough space to operate, the abdominal wall is elevated by inflating the cavity with gas, typically carbon dioxide. Other long, thin surgical instruments are then introduced through additional port sites, which can be used by the surgeon to operate. The placement of these port sites is carefully planned to allow optimal access to the surgical field.

Laparoscopic surgery has been further enhanced with the use of surgical robots. Using these systems, the surgeon moves the surgical instruments indirectly by controlling robotic arms, which are inserted into the operating field through small incisions. **Robot-assisted surgery** is now routinely used worldwide and has helped overcome some of the limitations of laparoscopy by enhancing the surgeon's dexterity. The robotic system is precise, provides the surgeon with a 3D view of the surgical field, and allows improved degree of rotation and manipulation of the surgical instruments. Several procedures such as prostatectomy and cholecystectomy can now be performed with this method.

Laparoendoscopic single-site surgery, also known as **single-port laparoscopy**, is the most recent advance in laparoscopic surgery. This method uses a single incision, usually umbilical, to introduce a port with several operating channels and can be performed with or without robotic assistance. Benefits include less postoperative pain, a faster recovery time, and an even better cosmetic result than traditional laparoscopic surgery.

ABDOMINAL WALL

The abdominal wall covers a large area. It is bounded superiorly by the xiphoid process and costal margins, posteriorly by the vertebral column, and inferiorly by the upper parts of the pelvic bones. Its layers consist of skin, superficial fascia (subcutaneous tissue), muscles and their associated deep fascias, extraperitoneal fascia, and parietal peritoneum (Fig. 4.24).

Superficial fascia

The superficial fascia of the abdominal wall (subcutaneous tissue of abdomen) is a layer of fatty connective tissue. It is usually a single layer similar to, and continuous with, the superficial fascia throughout other regions of the body. However, in the lower region of the anterior part of the abdominal wall, below the umbilicus, it forms two layers: a superficial fatty layer and a deeper membranous layer.

Superficial layer

The superficial fatty layer of superficial fascia (**Camper's fascia**) contains fat and varies in thickness (Fig. 4.25 and 4.26). It is continuous superficial to the inguinal ligament with the superficial fascia of the thigh and with a similar layer in the perineum.

In men, this superficial layer continues over the penis and, after losing its fat and fusing with the deeper layer of superficial fascia, continues into the scrotum where it forms a specialized fascial layer containing smooth muscle fibers (the **dartos fascia**). In women, this superficial layer retains some fat and is a component of the labia majora.

Deeper layer

The deeper membranous layer of superficial fascia (**Scarpa's fascia**) is thin and membranous, and contains little or no fat (see Fig. 4.25). Inferiorly, it continues into the thigh, but just below the inguinal ligament, it fuses with the deep fascia of the thigh (the **fascia lata**; Fig. 4.26). In the midline, it is firmly attached to the linea alba and the symphysis pubis. It continues into the anterior part of the perineum where it is firmly attached to the ischiopubic rami and to the posterior margin of the perineal membrane. Here, it is referred to as the **superficial perineal fascia** (**Colles' fascia**).

In men, the deeper membranous layer of superficial fascia blends with the superficial layer as they both pass over the penis, forming the superficial fascia of the penis, before they continue into the scrotum where they form the dartos fascia (Fig. 4.25). Also in men, extensions of the deeper membranous layer of superficial fascia attached to the pubic symphysis pass inferiorly onto the dorsum and

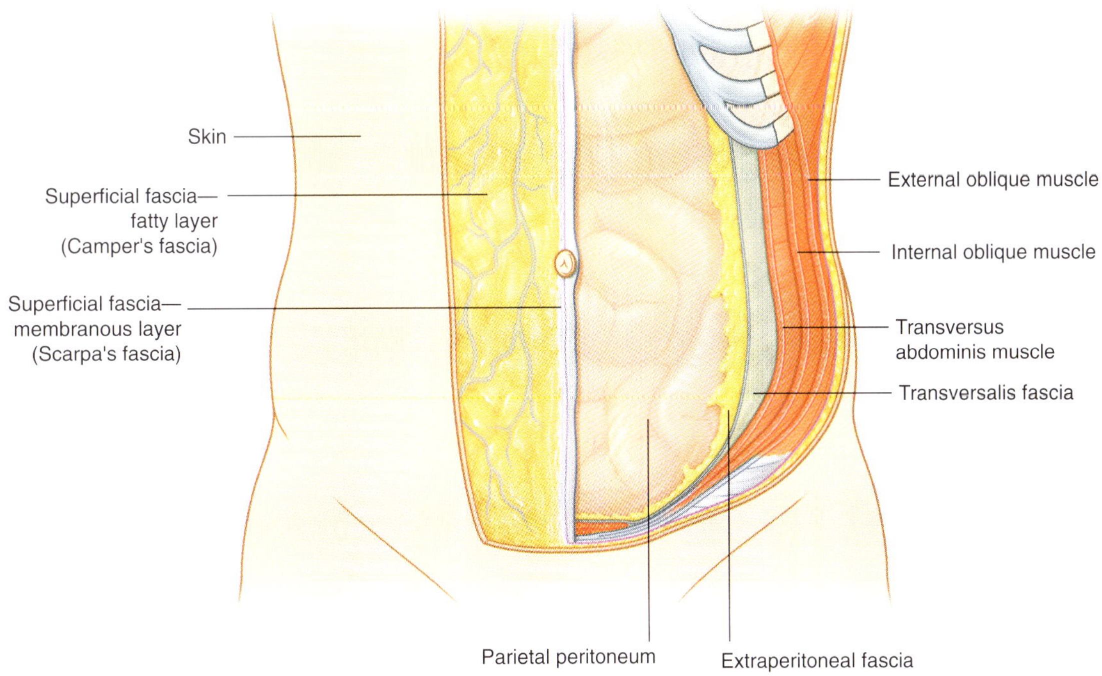

Fig. 4.24 Layers of the abdominal wall.

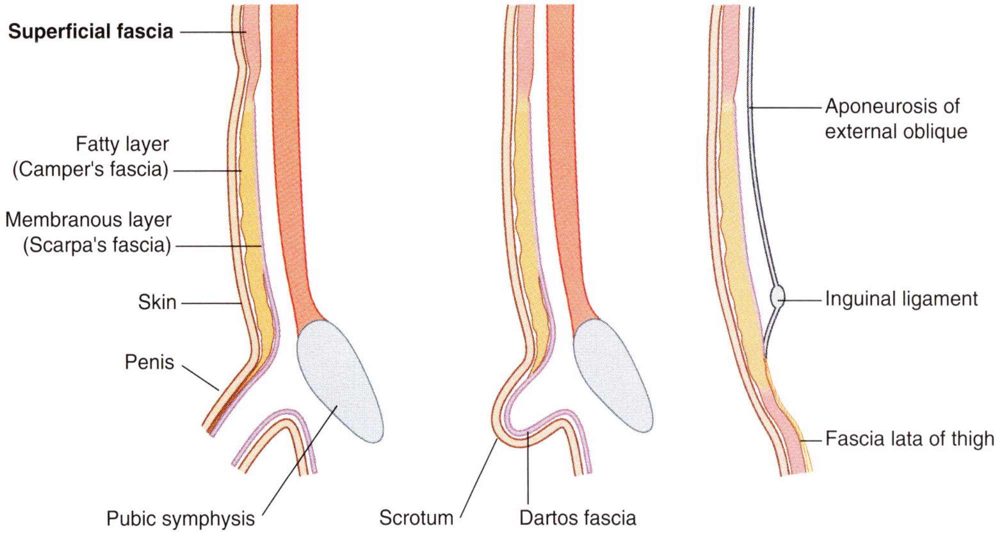

Fig. 4.25 Superficial fascia.

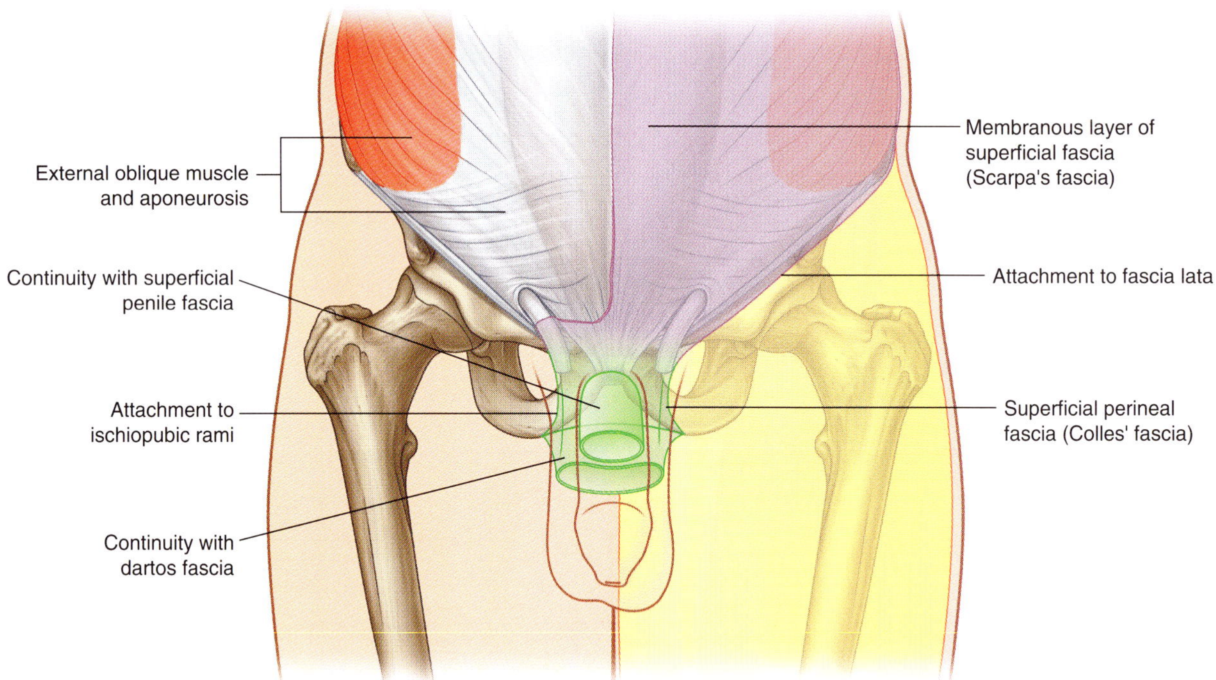

Fig. 4.26 Continuity of membranous layer of superficial fascia into other areas.

sides of the penis to form the **fundiform ligament of penis**. In women, the membranous layer of the superficial fascia continues into the labia majora and the anterior part of the perineum.

Anterolateral muscles

There are five muscles in the anterolateral group of abdominal wall muscles:

- Three flat muscles whose fibers begin posterolaterally, pass anteriorly, and are replaced by an aponeurosis as each muscle continues toward the midline—the external oblique, internal oblique, and transversus abdominis muscles.
- Two vertical muscles, near the midline, which are enclosed within a tendinous sheath formed by the aponeuroses of the flat muscles—the rectus abdominis and pyramidalis muscles.

Each of these five muscles has specific actions, but together the muscles are critical for the maintenance of many normal physiological functions (Fig. 4.3 and 4.4). By their positioning, they form a firm, but flexible, wall that keeps the abdominal viscera within the abdominal cavity, protects the viscera from injury, and helps maintain the position of the viscera in the erect posture against the action of gravity.

In addition, contraction of these muscles assists in both quiet and forced expiration by pushing the viscera upward (which helps push the relaxed diaphragm further into the thoracic cavity) and in coughing and vomiting.

All these muscles are also involved in any action that increases intraabdominal pressure, including parturition (childbirth), micturition (urination), and defecation (expulsion of feces from the rectum).

Flat muscles

External oblique

The most superficial of the three flat muscles in the anterolateral group of abdominal wall muscles is the **external oblique**, which is immediately deep to the superficial fascia (Fig. 4.27, Table 4.1). Its laterally placed muscle fibers pass in an inferomedial direction, while its large

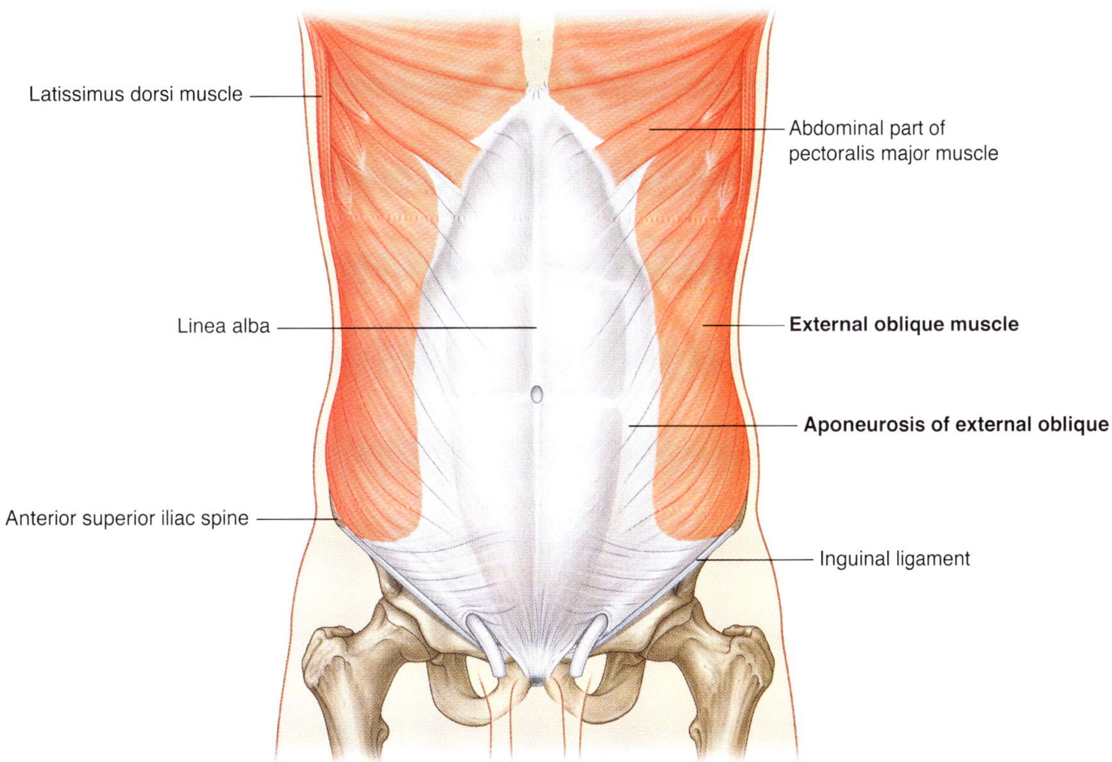

Fig. 4.27 External oblique muscle and its aponeurosis.

aponeurotic component covers the anterior part of the abdominal wall to the midline. Approaching the midline, the aponeuroses of both sides are entwined, forming the linea alba, which extends from the xiphoid process to the pubic symphysis.

Associated ligaments

The lower border of the external oblique aponeurosis forms the **inguinal ligament** on each side (Fig. 4.27). This thickened reinforced free edge of the external oblique aponeurosis passes between the anterior superior iliac spine laterally and the pubic tubercle medially (Fig. 4.28). It folds deep to itself forming a trough, which plays an important role in the formation of the inguinal canal.

Several other ligaments are also formed from extensions of the fibers at the medial end of the inguinal ligament:

- The **lacunar (Gimbernat's) ligament** is a crescent-shaped extension of fibers at the medial end of the inguinal ligament that passes backward to attach to the **pecten pubis** on the superior ramus of the pubic bone (Fig. 4.28, 4.29, and 4.50B).
- Additional fibers extend from the lacunar ligament along the pecten pubis of the pelvic brim to form the **pectineal (Cooper's) ligament**.

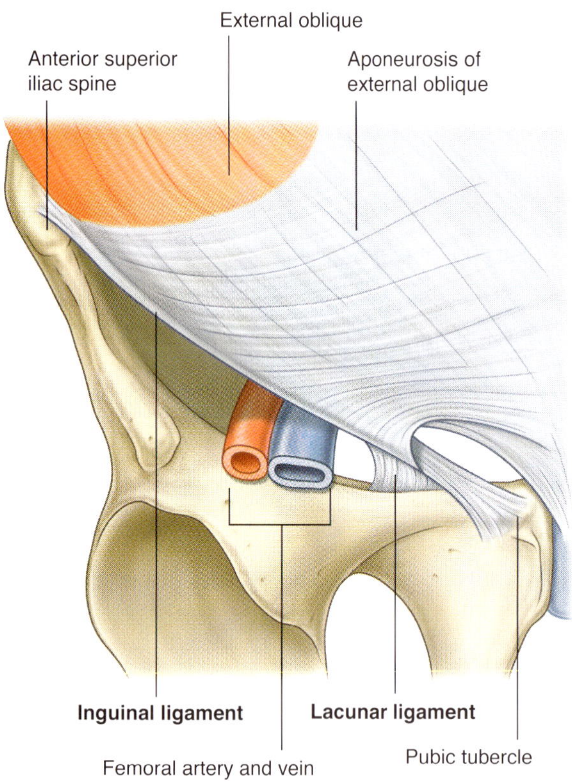

Fig. 4.28 Ligaments formed from the external oblique aponeurosis.

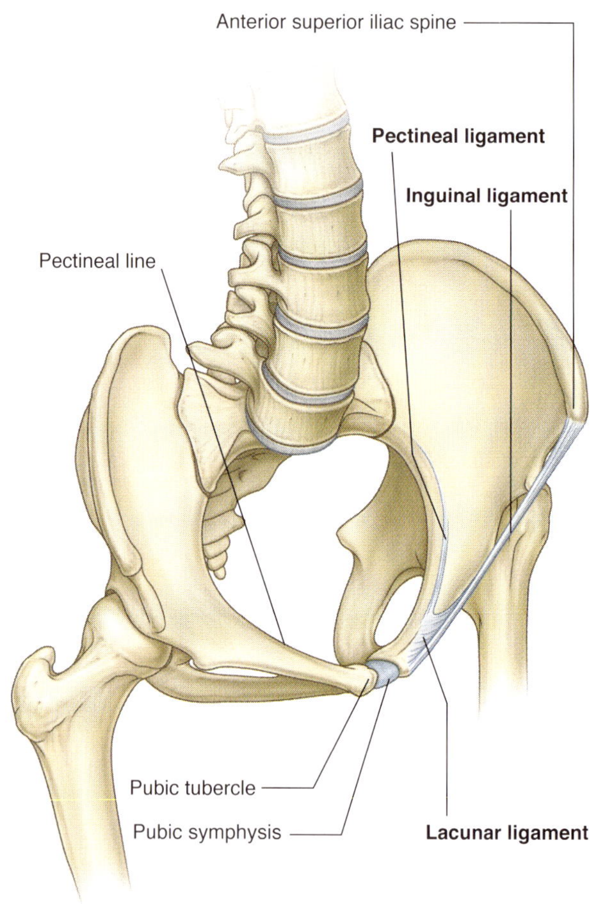

Fig. 4.29 Ligaments of the inguinal region.

Internal oblique

Deep to the external oblique muscle is the **internal oblique** muscle, which is the second of the three flat muscles (Fig. 4.30, Table 4.1). This muscle is smaller and thinner than the external oblique, with most of its muscle fibers passing in a superomedial direction. Its lateral muscular components end anteriorly as an aponeurosis that blends into the linea alba at the midline.

Transversus abdominis

Deep to the internal oblique muscle is the **transversus abdominis** muscle (Fig. 4.31, Table 4.1), so named because of the direction of most of its muscle fibers. It ends in an anterior aponeurosis, which blends with the linea alba at the midline.

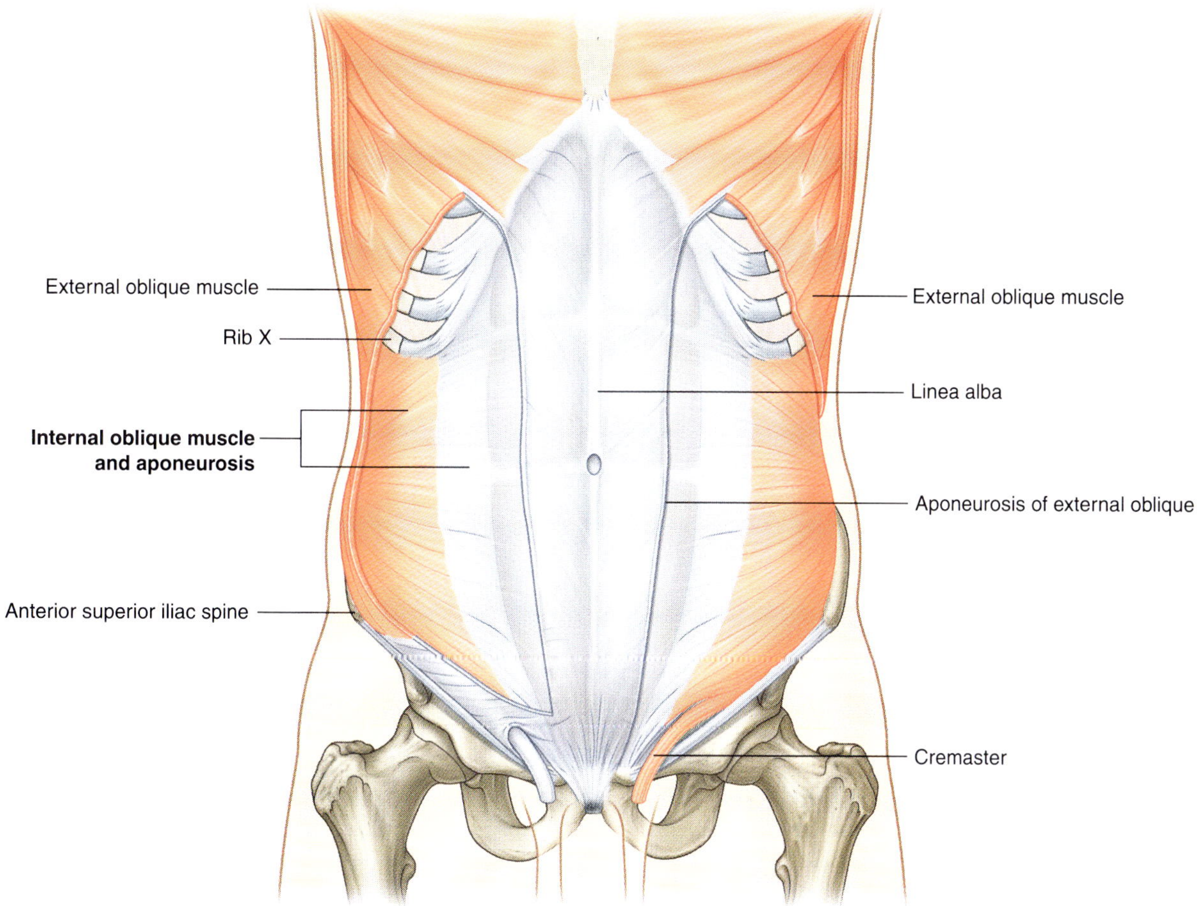

Fig. 4.30 Internal oblique muscle and its aponeurosis.

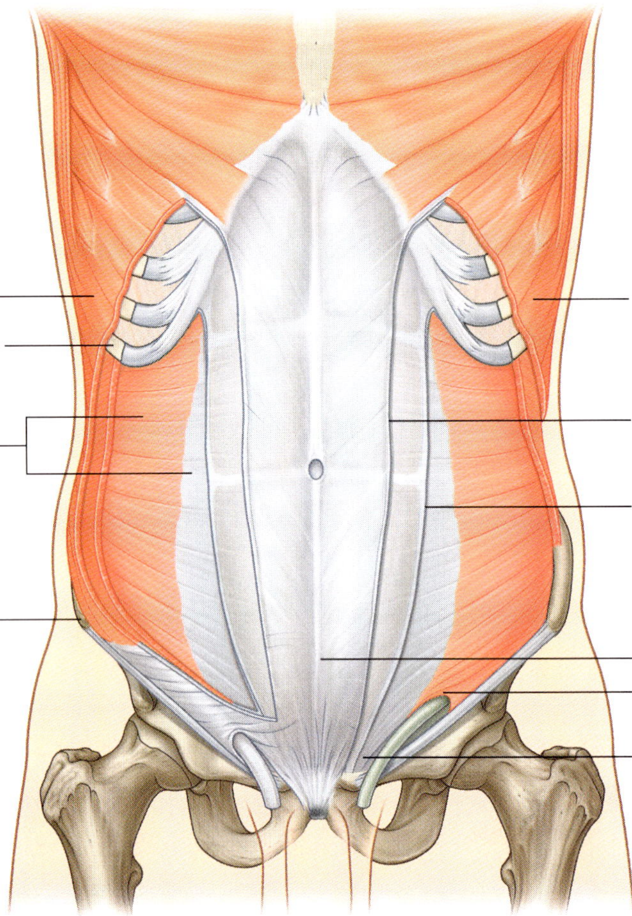

Fig. 4.31 Transversus abdominis muscle and its aponeurosis.

Transversalis fascia

Each of the three flat muscles is covered on its anterior and posterior surfaces by a layer of deep (or investing) fascia. In general, these layers are unremarkable except for the layer deep to the transversus abdominis muscle (the **transversalis fascia**), which is better developed.

The transversalis fascia is a continuous layer of deep fascia that lines the abdominal cavity and continues into the pelvic cavity. It crosses the midline anteriorly, associating with the transversalis fascia of the opposite side, and is continuous with the fascia on the inferior surface of the diaphragm. It is continuous posteriorly with the deep fascia covering the muscles of the posterior abdominal wall and attaches to the thoracolumbar fascia.

After attaching to the iliac crest, the transversalis fascia blends with the fascia covering the muscles associated with the upper regions of the pelvic bones and with similar fascia covering the muscles of the pelvic cavity. At this point, it is referred to as the **parietal pelvic** (or **endopelvic**) **fascia**.

There is therefore a continuous layer of deep fascia surrounding the abdominal cavity that is thick in some areas, thin in others, attached or free, and participates in the formation of specialized structures.

Vertical muscles

The two vertical muscles in the anterolateral group of abdominal wall muscles are the large rectus abdominis and the small pyramidalis (Fig. 4.32, Table 4.1).

Rectus abdominis

The **rectus abdominis** is a long, flat muscle and extends the length of the anterior abdominal wall. It is a paired muscle, separated in the midline by the linea alba, and it

Table 4.1 Abdominal wall muscles

Muscle	Origin	Insertion	Innervation	Function
External oblique	Muscular slips from the outer surfaces of the lower eight ribs (ribs V to XII)	Lateral lip of iliac crest; linea alba	Anterior rami of lower six thoracic spinal nerves (T7 to T12)	Compress abdominal contents; both muscles flex trunk; each muscle bends trunk to same side, turning anterior part of abdomen to opposite side
Internal oblique	Thoracolumbar fascia; iliac crest between origins of external and transversus; lateral two-thirds of inguinal ligament	Inferior border of the lower three or four ribs; linea alba; pubic crest and pectineal line	Anterior rami of lower six thoracic spinal nerves (T7 to T12) and L1	Compress abdominal contents; both muscles flex trunk; each muscle bends trunk and turns anterior part of abdomen to same side
Transversus abdominis	Thoracolumbar fascia; medial lip of iliac crest; lateral one-third of inguinal ligament; costal cartilages lower six ribs (ribs VII to XII)	Linea alba; pubic crest and pectineal line	Anterior rami of lower six thoracic spinal nerves (T7 to T12) and L1	Compress abdominal contents
Rectus abdominis	Pubic crest, pubic tubercle, and pubic symphysis	Costal cartilages of ribs V to VII; xiphoid process	Anterior rami of lower seven thoracic spinal nerves (T6 to T12)	Compress abdominal contents; flex vertebral column; tense abdominal wall
Pyramidalis	Front of pubis and pubic symphysis	Linea alba	Anterior ramus of T12	Tenses the linea alba

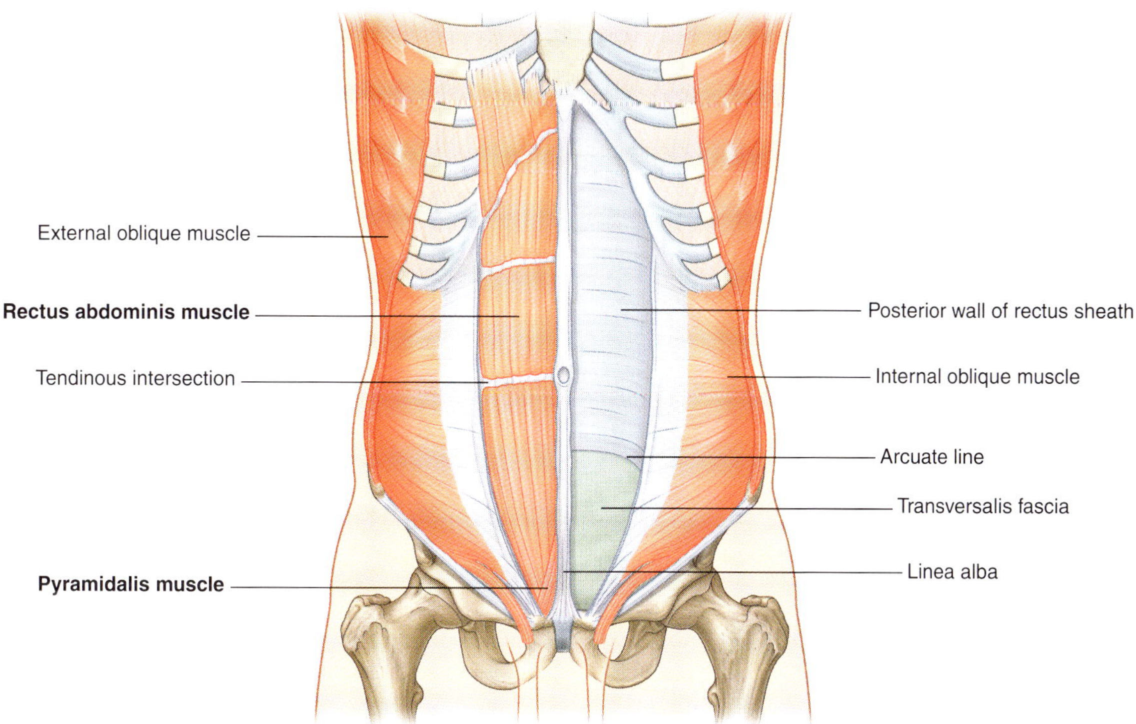

Fig. 4.32 Rectus abdominis and pyramidalis muscles.

widens and thins as it ascends from the pubic symphysis to the costal margin. Along its course, it is intersected by three or four transverse fibrous bands or **tendinous intersections** (Fig. 4.32). These are easily visible on individuals with a well-developed rectus abdominis.

Pyramidalis

The second vertical muscle is the **pyramidalis**. This small, triangular muscle, which may be absent, is anterior to the rectus abdominis and has its base on the pubis, and its apex is attached superiorly and medially to the linea alba (Fig. 4.32).

Rectus sheath

The rectus abdominis and pyramidalis muscles are enclosed in an aponeurotic tendinous sheath (the **rectus sheath**) formed by a unique layering of the aponeuroses of the external and internal oblique, and transversus abdominis muscles (Fig. 4.33).

The rectus sheath completely encloses the upper three-quarters of the rectus abdominis and covers the anterior surface of the lower one-quarter of the muscle. As no sheath covers the posterior surface of the lower quarter of the rectus abdominis muscle, the muscle at this point is in direct contact with the transversalis fascia.

The formation of the rectus sheath surrounding the upper three-quarters of the rectus abdominis muscle has the following pattern:

- The anterior wall consists of the aponeurosis of the external oblique and the anterior half of the aponeurosis of the internal oblique, which splits at the lateral margin of the rectus abdominis (Fig. 4.33A).
- The posterior wall of the rectus sheath consists of the posterior half of the aponeurosis of the internal oblique and the aponeurosis of the transversus abdominis.

At a point midway between the umbilicus and the pubic symphysis, corresponding to the beginning of the lower one-quarter of the rectus abdominis muscle, all of the aponeuroses pass anterior to the rectus muscle. There is no posterior wall of the rectus sheath and the anterior wall of the sheath consists of the aponeuroses of the external oblique, the internal oblique, and the transversus abdominis muscles. From this point inferiorly, the rectus abdominis muscle is in direct contact with the transversalis fascia. Marking this point of transition is an arch of fibers (the **arcuate line**; see Fig. 4.32), which is the lower free edge of the posterior wall of the rectus sheath.

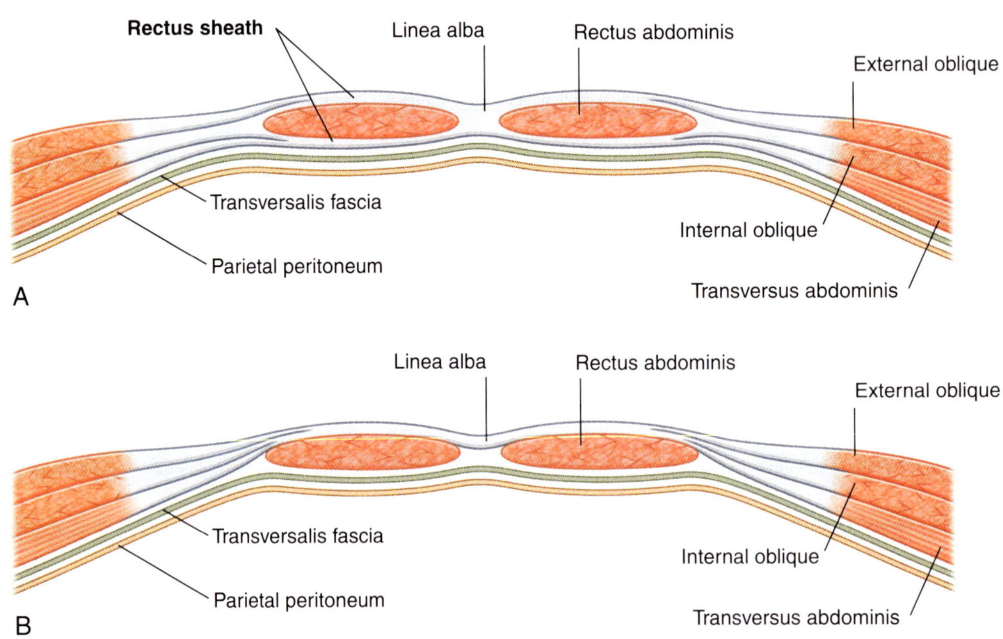

Fig. 4.33 Organization of the rectus sheath. **(A)** Transverse section through the upper three-quarters of the rectus sheath. **(B)** Transverse section through the lower one-quarter of the rectus sheath.

Extraperitoneal fascia

Deep to the transversalis fascia is a layer of connective tissue, the **extraperitoneal fascia**, which separates the transversalis fascia from the peritoneum (Fig. 4.34). Containing varying amounts of fat, this layer not only lines the abdominal cavity but also is continuous with a similar layer lining the pelvic cavity. It is abundant on the posterior abdominal wall, especially around the kidneys, continues over organs covered by peritoneal reflections, such as the ascending colon (see Fig. 4. 93), and, as the vasculature is located in this layer, extends into mesenteries with the blood vessels. Viscera in the extraperitoneal fascia are referred to as **retroperitoneal.**

In the description of specific surgical procedures, the terminology used to describe the extraperitoneal fascia is further modified. The fascia toward the anterior side of the body is described as preperitoneal (or, less commonly, properitoneal) and the fascia toward the posterior side of the body has been described as retroperitoneal (Fig. 4.35). Examples of the use of these terms would be the continuity of fat in the inguinal canal with the preperitoneal fat and a transabdominal preperitoneal laparoscopic repair of an inguinal hernia.

Peritoneum

Deep to the extraperitoneal fascia is the peritoneum (see Fig. 4.6 and 4.7). This thin serous membrane lines the walls of the abdominal cavity and, at various points, reflects onto the abdominal viscera, providing either a complete or a partial covering. The peritoneum lining the abdominal wall is the parietal peritoneum; the peritoneum covering the viscera is the visceral peritoneum.

The continuous lining of the abdominal walls by the parietal peritoneum forms a sac. This sac is closed in men but has two openings in women where the uterine tubes provide a passage to the outside. The closed sac in men and the semiclosed sac in women are called the peritoneal cavity.

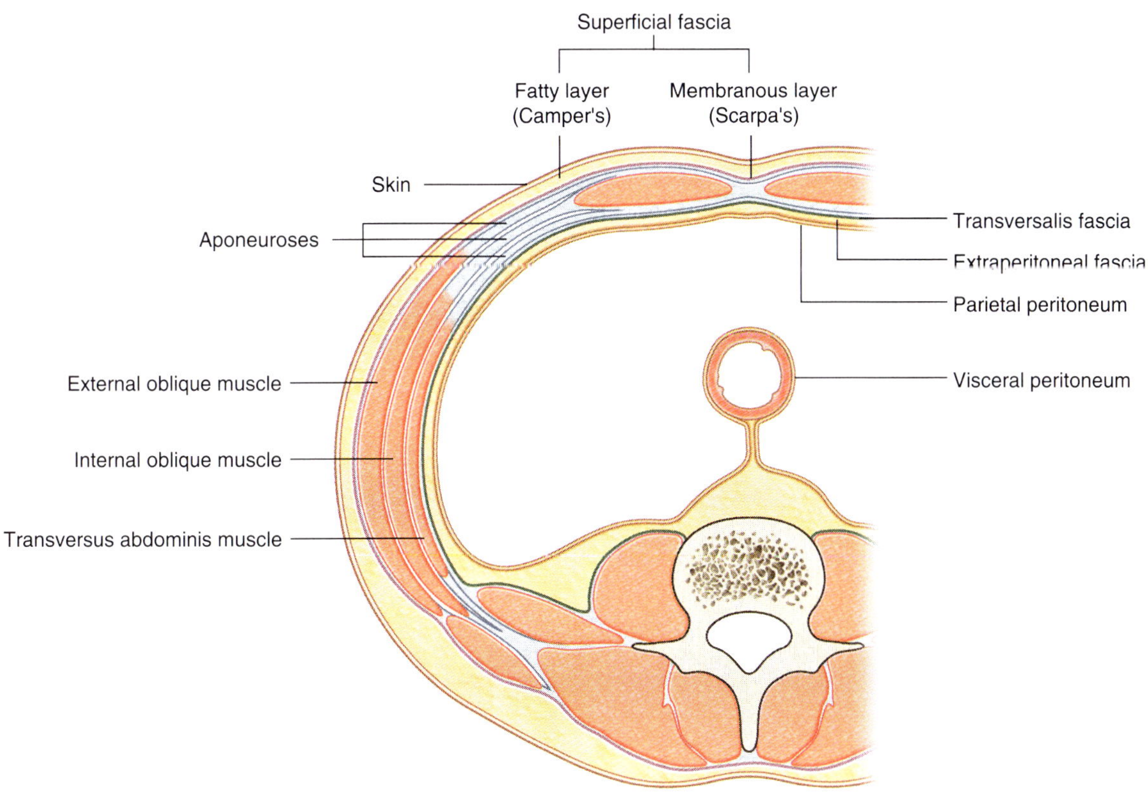

Fig. 4.34 Transverse section showing the layers of the abdominal wall.

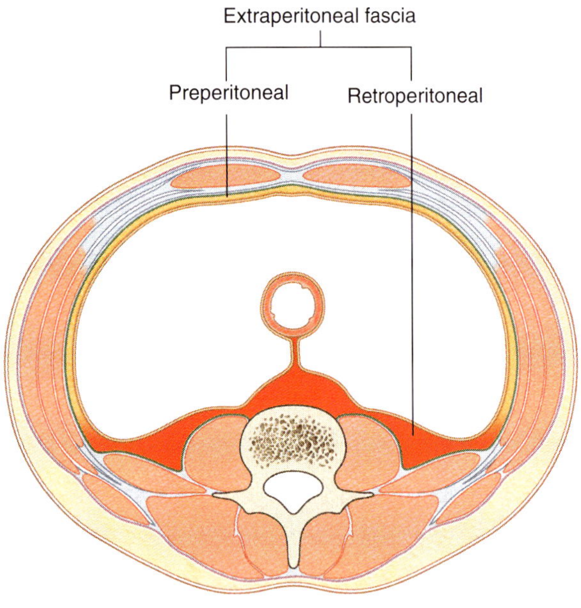

Fig. 4.35 Subdivisions of the extraperitoneal fascia.

Innervation

The skin, muscles, and parietal peritoneum of the anterolateral abdominal wall are supplied by T7 to T12 and L1 spinal nerves. The anterior rami of these spinal nerves pass around the body, from posterior to anterior, in an inferomedial direction (Fig. 4.36). As they proceed, they give off a lateral cutaneous branch and end as an anterior cutaneous branch.

The intercostal nerves (T7 to T11) leave their intercostal spaces, passing deep to the costal cartilages, and continue onto the anterolateral abdominal wall **between** the internal oblique and transversus abdominis muscles (Fig. 4.37). Reaching the lateral edge of the rectus sheath, they enter the rectus sheath and pass posterior to the lateral aspect of the rectus abdominis muscle. Approaching the midline, anterior cutaneous branches pass through the rectus abdominis muscle and the anterior wall of the rectus sheath to supply the skin.

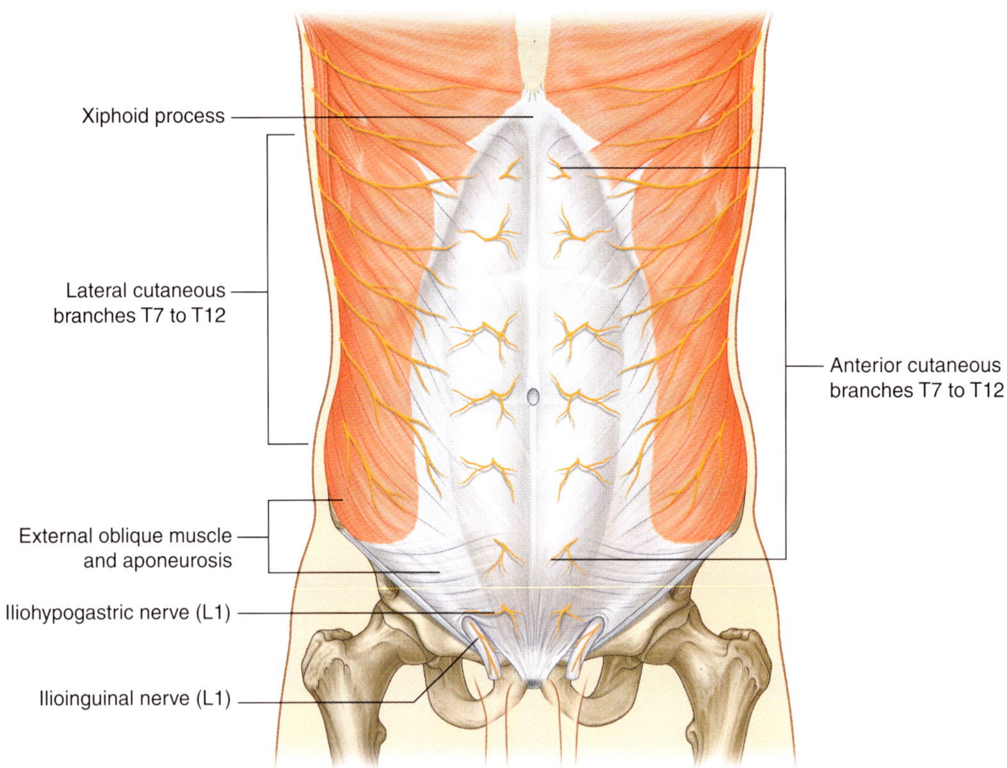

Fig. 4.36 Innervation of the anterolateral abdominal wall.

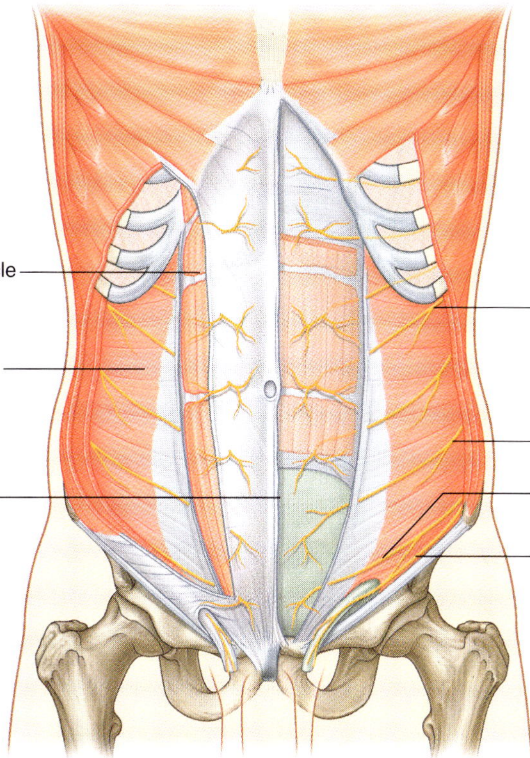

Fig. 4.37 Path taken by the nerves innervating the anterolateral abdominal wall.

Spinal nerve T12 (the **subcostal nerve**) follows a similar course as the intercostals. Branches of L1 (the **iliohypogastric nerve** and **ilioinguinal nerve**), which originate from the lumbar plexus, follow similar courses initially, but deviate from this pattern near their final destination.

Along their course, nerves T7 to T12 and L1 supply branches to the anterolateral abdominal wall muscles and the underlying parietal peritoneum. All terminate by supplying skin:

- Nerves T7 to T9 supply the skin from the xiphoid process to just above the umbilicus.
- T10 supplies the skin around the umbilicus.
- T11, T12, and L1 supply the skin from just below the umbilicus to, and including, the pubic region (Fig. 4.38).
- Additionally, the ilioinguinal nerve (a branch of L1) supplies the anterior surface of the scrotum or labia majora, and sends a small cutaneous branch to the thigh.

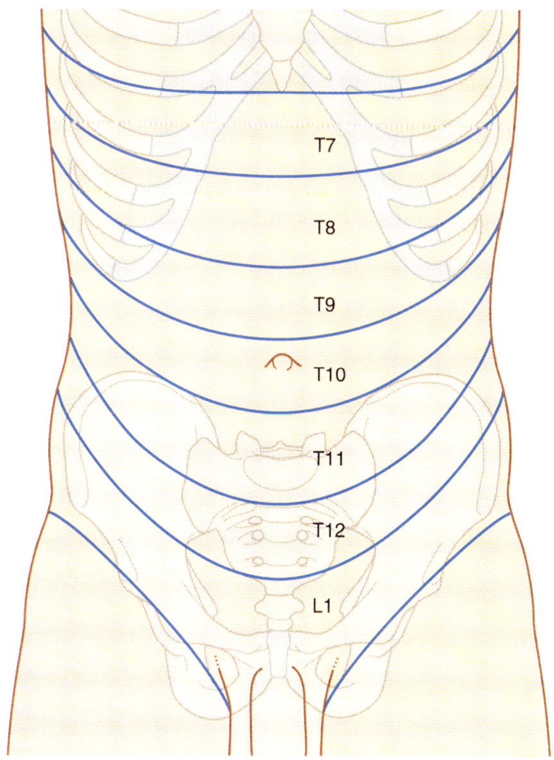

Fig. 4.38 Dermatomes of the anterolateral abdominal wall.

Arterial supply and venous drainage

Numerous blood vessels supply the anterolateral abdominal wall. Superficially:

- The superior part of the wall is supplied by branches from the **musculophrenic artery**, a terminal branch of the **internal thoracic artery**.
- The inferior part of the wall is supplied by the medially placed **superficial epigastric artery** and the laterally placed **superficial circumflex iliac artery**, both branches of the **femoral artery** (Fig. 4.39).

At a deeper level:

- The superior part of the wall is supplied by the **superior epigastric artery**, a terminal branch of the internal thoracic artery.
- The lateral part of the wall is supplied by branches of the **10th** and **11th intercostal arteries** and the **subcostal artery**.
- The inferior part of the wall is supplied by the medially placed **inferior epigastric artery** and the laterally placed **deep circumflex iliac artery**, both branches of the **external iliac artery**.

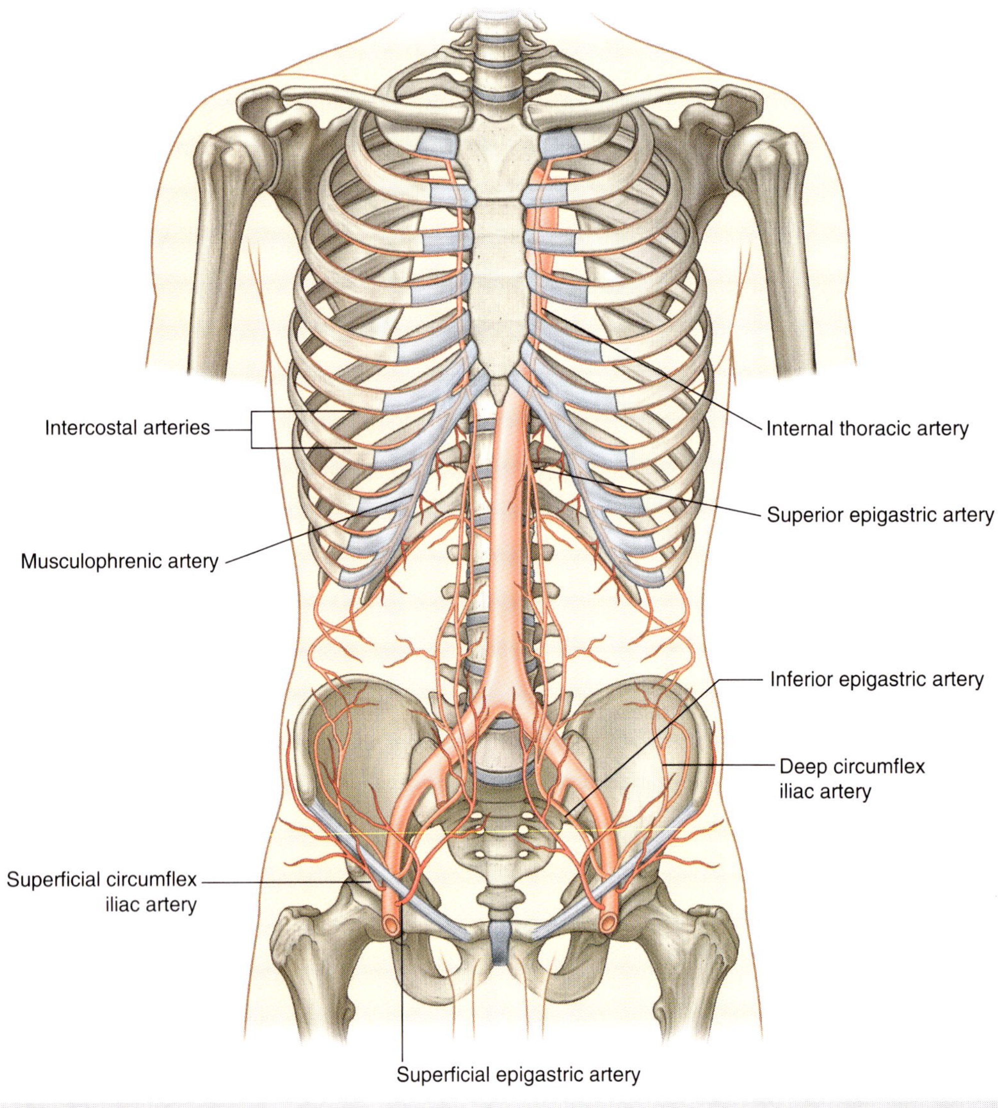

Fig. 4.39 Arterial supply to the anterolateral abdominal wall.

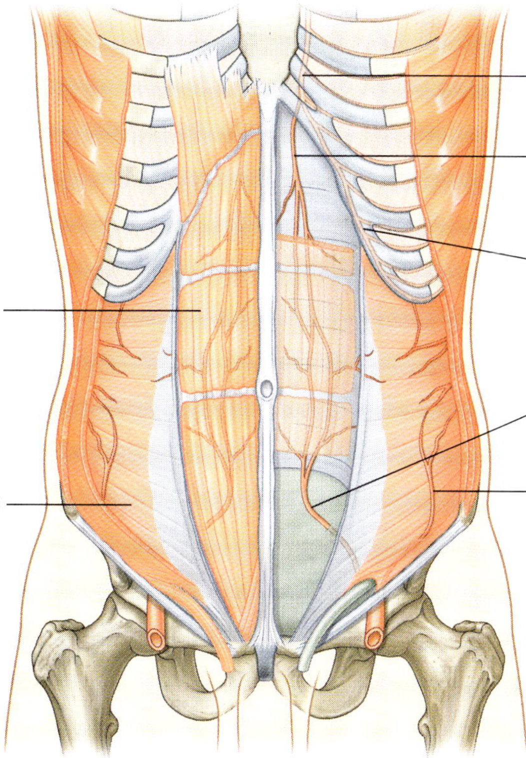

Fig. 4.40 Superior and inferior epigastric arteries.

The superior and inferior epigastric arteries both enter the rectus sheath. They are posterior to the rectus abdominis muscle throughout their course, and anastomose with each other (Fig. 4.40).

Veins of similar names follow the arteries and are responsible for venous drainage.

Lymphatic drainage

Lymphatic drainage of the anterolateral abdominal wall follows the basic principles of lymphatic drainage:

- Superficial lymphatics above the umbilicus pass in a superior direction to the **axillary nodes**, while drainage below the umbilicus passes in an inferior direction to the **superficial inguinal nodes.**
- Deep lymphatic drainage follows the deep arteries back to **parasternal nodes** along the internal thoracic artery, lumbar nodes along the abdominal aorta, and external iliac nodes along the external iliac artery.

GROIN

SET INDUCTION—CASE SCENARIO 2: INDIRECT INGUINAL HERNIA

An 8-year-old male presented at the surgery OPD with a swelling in the groin. It had descended into the scrotum, and there was an increase in size of the swelling when the patient coughed. Knowledge of the inguinal canal is needed to diagnose a patient as indirect inguinal hernia.

<table>
<tr><td rowspan="2">REMEMBER
[Recall Facts]</td><td colspan="3">OUTLINE 2. INGUINAL REGION—LEARNING OBJECTIVES
[By the end of this section the student should be able to:]</td><td colspan="2" rowspan="2">EVALUATE
[Explain Concepts]</td></tr>
<tr><td colspan="3">DEMONSTRATE AND ANALYZE RELATIONSHIPS
[Identify structures in a Prosected Specimen or Figure]</td></tr>
<tr><td rowspan="7">1. Describe the extent, boundaries, and contents of the inguinal canal
2. Explain the descent of the testis and the formation of the inguinal canal
3. Describe the formation of the deep and superficial inguinal rings
4. Describe the contents of the spermatic cord
5. Describe indirect and direct inguinal hernias
6. List the danger areas of the inguinal region
7. List the different types of hernias</td><td>Level I</td><td>Level II</td><td>Level III</td><td colspan="2" rowspan="2">■ Boundaries of inguinal canal
■ Direct and indirect inguinal hernia
■ Factors preventing inguinal hernia
■ Nerves involved in the cremasteric reflex</td></tr>
<tr><td rowspan="6">■ External oblique aponeurosis
■ Arching fibers of internal oblique and transverses abdominis muscle laterally
■ Spermatic cord in males and round ligament of uterus in females
■ Inguinal ligament
■ Fascia transversalis
■ Deep inguinal ring
■ Conjoint tendon
■ Ductus deferens
■ Testicular artery
■ Pampiniform plexus</td><td rowspan="6">■ Cremaster muscle
■ Ilioinguinal nerve
■ Genital branch of genitofemoral nerve</td><td rowspan="6">■ Lacunar ligament
■ Hesselbach's triangle
■ Reflected part of inguinal ligament
■ Artery to the ductus deferens
■ Cremasteric artery
■ Testicular plexus of sympathetic nerves</td></tr>
<tr><td colspan="2">EARLY CLINICAL EXPOSURE
[Apply Anatomical knowledge]</td></tr>
<tr><td>Surgical Anatomy/ Pathology/ Trauma</td><td>Imaging/ Surface Anatomy</td></tr>
<tr><td>■ Inguinal hernia
■ Types of hernia
■ Danger areas of inguinal region—triangle of doom, triangle of pain, and circle of death</td><td></td></tr>
<tr><td colspan="2">PROBLEM SOLVING/ CLINICAL CASES
[Interpret]</td></tr>
<tr><td colspan="2">■ Explain the reason for each of the coverings of a direct and an indirect inguinal hernia
■ Differentiate inguinal and femoral hernias</td></tr>
</table>

The groin (inguinal region) is the area of junction between the anterior abdominal wall and the thigh. In this area, the abdominal wall is weakened from changes that occur during development and a peritoneal sac or diverticulum, with or without abdominal contents, can therefore protrude through it, creating an inguinal hernia. This type of hernia can occur in both sexes, but it is most common in males.

The inherent weakness in the anterior abdominal wall in the groin is caused by changes that occur during the development of the gonads. Before the descent of the testes and ovaries from their initial position high in the posterior abdominal wall, a peritoneal outpouching (the processus vaginalis) forms (Fig. 4.41), protruding through the various layers of the anterior abdominal wall and acquiring coverings from each:

- The transversalis fascia forms its deepest covering (see Fig. 4.43).
- The second covering is formed by the musculature of the internal oblique, Fig. 4.41 (a covering from the transversus abdominis muscle is not acquired because the processus vaginalis passes under the arching fibers of the transversus abdominus muscle, Fig. 4.31).
- Its most superficial covering is the aponeurosis of the external oblique (Fig. 4.27).

As a result, the processus vaginalis is transformed into a tubular structure with multiple coverings from the layers of the anterior abdominal wall. This forms the basic structure of the **inguinal canal**.

The final event in this development is the descent of the testes into the scrotum or of the ovaries into the pelvic cavity. This process depends on the development of the gubernaculum, which extends from the inferior border of the developing gonad to the labioscrotal swellings (Fig. 4.41).

The processus vaginalis is immediately anterior to the gubernaculum within the inguinal canal.

In men, as the testes descend, the testes and their accompanying vessels, ducts, and nerves pass through the inguinal canal and are therefore surrounded by the same fascial layers of the abdominal wall. Testicular descent completes the formation of the spermatic cord in men.

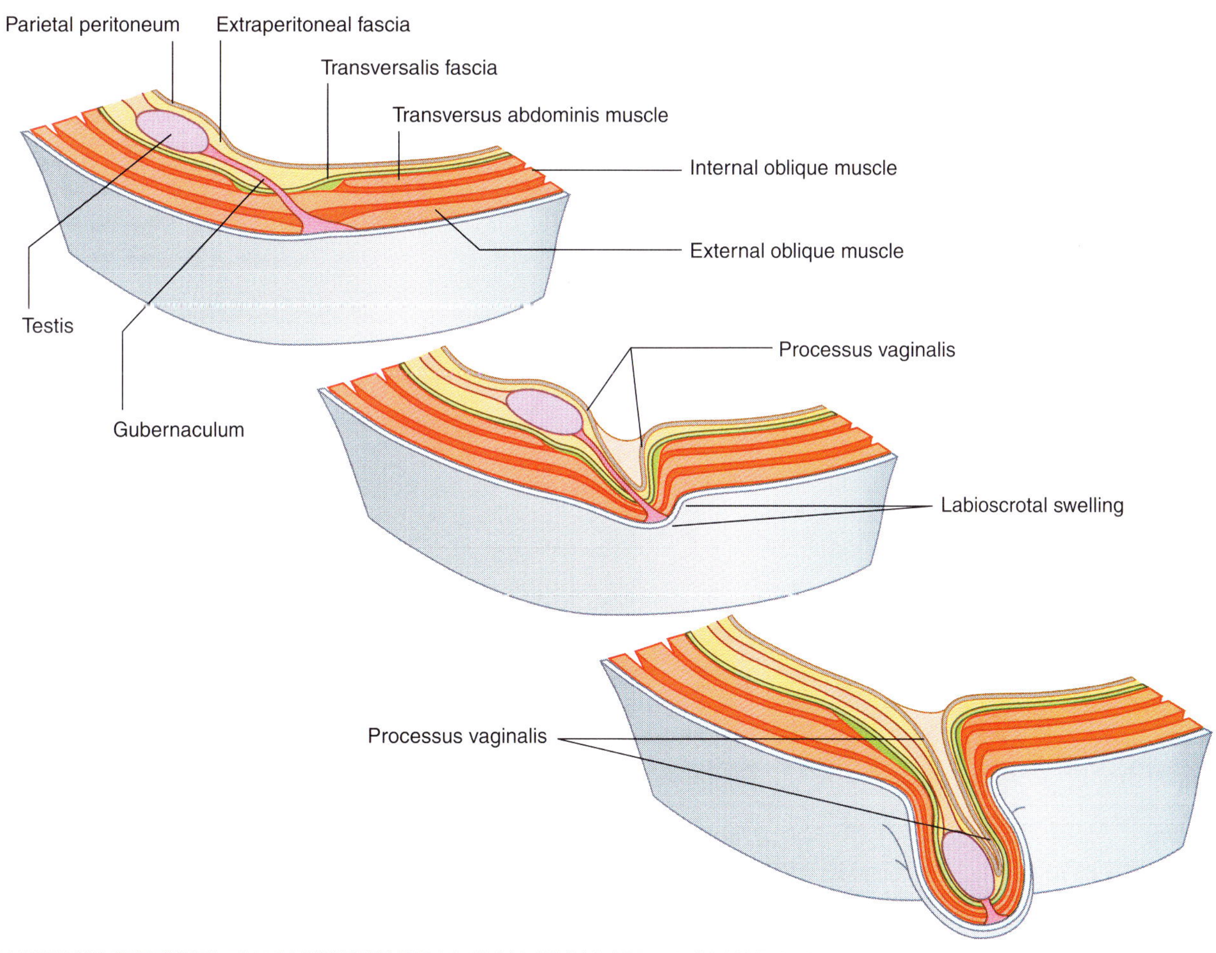

Fig. 4.41 Descent of the testis from week 7 (postfertilization) to birth.

In women, the ovaries descend into the pelvic cavity and become associated with the developing uterus. Therefore, the only remaining structure passing through the inguinal canal is the round ligament of the uterus, which is a remnant of the gubernaculum.

The development sequence is concluded in both sexes when the processus vaginalis obliterates. If this does not occur or is incomplete, a potential weakness exists in the anterior abdominal wall and an inguinal hernia may develop. In males, only proximal regions of the tunica vaginalis obliterate. The distal end expands to enclose most of the testis in the scrotum. In other words, the cavity of the tunica vaginalis in men forms as an extension of the developing peritoneal cavity that becomes separated off during development.

Inguinal canal

The inguinal canal is a slit-like passage that extends in a downward and medial direction, just above and parallel to the lower half of the inguinal ligament. It begins at the deep inguinal ring and continues for approximately 4 cm, ending at the superficial inguinal ring (Fig. 4.42). The contents of the canal are the genital branch of the genitofemoral nerve, the **spermatic cord** in men, and the round ligament of the uterus in women. Additionally, in both sexes, the ilioinguinal nerve passes through part of the canal, exiting through the superficial inguinal ring with the other contents.

Deep inguinal ring

The deep (internal) inguinal ring is the beginning of the inguinal canal and is at a point midway between the anterior superior iliac spine and the pubic symphysis (Fig. 4.43). It is just above the inguinal ligament and immediately lateral to the inferior epigastric vessels. Although sometimes referred to as a defect or opening in the transversalis fascia, it is actually the beginning of the tubular evagination of transversalis fascia that forms one of the coverings (the **internal spermatic fascia**) of the spermatic cord in men or the round ligament of the uterus in women.

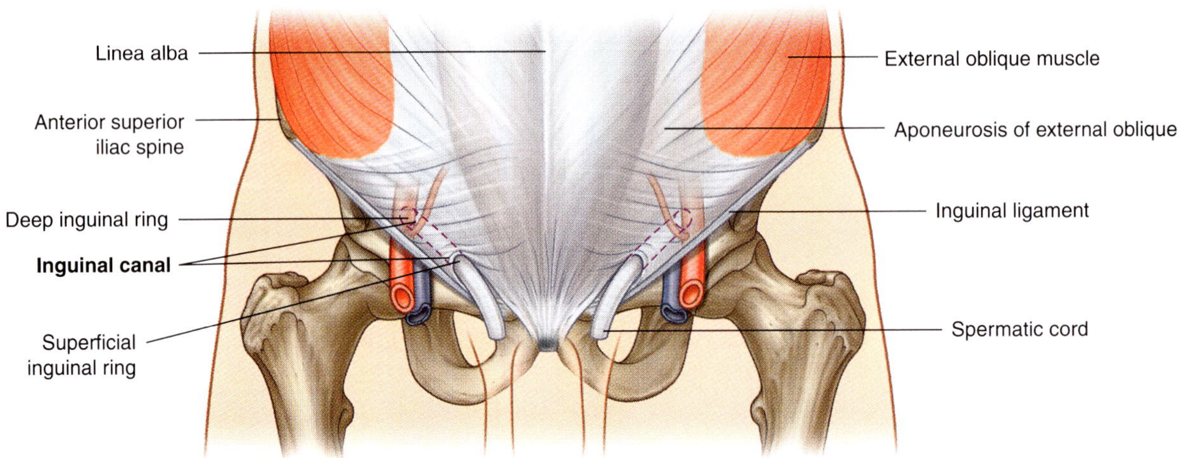

Fig. 4.42 Inguinal canal.

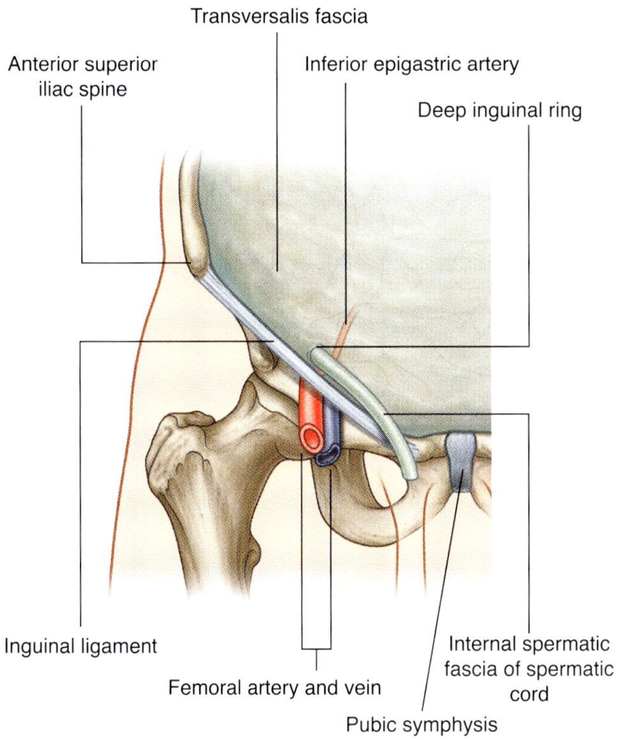

Fig. 4.43 Deep inguinal ring and the transversalis fascia.

Superficial inguinal ring

The superficial (external) inguinal ring is the end of the inguinal canal and is superior to the pubic tubercle (Fig. 4.44). It is a triangular opening in the aponeurosis of the external oblique, with its apex pointing superolaterally and its base formed by the pubic crest. The two remaining sides of the triangle (the **medial crus** and the **lateral crus**) are attached to the pubic symphysis and the pubic tubercle, respectively. At the apex of the triangle the two crura are held together by crossing (intercrural) fibers, which prevent further widening of the superficial ring.

As with the deep inguinal ring, the superficial inguinal ring is actually the beginning of the tubular evagination of the aponeurosis of the external oblique onto the structures traversing the inguinal canal and emerging from the superficial inguinal ring. This continuation of tissue over the spermatic cord is the **external spermatic fascia** (Fig. 4.27).

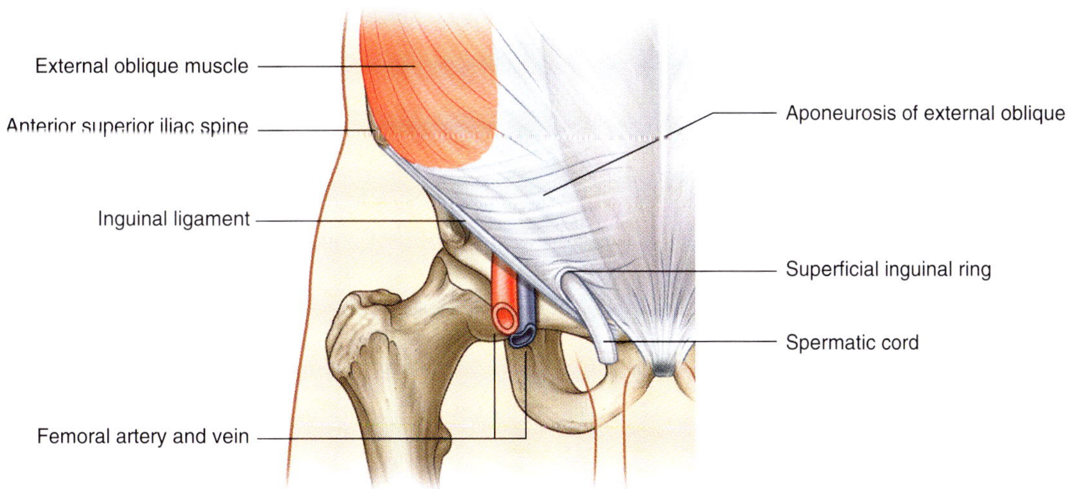

Fig. 4.44 Superficial inguinal ring and the aponeurosis of the external oblique.

Anterior wall

The anterior wall of the inguinal canal is formed along its entire length by the aponeurosis of the external oblique muscle (Fig. 4.44). It is also reinforced laterally by the lower fibers of the internal oblique that originate from the lateral two-thirds of the inguinal ligament (Fig. 4.45). This adds an additional covering over the deep inguinal ring, which is a potential point of weakness in the anterior abdominal wall. Furthermore, as the internal oblique muscle covers the deep inguinal ring, it also contributes a layer (the **cremasteric fascia** containing the **cremasteric muscle**) to the coverings of the structures traversing the inguinal canal (Fig. 4.30).

Posterior wall

The posterior wall of the inguinal canal is formed along its entire length by the transversalis fascia (see Fig. 4.43). It is reinforced along its medial one-third by the **conjoint tendon** (**inguinal falx**; Fig. 4.45). This tendon is the combined insertion of the transversus abdominis and internal oblique muscles into the pubic crest and pectineal line.

As with the internal oblique muscle's reinforcement of the area of the deep inguinal ring, the position of the conjoint tendon posterior to the superficial inguinal ring provides additional support to a potential point of weakness in the anterior abdominal wall.

Roof

The roof (superior wall) of the inguinal canal is formed by the arching fibers of the transversus abdominis and internal oblique muscles (Fig. 4.45 and 4.46). They pass from their lateral points of origin from the inguinal ligament to their common medial attachment as the conjoint tendon.

Floor

The floor (inferior wall) of the inguinal canal is formed by the medial one-half of the inguinal ligament. This rolled-under, free margin of the lowest part of the aponeurosis of the external oblique forms a gutter or trough on which the contents of the inguinal canal are positioned. The lacunar ligament reinforces most of the medial part of the gutter (Fig. 4.29).

Contents

The contents of the inguinal canal are

- The spermatic cord in men
- The round ligament of the uterus and genital branch of the genitofemoral nerve in women

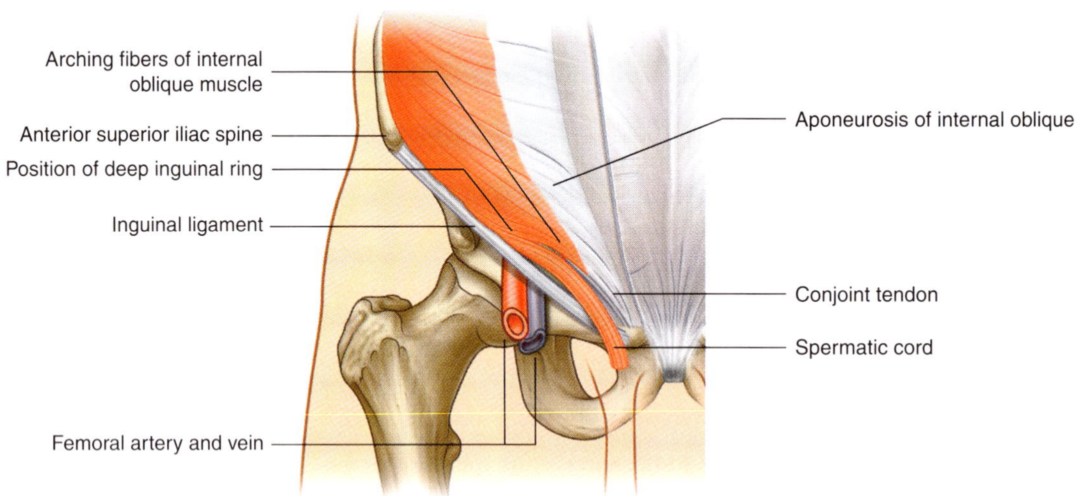

Fig. 4.45 Internal oblique muscle and the inguinal canal.

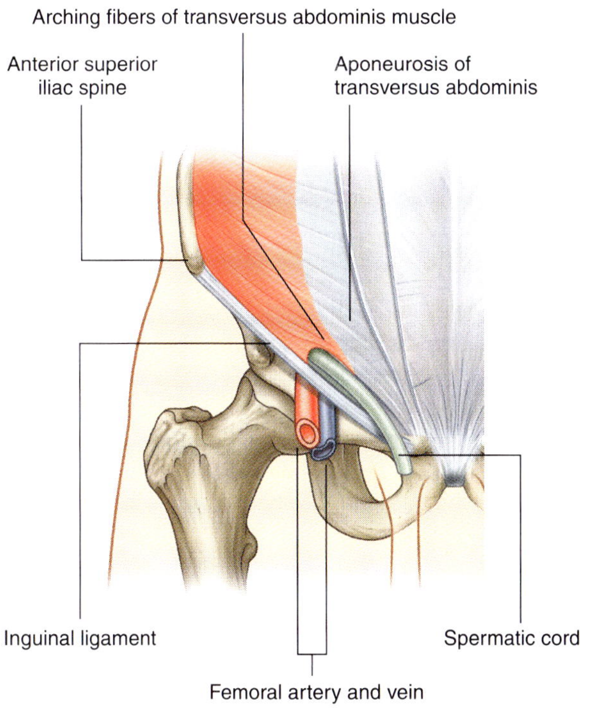

Fig. 4.46 Transversus abdominis muscle and the inguinal canal.

These structures enter the inguinal canal through the deep inguinal ring and exit it through the superficial inguinal ring.

Additionally, the ilioinguinal nerve (L1) passes through part of the inguinal canal. This nerve is a branch of the lumbar plexus, enters the abdominal wall posteriorly by piercing the internal surface of the transversus abdominis muscle, and continues through the layers of the anterior abdominal wall by piercing the internal oblique muscle. As it continues to pass inferomedially, it enters the inguinal canal. It continues down the canal to exit through the superficial inguinal ring (Fig. 4.37).

Spermatic cord

The spermatic cord begins to form proximally at the deep inguinal ring and consists of structures passing between the abdominopelvic cavities and the testis, and the three fascial coverings that enclose these structures (Fig. 4.47A).

The structures in the spermatic cord include:

- The ductus deferens
- The artery to the ductus deferens (from the inferior vesical artery)
- The testicular artery (from the abdominal aorta)
- The pampiniform plexus of veins (which converges at the deep inguinal ring to form the testicular veins)
- The cremasteric artery and vein (small vessels associated with the cremasteric fascia which are connected to the inferior epigastric vessels)
- The genital branch of the genitofemoral nerve (innervation to the cremasteric muscle)
- Sympathetic and visceral afferent nerve fibers
- Lymphatics draining the testis to the lumbar lymph nodes
- Remnants of the processus vaginalis

These structures enter the deep inguinal ring, proceed down the inguinal canal, and exit from the superficial inguinal ring, having acquired the three fascial coverings during their journey. This collection of structures and fascias continues into the scrotum where the structures connect with the testes and the fascias surround the testes.

Three fascias enclose the contents of the spermatic cord:

- The internal spermatic fascia, which is the deepest layer, arises from the transversalis fascia and is attached to the margins of the deep inguinal ring.
- The cremasteric fascia with the associated cremasteric muscle, which is the middle fascial layer, arises from the internal oblique muscle.
- The external spermatic fascia, which is the most superficial covering of the spermatic cord, arises from the aponeurosis of the external oblique muscle and is attached to the margins of the superficial inguinal ring (Fig. 4.47A).

Round ligament of the uterus

The round ligament of the uterus is a cord-like structure that passes from the uterus to the deep inguinal ring where it enters the inguinal canal (Fig. 4.47B). It passes down the inguinal canal and exits through the superficial inguinal ring. At this point, its structure is in the form of a few strands of tissue, which attach to the connective tissue associated with the labia majora. As it traverses the inguinal canal, it acquires the same coverings as the spermatic cord in men.

The round ligament of the uterus is the long distal part of the original gubernaculum in the fetus that extends from the ovary to the labioscrotal swellings. From its attachment to the uterus, a ligament continues to the ovary called the ligament of the ovary that develops from the short proximal part of the gubernaculum.

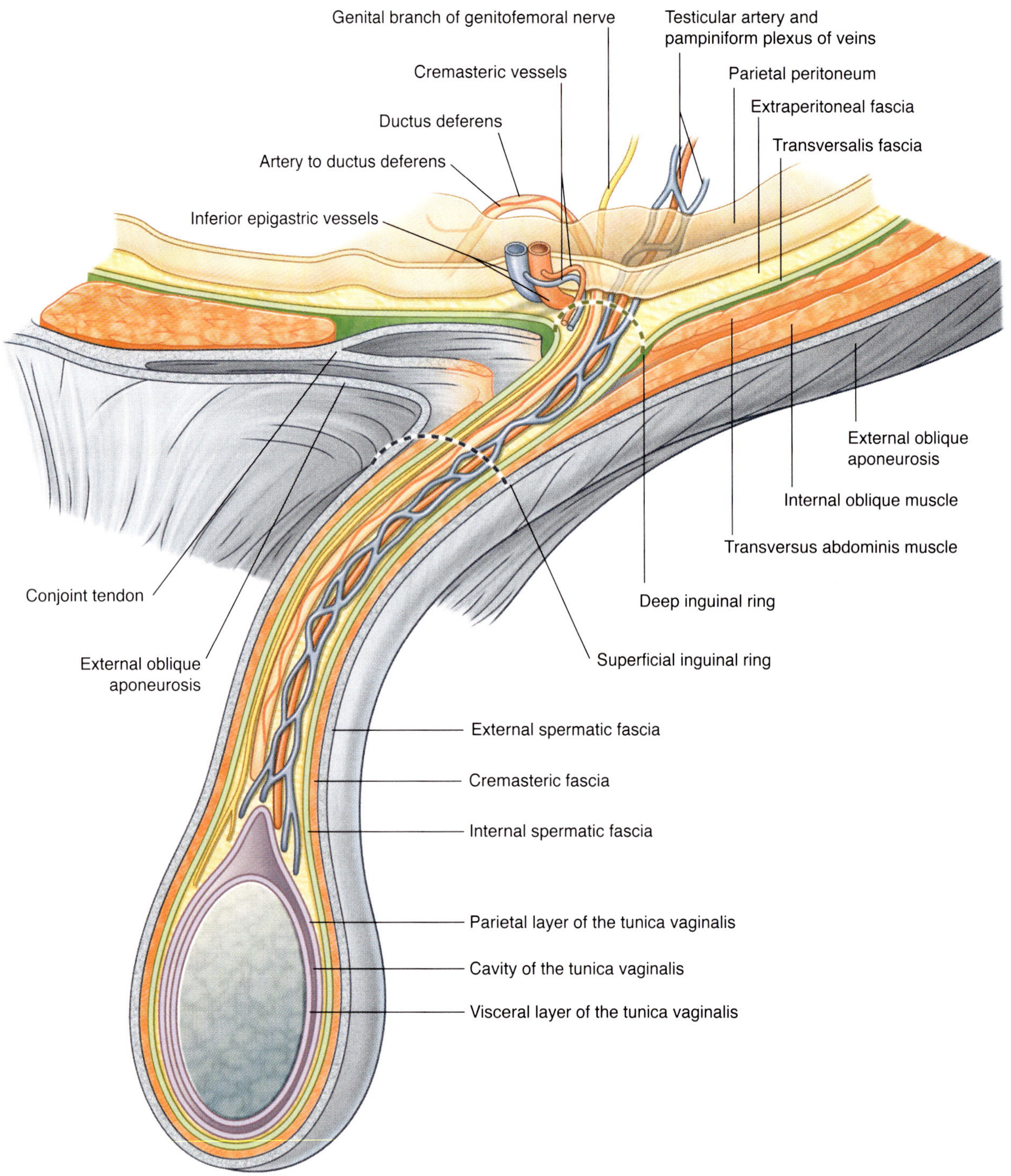

Fig. 4.47(A) Spermatic cord (men).

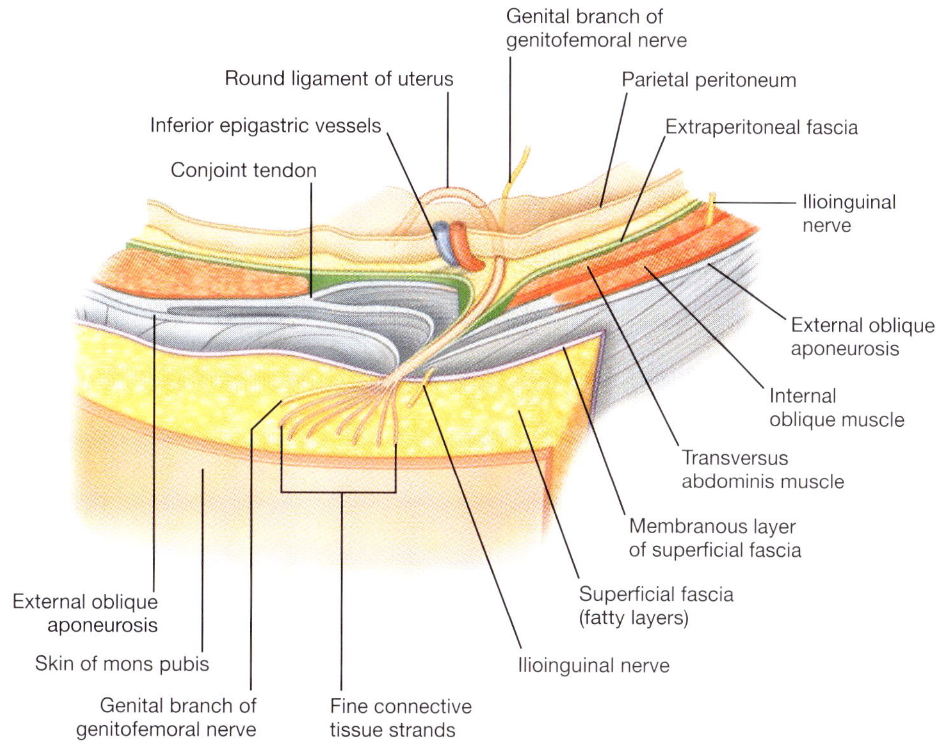

Fig. 4.47(B) Round ligament of uterus (women).

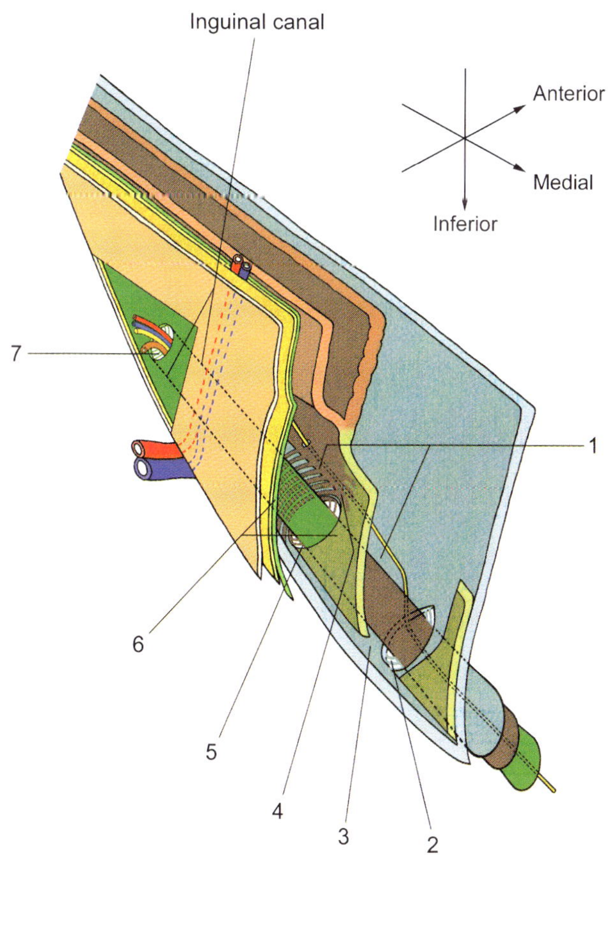

LD Fig. 4.47A.1 Left inguinal canal viewed from the posterior, medial and inferior aspect showing its walls and the coverings of the spermatic cord. Parts of the posterior wall have been removed.

Questions

LD Fig. 4.47A.1.A At each of the areas labelled 1, 3, 4, and 6, name the wall of the inguinal canal that is indicated and how it is formed at that location.

LD Fig. 4.47A.1.B At each of the areas labelled 2, 5, and 7, name the coverings of the spermatic cord and the structure from which it is derived.

LD Fig. 4.47.1C Which boundary of the inguinal triangle (Hesselbach's triangle) is not seen? How are the other boundaries formed? Why is this triangle important clinically?

Answers

LD Fig. 4.47A.1.A At 1, the anterior wall is formed by the internal oblique muscle and the aponeurosis of the external oblique; at 3, the floor is formed by the inguinal ligament; at 4, the roof is formed by the fibres of the internal oblique that arch from anterior to posterior; and at 6, the posterior wall is formed by the transversalis fascia and conjoint tendon.

LD Fig. 4.47A.1.B At 2, the external spermatic fascia is derived from the external oblique aponeurosis; at 5, the cremaster is derived from internal oblique; and at 7, the internal spermatic fascia is derived from the transversalis fascia.

LD Fig. 4.47.1C The medial boundary, which is formed by the lateral border of rectus abdominis is not seen.

The inferior boundary is formed by the inguinal ligament, and the medial boundary by the inferior epigastric vessels.

This triangle is the location where a direct inguinal hernia may occur if abdominal viscera push the posterior wall of the inguinal canal forwards into the inguinal canal.

Early clinical exposure

Cremasteric reflex

In men, the cremaster muscle and cremasteric fascia form the middle or second covering of the spermatic cord. This muscle and its associated fascia are supplied by the genital branch of the genitofemoral nerve (L1/L2). Contraction of this muscle and the resulting elevation of the testis can be stimulated by a reflex arc. Gently touching the skin at and around the anterior aspect of the superior part of the thigh stimulates the sensory fibers in the ilio-inguinal nerve. These sensory fibers enter the spinal cord at level L1. At this level, the sensory fibers stimulate the motor fibers carried in the genital branch of the genitofemoral nerve, which results in contraction of the cremaster muscle and elevation of the testis.

The cremasteric reflex is more active in children, tending to diminish with age. As with many reflexes, it may be absent in certain neurological disorders. Although it can be used for testing spinal cord function at level L1 in men, its clinical use is limited.

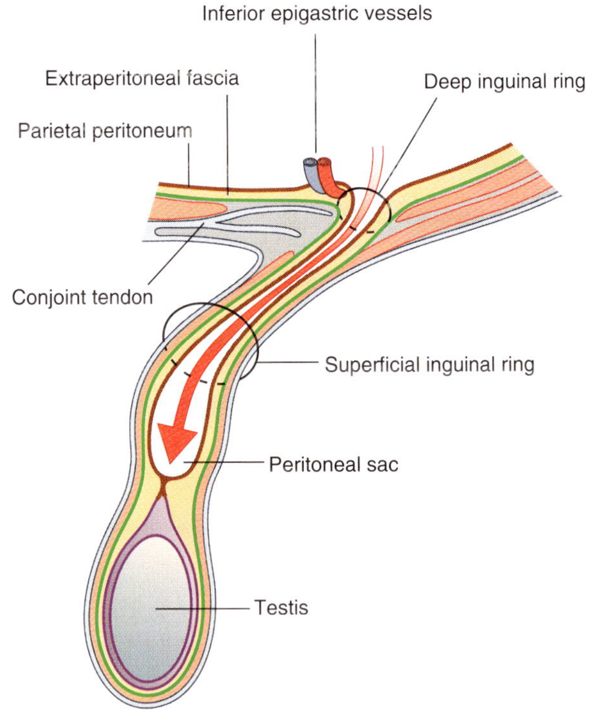

Fig. 4.48 Indirect inguinal hernia.

Inguinal hernias

An inguinal hernia is the protrusion or passage of a peritoneal sac, with or without abdominal contents, through a weakened part of the abdominal wall in the groin. It occurs because the peritoneal sac enters the inguinal canal either:

- Through the deep inguinal ring or
- Directly, through the posterior wall of the inguinal canal

Inguinal hernias are therefore classified as either indirect or direct.

Indirect inguinal hernias

The indirect inguinal hernia is the most common of the two types of inguinal hernia and is much more common in men than in women (Fig. 4.48). It occurs because some part, or all, of the embryonic processus vaginalis remains open or patent. It is therefore referred to as being congenital in origin.

The protruding peritoneal sac enters the inguinal canal by passing through the deep inguinal ring. The neck of the sac is the proximal part of the protrusion. It is located just lateral to the inferior epigastric vessels. The extent of its excursion down the inguinal canal depends on the amount of processus vaginalis that remains patent. If the entire processus vaginalis remains patent, the peritoneal sac may traverse the length of the inguinal canal, exit the superficial inguinal ring, and continue into the scrotum in men or the labia majus in women. In this case, the protruding peritoneal sac acquires the same three coverings as those associated with the spermatic cord in men or the round ligament of the uterus in women.

Direct inguinal hernias

A peritoneal sac that enters the medial end of the inguinal canal directly through a weakened posterior wall is a direct inguinal hernia (Fig. 4.49). It is usually described as acquired because it develops when abdominal musculature has been weakened, and is commonly seen in elderly men. The bulging and the neck of the hernia sac occur medial to the inferior epigastric vessels in the inguinal triangle (Hesselbach's triangle), which is bounded:

- Laterally by the inferior epigastric artery
- Medially by the rectus abdominis muscle
- Inferiorly by the inguinal ligament (Fig. 4.50A)

Internally, a thickening of the transversalis fascia (the iliopubic tract) follows the course of the inguinal ligament (Fig. 4.50A).

This type of inguinal hernia does not usually traverse the entire length of the inguinal canal. If it exits through the superficial inguinal ring, the peritoneal sac acquires a layer of external spermatic fascia and can extend, like an indirect hernia, into the scrotum.

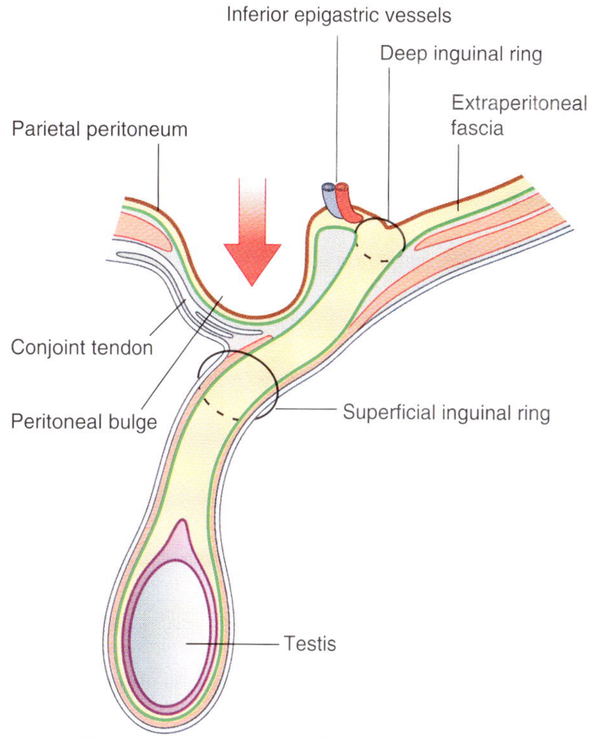

Fig. 4.49 Direct inguinal hernia.

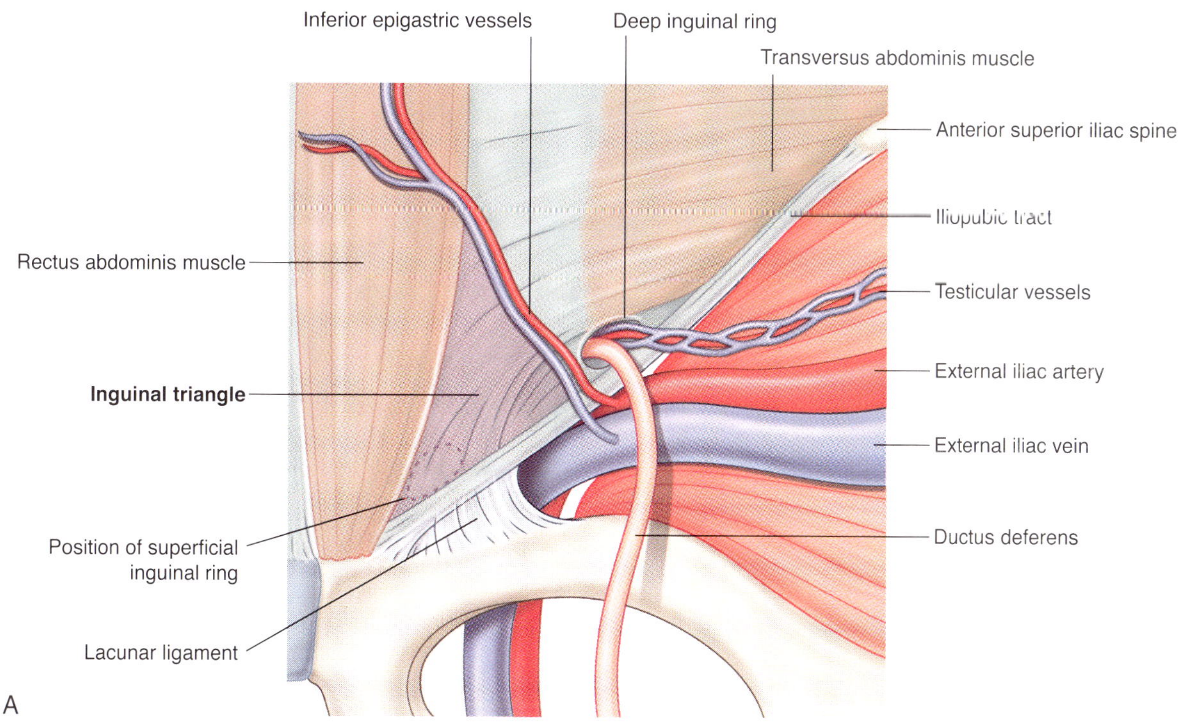

Fig. 4.50 Right inguinal triangle. **(A)** Internal view.

Continued

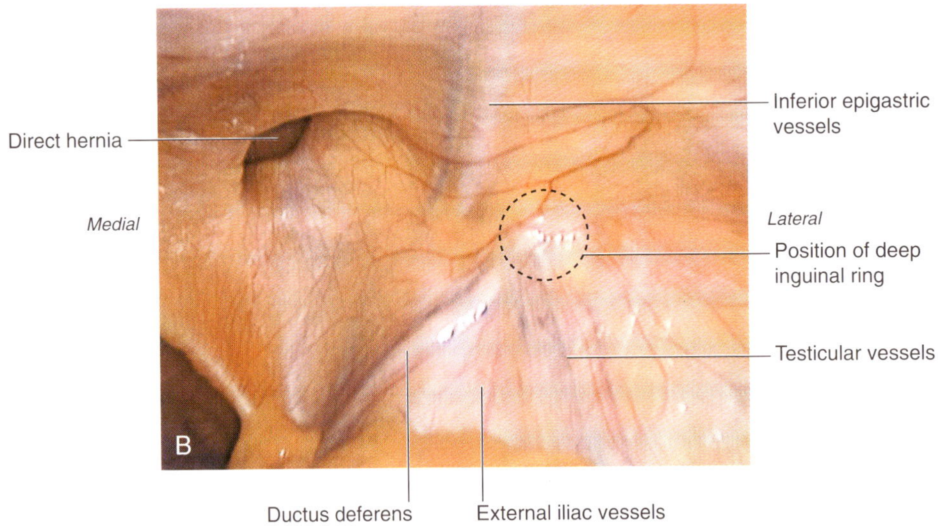

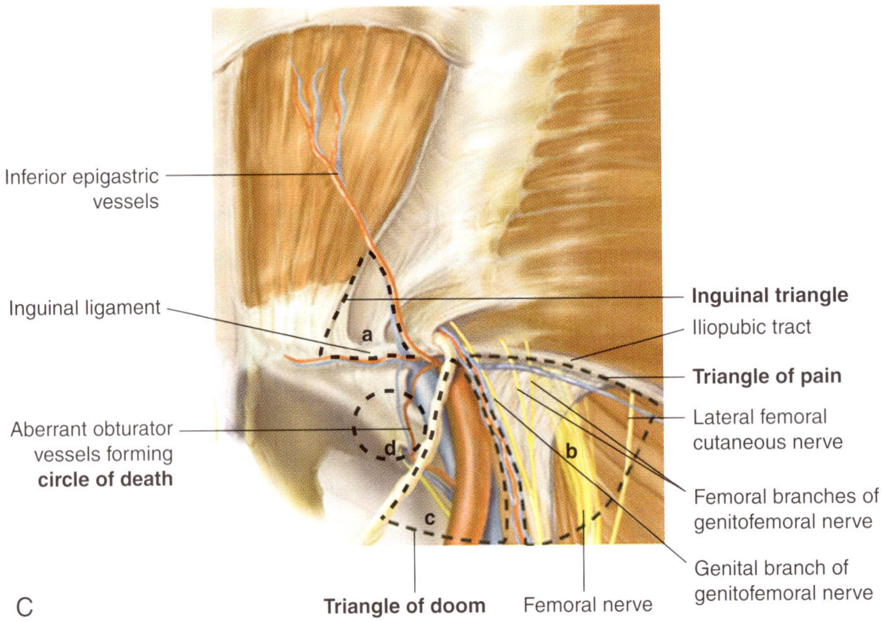

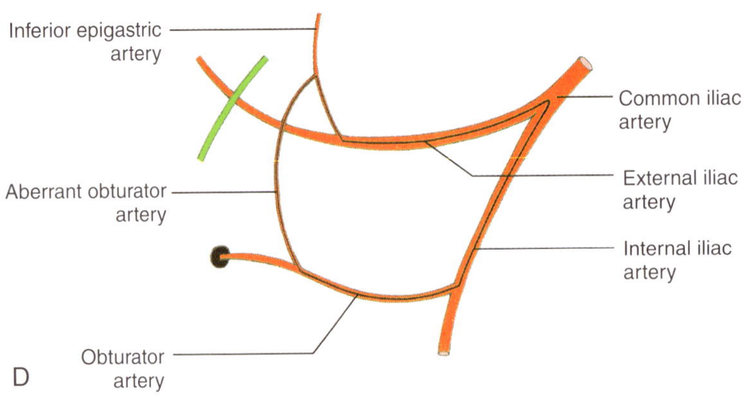

Fig. 4.50, cont'd **(B)** Laparoscopic view showing the parietal peritoneum still covering the area. **(C)** Laparoscopic view showing the (a) inguinal triangle, (b) triangle of doom, (c) triangle of pain, and (d) circle of death. **(D)** Lateral view showing the aberrant obturator artery forming the circle of death. *Source:* **(C)** Triangle for pain: JL Cameron, AM Cameron. Laparoscopic Inguinal Herniorrhaphy. 10ed. 2011.

Danger areas of the inguinal region

Three danger areas are of concern during surgery in the inguinal region, namely the triangle of doom, the triangle of pain, and circle of death. The apices of the two triangles are at the deep inguinal ring. Together, both these triangles form the quadrilateral of disaster and are separated by the gonadal vessels (Fig. 4.50C). If staples or sutures are placed in the triangle of doom, it can injure the external iliac vessels, which can be fatal; and if they are placed in the triangle of pain, it can injure the nerves present there and result in pain. Surgery in the region of the lacunar ligament may injure an artery which may be present (the aberrant obturator artery, which forms the circle of death), and can result in fatal hemorrhage. The **triangle of doom** is bounded medially by the ductus deferens, laterally by the gonadal vessels, and posteriorly by a reflection of peritoneum. The contents of the triangle include the external iliac vessels. The **triangle of pain** is bounded inferomedially by the gonadal vessels, superolaterally by the iliopubic tract, and posteriorly by a reflection of peritoneum. The contents of the triangle include the following nerves: femoral branch of genitofemoral nerve, anterior femoral cutaneous nerve, lateral femoral cutaneous nerve, and femoral nerve.

The **circle of death**, crown of death, or corona mortis is occasionally present if there is a large anastomosis between the inferior epigastric artery and the obturator artery (the aberrant obturator artery) behind the lacunar ligament. The circle of death is formed by the common iliac artery, external and internal iliac arteries, obturator artery, aberrant obturator artery, and inferior epigastric artery (Fig. 4.50D).

Early clinical exposure

Masses at the groin

Around the groin, there is a complex confluence of anatomical structures. Careful examination and good anatomical knowledge allows determination of the correct anatomical structure from which the mass arises and therefore the diagnosis. The most common masses in the groin are hernias.

The key to groin examination is determining the position of the inguinal ligament. The inguinal ligament passes between the anterior superior iliac spine laterally and the pubic tubercle medially. Inguinal hernias are above the inguinal ligament and are usually more apparent on standing. A visual assessment of the lump is necessary, bearing in mind the anatomical landmarks of the inguinal ligament.

In men, it is wise to examine the scrotum to check for a lump. If an abnormal mass is present, an inability to feel its upper edge suggests that it may originate from the inguinal canal and might be a hernia. On placing the hand over the lump and asking the patient to cough, the lump bulges outward.

An attempt should be made to reduce the swelling by applying gentle, firm pressure over the lump. If the lump is reducible, the hand should be withdrawn and careful observation will reveal recurrence of the mass.

The position of an abnormal mass in the groin relative to the pubic tubercle is very important, as are the presence of increased temperature and pain, which may represent early signs of strangulation or infection.

As a general rule:

- An inguinal hernia appears through the superficial inguinal ring **above** the pubic tubercle and crest.
- A femoral hernia (as described on page 452 below) is a protrusion through the femoral canal **where the neck of the hernial sac is inferior and lateral** to the pubic tubercle.

A hernia is the protrusion of a viscus, in part or in whole, through a normal or abnormal opening. The viscus usually carries a covering of parietal peritoneum, which forms the lining of the hernial sac.

Inguinal hernias

Hernias occur in a variety of regions. The commonest site is the groin. In some patients, inguinal hernias are present from birth (congenital) and are caused by the persistence of the processus vaginalis and the passage of viscera through the inguinal canal. Acquired hernias occur in older patients and causes include raised intraabdominal pressure (e.g., from repeated coughing associated with lung disease), damage to nerves of the anterior abdominal wall (e.g., from surgical abdominal incisions), and weakening of the walls of the inguinal canal.

One of the potential problems with hernias is that bowel and fat may become stuck within the hernial sac. This can cause appreciable pain and bowel obstruction, necessitating urgent surgery. Another potential risk is **strangulation** of the hernia, in which the blood supply to the bowel is cut off at the neck of the hernial sac, rendering the bowel ischemic and susceptible to perforation (Fig. 4.51A).

The hernial sac of an **indirect inguinal hernia** enters the deep inguinal ring and passes through the inguinal canal. If the hernia is large enough, the hernial sac may emerge through the superficial inguinal ring. In men, such a hernia may extend into the scrotum (Fig. 4.51B).

The hernial sac of a **direct inguinal hernia** pushes forward through the posterior wall of the inguinal canal immediately

Continued

Early clinical exposure—cont'd

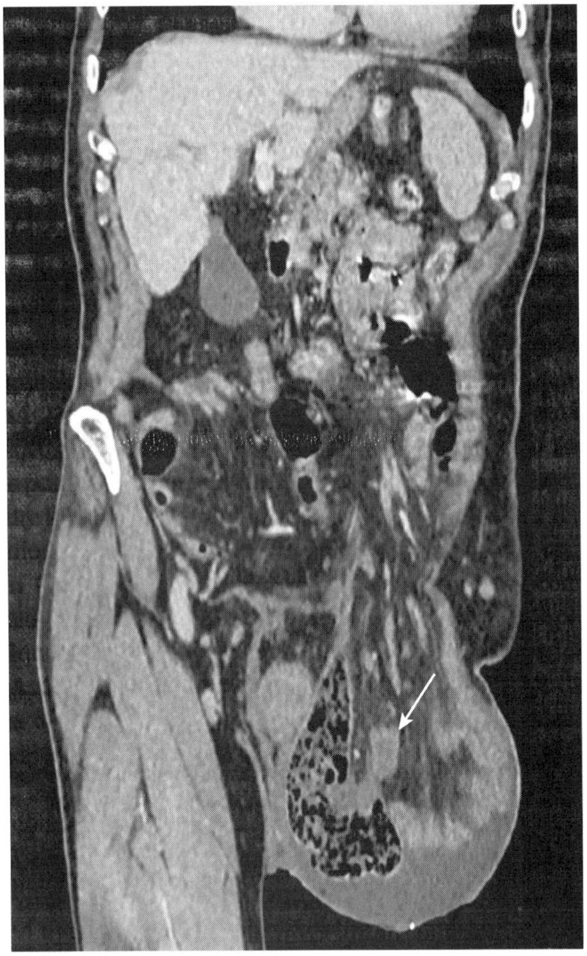

Fig. 4.51 (A) Coronal CT shows a large inguinal hernia containing loops of large and small bowel *(arrow)* on the left side of a male patient.

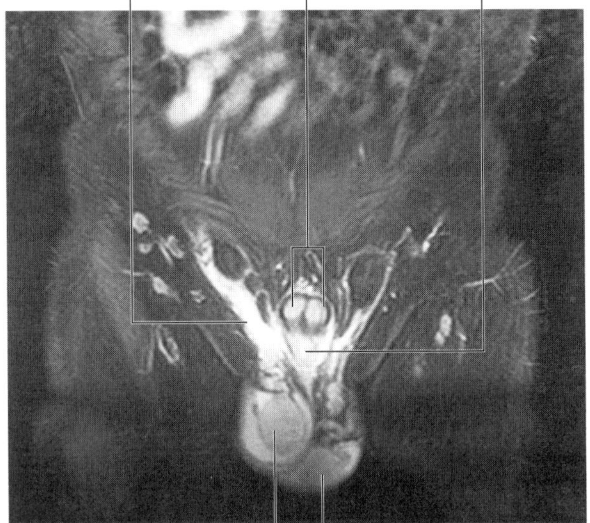

Fig. 4.51 (B) Right indirect inguinal hernia. T2, fat saturated, weighted magnetic resonance image in the coronal plane of a male groin.

posterior to the superficial inguinal ring. The hernia protrudes directly forward medial to the inferior epigastric vessels and through the superficial inguinal ring.

The differentiation between an indirect and a direct inguinal hernia is made during surgery when the inferior epigastric vessels are identified at the medial edge of the deep internal ring:

- An indirect hernial sac passes lateral to the inferior epigastric vessels.
- A direct hernia is medial to the inferior epigastric vessels.

Inguinal hernias occur more commonly in men than in women possibly because men have a much larger inguinal canal than women.

When the intraabdominal pressure increases, the mechanisms that **tend to prevent an inguinal hernia** include the following: (1) the arching fibers of internal oblique and transversus abdominis are pulled down while the inguinal ligament is pulled upward (shutter action); (2) the two pillars of the sling formed by condensations of the fascia transversalis (which extend superolaterally) at the deep inguinal ring are pulled together (shutter mechanism); (3) the anterior and posterior walls of the inguinal canal are pressed together, and where there is a deficiency in one wall, the opposite wall is strengthened (valvular mechanism); and (4) the spermatic cord is pulled upward tending to plug the inguinal canal (plugging mechanism).

Femoral hernias

A **femoral hernia** passes through the femoral canal and into the medial aspect of the anterior thigh. The femoral canal lies at the medial edge of the femoral sheath, which contains the femoral artery, femoral vein, and lymphatics. The neck of the femoral canal is extremely narrow and is prone to trapping bowel within the sac, so making this type of hernia irreducible and susceptible to bowel strangulation. Femoral

Early clinical exposure—cont'd

hernias are usually acquired, are not congenital, and most commonly occur in middle-aged and elderly populations. In addition, because women generally have wider pelvises than men, they tend to occur more commonly in women.

Sportsmen's groin/sportsmen's hernia

The groin can loosely be defined as the area where the leg meets the trunk near the midline. Here the abdominal muscles of the trunk blend in with the adductor muscles of the thigh, the medial end of the inguinal ligament attaches to the pubic tubercle, the pubic symphysis attaches the two pubic bones together, and the superficial (external) inguinal ring is present. It also is in and around this region where there is considerable translation of force during most athletic and sporting activities. Pain in the groin or pubic region can be due to numerous causes, which include inflammatory changes at the pubic symphysis, problems at the insertion of the rectus abdominis/adductor longus, and hernias.

Umbilical hernias

Umbilical hernias are rare. Occasionally, they are congenital and result from failure of the small bowel to return to the abdominal cavity from the umbilical cord during development. After birth, umbilical hernias may result from incomplete closure of the umbilicus (navel). Overall, most of these hernias close in the first year of life, and surgical repair is not generally attempted until later.

Paraumbilical hernias may occur in adults at and around the umbilicus and often have small necks, and so require surgical treatment.

Incisional hernias

Incisional hernias occur through a defect in a scar of a previous abdominal operation. Usually, the necks of these hernias are wide and do not therefore strangulate the viscera they contain.

Other hernias

An **internal hernia** is a protrusion of the viscera through the peritoneum or mesentery, but remaining within the abdominal cavity. It includes paraduodenal, pericecal, foramen of Winslow and intersigmoid hernias.

A **spigelian hernia** passes forward near the arcuate line and lateral to the lateral border of the rectus abdominis at the lower part of the posterior rectus sheath. It may appear as a tender mass on one side of the lower anterior abdominal wall.

Abdominopelvic cavity hernias can also develop in association with the pelvic walls, and sites include the obturator canal, the greater sciatic foramen and above and below the piriformis muscle.

Abdomen

ABDOMINAL VISCERA

Peritoneum

SET INDUCTION—CASE SCENARIO 3: PERITONITIS

A 40-year-old male was brought to the emergency department with a history of severe abdominal pain of sudden onset. On examination, he was found suffering from fever and rigidity of the anterior abdominal wall. A diagnosis of peritonitis was made after the X-ray showed pneumoperitoneum. Knowledge of the peritoneal cavity is needed to manage this case.

<table>
<tr><th rowspan="2">REMEMBER
[Recall Facts]</th><th colspan="3">OUTLINE 3. PERITONEUM—LEARNING OBJECTIVES
[By the end of this section the student should be able to:]</th><th colspan="2" rowspan="2">EVALUATE
[Explain Concepts]</th></tr>
<tr><th colspan="3">DEMONSTRATE AND ANALYZE RELATIONSHIPS
[Identify structures in a Prosected Specimen or Figure]</th></tr>
<tr><td rowspan="6">1. List the intraperitoneal and extraperitoneal organs
2. Describe the difference between primary and secondary retroperitoneal organs
3. Describe the innervations of the peritoneum
4. Describe briefly the difference between the greater sac and lesser sac
5. Mention the boundaries of the epiploic foramen
6. Name the omenta, mesenteries, and peritoneal ligaments
7. Name the parts of the greater and lesser omentum
8. Describe the transverse mesocolon and sigmoid mesocolon
9. Describe briefly the supracolic and infracolic compartments</td><td>Level I</td><td>Level II</td><td>Level III</td><td colspan="2" rowspan="2">■ Subdivision of peritoneal cavity into compartments
■ Formation of greater and lesser sacs and their communication through the epiploic foramen
■ Free edge of the ventral mesentery</td></tr>
<tr><td rowspan="5">■ Peritoneal cavity
■ Peritoneum:
  ■ Visceral
  ■ Parietal
■ Greater omentum
■ On the posterior aspect of the anterior abdominal wall observe:
  ■ Falciform ligament
  ■ Ligamentum teres
  ■ Median, medial, and lateral umbilical folds
■ Transverse colon and mesocolon
■ Compartments—supracolic and infracolic
■ Lesser omentum
■ Epiploic foramen and its boundaries
■ Greater sac
■ Lesser sac
■ Subdiaphragmatic spaces—hepatorenal pouch
■ Paracolic gutters</td><td rowspan="5">■ Right and left gastro-omental vessels</td><td rowspan="5"></td></tr>
<tr><th colspan="2">EARLY CLINICAL EXPOSURE
[Apply Anatomical knowledge]</th></tr>
<tr><th>Surgical Anatomy/ Pathology/ Trauma</th><th>Imaging/ Surface Anatomy</th></tr>
<tr><td>■ Ascites
■ Peritonitis
■ Peritoneal dialysis
■ Subphrenic spaces
■ Ventriculoperitoneal shunt
■ Pneumoperitoneum</td><td>Ultrasound examination to detect collections of fluid</td></tr>
<tr><td colspan="2">PROBLEM SOLVING/ CLINICAL CASES [Interpret]
■ Describe the applied anatomy of the subdiaphragmatic spaces</td></tr>
</table>

A thin membrane (the peritoneum) lines the walls of the abdominal cavity and covers much of the viscera. The parietal peritoneum lines the walls of the cavity and the visceral peritoneum covers the viscera. Between the parietal and visceral layers of peritoneum is a potential space (the peritoneal cavity). Abdominal viscera either are suspended in the peritoneal cavity by folds of peritoneum (**mesenteries**) or are outside the peritoneal cavity. Organs suspended in the cavity are referred to as intraperitoneal (Fig. 4.52 and 4.6); organs outside the peritoneal cavity, with only one surface or part of one surface covered by peritoneum, are retroperitoneal.

Intraperitoneal organs include the stomach, proximal 2 cm of the duodenum, jejunum, ileum, cecum, appendix, transverse colon, sigmoid colon, liver, gallbladder, tail of pancreas, and spleen. The **primary retroperitoneal organs** include the kidneys, ureter, and suprarenal. The **secondary retroperitoneal organs** include the duodenum (except the proximal 2 cm), ascending colon, descending colon, pancreas (except the tail), and the rectum.

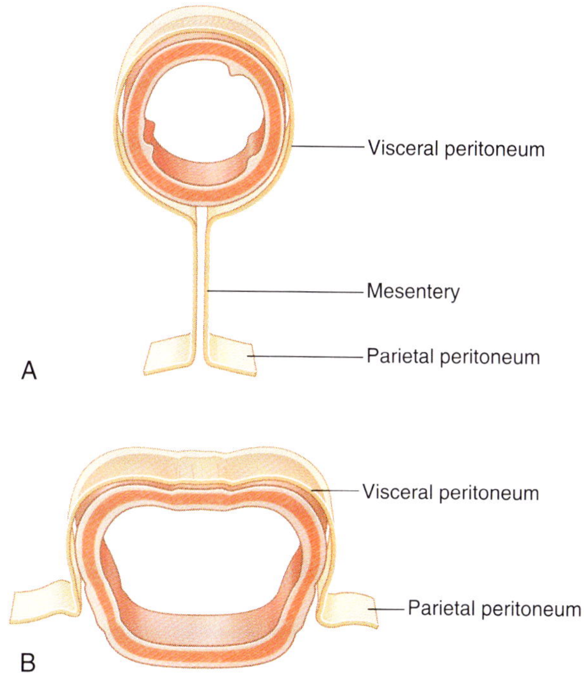

Fig. 4.52 **(A)** Intraperitoneal. **(B)** Retroperitoneal.

Innervation of the peritoneum

The parietal peritoneum associated with the abdominal wall is innervated by somatic afferents carried in branches of the associated spinal nerves and is therefore sensitive to well-localized pain. The visceral peritoneum is innervated by visceral afferents that accompany autonomic nerves (sympathetic and parasympathetic) back to the central nervous system. Activation of these fibers can lead to referred and poorly localized sensations of discomfort, and to reflex visceral motor activity.

Peritoneal cavity

The peritoneal cavity is subdivided into the greater sac and the omental bursa (lesser sac; Fig. 4.53).

- The **greater sac** accounts for most of the space in the peritoneal cavity, beginning superiorly at the diaphragm and continuing inferiorly into the pelvic cavity. It is entered once the parietal peritoneum has been penetrated.
- The **omental bursa** is a smaller subdivision of the peritoneal cavity posterior to the stomach and liver and is continuous with the greater sac through an opening, the omental (epiploic) foramen (Fig. 4.54A).

Surrounding the **omental** (epiploic) foramen or foramen of Winslow are numerous structures covered with peritoneum. They include the portal vein, hepatic artery proper, and bile duct anteriorly; the inferior vena cava posteriorly; the caudate lobe of the liver superiorly; and the first part of the duodenum inferiorly.

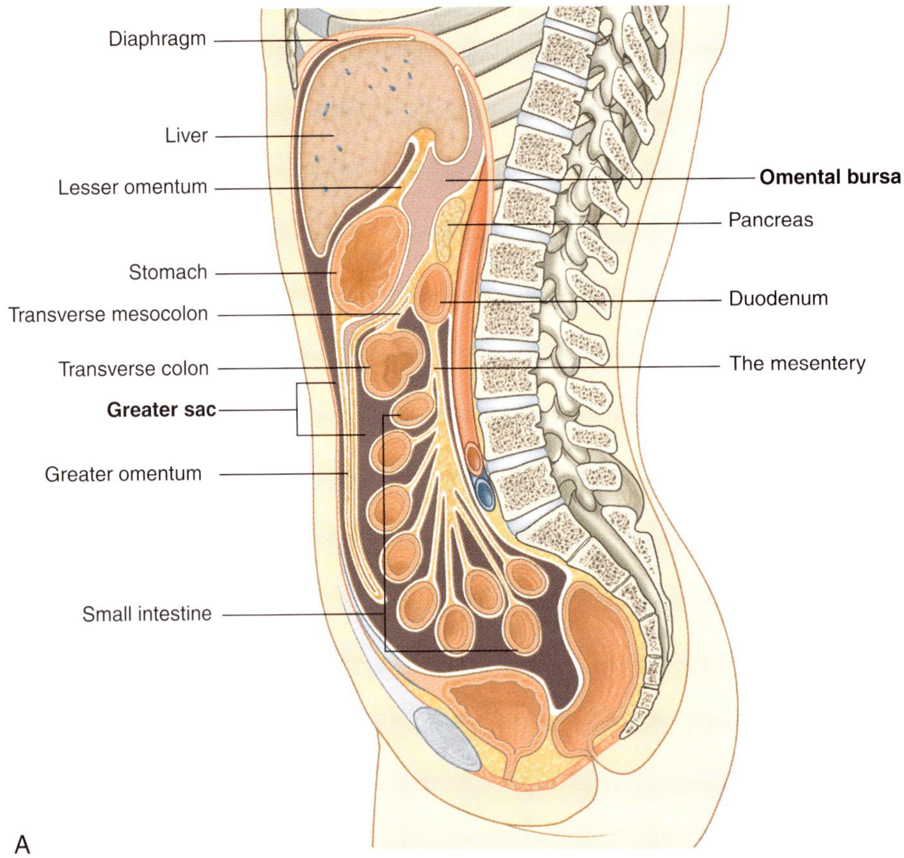

A

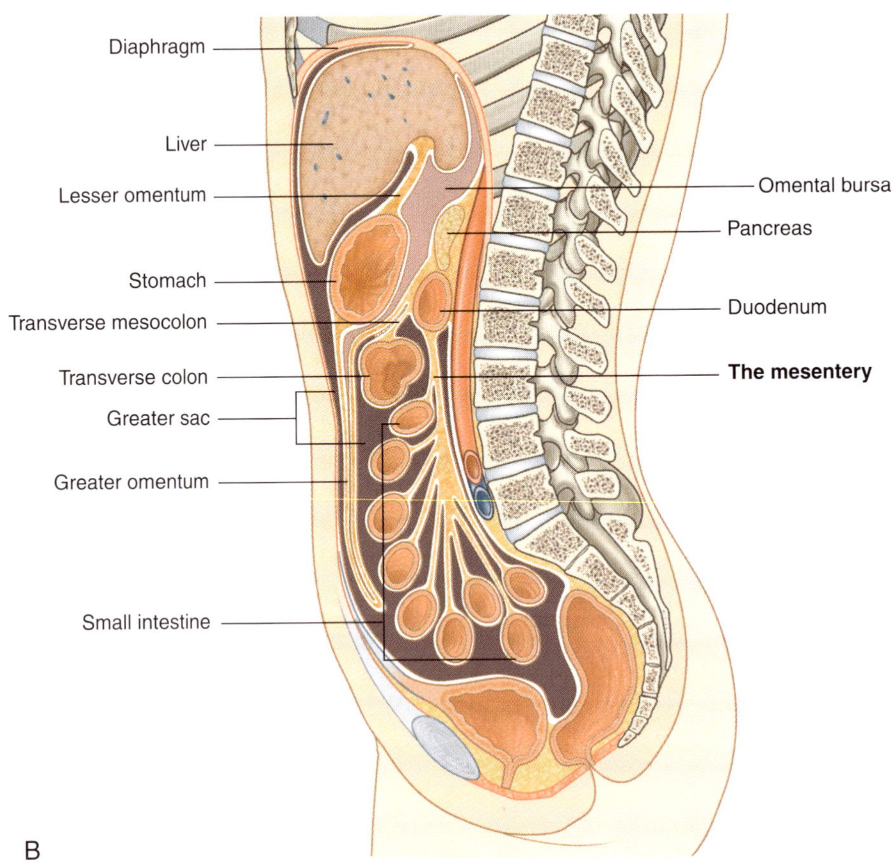

B

Fig. 4.53 **(A)** Greater and lesser sacs of the peritoneal cavity. **(B)** The mesentery.

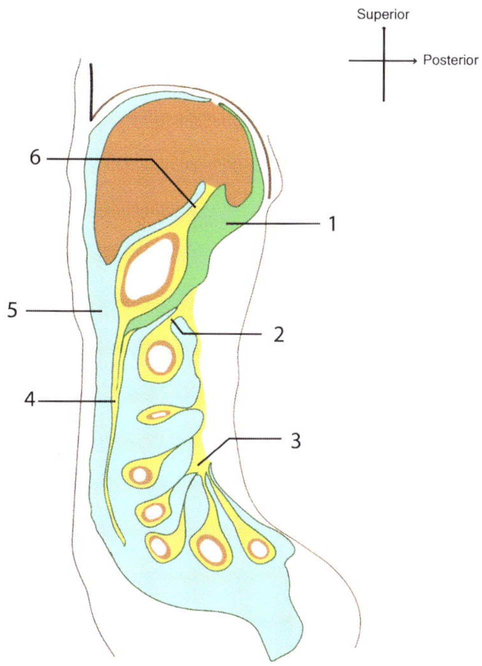

LD Fig. 4.53.1 Sagittal section showing the greater and lesser sacs.
Questions
LD Fig. 4.53.1A Name the labelled structures.
LD Fig. 4.53.1B What are the two main subdivisions of "5"?

Answers
LD Fig. 4.53.1A
1. Lesser sac
2. Transverse mesocolon
3. The mesentery
4. Greater omentum
5. Greater sac
6. Lesser omentum

LD Fig. 4.53.1B The main subdivisions of the greater sac are the supracolic and infracolic compartments.

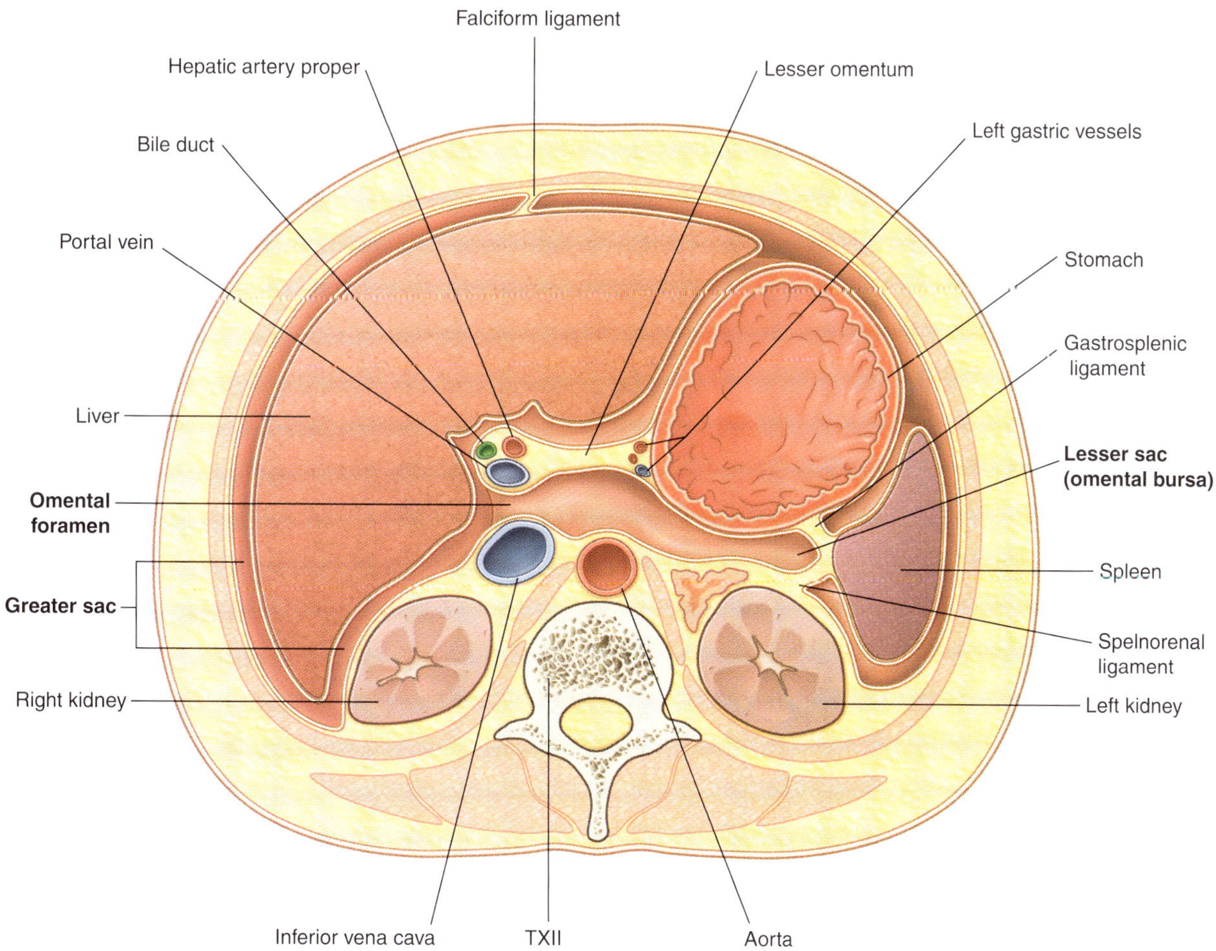

Fig. 4.54(A) Transverse section illustrating the continuity between the greater and lesser sacs through the omental (epiploic) foramen.

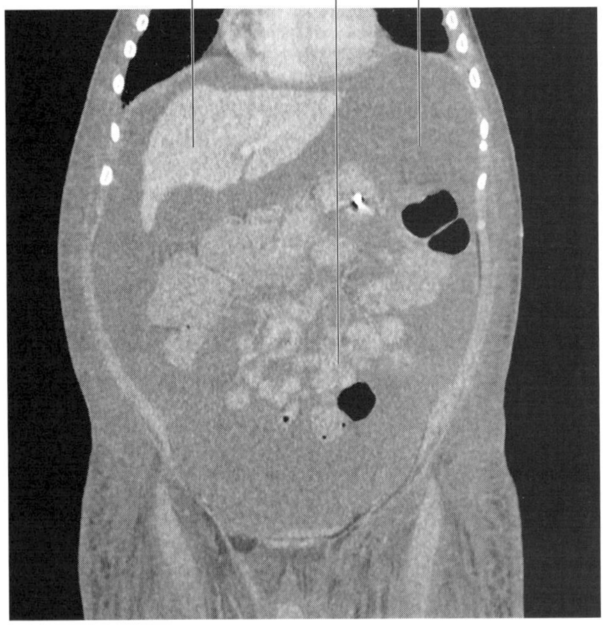

Fig. 4.54(B) Coronal CT shows ascites fluid in abdominal cavity.

Early clinical exposure

Peritoneum

A small volume of peritoneal fluid within the peritoneal cavity lubricates movement of the viscera suspended in the abdominal cavity. It is not detectable on any available imaging such as ultrasound or computed tomography (CT). In various pathological conditions (e.g., in liver cirrhosis, acute pancreatitis, or heart failure), the volume of peritoneal fluid can increase; this is known as ascites. In cases of high volume of free intraperitoneal fluid, marked abdominal distention can be observed (Fig. 4.54B).

The peritoneal space has a large surface area, which facilitates the spread of disease through the peritoneal cavity and over the bowel and visceral surfaces. Conversely, this large surface area can be used for administering certain types of treatment and a number of procedures.

Ventriculoperitoneal shunts

Patients with obstructive hydrocephalus (an excessive accumulation of cerebrospinal fluid within the cerebral ventricular system) require continuous drainage of this fluid. This is achieved by placing a fine-bore catheter through the skull into the cerebral ventricles and placing the extracranial part of the tube beneath the scalp and skin of the chest wall and then passing it through the abdominal wall into the peritoneal cavity. Cerebrospinal fluid drains through the tube into the peritoneal cavity, where it is absorbed.

Dialysis and peritoneal dialysis

People who develop renal failure require dialysis to live. There are two methods.

In the first method (**hemodialysis**), blood is taken from the circulation, dialyzed through a complex artificial membrane, and returned to the body. A high rate of blood flow is required to remove excess body fluid, exchange electrolytes, and remove noxious metabolites. To accomplish this, either an arteriovenous fistula is established surgically (by connecting an artery to a vein, usually in the upper limb, and requiring approximately 6 weeks to "mature") and is cannulated each time the patient returns for dialysis, or a large-bore cannula is placed into the right atrium, through which blood can be aspirated and returned.

In the second method of dialysis, the peritoneum is used as the dialysis membrane. The large surface area of the peritoneal cavity is an ideal dialysis membrane for fluid and electrolyte exchange. To accomplish dialysis, a small tube is inserted through the abdominal wall and dialysis fluid is injected into the peritoneal cavity. Electrolytes and molecules are exchanged across the peritoneum between the fluid and blood. Once dialysis is completed, the fluid is drained.

Peritoneal spread of disease

The large surface area of the peritoneal cavity allows infection and malignant disease to spread easily throughout the abdomen (Fig. 4.55A). If malignant cells enter the peritoneal cavity by direct invasion (e.g., from colon or ovarian cancer), spread may be rapid. Similarly, a surgeon excising a malignant tumor and releasing malignant cells into the peritoneal cavity may cause an appreciable worsening of the patient's prognosis. Infection can also spread across the large surface area.

Early clinical exposure—cont'd

The peritoneal cavity can also act as a barrier to, and container of, disease. Intraabdominal infection therefore tends to remain below the diaphragm rather than spread into other body cavities.

Perforated bowel

A perforated bowel (e.g., caused by a perforated duodenal ulcer) often leads to the release of gas into the peritoneal cavity (pneumoperitoneum). This free gas can be easily visualized on an erect chest radiograph—gas can be demonstrated in extremely small amounts beneath the diaphragm. A patient with severe abdominal pain and subdiaphragmatic free gas needs a laparotomy (Fig. 4.55B).

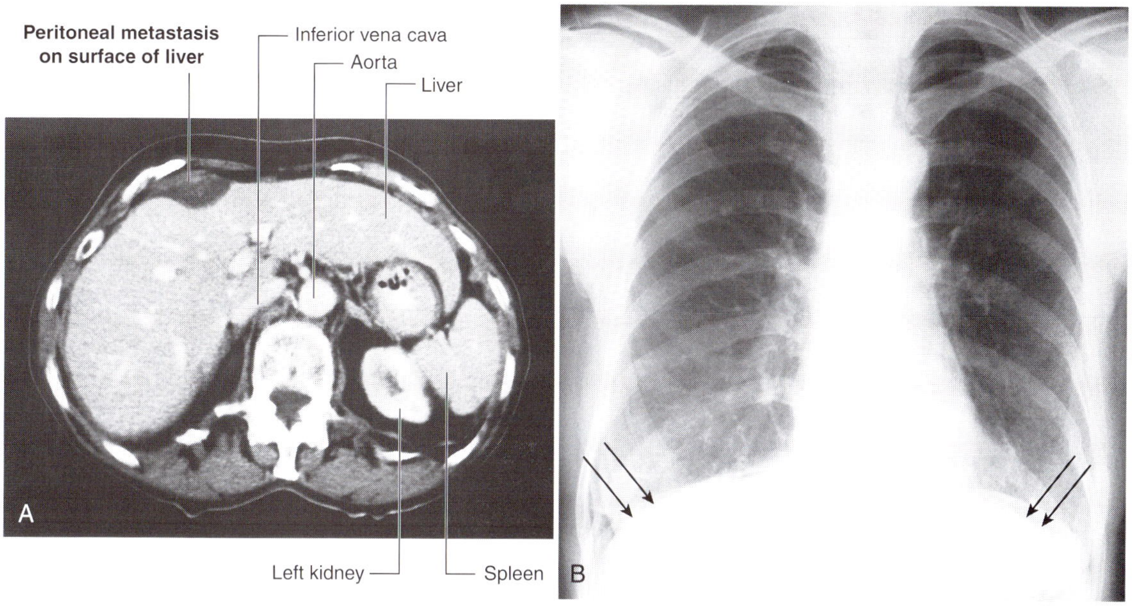

Fig. 4.55(A) Peritoneal metastasis on the surface of the liver. Computed tomogram in the axial plane of the upper abdomen. **(B)** X-ray showing free gas under the diaphragm (pneumoperitoneum) indicated by pointers.

Omenta, mesenteries, and ligaments

Throughout the peritoneal cavity, numerous peritoneal folds connect organs to each other or to the abdominal wall. These folds (omenta, mesenteries, and ligaments) develop from the original dorsal and ventral mesenteries, which suspend the developing gastrointestinal tract in the embryonic coelomic cavity. Some contain vessels and nerves supplying the viscera, while others help maintain the proper positioning of the viscera.

Omenta

The omenta consist of two layers of peritoneum, which pass from the stomach and the first part of the duodenum to other viscera:

- The greater omentum, derived from the dorsal mesentery
- The lesser omentum, derived from the ventral mesentery

Greater omentum

The **greater omentum** is a large, apron-like, peritoneal fold that attaches to the greater curvature of the stomach and the first part of the duodenum (Fig. 4.56). It drapes inferiorly over the transverse colon and the coils of the jejunum and ileum (see Fig. 4.53). Turning posteriorly, it ascends to associate with, and become adherent to, the peritoneum on the superior surface of the transverse colon (gastrocolic ligament). It is also adherent to the anterior layer of the transverse mesocolon before arriving at the posterior abdominal wall. The greater omentum also includes a part which extends to the spleen (gastrosplenic ligament) and a part attached to the diaphragm (gastrophrenic ligament).

Usually a thin membrane, the greater omentum always contains an accumulation of fat, which may become substantial in some individuals. Additionally, there are two arteries and accompanying veins, the **right** and **left gastro-omental vessels**, between this double-layered peritoneal apron just inferior to the greater curvature of the stomach (see Fig. 4.60).

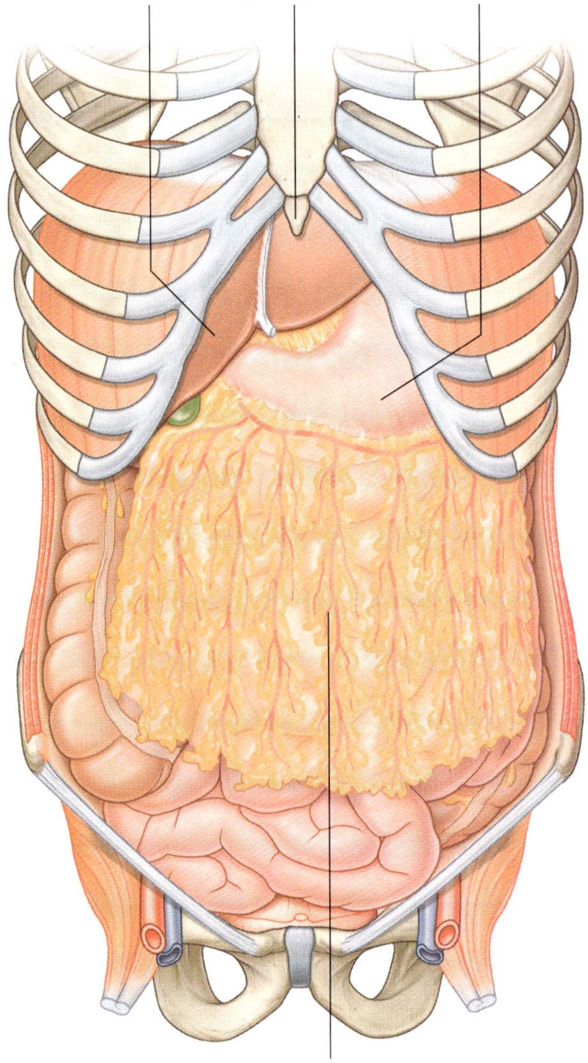

Fig. 4.56 Greater omentum.

Lesser omentum

The other two-layered peritoneal omentum is the **lesser omentum** (Fig. 4.57). It extends from the lesser curvature of the stomach and the first part of the duodenum to the inferior surface of the liver (Fig. 4.53 and 4.57).

It is a thin membrane continuous with the peritoneal coverings of the anterior and posterior surfaces of the stomach and the first part of the duodenum. It is divided into:

- A medial hepatogastric ligament, which passes between the stomach and liver
- A lateral hepatoduodenal ligament, which passes between the duodenum and liver (Fig. 4.57)

The hepatoduodenal ligament ends laterally as a free margin and serves as the anterior border of the omental foramen (Fig. 4.54A). It represents the lower free edge of the ventral mesentery (Fig. 4.17A). Enclosed in this free edge are the hepatic artery proper, the bile duct, and the portal vein. Additionally, the right and left gastric vessels are between the layers of the lesser omentum near the lesser curvature of the stomach.

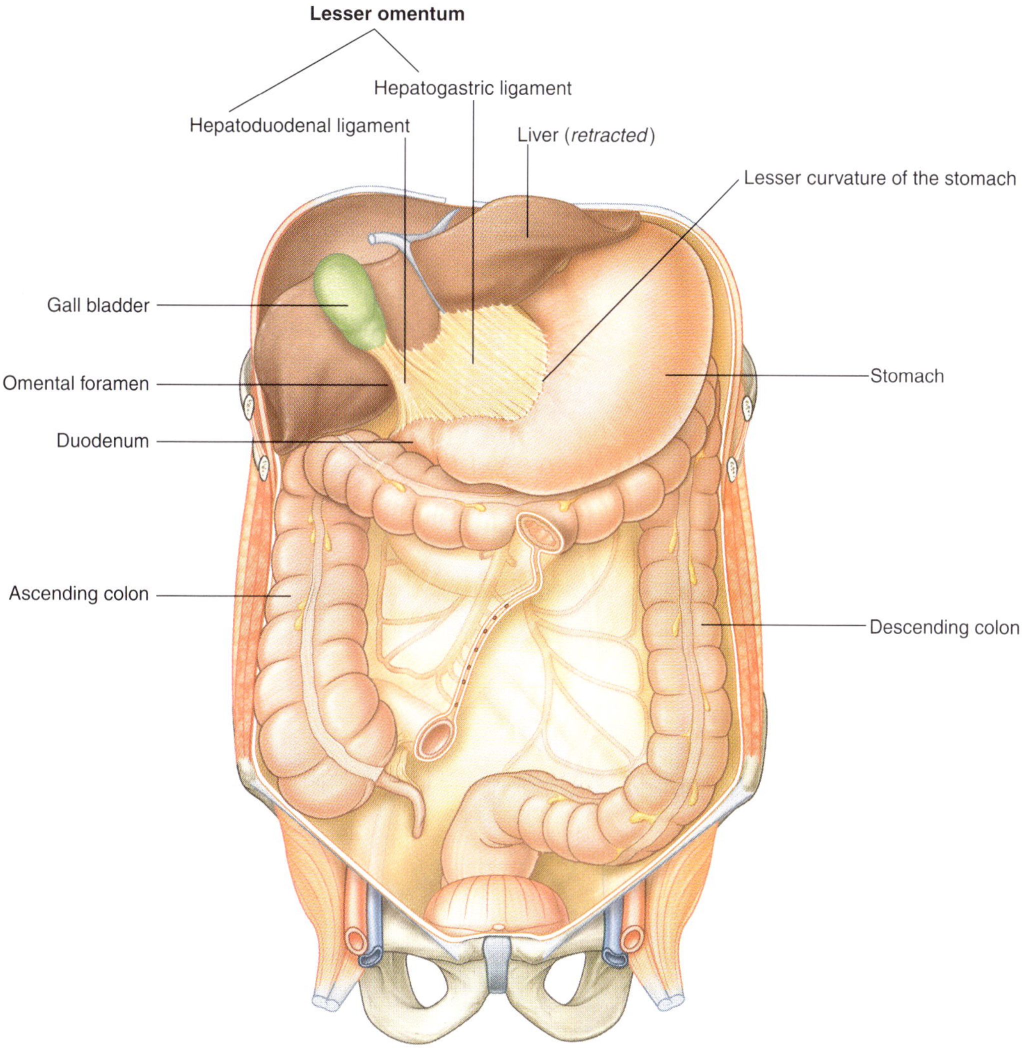

Fig. 4.57 Lesser omentum.

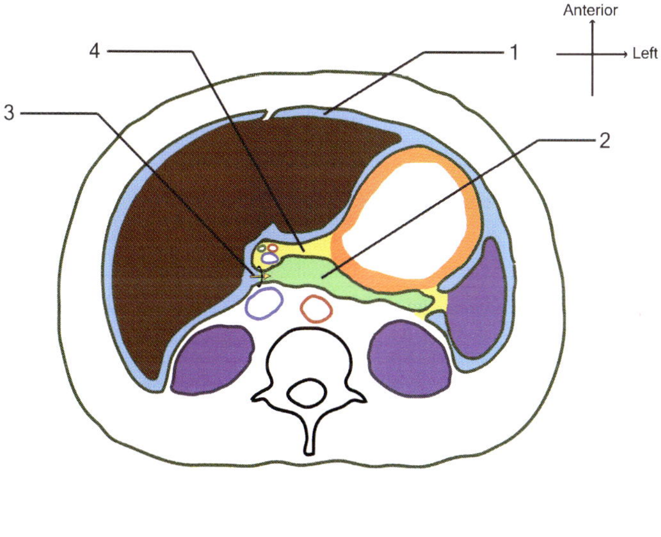

LD Fig. 4.57.1 Transverse section of the lesser sac at the level of the epiploic foramen.

Questions

LD Fig. 4.57A Name the labelled areas.

LD Fig. 4.57B Name two structures anterior to "2".

LD Fig. 4.57C Name two ligaments related to the left end of "2".

LD Fig. 4.57D List the anterior and posterior relations of "3".

LD Fig. 4.57E Name the structures seen here which are attached to the lesser and greater curvatures of the stomach.

Answers

LD Fig. 4.57A The labelled areas are:

1. Greater sac
2. Lesser sac
3. Epiploic foramen
4. Lesser omentum

LD Fig. 4.57B Two structures anterior to "2" are: Stomach and lesser omentum.

LD Fig. 4.57C Two ligaments at the left end of "2" are: Gastrosplenic and lienorenal ligaments.

LD Fig. 4.57D Anterior relations of "3" are the portal vein, bile duct and proper hepatic artery.

The posterior relation of "3" is the inferior vena cava.

LD Fig. 4.57E The lesser omentum is attached to the lesser curvature and the gastrosplenic ligament is attached to the greater omentum.

Early clinical exposure

The greater omentum

When a laparotomy is performed and the peritoneal cavity is opened, the first structure usually encountered is the greater omentum. This fatty double-layered vascular membrane hangs like an apron from the greater curvature of the stomach, drapes over the transverse colon, and lies freely suspended within the abdominal cavity. It is often referred to as the "**policeman of the abdomen**" because of its apparent ability to migrate to any inflamed area and wrap itself around the organ to wall off inflammation. When a part of bowel becomes inflamed, it ceases peristalsis. This aperistaltic area is referred to as a local paralytic ileus. The remaining noninflamed part of the bowel continues to move and "massages" the greater omentum to the region where there is no peristalsis. The localized inflammatory reaction spreads to the greater omentum, which then adheres to the diseased area of bowel.

The greater omentum is also an important site for metastatic tumor spread. Direct omental spread by a transcoelomic route is common for carcinoma of the ovary. As the metastases develop within the greater omentum, it becomes significantly thickened.

In CT imaging and during laparotomy, the thickened omentum is referred to as an "**omental cake**."

Mesenteries

Mesenteries are peritoneal folds that attach viscera to the posterior abdominal wall. They allow some movement and provide a conduit for vessels, nerves, and lymphatics to reach the viscera and include:

- The mesentery—associated with parts of the small intestine (Fig. 4.53)
- The transverse mesocolon—associated with the transverse colon
- The sigmoid mesocolon—associated with the sigmoid colon
- All of these are derivatives of the dorsal mesentery. The mesentery of the small and large intestine has recently been regarded as being contiguous, and a right and left mesocolon are described (Fig. 4.58B).

Mesentery

The mesentery is a large, fan-shaped, double-layered fold of peritoneum that connects the jejunum and ileum to the posterior abdominal wall (Fig. 4.58A). Its superior attachment is at the duodenojejunal junction, just to the left of the upper lumbar part of the vertebral column. It passes obliquely downward and to the right, ending at the ileocecal junction near the upper border of the right sacroiliac joint. In the fat between the two peritoneal layers of the mesentery are the arteries, veins, nerves, and lymphatics that supply the jejunum and ileum (Fig. 4.53B and 4.68).

Transverse mesocolon

The **transverse mesocolon** is a fold of peritoneum that connects the transverse colon to the posterior abdominal wall (Fig. 4.58). Its two layers of peritoneum leave the posterior abdominal wall across the anterior surface of the head and body of the pancreas and pass anteroinferiorly to surround the transverse colon (see Fig. 4.53A and 4.137). Between its layers are the arteries, veins, nerves, and lymphatics related to the transverse colon. The anterior

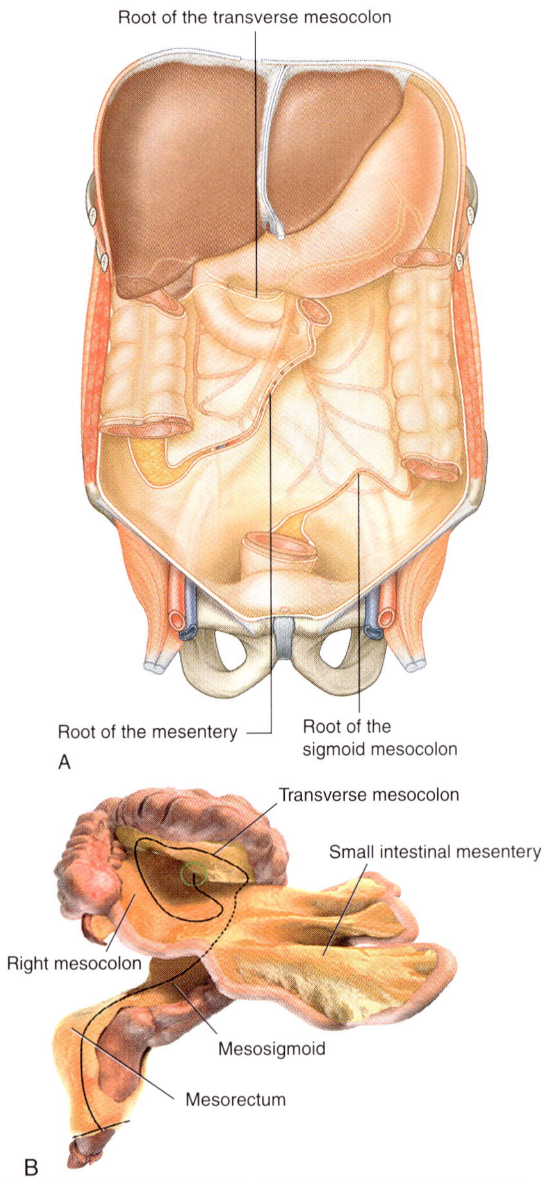

Fig. 4.58(A) Peritoneal reflections, forming mesenteries, outlined on the posterior abdominal wall. **(B)** Contiguity of the mesentery of the small intestine and colon that has been recently described. *Source:* **(B)** Special Credit "Reprinted with permission from Elsevier (The Lancet: 2016:1:238-247)".

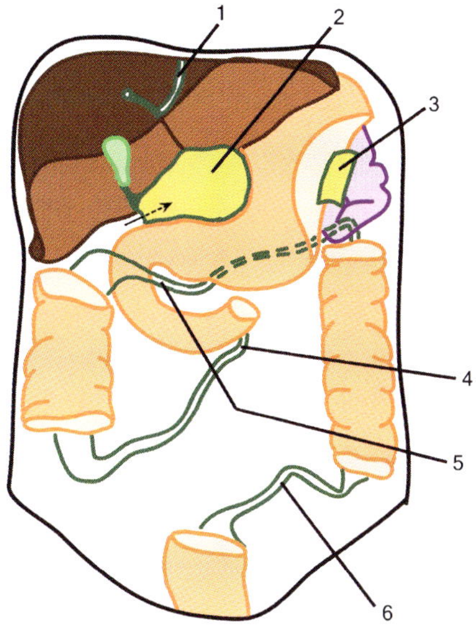

LD Fig. 4.58.1 Folds of mesentery and their attachments shown by reflecting the inferior border of the liver upwards and the left part of the stomach reflected to the right.

Questions

LD Fig. 4.58A Name the labelled areas.

LD Fig. 4.58B

What does the arrow indicate?

LD Fig. 4.58C

Discuss the attachment of the derivatives of the gut tube to the posterior abdominal wall.

Answers

LD Fig. 4.58A

1. Falciform ligament
2. Lesser omentum
3. Gastrosplenic ligament
4. Root of the mesentery
5. Root of the transverse mesocolon
6. Root of the sigmoid mesocolon

LD Fig. 4.58B The arrow indicates the epiploic foramen behind the free edge of the lesser omentum.

LD Fig. 4.58C The following derivatives of the gut tube are attached to the posterior abdominal wall, alternately with a mesentery and without a mesentery: stomach (via the greater omentum), duodenum, other parts of the small intestine (via the mesentery), ascending colon, transverse colon (via the transverse mesocolon), descending colon, sigmoid colon (via the sigmoid mesocolon), and rectum.

The description of the attachments via a mesentery as follows: the greater omentum is fused to the transverse mesocolon; the root of the mesentery is a straight line from the duodenojejunal junction to the ileocaecal junction; the root of the transverse mesocolon is a straight line from the right colic flexure to the left colic flexure; the root of the sigmoid colon is in the form of an inverted "V" and extends from the junction of the descending colon and sigmoid colon to the rectosigmoid junction.

While following the shape of the attachment on the posterior abdominal wall of some of the derivatives of the gut tube from proximal to distal, it is observed that it is in the shape of a question mark (?) starting from the duodenojejunal junction and extending along the intestinal tract till the rectum.

layer of the transverse mesocolon is adherent to the posterior layer of the greater omentum.

Sigmoid mesocolon

The **sigmoid mesocolon** is an inverted, V-shaped peritoneal fold that attaches the sigmoid colon to the abdominal wall (Fig. 4.58A and B). The apex of the V is near the division of the left common iliac artery into its internal and external branches, with the descending left limb of the inverted-V along the medial border of the left psoas major muscle and the right limb of the inverted-V descending into the pelvis to end at the level of vertebra SIII. The sigmoid and superior rectal vessels, along with the nerves and lymphatics associated with the sigmoid colon, pass through this peritoneal fold (see Fig. 4.84).

Ligaments

Peritoneal ligaments consist of two layers of peritoneum that connect two organs to each other or attach an organ to the body wall, and may form part of an omentum. They are usually named after the structures being connected. For example, the **splenorenal ligament** connects the left kidney to the spleen and the **gastrophrenic ligament** connects the stomach to the diaphragm.

Peritoneal folds include omenta, ligaments, and mesenteries. The folds are **underlined** below and the contents of the folds are listed in **brackets.** In addition to these contents, there are autonomic nerves, lymphatics, and fat.

Greater omentum includes (a) gastrophrenic ligament (right and left gastroepiploic vessels and fat), (b) gastrosplenic ligament (short gastric vessels and left gastro-omental vessels), and (c) splenorenal ligament (splenic vessels and tail of pancreas)

Lesser omentum includes (a) hepatogastric ligament (right and left gastric vessels) and (b) hepatoduodenal ligament (right free margin contains the hepatic artery, bile duct, and portal vein)

Falciform ligament (ligamentum teres), anterior and posterior coronary ligaments, right and left triangular ligaments

The mesentery (superior mesenteric vessels, jejunal and ileal vessels)

Transverse mesocolon (middle colic vessels and their branches and tributaries)

Sigmoid mesocolon (sigmoid and superior rectal vessels)

Mesoappendix (appendicular vessels)

The peritoneal cavity can be divided into two compartments, namely the supramesocolic (supracolic) and inframesocolic (infracolic) compartments by the transverse mesocolon, transverse colon, and greater omentum (Fig. 4.53A and 4.54A).

The supramesocolic compartment is between the diaphragm and the transverse mesocolon and can be divided into right and left supramesocolic spaces. The right supramesocolic space includes the right subphrenic space (between the diaphragm and the right lobe of liver, and between the falciform ligament and anterior layer of the coronary ligament), right subhepatic space (hepatorenal or Morrison's pouch between the inferior surface of right lobe of liver and the right kidney) and lesser sac (Fig. 4.53C). The left supramesocolic space includes the left subphrenic space (between the diaphragm and lateral segment of the left lobe of liver, and to the left of the falciform ligament), the left perihepatic space (gastrohepatic recess) and the left posterior subphrenic space (perisplenic space). Two extraperitoneal spaces: right (bare area of the liver) and left (anterior to the left kidney) are located outside the peritoneal cavity but are significant because they may be the site of fluid accumulation.

The inframesocolic compartment is located below the transverse mesocolon and is divided by the root of the mesentery into two spaces, namely right inframesocolic and left inframesocolic space (Fig. 4.58B). The right and left paracolic gutters are lateral to the ascending colon and descending colon. Generally, peritoneal infections may spread form one space to another.

Organs

SET INDUCTION—CASE SCENARIO 4: CANCER OF THE STOMACH

A 63-year-old female was brought to the surgery department with complaints of loss of weight and loss of appetite. On examination, a hard mass was felt in the epigastric region. A diagnosis of cancer of the stomach was made. Knowledge of the anatomy of the stomach including its blood supply and lymphatic drainage is needful to manage this case.

<table>
<tr><th rowspan="2">REMEMBER
[Recall Facts]</th><th colspan="3">OUTLINE 4. ABDOMINAL ESOPHAGUS AND STOMACH—LEARNING OBJECTIVES
[By the end of this section, the student should be able to:]</th><th colspan="2" rowspan="2">EVALUATE
[Explain Concepts]</th></tr>
<tr><th colspan="3">DEMONSTRATE AND ANALYZE RELATIONSHIPS
[Identify structures in a Prosected Specimen or Figure]</th></tr>
<tr><td rowspan="6">Abdominal esophagus
1. Describe the relation of the vagal trunks to the vagus nerves
2. Describe the blood supply of the abdominal part of the esophagus
Stomach
1. List the regions of the stomach
2. List the parts of the stomach
3. Describe the relations of the stomach
4. Describe the blood supply of the stomach
5. Describe the lymphatic drainage of the stomach
6. Describe the nerve supply of the stomach</td><td>Level I</td><td>Level II</td><td>Level III</td><td colspan="2" rowspan="2">■ Peritoneal relations
■ Blood supply
■ Nerve supply
■ Lymphatic drainage</td></tr>
<tr><td rowspan="5">■ Ends—cardiac and pyloric
■ Curvatures—greater and lesser
■ Parts—fundus, body, and pylorus
■ Surfaces—anterior and posterior</td><td rowspan="5">■ Cardiac notch
■ Incisura angularis
■ Pyloric part—antrum, canal, and pylorus
■ Structures forming stomach bed:
■ Left kidney and suprarenal gland
■ Pancreas
■ Left crus of diaphragm
■ Splenic artery
■ Transverse mesocolon
■ Anterior and posterior gastric branches of the vagi</td><td rowspan="5">■ Sulcus intermedius
■ Gastric triangle</td></tr>
<tr><td colspan="2">EARLY CLINICAL EXPOSURE
[Apply Anatomical Knowledge]</td></tr>
<tr><td>Surgical Anatomy/ Pathology/ Trauma</td><td>Imaging/ Surface Anatomy</td></tr>
<tr><td>■ Gastritis
■ Gastric ulcers
■ Pyloric stenosis
■ Gastrectomy
■ Vagotomy
■ Carcinoma of the stomach</td><td>■ Gastroscopy
■ Barium meal study</td></tr>
<tr><td colspan="2">PROBLEM SOLVING/ CLINICAL CASES
[Interpret]
■ Discuss the reasons for the various types of vagotomies
■ Discuss bariatric surgery</td></tr>
</table>

Abdominal esophagus

The abdominal esophagus represents the short distal part of the esophagus located in the abdominal cavity. Emerging through the right crus of the diaphragm, usually at the level of vertebra TX, it passes from the esophageal hiatus to the cardiac orifice of the stomach just left of the midline (Fig. 4.59). The normal acute angle between the abdominal esophagus and fundus of stomach at the esophagogastric junction is known as the angle of His. The acuteness of this angle is less in infants and this predisposes to gastroesophageal reflux.

Associated with the esophagus, as it enters the abdominal cavity, are the anterior and posterior vagal trunks (see Fig. 4.127):

- The **anterior vagal trunk** consists of several smaller trunks whose fibers mostly come from the left vagus nerve. Clockwise rotation of the foregut (along its long axis when viewed from above) occurs during development. This moves these trunks to the anterior surface of the esophagus.
- Similarly, the **posterior vagal trunk** consists of a single trunk whose fibers mostly come from the right vagus nerve, and rotational changes during development move this trunk to the posterior surface of the esophagus.

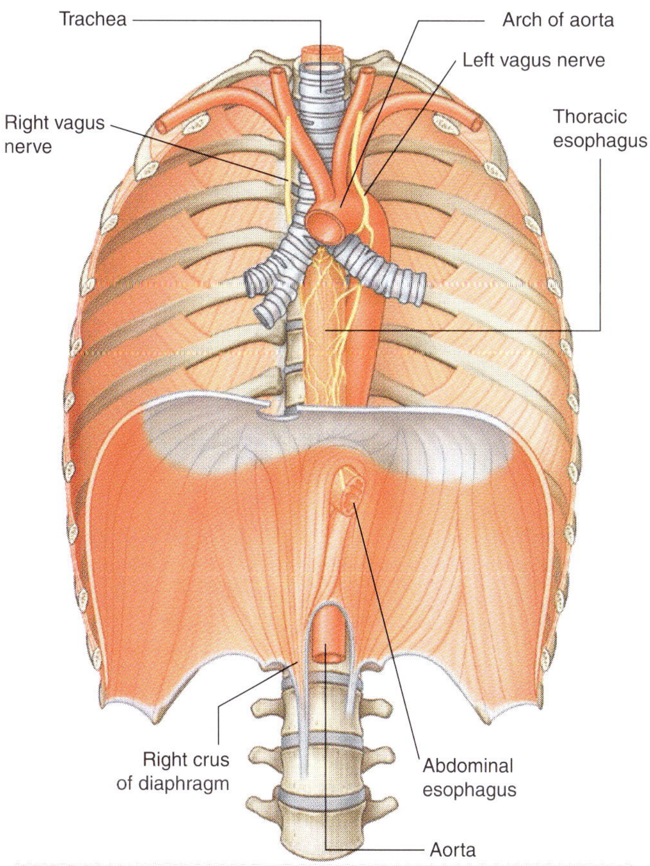

Fig. 4.59 Abdominal esophagus.

The arterial supply to the abdominal esophagus (Fig. 4.60) includes:

- Esophageal branches from the left gastric artery (from the celiac trunk)
- Esophageal branches from the left inferior phrenic artery (from the abdominal aorta, see also Fig. 4.132)

Stomach

The stomach is the most dilated part of the gastrointestinal tract and has a J-like shape (Fig. 4.61 and 4.62). Positioned between the abdominal esophagus and the small intestine, the stomach is in the epigastric, umbilical, and left hypochondrium regions of the abdomen (Fig. 4.23).

The stomach is divided into four regions:

- The cardia, which surrounds the opening of the esophagus into the stomach
- The fundus of the stomach, which is the area above the level of the cardial orifice
- The body of the stomach, which is the largest region of the stomach
- The pyloric part, which is divided into the pyloric antrum and pyloric canal and is the distal end of the stomach

The most distal portion of the pyloric part of the stomach is the **pylorus** (Fig. 4.61). It is marked on the surface of the organ by the **pyloric constriction** and contains a thickened ring of gastric circular muscle, the **pyloric sphincter**, that surrounds the distal opening of the stomach, the **pyloric orifice** (Fig. 4.61 and 4.62B). The pyloric orifice is just to the right of the midline in a plane that passes through the lower border of vertebra LI (the **transpyloric plane**).

Other features of the stomach include:

- The **greater curvature**, which is a point of attachment for the gastrophrenic and gastrosplenic ligaments and the greater omentum (Fig. 4.54A)
- The **lesser curvature**, which is a point of attachment for the lesser omentum
- The **cardial notch**, which is the superior angle created where the esophagus enters the stomach
- The **angular incisure**, which is a bend on the lesser curvature

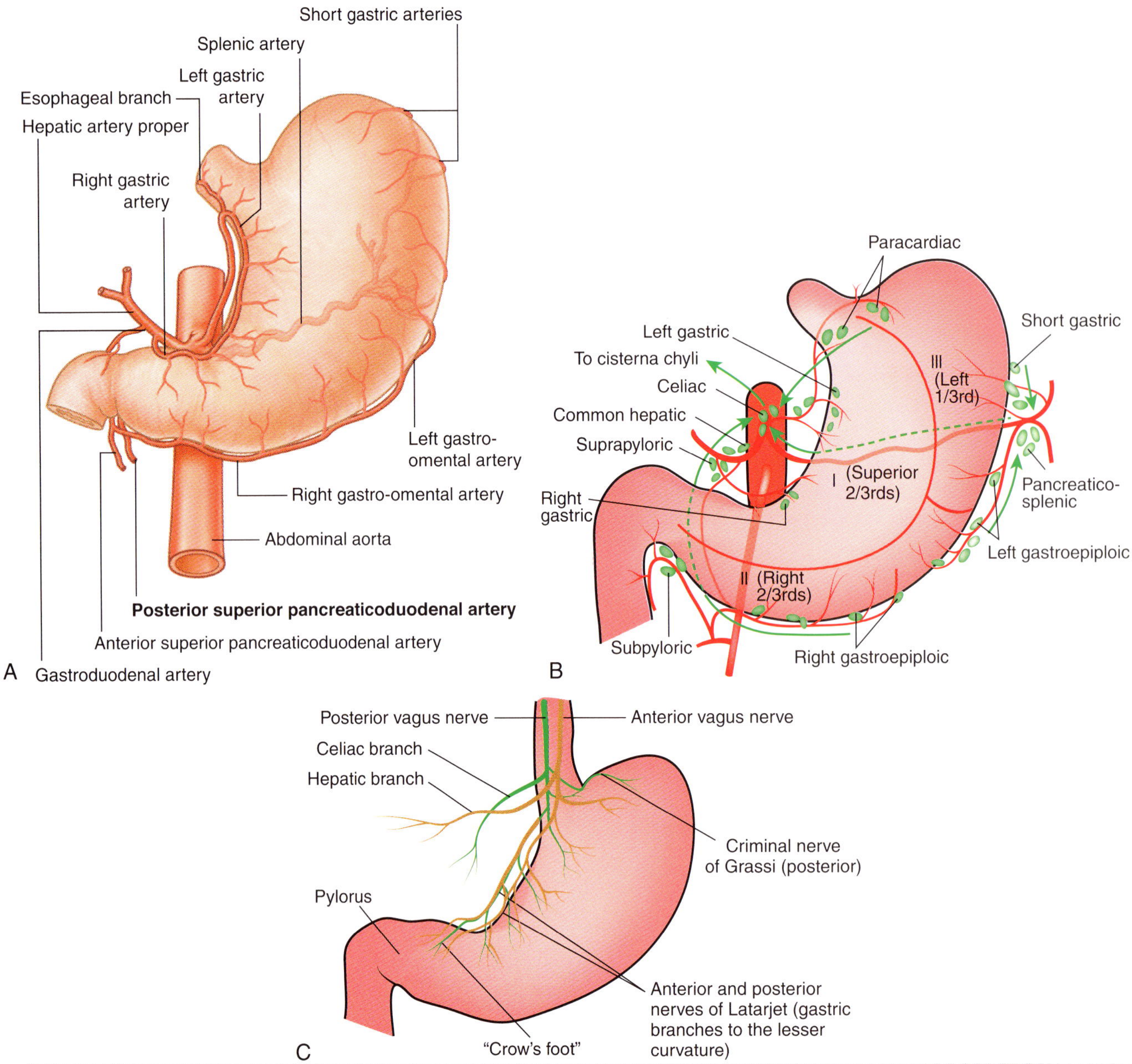

Fig. 4.60(A) Arterial supply. **(B)** Lymph node groups and their drainage. **(C)** Parasympathetic nerve supply to the abdominal esophagus and stomach.

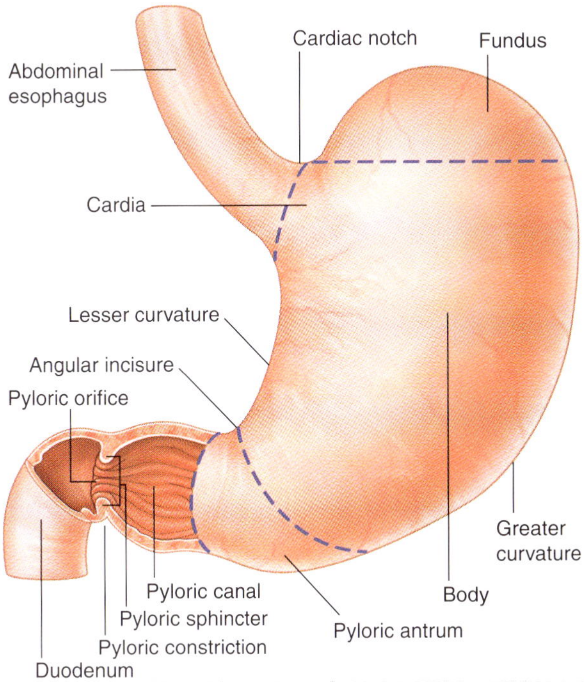

Fig. 4.61 Stomach.

Relations of the stomach

Anterior relations of the stomach include the left lobe of the liver, quadrate lobe of liver (to which the pylorus is related), diaphragm, rib cage, and anterior abdominal wall (Fig. 4.56).

Posterior relations of stomach (stomach bed) include the left kidney, left suprarenal, pancreas, splenic artery, transverse mesocolon, transverse colon, and diaphragm. These structures are separated from the stomach by the lesser sac (Fig. 4.63A and 4.76).

The arterial supply to the stomach (Fig. 4.60) includes:

- The left gastric artery from the celiac trunk
- The right gastric artery from the hepatic artery proper
- The right gastro-omental artery from the gastroduodenal artery
- The left gastro-omental artery from the splenic artery
- The posterior gastric artery from the splenic artery (variant and not always present)

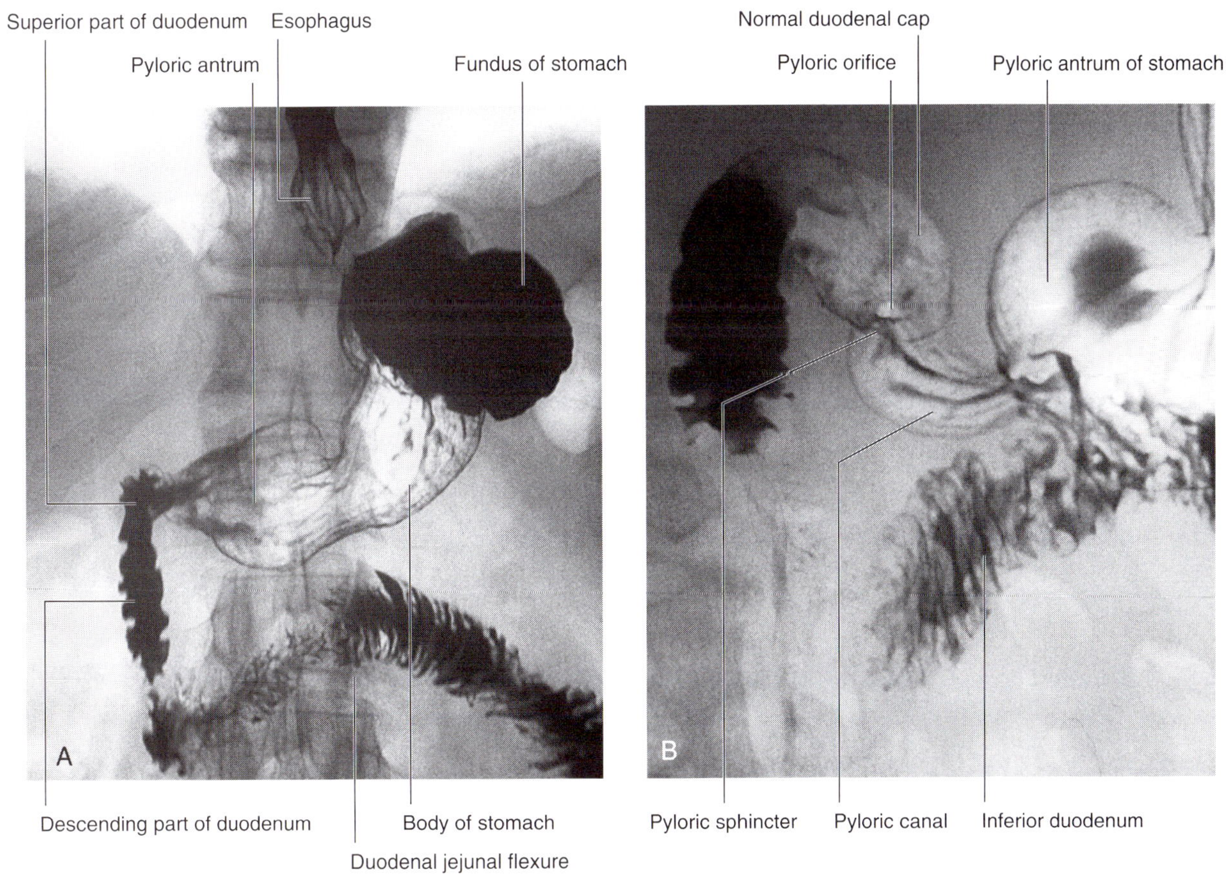

Fig. 4.62 Radiograph, using barium, showing the stomach and duodenum. **(A)** Double-contrast radiograph of the stomach. **(B)** Double-contrast radiograph showing the duodenal cap.

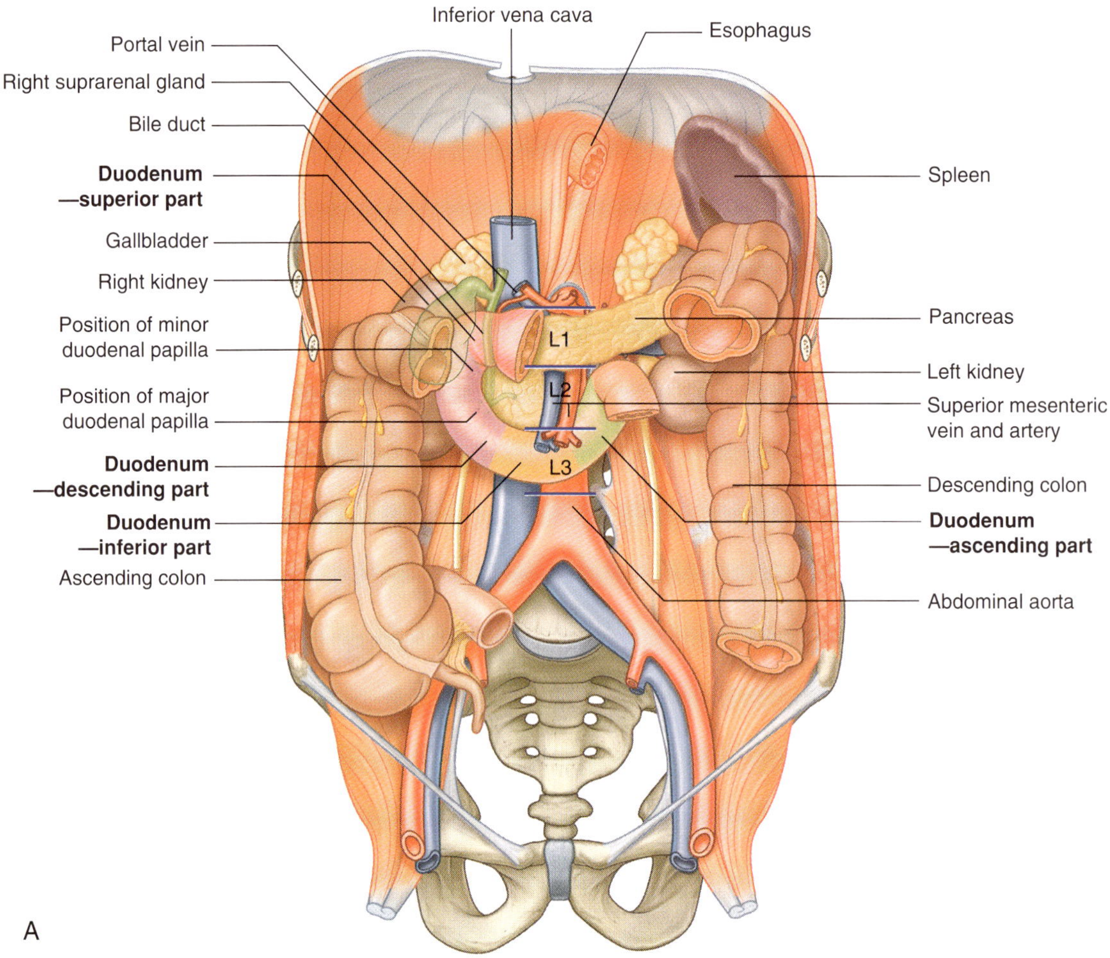

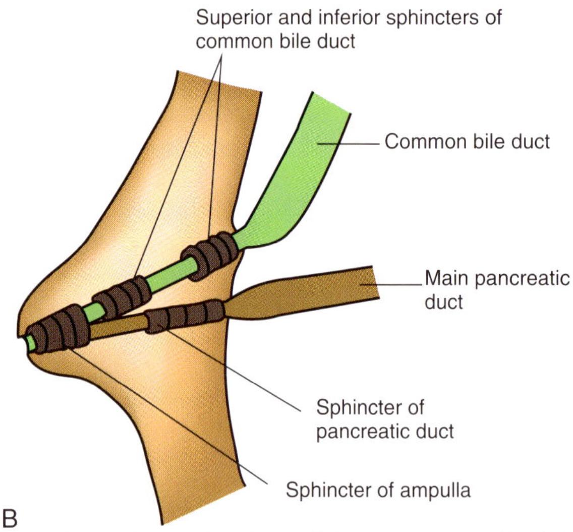

Fig. 4.63(A) Duodenum. **(B)** Sphincter of Boyden.

Early clinical exposure

Anastomosis between arteries to the stomach enables adequate blood supply to the stomach after surgical removal of part of the stomach to excise a cancerous growth.

The veins draining the stomach accompany the corresponding named arteries and drain into the superior mesenteric vein, splenic vein, or the portal vein.

Lymphatic drainage

The lymphatics follow the course of the arteries, and the lymph nodes that drain the stomach are the hepatic nodes, subpyloric nodes, gastric nodes, and the pancreaticosplenic nodes (Fig. 4.60B). The lymphatic drainage is from three areas. Area I is the superior two-thirds of the stomach which drains along the gastric arteries. Area II is the right two-thirds of the inferior one-third of the stomach which drains along the right gastro-omental artery. Area III is the left one-third of the inferior one-third which drains along the branches of the splenic artery.

Nerve supply

The **sympathetic supply** to the stomach is from T5 to T12 spinal segments through the sympathetic chain, greater and lesser splanchnic nerves and celiac plexus (see Fig. 4.125 and 4.126).

The **parasympathetic supply** to the stomach is from the vagus nerves. The anterior vagal trunk divides to give gastric branches, pyloric branches, and a hepatic branch. The gastric branch of the anterior vagal trunk supplying the lesser curvature diverges like a "crow's foot" and is known as the nerve of Latarjet.

The posterior vagal trunk divides into gastric branches and celiac branches. Since the vagus controls the acid secretion from the stomach, vagotomy (sectioning of the vagus nerves) may be done (it is rarely done now) in order to reduce acid secretion from the stomach. In truncal vagotomy, the anterior and posterior vagal trunks are cut, and thus pyloric and hepatic branches lose their function; in selective vagotomy, the hepatic and coeliac branches are spared and the gastric and pyloric branches are cut; and in highly selective (proximal or parietal cell) vagotomy, branches to the fundus and body of the stomach (which contain the parietal cells) are cut. The branch of the posterior vagal trunk that supplies the fundus and may escape notice during a highly selective vagotomy is referred to as the "criminal nerve of Grassi"(Fig. 4.60C).

The **visceral sensory fibers** follow the course of the sympathetics till the trunk of the spinal nerves, and then pass via the dorsal root ganglia to the corresponding spinal segments. The sensations of stretch and ischaemia are transmitted via this route.

Visceral sensory fibers from viscera in contact with the peritoneum which are said to be above the **pelvic pain line** (and in the case of the large intestine, the viscera above the middle of the sigmoid colon) pass with the sympathetic efferents. The visceral sensory fibers from structures below this line pass with the parasympathetic efferents (pelvic splanchnic nerves).

Small intestine

SET INDUCTION—CASE SCENARIO 5: PERFORATED DUODENAL ULCER

A 43-year-old male was brought to the emergency department with a history of severe pain in the abdomen. On examination, rigidity of the abdominal wall was found and investigations revealed that his hemoglobin was 5 g%. A diagnosis of ruptured duodenal ulcer with erosion of the superior pancreaticoduodenal artery was suspected. Knowledge of the anatomy of the small intestine is needed to manage this case.

<table>
<tr><th rowspan="2">REMEMBER
[Recall Facts]</th><th colspan="3">OUTLINE 5. SMALL INTESTINE—LEARNING OBJECTIVES
[By the end of this section, the student should be able to:]</th><th rowspan="2" colspan="2">EVALUATE
[Explain Concepts]</th></tr>
<tr><th colspan="3">DEMONSTRATE AND ANALYZE RELATIONSHIPS
[Identify structures in a Prosected Specimen or Figure]</th></tr>
<tr><td rowspan="6">1. Describe the location of the small intestine
2. Describe the features to distinguish the parts of the small intestine
3. Describe the attachments and contents of the mesentery
4. Describe the relations, blood supply, nerve supply, and lymphatics of the small intestine</td><td>Level I</td><td>Level II</td><td>Level III</td><td colspan="2">■ Differences between jejunum and ileum
■ Blood supply, nerve supply, and lymphatic drainage of jejunum and ileum
■ Parts of the duodenum and relation
■ Second part of duodenum</td></tr>
<tr><td rowspan="5">■ Mesentery
■ Root of mesentery
■ Superior mesenteric vessels and branches of superior mesenteric artery
■ Small intestine:
  ■ Duodenum
  ■ Jejunum
  ■ Ileum
■ Duodenum—situation, parts, important relations
■ Plica circularis and their distribution in jejunum and ileum
■ Payer's patches in ileum</td><td rowspan="5">■ Differences between jejunum and ileum in:
  ■ Fat distribution in the mesentery
  ■ Arterial arcades
  ■ "Windows" between vasa recta
■ Duodenojejunal flexure
■ Ileocecal junction
■ Differences in thickness of wall between jejunum and ileum</td><td rowspan="5">■ Duodenal fossae
■ Mesenteric group of lymph nodes
■ Suspensory ligament of Treitz</td><th colspan="2">EARLY CLINICAL EXPOSURE
[Apply Anatomical Knowledge]</th></tr>
<tr><th>Surgical Anatomy/ Pathology/ Trauma</th><th>Imaging/ Surface Anatomy</th></tr>
<tr><td>■ Duodenal ulcer
■ Duodenal cap in barium meal study
■ Enteritis
■ Paralytic ileus
■ Meckel's diverticulum</td><td>Barium meal follow through</td></tr>
<tr><th colspan="2">PROBLEM SOLVING/ CLINICAL CASES
[Interpret]</th></tr>
<tr><td colspan="2">■ Explain how knowledge of the direction of the root of the mesentery can help to determine the proximal segment of a loop of small intestine
■ Importance of the arterial anastomoses between arteries to the small intestine</td></tr>
</table>

The small intestine is the longest part of the gastrointestinal tract and extends from the pyloric orifice of the stomach to the ileocecal fold. This hollow tube, which is approximately 6–7 m long with a narrowing diameter from beginning to end, consists of the duodenum, the jejunum, and the ileum.

Duodenum

The first part of the small intestine is the duodenum. This C-shaped structure, adjacent to the head of the pancreas, is 20–25 cm long and is above the level of the umbilicus; its lumen is the widest part of the small intestine (Fig. 4.63A). It is retroperitoneal except for its beginning, which is connected to the liver by the hepatoduodenal ligament, a part of the lesser omentum (Fig. 4.57).

The duodenum is divided into four parts (Fig. 4.63A).

- The **superior part** (first part) extends from the pyloric orifice of the stomach to the neck of the gallbladder, is just to the right of the body of vertebra LI, and passes anterior to the bile duct, gastroduodenal artery, portal vein, and inferior vena cava. Clinically, the beginning of this part of the duodenum is referred to as the ampulla or **duodenal cap**, and most duodenal ulcers occur in this part of the duodenum.
- The **descending part** (second part) of the duodenum is just to the right of midline and extends from the neck of the gallbladder to the lower border of vertebra LIII. Its anterior surface is crossed by the transverse colon, posterior to it is the right kidney, and medial to it is the head of the pancreas. This part of the duodenum contains the **major duodenal papilla**, which is the common entrance for the bile and pancreatic ducts, and the **minor duodenal papilla**, which is the entrance for the accessory pancreatic duct. The common bile duct and the pancreatic duct form a common channel that contains a dilated segment known as hepatopancreatic ampulla (of Vater). The major duodenal papilla is situated 8–10 cm distal to the pylorus on the posteromedial wall. Superior to the major duodenal papillae is an arched mucosal fold called "Monk's hood." There is a longitudinal mucosal fold which extends downward from the major duodenal papilla. The junction of the foregut and the midgut is immediately below the major duodenal papilla. The intramural portions of the common bile duct, main pancreatic duct, and the hepatopancreatic ampulla are surrounded by a circular and spiral smooth muscle coat that forms a sphincter complex known as the sphincter of Boyden. It is composed of four sphincters, namely superior choledochal sphincter, inferior choledochal sphincter, sphincter ampullae (sphincter of Oddi), and pancreatic sphincter (Fig. 4.63B). Endoscopic retrograde cholangiopancreatography (ERCP) enables a physician to visualize the bile ducts and pancreatic ducts. Magnetic resonance cholangiopancreatography (MRCP) makes use of magnetic resonance imaging (MRI) to visualize these ducts. The **inferior part (**third part) of the duodenum is the longest section, and passes anterior to the inferior vena cava, the aorta, and the vertebral column (Fig. 4.62B and 4.63A). It is crossed anteriorly by the superior mesenteric artery and vein.
- The **ascending part** (fourth part) of the duodenum passes upward on, or to the left of, the aorta to approximately the upper border of vertebra LII and terminates at the **duodenojejunal flexure**.

This duodenojejunal flexure is surrounded by a fold of peritoneum. It is connected to the connective tissue around the origins of the celiac artery and superior mesenteric artery by muscle fibers called the **suspensory muscle (ligament) of duodenum (ligament of Treitz)** (Fig. 4.58B).

The arterial supply to the duodenum (Fig. 4.64) includes branches from the:

- Gastroduodenal artery

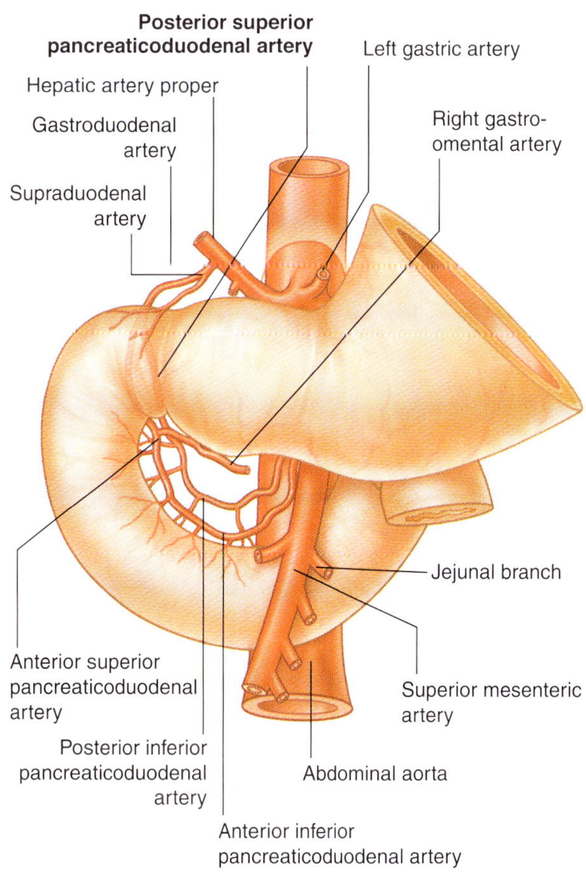

Fig. 4.64 Arterial supply to the duodenum.

- Supraduodenal artery from the gastroduodenal artery
- Anterior superior pancreaticoduodenal artery (from the gastroduodenal artery)
- Posterior superior pancreaticoduodenal artery (from the gastroduodenal artery)
- Anterior inferior pancreaticoduodenal artery (from the inferior pancreaticoduodenal artery—a branch of the superior mesenteric artery)
- Posterior inferior pancreaticoduodenal artery (from the inferior pancreaticoduodenal artery—a branch of the superior mesenteric artery)
- First jejunal branch from the superior mesenteric artery

Jejunum

The jejunum and ileum make up the last two sections of the small intestine (Fig. 4.65). The jejunum represents the proximal two-fifths. It is mostly in the left upper quadrant of the abdomen and is larger in diameter and has a thicker wall than the ileum. Additionally, the inner mucosal lining of the jejunum is characterized by prominent folds that circle the lumen (plicae circulares), which are more numerous here than in the ileum, and in a barium meal this causes the typical feathery appearance that characterizes the jejunum. The less prominent arterial arcades and longer vasa recta (straight arteries) compared to those of the ileum are a unique characteristic of the jejunum (Fig. 4.66). The lumen of the jejunum is usually larger, and the wall thicker than in the ileum. The arterial supply to the jejunum includes jejunal arteries from the superior mesenteric artery.

Ileum

The ileum makes up the distal three-fifths of the small intestine and is mostly in the right lower quadrant. Compared to the jejunum, the ileum has thinner walls, fewer and less prominent mucosal folds (plicae circulares), shorter vasa recta, more mesenteric fat, and more arterial arcades (Fig. 4.66).

The ileum opens into the large intestine, where the cecum and ascending colon join together. Two flaps projecting into the lumen of the large intestine (the **ileocecal fold**) surround the opening (Fig. 4.67). The flaps of the ileocecal fold come together at their end, forming ridges. Musculature from the ileum continues into each flap, forming a sphincter.

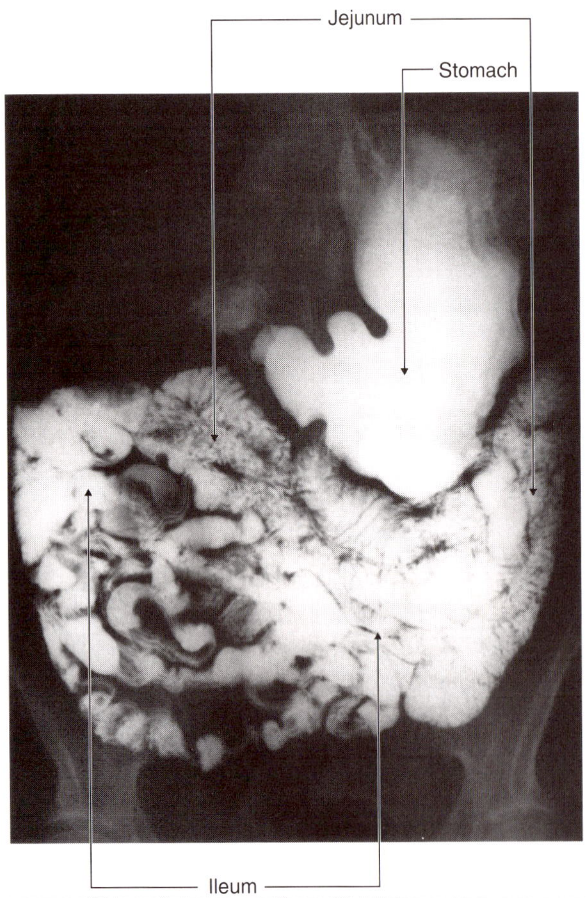

Fig. 4.65 Radiograph, using barium, showing the jejunum and ileum.

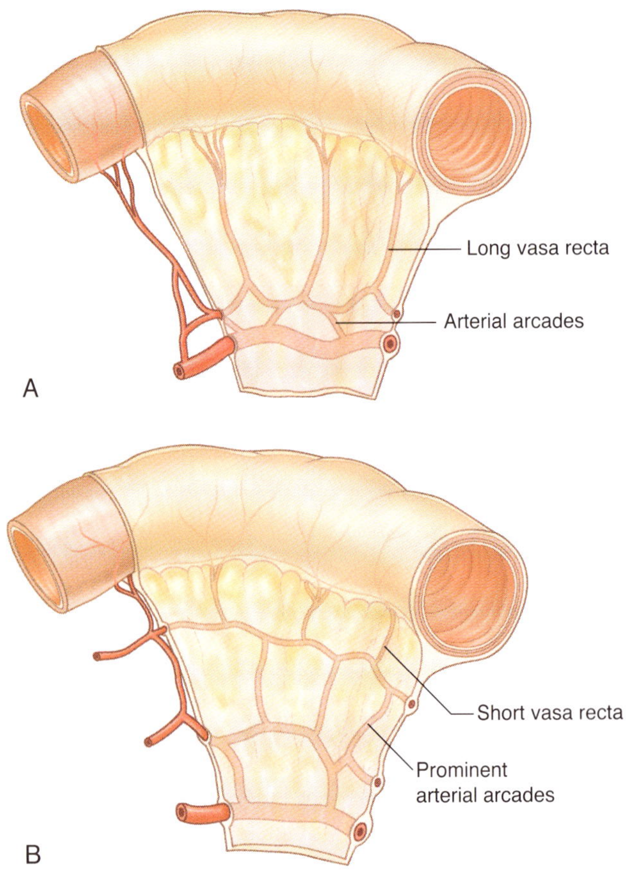

Fig. 4.66 Differences in the arterial supply to the small intestine. **(A)** Jejunum. **(B)** Ileum.

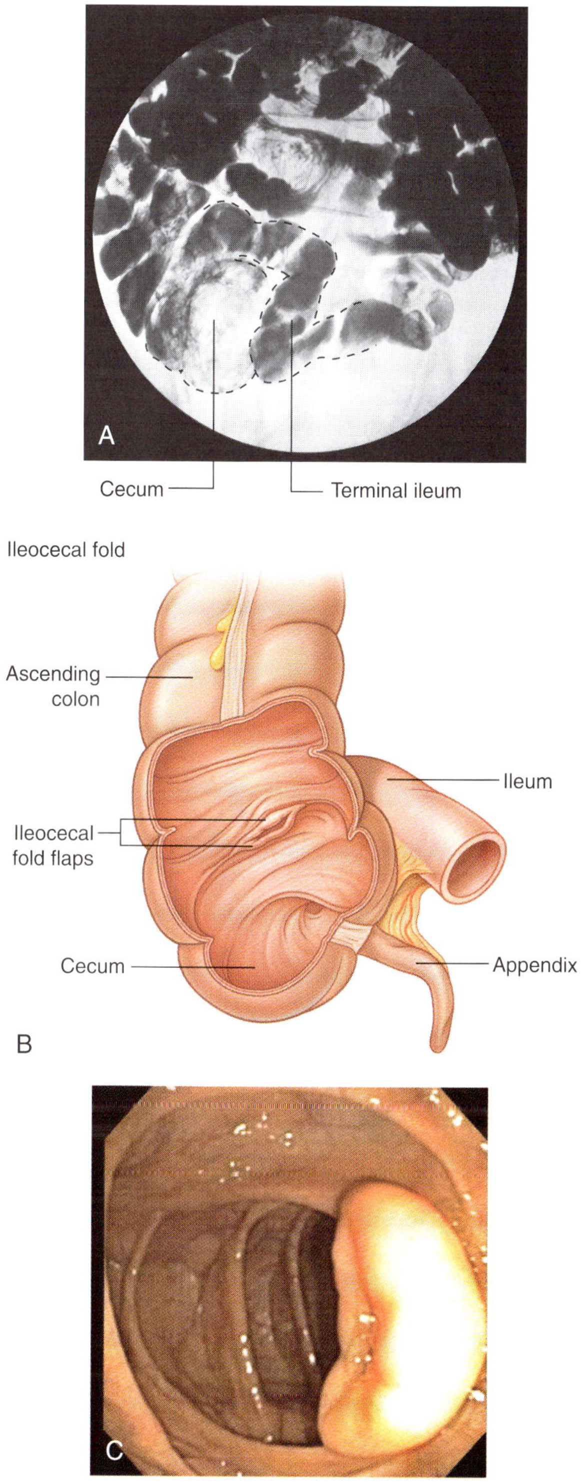

Fig. 4.67 Ileocecal junction. **(A)** Radiograph showing ileocecal junction. **(B)** Illustration showing ileocecal junction and the ileocecal fold. **(C)** Endoscopic image of the ileocecal fold.

Possible functions of the ileocecal fold include preventing reflux from the cecum to the ileum, and regulating the passage of contents from the ileum to the cecum.

The arterial supply to the ileum (Fig. 4.68) includes:

- Ileal arteries from the superior mesenteric artery
- An ileal branch from the ileocolic artery (from the superior mesenteric artery, see also Fig. 4.84)

Early clinical exposure

Epithelial transition between the abdominal esophagus and stomach

The gastroesophageal junction is demarcated by a transition from one epithelial type to another epithelial type. In some people, the histological junction does not lie at the physiological gastroesophageal junction (lower esophageal sphincter) but is in the lower one-third of the esophagus. This may predispose these people to esophageal ulceration and is also associated with an increased risk of adenocarcinoma (Fig. 4.70).

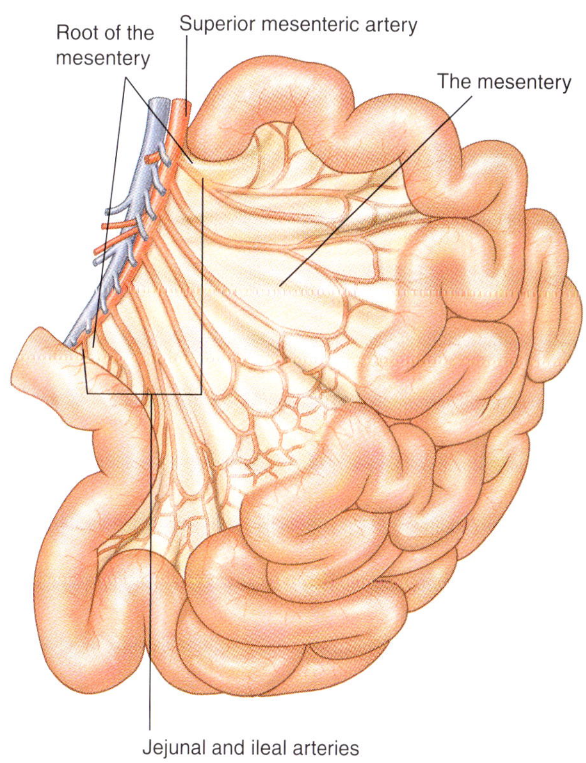

Fig. 4.68 Arterial supply to the ileum.

Early clinical exposure

Duodenal ulceration

Duodenal ulcers usually occur in the superior part of the duodenum and are much less common than they were 50 years ago. At first, there was no treatment and patients died from hemorrhage or peritonitis. As surgical techniques developed, patients with duodenal ulcers were subjected to extensive upper gastrointestinal surgery to prevent ulcer recurrence and for some patients the treatment was dangerous. As knowledge and understanding of the mechanisms for acid secretion in the stomach increased, drugs were developed to block acid stimulation and secretion indirectly (**histamine H_2-receptor antagonists**) and these have significantly reduced the morbidity and mortality rates of this disease. Pharmacological therapy can now directly inhibit the cells of the stomach that produce acid with, for example, **proton pump inhibitors**. Patients are also screened for the bacteria ***Helicobacter pylori,*** which when eradicated (by antibiotic treatment) significantly reduces duodenal ulcer formation.

Anatomically, duodenal ulcers tend to occur either anteriorly or posteriorly.

Posterior duodenal ulcers erode either directly onto the gastroduodenal artery or, more commonly, onto the **posterior superior pancreaticoduodenal artery** (Fig. 4.64), which can produce torrential hemorrhage, which may be fatal in some patients. Treatment may involve extensive upper abdominal surgery with ligation of the vessels or by **endovascular means** whereby the radiologist may place a very fine catheter retrogradely from the femoral artery into the celiac artery. The common hepatic artery and the gastroduodenal artery are cannulated and the bleeding area may be blocked using small coils, which stem the flow of blood.

Anterior duodenal ulcers erode into the peritoneal cavity, causing **peritonitis**. This intense inflammatory reaction and the local lack of peristalsis (ileus) promote adhesion of the greater omentum, which attempts to seal off the perforation. The stomach and duodenum usually contain considerable amounts of gas, which enters the peritoneal cavity and can be observed on a chest radiograph of an erect patient as **subdiaphragmatic free gas** (Fig. 4.55B). In most instances, treatment for the ulcer is surgical.

Early clinical exposure

Examination of the upper gastrointestinal tract

It is often necessary to examine the esophagus, stomach, duodenum, and proximal jejunum for disease. After taking an appropriate history and examining the patient, most physicians arrange a series of simple blood tests to look for bleeding, inflammation, and tumors. The next steps in the investigation assess the three components of any loop of bowel, namely, the lumen, the wall, and masses extrinsic to the bowel, which may compress or erode into it.

Examination of the bowel lumen

Barium sulfate solutions may be swallowed by the patient and can be visualized using an X-ray fluoroscopy unit. The lumen can be examined for masses (e.g., polyps and tumors) and peristaltic waves can be assessed. Patients may also be given carbon dioxide–releasing granules to fill the stomach so that the barium thinly coats the mucosa, resulting in images displaying fine mucosal detail. These tests are relatively simple and can be used to image the esophagus, stomach, duodenum, and small bowel.

Examination of the bowel wall and extrinsic masses

Endoscopy is a minimally invasive diagnostic medical procedure that can be used to assess the interior surfaces of an organ by inserting a tube into the body. The instrument is typically made of a flexible plastic material through which a light source and eyepiece are attached at one end. Some systems allow passage of small instruments through the main bore of the endoscope to obtain biopsies and to also undertake small procedures (e.g., the removal of polyps).

In gastrointestinal and abdominal medicine an endoscope is used to assess the esophagus, stomach, duodenum, and proximal small bowel (Fig. 4.69–4.72). The tube is swallowed by the patient under light sedation and is extremely well tolerated.

Assessment of the colon is performed by passage of the tube through the anus and into the rectum.

The endoscope is then advanced via the colon to the cecum and sometimes to the terminal ileum. The patient

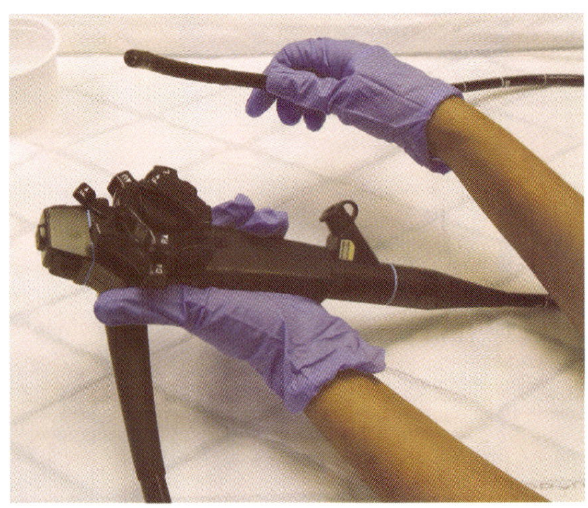

Fig. 4.69 The endoscope is a flexible plastic tube that can be controlled from the proximal end. Through a side portal various devices can be inserted, which run through the endoscope and can be used to obtain biopsies and to perform minor endoluminal surgical procedures (e.g., excision of polyps).

Early clinical exposure—cont'd

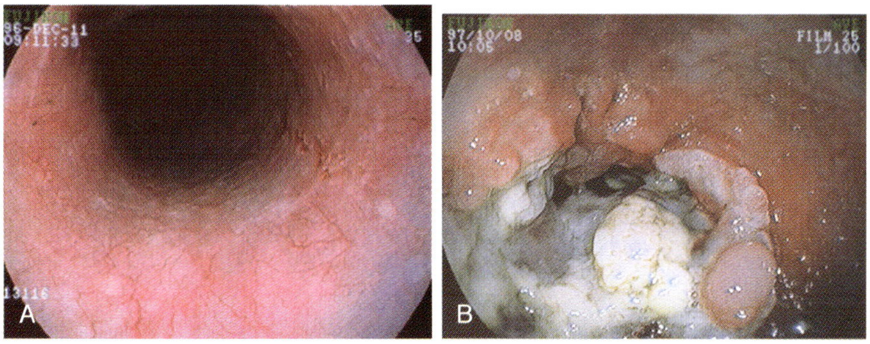

Fig. 4.70 Endoscopic images of the gastroesophageal junction. **(A)** Normal. **(B)** Esophageal cancer at gastroesophageal junction.

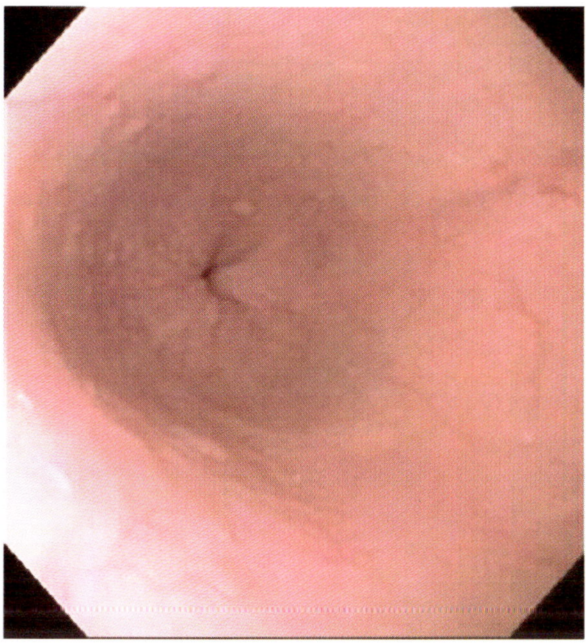

Fig. 4.71 Endoscopic image of the pyloric antrum of the stomach looking toward the pylorus.

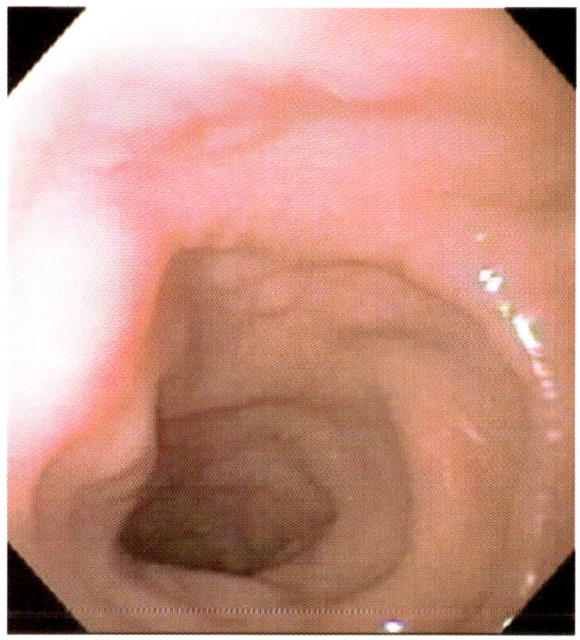

Fig. 4.72 Endoscopic image showing normal appearance of the second part of the duodenum.

undergoes bowel preparation before the examination to allow good visualization of the entire large bowel. Specially designed solutions are taken orally to help clear the bowel of fecal material. Air, water, and suction may be used during the examination to improve visualization. Biopsies, polyp removal, cauterization of bleeding, and stent placement can also be performed using additional instruments that can be passed through special openings in the colonoscope.

Cross-sectional imaging using CT or magnetic resonance is another way to assess the bowel lumen and wall. Magnetic resonance is particularly useful in assessment of the small bowel because it allows dynamic assessment of bowel distention and motility and provides good visualization of segmental or continuous bowel wall thickening and mural or mucosal ulcerations and also can demonstrate increased vascularity of the small bowel mesentery (Fig. 4.72A). It is usually performed in patients with inflammatory bowel diseases, such as Crohn's disease.

CT colonography

CT colonography (also called virtual colonoscopy or CT pneumocolon) is an alternative way to visualize and assess the colon for abnormal lesions such as polyps or strictures with the use of spiral CT to produce high-resolution 3D views of the large bowel. It is less invasive than traditional colonoscopy, but to achieve good-quality images the patient needs to take bowel preparations to ensure bowel cleansing, and the colon needs to be insufflated with CO_2. Different clinical situations and the particular investigations that are recommended for them are as follows: if a tumor is present (Fig. 4.72B), both CT and MRI; to assess regional disease, MRI; abnormal lymph nodes, MRI, CT; and distant metastases, CT.

Continued

Early clinical exposure—cont'd

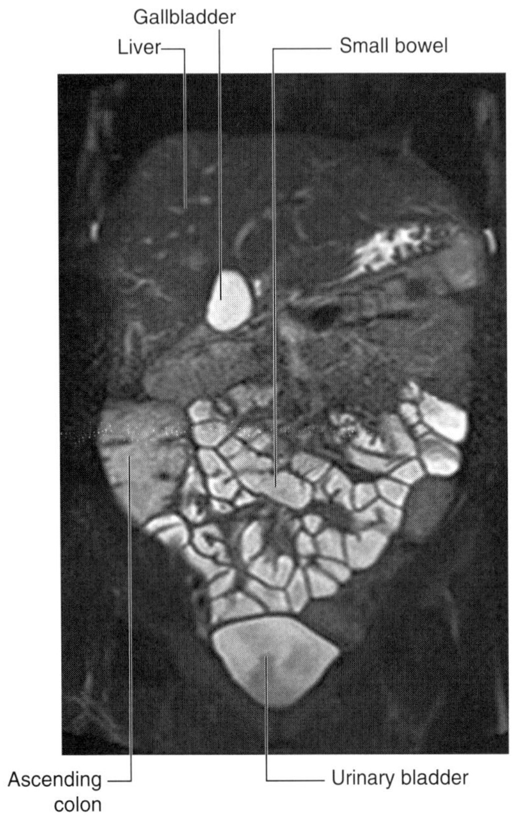

Fig. 4.72(A) Small bowel visualization using MRI in coronal plane.

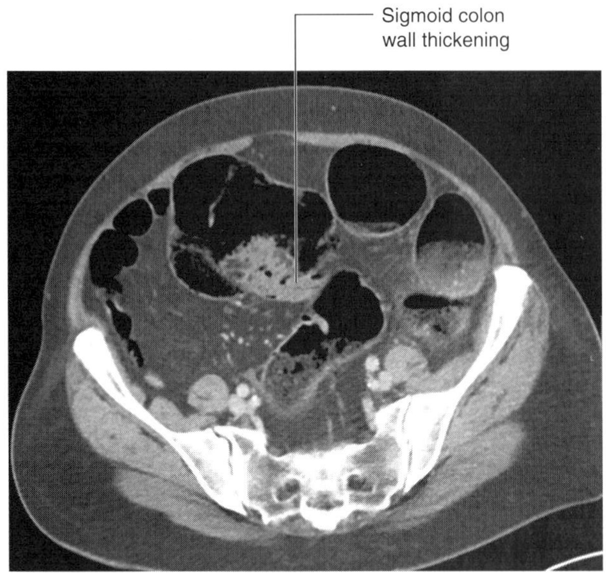

Fig. 4.72(B) Axial CT shows sigmoid colon wall thickening caused by tumor.

Early clinical exposure

Meckel's diverticulum

A Meckel's diverticulum (Fig. 4.73) is the remnant of the proximal part of the yolk stalk (vitelline duct) that extends into the umbilical cord in the embryo and lies on the antimesenteric border of the ileum. It appears as a blind-ended tubular outgrowth of bowel. Although it is an uncommon finding (occurring in approximately 2% of the population), it is always important to consider the diagnosis of Meckel's diverticulum because it does produce symptoms (which may mimic appendicitis) in a small number of patients. Conditions in which it may be involved include hemorrhage, intussusception, diverticulitis, ulceration, and obstruction.

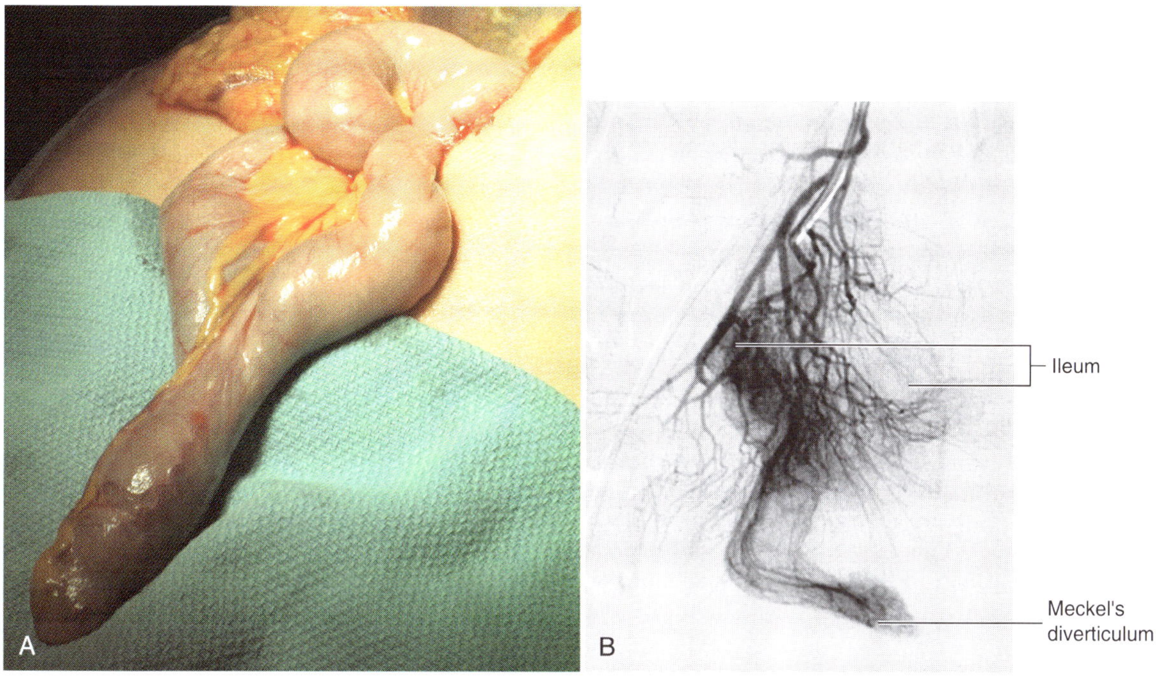

Fig. 4.73 Vasculature associated with a Meckel's diverticulum. **(A)** Surgical image of Meckel's diverticulum. **(B)** Digital subtraction angiography.

Early clinical exposure

Computed tomography scanning and magnetic resonance imaging

These imaging techniques can provide important information about the wall of the bowel that may not be obtained from barium or endoscopic studies. Thickening of the wall may indicate inflammatory change or tumor and is always regarded with suspicion. If a tumor is demonstrated, the locoregional spread can be assessed, along with lymphadenopathy and metastatic spread.

Advanced imaging methods

Endoscopic ultrasound (EUS) uses a small ultrasound device placed on the end of the endoscope to assess the upper gastrointestinal tract. It can produce extremely high-powered views of the mucosa and submucosa and therefore show whether a tumor is resectable. It also provides guidance to the clinician when taking a biopsy.

Early clinical exposure

Carcinoma of the stomach

Carcinoma of the stomach is a common gastrointestinal malignancy. Chronic gastric inflammation (gastritis), pernicious anemia, and polyps predispose to the development of this aggressive cancer, which is usually not diagnosed until late in the course of the disease. Symptoms include vague epigastric pain, early fullness with eating, bleeding leading to chronic anemia, and obstruction.

The diagnosis may be made using barium sulfate (barium swallow), conventional radiology or endoscopy (which allows a biopsy to be obtained at the same time). Ultrasound scanning is used to check the liver for metastatic spread, and, if negative, CT is carried out to assess for surgical resectability. If carcinoma of the stomach is diagnosed early, a curative surgical resection is possible. However, because most patients do not seek treatment until late in the disease, the overall 5-year survival rate is between 5% and 20%, with a mean survival time of between 5 and 8 months.

Large intestine

SET INDUCTION—CASE SCENARIO 6: APPENDICITIS

A 25-year-old female was brought to the emergency department with complaints of fever, vomiting, and severe abdominal pain for 7 hours which was initially located at the umbilical region and later was located in the right iliac fossa. On examination, maximal tenderness was found over McBurney's point. A diagnosis of acute appendicitis was made. Knowledge of the anatomy of the large intestine is needed to manage this case.

OUTLINE 6. LARGE INTESTINE—LEARNING OBJECTIVES [By the end of this section, the student should be able to:]

REMEMBER [Recall Facts]	DEMONSTRATE AND ANALYZE RELATIONSHIPS [Identify structures in a Prosected Specimen or Figure]			EVALUATE [Explain Concepts]
	Level I	**Level II**	**Level III**	

1. List the parts of the large intestine and describe the location where each part begins and ends
2. Describe briefly the relations of the cecum
3. Describe the peritoneal folds in relation to the cecum and appendix
4. Describe the differences between small intestine and large intestine
5. Describe the relations, blood supply, nerve supply, and lymphatic drainage of the large intestine
	■ Branches of superior mesenteric artery:
	  ■ Ileocol-ic
	  ■ Middle colic
	  ■ Right colic
	■ Inferior mesenteric vessels
	■ Branches of inferior mesenteric artery:
	  ■ Left colic
	  ■ Sigmoid
	■ Parts of large intestine
	■ Features—taeniae coli, haustrations, appendices epiploicae
	■ Transverse mesocolon with middle colic vessels
	■ Ileocecal and appendicular orifices
		■ Marginal artery of Drummond
		■ Position of appendix
		■ Mesoappendix with appendicular vessels
		■ Ileocecal valve
		■ Posterior relations of cecum, ascending, and descending colon
			■ Mesenteric group of lymph nodes	■ Posterior relations of cecum, ascending and descending colon
				■ Positions of appendix
				■ Blood supply, nerve supply, and lymphatic drainage of the large intestine

EARLY CLINICAL EXPOSURE [Apply Anatomical Knowledge]	
Surgical Anatomy/ Pathology/ Trauma	**Imaging/ Surface Anatomy**
■ Appendicitis ■ Appendectomy ■ Carcinoma of the colon ■ Colectomy ■ Intussusception ■ Volvulus ■ Ostomies ■ Diverticular disease	■ Barium enema ■ Colonoscopy ■ McBurney's point
PROBLEM SOLVING/ CLINICAL CASES [Interpret]	
■ Discuss the basis for the pain felt in appendicitis ■ Surgical implication of the lack of blood vessels in the lateral paracolic gutters ■ Importance of the arterial anastomoses between blood vessels to the large intestine	

The large intestine extends from the distal end of the ileum to the anus, a distance of approximately 1.5 m in adults. It absorbs fluids and salts from the gut contents, thus forming feces, and consists of the cecum, appendix, colon, rectum, and anal canal (Fig. 4.74 and 4.75).

Beginning in the right groin as the cecum, with its associated appendix, the large intestine continues upward as the **ascending colon** through the right flank and into the right hypochondrium (Fig. 4.76). Just below the liver, it bends to the left, forming the **right colic flexure** (**hepatic flexure**), and crosses the abdomen as the **transverse colon** to the left hypochondrium. At this position, just below the spleen, the large intestine bends downward, forming the **left colic flexure** (**splenic flexure**), and continues as the **descending colon** through the left flank and into the left groin.

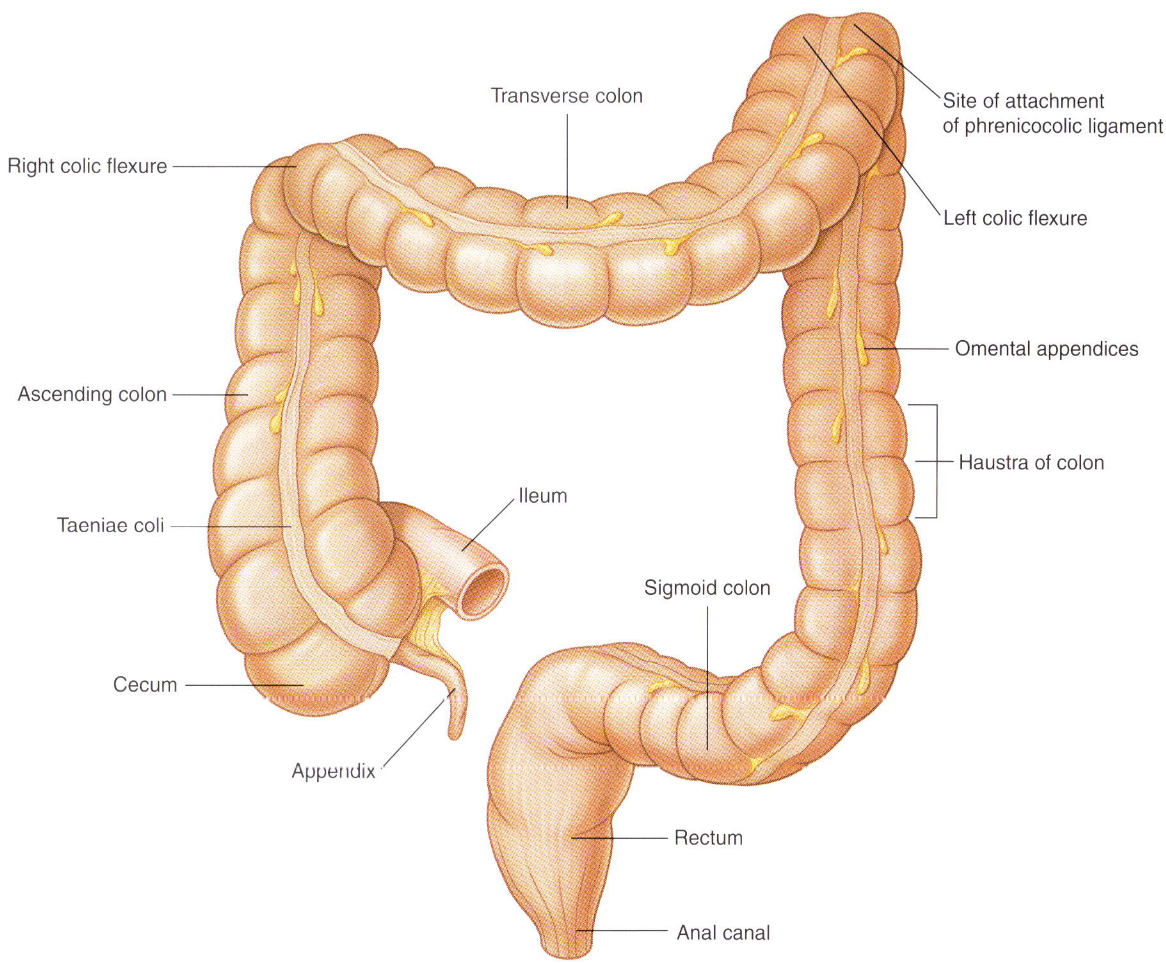

Fig. 4.74 Large intestine.

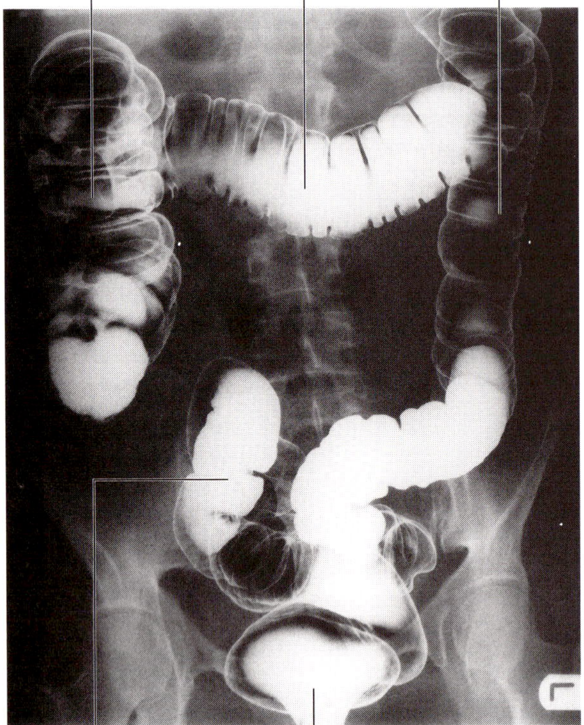

Fig. 4.75 Radiograph, using barium, showing the large intestine.

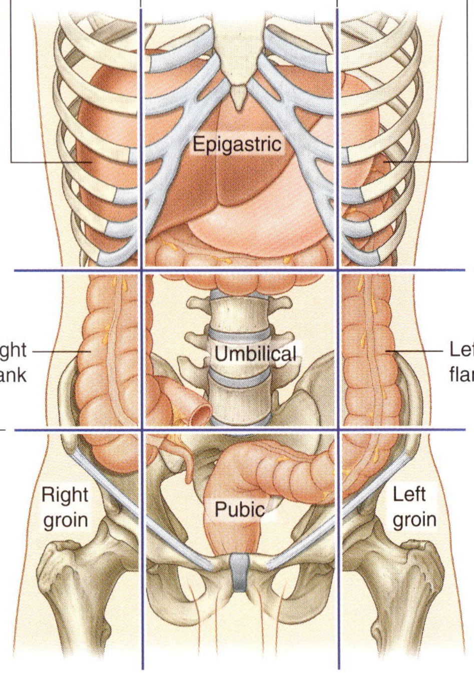

Fig. 4.76 Position of the large intestine in the nine-region organizational pattern.

It enters the upper part of the pelvic cavity as the sigmoid colon, continues on the posterior wall of the pelvic cavity as the rectum, and terminates as the anal canal.

The general characteristics of most of the large intestine (Fig. 4.74) are as follows:

- Its large internal diameter compared to that of the small intestine.
- Peritoneal-covered accumulations of fat (the **omental appendices**) are associated with the colon.
- The segregation of longitudinal muscle in its walls into three narrow bands (the **taeniae coli)**, which are observed in the cecum and colon.
- The sacculations of the colon (the **haustra of the colon**).

Cecum and appendix

The **cecum** is the first part of the large intestine (Fig. 4.67B and 4.77A). It is inferior to the ileocecal opening and in the right iliac fossa. It is an intraperitoneal structure because of its mobility, not because of its suspension by a mesentery.

The cecum is continuous with the ascending colon at the entrance of the ileum and is usually in contact with the anterior abdominal wall. It may extend below the pelvic brim to lie in the true pelvis. The appendix is attached to the posteromedial wall of the cecum, just inferior to the end of the ileum (Fig. 4.77A). The interior of the cecum presents two orifices, namely the ileocecal orifice and the appendicular orifice. The ileocecal orifice is located on the posteromedial aspect of the cecum and is guarded by the ileocecal valve. The appendicular orifice is located below the ileocecal orifice and is guarded by valve of Gerlach. The peritoneal fold between the terminal ileum and the anterior layer of mesoappendix is known as the **inferior ileocecal fold** or "bloodless fold of Treves." Above the ileocecal junction is the **superior ileocecal fold** or vascular fold of the cecum (Fig. 4.77B)

The **appendix** is a narrow, hollow, blind-ended tube connected to the cecum. It has large aggregations of lymphoid tissue in its walls and is suspended from the terminal ileum by the **mesoappendix** (Fig. 4.78), which contains the **appendicular vessels**. Its point of attachment to the cecum is located at the point of convergence of the three taeniae at the base of the appendix. The location of the rest of the appendix varies considerably (Fig. 4.79). It may be:

- Posterior to the cecum or posterior to the cecum and lower ascending colon, in a retrocecal or retrocolic position

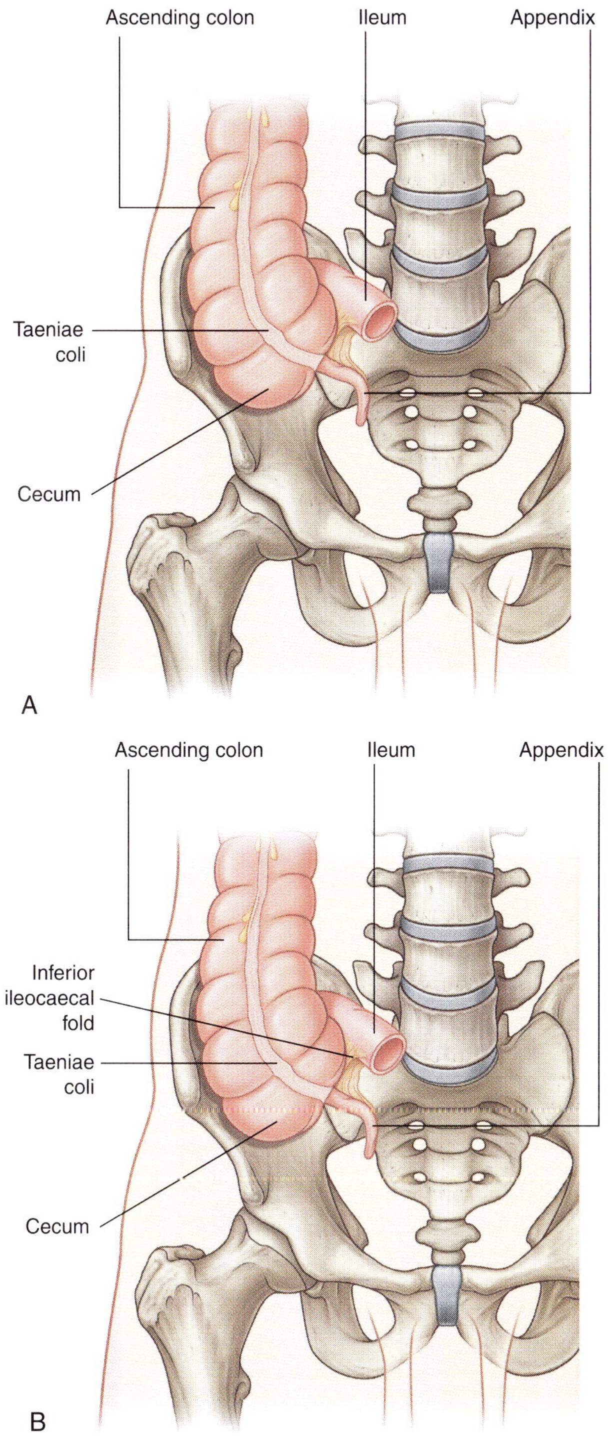

Fig. 4.77(A) Cecum and appendix. **(B)** Peritoneal folds related to the ileocecal junction.

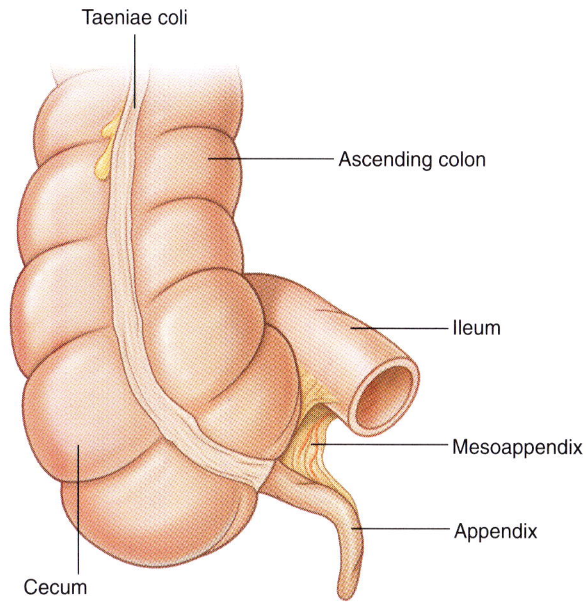

Fig. 4.78 Mesoappendix and appendicular vessels.

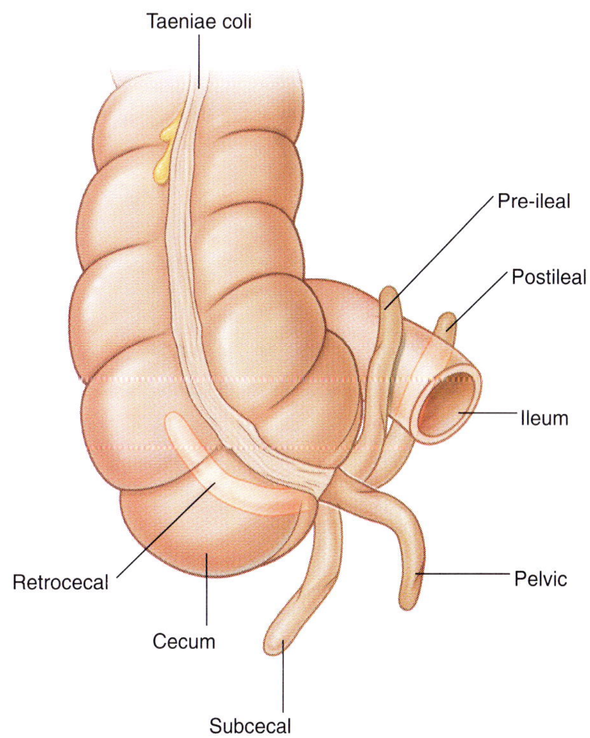

Fig. 4.79 Positions of the appendix.

- Suspended over the pelvic brim in a pelvic or descending position
- Below the cecum in a subcecal location
- Anterior to the terminal ileum, possibly contacting the anterior abdominal wall, in a pre-ileal position or posterior to the terminal ileum in a postileal position

The surface projection of the base of the appendix is at the junction of the lateral and middle one-third of a line from the anterior superior iliac spine to the umbilicus (McBurney's point). People with appendicitis may describe pain at or near this location. It is the site of maximum sensitivity to pain on touching (tenderness).

The arterial supply to the cecum and appendix (Fig. 4.80) includes:

- The anterior cecal artery from the ileocolic artery (from the superior mesenteric artery)
- The posterior cecal artery from the ileocolic artery (from the superior mesenteric artery)
- The appendicular artery from the ileocolic artery (from the superior mesenteric artery)

An accessory appendicular artery (artery of Seshachalam) is a branch of the posterior cecal artery that may be present in the mesoappendix.

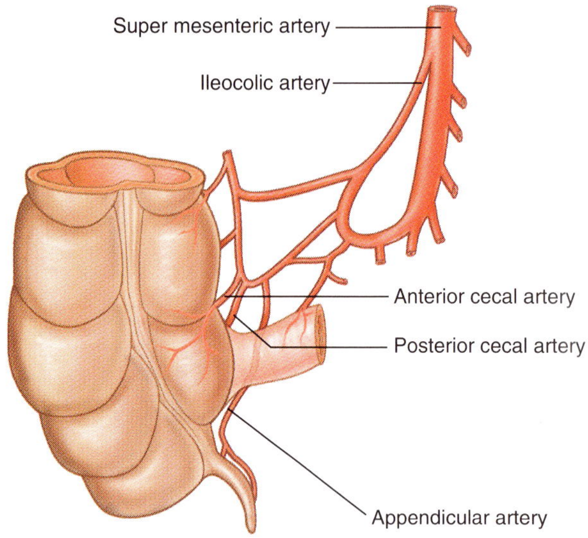

Fig. 4.80 Arterial supply to the cecum and appendix.

Early clinical exposure

Appendicitis

Acute appendicitis is an abdominal emergency. It usually occurs when the appendix is obstructed by either a fecalith or enlargement of the lymphoid nodules. Within the obstructed appendix, bacteria proliferate and invade the appendix wall, which becomes damaged by pressure necrosis. In some instances, this may resolve spontaneously; in other cases, inflammatory change (Fig. 4.81A and B) continues and perforation ensues, which may lead to localized or generalized peritonitis.

Most patients with acute appendicitis have localized tenderness in the right groin. Initially, the pain begins as a central, periumbilical, colicky type of pain, which tends to come and go. After 6–10 hours, the pain tends to localize in the right iliac fossa and becomes constant. Patients may develop a fever, nausea, and vomiting. The etiology of the pain for appendicitis is described in Case 1 of Chapter 1, p. 57.

The treatment for appendicitis is appendectomy.

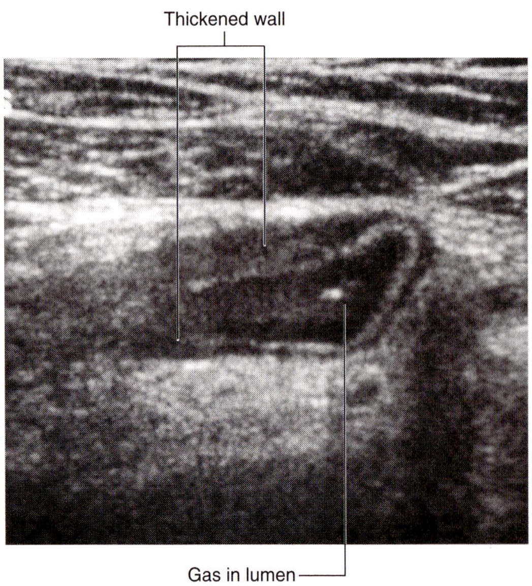

Fig. 4.81(A) Inflamed appendix. Ultrasound scan.

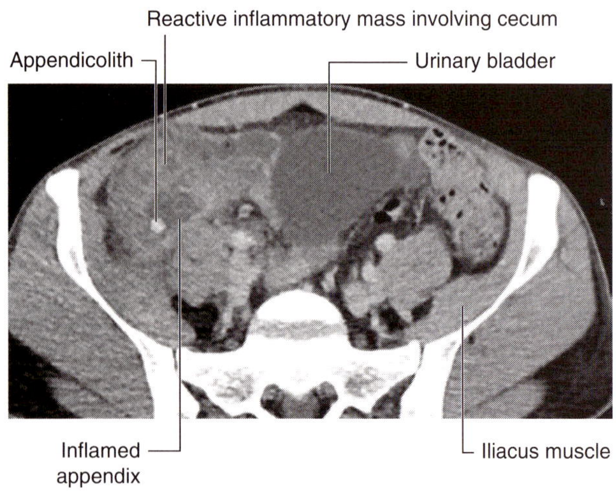

Fig. 4.81(B) Axial CT shows inflamed appendix.

Colon

The colon extends superiorly from the cecum and consists of the ascending, transverse, descending, and sigmoid colon (Fig. 4.82). Its ascending and descending segments are (secondarily) retroperitoneal and its transverse and sigmoid segments are intraperitoneal.

At the junction of the ascending and transverse colon is the right colic flexure, which is just inferior to the right lobe of the liver (Fig. 4.83). A similar, but more acute bend (the left colic flexure) occurs at the junction of the transverse and descending colon. This bend is just inferior to the spleen, is higher and more posterior than the right colic flexure, and is attached to the diaphragm by the phrenicocolic ligament (see Fig. 4.103).

Immediately lateral to the ascending and descending colon are the **right** and **left paracolic gutters** (Fig. 4.82). These depressions are formed between the lateral margins of the ascending and descending colon and the posterolateral abdominal wall and are gutters through which material can pass from one region of the peritoneal cavity to another. Because major vessels and lymphatics are on the medial or posteromedial sides of the ascending and descending colon, a relatively blood-free mobilization of the ascending and descending colon is possible by cutting the peritoneum along these lateral paracolic gutters.

The final segment of the colon (the sigmoid colon) begins above the pelvic inlet and extends to the level of vertebra SIII, where it is continuous with the rectum (Fig. 4.82). This S-shaped structure is quite mobile except at its beginning, where it continues from the descending colon, and at its end, where it continues as the rectum. Between these points, it is suspended by the sigmoid mesocolon.

The arterial supply to the ascending colon (Fig. 4.84) includes:

- The colic branch from the ileocolic artery (from the superior mesenteric artery, Fig. 4.80)
- The anterior cecal artery from the ileocolic artery (from the superior mesenteric artery)
- The posterior cecal artery from the ileocolic artery (from the superior mesenteric artery)
- The right colic artery from the superior mesenteric artery

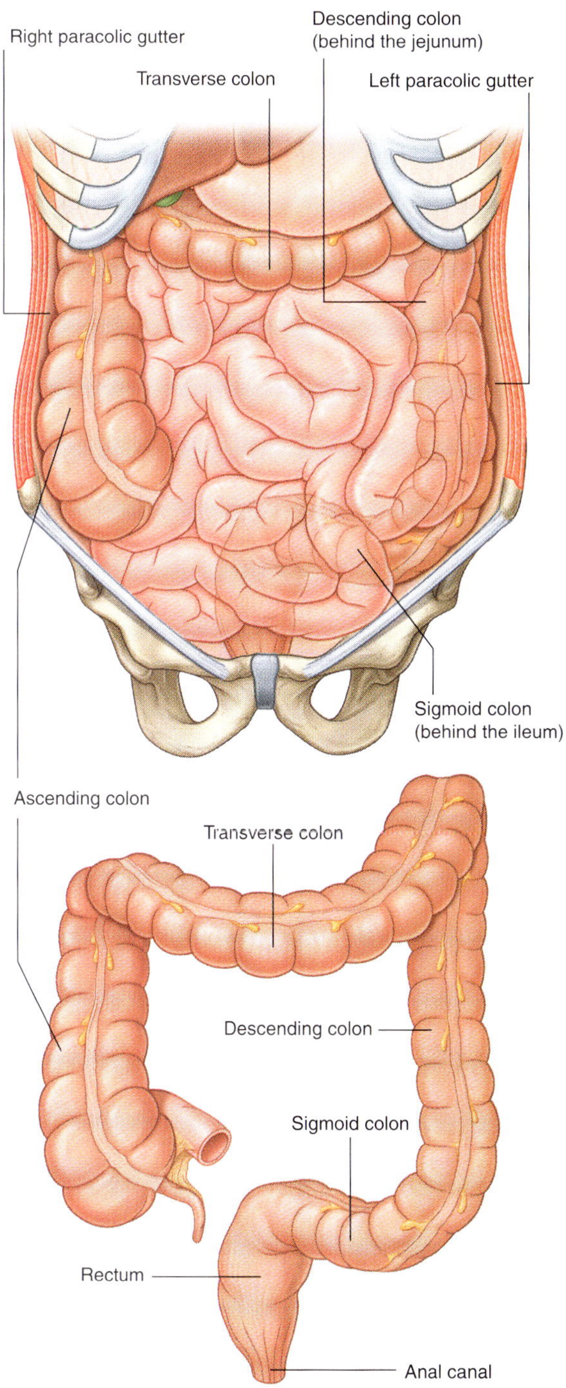

Fig. 4.82 Colon.

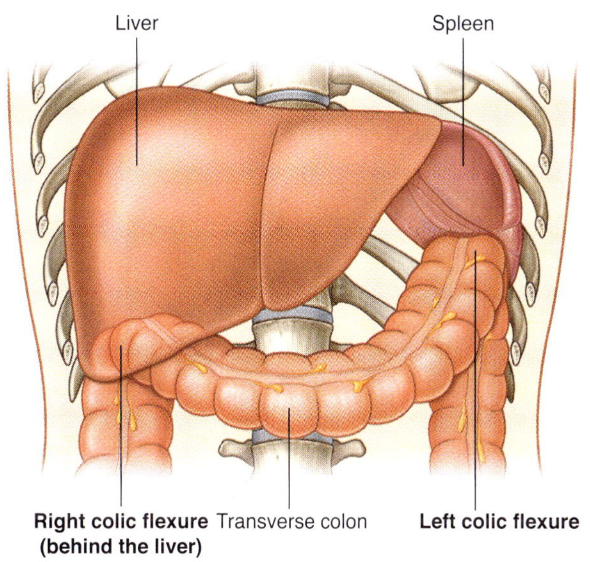

Fig. 4.83 Right and left colic flexures.

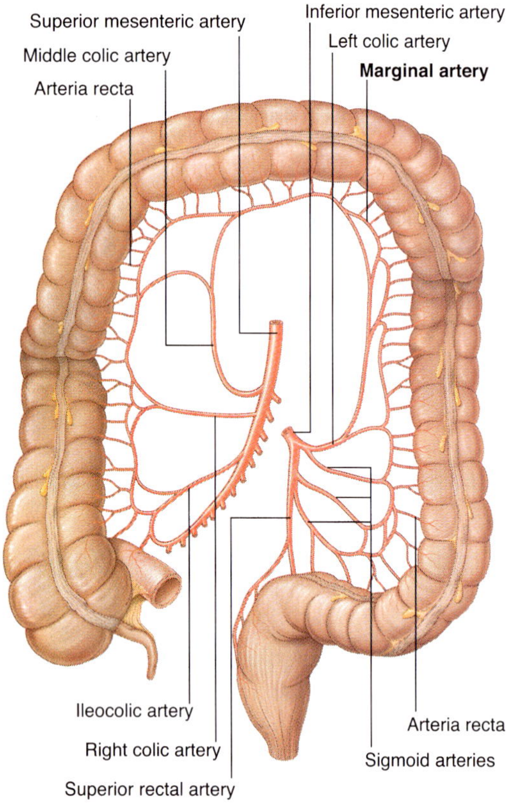

Fig. 4.84 Arterial supply to the colon.

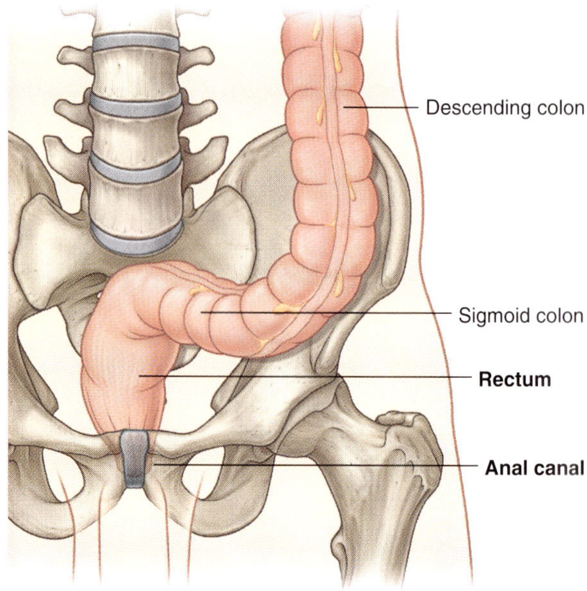

Fig. 4.85 Rectum and anal canal.

The arterial supply to the transverse colon (Fig. 4.84) includes:

- The right colic artery from the superior mesenteric artery
- The middle colic artery from the superior mesenteric artery
- The left colic artery from the inferior mesenteric artery

The arterial supply to the descending colon (Fig. 4.84) includes the left colic artery from the inferior mesenteric artery.

The arterial supply to the sigmoid colon (Fig. 4.84) includes sigmoidal arteries from the inferior mesenteric artery.

Rectum and anal canal

Extending from the sigmoid colon is the rectum (Fig. 4.85). The **rectosigmoid junction** is usually described as being at the level of vertebra SIII or at the end of the sigmoid mesocolon because the rectum is a retroperitoneal structure.

The arterial supply to the rectum and anal canal (Fig. 4.86) includes:

- The superior rectal artery from the inferior mesenteric artery
- The middle rectal artery from the internal iliac artery
- The inferior rectal artery from the internal pudendal artery (from the internal iliac artery)

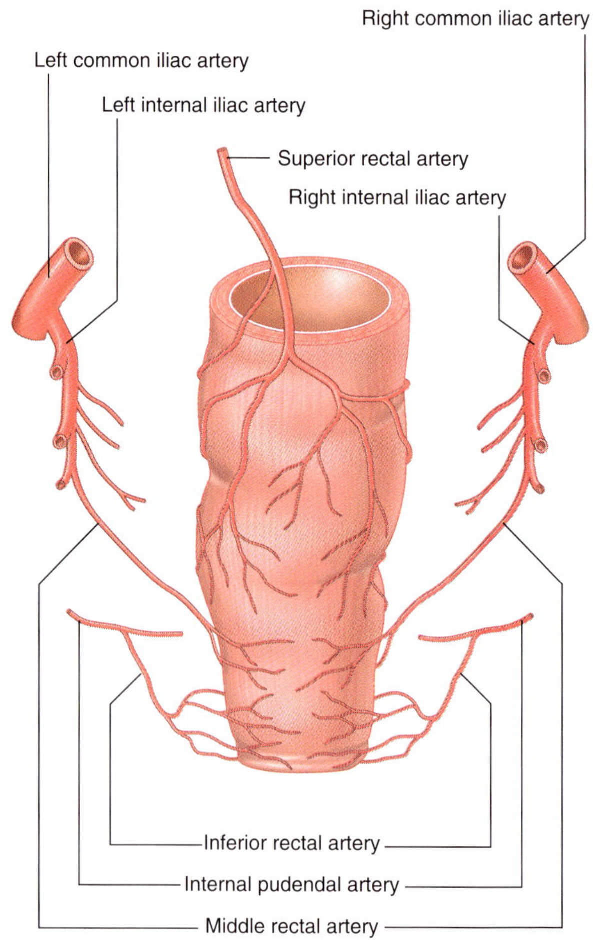

Fig. 4.86 Arterial supply to the rectum and anal canal. Posterior view.

Early clinical exposure

Congenital disorders of the gastrointestinal tract

The normal positions of the abdominal viscera result from a complex series of rotations that the gut tube undergoes and from the growth of the abdominal cavity to accommodate changes in the size of the developing organs. A number of developmental anomalies can occur during gut development, many of which appear in the neonate or infant, and some of which are surgical emergencies. Occasionally, such disorders are diagnosed only in adults.

Malrotation and midgut volvulus

Malrotation is incomplete rotation and fixation of the midgut after it has passed from the umbilical sac and returned to the abdominal coelom (Fig. 4.87 and 4.88). The proximal attachment of the small bowel mesentery begins at the **suspensory muscle of duodenum (ligament of Treitz)**, which determines the position of the duodenojejunal junction (Fig. 4.63C). The mesentery of the small bowel ends at the level of the ileocecal junction in the right lower quadrant. This long line of fixation of the mesentery prevents accidental twists of the gut (Fig. 4.57).

If the duodenojejunal flexure or the cecum does not end up in its usual site, the posterior attachment of the small bowel mesentery is shorter than normal, which permits twisting of the small bowel around the axis of the superior mesenteric artery. Twisting of the bowel, in general, is termed **volvulus**. Volvulus of the small bowel may lead to a reduction of blood flow and infarction.

In some patients, the cecum ends up in the midabdomen. From the cecum and the right side of the colon, a series of peritoneal folds (**Ladd's bands**) develops that extends to the right undersurface of the liver and compresses the duodenum. A small bowel volvulus may then occur as well as duodenal obstruction. Emergency surgery may be necessary to divide the bands.

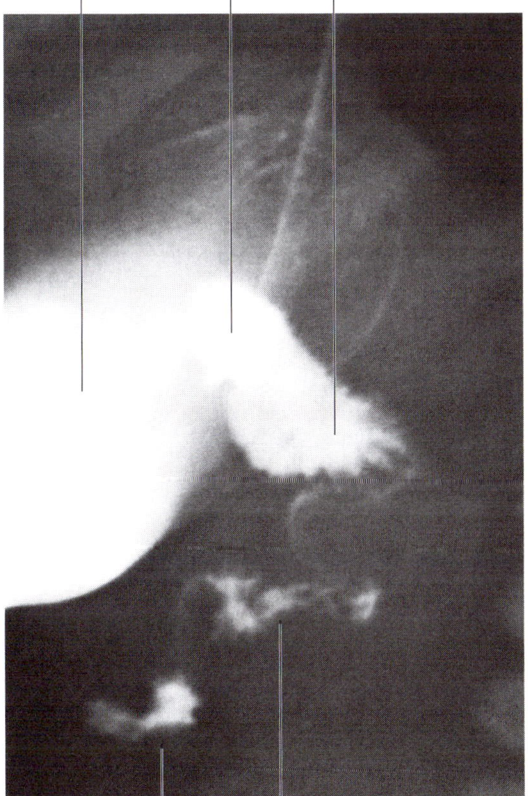

Fig. 4.87 Small bowel malrotation and volvulus. Radiograph of stomach, duodenum, and upper jejunum using barium sulfate.

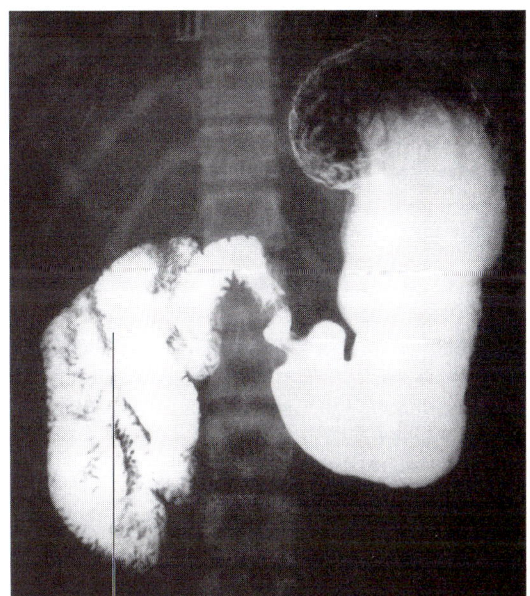

Fig. 4.88 Small bowel malrotation. Radiograph of stomach, duodenum, and jejunum using barium sulfate.

Early clinical exposure

Bowel obstruction

A bowel obstruction can be either functional or due to a true obstruction. Mechanical obstruction is caused by an intraluminal, mural, or extrinsic mass which can be secondary to a foreign body, obstructing tumor in the wall, or extrinsic compression from an adhesion, or embryological band (Fig. 4.89A).

A functional obstruction is usually due to an inability of the bowel to peristalse, which again has a number of causes, and most frequently is a postsurgical state due to excessive intraoperative bowel handling. Other causes may well include abnormality of electrolytes (e.g., low sodium and potassium) rendering the bowel paralyzed until correction has occurred.

The signs and symptoms of obstruction depend on the level at which the obstruction has occurred. The primary symptom is central abdominal, intermittent, colicky pain as the peristaltic waves try to overcome the obstruction. Abdominal distention will occur if it is a low obstruction (distal), allowing more proximal loops of bowel to fill with fluid. A high obstruction (in the proximal small bowel) may not produce abdominal distention.

Vomiting and absolute constipation, including the inability to pass flatus, will ensue.

Early diagnosis is important because considerable fluid and electrolytes enter the bowel lumen and fail to be reabsorbed, which produces dehydration and electrolyte abnormalities. Furthermore, the bowel continues to distend, compromising the blood supply within the bowel wall, which may lead to ischemia and perforation. The symptoms and signs are variable and depend on the level of obstruction.

Small bowel obstruction is typically caused by adhesions following previous surgery, and history should always be sought for any operations or abdominal interventions (e.g., previous appendectomy). Other causes include bowel passing into hernias (e.g., inguinal) and bowel twisting on its own mesentery (volvulus). Examination of hernial orifices is mandatory in patients with bowel obstruction (Fig. 4.89B).

Large bowel obstruction is commonly caused by a tumor. Other potential causes include hernias and inflammatory diverticular disease of the sigmoid colon (Fig. 4.89C).

The treatment is intravenous replacement of fluid and electrolytes, analgesia, and relief of obstruction. The passage of a nasogastric tube allows aspiration of fluid from the stomach. In many instances, small bowel obstruction, typically secondary to adhesions, will settle with nonoperative management. Large bowel obstruction may require an urgent operation to remove the obstructing lesion using a colonic stent (Fig. 4.90), or a temporary bypass procedure (e.g., defunctioning colostomy).

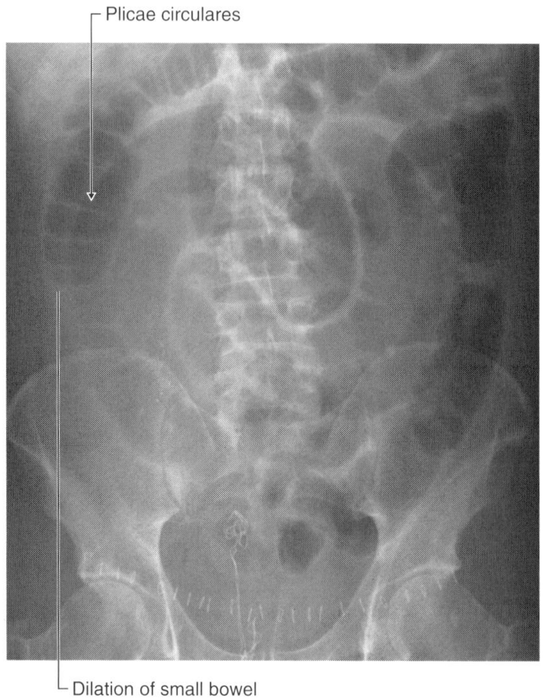

Fig. 4.89 (A) This radiograph of the abdomen, anteroposterior view, demonstrates a number of dilated loops of small bowel. Small bowel can be identified by the plicae circulares that pass from wall to wall as indicated. The large bowel is not dilated. The cause of the small bowel dilatation is an adhesion after pelvic surgery.

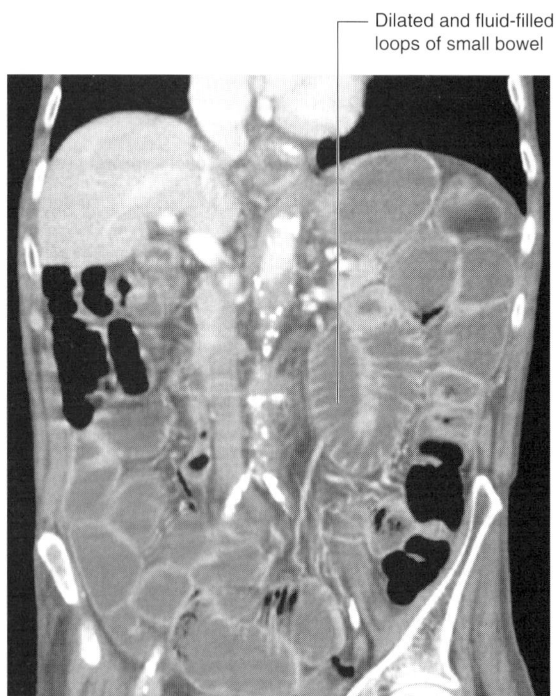

Fig. 4.89 (B) Coronal CT demonstrates dilated and fluid-filled loops of small bowel in patient with small bowel obstruction.

Early clinical exposure—cont'd

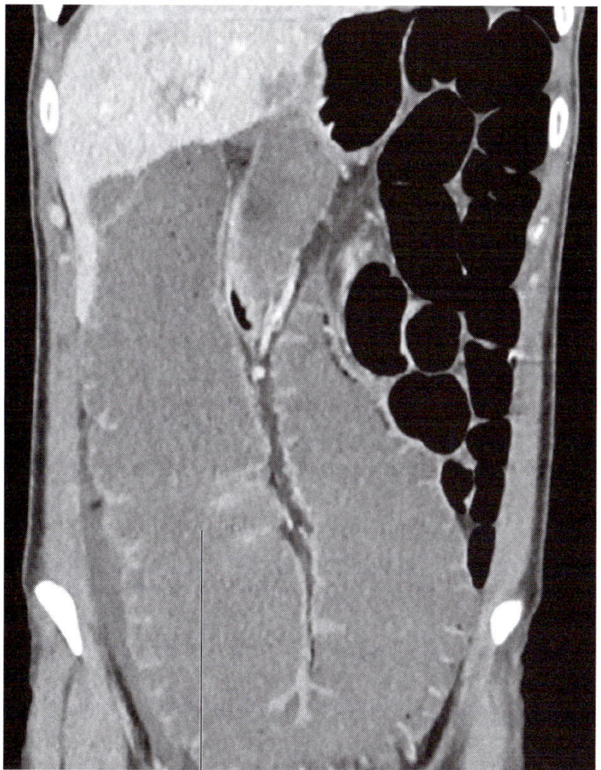

Fig. 4.89 (C) Coronal CT of abdomen shows fluid-filled and dilated ascending and transverse colon in patient with large bowel obstruction.

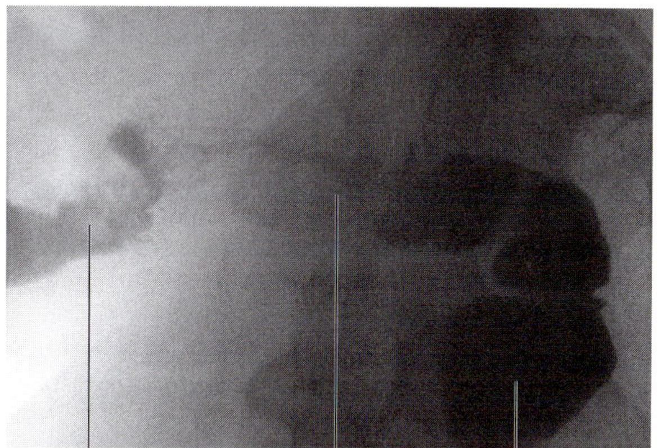

Fig. 4.90 This oblique radiograph demonstrates contrast passing through a colonic stent that has been placed to relieve bowel obstruction prior to surgery.

Early clinical exposure

Diverticular disease

Diverticular disease is the development of multiple colonic diverticula, predominantly throughout the sigmoid colon, though the whole colon may be affected (Fig. 4.91A). The sigmoid colon has the smallest diameter of any portion of the colon and is therefore the site where intraluminal pressure is potentially the highest. Poor dietary fiber intake and obesity are also linked to diverticular disease.

The presence of multiple diverticula does not necessarily mean the patient requires any treatment. Moreover, many patients have no other symptoms or signs.

Patients tend to develop symptoms and signs when the neck of the diverticulum becomes obstructed by feces and becomes infected. Inflammation may spread along the wall, causing abdominal pain. When the sigmoid colon becomes inflamed (diverticulitis), abdominal pain and fever ensue (Fig. 4.91B).

Because of the anatomical position of the sigmoid colon, there are a number of complications that may occur. The diverticula can perforate to form an abscess in the pelvis. The inflammation may produce an inflammatory mass, obstructing the left ureter. Inflammation may also spread to the bladder, producing a fistula between the sigmoid colon and the bladder. In these circumstances, patients may develop a urinary tract infection and rarely have fecal material and gas passing per urethra.

The diagnosis is based upon clinical examination and often CT scanning. In the first instance, patients will be treated with antibiotic therapy; however, a surgical resection may be necessary if symptoms persist.

Continued

Early clinical exposure—cont'd

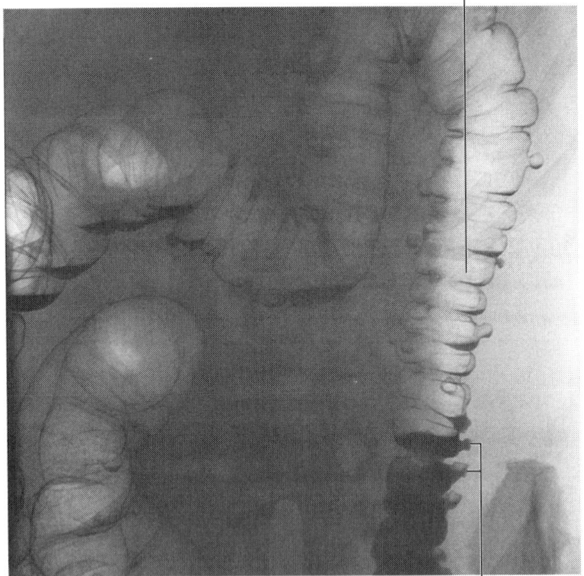

Fig. 4.91(A) This double-contrast barium enema demonstrates numerous small outpouchings throughout the distal large bowel predominantly within the descending colon and the sigmoid colon. These small outpouchings are diverticula, and in most instances remain quiescent.

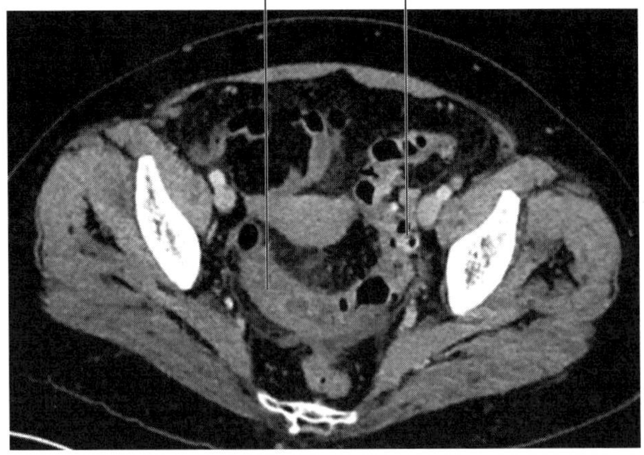

Fig. 4.91(B) Axial CT of inflamed sigmoid colon in patient with diverticulitis.

Early clinical exposure

Ostomies

It is occasionally necessary to surgically externalize bowel to the anterior abdominal wall. Externalization of bowel plays an important role in patient management. These extraanatomical bypass procedures are based on anatomical knowledge and in many instances are life saving.

Gastrostomy

Gastrostomy is performed when the stomach is attached to the anterior abdominal wall and a tube is placed through the skin into the stomach. Typically this is performed to feed the patient when it is impossible to take food and fluid orally (e.g., complex head and neck cancer). The procedure can be performed either surgically or through a direct needlestick puncture under sedation in the anterior abdominal wall.

Jejunostomy

Similarly the jejunum can be brought to the anterior abdominal wall and fixed. The jejunostomy is used as a site where a feeding tube is placed through the anterior abdominal wall into the efferent part of the jejunum to enable flow in the direction of peristalsis.

Ileostomy

An ileostomy is performed when small bowel contents need to be diverted from the distal bowel. An ileostomy is often performed to protect a distal surgical anastomosis, such as in the colon to allow healing after surgery.

Colostomy

There are a number of instances when a colostomy may be necessary. In many circumstances, it is performed to protect the distal large bowel after surgery. A further indication would include large bowel obstruction with imminent perforation wherein a colostomy allows decompression of the bowel and its contents. This is a safe and temporary procedure performed when the patient is too unwell for extensive bowel surgery. It is relatively straightforward and carries reduced risk, preventing significant morbidity and mortality.

Early clinical exposure—cont'd

An **end colostomy** is necessary when the patient has undergone a surgical resection of the rectum and anus (typically for cancer).

Ileal conduit

An ileal conduit is an extraanatomical procedure and is performed after resection of the bladder for tumor. In this situation, a short segment of small bowel is identified. The bowel is divided twice to produce a 20-cm segment of small bowel on its own mesentery. This isolated segment of bowel is used as a conduit. The remaining bowel is joined together. The proximal end is anastomosed to the ureters, and the distal end is anastomosed to the anterior abdominal wall. Hence, urine passes from the kidneys into the ureters and through the short segment of small bowel to the anterior abdominal wall.

When patients have an ileostomy, colostomy, or ileal conduit, it is necessary for them to fix a collecting bag onto the anterior abdominal wall. Contrary to one's initial thoughts, these bags are tolerated extremely well by most patients and allow patients to live a nearly normal and healthy life.

Liver

SET INDUCTION—CASE SCENARIO: 7 HEPATIC CANCER

A 62-year-old male was brought to the surgery OPD with complaints of loss of appetite, loss of weight, and a mass felt in the epigastrium. He was diagnosed with primary cancer of the liver, and a segmentectomy was planned. Knowledge of the liver is needed to manage this case.

REMEMBER [Recall Facts]	**OUTLINE 7. LIVER AND GALLBLADDER—LEARNING OBJECTIVES [By the end of this section, the student should be able to:]** **DEMONSTRATE AND ANALYZE RELATIONSHIPS [Identify structures in a Prosected Specimen or Figure]**			**EVALUATE [Explain Concepts]**
	Level I	**Level II**	**Level III**	
1. Describe the surfaces and relations of the liver 2. Describe the ligaments attached to the liver 3. Describe the functional and traditional lobes of the liver 4. Describe the segments of the liver 5. Describe the parts, functions, and relations of the gallbladder	■ Gallbladder—parts (fundus, body, and neck) ■ Fossa for the gallbladder ■ Cystic duct ■ Common hepatic duct ■ Hepatic artery proper ■ Portal vein ■ Liver: ■ Anatomical position ■ Anatomical lobes (right, left, caudate, and quadrate) ■ Physiological lobes (right and left) ■ Surfaces (diaphragmatic and visceral) ■ Borders (inferior) ■ Fissures (for ligamentum teres and venosum) ■ Relations of visceral surface ■ Ligaments (teres, coronary, and triangular) ■ Bare area	■ Important relations of the gallbladder ■ Hepatocystic triangle ■ Calot's triangle ■ Cystic artery ■ Right and left branches of the hepatic duct, hepatic artery proper, and portal vein	■ Liver: ■ Tuber omentale ■ Caudate and papillary processes	■ Bare area of liver ■ Peritoneal recesses of liver ■ Relations of visceral surface of the liver ■ Blood supply and vascular segments of the liver ■ Lymphatic drainage of liver

EARLY CLINICAL EXPOSURE [Apply Anatomical Knowledge]	
Surgical Anatomy/ Pathology/ Trauma	**Imaging/ Surface Anatomy**
■ Hepatitis ■ Cirrhosis ■ Liver biopsy ■ Hepatorenal pouch of Morrison ■ Cholecystitis ■ Gallstones ■ Calot's triangle	■ Cholecystogram ■ Palpation of the liver

PROBLEM SOLVING/ CLINICAL CASES [Interpret]
■ Discuss the basis for hepatic segmentectomy ■ Discuss the pain felt in cholecystitis

The liver is the largest visceral organ in the body and is primarily in the right hypochondrium and epigastric region, extending into the left hypochondrium (or in the right upper quadrant, extending into the left upper quadrant) (Fig. 4.92).

Surfaces of the liver include:

- A **diaphragmatic surface** in the anterior, superior, and posterior directions
- A **visceral surface** in the inferior direction (Fig. 4.93)

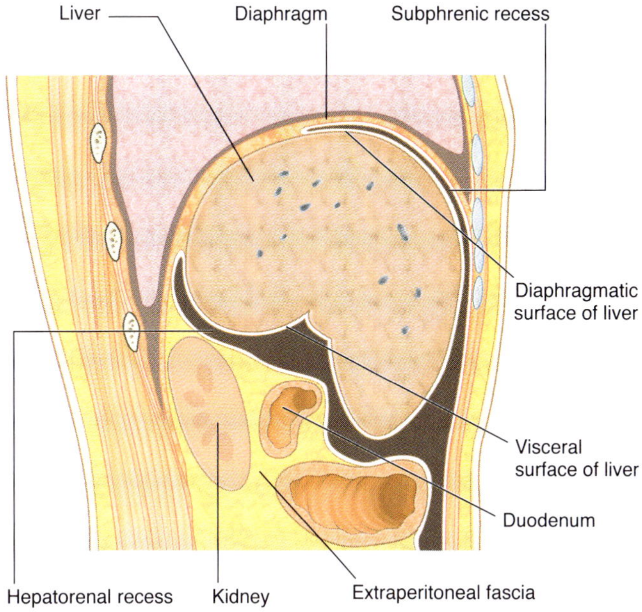

Fig. 4.93 Surfaces of the liver and recesses associated with the liver.

Diaphragmatic surface

The diaphragmatic surface of the liver, is smooth and domed, and lies against the inferior surface of the diaphragm (Fig. 4.94). Associated with it are the subphrenic and hepatorenal recesses (Fig. 4.93):

- The **subphrenic recess** separates the diaphragmatic surface of the liver from the diaphragm and is divided into right and left areas by the **falciform ligament**, a structure derived from the ventral mesentery in the embryo.
- The hepatorenal recess is a part of the peritoneal cavity on the right side between the liver and the right kidney and right suprarenal gland.

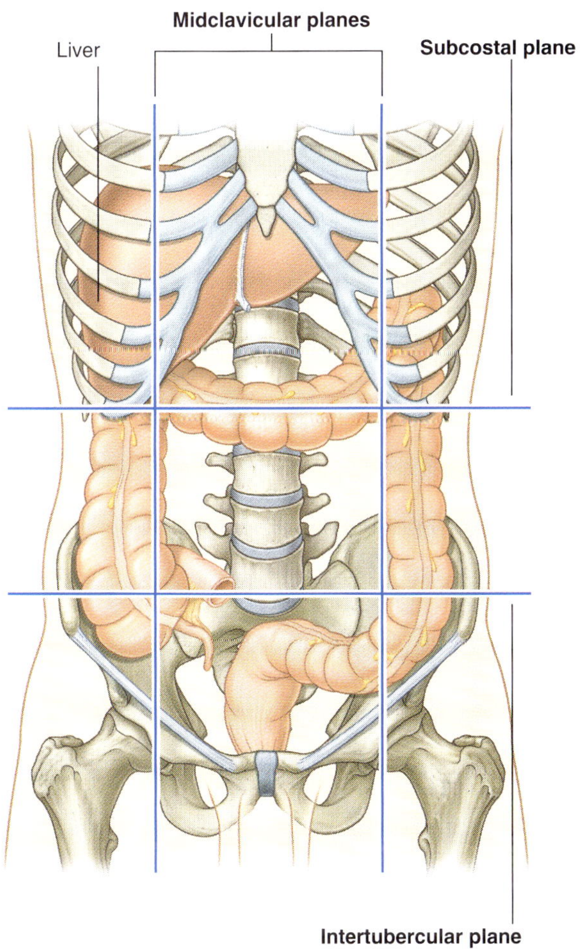

Fig. 4.92 Position of the liver in the abdomen.

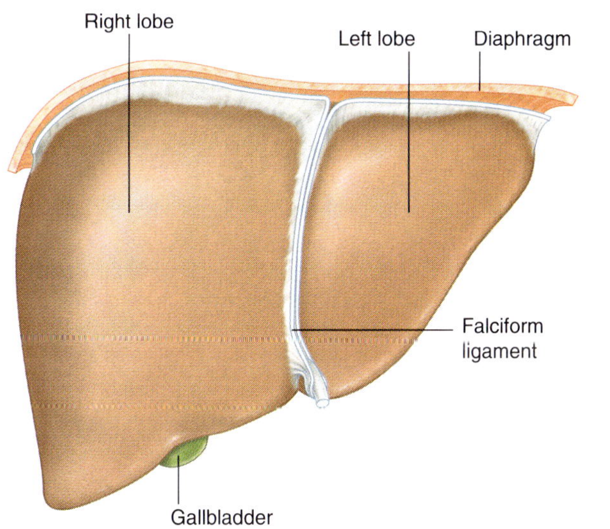

Fig. 4.94 Diaphragmatic surface of the liver.

The subphrenic and hepatorenal recesses are continuous anteriorly.

Visceral surface

The visceral surface of the liver is covered with visceral peritoneum except in the **fossa for the** gallbladder and at the **porta hepatis** (gateway to the liver; Fig. 4.95). Structures related to this surface include the following (Fig. 4.96):

- Esophagus
- Right anterior part of the stomach
- Superior part of the duodenum (related to the body of the gallbladder)
- Lesser omentum
- Gallbladder
- Right colic flexure
- Transverse colon (related to fundus of the gallbladder)
- Right kidney
- Right suprarenal gland

The **porta hepatis** serves as the point of entry into the liver for the hepatic arteries and the portal vein, and the exit point for the hepatic ducts (Fig. 4.95).

Associated ligaments

The liver is attached to the anterior abdominal wall by the **falciform ligament** and, except for a small area of the liver which lies directly against the diaphragm (the

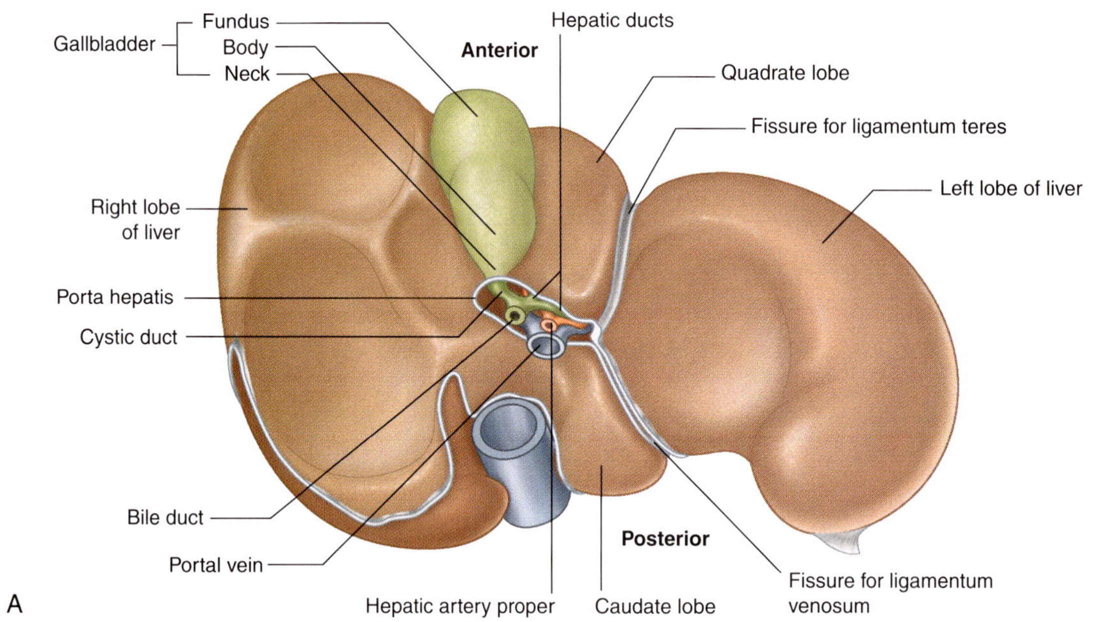

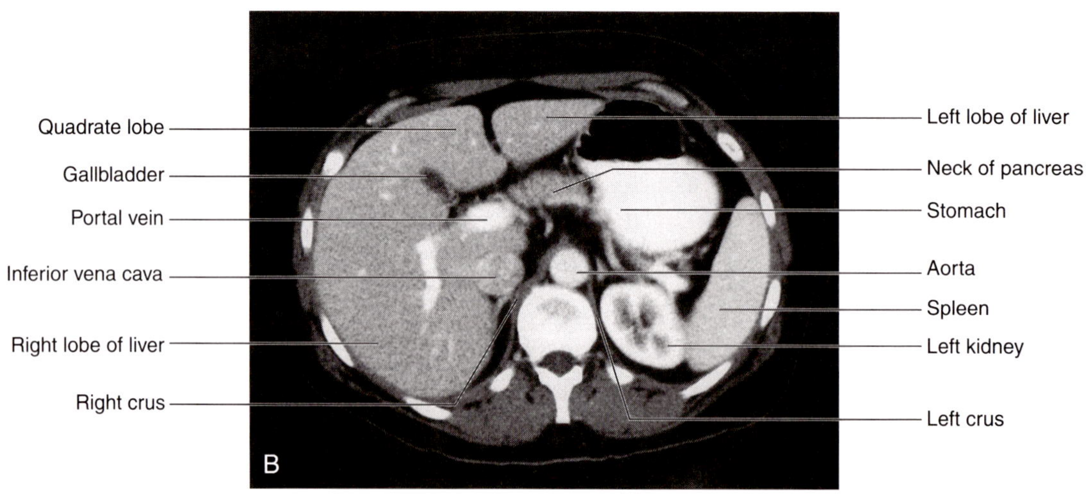

Fig. 4.95 Visceral surface of the liver. **(A)** Illustration. **(B)** Abdominal computed tomogram, with contrast, in the axial plane.

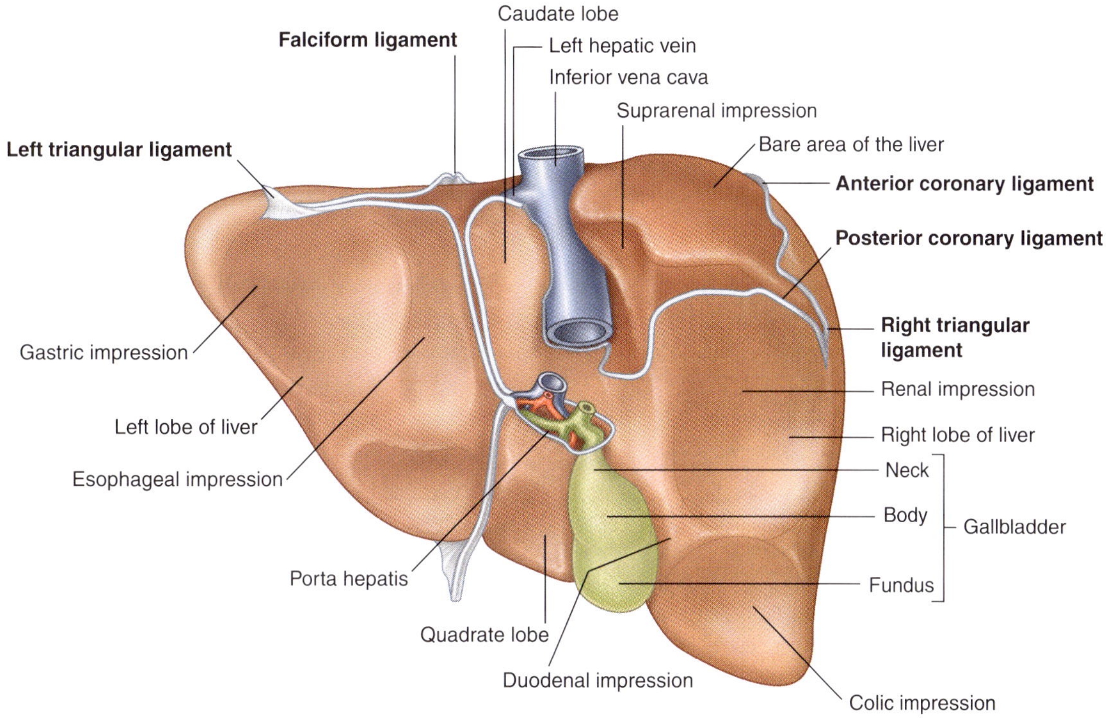

Fig. 4.96 Posterior view of the bare area of the liver and associated ligaments.

bare area), the liver is almost completely surrounded by visceral peritoneum (Fig. 4.96). Additional folds of peritoneum connect the liver to the stomach (**hepatogastric ligament,** Fig. 4.57), the duodenum (**hepatoduodenal ligament**) and the diaphragm (**right** and **left triangular ligaments** and **anterior** and **posterior coronary ligaments**).

The bare area of the liver is a part of the liver on the diaphragmatic surface where there is no intervening peritoneum between the liver and the diaphragm (Fig. 4.96):

- The anterior boundary of the bare area is indicated by a reflection of peritoneum—the anterior coronary ligament.
- The posterior boundary of the bare area is indicated by a reflection of peritoneum—the posterior coronary ligament.
- Where the coronary ligaments come together laterally, they form the right triangular ligament.

Lobes

The liver is divided into right and left functional lobes by a line passing through the fossae for the gallbladder and the inferior vena cava (Cantlie's line) (Fig. 4.95). The middle hepatic vein lies in this line. The Couinaud classification divides the liver into eight independent functional units called segments (see Fig. 4.107). Segment I is the caudate lobe and segment VIII is only visible on the diaphragmatic surface. Hepatic veins are at the periphery of each segment. At the center of each segment are branches of the portal veins, hepatic arteries, and hepatic ducts.

Traditionally, the liver has been divided into right and left lobes by the falciform ligament and the fissure for ligamentum teres and the fissure for ligamentum venosum. The **right lobe of the liver** is the largest lobe, whereas the **left lobe of the liver** is smaller. The quadrate and caudate lobes are described as a part of the right lobe of the liver but functionally they are distinct.

- The **quadrate lobe** is visible on the anterior part of the visceral surface of the liver and posteriorly is in contact with the pylorus of the stomach. It is bounded on the left by the fissure for the ligamentum teres and on the right by the fossa for the gallbladder. Functionally, it is part of the left functional lobe of the liver.
- The **caudate lobe** is visible on the posterior part of the visceral surface of the liver. It is bounded on the left by the fissure for the ligamentum venosum and on the right by the groove for the inferior vena cava. Functionally, it is separate from the right and the left functional lobes of the liver and has separate veins which drain to the inferior vena cava.

The fissure of Ganz or Rouviere's sulcus is a fissure on the visceral surface of the liver anterior to segment I that is seen clearly during posterior dissection during laparoscopic cholecystectomy. It runs transversely inferior to the caudate process at the level of the porta hepatis where the right posterior pedicle enters the liver. It serves as an important landmark in cholecystectomy to avoid bile duct injury.

The arterial supply to the liver includes:

- The right hepatic artery from the hepatic artery proper (a branch of the common hepatic artery from the celiac trunk)
- The left hepatic artery from the hepatic artery proper (a branch of the common hepatic artery from the celiac trunk)

Gallbladder

The **gallbladder** is a pear-shaped sac lying on the visceral surface of the right lobe of the liver in a fossa to the right of the quadrate lobe (Fig. 4.95). It has:

- A rounded end (**fundus of the gallbladder**), which may project from the inferior border of the liver
- A major part in the fossa (**body of the gallbladder**), which may lie against the transverse colon and the superior part of the duodenum
- A narrow part (**neck of the gallbladder**) with mucosal folds forming the spiral fold. Hartmann's pouch is a small outpouching at the junction of the body and neck of the gallbladder

The arterial supply to the gallbladder (Fig. 4.97) is the cystic artery from the right hepatic artery (a branch of the hepatic artery proper). The hepatocystic or hepatobiliary triangle is bounded by the cystic duct on the right, common hepatic duct on the left, and the visceral surface of the liver superiorly. It contains the cystic artery and the cystic lymph node (of Lund). In the original description of Calot's triangle, the superior boundary was the cystic artery. Variations are common in this area. The gallbladder receives, concentrates, and stores bile from the liver.

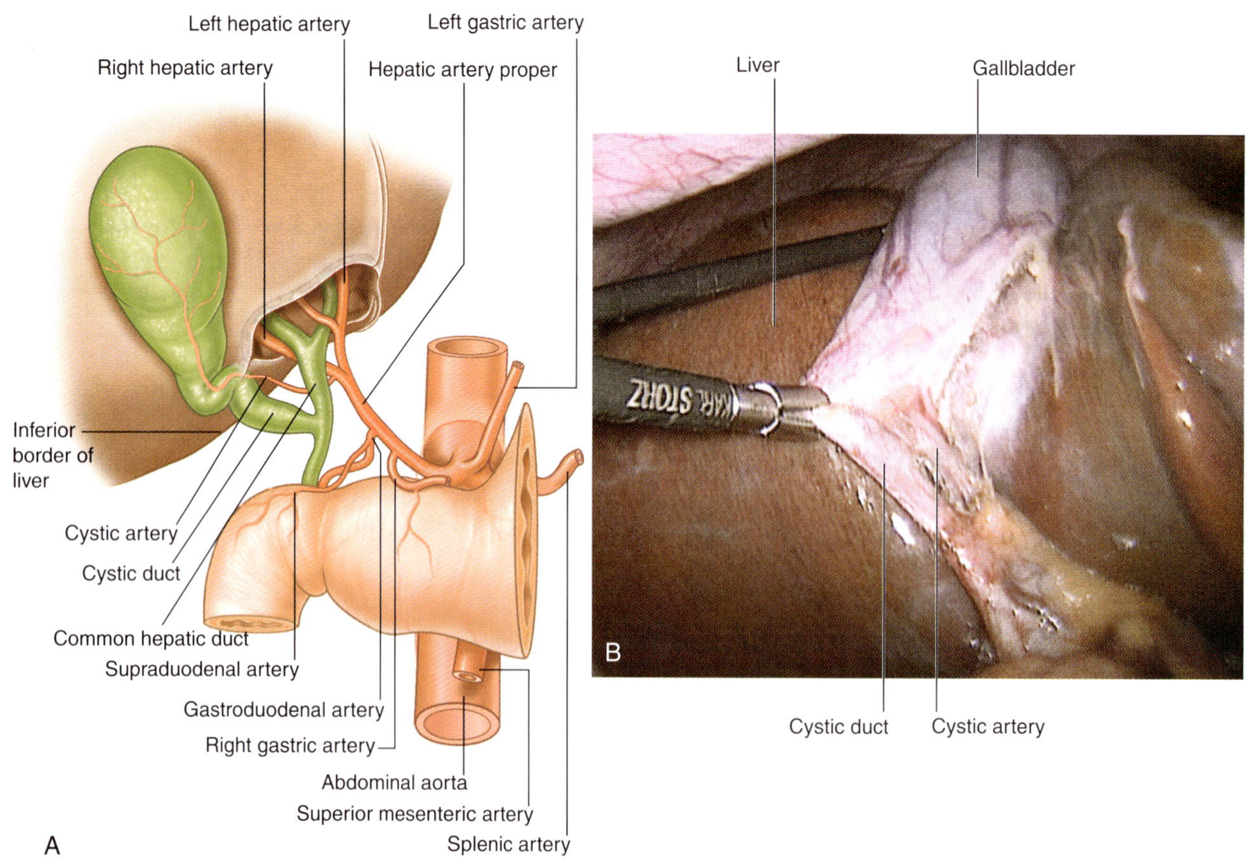

Fig. 4.97 Arterial supply to the liver and gallbladder. **(A)** Schematic. **(B)** Laparoscopic surgical view of cystic duct and cystic artery.

Pancreas

SET INDUCTION—CASE SCENARIO 8A: ANNULAR PANCREAS

An ultrasound was done during a routine prenatal checkup in an obstetric OPD for a 23-year-old pregnant female with 8-month gestation when it was noted that there was an increase in size of the abdomen more than was expected. A diagnosis of polyhydramnios was made and the cause was an annular pancreas in the fetus. Knowledge of the anatomy of the pancreas is needed to manage this case.

SET INDUCTION—CASE SCENARIO 8B: RUPTURED SPLEEN

A 25-year-old male was brought to the emergency department with complaints of a road traffic accident. He had a bruise superficial to his left rib X and severe pallor. A diagnosis of a ruptured spleen was made. Knowledge of the spleen is needed to manage this case.

<table>
<tr><th rowspan="2">REMEMBER
[Recall Facts]</th><th colspan="3">OUTLINE 8. PANCREAS AND SPLEEN—LEARNING OBJECTIVES
[By the end of this section, the student should be able to:]</th><th colspan="2" rowspan="2">EVALUATE
[Explain Concepts]</th></tr>
<tr><th colspan="3">DEMONSTRATE AND ANALYZE RELATIONSHIPS
[Identify structures in a Prosected Specimen or Figure]</th></tr>
<tr><td rowspan="6">Pancreas
1. Describe the ducts of the pancreas
2. Describe the arterial supply of the pancreas
3. Describe the termination of the biliary and pancreatic ducts
Spleen
1. Describe the ligaments attached to the spleen
2. List the relations of the spleen</td><td>Level I</td><td>Level II</td><td>Level III</td><td colspan="2">■ Peritoneal reflections of the spleen
■ Ligaments of the spleen</td></tr>
<tr><td rowspan="5">Pancreas
■ Situation, parts, surfaces, borders, important relations
■ Splenic vessels
■ Formation of portal vein
■ Origin of superior mesenteric artery
■ Common bile duct
■ Main pancreatic duct (of Wirsung)
■ Major duodenal papilla
Spleen
■ Anatomical position
■ Ends—anterior (lateral) and posterior (medial)
■ Borders—superior, inferior, and intermediate
■ Surfaces—diaphragmatic and visceral; Impressions—gastric, renal, colic, and pancreatic
■ Gastrosplenic ligament
■ Lienorenal ligament</td><td rowspan="5">■ Superior and inferior pancreaticoduodenal arteries
■ Inferior mesenteric vein
■ Accessory pancreatic duct (of Santorini)
■ Minor duodenal papilla
■ Short gastric vessels
■ Left gastro-omental vessels
■ Splenic notch</td><td rowspan="5"></td><td colspan="2">EARLY CLINICAL EXPOSURE
[Apply Anatomical Knowledge]</td></tr>
<tr><td>Surgical Anatomy/ Pathology/ Trauma</td><td>Imaging/ Surface Anatomy</td></tr>
<tr><td>■ Acute and chronic pancreatitis
■ Carcinoma of pancreas
■ Obstructive jaundice
■ Portal hypertension and portocaval shunts
■ Splenomegaly
■ Splenic rupture
■ Splenectomy
■ Splenic puncture</td><td>■ ERCP—endoscopic retrograde cholangiopancreatography
■ Palpation of the spleen</td></tr>
<tr><td colspan="2">PROBLEM SOLVING/CLINICAL CASES
[Interpret]</td></tr>
<tr><td colspan="2">■ Why is cancer of the pancreas described as the "silent killer"?
■ How is it possible to arrest bleeding from the liver?</td></tr>
</table>

The pancreas lies mostly posterior to the stomach (Fig. 4.98 and 4.99). It extends across the posterior abdominal wall from the duodenum, on the right, to the spleen, on the left.

The pancreas is (secondarily) retroperitoneal except for a small part of its tail and consists of a head, uncinate process, neck, body, and tail.

- The **head of the pancreas** lies within the C-shaped concavity of the duodenum. Osler described it as an "abdominal organ of romance" based on its location, as the head of pancreas is folded in the arms of the duodenum.
- Projecting from the lower part of the head is the **uncinate process**, which passes posterior to the superior mesenteric vessels.

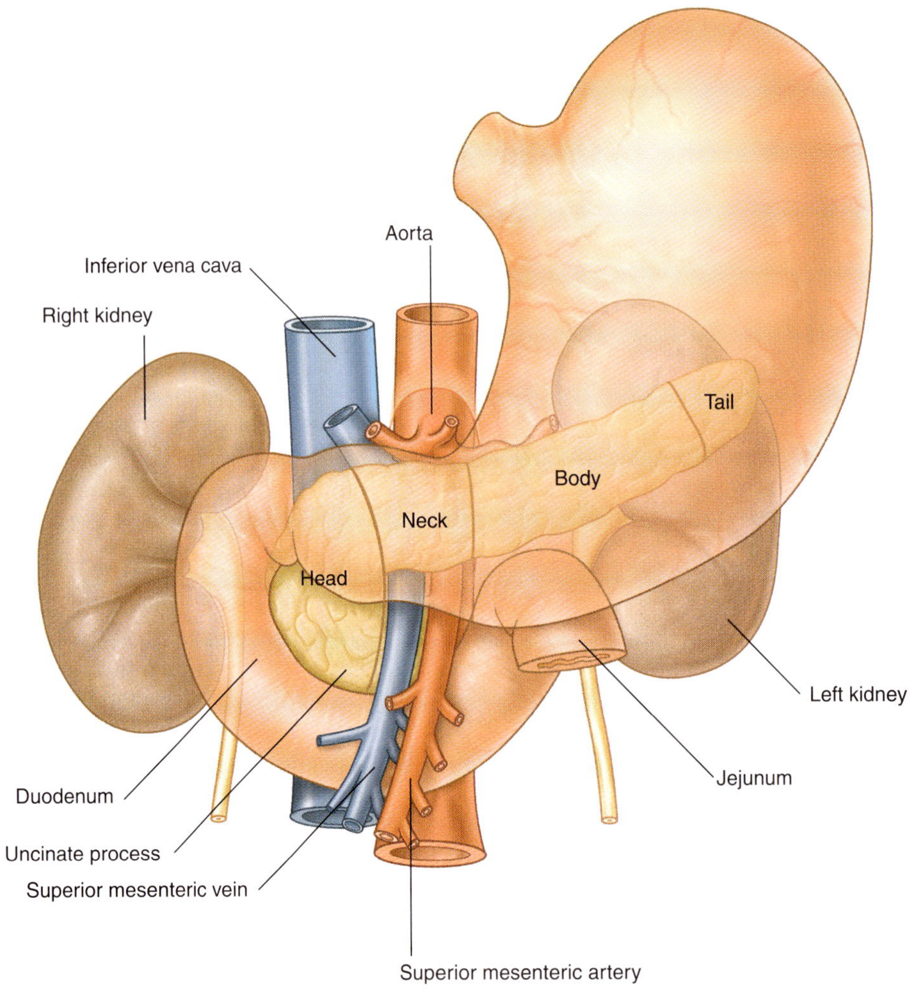

Fig. 4.98 Pancreas.

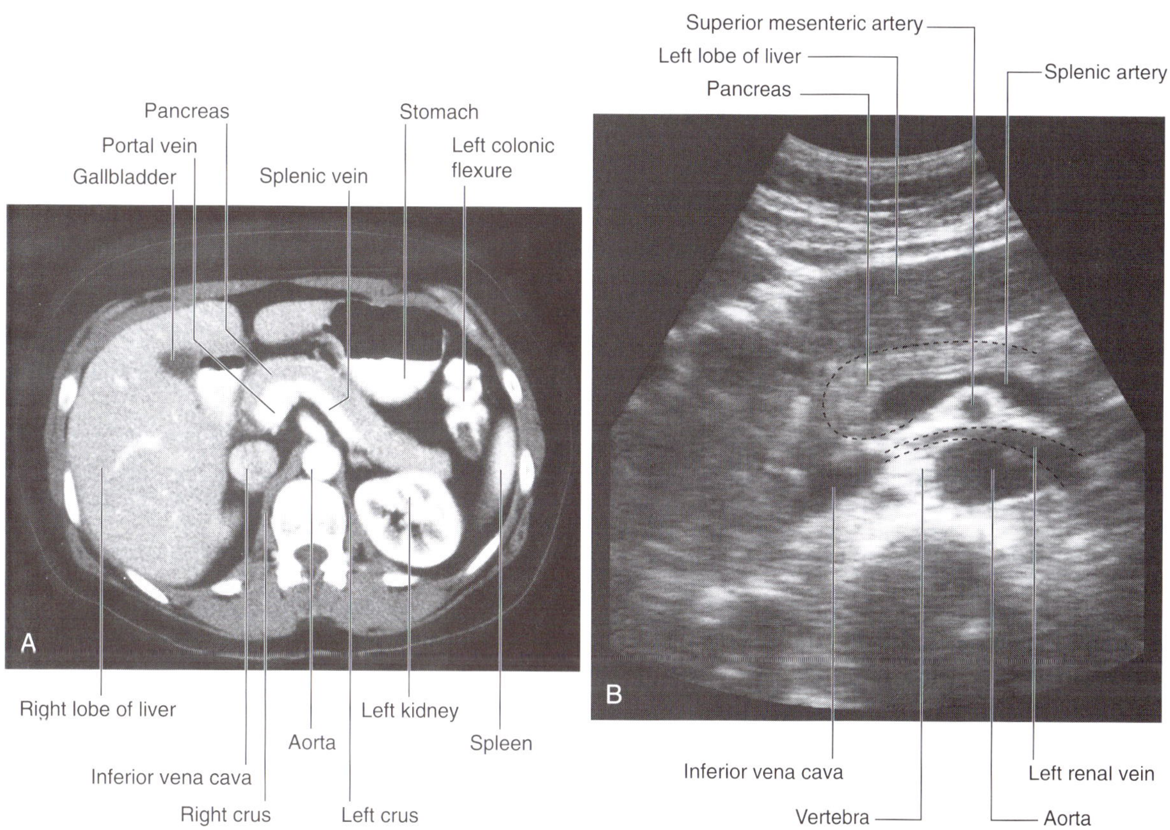

Fig. 4.99 Abdominal images. **(A)** Abdominal computed tomogram, with contrast, in the axial plane. **(B)** Abdominal ultrasound scan.

- The **neck of the pancreas** is anterior to the superior mesenteric vessels. Posterior to the neck of the pancreas, the superior mesenteric and splenic veins join to form the portal vein.
- The **body of the pancreas** is elongate and extends from the neck to the tail of the pancreas.
- The **tail of the pancreas** passes between layers of the splenorenal ligament (Fig. 4.54A).

The main **pancreatic duct (duct of Wirsung)** begins in the tail of the pancreas (Fig. 4.100). It passes to the right through the body of the pancreas and, after entering the head of the pancreas, turns inferiorly. In the lower part of the head of the pancreas, the pancreatic duct joins the bile duct. The joining of these two structures forms the **hepatopancreatic ampulla** (ampulla of Vater), which enters the descending (second) part of the duodenum at the **major duodenal papilla**. Surrounding the ampulla is the **sphincter of ampulla** (sphincter of Oddi), which is a collection of smooth muscles.

The **accessory pancreatic duct or (duct of Santorini)** empties into the duodenum just above the major duodenal papilla at the **minor duodenal papilla** (Fig. 4.100). If the accessory duct is followed from the minor papilla into the head of the pancreas, a branch point is discovered:

- One branch continues to the left, through the head of the pancreas, and may connect with the main pancreatic duct at the point where it turns inferiorly.
- A second branch descends into the lower part of the head of the pancreas, anterior to the pancreatic duct, and ends in the uncinate process.

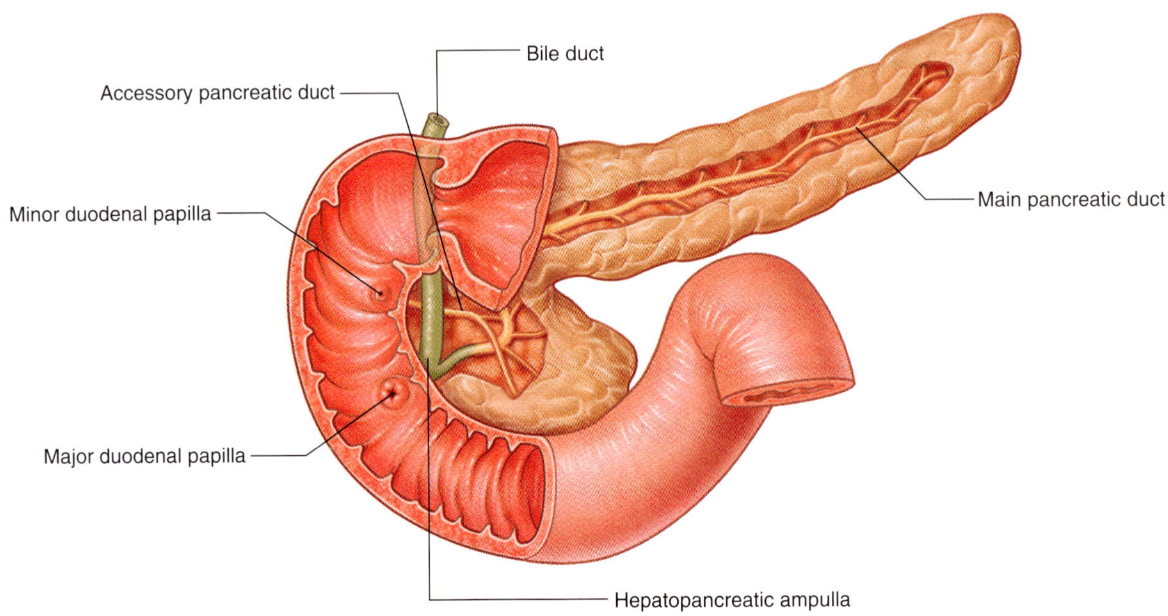

Fig. 4.100 Pancreatic duct system.

The main and accessory pancreatic ducts usually communicate with each other. The presence of these two ducts reflects the embryological origin of the pancreas from dorsal and ventral pancreatic buds from the foregut.

The arterial supply to the pancreas (Fig. 4.101 and 4.113) includes the:

- Gastroduodenal artery from the common hepatic artery (a branch of the celiac trunk)
- Anterior superior pancreaticoduodenal artery from the gastroduodenal artery
- Posterior superior pancreaticoduodenal artery from the gastroduodenal artery
- Dorsal pancreatic artery from the splenic artery
- Great (greater) pancreatic artery from the splenic artery
- Anterior inferior pancreaticoduodenal artery from the inferior pancreaticoduodenal artery (a branch of the superior mesenteric artery)
- Posterior inferior pancreaticoduodenal artery from the inferior pancreaticoduodenal artery (a branch of the superior mesenteric artery)

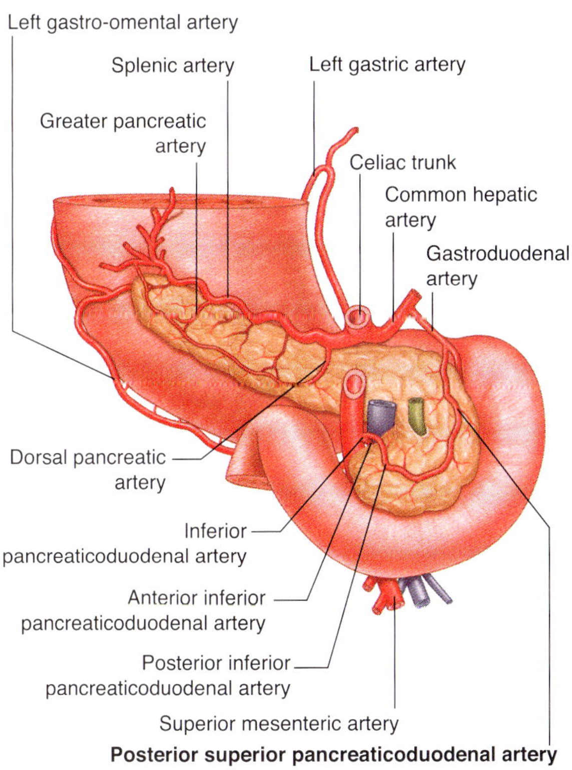

Fig. 4.101 Arterial supply to the pancreas. Posterior view.

Kirk's arterial arcade in the pancreas is formed by an anastomosis of the right branch of the dorsal pancreatic artery with a branch of the gastroduodenal artery.

Early clinical exposure

Annular pancreas

The pancreas develops from ventral and dorsal pancreatic buds from the foregut. The dorsal bud forms most of the head, neck, and body of the pancreas. The ventral bud rotates around the bile duct to form part of the head and the uncinate process. If the ventral bud splits (becomes bifid), the two segments may encircle the duodenum. The duodenum is therefore constricted and may even undergo atresia, and be absent at birth because of developmental problems. After birth, the child may fail to thrive and may vomit due to poor gastric emptying.

Sometimes an annular pancreas is diagnosed in utero by ultrasound scanning. The obstruction of the duodenum may prevent the fetus from swallowing enough amniotic fluid, which may increase the overall volume of amniotic fluid in the amniotic sac surrounding the fetus (**polyhydramnios**).

Early clinical exposure

Pancreatic cancer

Pancreatic cancer accounts for a significant number of deaths and is often referred to as the "silent killer." Malignant tumors of the pancreas may occur anywhere within the pancreas but are most frequent within the head and the neck. There are a number of nonspecific findings in patients with pancreatic cancer, including upper abdominal pain, loss of appetite, and weight loss. Depending on the exact site of the cancer, obstruction of the bile duct may occur, which can produce **obstructive jaundice**. Although surgery is indicated in patients where there is a possibility of cure, most detected cancers have typically spread locally, invading the portal vein and superior mesenteric vessels, and may extend into the porta hepatis. Lymph node spread also is common and these factors would preclude curative surgery.

Given the position of the pancreas, a surgical resection is a complex procedure involving resection of the region of pancreatic tumor usually with part of the duodenum, necessitating a complex bypass procedure.

Duct system for bile

The duct system for the passage of bile extends from the liver, connects with the gallbladder, and empties into the descending part of the duodenum (Fig. 4.102). The coalescence of ducts begins in the liver parenchyma and continues until the **right** and **left hepatic ducts** are formed. These drain the respective lobes of the liver.

The two hepatic ducts combine to form the **common hepatic duct**, which runs near the liver, with the hepatic artery proper and portal vein in the free margin of the lesser omentum.

As the common hepatic duct continues to descend, it is joined by the **cystic duct** from the gallbladder. This completes the formation of the **bile duct**. At this point, the bile duct lies to the right of the hepatic artery proper and usually to the right of, and anterior to, the portal vein in the free margin of the lesser omentum. The **omental foramen** is posterior to these structures at this point (Fig. 4.54A). Bleeding from the liver can be controlled by compressing the hepatoduodenal ligament (Pringle's maneuver). This ligament contains the hepatic artery and portal vein.

The bile duct continues to descend, passing posterior to the superior part of the duodenum before joining with the main pancreatic duct to enter the descending part of the duodenum at the major duodenal papilla (Fig. 4.102).

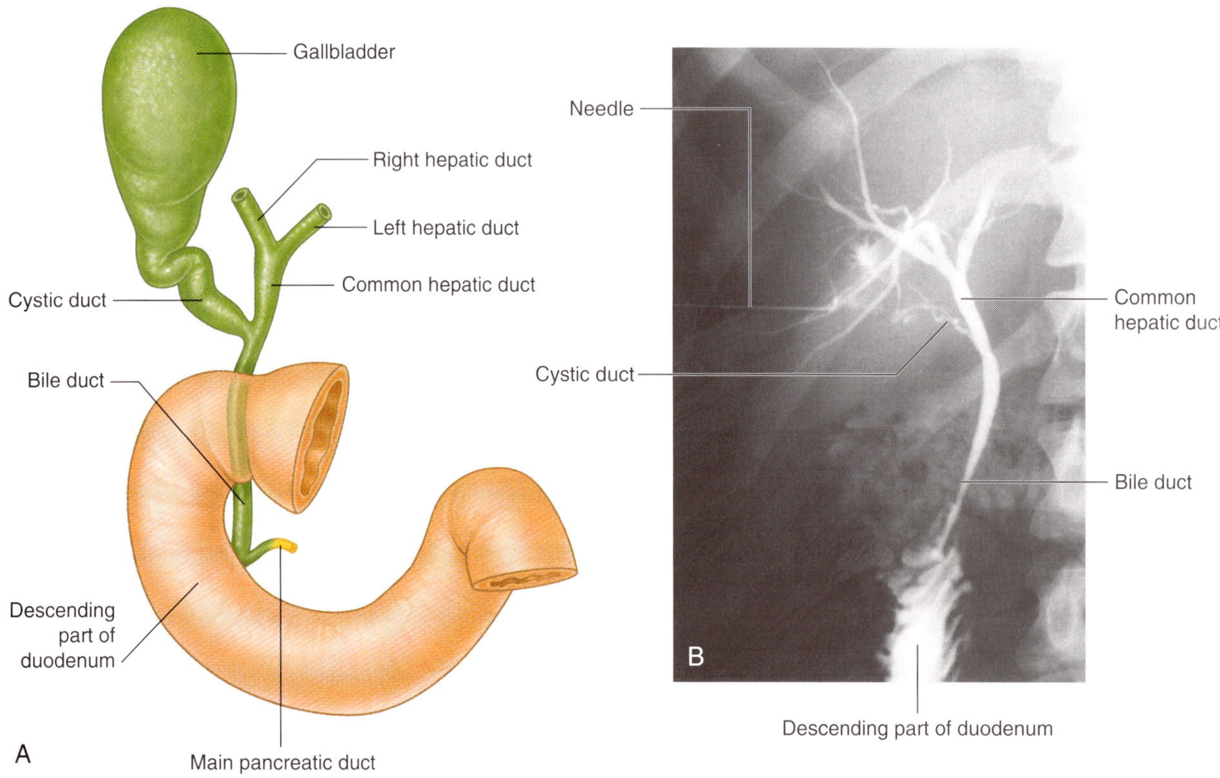

Fig. 4.102 Bile drainage. **(A)** Duct system for passage of bile. **(B)** Percutaneous transhepatic cholangiogram demonstrating the bile duct system.

Spleen

SET INDUCTION—CASE SCENARIO 9: PORTAL HYPERTENSION

A 56-year-old male who was a chronic alcoholic was brought to the emergency department with a history of unconsciousness for 2 hours after vomiting fresh blood. On examination, he was found to have a grossly distended abdomen with veins radiating from the umbilicus. A diagnosis of portal hypertension with ruptured esophageal varices was made. Knowledge of the blood supply of the abdominal viscera is needed to manage this case.

<table>
<tr><td rowspan="2">REMEMBER
[Recall Facts]</td><td colspan="3">OUTLINE 9. VESSELS AND NERVES OF THE GASTROINTESTINAL TRACT—LEARNING OBJECTIVES
[By the end of this section, the student should be able to:]</td><td colspan="2" rowspan="2">EVALUATE
[Explain Concepts]</td></tr>
<tr><td colspan="3">DEMONSTRATE AND ANALYZE RELATIONSHIPS
[Identify structures in a Prosected Specimen or Figure]</td></tr>
<tr><td rowspan="7">Arteries
1. List the unpaired branches of the abdominal aorta
2. Describe the course and branches of the coeliac, superior mesenteric, and inferior mesenteric arteries
3. Describe the course and branches of the left gastric, splenic, and common hepatic arteries
Veins
1. Describe the course and tributaries of the portal vein
2. Describe the course and tributaries of the splenic vein
3. Describe the course and tributaries of the superior mesenteric vein
Lymphatics
1. Name the preaortic lymph nodes
2. Describe the tributaries of the cisterna chyli
Nerves
1. Describe the sympathetic trunk and splanchnic nerves
2. Describe the abdominal prevertebral plexuses and ganglia
3. Describe the vagus, pelvic splanchnic nerves, and the enteric nervous system</td><td>Level I</td><td>Level II</td><td>Level III</td><td colspan="2" rowspan="2">■ Arterial anastomoses between the unpaired branches of the aorta
■ Formation of the portal vein</td></tr>
<tr><td rowspan="6">■ Unpaired branches of the aorta
■ Coeliac artery and its branches—left gastric
■ Superior mesenteric artery and its branches—jejunal, ileal, middle colic, right colic, ileocolic arteries
■ Inferior mesenteric artery and its branches—left colic, sigmoidal, and superior rectal arteries
■ Portal vein and its tributaries
■ Cisterna chyli
■ Thoracic duct
■ Sympathetic trunk
■ Splanchnic nerves</td><td rowspan="6">■ Superior and inferior pancreaticoduodenal arteries</td><td rowspan="6">■ Marginal artery of Drummond</td></tr>
<tr><td colspan="2">EARLY CLINICAL EXPOSURE
[Apply Anatomical Knowledge]</td></tr>
<tr><td>Surgical Anatomy/ Pathology/ Trauma</td><td>Imaging/ Surface Anatomy</td></tr>
<tr><td>■ Watershed areas in arterial supply of the gastrointestinal tract
■ Narrowing of the openings of the coeliac and superior mesenteric arteries
■ Sites of portosystemic anastomosis</td><td>■ Digital subtraction imaging</td></tr>
<tr><td colspan="2">PROBLEM SOLVING/CLINICAL CASES
[Interpret]</td></tr>
<tr><td colspan="2">■ Discuss the reason for ischemia of the splenic flexure of the colon
■ Discuss the cause of the manifestations of portal hypertension
■ Differentiate between sympathetic and parasympathetic splanchnic nerves</td></tr>
</table>

The spleen develops as part of the vascular system in the part of the dorsal mesentery that suspends the developing stomach from the body wall (Fig. 4.13). In the adult, the spleen lies against the diaphragm, in the area of rib IX to rib XI (Fig. 4.103). It is therefore in the left upper quadrant, or left hypochondrium, of the abdomen.

The spleen is connected to the:

- Greater curvature of the stomach by the gastrosplenic ligament, which contains the short gastric and left gastro-omental vessels
- Left kidney by the splenorenal ligament (Fig. 4.104), which contains the splenic vessels

The gastrosplenic ligament is part of the greater omentum.

The spleen is surrounded by visceral peritoneum except in the area of the hilum on the visceral surface of the spleen (Fig. 4.105). The **splenic hilum** is the entry and exit point for the splenic vessels, which lie in peritoneal ligaments. Occasionally the tail of the pancreas reaches the splenic hilum. The relations of the visceral surface are illustrated in Fig. 4.103–4.105.

The arterial supply to the spleen (Fig. 4.106) is the splenic artery from the celiac trunk.

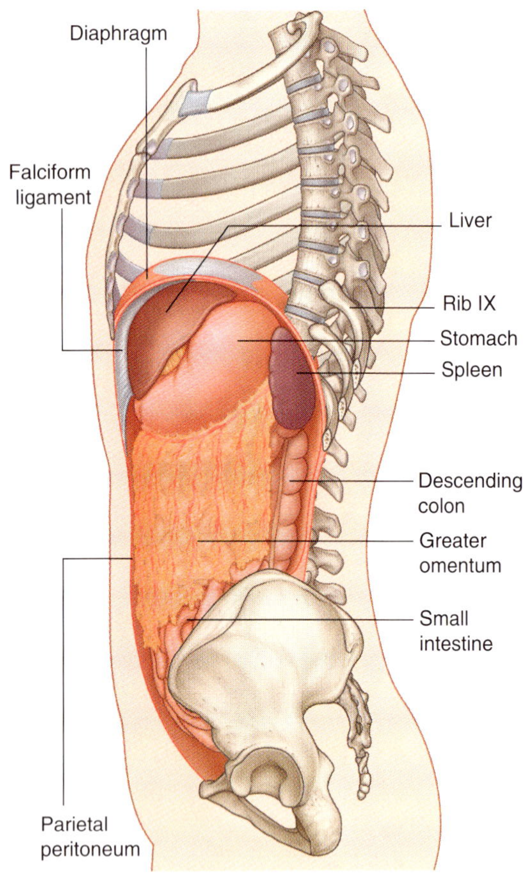

Fig. 4.103 Spleen.

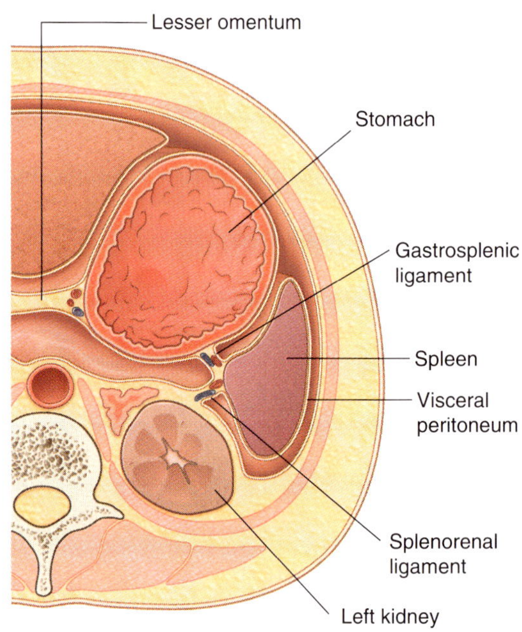

Fig. 4.104 Splenic ligaments and related vasculature.

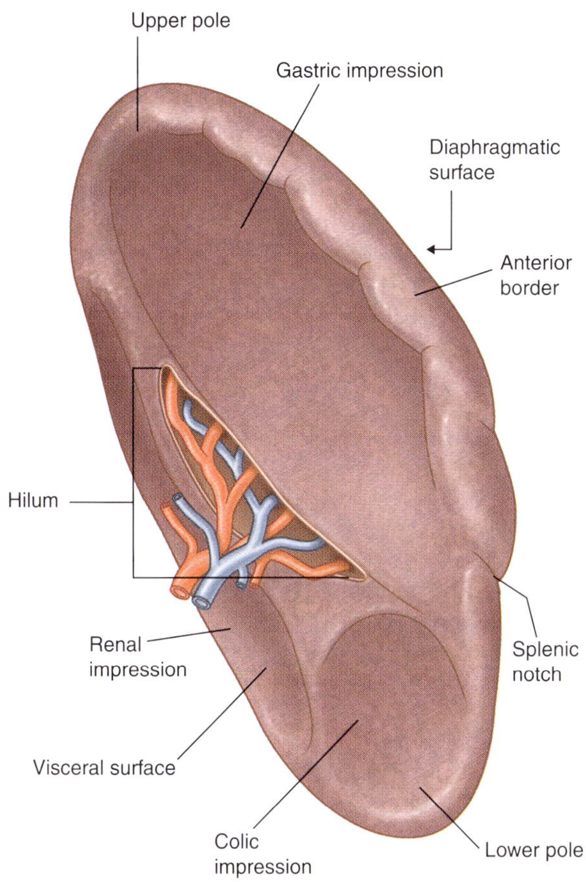

Fig. 4.105 Surfaces and hilum of the spleen.

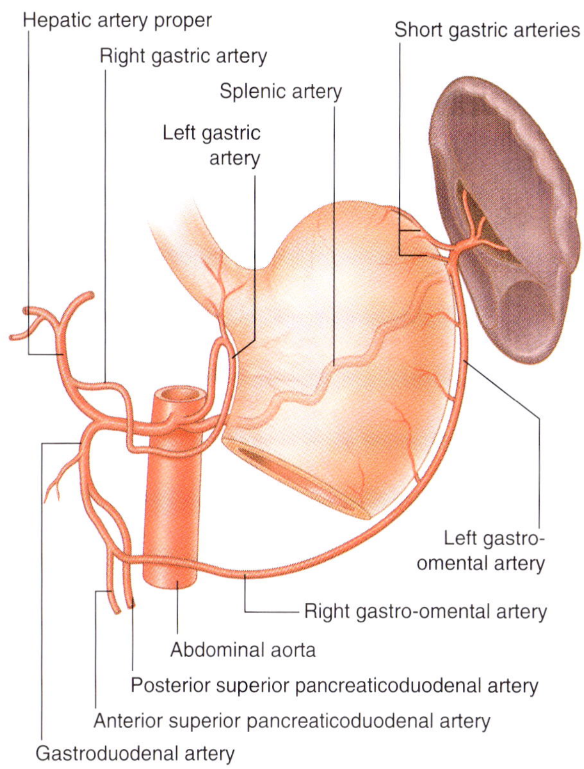

Fig. 4.106 Arterial supply to the spleen.

Early clinical exposure

Segmental anatomy of the liver

For many years, the segmental anatomy of the liver was of little importance. However, since the development of liver resection surgery, the size, shape, and segmental anatomy of the liver have become clinically important, especially with regard to liver resection for metastatic disease. Indeed, with detailed knowledge of the segments, curative surgery can be performed in patients with tumor metastases.

The liver is divided by the **principal plane**, which divides the organ into halves of approximately equal size. This imaginary line is defined by a parasagittal line that passes from the gallbladder fossa to the inferior vena cava. It is in this plane that the middle hepatic vein is found. Importantly, the principal plane divides the left half of the liver from the right half. The traditionally described lobes of the liver are unequal in size and bear only little relevance to operative anatomy.

The eight-segment anatomy of the liver relates to the hepatic arterial, portal, and biliary drainage of these segments (Fig. 4.107). The left hepatic vein separates the medial and lateral segments. Then right hepatic vein separates the anterior and posterior segments. The portal vein separates the upper and lower segments.

The caudate lobe is defined as segment I, and the remaining segments are numbered in a clockwise fashion up to segment VIII. The features are extremely consistent between individuals.

From a surgical perspective, a right hepatectomy would involve division of the liver in the principal plane in which segments V, VI, VII, and VIII would be removed, leaving segments I, II, III, and IV.

Continued

Early clinical exposure—cont'd

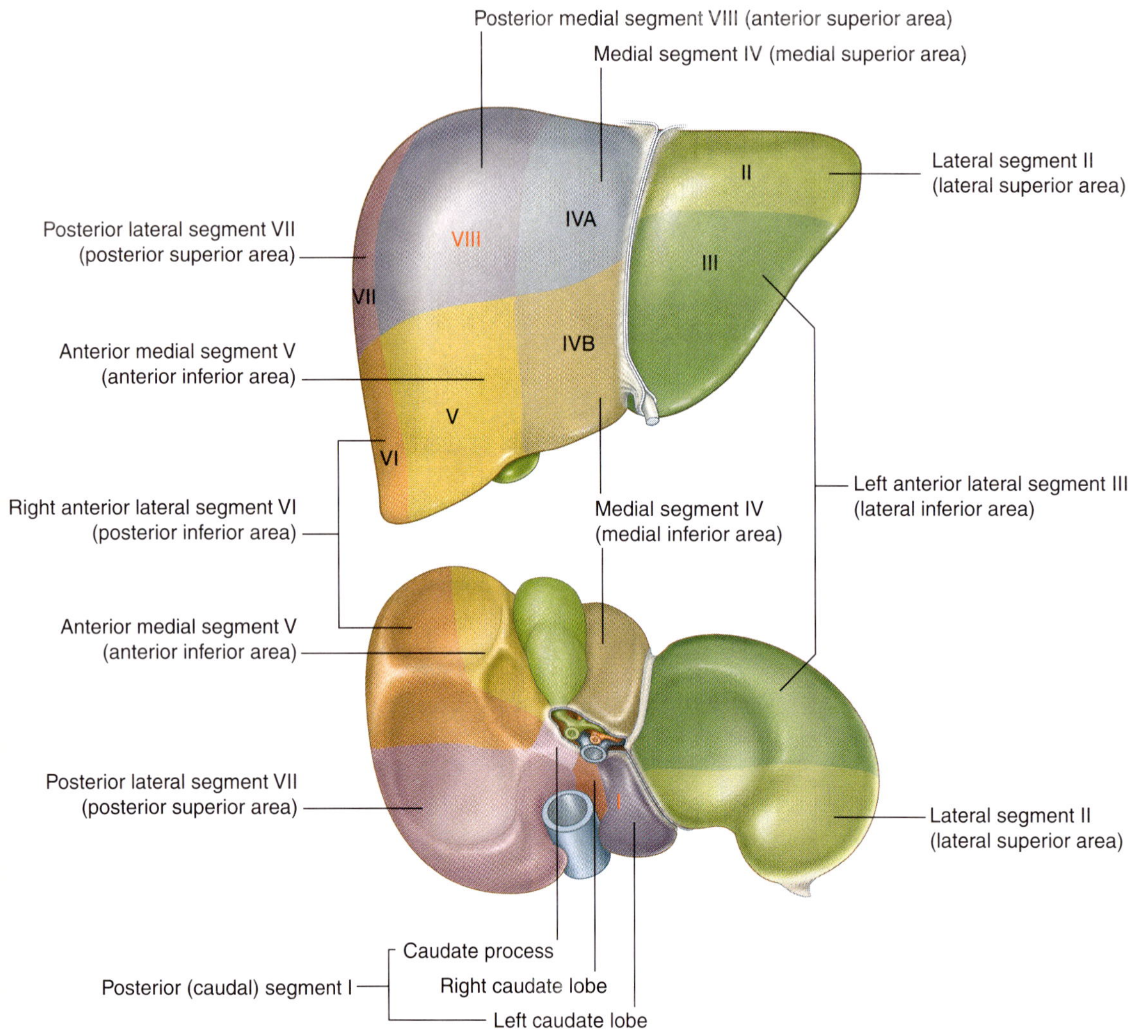

Fig. 4.107 Division of the liver into segments based upon the distribution of the bile ducts and hepatic vessels (Couinaud's segments). The segments labelled in red (unlike the other segments) are visible on only one surface, either the diaphragmatic or visceral surface.

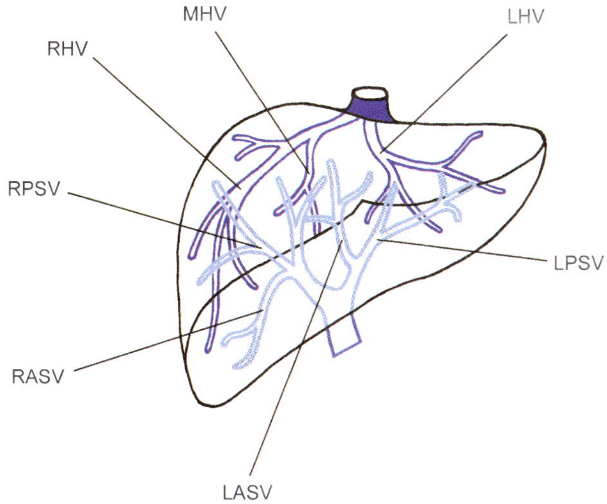

LD Fig. 4.107.1 Veins of the liver and subdivisions of the liver

Questions

LD Fig. 4.107.1A List the four main branches of the portal vein labelled as RASV, RPSV, LASV, and LPSV.

LD Fig. 4.107.1B How is the liver divided into four portal sectors?

LD Fig. 4.107.1C Name the three hepatic veins (tributaries of the hepatic vein) labelled as RHV, MHV, and LHV?

LD Fig. 4.107.1D Where do the three hepatic veins lie?

LD Fig. 4.107.1E What supplies the subsectors of the liver?

LD Fig. 4.107.1F Mention an example of parts of the liver supplied by first, second, and third order divisions of the hepatic ducts and hepatic arteries which can be surgically removed.

Answers

LD Fig. 4.107.1A The four main branches of the portal vein are right anterior (medial) sectoral vein, right posterior (lateral) sectoral vein, left anterior (medial) sectoral vein, and left posterior (lateral) sectoral vein.

LD Fig. 4.107.1B The liver is divided into four portal sectors each of which is supplied by one of the four main branches of the portal vein. These branches are the lateral and medial branches of the right branch of the portal vein; and the lateral and medial branches of the left branch of the portal vein.

LD Fig. 4.107.1C The three hepatic veins are the right hepatic vein, middle hepatic vein, and left hepatic vein.

LD Fig. 4.107.1D The right, left, and middle hepatic veins, which lie in the right, main, and left portal fissures.

LD Fig. 4.107.1E The subsectors of the liver are supplied by the contents of the vascular biliary sheaths.

LD Fig. 4.107.1F Examples of surgically resections of parts of the liver supplied by first-, second-, and third-order divisions of the hepatic ducts and hepatic arteries are left hepatectomy (segments 2, 3, and 4), left lateral sectionectomy (segments 2 and 3), and segmentectomy (segment 3), respectively.

Early clinical exposure

Gallstones

Gallstones are present in approximately 10% of people over the age of 40 and are more common in women. They consist of a variety of components but are predominantly a mixture of cholesterol and bile pigment. They may undergo calcification, which can be demonstrated on plain radiographs. Gallstones may be visualized incidentally as part of a routine abdominal ultrasound scan (Fig. 4.108A) or on a plain radiograph. The easiest way to confirm the presence of gallstones is by performing a fasting ultrasound examination of the gallbladder. The patient refrains from eating for 6 hours to ensure the gallbladder is well distended and there is little shadowing from overlying bowel gas. The examination may also identify bile duct dilatation and the presence of cholecystitis. MRCP is another way to image the gallbladder and biliary tree. MRCP uses fluid present in the bile ducts and in the pancreatic duct as a contrast agent to show stones as well as filling defects within the gallbladder and intrahepatic or extrahepatic bile ducts. It can demonstrate strictures in the biliary tree and can also be used to visualize liver and pancreatic anatomy (Fig. 4.108B). From time to time, gallstones impact in the region of Hartmann's pouch, which is a bulbous region of the neck of the gallbladder. When the gallstone lodges in this area, the gallbladder cannot empty normally and contractions of the gallbladder wall produce severe pain. If this persists, a cholecystectomy (removal of the gallbladder) may be necessary.

Sometimes the gallbladder may become inflamed (cholecystitis). If the inflammation involves the related parietal peritoneum of the diaphragm, pain may not only occur in the right upper quadrant of the abdomen but also be referred to the shoulder on the right side. This referred pain is due to the innervation of the visceral peritoneum of the diaphragm by spinal cord levels (C3 to C5) that also innervate skin over the shoulder. In this case, one somatic sensory region of low sensory output (diaphragm) is referred to another somatic sensory region of high sensory output (dermatomes).

From time to time, small gallstones pass into the bile duct and are trapped in the region of the sphincter of the

Continued

Early clinical exposure—cont'd

ampulla, which obstructs the flow of bile into the duodenum. This, in turn, produces jaundice.

ERCP

ERCP can be undertaken to remove obstructing gallstones within the biliary tree. This procedure combines endoluminal endoscopy with fluoroscopy to diagnose and treat

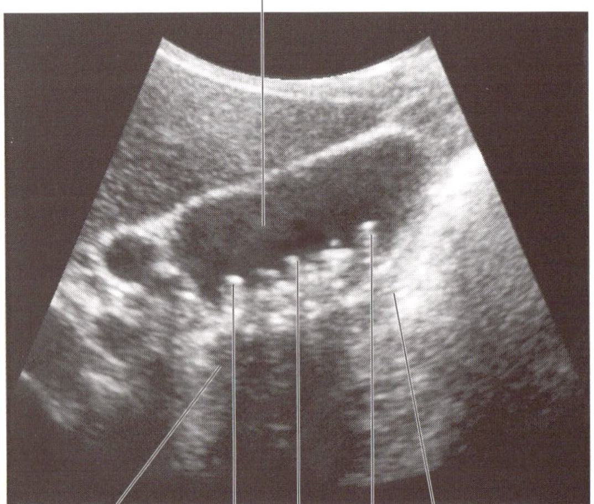

Fig. 4.108(A) Gallbladder containing multiple stones. Ultrasound scan.

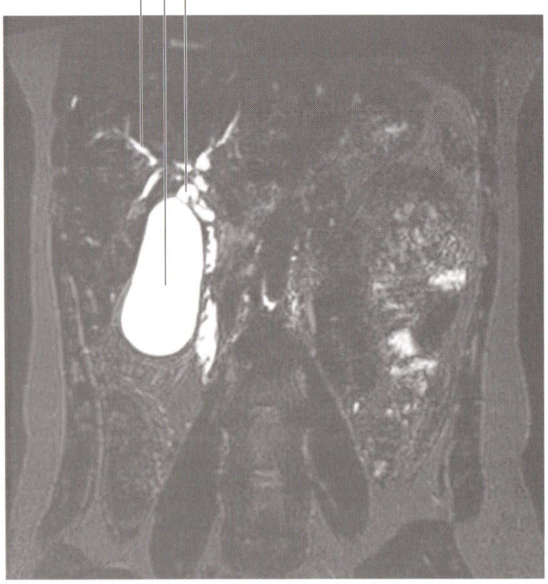

Fig. 4.108(B) Magnetic resonance cholangiopancreatography (MRCP) in the coronal plane.

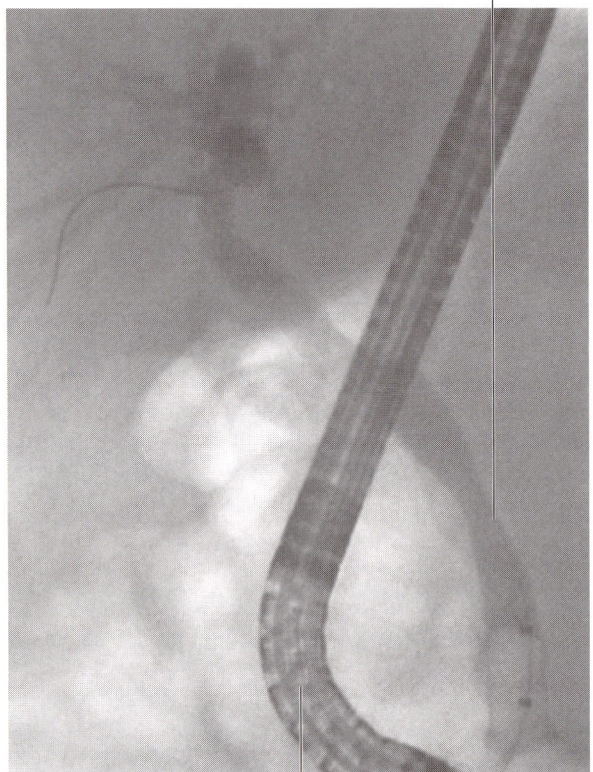

Fig. 4.108(C) Endoscopic retrograde cholangiopancreatography (ERCP) of biliary system.

problems in the biliary and pancreatic ducts. An endoscope with a side-viewing optical system is advanced through the esophagus and stomach and placed in the second part of the duodenum where the major papilla (the ampulla of Vater) is identified. This is where the pancreatic duct converges with the common bile duct. The papilla is initially examined for possible abnormalities (stuck stone or malignant growth) and a biopsy may be taken if necessary. Then either the bile duct or pancreatic duct is cannulated and a small amount of radiopaque contrast medium is injected to visualize either the bile duct (cholangiogram) or pancreatic duct (pancreatogram) (Fig. 4.108C). If a stone is present, it can be removed with a stone basket or an extraction balloon. Usually, a sphincterotomy is performed before stone removal to ease its passage through the distal bile duct.

In cases of biliary tree obstruction caused by benign or malignant strictures, a stent can be placed into the common bile duct or into one of the main hepatic ducts to allow opening of the narrowed segment. The patency of the newly inserted stent is confirmed by instillation of more contrast medium to demonstrate free flow of contrast through the stent.

Early clinical exposure

Jaundice

Jaundice is a yellow discoloration of the skin caused by excess bile pigment (bilirubin) within the plasma. The yellow color is best appreciated by looking at the normally white sclerae of the eyes, which turn yellow.

The extent of the elevation of the bile pigments and the duration for which they have been elevated account for the severity of jaundice.

Simplified explanation to understanding the types of jaundice and their anatomical causes

When red blood cells are destroyed by the reticuloendothelial system, the iron from the hemoglobin molecule is recycled, whereas the porphyrin ring (globin) compounds are broken down to form fat-soluble bilirubin. On reaching the liver via the bloodstream, the fat-soluble bilirubin is converted to a water-soluble form of bilirubin. This water-soluble bilirubin is secreted into the biliary tree and then in turn into the bowel, where it forms the dark color of the stool.

Prehepatic jaundice

This type of jaundice is usually produced by conditions where there is an excessive breakdown of red blood cells (e.g., in incompatible blood transfusion and hemolytic anemia).

Hepatic jaundice

The complex biochemical reactions for converting fat-soluble bilirubin into water-soluble bilirubin may be affected by inflammatory change within the liver (e.g., from hepatitis or chronic liver disease, such as liver cirrhosis) and poisons (e.g., paracetamol overdose).

Posthepatic jaundice

Any obstruction of the biliary tree can produce jaundice, but the two most common causes are gallstones within the bile duct and an obstructing tumor at the head of the pancreas.

Early clinical exposure

Spleen disorders

From a clinical point of view, there are two main categories of spleen disorders: rupture and enlargement.

Splenic rupture

This tends to occur when there is localized trauma to the left upper quadrant. It may be associated with left lower rib fractures. Because the spleen has such an extremely thin capsule, it is susceptible to injury even when there is no damage to surrounding structures, and because the spleen is highly vascular, when ruptured, it bleeds profusely into the peritoneal cavity. Splenic rupture should always be suspected with blunt abdominal injury. Current treatments preserve as much of the spleen as possible, but some patients require splenectomy.

Splenic enlargement

The spleen is an organ of the reticuloendothelial system involved in hematopoiesis and immunological surveillance. Diseases that affect the reticuloendothelial system (e.g., leukemia or lymphoma) may produce generalized lymphadenopathy and enlargement of the spleen (splenomegaly) (Fig. 4.109). The spleen often enlarges when performing its normal physiological functions, such as when clearing microorganisms and particulates from the circulation, producing increased antibodies in the course of sepsis, or removing deficient or destroyed erythrocytes (e.g., in thalassemia and spherocytosis). Splenomegaly may also be a result of increased venous pressure caused by congestive heart failure, splenic vein thrombosis, or portal hypertension. An enlarged spleen is prone to rupture. An enlarged spleen may be palpated in the left upper quadrant of the abdomen. Further enlargement of the spleen is downward and to the right toward the right lower quadrant. The long axis of the spleen is parallel to rib X (see Fig. 4.171).

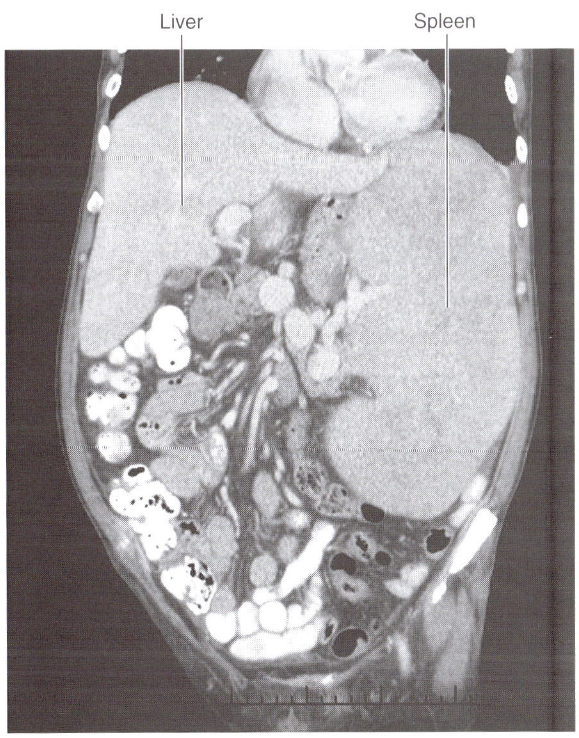

Fig. 4.109 Coronal CT of the abdomen containing a massively enlarged spleen (splenomegaly).

Arterial supply

The **abdominal aorta** begins at the aortic hiatus of the diaphragm, anterior to the lower border of vertebra TXII (Fig. 4.110). It descends through the abdomen, anterior to the vertebral bodies, and by the time it ends at the level of vertebra LIV, it is slightly to the left of midline. The terminal branches of the abdominal aorta are the two **common iliac arteries**.

Anterior branches of the abdominal aorta

The abdominal aorta has anterior, lateral, and posterior branches as it passes through the abdominal cavity. The three anterior branches supply the gastrointestinal viscera: the **celiac trunk** and the **superior mesenteric** and **inferior mesenteric arteries** (Fig. 4.110).

The primitive gut tube can be divided into foregut, midgut, and hindgut regions. The boundaries of these regions

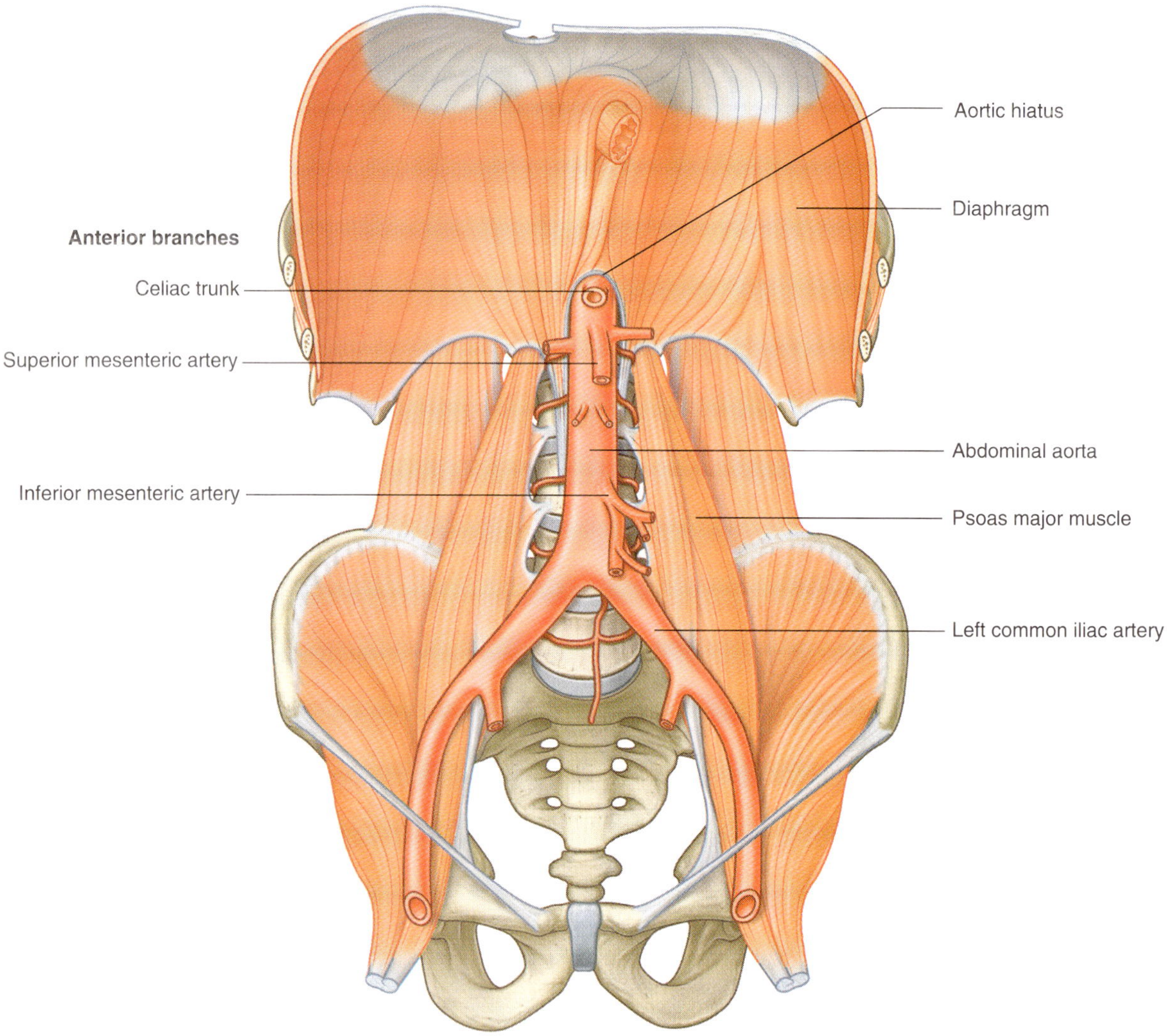

Fig. 4.110 Anterior branches of the abdominal aorta.

are directly related to the areas of distribution of the three anterior branches of the abdominal aorta (Fig. 4.111).

- The **foregut** begins with the abdominal esophagus and ends just inferior to the major duodenal papilla, midway along the descending part of the duodenum. It includes the abdominal esophagus, stomach, duodenum (superior to the major papilla), liver, pancreas, and gallbladder. The spleen also develops in relation to the foregut region. The foregut is supplied by the celiac trunk.

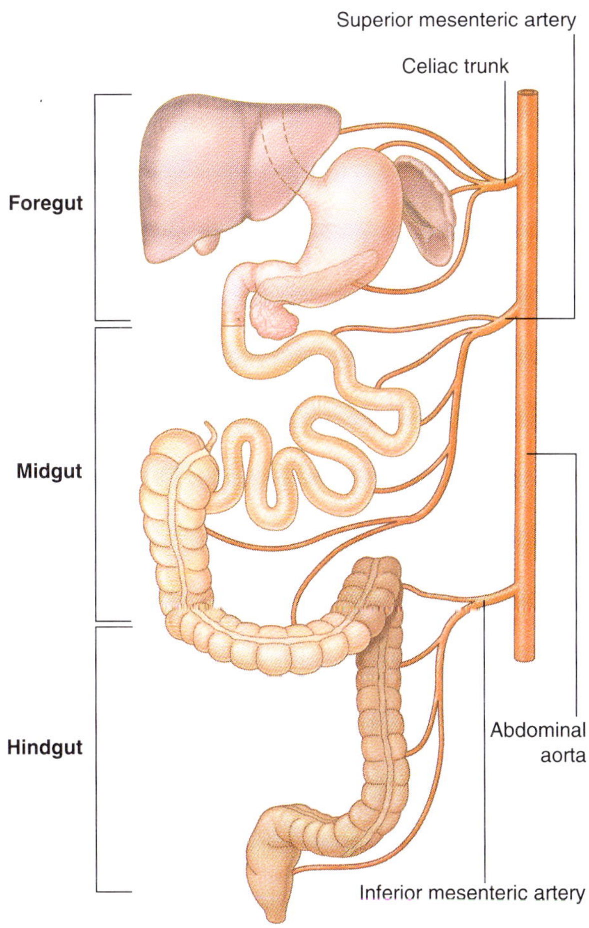

Fig. 4.111 Divisions of the gastrointestinal tract into foregut, midgut, and hindgut, summarizing the primary arterial supply to each segment.

- The **midgut** begins just inferior to the major duodenal papilla, in the descending part of the duodenum, and ends at the junction between the proximal two-thirds and distal one-third of the transverse colon. It includes the duodenum (inferior to the major duodenal papilla), jejunum, ileum, cecum, appendix, ascending colon, and right two-thirds of the transverse colon. The midgut is supplied by the superior mesenteric artery (Fig. 4.111).
- The **hindgut** begins at the junction between the proximal two-thirds and distal one-third of the transverse colon and ends midway through the anal canal. It includes the left one-third of the transverse colon, descending colon, sigmoid colon, rectum, and upper part of the anal canal, above the pectinate line. The hindgut is supplied by the inferior mesenteric artery (Fig. 4.111).

Celiac trunk

The celiac trunk is the anterior branch of the abdominal aorta supplying the foregut. It arises from the abdominal aorta immediately below the aortic hiatus of the diaphragm (Fig. 4.112), anterior to the upper part of vertebra LI. It immediately divides into the left gastric, splenic, and common hepatic arteries (Flowchart 4.1).

Left gastric artery

The **left gastric artery** is the smallest branch of the celiac trunk. It ascends to the cardioesophageal junction and sends **esophageal branches** upward to the abdominal part of the esophagus (Fig. 4.112). Some of these branches continue through the esophageal hiatus of the diaphragm and anastomose with esophageal branches from the thoracic aorta. The left gastric artery itself turns to the right and descends along the lesser curvature of the stomach in the lesser omentum. It supplies both surfaces of the stomach in this area and anastomoses with the right gastric artery.

Splenic artery

The **splenic artery**, the largest branch of the celiac trunk, takes a tortuous course to the left along the superior border of the pancreas (Fig. 4.112). It travels in the splenorenal ligament and divides into numerous branches, which enter the hilum of the spleen. As the splenic artery passes along the superior border of the pancreas, it gives off

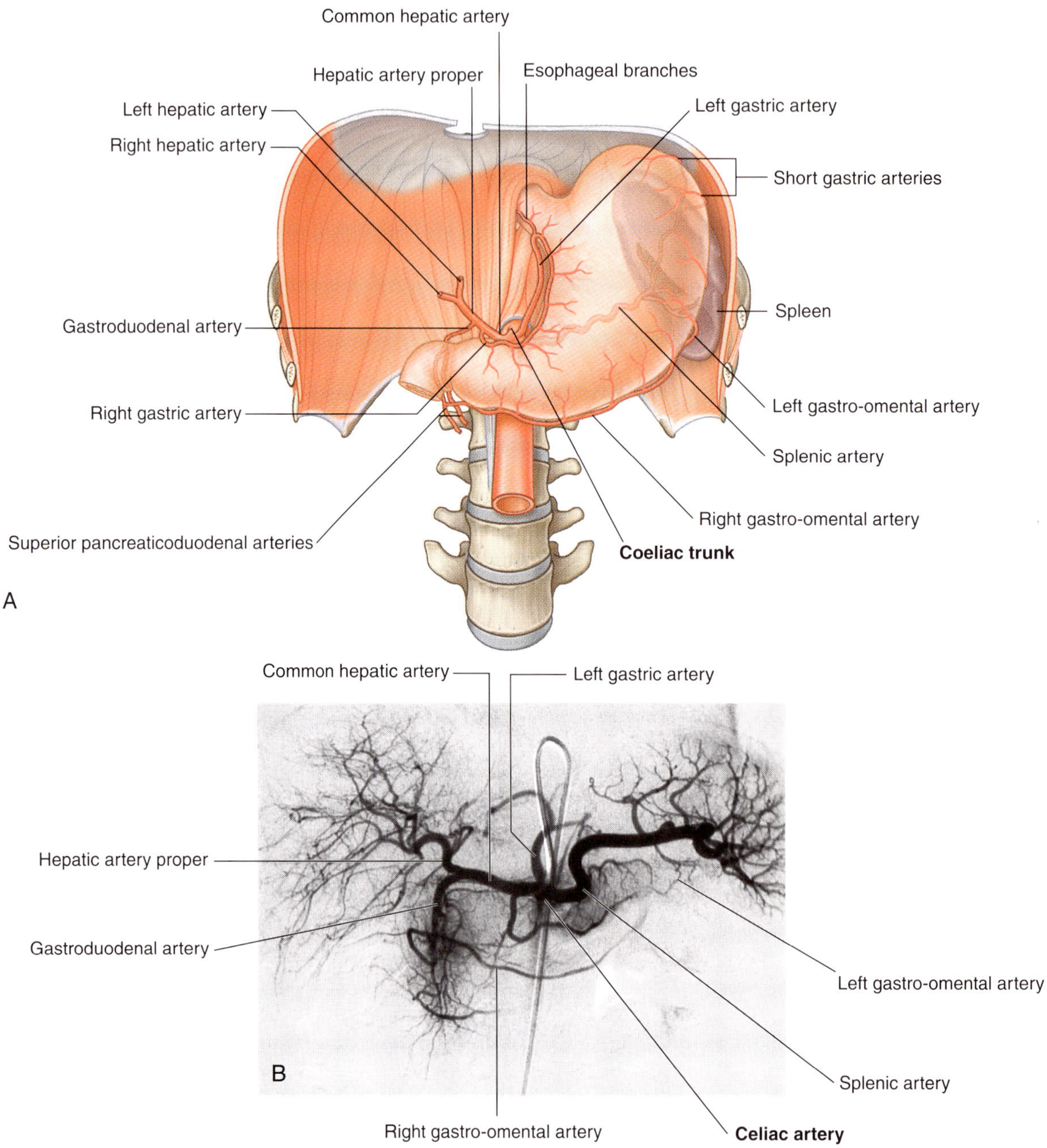

Fig. 4.112 Celiac trunk. **(A)** Distribution of the celiac trunk. **(B)** Digital subtraction angiography of the celiac trunk and its branches.

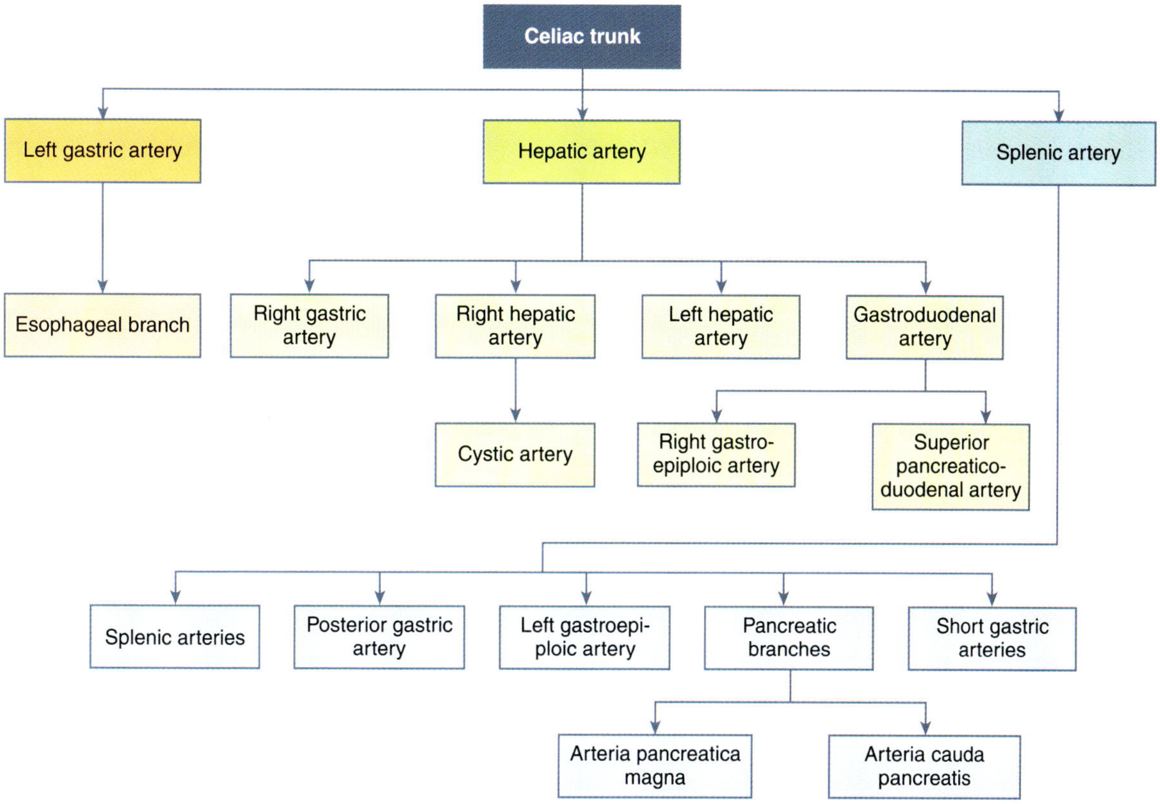

Flowchart 4.1 Branches of celiac trunk.

numerous small branches to supply the neck, body, and tail of the pancreas (Fig. 4.113).

Approaching the spleen, the splenic artery gives off **short gastric arteries**, which pass through the gastrosplenic ligament to supply the fundus of the stomach. It also gives off the **left gastro-omental artery**, which runs to the right along the greater curvature of the stomach, and anastomoses with the right gastro-omental artery.

Common hepatic artery

The **common hepatic artery** is a medium-sized branch of the celiac trunk that runs to the right and divides into its two terminal branches, the **hepatic artery proper** and the **gastroduodenal artery** (Fig. 4.112 and 4.113).

The hepatic artery proper ascends toward the liver in the free edge of the lesser omentum (Fig. 4.54A). It runs to the left of the bile duct and anterior to the portal vein, and divides into the **right** and **left hepatic arteries** near the porta hepatis (Fig. 4.114).

As the right hepatic artery nears the liver, it gives off the cystic artery to the gallbladder.

The gastroduodenal artery may give off the **supraduodenal artery** and does give off the **posterior superior pancreaticoduodenal artery** near the upper border of the superior part of the duodenum. This artery may be eroded by a posterior duodenal ulcer. After these branches, the gastroduodenal artery continues descending posterior to the superior part of the duodenum. Reaching the lower border of the superior part of the duodenum, the gastroduodenal artery divides into its terminal branches, the **right gastro-omental artery** and the **anterior superior pancreaticoduodenal artery** (Fig. 4.113).

The right gastro-omental artery passes to the left, along the greater curvature of the stomach, eventually anastomosing with the left gastro-omental artery from the splenic artery (Fig. 4.112). The right gastro-omental artery sends branches to both surfaces of the stomach and additional branches descend into the greater omentum (Fig. 4.56).

The anterior superior pancreaticoduodenal artery descends and, along with the posterior superior pancreaticoduodenal artery, supplies the head of the pancreas and the duodenum (Fig. 4.113). These vessels eventually anastomose with the anterior and posterior branches of the inferior pancreaticoduodenal artery.

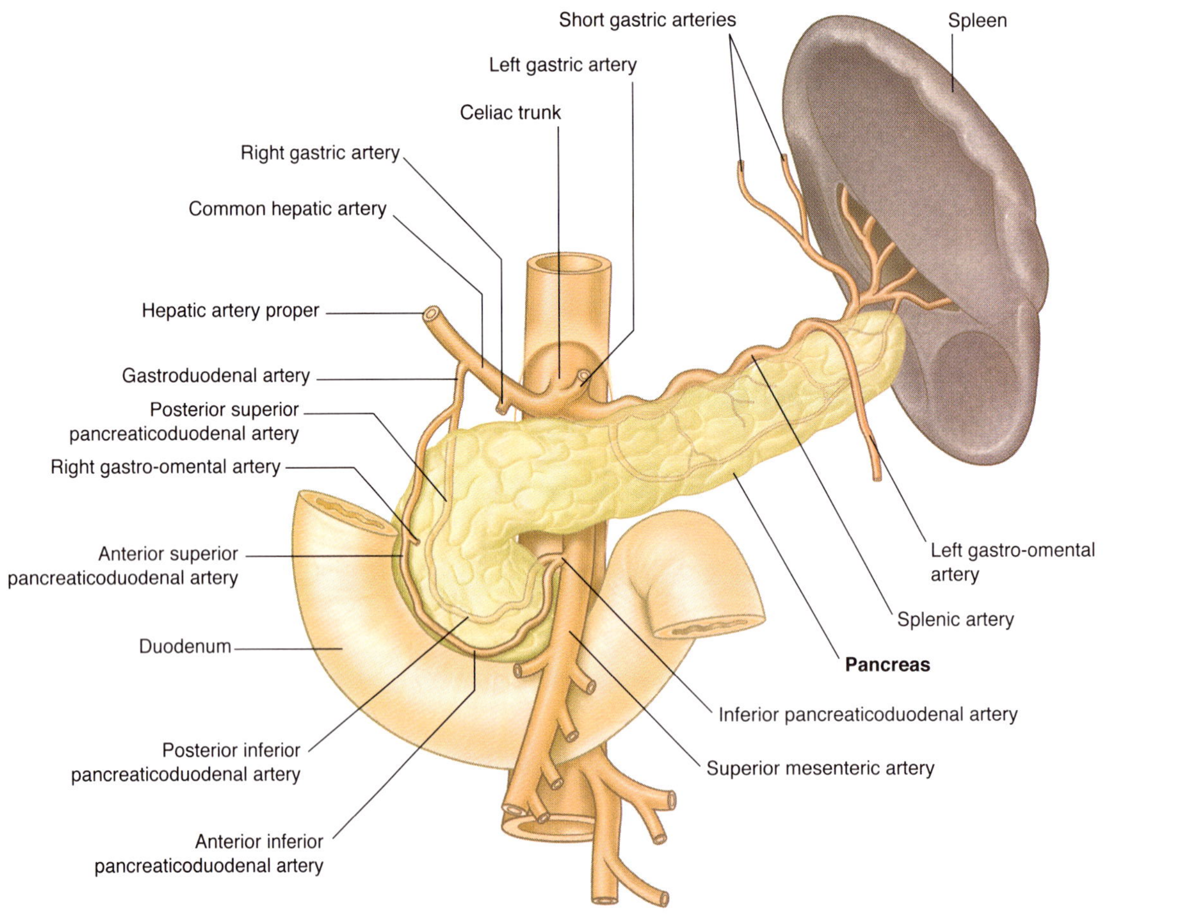

Fig. 4.113 Arterial supply to the pancreas.

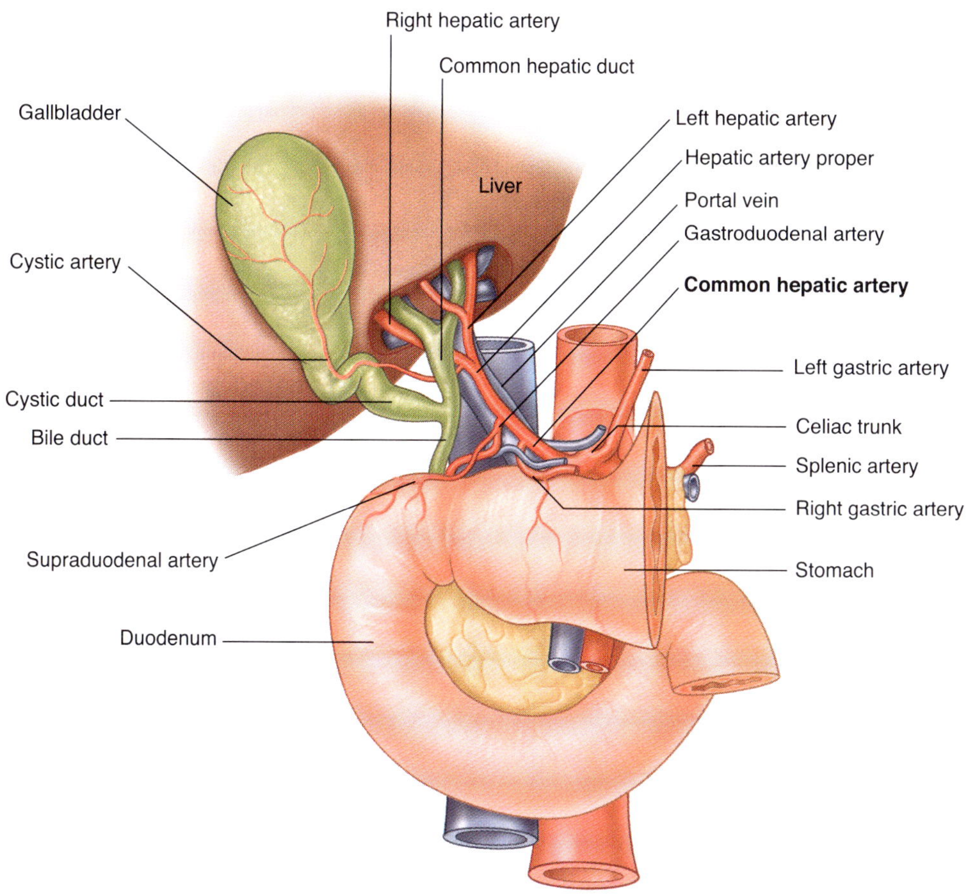

Fig. 4.114 Distribution of the common hepatic artery.

Superior mesenteric artery

The superior mesenteric artery is the anterior branch of the abdominal aorta supplying the midgut. It arises from the abdominal aorta immediately below the celiac artery (Fig. 4.115), anterior to the lower part of vertebra LI.

The superior mesenteric artery is crossed anteriorly by the splenic vein and the neck of the pancreas. Posterior to the artery are the left renal vein, the uncinate process of the pancreas, and the inferior part of the duodenum. After giving off its first branch (the **inferior pancreaticoduodenal artery**), the superior mesenteric artery gives off **jejunal** and **ileal arteries** on its left (Fig. 4.115). Branching from the right side of the main trunk of the superior mesenteric artery are three vessels—the **middle colic, right colic**, and **ileocolic arteries**—which supply the terminal ileum, cecum, ascending colon, and two-thirds of the transverse colon (Flowchart 4.2).

Inferior pancreaticoduodenal artery

The inferior pancreaticoduodenal artery is the first branch of the superior mesenteric artery. It divides immediately into anterior and posterior branches, which ascend on the corresponding sides of the head of the pancreas. Superiorly, these arteries anastomose with anterior and posterior superior pancreaticoduodenal arteries (see Fig. 4.114 and 4.115). This arterial network supplies the head and uncinate process of the pancreas and the duodenum.

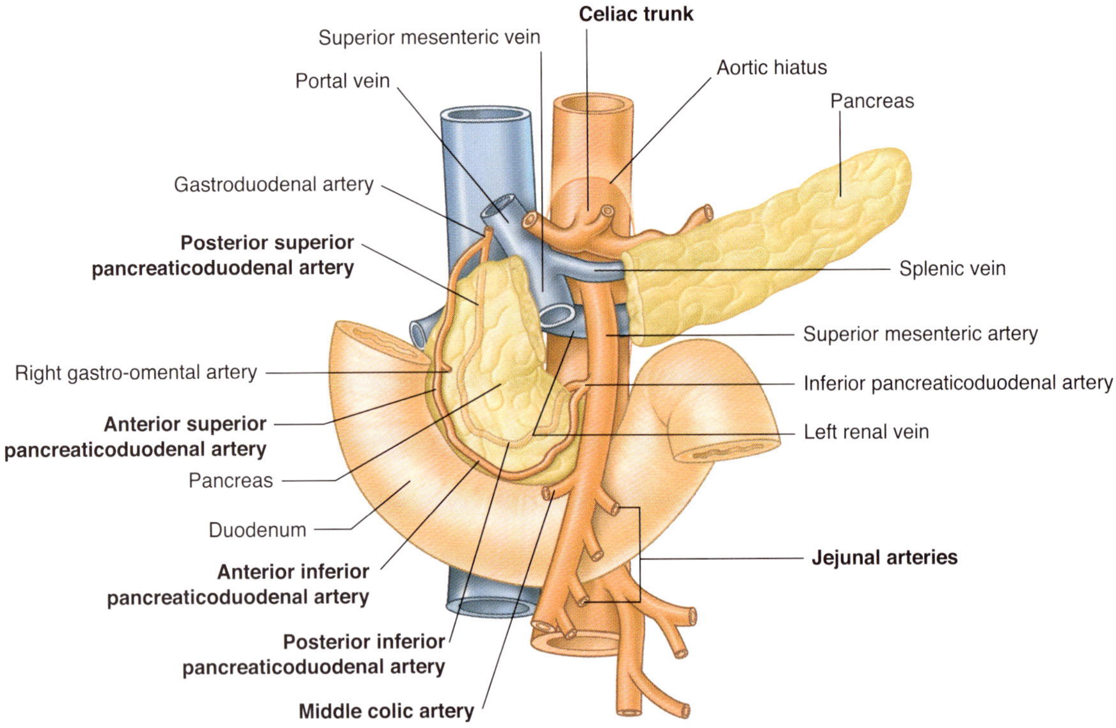

Fig. 4.115 Initial branching and relationships of the superior mesenteric artery.

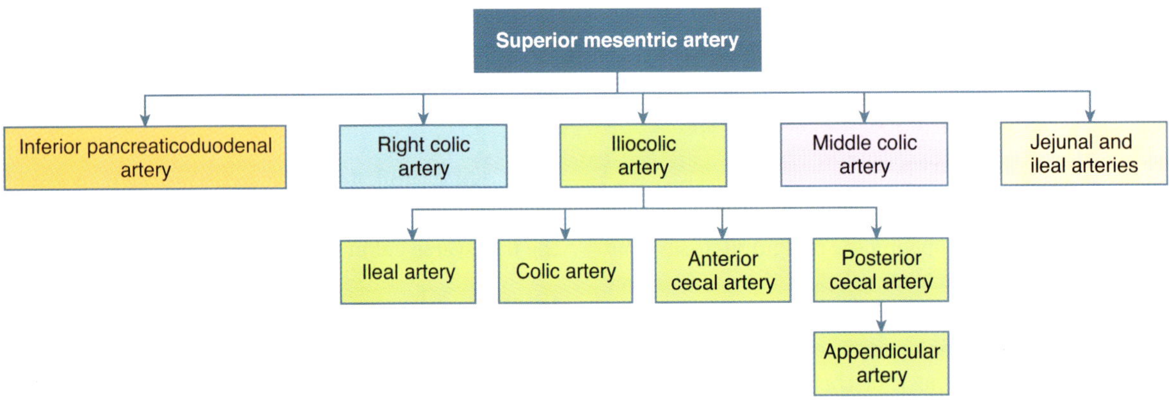

Flowchart 4.2 Branches of superior mesenteric artery.

Jejunal and ileal arteries

Distal to the inferior pancreaticoduodenal artery, the superior mesenteric artery gives off numerous branches. Arising on the left is a large number of jejunal and ileal arteries supplying the jejunum and most of the ileum (Fig. 4.116). These branches leave the main trunk of the artery, pass between two layers of the mesentery, and form anastomosing arches or arcades as they pass outward to supply the small intestine. The number of arterial arcades increases distally along the gut (Fig. 4.66).

There may be single and then double arcades in the area of the jejunum, with a continued increase in the number

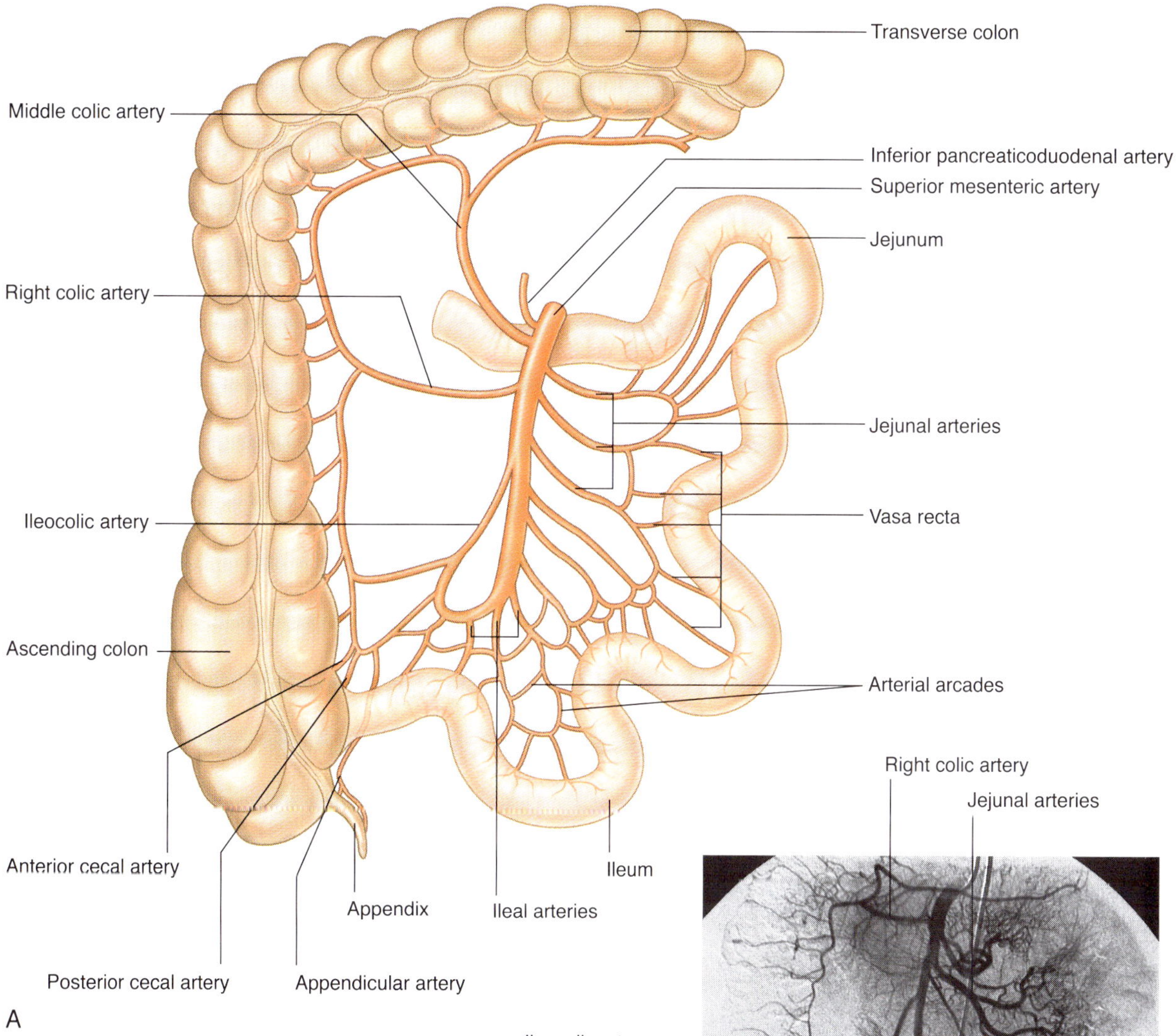

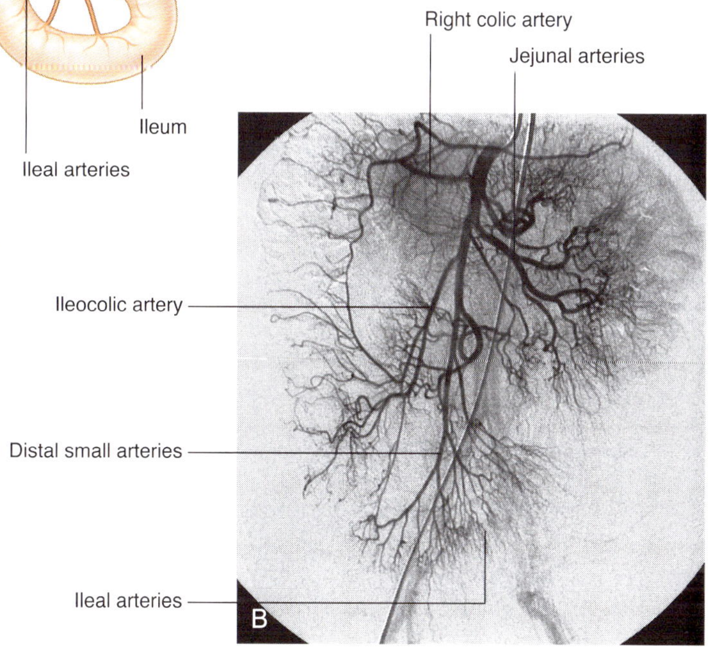

Fig. 4.116 Superior mesenteric artery. **(A)** Distribution of the superior mesenteric artery. **(B)** Digital subtraction angiography of the superior mesenteric artery and its branches.

of arcades moving into and through the area of the ileum. Extending from the terminal arcade are vasa recta (straight arteries), which provide the final direct vascular supply to the walls of the small intestine. The **vasa recta** supplying the jejunum are usually long and close together, forming narrow windows visible in the mesentery. The vasa recta supplying the ileum are generally short and far apart, forming low broad windows.

Middle colic artery

The middle colic artery is the first of the three branches from the right side of the main trunk of the superior mesenteric artery (Fig. 4.116). It arises at the point where the superior mesenteric artery emerges at the lower border of the pancreas. The middle colic artery passes into the transverse mesocolon (Fig. 4.53B) and divides into right and left branches. The right branch anastomoses with the right colic artery while the left branch anastomoses with the left colic artery, which is a branch of the inferior mesenteric artery.

Right colic artery

Continuing distally along the main trunk of the superior mesenteric artery, the right colic artery is the second of the three branches from the right side of the main trunk of the superior mesenteric artery (Fig. 4.116). It is an inconsistent branch, and passes to the right in a retroperitoneal position to supply the ascending colon. Nearing the colon, it divides into a descending branch, which anastomoses with the ileocolic artery, and an ascending branch, which anastomoses with the middle colic artery.

Ileocolic artery

The final branch arising from the right side of the superior mesenteric artery is the ileocolic artery (Fig. 4.116). This passes downward and to the right toward the right iliac fossa where it divides into superior and inferior branches:

- The superior branch passes upward along the ascending colon to anastomose with the right colic artery.
- The inferior branch continues toward the ileocolic junction, dividing into **colic, cecal, appendicular**, and **ileal branches** (Fig. 4.116).

The specific pattern of distribution and origin of these branches is variable:

- The colic branch crosses to the ascending colon and passes upward to supply the first part of the ascending colon.
- Anterior and posterior cecal branches, arising either as a common trunk or as separate branches, supply corresponding sides of the cecum.
- The appendicular branch enters the free margin of and supplies the mesoappendix and the appendix.
- The ileal branch passes to the left and ascends to supply the final part of the ileum before anastomosing with the superior mesenteric artery.

Inferior mesenteric artery

The inferior mesenteric artery is the anterior branch of the abdominal aorta that supplies the hindgut. It is the smallest of the three anterior branches of the abdominal aorta and arises anterior to the body of vertebra LIII. Initially, the inferior mesenteric artery descends anterior to the aorta and then passes to the left as it continues inferiorly (Fig. 4.117A). Its branches include the **left colic artery, several sigmoid arteries**, and the **superior rectal artery (**Flowchart 4.3**)**.

Left colic artery

The left colic artery is the first branch of the inferior mesenteric artery (Fig. 4.117A). It ascends retroperitoneally, dividing into ascending and descending branches:

- The ascending branch passes anterior to the left kidney, then enters the transverse mesocolon, and passes superiorly to supply the upper part of the descending colon and the distal part of the transverse colon; it anastomoses with branches of the middle colic artery (Fig. 4.84).

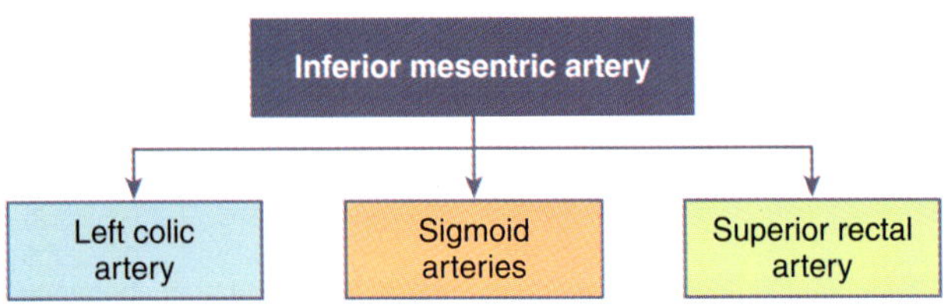

Flowchart 4.3 Branches of inferior mesenteric artery.

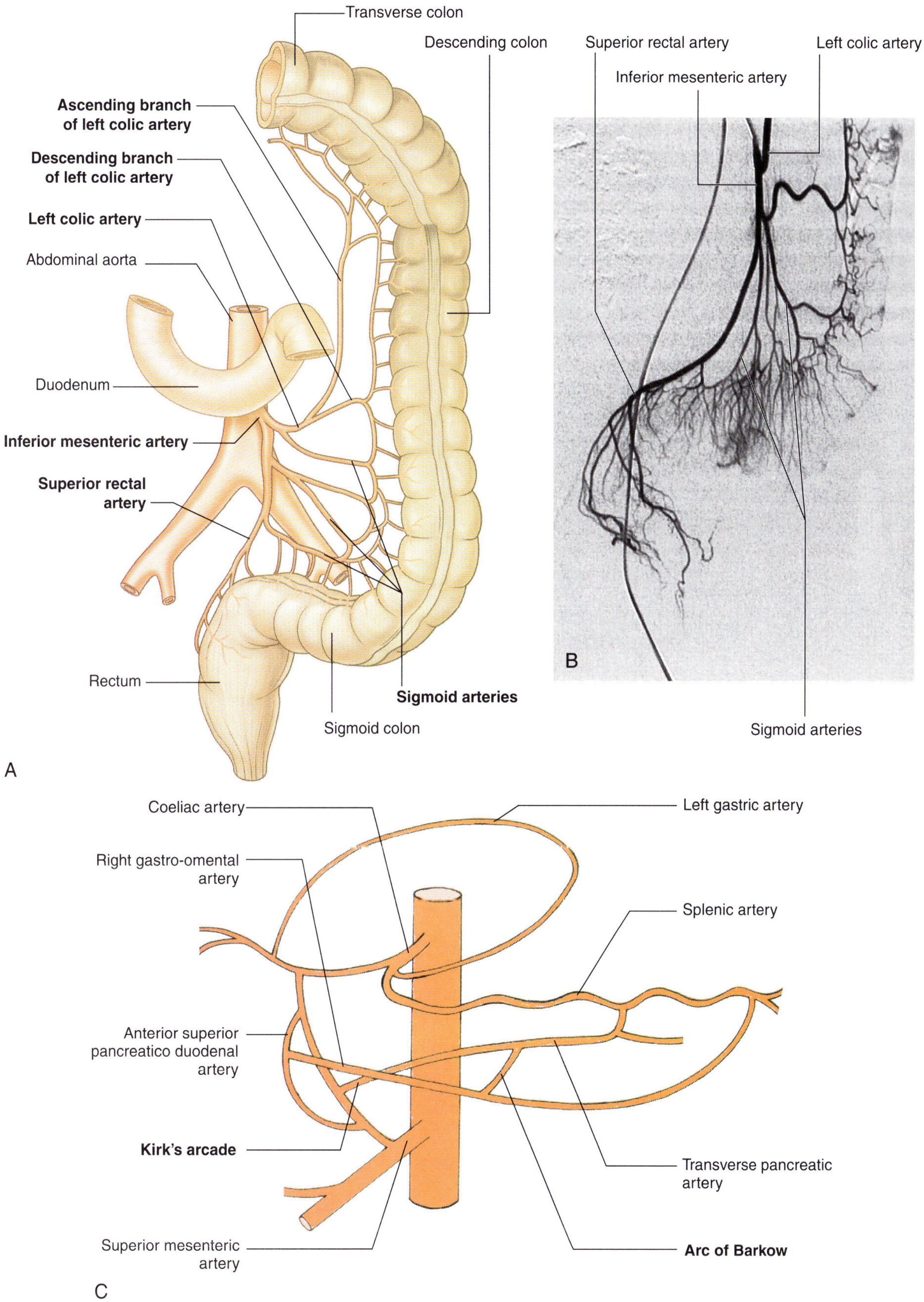

Fig. 4.117 Inferior mesenteric artery. **(A)** Distribution of the inferior mesenteric artery. **(B)** Digital subtraction angiography (DSA) of the inferior mesenteric artery and its branches. **(C)** Arcade of Kirk and arch of Barkow.

Continued

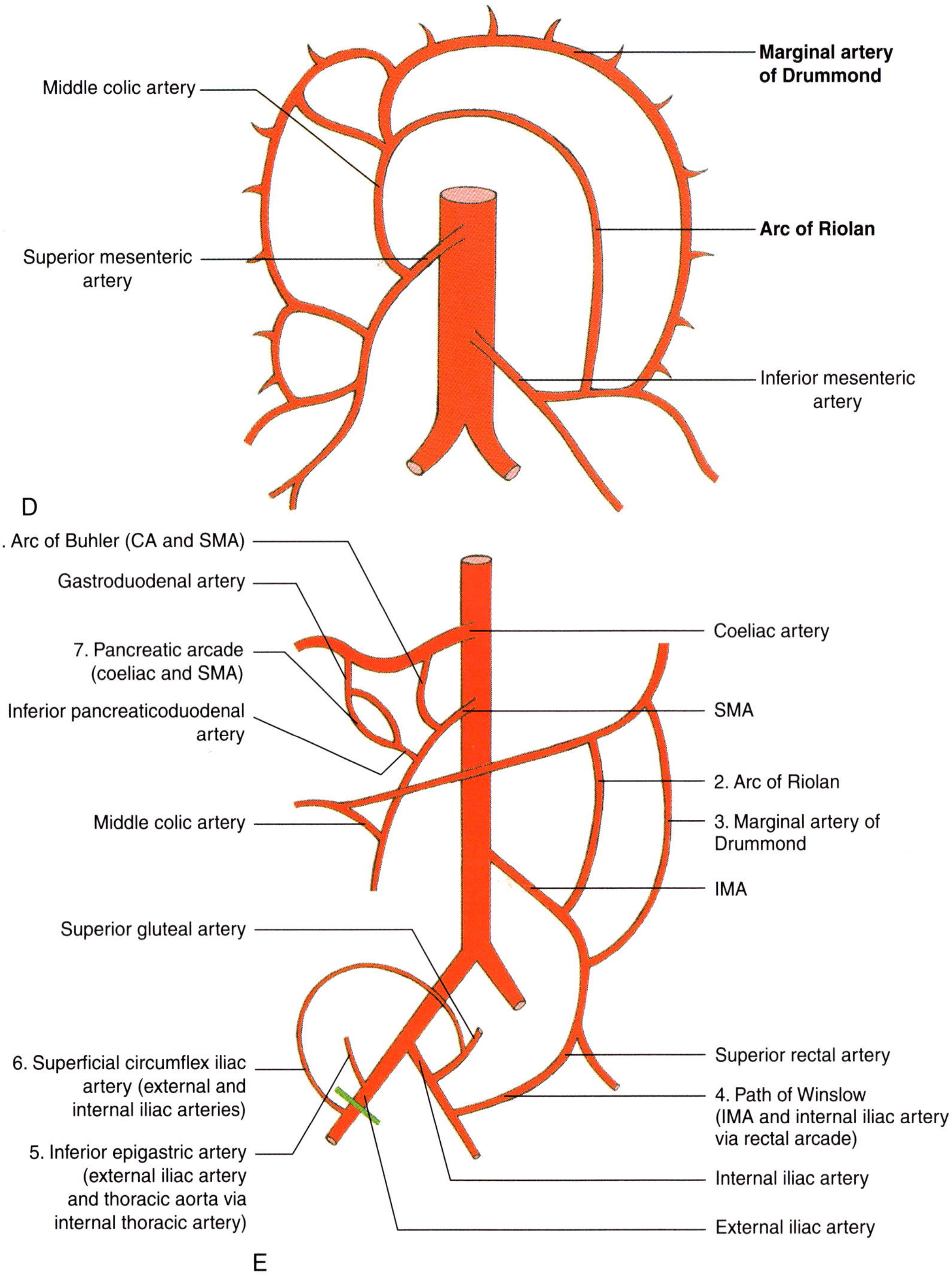

Fig. 4.117, cont'd (D) Arch of Riolan and marginal artery of Drummond. **(E)** Overview of various arterial anastomoses. (1) Arc of Buhler, (2) arc of Riolan (medial), (3) marginal artery of Drummond (lateral), (4) path of Winslow, (5) inferior epigastric artery, (6) superficial circumflex iliac artery, and (7) pancreatic arcade. CA, coeliac artery; SMA, superior mesenteric artery; IMA, inferior mesenteric artery.

- The descending branch passes inferiorly, supplying the lower part of the descending colon, and anastomoses with the first sigmoid artery.

Sigmoid arteries

The sigmoid arteries consist of two to four branches, which descend to the left, in the sigmoid mesocolon, to supply the lowest part of the descending colon and the sigmoid colon (Fig. 4.117A). These branches anastomose superiorly with branches from the left colic artery and inferiorly with branches from the superior rectal artery.

Superior rectal artery

The terminal branch of the inferior mesenteric artery is the superior rectal artery (Fig. 4.117A and B). This vessel descends into the pelvic cavity in the sigmoid mesocolon, crossing the left common iliac vessels. Opposite vertebra SIII, the superior rectal artery divides. The two terminal branches descend on each side of the rectum, dividing into smaller branches in the wall of the rectum. These smaller branches continue inferiorly to the level of the internal anal sphincter, anastomosing along the way with branches from the middle rectal arteries (from the internal iliac artery) and the inferior rectal arteries (from the internal pudendal artery).

Mesenteric anastomoses

The right transverse branches of the dorsal pancreatic artery anastomose with the anterior and posterior pancreaticoduodenal arcades to form **Kirk's arcade** (Fig. 4.117C). The **arc of Buhler** refers to an inconsistent artery that **directly** connects the celiac axis and the superior mesenteric artery. The arc of Barkow refers to the collateral pathway between the celiac axis and the superior mesenteric artery in the greater omentum. The right and left gastro-omental arteries, branches of the gastroduodenal and splenic artery, respectively, give branches to supply the greater omentum. The posterior epiploic arteries of the transverse pancreatic and the middle colic arteries supply the greater omentum and join the gastro-omental arteries to form the **arc of Barkow** (Fig. 4.117C). Sudeck's critical point at the rectosigmoid junction is described as the point of origin of the last sigmoid arterial branch, originating from the inferior mesenteric artery.

The **arc of Riolan**, also known as the mesenteric meandering artery (of Moskowitz) or central anastomotic mesenteric artery, is an arterial anastomosis between the superior and inferior mesenteric arteries via the middle colic artery (Fig. 4.117D).

The **marginal artery of Drummond,** also known as the marginal artery of the colon, is a continuous arterial arcade along the inner border of the colon formed by the anastomoses of the terminal branches of the superior mesenteric artery and inferior mesenteric artery (Flowchart 4.4).

Griffiths point (or Griffiths' critical point) is the site of watershed anastomosis between the ascending left colic artery and the marginal artery of Drummond occurring in the region of the splenic flexure (Fig. 4.117E).

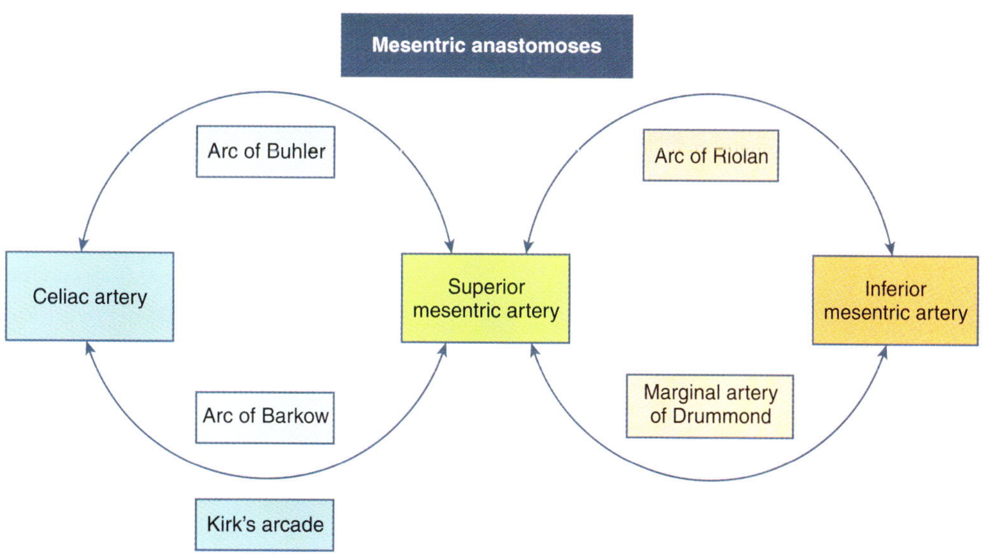

Flowchart 4.4 Mesenteric anastomoses.

Early clinical exposure

Vascular supply to the gastrointestinal system

The abdominal parts of the gastrointestinal system are supplied mainly by the celiac trunk and the superior mesenteric and inferior mesenteric arteries (Fig. 4.118):

- The celiac trunk supplies the lower esophagus, stomach, superior part of the duodenum, and proximal half of the descending part of the duodenum.
- The superior mesenteric artery supplies the rest of the duodenum, the jejunum, the ileum, the ascending colon, and the proximal two-thirds of the transverse colon.
- The inferior mesenteric artery supplies the rest of the transverse colon, the descending colon, the sigmoid colon, and most of the rectum.

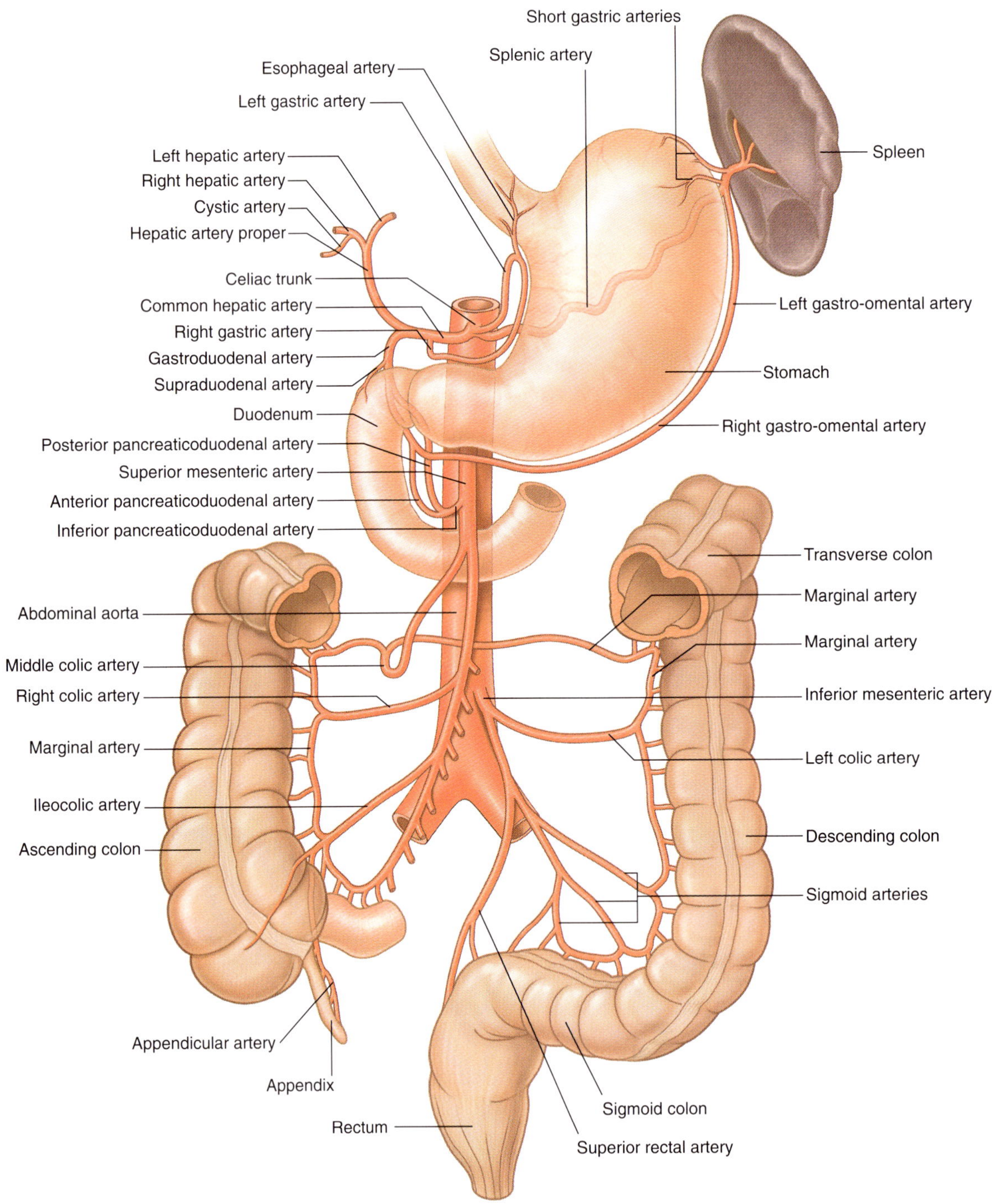

Fig. 4.118 Arterial supply to the abdominal parts of the gastrointestinal system and to the spleen.

Early clinical exposure—cont'd

Along the descending part of the duodenum, there is a potential watershed area between the celiac trunk blood supply and the superior mesenteric arterial blood supply. It is unusual for this area to become ischemic, whereas the watershed area between the superior mesenteric artery and the inferior mesenteric artery, near the splenic flexure, is extremely vulnerable to ischemia.

In certain disease states, the region of the splenic flexure of the colon can become ischemic. When this occurs, the mucosa sloughs off, rendering the patient susceptible to infection and perforation of the large bowel, which then requires urgent surgical attention.

Arteriosclerosis may occur throughout the abdominal aorta and at the openings of the celiac trunk and the superior mesenteric and inferior mesenteric arteries. Not infrequently, the inferior mesenteric artery becomes occluded. Interestingly, many of these patients do not suffer any complications, because anastomoses between the right, middle, and left colic arteries gradually enlarge, forming a continuous **marginal artery**. The distal large bowel therefore becomes supplied by this enlarged marginal artery (marginal artery of Drummond), which replaces the blood supply of the inferior mesenteric artery (Fig. 4.119).

If the openings of the celiac trunk and superior mesenteric artery become narrowed, the blood supply to the gut is diminished. After a heavy meal, the oxygen demand of the bowel therefore outstrips the limited supply of blood through the stenosed vessels, resulting in severe pain and discomfort (**mesenteric angina**). Patients with this condition tend not to eat because of the pain and rapidly lose weight. The diagnosis is determined by aortic angiography, and the stenoses of the celiac trunk and superior mesenteric artery are best appreciated in the lateral view.

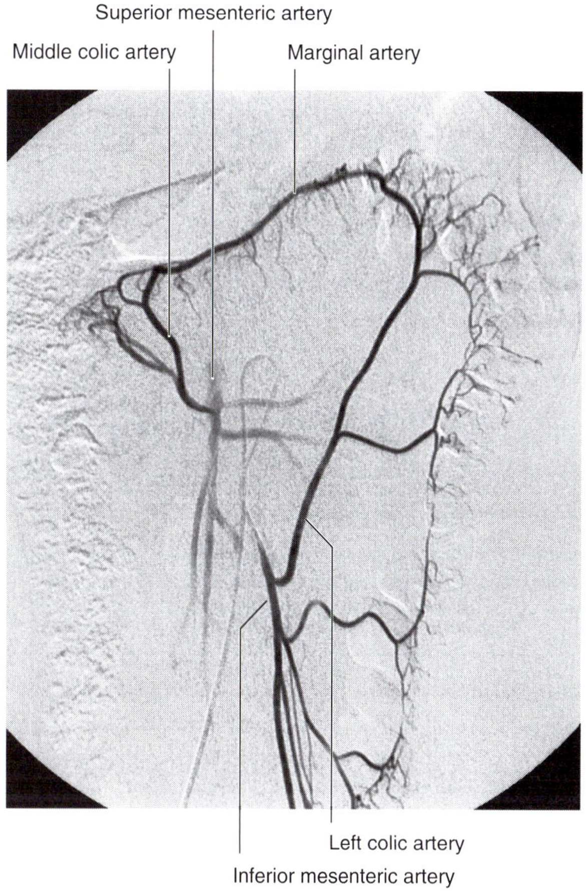

Fig. 4.119 Enlarged marginal artery connecting the superior and inferior mesenteric arteries. Digital subtraction angiogram.

Venous drainage

Venous drainage of the spleen, pancreas, gallbladder, and abdominal part of the gastrointestinal tract, except for the inferior part of the rectum, is through the portal system of veins, which deliver blood from these structures to the liver. Once blood passes through the hepatic sinusoids, it passes through progressively larger veins until it enters the hepatic veins, which return the venous blood to the inferior vena cava just inferior to the diaphragm.

Portal vein

The **portal vein** is the final common pathway for the transport of venous blood from the spleen, pancreas, gallbladder, and abdominal part of the gastrointestinal tract. It is formed by the union of the **splenic vein** and the **superior mesenteric vein** posterior to the neck of the pancreas at the level of vertebra LII (Fig. 4.120).

Ascending toward the liver, the portal vein passes posterior to the superior part of the duodenum and enters the right margin of the lesser omentum. As it passes through this part of the lesser omentum, it is anterior to the omental foramen and posterior to both the bile duct, which is slightly to its right, and the hepatic artery proper, which is slightly to its left (see Fig. 4.54A and Fig. 4.114).

On approaching the liver, the portal vein divides into **right** and **left branches**, which enter the liver parenchyma. Tributaries to the portal vein include:

- **Right** and **left gastric veins** draining the lesser curvature of the stomach and abdominal esophagus
- **Cystic veins** from the gallbladder
- The **paraumbilical veins**, which accompany the obliterated umbilical vein and connect to veins on the anterior abdominal wall (see Fig. 4.122)

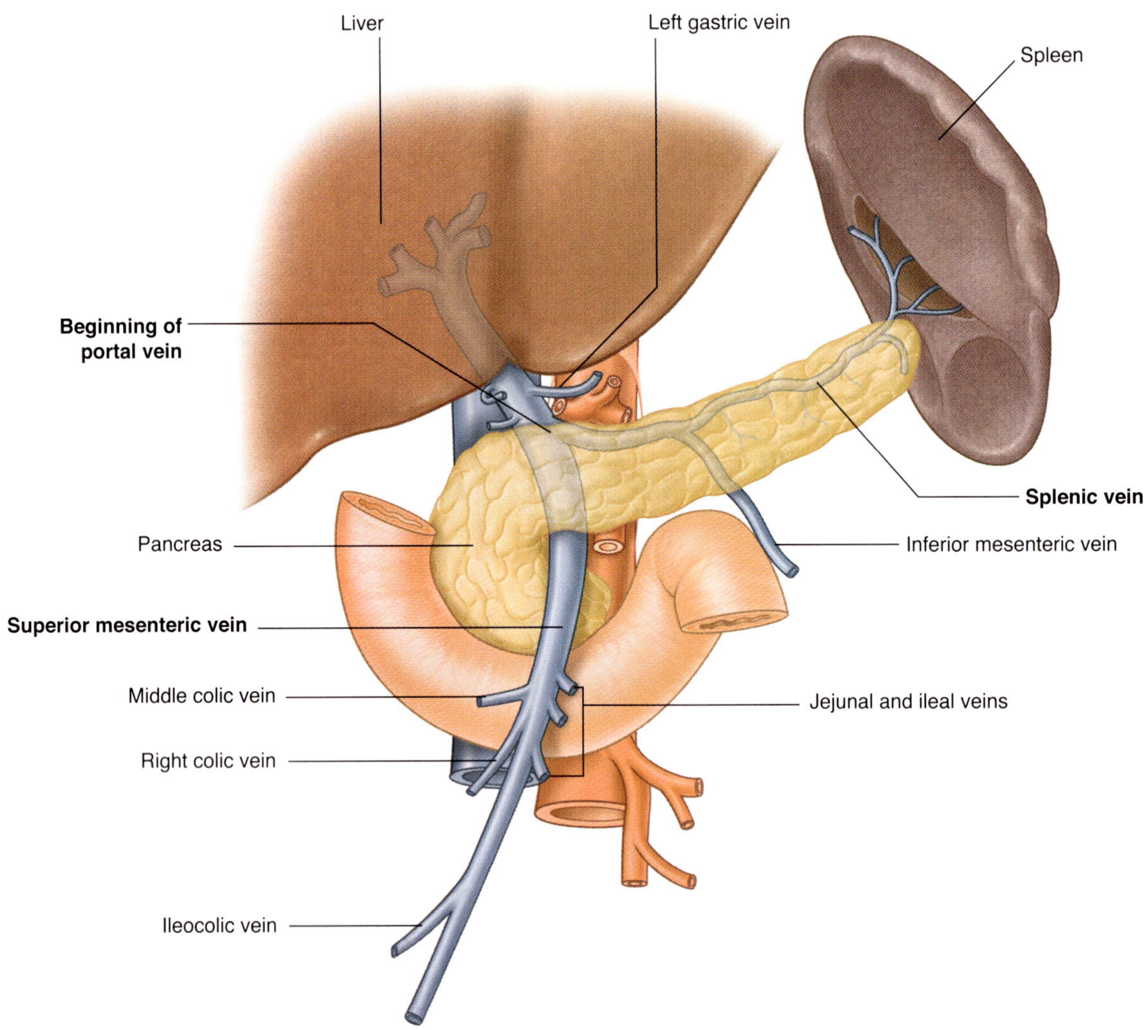

Fig. 4.120 Portal vein.

Splenic vein

The splenic vein forms from numerous smaller vessels leaving the hilum of the spleen (Fig. 4.121). It passes to the right, passing through the splenorenal ligament with the splenic artery and the tail of the pancreas (Fig. 4.54A). Continuing to the right, the large, straight splenic vein is in contact with the body of the pancreas as it crosses the posterior abdominal wall. Posterior to the neck of the pancreas, the splenic vein joins the superior mesenteric vein to form the portal vein.

Tributaries to the splenic vein include:

- **Short gastric veins** from the fundus and left part of the greater curvature of the stomach
- The **left gastro-omental vein** from the greater curvature of the stomach
- **Pancreatic veins** draining the body and tail of the pancreas
- Usually the **inferior mesenteric vein**

Superior mesenteric vein

The superior mesenteric vein drains blood from the small intestine, cecum, ascending colon, and transverse colon (Fig. 4.121). It begins in the right iliac fossa as veins draining the terminal ileum, cecum, and appendix join, and ascends in the mesentery to the right of the superior mesenteric artery.

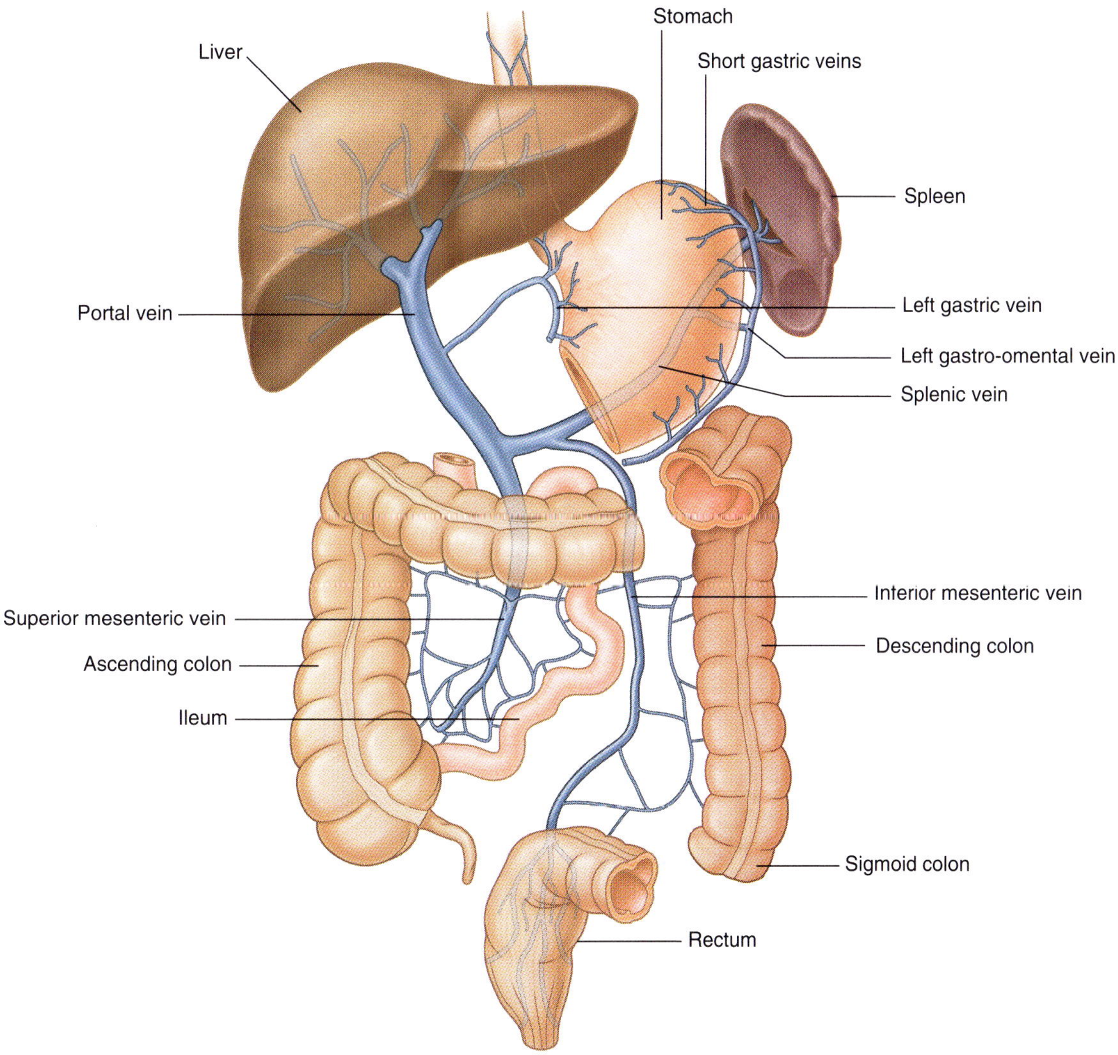

Fig. 4.121 Venous drainage of the abdominal portion of the gastrointestinal tract.

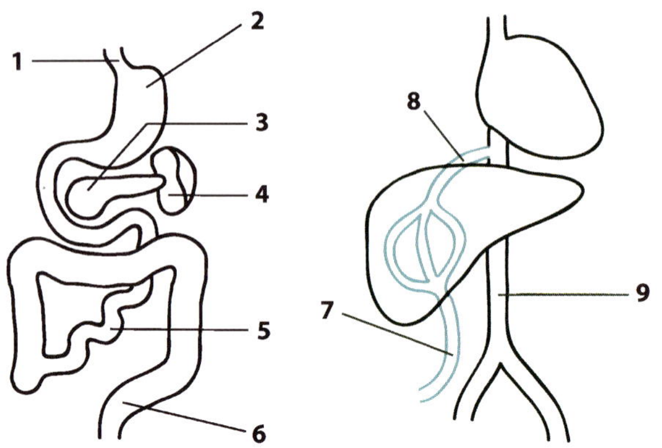

LD Fig. 4.121.1 Schematic diagram of the venous drainage of parts of the alimentary system

Questions

LD Fig. 4.121.1A Name the labelled structures which drain to the structure labelled 7.

LD Fig. 4.121.1B Name the structures labelled 7, 8, and 9.

Answers

LD Fig. 4.121.1A

1. Oesophagus
2. Stomach
3. Pancreas
4. Spleen
5. Small intestine
6. Large intestine

LD Fig. 4.121.1B 7. Portal vein

8. Hepatic vein
9. Inferior vena cava

Posterior to the neck of the pancreas, the superior mesenteric vein joins the splenic vein to form the portal vein.

As a corresponding vein accompanies each branch of the superior mesenteric artery, tributaries to the superior mesenteric vein include jejunal, ileal, ileocolic, right colic, and middle colic veins. Additional tributaries include:

- The **right gastro-omental vein**, draining the right part of the greater curvature of the stomach
- The **anterior** and **posterior inferior pancreaticoduodenal veins**, which pass alongside the arteries of the same name; the anterior superior pancreaticoduodenal vein usually empties into the right gastro-omental vein, and the posterior superior pancreaticoduodenal vein usually empties directly into the portal vein

Inferior mesenteric vein

The **inferior mesenteric vein** drains blood from the rectum, sigmoid colon, descending colon, and **splenic flexure** (Fig. 4.121). It begins as a continuation of the **superior rectal vein** and ascends, receiving the sigmoid veins and the **left colic vein**. All these veins accompany arteries of the same name. Continuing to ascend, the inferior mesenteric vein passes to the left of the duodenojejunal flexure and then posterior to the body of the pancreas and usually joins the splenic vein. Occasionally, it ends at the junction of the splenic and superior mesenteric veins or joins the superior mesenteric vein.

Early clinical exposure

Hepatic cirrhosis

Cirrhosis is a complex disorder of the liver, the diagnosis of which is confirmed histologically. When a diagnosis is suspected, a liver biopsy is necessary.

Cirrhosis is characterized by widespread hepatic fibrosis interspersed with areas of nodular regeneration and abnormal reconstruction of preexisting lobular architecture. The presence of cirrhosis implies previous or continuing liver cell damage.

The etiology of cirrhosis is complex and includes toxins (alcohol), viral inflammation, biliary obstruction, vascular outlet obstruction, nutritional (malnutrition) causes, and inherited anatomical and metabolic disorders.

As the cirrhosis progresses, the intrahepatic vasculature is distorted, which in turn leads to increased pressure in the portal vein and its draining tributaries (portal hypertension). Portal hypertension produces increased pressure in the splenic venules, leading to **splenic enlargement**. At the sites of portosystemic anastomosis (Fig. 4.122), large dilated veins (varices) develop. These veins are susceptible to bleeding and may produce marked blood loss, which in some instances can be fatal.

The liver is responsible for the production of numerous proteins, including those of the clotting cascade. Any disorder of the liver (including infection and cirrhosis) may decrease the production of these proteins and so **prevent adequate blood clotting**. Patients with severe cirrhosis of the liver have a significant risk of serious bleeding, even from small cuts; in addition, when varices rupture, there is a danger of rapid exsanguination.

As the liver progressively fails, the patient develops **salt and water retention**, which produces skin and subcutaneous edema. Fluid (ascites) is also retained in the peritoneal cavity, which can hold many liters.

The poorly functioning liver cells (hepatocytes) are unable to break down blood and blood products, leading to an increase in the serum bilirubin level, which manifests as **jaundice**.

With the failure of normal liver metabolism, toxic metabolic by-products do not convert to nontoxic metabolites.

Early clinical exposure—cont'd

This buildup of noxious compounds is made worse by the numerous portosystemic shunts, which allow the toxic metabolites to bypass the liver. Patients may develop severe **neurological features**, which may lead to epileptic fits, dementia, and irreversible neurological damage.

Hepatic encephalopathy is one of the urgent criteria for liver transplantation; if the condition is not reversed, it leads to irreversible neurological damage and death.

Portosystemic anastomosis

The hepatic portal system drains blood from the visceral organs of the abdomen to the liver. In normal individuals, 100% of the portal venous blood flow can be recovered from the hepatic veins, whereas in patients with elevated portal vein pressure (e.g., from cirrhosis), there is significantly less blood flow to the liver. The rest of the blood enters collateral channels, which drain into the systemic circulation at specific points (Fig. 4.19 and 4.122). The largest of these collaterals occur at:

- The gastroesophageal junction around the cardia of the stomach—where the left gastric vein and its tributaries form a portosystemic anastomosis with tributaries to the azygos system of veins of the caval system
- The anus—the superior rectal vein of the portal system anastomoses with the middle and inferior rectal veins of the systemic venous system
- The anterior abdominal wall around the umbilicus—the paraumbilical veins anastomose with veins on the anterior abdominal wall

When the pressure in the portal vein is elevated, venous enlargement (varices) tend to occur at and around the sites of portosystemic anastomoses and these enlarged veins are called:

- Hemorrhoids at the anorectal junction
- Esophageal varices at the gastroesophageal junction
- Caput medusae at the umbilicus

Esophageal varices are susceptible to trauma and, once damaged, may bleed profusely, requiring urgent surgical intervention.

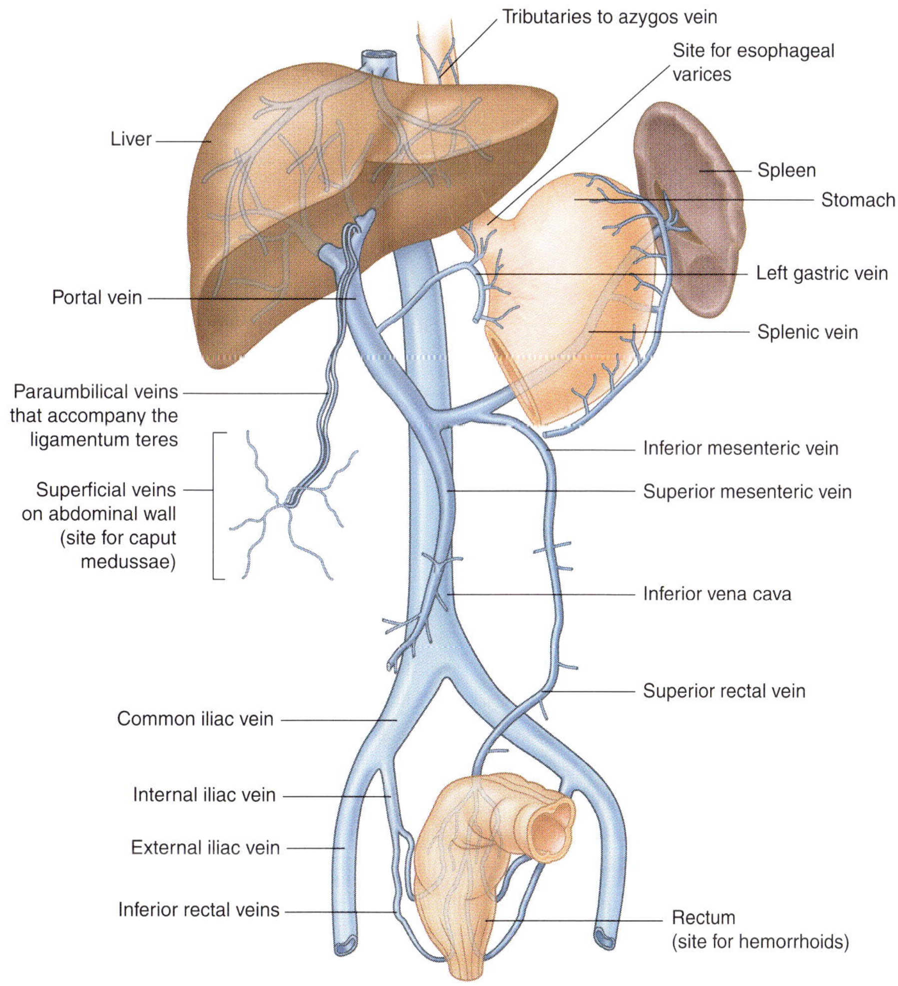

Fig. 4.122 Portosystemic anastomoses.

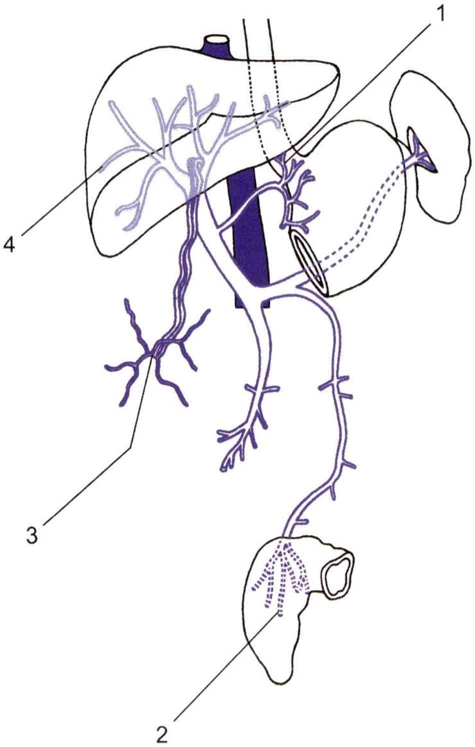

LD Fig. 4.122.1 Sites of portosystemic anastomosis.

Questions

LD Fig. 4.122.1A Name the locations indicated by the labels 1–4 and list the portal and the systemic tributaries which anastomose there.

LD Fig. 4.122.1B Discuss a way to recap the location of the sites of portosystemic anastomosis.

Answers

LD Fig. 4.122.1A

1. At the lower end of oesophagus, the oesophageal tributaries of the left gastric vein anastomose with those of the left accessory hemiazygos vein.
2. At the anterior abdominal wall, the paraumbilical veins anastomose with the superficial veins of the anterior abdominal wall.
3. At the rectum, the superior rectal vein anastomoses with both the middle and inferior rectal veins.
4. At the bare area of the liver, the branches of the portal vein anastomose with the tributaries of the inferior vena cava.

LD Fig. 4.122.1B The locations are roughly located at the superior, inferior, anterior, and posterior parts of the abdominal cavity.

Lymphatics

Lymphatic drainage of the abdominal part of the gastrointestinal tract, as low as the inferior part of the rectum, as well as the spleen, pancreas, gallbladder, and liver, is through vessels and nodes that eventually end in large collections of **preaortic lymph nodes** at the origins of the three anterior branches of the abdominal aorta, which supply these structures. These collections are therefore referred to as the **celiac, superior mesenteric**, and **inferior mesenteric** groups of preaortic lymph nodes. Lymph from viscera is supplied by three routes:

- The celiac trunk (i.e., structures that are part of the abdominal foregut) drains to preaortic nodes near the origin of the celiac trunk (Fig. 4.123)—these celiac nodes also receive lymph from the superior mesenteric and inferior mesenteric groups of preaortic nodes, and lymph from the celiac nodes enters the **cisterna chyli** (Fig. 6.95)
- The superior mesenteric artery (i.e., structures that are part of the abdominal midgut) drains to preaortic nodes near the origin of the superior mesenteric artery (Fig. 4.123)—these superior mesenteric nodes also receive lymph from the inferior mesenteric groups of preaortic nodes, and lymph from the superior mesenteric nodes drains to the celiac nodes.
- The inferior mesenteric artery (i.e., structures that are part of the hindgut) drains to preaortic nodes near the origin of the inferior mesenteric artery (Fig. 4.123), and lymph from the inferior mesenteric nodes drains to the superior mesenteric nodes.

Innervation

Abdominal viscera are innervated by both extrinsic and intrinsic components of the nervous system:

- Extrinsic innervation involves receiving motor impulses from, and sending sensory information to, the central nervous system.
- Intrinsic innervation involves the regulation of digestive tract activities by a generally independent network of sensory and motor neurons (the enteric nervous system).

Abdominal viscera receiving extrinsic innervation include the abdominal part of the gastrointestinal tract, the spleen, the pancreas, the gallbladder, and the liver. These viscera send sensory information back to the central nervous system through visceral afferent fibers and receive motor impulses from the central nervous system through visceral efferent fibers.

The visceral efferent fibers are part of the sympathetic and parasympathetic parts of the autonomic division of the peripheral nervous system.

Structural components serving as conduits for these afferent and efferent fibers include posterior and anterior

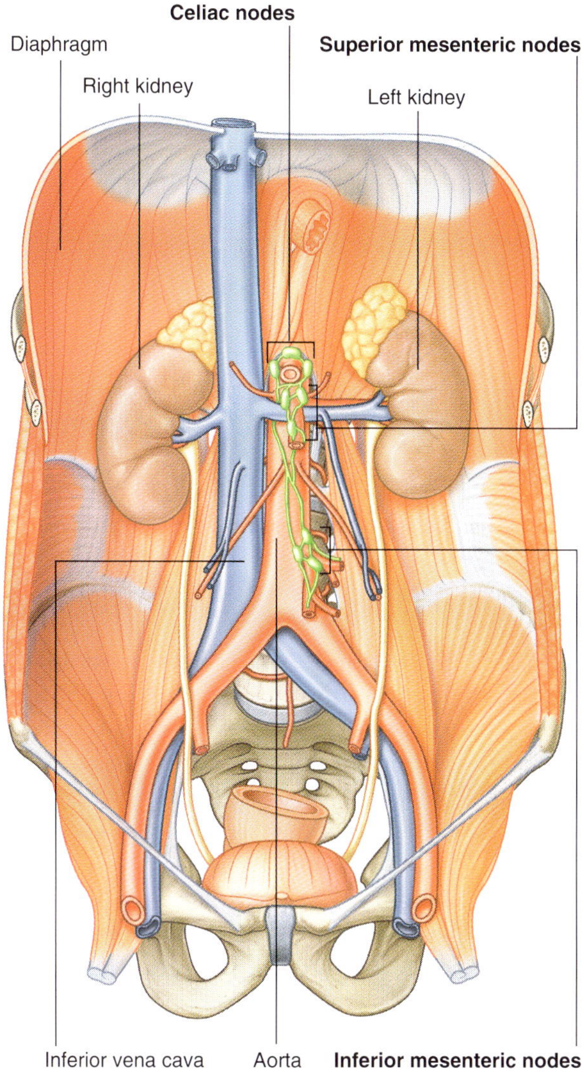

Fig. 4.123 Lymphatic drainage of the abdominal portion of the gastrointestinal tract.

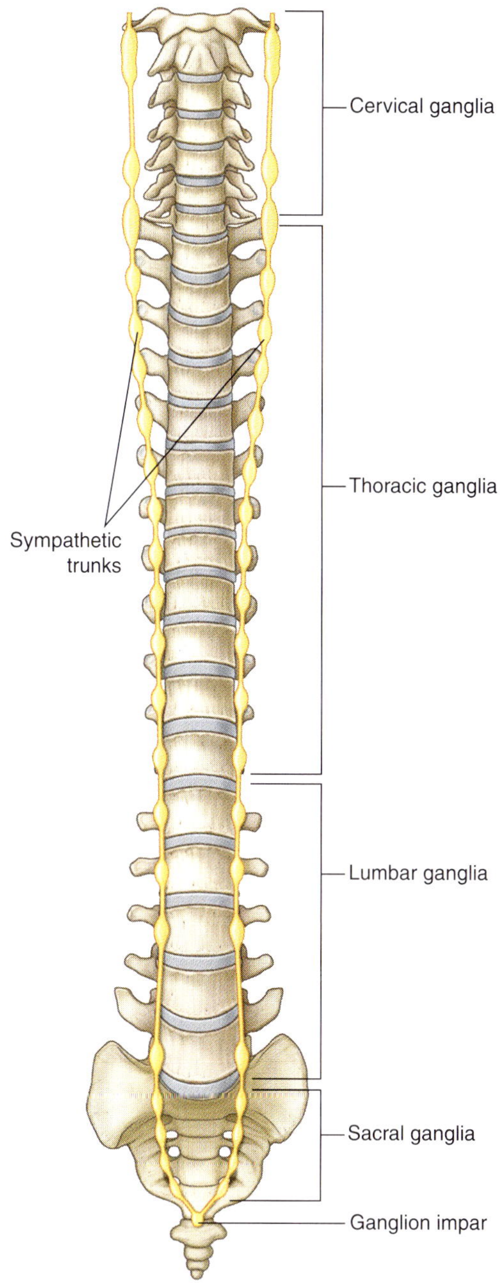

Fig. 4.124 Sympathetic trunks.

roots of the spinal cord, respectively, spinal nerves, anterior rami, white and gray rami communicantes, the sympathetic trunks, splanchnic nerves carrying sympathetic fibers (thoracic, lumbar, and sacral), the vagus nerves [X], parasympathetic fibers (pelvic), the prevertebral plexus and related ganglia.

The enteric nervous system consists of motor and sensory neurons in two interconnected plexuses in the walls of the gastrointestinal tract. These neurons control the coordinated contraction and relaxation of intestinal smooth muscle and regulate gastric secretion and blood flow.

Sympathetic trunks

The sympathetic trunks are two parallel nerve cords extending on either side of the vertebral column from the base of the skull to the coccyx (Fig. 4.124). As they pass through the neck, they lie posterior to the carotid sheath. In the upper thorax, they are anterior to the necks of the ribs, while in the lower thorax they are on the lateral aspect of the vertebral bodies. In the abdomen, they are anterolateral to the lumbar vertebral bodies and, continuing into the pelvis, they are anterior to the sacrum. The two sympathetic trunks come together anterior to the coccyx to form the **ganglion impar**.

Throughout the extent of the sympathetic trunks, small raised areas are visible. These collections of neuronal cell bodies outside the CNS are the paravertebral sympathetic ganglia. There are usually:

- Three ganglia in the cervical region
- Eleven or 12 ganglia in the thoracic region
- Four ganglia in the lumbar region
- Four or five ganglia in the sacral region
- The ganglion impar anterior to the coccyx (Fig. 4.124)

The ganglia and trunks are connected to adjacent spinal nerves by gray rami communicantes throughout the length of the sympathetic trunk and by white rami communicantes in the thoracic and upper lumbar parts of the trunk (T1 to L2). Neuronal fibers found in the sympathetic trunks include **preganglionic** and **postganglionic sympathetic fibers** and **visceral afferent fibers**.

Splanchnic nerves

The splanchnic nerves are important components in the innervation of the abdominal viscera. They pass from the sympathetic trunk or sympathetic ganglia associated with the trunk, to the prevertebral plexus and ganglia anterior to the abdominal aorta.

There are two different types of splanchnic nerves, depending on the type of visceral efferent fiber they are carrying:

- The thoracic, lumbar, and sacral splanchnic nerves carry preganglionic sympathetic fibers from the sympathetic trunk to ganglia in the **prevertebral plexus**, and also visceral afferent fibers.
- The pelvic splanchnic nerves (parasympathetic root) carry preganglionic parasympathetic fibers from anterior rami of S2, S3, and S4 spinal nerves to an extension of the prevertebral plexus in the pelvis (the **inferior hypogastric plexus** or **pelvic plexus**).

Thoracic splanchnic nerves

Three **thoracic splanchnic nerves** pass from sympathetic ganglia along the sympathetic trunk in the thorax to the prevertebral plexus and ganglia associated with the abdominal aorta in the abdomen (Fig. 4.125):

- The greater splanchnic nerve arises from the fifth to the ninth (or 10th) thoracic ganglia and travels to the celiac ganglion in the abdomen (a prevertebral ganglion associated with the celiac trunk).
- The lesser splanchnic nerve arises from the ninth and 10th (or 10th and 11th) thoracic ganglia and travels to the aorticorenal ganglion.
- The least splanchnic nerve, when present, arises from the 12th thoracic ganglion and travels to the renal plexus.

Lumbar and sacral splanchnic nerves

There are usually two to four **lumbar splanchnic nerves**, which pass from the lumbar part of the sympathetic trunk or associated ganglia and enter the prevertebral plexus (Fig. 4.125).

Similarly, the **sacral splanchnic nerves** pass from the sacral part of the sympathetic trunk or associated ganglia and enter the inferior hypogastric plexus, which is an extension of the prevertebral plexus into the pelvis.

Pelvic splanchnic nerves

The **pelvic splanchnic nerves** (**parasympathetic root**) are unique. They are the only splanchnic nerves that carry parasympathetic fibers. In other words, they do not originate from the sympathetic trunks. Rather, they originate directly from the anterior rami of S2 to S4. Preganglionic parasympathetic fibers originating in the sacral spinal cord pass from the S2 to S4 spinal nerves to the inferior hypogastric plexus (Fig. 4.125). Once in this plexus, some of these fibers pass upward, enter the abdominal prevertebral plexus, and distribute with the arteries supplying the hindgut. This provides the pathway for innervation of the distal one-third of the transverse colon, the descending colon, and the sigmoid colon by preganglionic parasympathetic fibers.

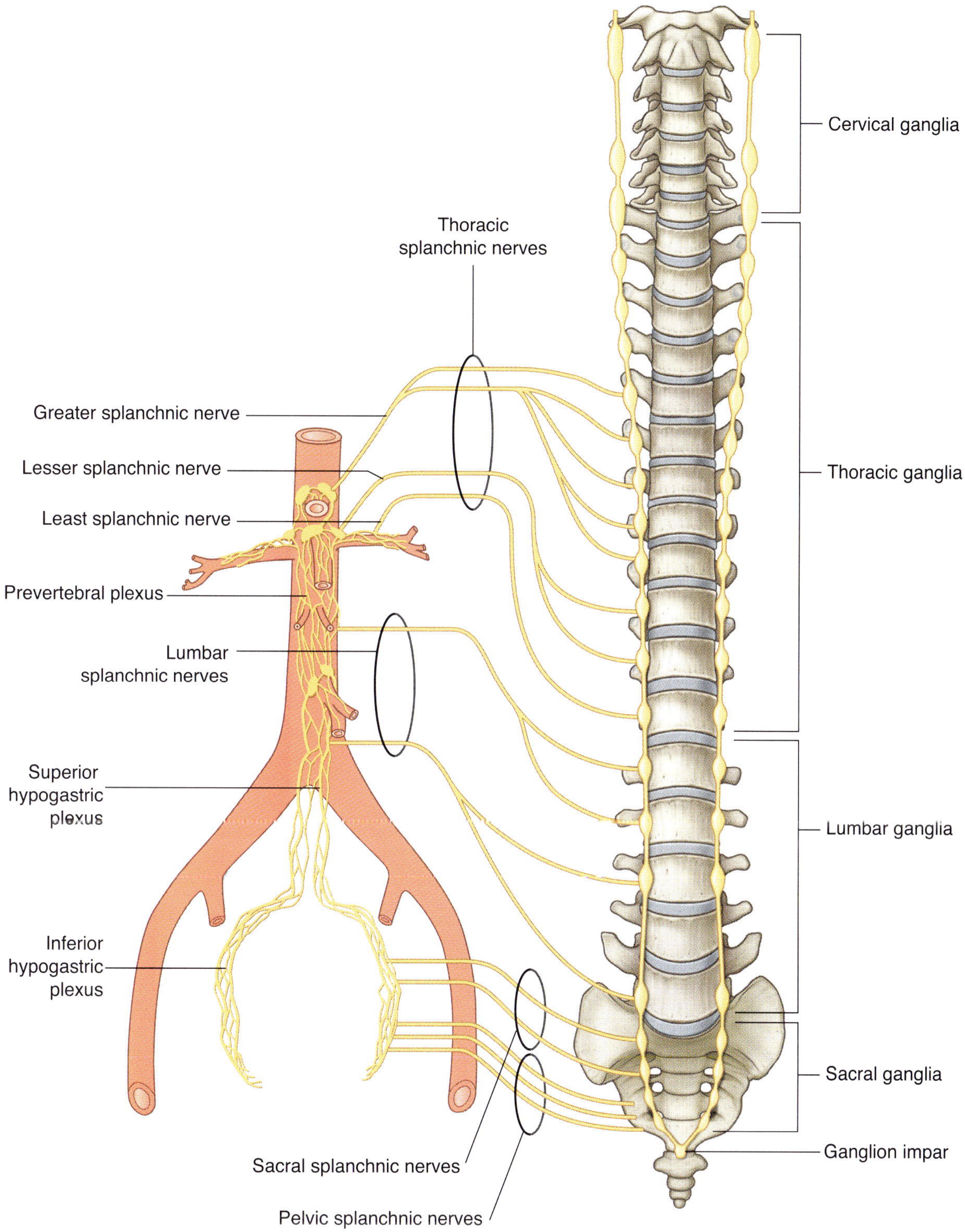

Fig. 4.125 Splanchnic nerves.

Abdominal prevertebral plexus and ganglia

The abdominal prevertebral plexus is a collection of nerve fibers that partly surround the abdominal aorta and is continuous onto its major branches. Scattered throughout the length of the abdominal prevertebral plexus are cell bodies of postganglionic sympathetic fibers. Some of these cell bodies are organized into distinct ganglia, while others are more random in their distribution. The ganglia are usually associated with specific branches of the abdominal aorta and named after these branches.

The three major divisions of the abdominal prevertebral plexus and associated ganglia are the celiac, aortic, and superior hypogastric plexuses (Fig. 4.126).

- The celiac plexus is the large accumulation of nerve fibers and ganglia associated with the roots of the celiac trunk and superior mesenteric artery immediately below the aortic hiatus of the diaphragm. Ganglia associated with the celiac plexus include two celiac ganglia, a single superior mesenteric ganglion, and two aorticorenal ganglia.
- The aortic plexus consists of nerve fibers and associated ganglia on the anterior and lateral surfaces of the abdominal aorta extending from just below the origin of the superior mesenteric artery to the bifurcation of the aorta into the two common iliac arteries. The major ganglion in this plexus is the inferior mesenteric ganglion at the root of the inferior mesenteric artery.
- The superior hypogastric plexus contains numerous small ganglia and is the final part of the abdominal prevertebral plexus before the prevertebral plexus continues into the pelvic cavity.

Each of these major plexuses gives origin to a number of secondary plexuses, which may also contain small ganglia. These plexuses are usually named after the vessels with which they are associated. For example, the celiac plexus is usually described as giving origin to the superior mesenteric plexus and the renal plexus, as well as other plexuses that extend out along the various branches of the celiac trunk. Similarly, the aortic plexus has secondary plexuses consisting of the inferior mesenteric plexus, the spermatic plexus, and the external iliac plexus.

Inferiorly, the superior hypogastric plexus divides into the **hypogastric nerves**, which descend into the pelvis and contribute to the formation of the inferior hypogastric or pelvic plexus (Fig. 4.126).

The abdominal prevertebral plexus receives:

- Preganglionic parasympathetic and visceral afferent fibers from the vagus nerves [X]
- Preganglionic sympathetic and visceral afferent fibers from the thoracic and lumbar splanchnic nerves
- Preganglionic parasympathetic fibers from the pelvic splanchnic nerves

Parasympathetic innervation

Parasympathetic innervation of the abdominal part of the gastrointestinal tract and of the spleen, pancreas, gallbladder, and liver is from two sources—the vagus nerves [X] and the pelvic splanchnic nerves.

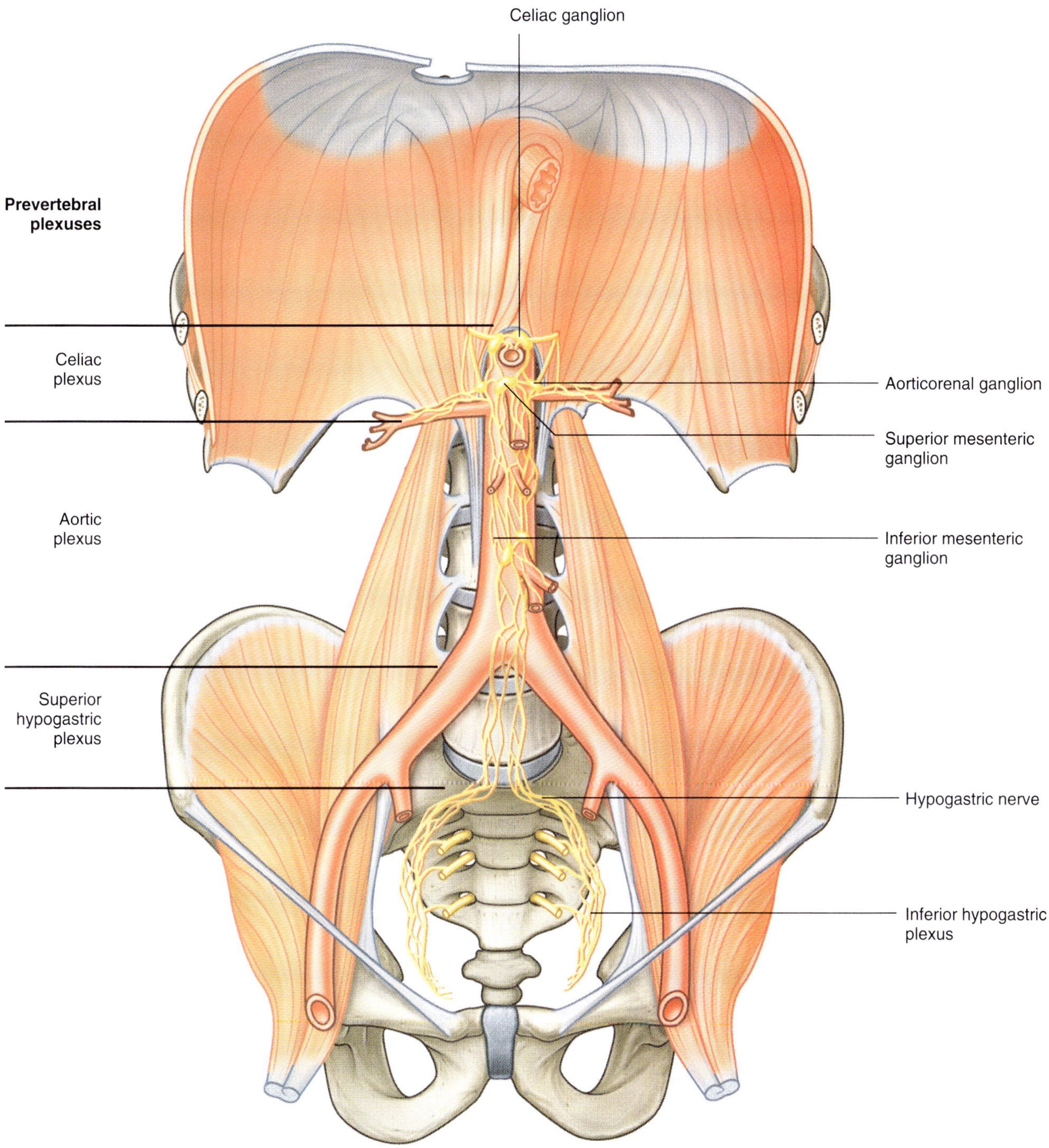

Fig. 4.126 Abdominal prevertebral plexus and ganglia.

Vagus nerves

The **vagus nerves** [X] enter the abdomen associated with the esophagus as the esophagus passes through the diaphragm (Fig. 4.127) and provide parasympathetic innervation to the foregut and midgut.

After entering the abdomen as the **anterior** and **posterior vagal trunks**, they send branches to the abdominal prevertebral plexus. These branches contain preganglionic parasympathetic fibers and visceral afferent fibers, which are distributed with the other components of the prevertebral plexus along the branches of the abdominal aorta.

Pelvic splanchnic nerves

The **pelvic splanchnic nerves**, carrying preganglionic parasympathetic fibers from S2 to S4 spinal cord levels, enter the inferior hypogastric plexus in the pelvis. Some of these fibers pass upward into the inferior mesenteric part of the prevertebral plexus in the abdomen (Fig. 4.127). Once there, these fibers are distributed with branches of the inferior mesenteric artery and provide parasympathetic innervation to the hindgut.

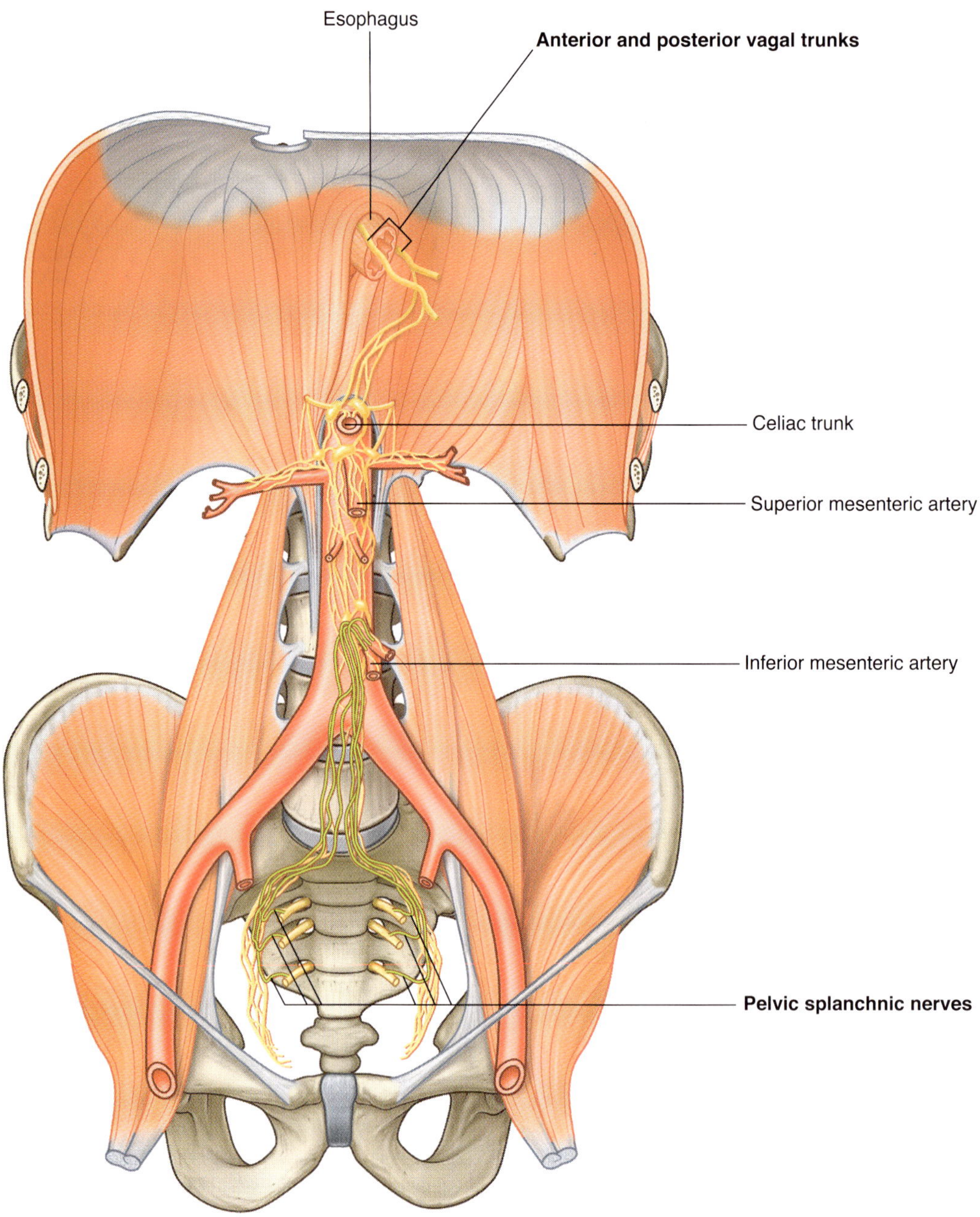

Fig. 4.127 Parasympathetic innervation of the abdominal portion of the gastrointestinal tract.

Enteric system

The enteric system is a division of the visceral part of the nervous system and is a local neuronal circuit in the wall of the gastrointestinal tract. It consists of motor and sensory neurons organized into two interconnected plexuses (the **myenteric** and **submucosal plexuses**) between the layers of the gastrointestinal wall, and the associated nerve fibers that pass between the plexuses and from the plexuses to the adjacent tissue (Fig. 4.128).

The enteric system regulates and coordinates numerous gastrointestinal tract activities, including gastric secretory activity, gastrointestinal blood flow, and the contraction and relaxation cycles of smooth muscle (**peristalsis**).

Although the enteric system is generally independent of the central nervous system, it does receive input from postganglionic sympathetic and preganglionic parasympathetic neurons that modifies its activities.

Sympathetic innervation of the stomach

The pathway of sympathetic innervation of the stomach is as follows:

- A preganglionic sympathetic fiber originating at the T6 level of the spinal cord enters an anterior root to leave the spinal cord (Fig. 1.47).
- At the level of the intervertebral foramen, the anterior root (which contains the preganglionic fiber) and a posterior root join to form a spinal nerve.
- Outside the vertebral column, the preganglionic fiber leaves the anterior ramus of the spinal nerve through the white ramus communicans.
- The white ramus communicans, containing the preganglionic fiber, connects to the sympathetic trunk.
- Entering the sympathetic trunk, the preganglionic fiber does not synapse but passes through the trunk and enters the greater splanchnic nerve.
- The greater splanchnic nerve passes through the crura of the diaphragm and enters the celiac ganglion.
- In the celiac ganglion, the preganglionic fiber synapses with a postganglionic neuron.
- The postganglionic fiber joins the plexus of nerve fibers surrounding the celiac trunk and continues along its branches.
- The postganglionic fiber travels through the plexus of nerves accompanying the branches of the celiac trunk supplying the stomach and eventually reaches its point of distribution.
- This input from the sympathetic system may modify the activities of the gastrointestinal tract controlled by the enteric nervous system.

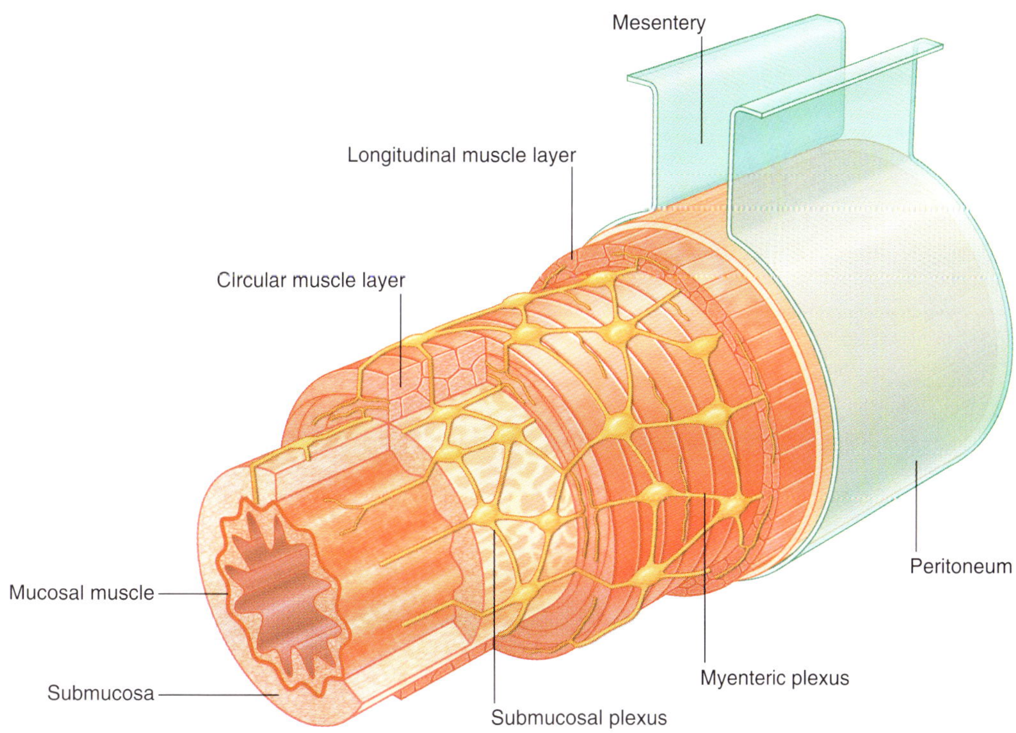

Fig. 4.128 The enteric system.

Early clinical exposure

Surgery for obesity

Surgery for obesity is also known as weight loss surgery and **bariatric surgery**. This type of surgery has become increasingly popular over the last few years for patients who are unable to achieve significant weight loss through appropriate diet modification and exercise programs. It is often regarded as a last resort. Importantly, we have to recognize the increasing medical impact that overweight patients pose. With obesity, the patient is more likely to develop diabetes and cardiovascular problems and may suffer from increased general health disorders. All of these have a significant impact on health care budgeting and are regarded as serious conditions for the "health of a nation."

There are a number of surgical options to treat obesity. Surgery for patients who are morbidly obese can be categorized into two main groups: malabsorptive procedures and restrictive procedures.

Malabsorptive procedures

There are a variety of bypass procedures that produce a malabsorption state, preventing further weight gain and also producing weight loss. There are complications, which may include anemia, osteoporosis, and diarrhea (e.g., jejunoileal bypass).

Predominantly restrictive procedures

Restrictive procedures involve placing a band or stapling in or around the stomach to decrease the size of this organ. This reduction produces an earlier feeling of satiety and prevents the patient from overeating.

Combination procedure

Probably the most popular procedure currently in the USA, this procedure involves stapling the proximal stomach and joining a loop of small bowel to the small gastric remnant.

Any overweight patient undergoing surgery faces significant risk and increased morbidity, with mortality rates from 1% to 5%.

POSTERIOR ABDOMINAL REGION

SET INDUCTION—CASE SCENARIO 10A: PSOAS ABSCESS

An 84-year-old male was brought to the surgery OPD with complaints of a swelling in the right groin for 2 months and low-grade fever for 2 months. A diagnosis of psoas abscess due to tuberculosis was made. Knowledge of the anatomy of the psoas sheath is needed to manage this case.

SET INDUCTION—CLINICAL SCENARIO 10B: PARALYSIS OF THE DIAPHRAGM

A 34-year-old female was undergoing a lymph node biopsy to remove an enlarged lymph node in the neck. After the surgery, it was noted that she had difficulty breathing, and there was weakness of the hemidiaphragm on the side that the surgery was done. Knowledge of the motor nerve supply of the diaphragm is needed to manage this case.

REMEMBER [Recall Facts]	**OUTLINE 10. POSTERIOR ABDOMINAL REGION 1, AND DIAPHRAGM—LEARNING OBJECTIVES [By the end of this section, the student should be able to:]**			**EVALUATE [Explain Concepts]**
	DEMONSTRATE AND ANALYZE RELATIONSHIPS [Identify structures in a Prosected Specimen or Figure]			
	Level I	**Level II**	**Level III**	
1. List the bones and muscles that form the posterior abdominal wall 2. Describe the origin, insertion, nerve supply, and action of the muscles of the posterior abdominal wall and the diaphragm 3. List the openings in the diaphragm, and mention the structures passing through them	▪ Psoas major ▪ Quadratus lumborum ▪ Iliacus ▪ Nerves—iliohypogastric, ilioinguinal, femoral, obturator, lumbosacral trunk Diaphragm: ▪ Parts—right and left domes, central tendon ▪ Origin—sternal, costal, lumbar—crura, medial and lateral arcuate ligaments ▪ Caval opening (in central tendon) ▪ Esophageal opening (in right crus) ▪ Aortic opening (behind median arcuate ligament) ▪ Phrenic nerves	▪ Psoas fascia ▪ Fascia iliaca ▪ Anterior layer of thoracolumbar fascia ▪ Subcostal nerve ▪ Genitofemoral ▪ Lateral cutaneous nerve of the thigh Diaphragm: ▪ Median arcuate ligament ▪ Other structures passing through major openings ▪ Openings for—superior epigastric vessels, subcostal vessels and nerves, sympathetic trunk, splanchnic nerves	▪ Psoas minor ▪ Medial arcuate ligament ▪ Lateral arcuate ligament ▪ Triangle of Marcille ▪ Branches of iliolumbar artery Diaphragm: ▪ Openings for—musculophrenic vessels, lower five intercostal nerves, hemiazygos vein	▪ Origin of diaphragm ▪ Actions of diaphragm **EARLY CLINICAL EXPOSURE [Apply Anatomical Knowledge]** **Surgical Anatomy/ Pathology/ Trauma**: ▪ Psoas abscess ▪ Meralgia paresthetica ▪ Psoas abscess ▪ Diaphragmatic hernia **Imaging/ Surface Anatomy** **PROBLEM SOLVING/ CLINICAL CASES [Interpret]** ▪ Describe the hernias that can occur through the diaphragm

The posterior abdominal region is posterior to the abdominal part of the gastrointestinal tract, the spleen, and the pancreas (Fig. 4.129). This area, bounded by bones and muscles making up the posterior abdominal wall, contains numerous structures that not only are directly involved in the activities of the abdominal contents but also use this area as a conduit between body regions. Examples include the abdominal aorta and its associated nerve plexuses, the inferior vena cava, the sympathetic trunks, and lymphatics. There are also structures originating in this area that are critical to the normal function of other regions of the body (i.e., the lumbar plexus of nerves), and there are organs that associate with this area during development and remain in it in the adult (i.e., the kidneys and suprarenal glands).

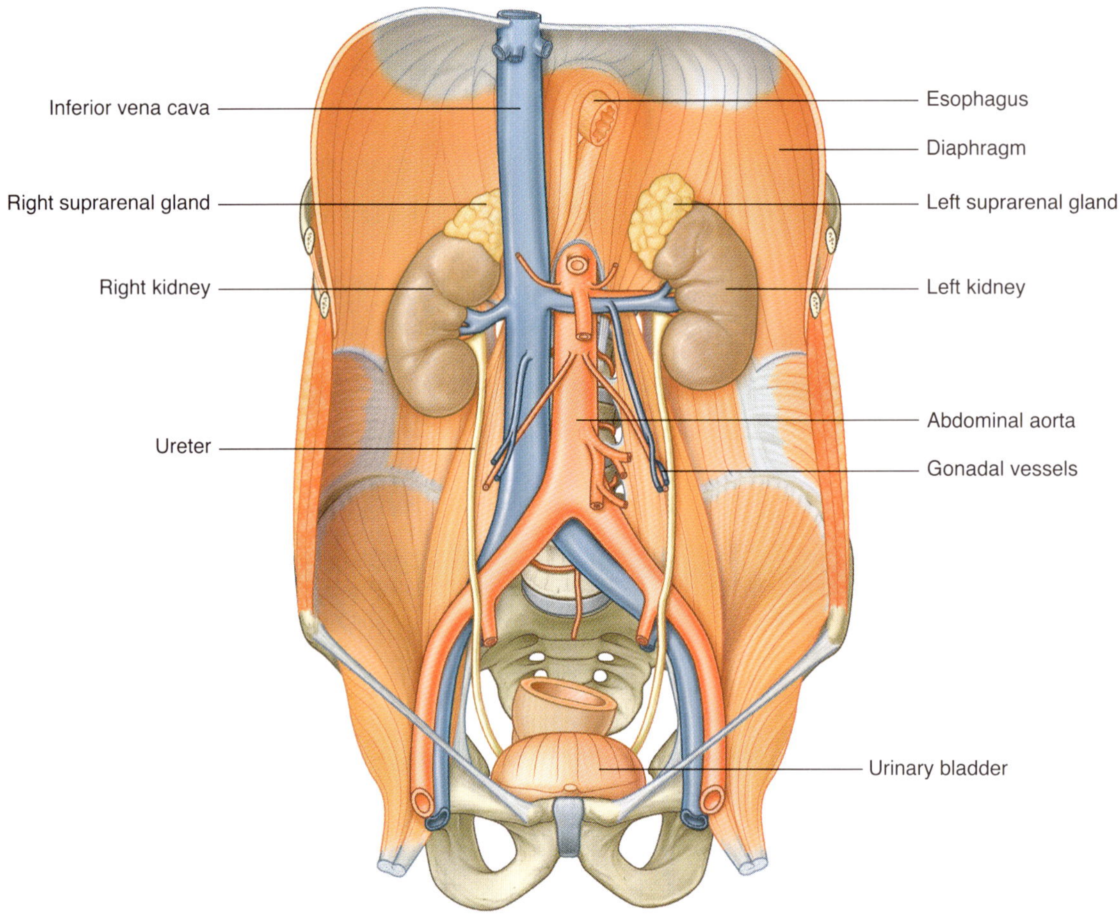

Fig. 4.129 Posterior abdominal region.

Posterior abdominal wall

Bones

Lumbar vertebrae and the sacrum

Projecting into the midline of the posterior abdominal area are the bodies of the five lumbar vertebrae (Fig. 4.130). The prominence of these structures in this region is due to the secondary curvature (a forward convexity) of the lumbar part of the vertebral column (see Fig. 2.2).

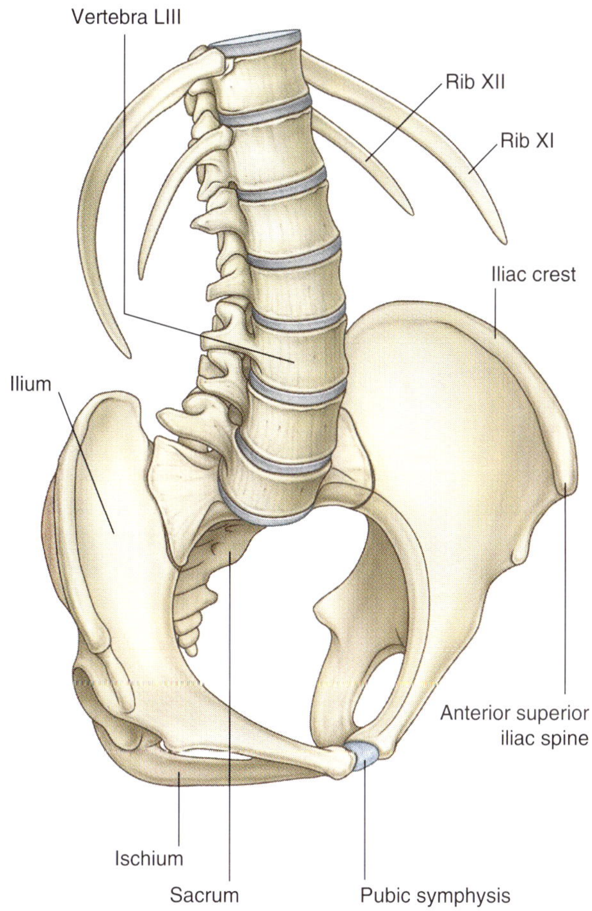

Fig. 4.130 Osteology of the posterior abdominal wall.

The lumbar vertebrae can be distinguished from cervical and thoracic vertebrae because of their size. They do not contain foramina transversaria or costal facets on the body of the vertebrae (see Fig. 2.20). They are much larger than any other vertebrae in any other region. The vertebral bodies are massive and progressively increase in size from vertebra LI to LV. The pedicles are short and stocky, the transverse processes are long and slender, and the spinous processes are large and stubby. The articular processes are large and oriented medially and laterally, which promotes flexion and extension but prevents lateral rotation in this part of the vertebral column.

Between each lumbar vertebra is an intervertebral disc, which completes this part of the midline boundary of the posterior abdominal wall.

The midline boundary of the posterior abdominal wall, inferior to the lumbar vertebrae, consists of the upper margin of the sacrum (Fig. 4.130). The sacrum is formed by the fusion of the five sacral vertebrae into a single, wedge-shaped bony structure that is broad superiorly and narrows inferiorly. Its concave anterior surface and its convex posterior surface contain anterior and posterior sacral foramina for the anterior and posterior rami of spinal nerves to pass through.

Pelvic bones

The **ilia**, which are components of each pelvic bone, attach laterally to the sacrum at the sacroiliac joints (Fig. 4.130). The upper part of each ilium expands outward into a thin wing-like area (the **iliac fossa**). The medial side of this region of each iliac bone, and the related muscles, are components of the posterior abdominal wall.

Ribs

Superiorly, ribs XI and XII complete the bony framework of the posterior abdominal wall (Fig. 4.130). These ribs are unique in that they do not articulate with the sternum or other ribs, they have a single articular facet on their heads, and they do not have necks or tubercles.

Rib XI is posterior to the superior part of the left kidney, and rib XII is posterior to the superior part of both kidneys. Also, rib XII serves as a point of attachment for numerous muscles and ligaments.

Muscles

Muscles forming the medial, lateral, inferior, and superior boundaries of the posterior abdominal region fill in the bony framework of the posterior abdominal wall (Table 4.2). Medially are the psoas major and minor muscles, laterally is the quadratus lumborum muscle, inferiorly is the iliacus muscle, and superiorly is the diaphragm (Fig. 4.131 and 4.132).

Psoas major and minor

Medially, the **psoas major** muscles cover the anterolateral surface of the bodies of the lumbar vertebrae, filling in the space between the vertebral bodies and the transverse processes (Fig. 4.131). Each of these muscles arises from the bodies of vertebra TXII and all five lumbar vertebrae, from the intervertebral discs between each vertebra, and from the transverse processes of the lumbar vertebrae. Passing inferiorly along the pelvic brim, each muscle continues into the anterior thigh, under the inguinal ligament, to attach to the lesser trochanter of the femur.

The psoas major muscle flexes the thigh at the hip joint when the trunk is stabilized and flexes the trunk against gravity when the body is supine. It is innervated by anterior rami of nerves L1 to L3. The **triangle of Marcille** is bounded medially by L5 vertebra, laterally by the medial border of the psoas major and inferiorly by the ala of the sacrum. In the floor of the triangle is the iliolumbar ligament, and the triangle contains the iliolumbar artery between the lumbosacral trunk medially and the obturator nerve laterally. Lateral to the triangle is the sympathetic trunk medially and the genitofemoral nerve laterally (see Fig. 4.161 and 5.63).

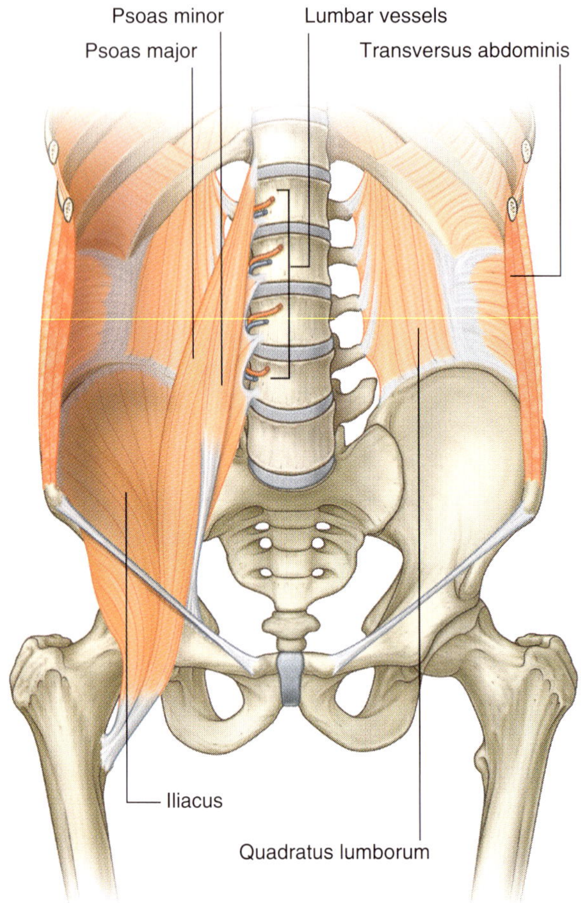

Fig. 4.131 Muscles of the posterior abdominal wall.

Table 4.2 Posterior abdominal wall muscles

Muscle	Origin	Insertion	Innervation	Function
Psoas major	Lateral surface of bodies of TXII to LV vertebrae, transverse processes of the lumbar vertebrae, and the intervertebral discs between TXII to LV vertebrae	Lesser trochanter of the femur	Anterior rami of L1 to L3	Flexion of thigh at hip joint
Psoas minor	Lateral surface of bodies of TXII and LI vertebrae and intervening intervertebral disc	Pectineal line of the pelvic brim and iliopubic eminence	Anterior rami of L1	Weak flexion of lumbar vertebral column
Quadratus lumborum	Transverse process of LV vertebra, iliolumbar ligament, and iliac crest	Transverse processes of LI to LIV vertebrae and inferior border of rib XII	Anterior rami of T12 and L1 to L4	Depress and stabilize rib XII and lateral bending of the trunk
Iliacus	Upper two-thirds of iliac fossa, anterior sacroiliac and iliolumbar ligaments, and upper lateral surface of sacrum	Lesser trochanter of femur	Femoral nerve (L2 to L4)	Flexion of thigh at hip joint

Associated with the psoas major muscle is the **psoas minor** muscle, which is sometimes absent. Lying on the surface of the psoas major when present, this slender muscle arises from vertebrae TXII and LI and the intervening intervertebral disc; its long tendon inserts into the pectineal line of the pelvic brim and the iliopubic eminence.

The psoas minor is a weak flexor of the lumbar vertebral column and is innervated by the anterior ramus of nerve L1.

Quadratus lumborum

Laterally, the quadratus lumborum muscles fill the space between rib XII and the iliac crest on both sides of the vertebral column (Fig. 4.131). They are overlapped medially by the psoas major muscles; along their lateral borders are the transversus abdominis muscles.

Each quadratus lumborum muscle arises from the transverse process of vertebra LV, the iliolumbar ligament, and the adjoining part of the iliac crest. The muscle attaches superiorly to the transverse process of the first four lumbar vertebrae and the inferior border of rib XII.

The quadratus lumborum muscles depress and stabilize rib XII and contribute to lateral bending of the trunk. Acting together, the muscles may extend the lumbar part of the vertebral column. They are innervated by anterior rami of T12 and L1 to L4 spinal nerves.

Iliacus

Inferiorly, an **iliacus** muscle fills the iliac fossa on each side (Fig. 4.131). From this expansive origin covering the iliac fossa, the muscle passes inferiorly, joins with the psoas major muscle, and attaches to the lesser trochanter of the femur. As they pass into the thigh, these combined muscles are referred to as the **iliopsoas** muscle.

Like the psoas major muscle, the iliacus flexes the thigh at the hip joint when the trunk is stabilized and flexes the trunk against gravity when the body is supine. It is innervated by the femoral nerve.

Diaphragm

Superiorly, the diaphragm forms the boundary of the posterior abdominal region. This musculotendinous sheet also separates the abdominal cavity from the thoracic cavity.

Structurally, the diaphragm consists of a central tendinous part into which the circumferentially arranged muscle fibers attach (Fig. 4.132). The diaphragm is anchored to the lumbar vertebrae by musculotendinous crura,

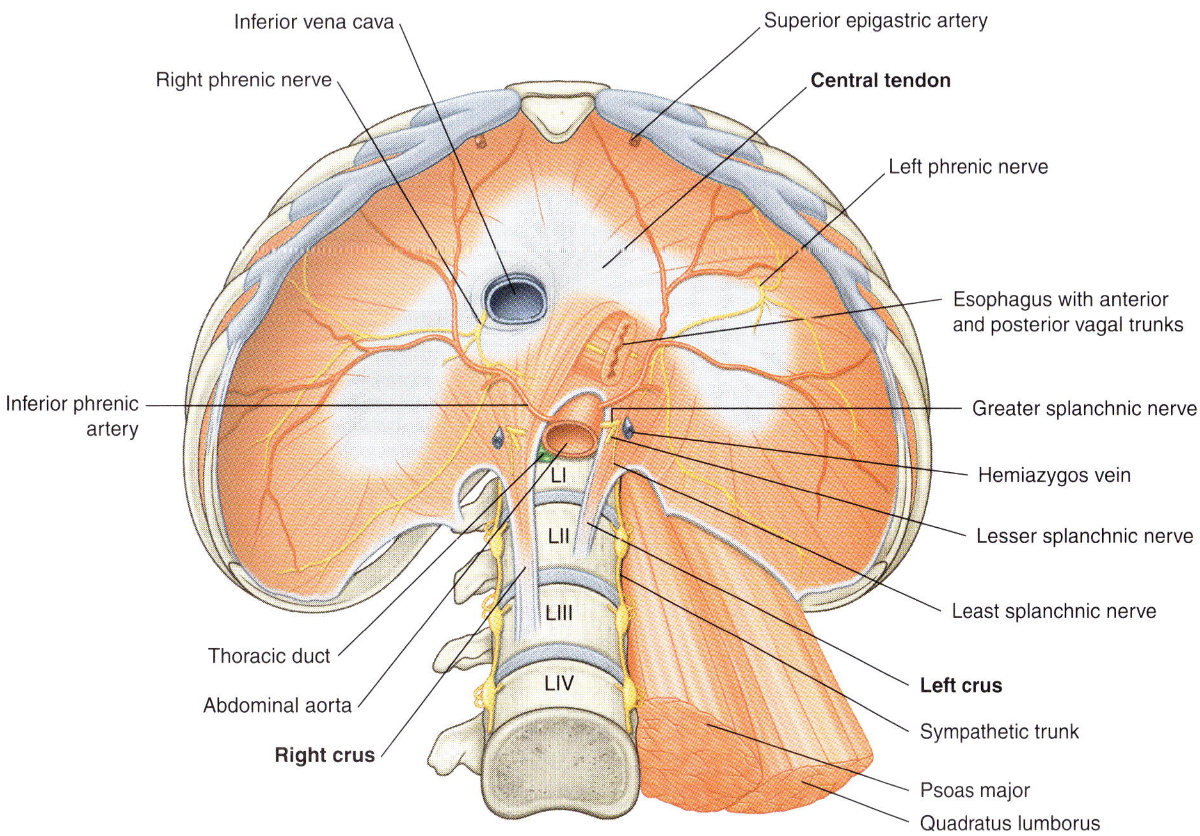

Fig. 4.132 Diaphragm.

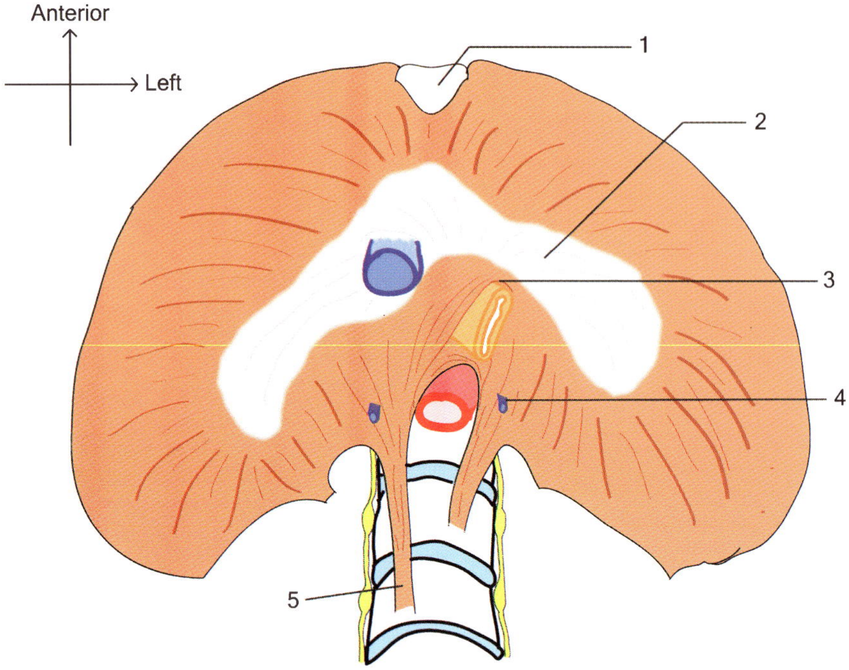

LD Fig. 4.132.1 The diaphragm

Questions

LD Fig. 4.132.1

A. Name the labelled structures.
B. What is the origin and insertion of the diaphragm?
C. What is a clinical correlate of the developmental origin of the diaphragm?
D. What are the structures that pass through the major openings of the diaphragm?
E. Describe a mnemonic that can be used to remember the vertebral levels of these major openings?
F. What passes through each of the minor openings in the diaphragm and where are they located?

Answers

LD Fig. 4.132.1A The structures indicated by the labels are

1. Sternum
2. Central tendon
3. Oesophageal opening
4. Hemiazygos vein
5. Right crus of the diaphragm

LD Fig. 4.132.1B The origin of the diaphragm is (i) sternal—from the xiphoid process of the sternum, (ii) costal—from the inner aspect of the lower six costal cartilages and ribs, and (iii) vertebral—from the median, medial, and lateral arcuate ligaments, and the crura from the lumbar vertebrae (L1 to L3 on the right, and L1 to L2 on the left). The insertion of the diaphragm is the central tendon of the diaphragm.

which blend with the anterior longitudinal ligament of the vertebral column:

- The right crus is the longest and broadest of the crura and is attached to the bodies of vertebrae LI to LIII and the intervening intervertebral discs (Fig. 4.133).
- Similarly, the left crus is attached to vertebrae LI and LII and the associated intervertebral disc.

The crura are connected across the midline by a tendinous arch (the **median arcuate ligament**), which passes anterior to the aorta (Fig. 4.133).

Lateral to the crura, a second tendinous arch is formed by the fascia covering the upper part of the psoas major muscle. This is the **medial arcuate ligament**, which is attached medially to the sides of vertebrae LI and LII and laterally to the transverse process of vertebra LI (Fig. 4.133).

A third tendinous arch, the **lateral arcuate ligament**, is formed by a thickening in the fascia that covers the quadratus lumborum. It is attached medially to the transverse process of vertebra LI and laterally to rib XII (Fig. 4.133).

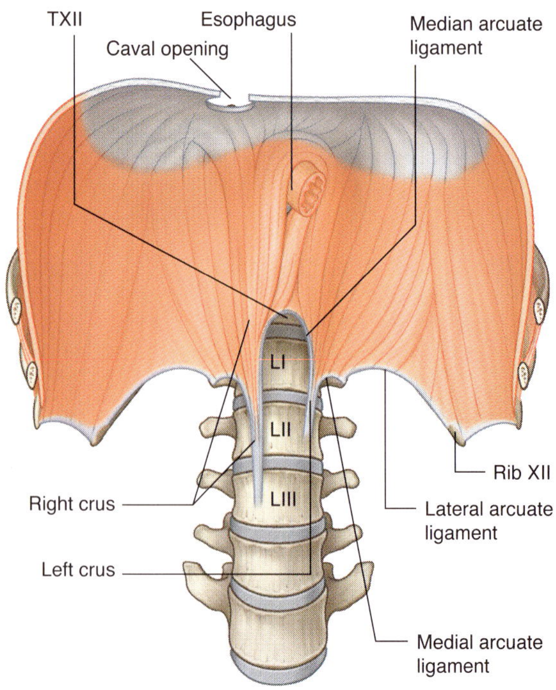

Fig. 4.133 Crura of the diaphragm.

The medial and lateral arcuate ligaments serve as points of origin for some of the muscular components of the diaphragm.

Structures passing through or around the diaphragm

Numerous structures pass through or around the diaphragm (Fig. 4.132):

- The aorta passes posterior to the diaphragm and anterior to the vertebral bodies at the lower level of vertebra TXII; it is between the two crura of the diaphragm and posterior to the median arcuate ligament, just to the left of midline.
- Accompanying the aorta through the aortic hiatus is the thoracic duct and, sometimes, the azygos vein.
- The esophagus passes through the musculature of the right crus of the diaphragm at the level of vertebra TX, just to the left of the aortic hiatus.
- Passing through the esophageal hiatus with the esophagus are the anterior and posterior vagal trunks, the esophageal branches and tributaries of the left gastric artery and vein, and a few lymphatic vessels.
- The third large opening in the diaphragm is the caval opening, through which the inferior vena cava passes from the abdominal cavity to the thoracic cavity (Fig. 4.132) at approximately vertebra TVIII in the central tendinous part of the diaphragm.
- Accompanying the inferior vena cava through the caval opening is the right phrenic nerve.
- The left phrenic nerve passes through the muscular part of the diaphragm just anterior to the central tendon on the left side.

Additional structures pass through small openings either in or just outside the diaphragm as they pass from the thoracic cavity to the abdominal cavity (Fig. 4.132):

- The greater, lesser, and least (when present) splanchnic nerves pass through the crura, on either side.
- The hemiazygos vein passes through the left crus.
- Passing posterior to the medial arcuate ligament, on either side, are the sympathetic trunks.
- Passing anterior to the diaphragm, just deep to the ribs, are the superior epigastric vessels.
- Other vessels and nerves (i.e., the musculophrenic vessels and intercostal nerves) also pass through the diaphragm at various points.

Domes

The classic appearance of the right and left domes of the diaphragm is caused by the underlying abdominal contents pushing these lateral areas upward, and by the fibrous pericardium, which is attached centrally, causing a flattening of the diaphragm in this area (Fig. 4.134).

The domes are produced by:

- The liver on the right, with some contribution from the right kidney and the right suprarenal gland
- The fundus of the stomach and spleen on the left, with contributions from the left kidney and the left suprarenal gland

Although the height of these domes varies during breathing, a reasonable estimate in normal expiration places the left dome at the fifth intercostal space and the right dome at rib V. This is important to remember when percussing the thorax.

During inspiration, the muscular part of the diaphragm contracts, causing the central tendon of the diaphragm to be drawn inferiorly. This results in some flattening of the domes, enlargement of the thoracic cavity, and a reduction in intrathoracic pressure. The physiological effect of these changes is that air enters the lungs and venous return to the heart is enhanced.

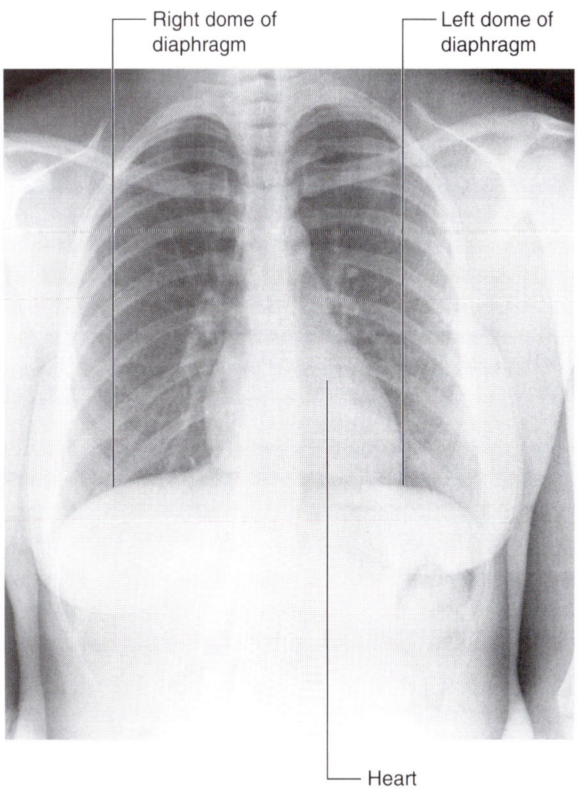

Fig. 4.134 Right and left domes of the diaphragm. Chest radiograph.

Blood supply

There is blood supply to the diaphragm on its superior and inferior surfaces:

- Superiorly, the musculophrenic and pericardiacophrenic arteries, both branches of the internal thoracic artery, and the superior phrenic artery, a branch of the thoracic aorta, supply the diaphragm.
- Inferiorly, the inferior phrenic arteries, branches of the abdominal aorta, supply the diaphragm (see Fig. 4.132).

Venous drainage is through companion veins to these arteries.

Innervation

Innervation of the diaphragm is primarily by the **phrenic nerves**. These nerves, from the C3 to C5 spinal cord levels, provide all motor innervation to the diaphragm and sensory fibers to the central part. They pass through the thoracic cavity, between the mediastinal pleura and the pericardium, to the superior surface of the diaphragm. At this point, the right phrenic nerve accompanies the inferior vena cava through the diaphragm and the left phrenic nerve passes through the diaphragm by itself (see Fig. 4.132). Additional sensory fibers are supplied to the peripheral areas of the diaphragm by the lower six thoracic nerves.

Early clinical exposure

Psoas abscess

The psoas muscle sheath is of greater importance than any other muscle sheath. The psoas muscle and its sheath arise not only from the lumbar vertebrae but also from the intervertebral discs between each vertebra. This disc origin is of critical importance. In certain types of infection, the intervertebral disc is preferentially affected (e.g., tuberculosis and salmonella discitis). As the infection of the disc develops, the infection spreads anteriorly and anterolaterally. In the anterolateral position, the infection passes into the psoas muscle sheath, and spreads within the muscle and sheath, and may appear below the inguinal ligament as a mass.

Early clinical exposure

Diaphragmatic hernias

To understand why a hernia occurs through the diaphragm, it is necessary to consider the embryology of the diaphragm.

The diaphragm is developed from four structures—the septum transversum, the posterior esophageal mesentery, the pleuroperitoneal membrane, and the peripheral rim of mesoderm from the body wall—which eventually fuse together, so separating the abdominal cavity from the thoracic cavity. The septum transversum forms the central tendon, which develops from a mesodermal origin in front of the embryo's head and then moves to its more adult position during formation of the head fold.

Fusion of the various components of the diaphragm may fail, and hernias may occur through the failed points of fusion (Fig. 4.135). The commonest sites are

- Between the xiphoid process and the costal margins on the right (Morgagni's hernia)
- Through an opening on the left when the pleuroperitoneal membrane fails to close the pericardioperitoneal canal (Bochdalek's hernia)

Hernias may also occur through the central tendon and through a congenitally large esophageal hiatus.

Morgagni's and Bochdalek's hernias tend to appear at or around the time of birth or in early infancy. They allow abdominal bowel to enter the thoracic cavity, which may compress the lungs and reduce respiratory function. Most of these hernias require surgical closure of the diaphragmatic defect.

Occasionally, small defects within the diaphragm fail to permit bowel through, but do allow free movement of fluid. Patients with ascites may develop pleural effusions, while patients with pleural effusions may develop ascites when these defects are present.

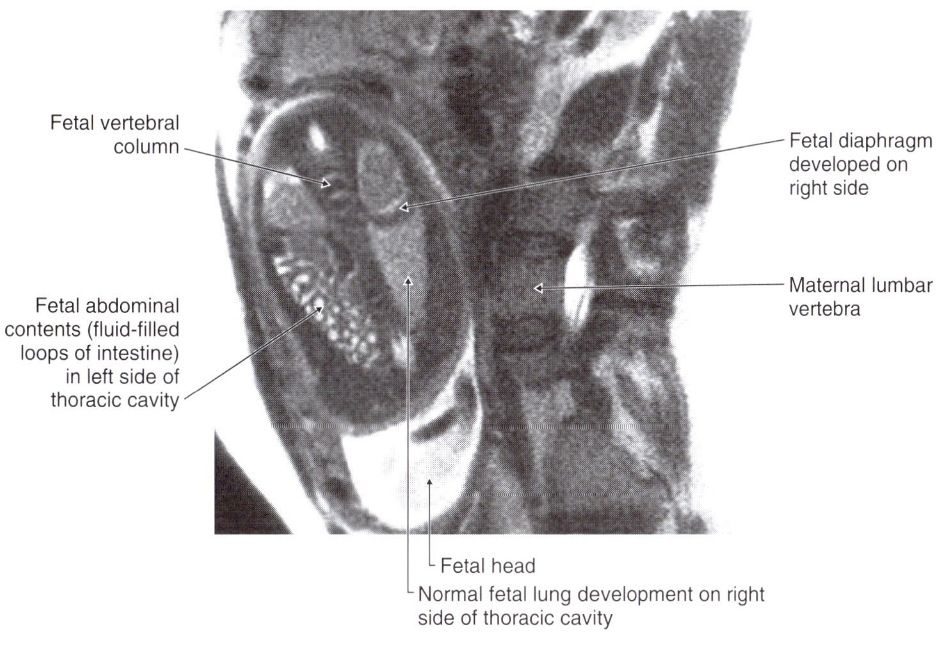

Fig. 4.135 Fetal diaphragmatic hernia in utero; T2-weighted MR image; fetus in coronal plane, mother in sagittal plane.

Early clinical exposure

Hiatus hernia

At the level of the esophageal hiatus, the diaphragm may be lax, allowing the fundus of the stomach to herniate into the posterior mediastinum (Fig. 4.136 A and B). This is also called a sliding hiatus hernia, where the esophagogastric junction is above the diaphragm. This typically causes symptoms of acid reflux. Ulceration may occur and may produce bleeding and anemia. The diagnosis is usually made by barium studies or endoscopy (Fig. 4.136). Treatment in the first instance is by medical management, although surgery may be necessary. Another type of hiatus hernia is a paraesophageal hernia, where the fundus of the stomach herniates parallel to the esophagus and the esophagogastric junction is below the diaphragm. This type is rarer, and may cause ischemia to the stomach.

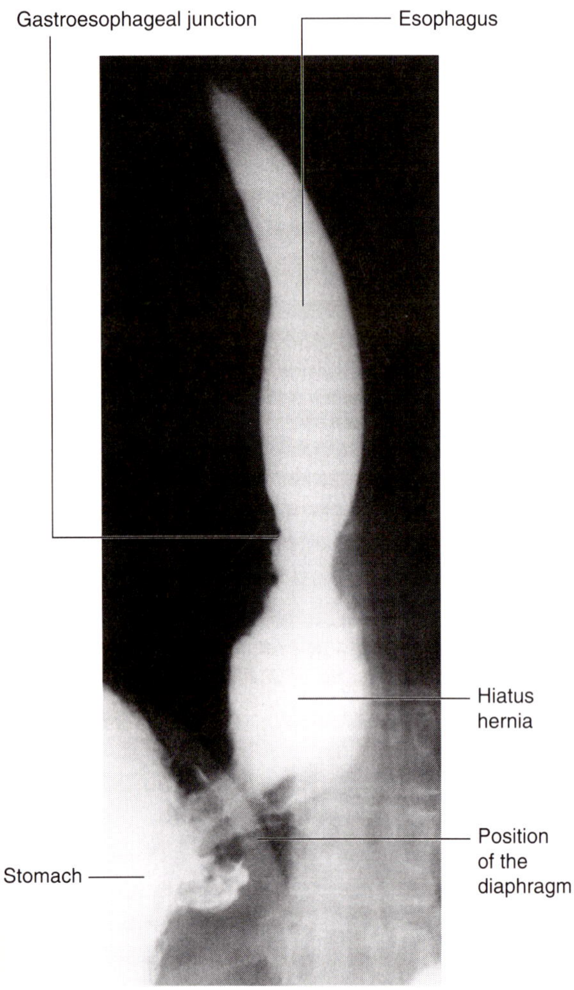

Fig. 4.136(A) Lower esophagus and upper stomach showing a hiatus hernia. Radiograph using barium sulfate.

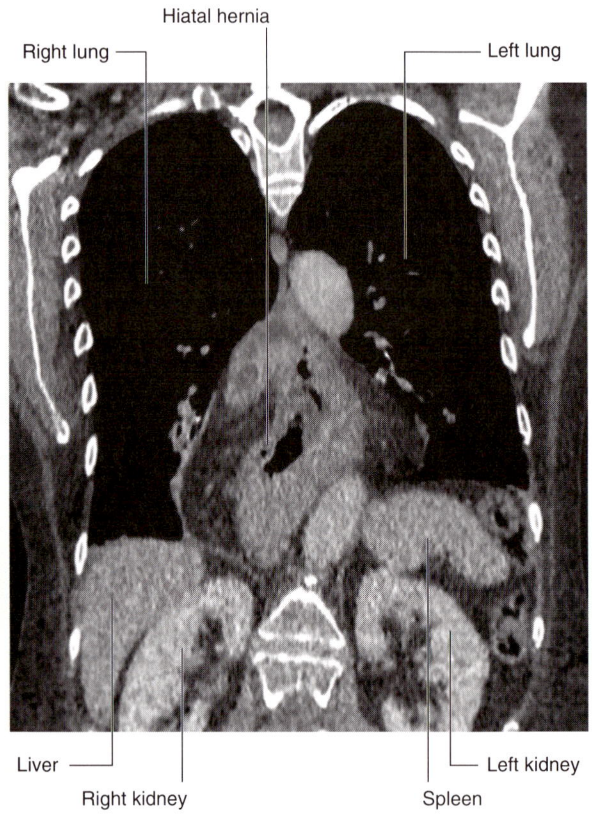

Fig. 4.136(B) Coronal CT of hiatal hernia.

Viscera

Kidneys

SET INDUCTION—CASE SCENARIO 11: URETERIC STONES

A 25-year-old male was brought to the surgery OPD with a history of sudden onset of pain on the side of the abdomen which appeared to spread to the groin. A diagnosis of ureteric stones was made. Knowledge of the anatomy of the ureter is needed to manage this case

REMEMBER [Recall Facts]	OUTLINE 11. KIDNEY, URETER, AND SUPRARENAL GLANDS—LEARNING OBJECTIVES [By the end of this section, the student should be able to:] DEMONSTRATE AND ANALYZE RELATIONSHIPS [Identify structures in a Prosected Specimen or Figure]			EVALUATE [Explain Concepts]
	Level I	**Level II**	**Level III**	

1. Describe the position and relations of the kidneys
2. Describe the coverings of the kidneys
3. Describe the internal structure of the kidney
4. Name the arterial segments of the kidney
5. List the sites of constrictions of the ureter
6. Mention the relations of the abdominal and pelvic parts of the ureter
7. Describe the arterial supply of the ureter
8. Describe the relations and blood supply of the suprarenal glands
	■ Coverings of kidney—fibrous capsule, perinephric fat, renal fascia, paranephric fat
	■ Kidneys—location, anatomical position and side determination, borders (medial and lateral), hilum, surfaces (anterior and posterior) and their relations, cortex, medulla, major and minor calyces, pelvis of ureter
	■ Ureter—course, relations, sites of constrictions
	■ Suprarenal glands—location, shape, important relations
		■ Branches of renal arteries
		■ Tributaries of renal veins
		■ Kidneys:
		  ■ Renal angle
		  ■ Renal columns and cortical arches in cortex
		  ■ Pyramids in medulla
		■ Suprarenal glands
		  ■ Suprarenal arteries and vein
			Kidneys:
			  ■ Morris' parallelogram
			  ■ Brodel's line
			  ■ Medullary rays and convoluted part in cortical arches
			  ■ Lobe and lobule of kidney
			■ Suprarenal glands:
			  ■ Surfaces
			  ■ Borders
				■ Anterior and posterior relations of kidneys
				■ Important relations of ureter and sites of constriction
				■ Important relations of suprarenal glands
				■ Blood supply of suprarenal glands

EARLY CLINICAL EXPOSURE [Apply Anatomical Knowledge]	
Surgical Anatomy/ Pathology/ Trauma	**Imaging/ Surface Anatomy**
■ Renal and ureteric colic ■ Posterior surgical approach to kidney ■ Renal transplantation ■ Venous extension of renal cell tumors ■ Nephrostomy	■ Intravenous urogram ■ Ultrasound ■ Computer tomography ■ Dimercaptosuccinic acid (DMSA) scintigraphy

PROBLEM SOLVING/ CLINICAL CASES [Interpret]
■ Discuss the basis for removal of one arterial segment of the kidney ■ What is the clinical importance of the constrictions of the ureter?

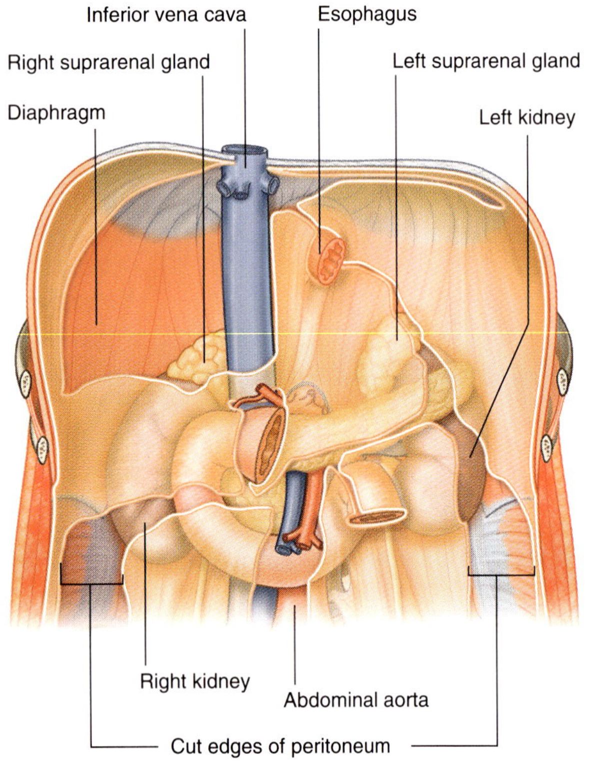

Fig. 4.137 Retroperitoneal position of the kidneys in the posterior abdominal region.

The bean-shaped kidneys are retroperitoneal in the posterior abdominal region (Fig. 4.137). They lie in the extraperitoneal connective tissue immediately lateral to the vertebral column. In the supine position, the kidneys extend from approximately vertebra TXII superiorly to vertebra LIII inferiorly, with the right kidney somewhat lower than the left because of its relationship with the liver. Although they are similar in size and shape, the left kidney is a longer and more slender organ than the right kidney, and nearer to the midline.

Relationships to other structures

The anterior surface of the right kidney is related to numerous structures. Some are separated from the kidney by a layer of peritoneum and some lie directly against the kidney (Fig. 4.138):

- A small part of the superior pole is covered by the right suprarenal gland.
- More inferiorly, a large part of the rest of the upper part of the anterior surface is against the liver and is separated from it by a layer of peritoneum.
- Medially, the descending part of the duodenum is retroperitoneal and contacts the kidney.
- The inferior pole of the kidney, on its lateral side, is directly associated with the right colic flexure and, on its medial side, is covered by a segment of the intraperitoneal small intestine.

The anterior surface of the left kidney is also related to numerous structures, some with an intervening layer of peritoneum and some directly against the kidney (Fig. 4.138):

- A small part of the superior pole, on its medial side, is covered by the left suprarenal gland.

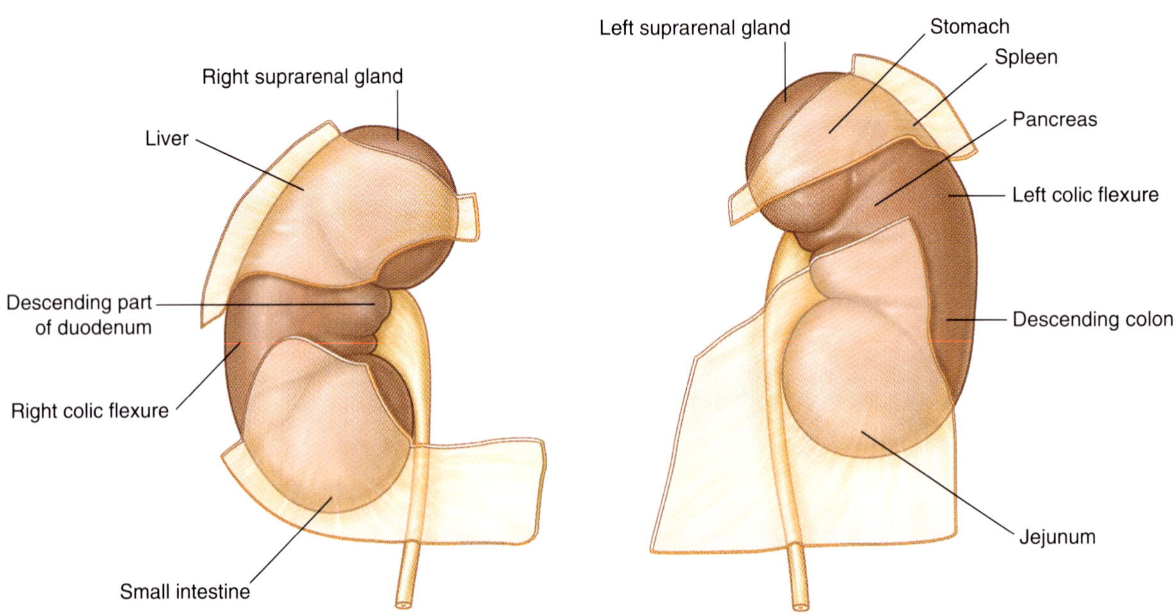

Fig. 4.138 Structures related to the anterior surface of each kidney.

- The rest of the superior pole is covered by the intraperitoneal stomach and spleen.
- More inferiorly, the retroperitoneal pancreas covers the middle part of the kidney.
- On its lateral side, the lower half of the kidney is covered by the left colic flexure and the beginning of the descending colon, and, on its medial side, by the parts of the intraperitoneal jejunum.

Posteriorly, the right and left kidneys are related to similar structures (Fig. 4.139). Superiorly is the diaphragm and inferior to this, moving in a medial to lateral direction, are the psoas major, quadratus lumborum, and transversus abdominis muscles.

The superior pole of the right kidney is anterior to rib XII, while the same region of the left kidney is anterior to ribs XI and XII. The pleural sacs and specifically, the costodiaphragmatic recesses therefore extend posterior to the kidneys.

Also passing posterior to the kidneys are the subcostal vessels and nerves and the iliohypogastric and ilioinguinal nerves (see Fig. 4.161).

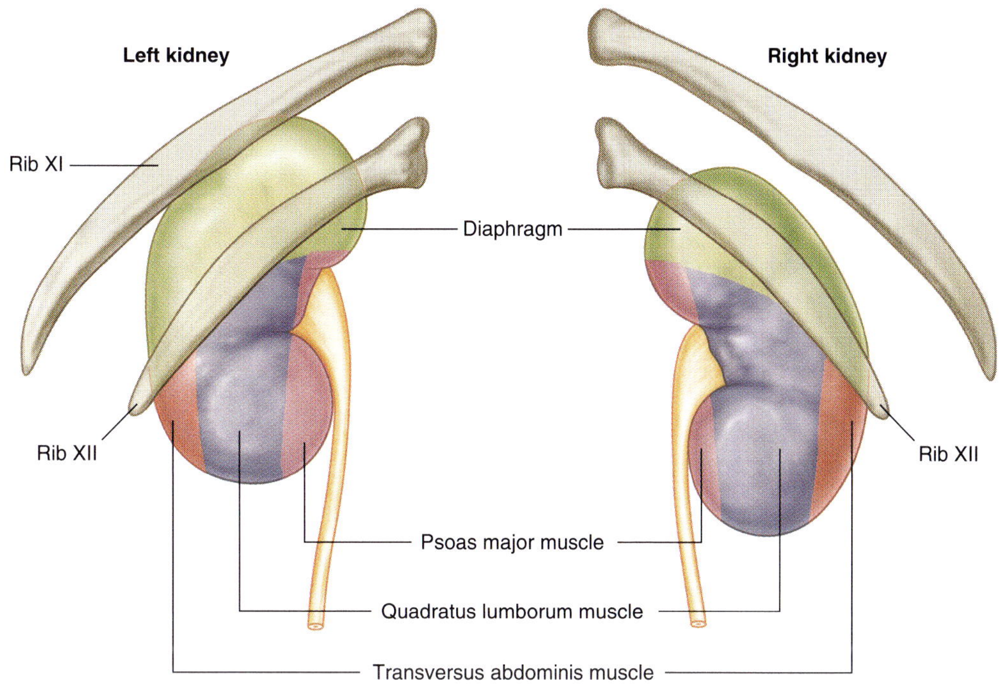

Fig. 4.139 Structures related to the posterior surface of each kidney.

Renal fat and fascia

The kidneys are enclosed in and associated with a unique arrangement of fascia and fat. Immediately outside the renal capsule, there is an accumulation of extraperitoneal fat—the **perinephric fat** (**perirenal fat**), which completely surrounds the kidney (Fig. 4.140). Enclosing the perinephric fat is a membranous condensation of the extraperitoneal fascia (the **renal fascia or Gerota's fascia**). The suprarenal glands are also enclosed in this fascial compartment, usually separated from the kidneys by a thin septum. The renal fascia must be incised in any surgical approach to this organ.

At the lateral margins of each kidney, the anterior and posterior layers of the renal fascia fuse (Fig. 4.140). This fused layer may connect with the transversalis fascia on the lateral abdominal wall.

Above each suprarenal gland, the anterior and posterior layers of the renal fascia fuse and blend with the fascia that covers the diaphragm.

Medially, the anterior layer of the renal fascia continues over the vessels in the hilum and fuses with the connective tissue associated with the abdominal aorta and the inferior vena cava (Fig. 4.140). In some cases, the anterior layer may cross the midline to the opposite side and blend with its companion layer.

The posterior layer of the renal fascia passes medially between the kidney and the fascia covering the quadratus lumborum muscle to fuse with the fascia covering the psoas major muscle.

Inferiorly, the anterior and posterior layers of the renal fascia enclose the ureters.

In addition to perinephric fat and the renal fascia, a final layer of **paranephric fat (pararenal fat)** (Fig. 4.140) accumulates posterior and posterolateral to each kidney.

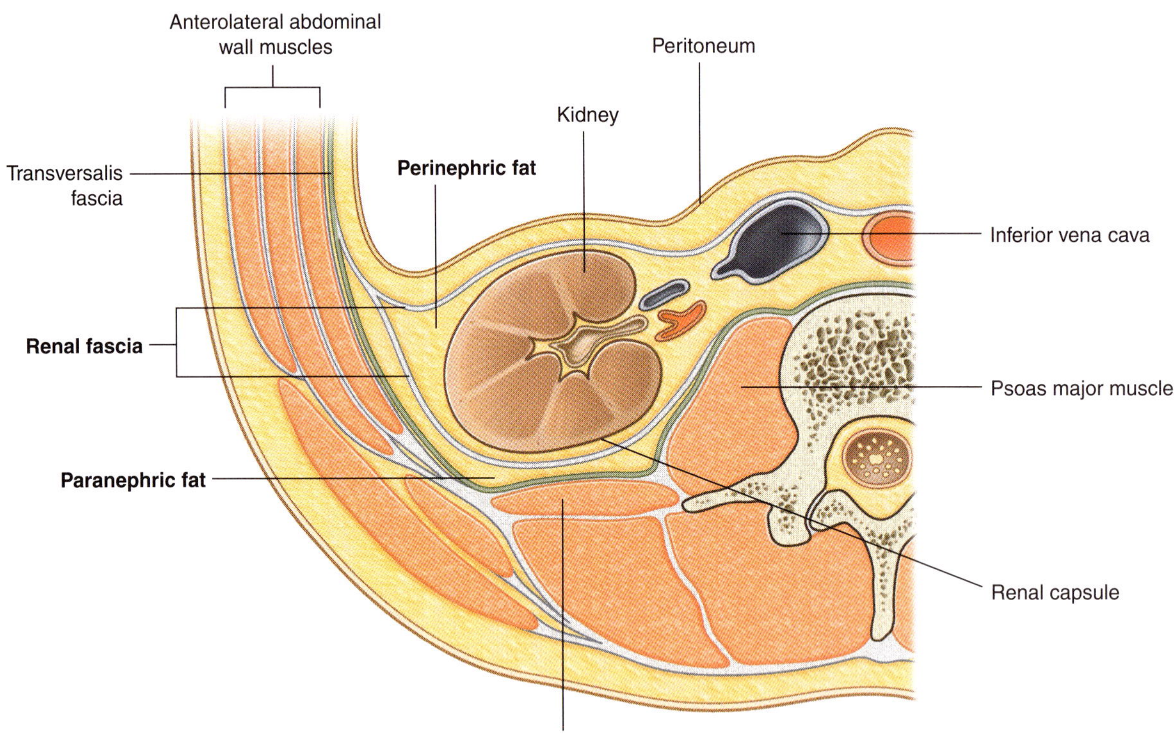

Fig. 4.140 Organization of fat and fascia surrounding the kidney.

Kidney structure

Each kidney has a smooth anterior and posterior surface covered by a fibrous capsule, which is easily removable except during disease.

Each kidney has two poles (upper and lower), two borders (medial and lateral), and two surfaces (anterior and posterior) and is 10–14 cm in length and 5–7 cm in width. The anterior surface of the right kidney is related to the liver, second part of duodenum, right suprarenal, ascending colon, right colic flexure, and right suprarenal gland. The anterior surface of the left kidney is related to the spleen, stomach, pancreas, descending colon, splenic flexure, and loops of jejunum (Fig. 4.63 and 4.138).

The posterior surface of each kidney is related to the psoas major, quadratus lumborum, transversus abdominis, diaphragm, ribs XI and XII, subcostal nerve, iliohypogastric nerve, and ilioinguinal nerve (Fig. 4.139 and 4.161). The renal angle is the angle formed between the inferior border of rib XII and the lateral border of erector spinae.

On the medial margin of each kidney is the **hilum of the kidney**, which is a deep vertical slit through which renal vessels, lymphatics, and nerves enter and leave the substance of the kidney (Fig. 4.141). Internally, the hilum is continuous with the renal sinus. Perinephric fat continues into the hilum and sinus and surrounds all structures.

Each kidney consists of an outer **renal cortex** and an inner renal medulla. The renal cortex is a continuous band of pale tissue that completely surrounds the renal medulla. Extensions of the renal cortex (the **renal columns**) project into the inner aspect of the kidney, dividing the renal medulla into discontinuous aggregations of triangular-shaped tissue (the **renal pyramids**).

The bases of the renal pyramids are directed outward, toward the renal cortex, while the apex of each renal pyramid projects inward, toward the **renal sinus**. The apical projection (**renal papilla**) is surrounded by a **minor calyx**.

The minor calices receive urine and represent the proximal parts of the tube that will eventually form the ureter (Fig. 4.141). In the renal sinus, several minor calices unite to form a **major calyx**, and two or three major calices unite to form the **renal pelvis**, which is the funnel-shaped superior end of the ureters.

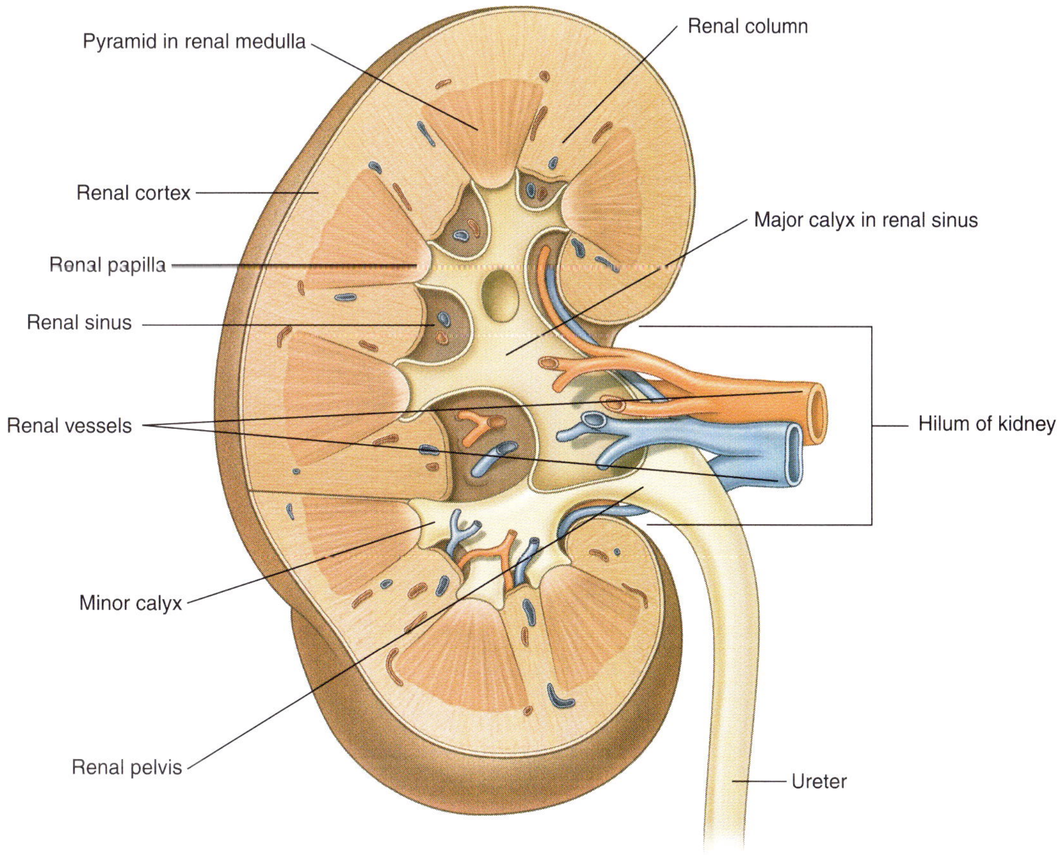

Fig. 4.141 Internal structure of the kidney.

Renal vasculature and lymphatics

A single large **renal artery**, a lateral branch of the abdominal aorta, supplies each kidney. These vessels usually arise just inferior to the origin of the superior mesenteric artery between vertebrae LI and LII (Fig. 4.142A). The **left renal artery** usually arises a little higher than the right, and the **right renal artery** is longer and passes posterior to the inferior vena cava.

As each renal artery approaches the renal hilum, it divides into anterior and posterior branches, which supply the renal parenchyma. There are five **arterial segments** of the kidney, each of which is supplied by a segmental artery, which is an end artery. The apical segment is the upper pole, and the inferior segment is the lower pole. The middle segment lies between the superior and inferior segments on the anterior aspect. Knowledge of the vascular anatomy of the kidney is important to perform a partial nephrectomy for renal cell cancers in order to avoid compromising the vascular supply to the remaining renal tissue (Fig. 4.142B). Accessory renal arteries are common. They originate from the lateral aspect of the abdominal aorta, either above or below the primary renal arteries, enter the hilum with the primary arteries or pass directly into the kidney at some other level, and are commonly called **extrahilar arteries**.

The bloodless line of Brodel is a relatively avascular plane in the posterolateral aspect of kidney between the anterior and posterior segmental arteries. It is a suitable site for an incision, though planned radial or intersegmental incisions are preferable.

Multiple renal veins contribute to the formation of the **left** and **right renal veins**, both of which are anterior to the renal arteries (Fig. 4.142A). The left renal vein is three times longer than the right renal vein. The renal collar is an accessory left renal vein that passes posterior to the aorta in addition to the normal left renal vein that passes anterior to the aorta before joining the inferior vena cava. Importantly, the longer left renal vein crosses the midline anterior to the abdominal aorta and posterior to the superior mesenteric artery and can be compressed by an aneurysm in either of these two vessels (nutcracker phenomenon) which may manifest as renal vein entrapment syndrome (Fig. 4.142C). This should be differentiated from superior mesenteric artery syndrome, which is compression of the third part of the duodenum between the superior mesenteric artery and abdominal aorta.

The lymphatic drainage of each kidney is to the **lateral aortic (lumbar) nodes** around the origin of the renal artery.

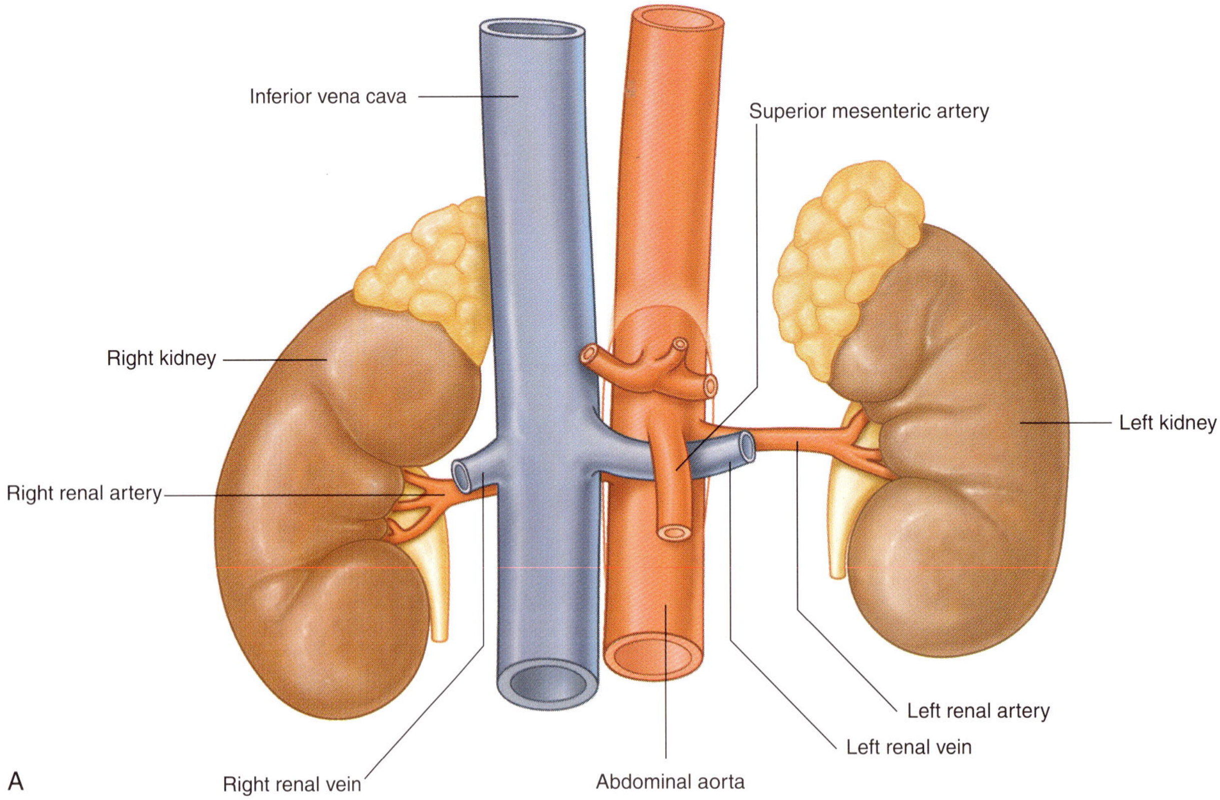

Fig. 4.142 (A) Renal vasculature.

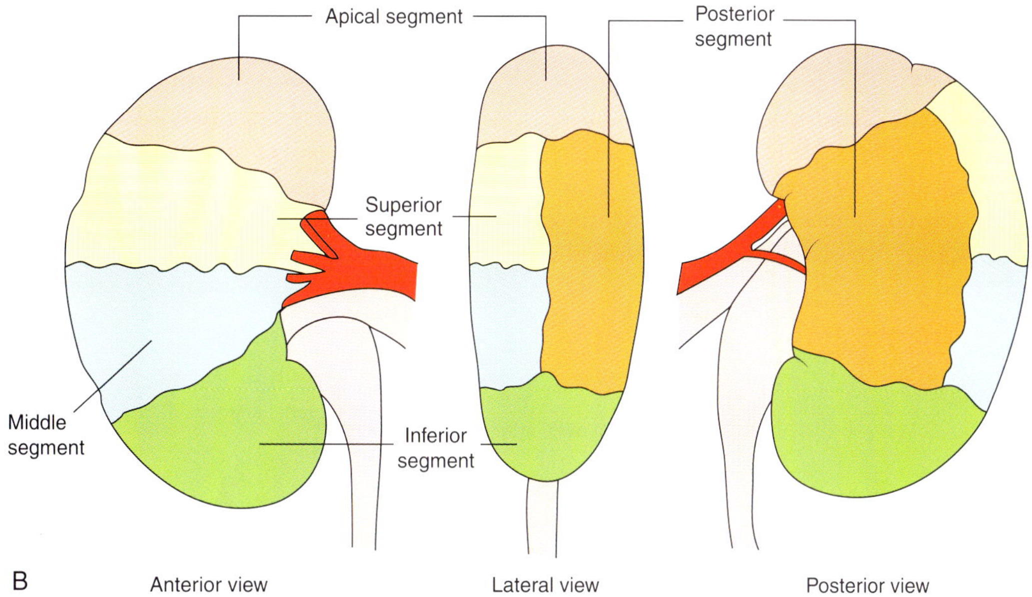

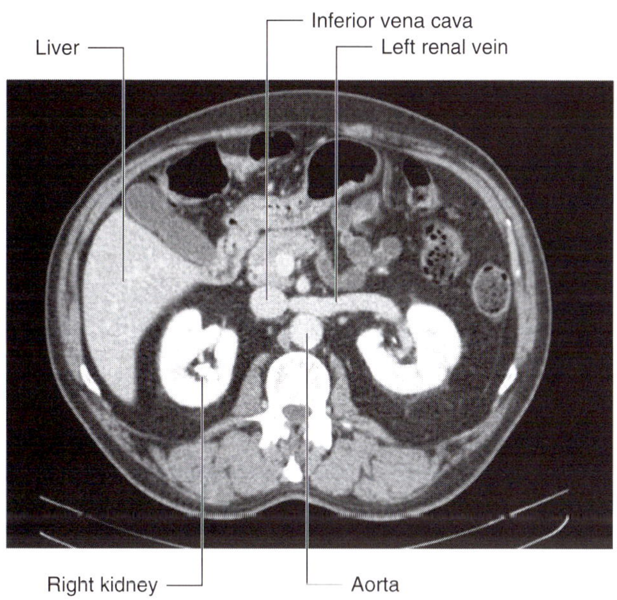

Fig. 4.142, cont'd(B) Arterial segments of the kidney. **(C)** CT image showing long left renal vein crossing the midline.

Ureters

The ureters are muscular tubes that transport urine from the kidneys to the bladder. They are continuous superiorly with the renal pelvis, which is a funnel-shaped structure in the renal sinus. The renal pelvis is formed from a condensation of two or three major calices, which in turn are formed by the condensation of several minor calices (see Fig. 4.141). The minor calices surround a renal papilla.

The renal pelvis narrows as it passes inferiorly through the hilum of the kidney and becomes continuous with the ureter at the **ureteropelvic junction** (Fig. 4.143A). Inferior to this junction, the ureters descend retroperitoneally on the medial aspect of the psoas major muscle and lateral to the tips of the lumbar vertebrae. At the pelvic brim, the ureters cross either the end of the common iliac artery or the beginning of the external iliac artery, enter the pelvic cavity, and continue their journey to the bladder.

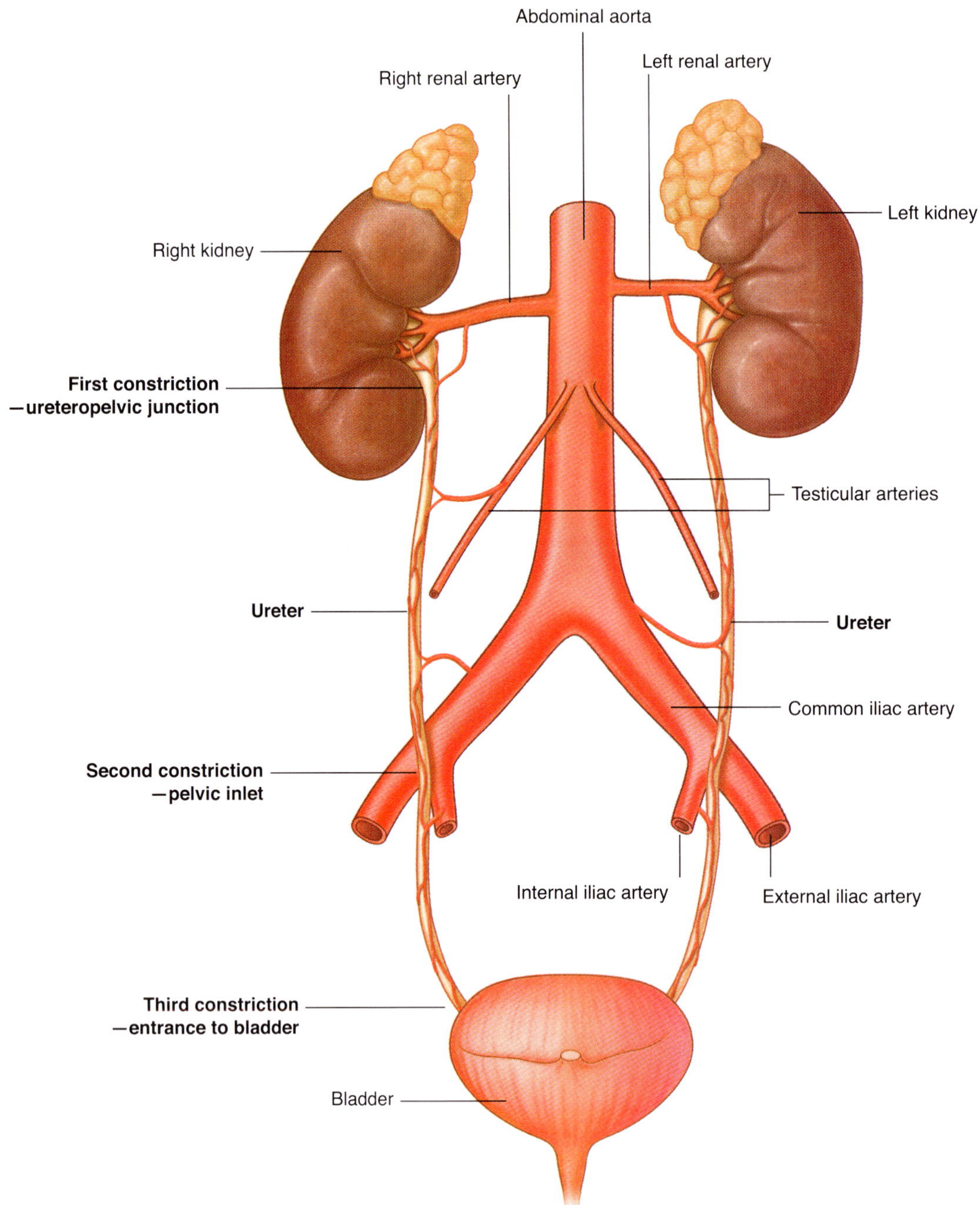

Fig. 4.143(A) Ureters.

The abdominal part of ureter crosses anterior to the genitofemoral nerve and is crossed by the testicular or ovarian vessels. The right ureter is covered by the duodenum (second part). At the apex of the pelvic mesocolon is the intersigmoid fossa which serves as a valuable landmark to identify the left ureter.

The pelvic part of ureter is crossed by the obliterated umbilical arteries in both males and females. In males, the ductus deferens crosses anterior to the ureter. In females, the ureter is located inferior to the broad ligament and uterine vessels. A mnemonic for this important relation is "water under the bridge"—as the ureter passes forward it lies below the uterine vessels which run transversely. Finally the ureter enters the urinary bladder by passing obliquely through its wall (Fig. 5.58A).

At three points along their course the ureters are constricted (Fig. 4.143A):

- The first point is at the ureteropelvic junction.
- The second point is where the ureters cross the common iliac vessels at the pelvic brim.
- The third point is where the ureters enter the wall of the bladder.

Kidney stones can become lodged at these constrictions.

Ureteric vasculature and lymphatics

The ureters receive arterial branches from adjacent vessels as they pass toward the bladder (Fig. 4.143A):

- The renal arteries supply the upper end.
- The middle part may receive branches from the abdominal aorta, the testicular or ovarian arteries, and the common iliac arteries.
- In the pelvic cavity, the ureters are supplied by one or more arteries from branches of the internal iliac arteries.

In all cases, arteries reaching the ureters divide into ascending and descending branches, which form longitudinal anastomoses.

Lymphatic drainage of the ureters follows a pattern similar to that of the arterial supply. Lymph from:

- The upper part of each ureter drains to the lateral aortic (lumbar) nodes
- The middle part of each ureter drains to lymph nodes associated with the common iliac vessels
- The inferior part of each ureter drains to lymph nodes associated with the external and internal iliac vessels

Ureteric innervation

Ureteric innervation is from the renal, aortic, superior hypogastric, and inferior hypogastric plexuses through nerves that follow the blood vessels.

Visceral efferent fibers come from both sympathetic and parasympathetic sources, whereas visceral afferent fibers return to T11 to L2 spinal cord levels. Ureteric pain, which is usually related to distention of the ureter, is therefore referred to cutaneous areas supplied by T11 to L2 spinal cord levels. These areas would most likely include the posterior and lateral abdominal wall below the ribs and above the iliac crest, the pubic region, the scrotum in males, the labia majora in females, and the proximal anterior aspect of the thigh (Fig. 1.39).

Early clinical exposure

Urinary tract stones

Urinary tract stones (calculi) occur more frequently in men than in women, are most common in people aged between 20 and 60 years, and are usually associated with sedentary lifestyles. The stones are polycrystalline aggregates of calcium, phosphate, oxalate, urate, and other soluble salts within an organic matrix. The urine becomes saturated with these salts, and small variations in the pH cause the salts to precipitate.

Typically the patient has pain that radiates from the infrascapular region (loin) into the groin, and even into the scrotum or labia majora. Blood in the urine (**hematuria**) may also be noticed.

Infection must be excluded because certain species of bacteria are commonly associated with urinary tract stones.

The complications of urinary tract stones include infection, urinary obstruction, and renal failure. Stones may also develop within the bladder and produce marked irritation, causing pain and discomfort.

The diagnosis of urinary tract stones is based upon history and examination. Stones are often visible on abdominal radiographs. Special investigations include ultrasound scanning, which may demonstrate the dilated renal pelvis and calices when the urinary system is obstructed. This is the preferred way of imaging in pregnant women or when clinical suspicion is low.

Continued

Early clinical exposure—cont'd

- Low-dose CT of the urinary tract (CT KUB), which allows the detection of even smaller stones, shows the exact level of obstruction and, based on the size, density, and location of the stone, can help the urologist plan a procedure to remove the stone if necessary (extracorporeal shock wave lithotripsy versus ureteroscopy, percutaneous nephrolithotomy, or, extremely rare these days, open surgery) (Fig. 4.143B).
- An intravenous urogram (IVU), which will demonstrate the obstruction, pinpoint the exact level of the stone is currently less often used because access to low-dose CT KUB has increased.

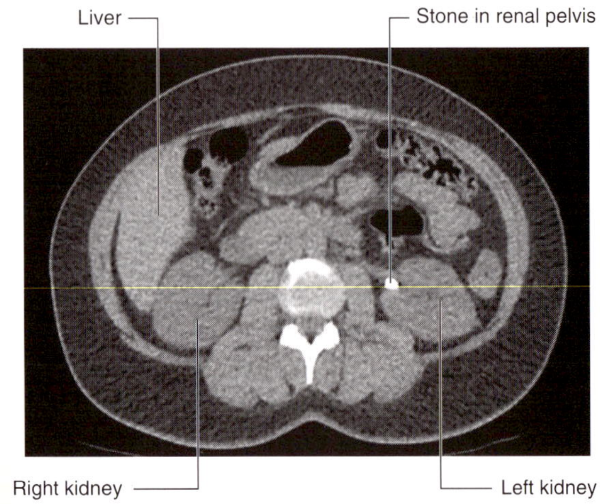

Fig. 4.143(B) Low-dose axial CT of urinary tract (CT KUB) displays stone in left renal pelvis.

Early clinical exposure

Urinary tract cancer

Most tumors that arise in the kidney are renal cell carcinomas. These tumors develop from the proximal tubular epithelium. Approximately 5% of tumors within the kidney are transitional cell tumors, which arise from the urothelium of the renal pelvis. Most patients typically have blood in the urine (hematuria), pain in the infrascapular region (loin), and a mass.

Renal cell tumors (Fig. 4.144 and 4.145) are unusual because they not only grow outward from the kidney, invading the fat and fascia, but also spread into the renal vein. This **venous extension** is rare for any other type of tumor, so, when seen, renal cell carcinoma should be suspected. In addition, the tumor may spread along the renal vein and into the inferior vena cava, and in rare cases can grow into the right atrium across the tricuspid valve and into the pulmonary artery.

Treatment for most renal cancers is surgical removal, even when metastatic spread is present, because some patients show regression of metastases.

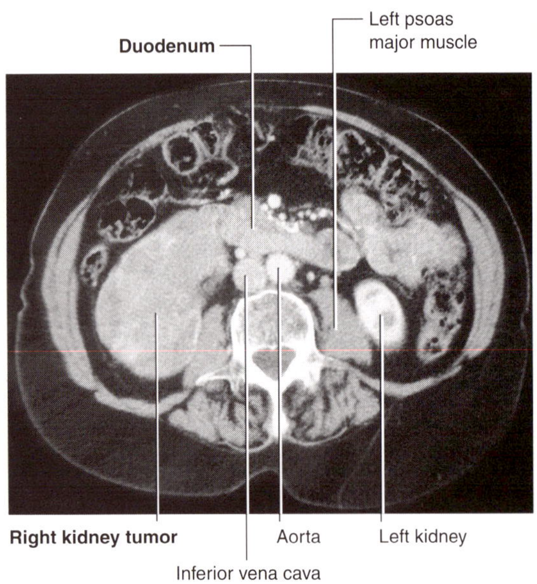

Fig. 4.144 Tumor in the right kidney growing toward, and possibly invading, the duodenum. Computed tomogram in the axial plane.

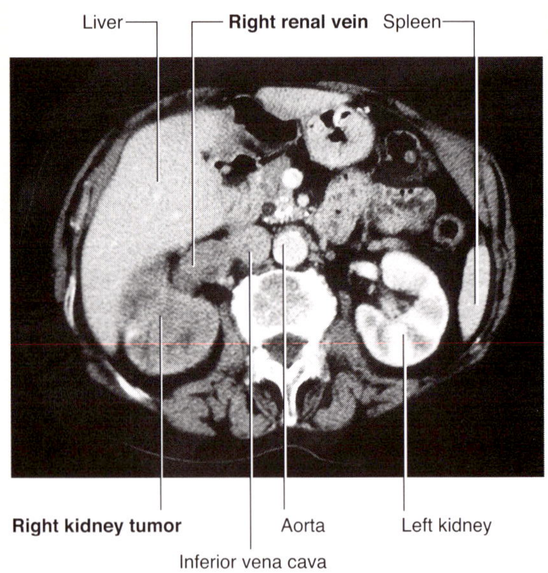

Fig. 4.145 Tumor in the right kidney spreading into the right renal vein. Computed tomogram in the axial plane.

Early clinical exposure—cont'd

Transitional cell carcinoma arises from the urothelium. The urothelium is present from the calices to the urethra and behaves as a "single unit." Therefore, when patients develop transitional carcinomas within the bladder, similar tumors may also be present within upper parts of the urinary tract. In patients with bladder cancer, the whole of the urinary tract must always be investigated to exclude the possibility of other tumors (Fig. 4.146). This is currently achieved by performing a dual-phase CT urogram that allows visualization of the renal parenchyma and the collecting system at the same time.

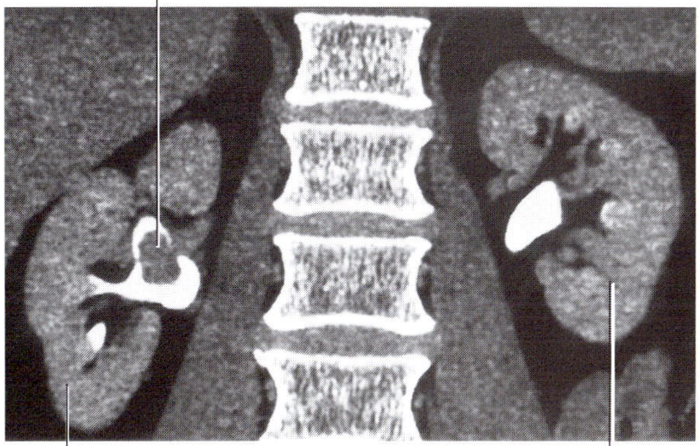

Fig. 4.146 Transitional cell carcinoma in the pelvis of the right kidney. Coronal computed tomogram reconstruction.

Early clinical exposure

Nephrostomy

A nephrostomy is a procedure where a tube is placed through the lateral or posterior abdominal wall into the renal cortex to lie within the renal pelvis. The function of this tube is to allow drainage of urine from the renal pelvis through the tube externally (Fig. 4.147).

The kidneys are situated on the posterior abdominal wall, and in thin healthy subjects may be only up to 2–3 cm from the skin. Access to the kidney is relatively straightforward, because the kidney can be easily visualized under ultrasound guidance. Using local anesthetic, a needle can be placed, under ultrasound direction, through the skin into the renal cortex and into the renal pelvis. A series of wires and tubes can be passed through the needle to position the drainage catheter.

The indications for such a procedure are many. In patients with distal ureteric obstruction the back pressure of urine within the ureters and the kidney significantly impairs the function of the kidney. This will produce renal failure and ultimately death. Furthermore, a dilated obstructed system is also susceptible to infection. In many cases, there is not only obstruction producing renal failure but also infected urine within the system.

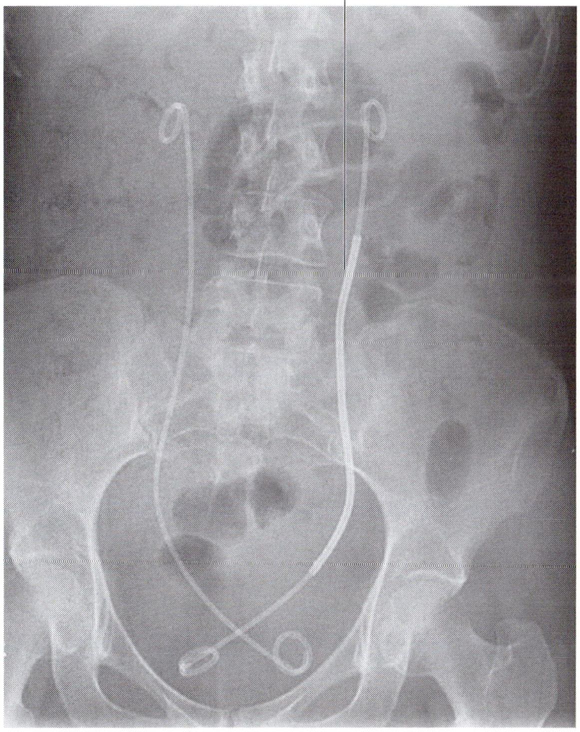

Fig. 4.147 This radiograph demonstrates a double-J stent (anteroposterior view). J-shaped curls at the two ends prevent the tube from migrating. The superior aspect of the double-J stent is situated within the renal pelvis. The stent passes through the ureter, describing the path of the ureter, and the tip of the double-J stent is projected over the bladder, which appears as a slightly dense area on the radiograph.

Early clinical exposure

Kidney transplant

Kidney transplantation began in the USA in the 1950s. Since the first transplant, the major problem for kidney transplantation has been tissue rejection. A number of years have passed since this initial procedure and there have been significant breakthroughs in transplant rejection medicine. Renal transplantation is now a common procedure undertaken in patients with end-stage renal failure.

Transplant kidneys are obtained from either living or deceased donors. The living donors are carefully assessed, because harvesting a kidney from a normal healthy individual, even with modern-day medicine, carries a small risk.

Deceased kidney donors are brain dead or have suffered cardiac death. The donor kidney is harvested with a small cuff of aortic and venous tissue. The ureter is also harvested.

An ideal place to situate the transplant kidney is in the left or the right iliac fossa (Fig. 4.148). A curvilinear incision is made paralleling the iliac crest and pubic symphysis. The external oblique muscle, internal oblique muscle, transversus abdominis muscle, and transversalis fascia are divided. The surgeon identifies the parietal peritoneum but does not enter the peritoneal cavity. The parietal peritoneum is medially retracted to reveal the external iliac artery, external iliac vein, and bladder. In some instances, the internal iliac artery of the recipient is mobilized and anastomosed directly as an end-to-end procedure onto the renal artery of the donor kidney. Similarly the internal iliac vein is anastomosed to the donor vein. In the presence of a small aortic cuff of tissue, the donor artery is anastomosed to the recipient external iliac artery and similarly for the venous anastomosis. The ureter is easily tunneled obliquely through the bladder wall with a straightforward anastomosis.

The left and right iliac fossae are ideal locations for the transplant kidney because a new space can be created without compromise to other structures. The great advantage of this procedure is the proximity to the anterior abdominal wall, which permits easy ultrasound visualization of the kidney and Doppler vascular assessment. Furthermore, in this position, biopsies are easily obtained. The extraperitoneal approach enables patients to make a swift recovery.

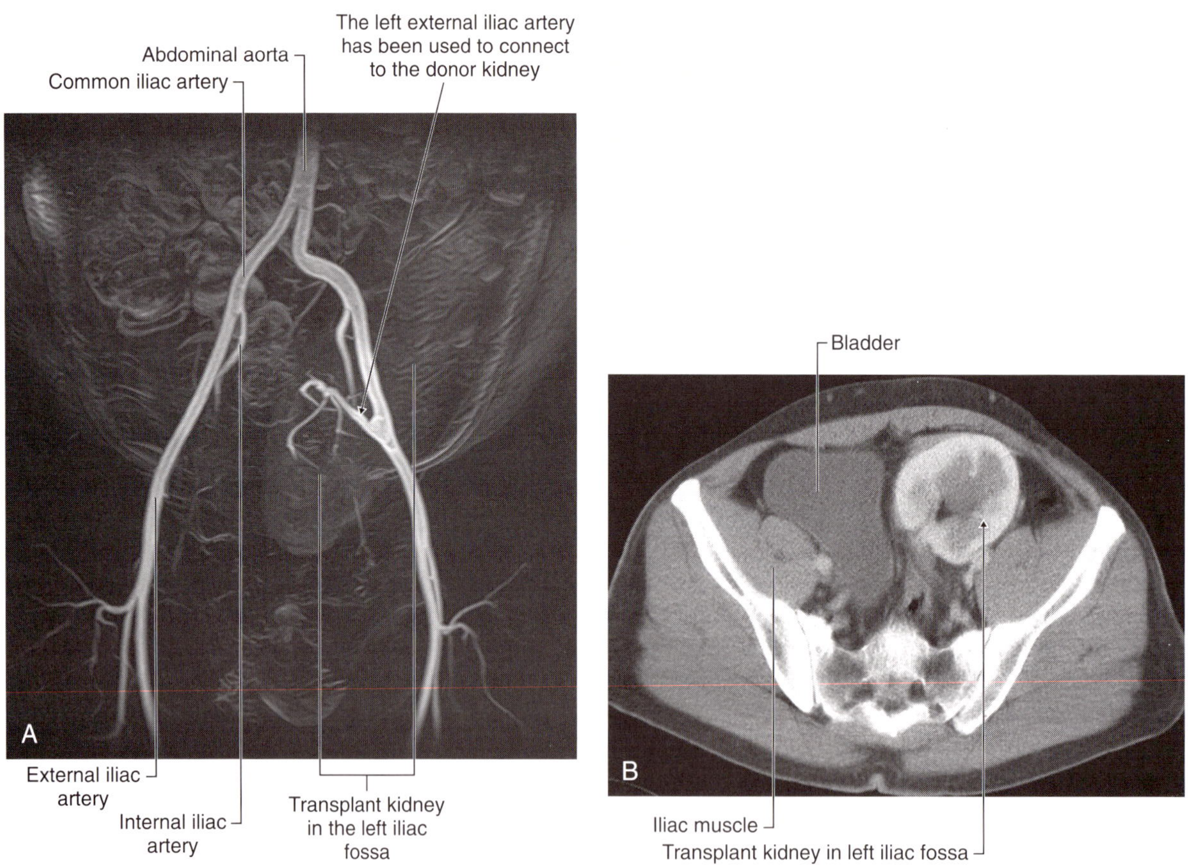

Fig. 4.148 Kidney transplant. **(A)** This image demonstrates an MR angiogram of the bifurcation of the aorta. Attaching to the left external iliac artery is the donor artery for a kidney that has been transplanted into the left iliac fossa. **(B)** Abdominal computed tomogram, in the axial plane, showing the transplanted kidney in the left iliac fossa.

Early clinical exposure

Investigation of the urinary tract

After an appropriate history and examination of the patient, including a digital rectal examination to assess the prostate in men, special investigations are required.

Cystoscopy

Cystoscopy is a technique that allows visualization of the urinary bladder and urethra using an optical system attached to a flexible or rigid tube (cystoscope). Images are displayed on a monitor, as done in other endoscopic studies. Biopsies, bladder stone removal, removal of foreign bodies from the bladder, and bleeding cauterization can be performed during cystoscopy. Cystoscopy is helpful in establishing the causes of macroscopic and microscopic hematuria, assessing bladder and urethral diverticula and fistulas, as well as serving as a tool to investigate patients with voiding problems.

Intravenous urogram

An IVU is one of the most important and commonly carried out radiological investigations (Fig. 4.149). The patient is injected intravenously with iodinated contrast medium. Most contrast media contain three iodine atoms spaced around a benzene ring. The relatively high atomic number of iodine compared to the atomic number of carbon, hydrogen, and oxygen, attenuates the radiation beam. After intravenous injection, contrast media are excreted predominantly by glomerular filtration, although some are secreted by the renal tubules. This allows visualization of the collecting system as well as the ureters and bladder.

Ultrasound

Ultrasound can be used to assess kidney size and the size of the calices, which may be dilated when obstructed. Although the ureters are poorly visualized using ultrasound, the bladder can be easily seen when full. Ultrasound measurements of bladder volume can be obtained before and after micturition.

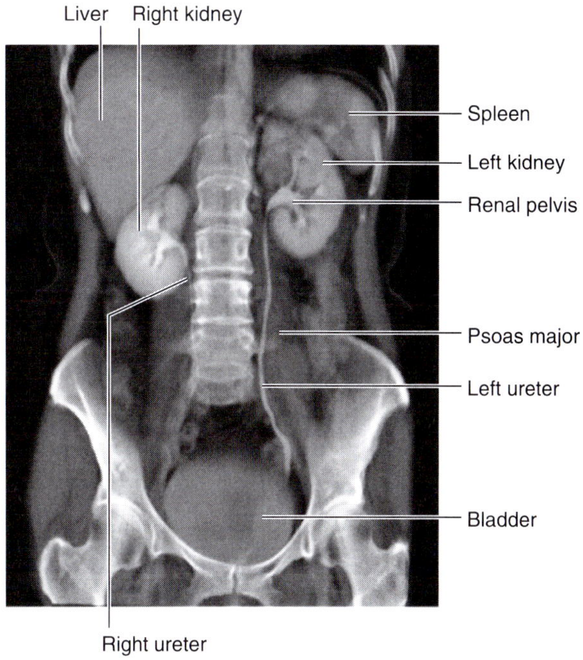

Fig. 4.149 Coronal view of 3D urogram using multidetector computed tomography.

Computed tomography

CT can be used to assess the kidneys, ureters, bladder, and adjacent structures and is a powerful tool for staging primary urinary tract tumors.

Nuclear medicine

Nuclear medicine is an extremely useful tool for investigating the urinary tract because radioisotope compounds can be used to estimate renal cell mass and function and assess the parenchyma for renal scarring (dimercaptosuccinic acid (DMSA) scintigraphy). These tests are often very useful in children when renal scarring and reflux disease is suspected.

Suprarenal glands

The suprarenal glands are associated with the superior pole of each kidney (Fig. 4.150). They consist of an outer cortex and an inner medulla. The right gland is shaped like a pyramid, whereas the left gland is semilunar in shape and the larger of the two.

Anterior to the right suprarenal gland is part of the right lobe of the liver and the inferior vena cava, whereas anterior to the left suprarenal gland is part of the stomach, pancreas, and, on occasion, the spleen. Parts of the diaphragm are posterior to both glands.

The suprarenal glands are surrounded by the perinephric fat and enclosed in the renal fascia, though a thin septum separates each gland from its associated kidney.

Suprarenal vasculature

The arterial supply to the suprarenal glands is extensive and arises from three primary sources (Fig. 4.150):

- As the bilateral inferior phrenic arteries pass upward from the abdominal aorta to the diaphragm, they give off multiple branches (superior suprarenal arteries) to the suprarenal glands.
- A middle branch (middle suprarenal artery) to the suprarenal glands usually arises directly from the abdominal aorta.
- Inferior branches (inferior suprarenal arteries) from the renal arteries pass upward to the suprarenal glands.

In contrast to this multiple arterial supply is the venous drainage, which usually consists of a single vein leaving the hilum of each gland. On the right side, the **right suprarenal vein** is short and almost immediately enters the inferior vena cava, while on the left side, the **left suprarenal vein** passes inferiorly to enter the left renal vein.

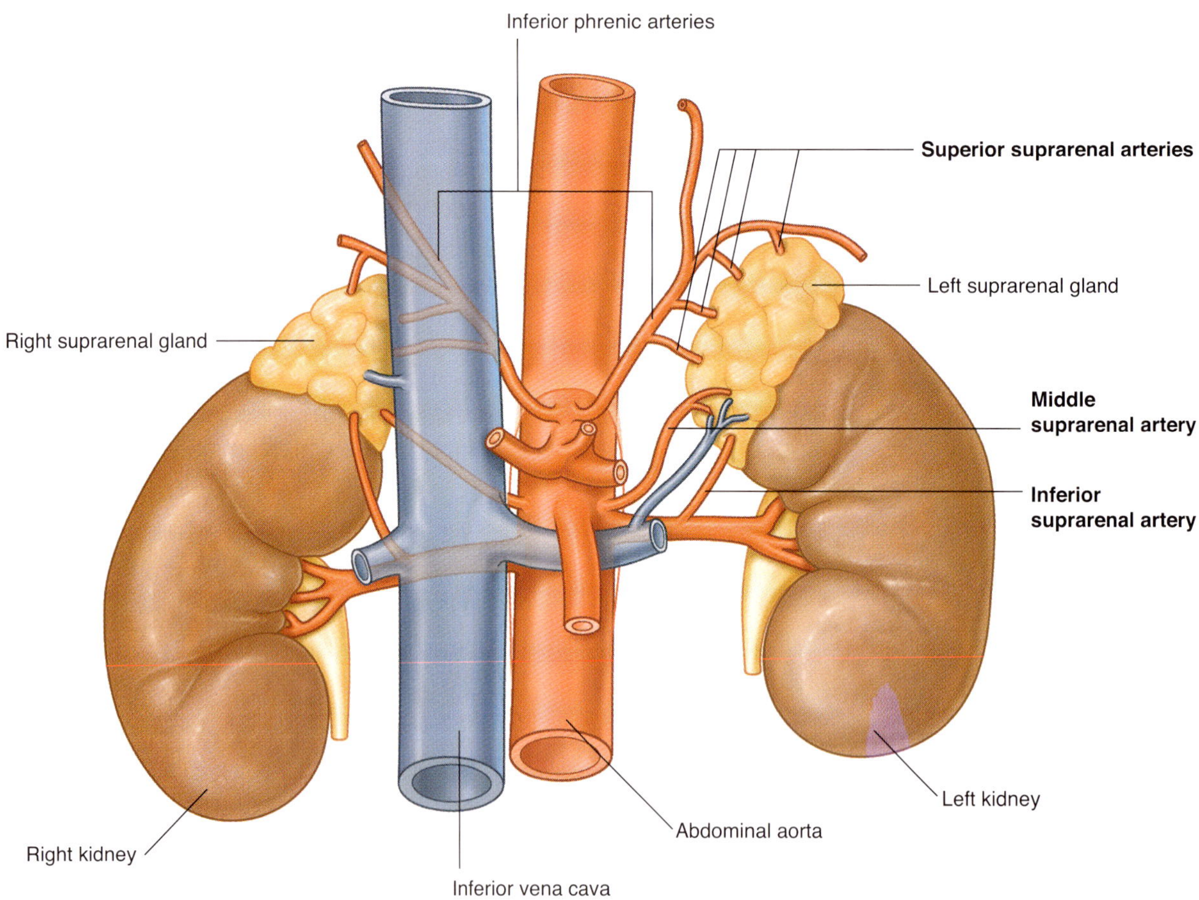

Fig. 4.150 Arterial supply to the suprarenal glands.

Vasculature

SET INDUCTION—CASE SCENARIO 12: ENLARGED SUPERFICIAL INGUINAL RING

A 46-year-old male was seen in the surgery OPD with complaints of a swelling in the groin that had extended to the scrotum when the patient stood and coughed. The surgeon asked the intern if the superficial inguinal ring was enlarged. Knowledge of the method to locate the superficial inguinal ring is needed to manage this case.

<table>
<tr><td rowspan="2">REMEMBER
[Recall Facts]</td><td colspan="3">OUTLINE 12. POSTERIOR ABDOMINAL REGION 2 AND SURFACE ANATOMY—LEARNING OBJECTIVES
[By the end of this section, the student should be able to:]</td><td colspan="2" rowspan="2">EVALUATE
[Explain Concepts]</td></tr>
<tr><td colspan="3">DEMONSTRATE AND ANALYZE RELATIONSHIPS
[Identify structures in a Prosected Specimen or Figure]</td></tr>
<tr><td rowspan="6">1. List the branches of the abdominal aorta
2. List the tributaries of the inferior vena cava
3. List the areas drained by the paraaortic (lumbar) lymph nodes
4. Name the prevertebral ganglia
5. Describe the lumbar plexus
6. Describe the method to locate the superficial inguinal ring in the male
7. Describe the method to locate the lumbar vertebral levels
8. Describe the location of the kidneys and spleen
9. Describe surface regions to which pain from the gut is referred</td><td rowspan="6">Level I
■ Abdominal aorta and its branches
■ Inferior vena cava and its tributaries
■ Sympathetic trunk</td><td rowspan="6">Level II
■ Important relations of abdominal aorta
■ Azygos vein
■ Cisterna chyli and continuation upward as thoracic duct
■ Important relations of inferior vena cava</td><td rowspan="6">Level III
■ Pre- and para-aortic groups of lymph nodes</td><td colspan="2">■ Arrangement of fascia on the posterior abdominal wall
■ Lymphatic drainage of abdomen
■ Course of important branches of lumbar plexus</td></tr>
<tr><td colspan="2">EARLY CLINICAL EXPOSURE
[Apply Anatomical Knowledge]</td></tr>
<tr><td>Surgical Anatomy/ Pathology/Trauma</td><td>Imaging/ Surface Anatomy</td></tr>
<tr><td>■ Inferior vena caval obstruction
■ Spine
■ Compression of the left common iliac vein by the right common iliac artery</td><td></td></tr>
<tr><td colspan="2">PROBLEM SOLVING/ CLINICAL CASES
[Interpret]</td></tr>
<tr><td colspan="2">■ Describe how the ascending lumbar vein is a collateral for the inferior vena cava
■ Describe the route for retroperitoneal lymph node surgery</td></tr>
</table>

Abdominal aorta

The abdominal aorta begins at the aortic hiatus of the diaphragm as a midline structure at approximately the lower level of vertebra TXII (Fig. 4.151). It passes downward on the anterior surface of the bodies of vertebrae LI to LIV, ending just to the left of midline at the lower level of vertebra LIV. At this point, it divides into the **right** and **left common iliac arteries**. This bifurcation can be visualized on the anterior abdominal wall as a point approximately 2.5 cm below the umbilicus or even with a line extending between the highest points of the iliac crest.

As the abdominal aorta passes through the posterior abdominal region, the prevertebral plexus of nerves and ganglia covers its anterior surface. It is also related to numerous other structures:

- Anterior to the abdominal aorta, as it descends, are the pancreas and splenic vein (Fig. 4.120), the left renal vein, and the inferior part of the duodenum.
- Several lumbar veins cross it posteriorly as they pass to the inferior vena cava (see Fig. 4.154).
- On its right side are the cisterna chyli (see Fig. 4.155), thoracic duct, azygos vein, right crus of the diaphragm, and the inferior vena cava.
- On its left side is the left crus of the diaphragm.

Branches of the abdominal aorta (Table 4.3) can be classified as:

- Visceral branches supplying organs
- Posterior branches supplying the diaphragm or body wall
- Terminal branches

Visceral branches

The visceral branches are either unpaired or paired vessels.

The three unpaired visceral branches that arise from the anterior surface of the abdominal aorta (Fig. 4.151) are

- The celiac trunk, which supplies the abdominal foregut
- The superior mesenteric artery, which supplies the abdominal midgut

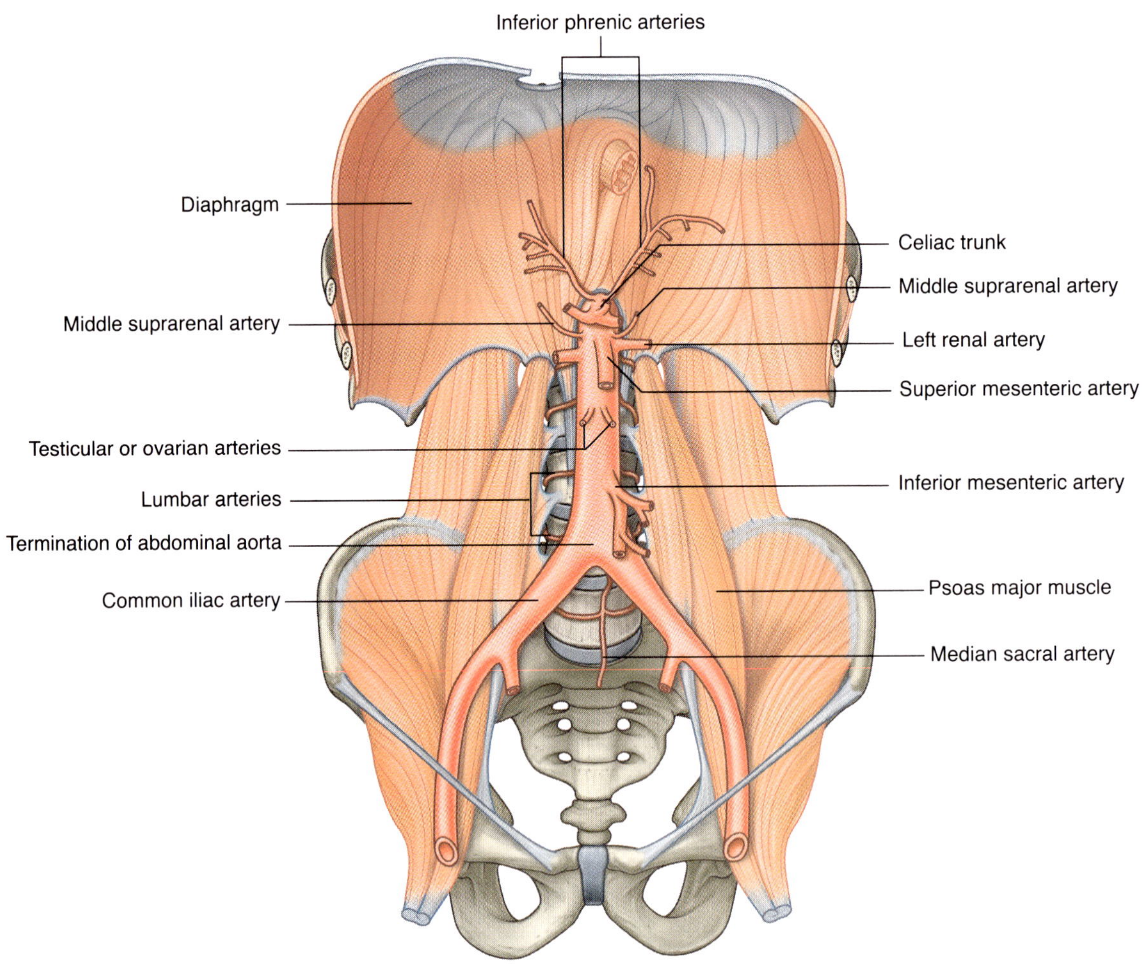

Fig. 4.151 Abdominal aorta.

Table 4.3 Branches of the abdominal aorta

Artery	Branch	Origin	Parts supplied
Celiac trunk	Anterior	Immediately inferior to the aortic hiatus of the diaphragm	Abdominal foregut
Superior mesenteric artery	Anterior	Immediately inferior to the celiac trunk	Abdominal midgut
Inferior mesenteric artery	Anterior	Inferior to the renal arteries	Abdominal hindgut
Middle suprarenal arteries	Lateral	Immediately superior to the renal arteries	Suprarenal glands
Renal arteries	Lateral	Immediately inferior to the superior mesenteric artery	Kidneys
Testicular or ovarian arteries	Paired anterior	Inferior to the renal arteries	Testes in male and ovaries in female
Inferior phrenic arteries	Lateral	Immediately inferior to the aortic hiatus	Diaphragm
Lumbar arteries	Posterior	Usually four pairs	Posterior abdominal wall and spinal cord
Median sacral artery	Posterior	Just superior to the aortic bifurcation, passes inferiorly across lumbar vertebrae, sacrum, and coccyx	
Common iliac arteries	Terminal	Bifurcation usually occurs at the level of LIV vertebra	

- The inferior mesenteric artery, which supplies the abdominal hindgut

The paired visceral branches of the abdominal aorta (Fig. 4.151) include:

- The middle suprarenal arteries—small, lateral branches of the abdominal aorta arising just above the renal arteries that are part of the multiple arterial supply to the suprarenal gland
- The renal arteries—lateral branches of the abdominal aorta that arise just inferior to the origin of the superior mesenteric artery between vertebrae LI and LII, and supply the kidneys
- The testicular or ovarian arteries—anterior branches of the abdominal aorta that arise below the origin of the renal arteries, and pass downward and laterally on the anterior surface of the psoas major muscle

Posterior branches

The posterior branches of the abdominal aorta are vessels supplying the diaphragm or body wall. They consist of the inferior phrenic arteries, the lumbar arteries, and the median sacral artery (Fig. 4.151).

Inferior phrenic arteries

The **inferior phrenic arteries** arise immediately inferior to the aortic hiatus of the diaphragm either directly from the abdominal aorta, as a common trunk from the abdominal aorta, or from the base of the celiac trunk (Fig. 4.151). Whatever their origin, they pass upward, provide some arterial supply to the suprarenal gland, and continue onto the inferior surface of the diaphragm.

Lumbar arteries

There are usually four pairs of **lumbar arteries** arising from the posterior surface of the abdominal aorta (Fig. 4.151). They run laterally and posteriorly over the bodies of the lumbar vertebrae, continue laterally, passing posterior to the sympathetic trunks and between the transverse processes of adjacent lumbar vertebrae, and reach the abdominal wall. From this point onward, they demonstrate a branching pattern similar to a posterior intercostal artery, which includes providing segmental branches that supply the spinal cord.

Median sacral artery

The final posterior branch is the **median sacral artery** (Fig. 4.151). This vessel arises from the posterior surface of the abdominal aorta just superior to the bifurcation and passes in an inferior direction, first over the anterior surface of the lower lumbar vertebrae and then over the anterior surface of the sacrum and coccyx.

Early clinical exposure

Abdominal aortic stent graft

An abdominal aortic aneurysm is a dilatation of the aorta and generally tends to occur in the infrarenal region (the region at or below the renal arteries). As the aorta expands, the risk of rupture increases, and it is now generally accepted that when an aneurysm reaches 5.5 cm or greater, an operation will significantly benefit the patient.

With the aging population, the number of abdominal aortic aneurysms is increasing. Moreover, with the increasing use of imaging techniques a number of abdominal aortic aneurysms are identified in asymptomatic patients.

For many years, the standard treatment for repair was an open operative technique, which involved a large incision from the xiphoid process of the sternum to the symphysis pubis and dissection of the aneurysm. The aneurysm was excised and a tubular woven graft was sewn into place. Recovery would take a number of days, even weeks, and most patients would be placed in the intensive care unit after the operation.

Further developments and modern techniques have led to a new type of procedure being performed to treat abdominal aortic aneurysms: the endovascular graft—placing a graft in the aortic aneurysm and lining the dilated vessel is not new and was first described over 10 years ago. Since the original description the devices have been modified on a number of occasions (Fig. 4.152).

The technique involves surgically dissecting the femoral artery below the inguinal ligament. A small incision is made in the femoral artery and the preloaded compressed graft with metal support struts is passed on a large catheter into the abdominal aorta through the femoral artery. Using X-ray for guidance, the graft is opened, lining the inside of the aorta. Limb attachments are made to the graft that extend into the common iliac arteries. This bifurcated tube device effectively excludes the abdominal aortic aneurysm.

This type of device is not suitable for all patients. Patients who receive this device do not need to go to the intensive care unit. Many patients leave the hospital within 24–48 hours. Importantly, this device can be used for patients who were deemed unfit for open surgical repair.

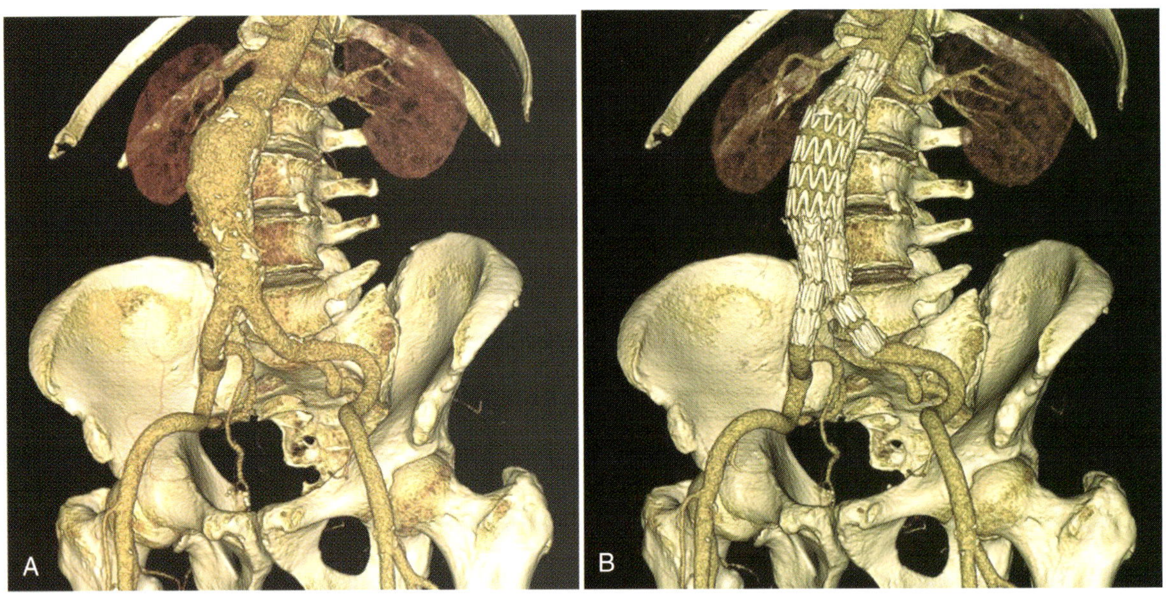

Fig. 4.152 Volume-rendered reconstruction using multidetector computed tomography of a patient with an infrarenal abdominal aortic aneurysm before **(A)** and after **(B)** endovascular aneurysm repair. Note the image only demonstrates the intraluminal contrast and not the entire vessel. White patches in the aorta represent intramural calcium.

Inferior vena cava

The inferior vena cava returns blood from all structures below the diaphragm to the right atrium of the heart. It is formed when the two common iliac veins come together at the level of vertebra LV, just to the right of midline. It ascends through the posterior abdominal region anterior to the vertebral column immediately to the right of the abdominal aorta (Fig. 4.153), continues in a superior direction, and leaves the abdomen by piercing the central tendon of the diaphragm at the level of vertebra TVIII.

During its course, the anterior surface of the inferior vena cava is crossed by the right common iliac artery, the root of the mesentery (Fig. 4.58A), the right testicular or ovarian artery, the inferior part of the duodenum, the head of the pancreas, the superior part of the duodenum, the bile duct, the portal vein (Fig. 4.114), and the liver, which overlaps and on occasion completely surrounds the vena cava (Fig. 4.153). The tributaries to the inferior vena cava include the:

- Common iliac veins
- Lumbar veins
- Right testicular or ovarian vein (Fig. 4.153)
- Renal veins

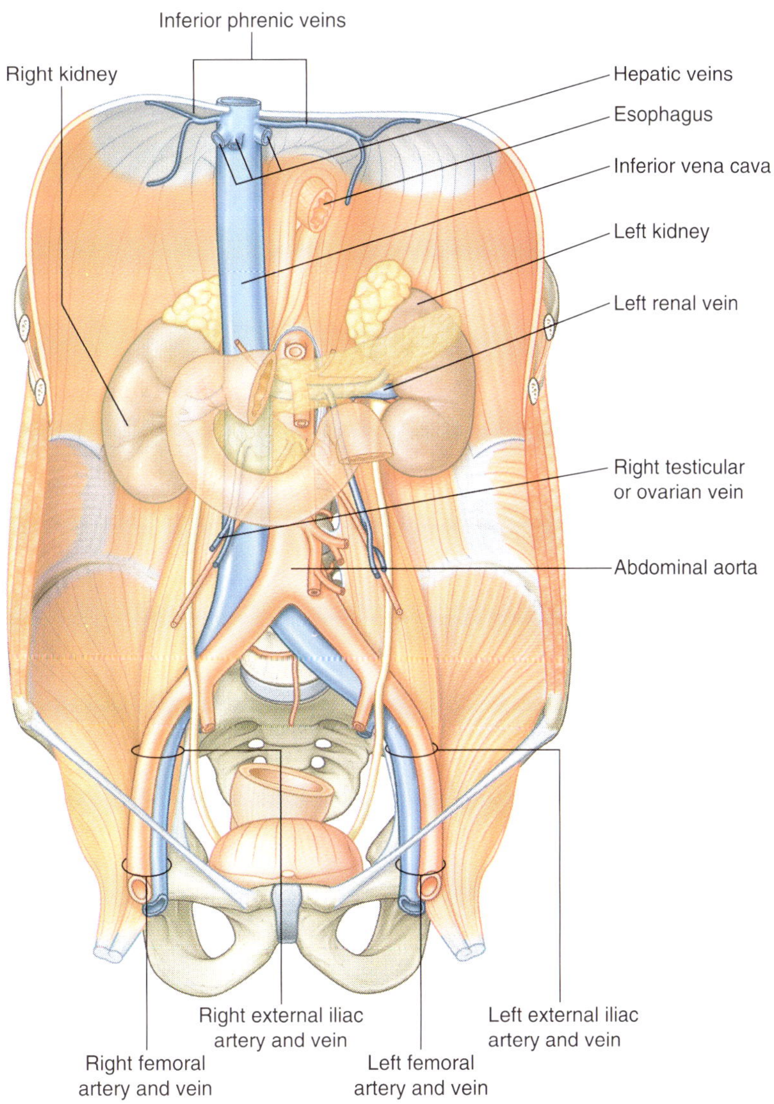

Fig. 4.153 Inferior vena cava.

- Right suprarenal vein (Fig. 4.150)
- Inferior phrenic veins
- Hepatic veins

There are no tributaries from the abdominal part of the gastrointestinal tract, the spleen, the pancreas, or the gallbladder, because veins from these structures are components of the portal venous system, which first passes through the liver.

Of the venous tributaries mentioned above, the **lumbar veins** are unique in their connections and deserve special attention. Not all of the lumbar veins drain directly into the inferior vena cava (Fig. 4.154):

- The fifth lumbar vein generally drains into the iliolumbar vein, a tributary of the common iliac vein.
- The third and fourth lumbar veins usually drain into the inferior vena cava.
- The first and second lumbar veins may empty into the ascending lumbar veins.

The **ascending lumbar veins** are long, anastomosing venous channels that connect the common iliac, iliolumbar, and lumbar veins with the azygos and hemiazygos veins of the thorax (Fig. 4.154).

If the inferior vena cava becomes blocked, the ascending lumbar veins become important collateral channels between the lower and upper parts of the body.

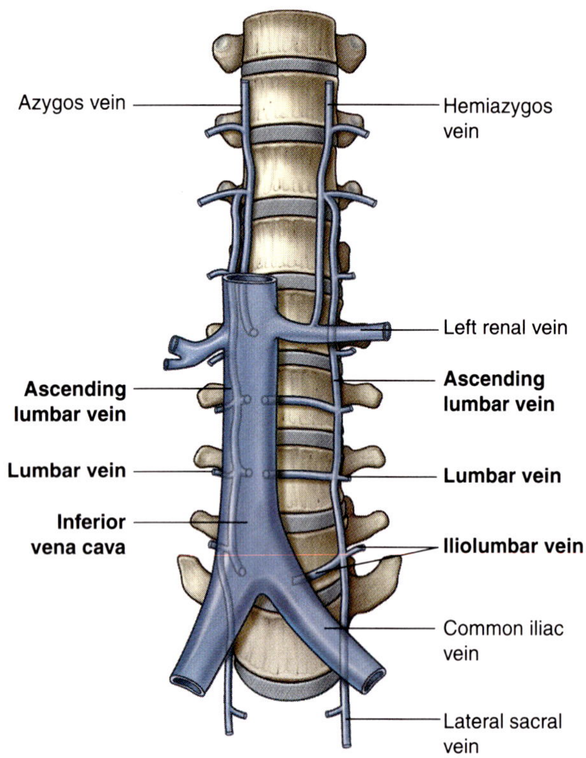

Fig. 4.154 Lumbar veins.

Early clinical exposure

Inferior vena cava filter

Deep vein thrombosis is a potentially fatal condition where a clot (thrombus) is formed in the deep venous system of the legs and the veins of the pelvis. Virchow described the reasons for thrombus formation as decreased blood flow, abnormality of the constituents of blood, and abnormalities of the vessel wall. Common predisposing factors include hospitalization and surgery, the oral contraceptive pill, smoking, and air travel. Other factors include clotting abnormalities (e.g., protein S and protein C deficiency).

The diagnosis of deep vein thrombosis may be difficult to establish, with symptoms including leg swelling and pain and discomfort in the calf. It may also be an incidental finding.

In practice, patients with suspected deep vein thrombosis undergo a D-dimer blood test, which measures levels of a fibrin degradation product. If this is positive, there is a high association with deep vein thrombosis.

The consequences of deep vein thrombosis are twofold. Occasionally, the clot may dislodge and pass into the venous system through the right side of the heart and into the main pulmonary arteries. If the clots are of significant size they obstruct blood flow to the lung and may produce instantaneous death. Secondary complications include destruction of the normal valvular system in the legs, which may lead to venous incompetency and chronic leg swelling with ulceration.

The management for deep vein thrombosis includes prevention. In order to prevent deep vein thrombosis, patients are optimized by removing all potential risk factors. Subcutaneous heparin may be injected and the patient wears compression stockings to prevent venous stasis while in the hospital.

In certain situations, it is not possible to optimize the patient with prophylactic treatment, and it may be necessary to insert a filter into the inferior vena cava that traps any large clots. It may be removed after the risk period has ended.

The right common iliac artery may rarely compress the left common iliac vein (Fig. 4.153) causing May–Thurner syndrome, or **iliac vein compression syndrome** (IVCS), and result in iliofemoral **deep venous thrombosis** (DVT).

Lymphatic system

Lymphatic drainage from most deep structures and regions of the body below the diaphragm converges mainly on collections of lymph nodes and vessels associated with the major blood vessels of the posterior abdominal region (Fig. 4.155). The lymph then predominantly drains into the thoracic duct. Major lymphatic channels that drain different regions of the body as a whole are summarized in Table 4.4 (also see Chapter 1, p. 36, for discussion of lymphatics in general).

Preaortic and lateral aortic or lumbar nodes (paraaortic nodes)

Approaching the aortic bifurcation, the collections of lymphatics associated with the two common iliac arteries and veins merge, and multiple groups of lymphatic vessels and

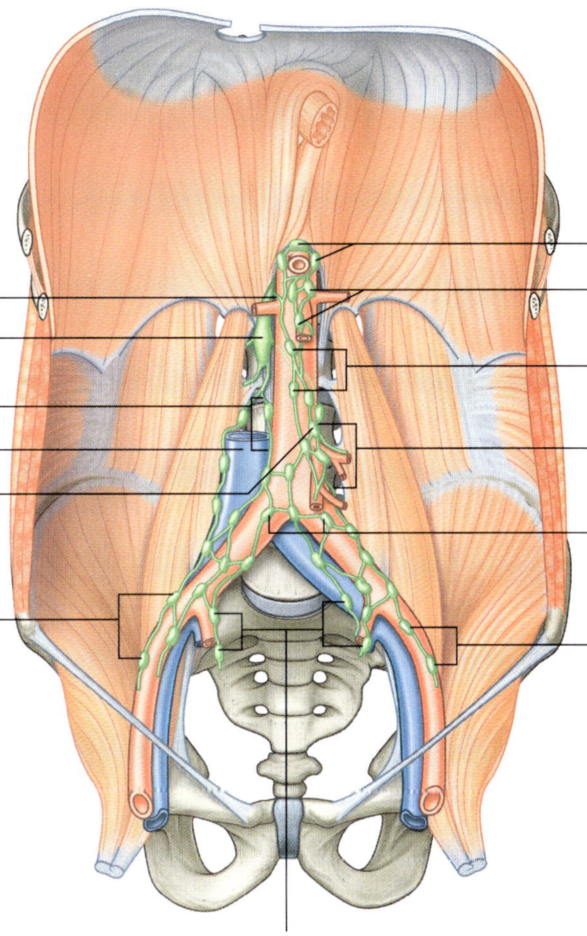

Fig. 4.155 Abdominal lymphatics.

Table 4.4 Lymphatic drainage (Fig. 1.31)

Lymphatic vessel	Area drained
Right jugular trunk	Right side of head and neck
Left jugular trunk	Left side of head and neck
Right subclavian trunk	Right upper limb, superficial regions of thoracic and upper abdominal walls
Left subclavian trunk	Left upper limb, superficial regions of thoracic and upper abdominal walls
Right bronchomediastinal trunk	Right lung and bronchi, mediastinal structures, thoracic wall
Left bronchomediastinal trunk	Left lung and bronchi, mediastinal structures, thoracic wall
Thoracic duct	Lower limbs, abdominal walls and viscera, pelvic walls and viscera, thoracic wall

nodes associated with the abdominal aorta and inferior vena cava pass superiorly. These collections may be subdivided into **preaortic nodes**, which are anterior to the abdominal aorta, and **right** and **left lateral aortic** or **lumbar nodes** (**paraaortic nodes**), which are positioned on either side of the abdominal aorta (Fig. 4.155).

As these collections of lymphatics pass through the posterior abdominal region, they continue to collect lymph from a variety of structures. The lateral aortic or lumbar lymph nodes (paraaortic nodes) receive lymphatics from the body wall, the kidneys, the suprarenal glands, and the testes or ovaries.

The preaortic nodes are organized around the three anterior branches of the abdominal aorta that supply the abdominal part of the gastrointestinal tract, as well as the spleen, pancreas, gallbladder, and liver. They are divided into celiac, superior mesenteric, and inferior mesenteric nodes, and receive lymph from the organs supplied by the similarly named arteries.

Finally, the lateral aortic or lumbar nodes form the right and left lumbar trunks, whereas the preaortic nodes form the intestinal trunk (Fig. 4.155). These trunks come together and form a confluence that, at times, appears as a saccular dilation (the cisterna chyli). This confluence of lymph trunks is posterior to the right side of the abdominal aorta and anterior to the bodies of vertebrae LI and LII. It marks the beginning of the thoracic duct.

Early clinical exposure

Retroperitoneal lymph node surgery

From a clinical perspective, retroperitoneal lymph nodes are arranged in two groups. The preaortic lymph node group drains lymph from the embryological midline structures, such as the liver, bowel, and pancreas. The paraaortic lymph node group (the lateral aortic or lumbar nodes), on either side of the aorta, drains lymph from bilateral structures, such as the kidneys and adrenal glands. Organs embryologically derived from the posterior abdominal wall also drain lymph to these nodes. These organs include the ovaries and the testes (importantly, the testes do not drain lymph to the inguinal regions).

In general, lymphatic drainage follows standard predictable routes; however, in the presence of disease, alternate routes of lymphatic drainage will occur.

There are a number of causes for enlarged retroperitoneal lymph nodes. In the adult, massively enlarged lymph nodes are a feature of lymphoma, and smaller lymph node enlargement is observed in the presence of infection and metastatic malignant spread of disease (e.g., colon cancer).

The treatment for malignant lymph node disease is based upon a number of factors, including the site of the primary tumor (e.g., bowel) and its histological cell type. Normally, the primary tumor is surgically removed and the lymph node spread and metastatic organ spread (e.g., to the liver and the lungs) are often treated with chemotherapy and radiotherapy.

In certain instances, it may be considered appropriate to resect the lymph nodes in the retroperitoneum (e.g., for testicular cancer).

The surgical approach to retroperitoneal lymph node resection involves a paramedian incision in the midclavicular line. The three layers of the anterolateral abdominal wall (external oblique, internal oblique, and transversus abdominis) are opened and the transversalis fascia is divided. The next structure the surgeon sees is the parietal peritoneum. Instead of entering the parietal peritoneum, which is standard procedure for most intraabdominal operations, the surgeon gently pushes the parietal peritoneum toward the midline, which moves the intraabdominal contents and allows a clear view of the retroperitoneal structures. On the left, the paraaortic lymph node group is easily demonstrated, with a clear view of the abdominal aorta and kidney. On the right, the inferior vena cava is demonstrated and has to be retracted to access the right paraaortic lymph node chain.

The procedure of retroperitoneal lymph node dissection is extremely well tolerated and lacks the problems of entering the peritoneal cavity (e.g., paralytic ileus). Unfortunately, a complication of a vertical incision in the midclavicular line is division of the segmental nerve supply to the rectus abdominis muscle. This produces muscle atrophy and asymmetrical proportions of the anterior abdominal wall.

Nervous system in the posterior abdominal region

Several important components of the nervous system are in the posterior abdominal region. These include the sympathetic trunks and associated splanchnic nerves, the plexus of nerves and ganglia associated with the abdominal aorta, and the lumbar plexus of nerves.

Sympathetic trunks and splanchnic nerves

The sympathetic trunks pass through the posterior abdominal region anterolateral to the lumbar vertebral bodies, before continuing across the sacral promontory and into the pelvic cavity (Fig. 4.156). Along their course, small enlargements are visible. These represent collections of neuronal cell bodies—primarily postganglionic neuronal cell bodies—which are located outside the central nervous system. They are sympathetic paravertebral ganglia. There are usually four ganglia along the sympathetic trunks in the posterior abdominal region.

Also associated with the sympathetic trunks in the posterior abdominal region are the lumbar splanchnic nerves (Fig. 4.156). These components of the nervous system pass from the sympathetic trunks to the plexus of nerves and ganglia associated with the abdominal aorta. Usually two to four lumbar splanchnic nerves carry preganglionic sympathetic fibers and visceral afferent fibers. Lumbar sympathectomy may be done for intractable sweating of the lower limbs.

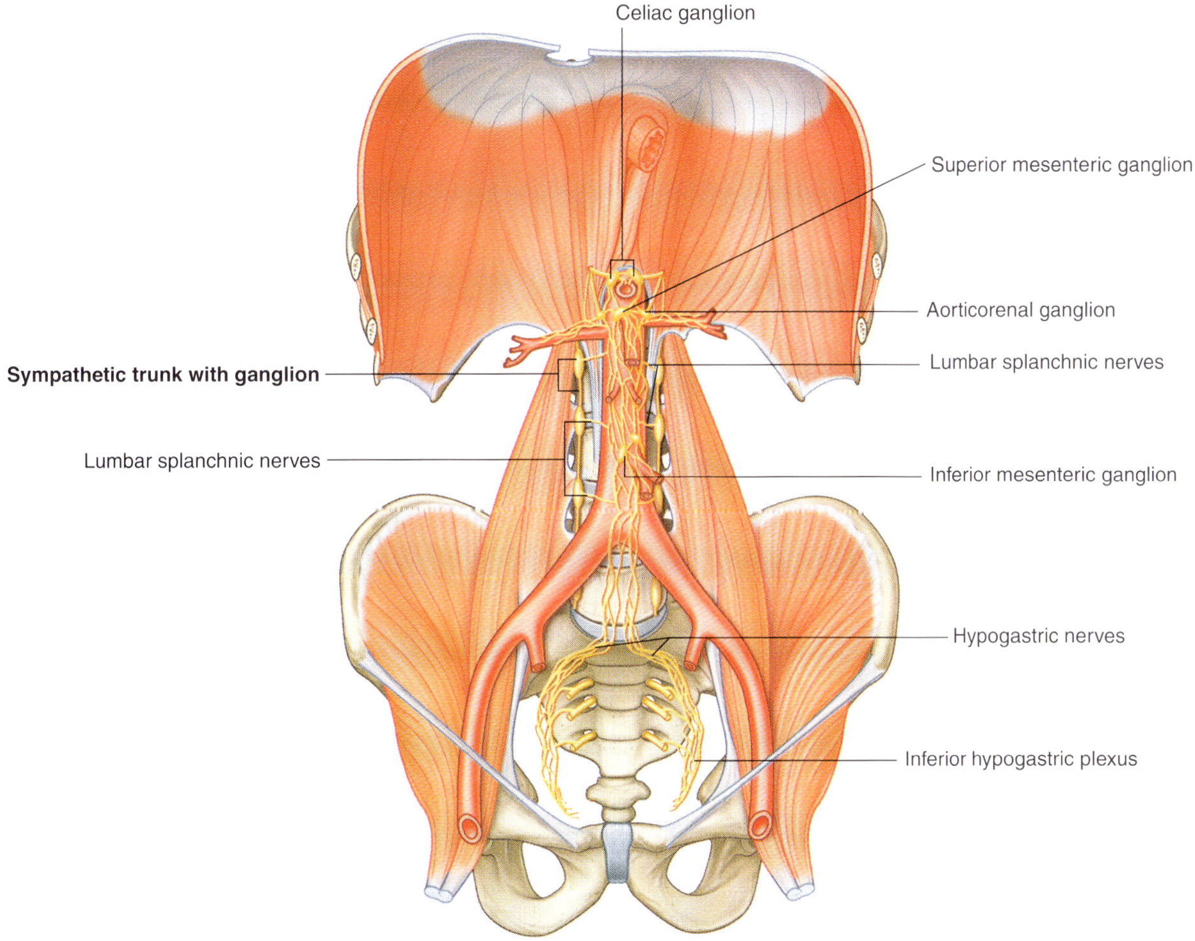

Fig. 4.156 Sympathetic trunks passing through the posterior abdominal region.

Abdominal prevertebral plexus and ganglia

The abdominal prevertebral plexus is a network of nerve fibers surrounding the abdominal aorta. It extends from the aortic hiatus of the diaphragm to the bifurcation of the aorta into the right and left common iliac arteries. Along its route, it is subdivided into smaller, named plexuses (Fig. 4.157):

- Beginning at the diaphragm and moving inferiorly, the initial accumulation of nerve fibers is referred to as the celiac plexus—this subdivision includes nerve fibers associated with the roots of the celiac trunk and superior mesenteric artery.
- Continuing inferiorly, the plexus of nerve fibers extending from just below the superior mesenteric artery to the aortic bifurcation is the abdominal aortic plexus (Fig. 4.157).
- At the bifurcation of the abdominal aorta, the abdominal prevertebral plexus continues inferiorly as the superior hypogastric plexus.

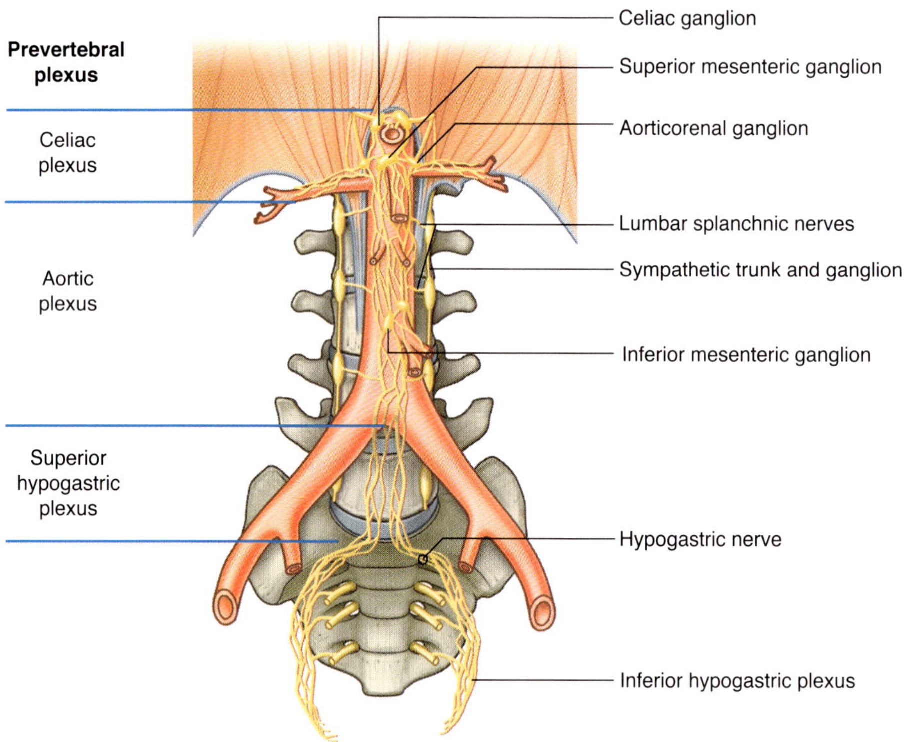

Fig. 4.157 Prevertebral plexus and ganglia in the posterior abdominal region.

Throughout its length, the abdominal prevertebral plexus is a conduit for:

- Preganglionic sympathetic and visceral afferent fibers from the thoracic and lumbar splanchnic nerves
- Preganglionic parasympathetic and visceral afferent fibers from the vagus nerves [X]
- Preganglionic parasympathetic fibers from the pelvic splanchnic nerves (Fig. 4.158)

Associated with the abdominal prevertebral plexus are clumps of nervous tissue (the **prevertebral ganglia**), which are collections of postganglionic sympathetic neuronal cell bodies in recognizable aggregations along the abdominal prevertebral plexus; they are usually named after the nearest branch of the abdominal aorta. They are therefore referred to as **celiac, superior mesenteric, aorticorenal,** and **inferior mesenteric ganglia** (Fig. 4.159). These structures, along with the abdominal prevertebral plexus, play a critical role in the innervation of the abdominal viscera.

Common sites for pain referred from the abdominal viscera and from the heart are given in Table 4.5.

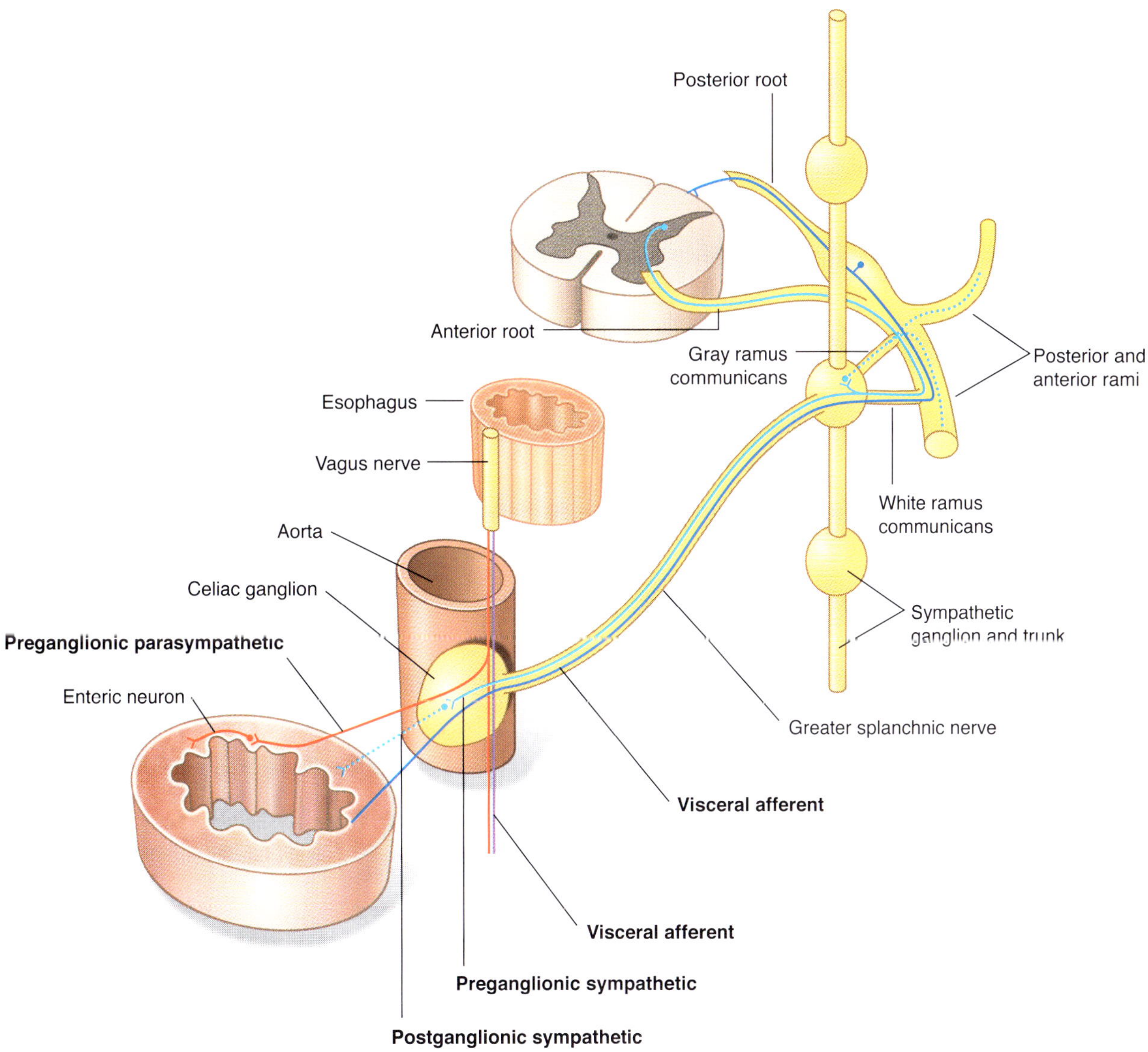

Fig. 4.158 Nerve fibers passing through the abdominal prevertebral plexus and ganglia.

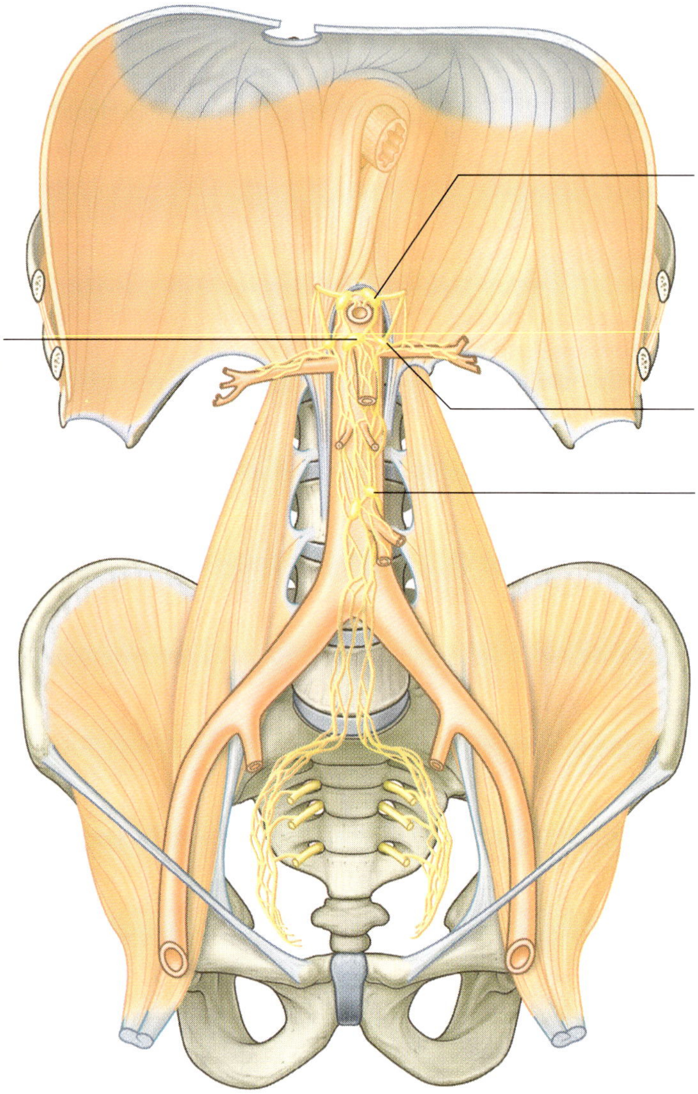

Fig. 4.159 Prevertebral ganglia associated with the prevertebral plexus.

Table 4.5 Referred pain pathways (visceral afferents) (Fig. 1.39)

Organ	Afferent pathway	Spinal cord level	Referral area
Heart	Thoracic splanchnic nerves	T1 to T4	Upper thorax and medial arm
Foregut (organs supplied by celiac trunk)	Greater splanchnic nerve	T5 to T9 (or T10)	Lower thorax and epigastric region
Midgut (organs supplied by superior mesenteric artery)	Lesser splanchnic nerve	T9, T10 (or T10, T11)	Umbilical region
Kidneys and upper ureter	Least splanchnic nerve	T12	Flanks (lateral regions)
Hindgut (organs supplied by inferior mesenteric artery) and lower ureter	Lumbar splanchnic nerves	L1, L2	Pubic region, lateral and anterior thighs, and groin

Lumbar plexus

The lumbar plexus is formed by the anterior rami of nerves L1 to L3 and most of the anterior ramus of L4 (Fig. 4.160; Table 4.6). It also receives a contribution from the T12 (subcostal) nerve.

Branches of the lumbar plexus include the iliohypogastric, ilioinguinal, and genitofemoral nerves lateral cutaneous nerve of the thigh (lateral femoral cutaneous) and femoral and obturator nerves. The lumbar plexus is located in the substance of the psoas major muscle anterior to its attachment to the transverse processes of the lumbar vertebrae (Fig. 4.161). Therefore, relative to the psoas major muscle, the various branches emerge:

- Anterior—genitofemoral nerve
- Medial—obturator nerve
- Lateral—iliohypogastric, ilioinguinal, and femoral nerves and the lateral cutaneous nerve of the thigh

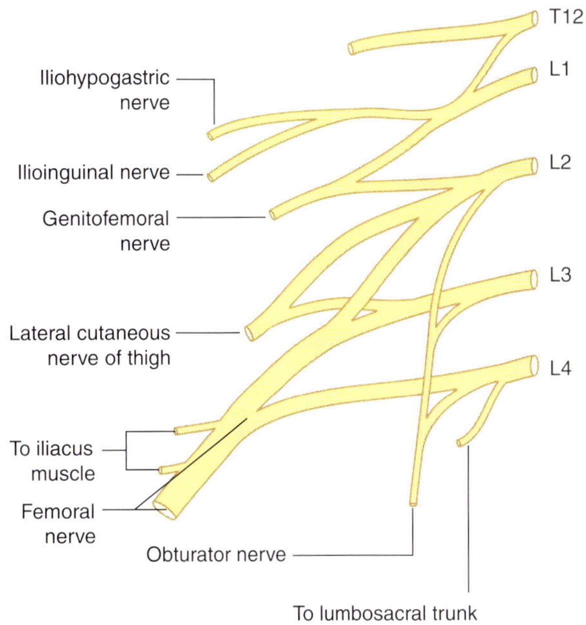

Fig. 4.160 Lumbar plexus.

Iliohypogastric and ilioinguinal nerves (L1)

The iliohypogastric and ilioinguinal nerves arise as a single trunk from the anterior ramus of nerve L1 (Fig. 4.160). Either before or soon after emerging from the lateral border of the psoas major muscle, this single trunk divides into the iliohypogastric and the ilioinguinal nerves.

Table 4.6 Branches of the lumbar plexus (Fig. 3.19 and 4.39)

Branch	Origin	Spinal segments	Function: motor	Function: sensory
Iliohypogastric	Anterior ramus L1	L1	Internal oblique and transversus abdominis	Posterolateral gluteal skin and skin in pubic region
Ilioinguinal	Anterior ramus L1	L1	Internal oblique and transversus abdominis	Skin in the upper medial thigh, and either the skin over the root of the penis and anterior scrotum or the mons pubis and labium majus
Genitofemoral	Anterior rami L1 and L2	L1, L2	Genital branch—male cremasteric muscle	Genital branch—skin of anterior scrotum or skin of mons pubis and labium majus; femoral branch—skin of upper anterior thigh
Lateral cutaneous nerve of thigh	Anterior rami L2 and L3	L2, L3		Skin on anterior and lateral thigh to the knee
Obturator	Anterior rami L2 to L4	L2 to L4	Obturator externus, pectineus, and muscles in medial compartment of thigh	Skin on medial aspect of the thigh
Femoral	Anterior rami L2 to L4	L2 to L4	Iliacus, pectineus, and muscles in anterior compartment of thigh	Skin on anterior thigh and medial surface of leg

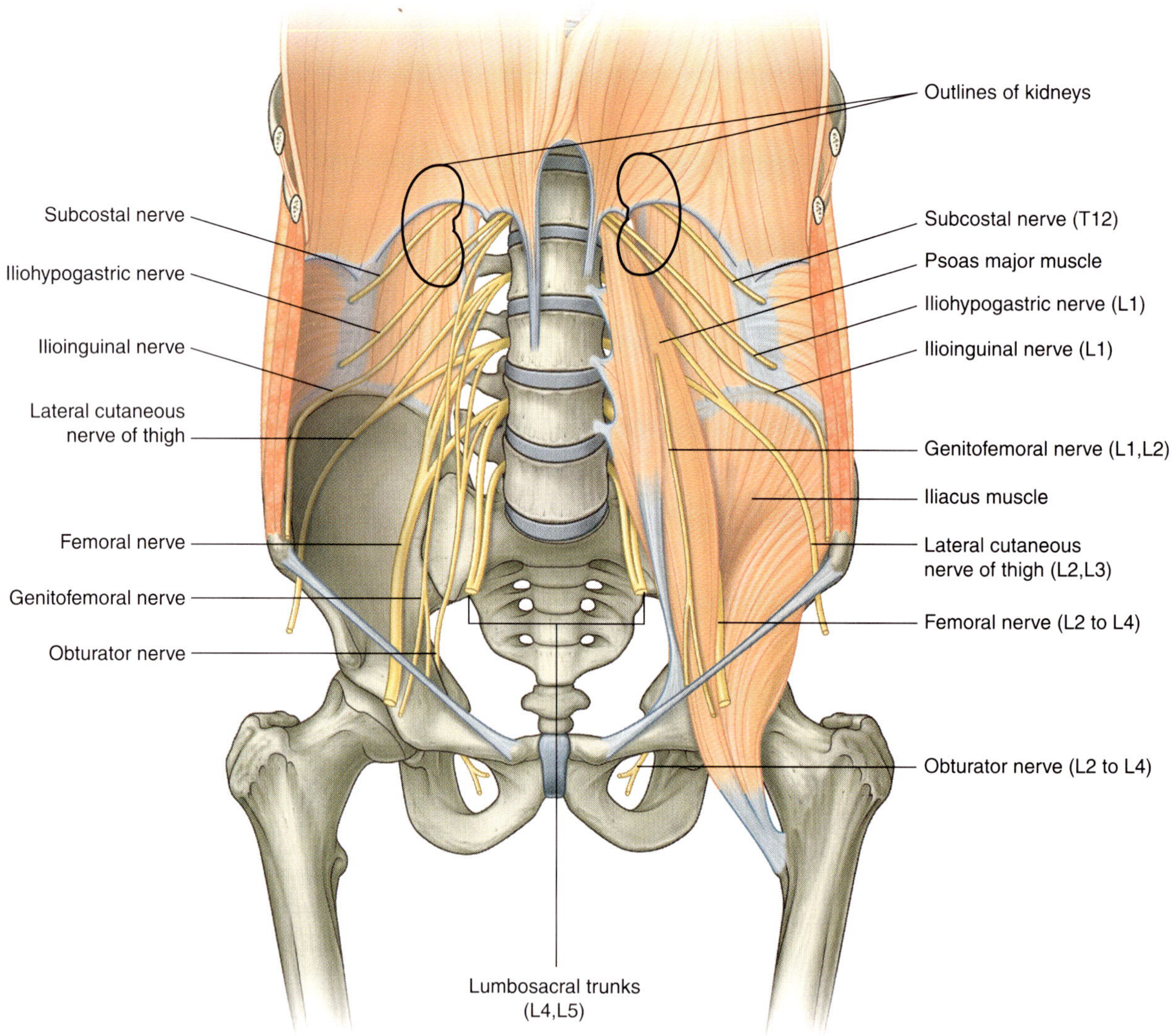

Fig. 4.161 Lumbar plexus in the posterior abdominal region.

Iliohypogastric nerve

The **iliohypogastric nerve** passes across the anterior surface of the quadratus lumborum muscle, posterior to the kidney (Fig. 4.161). It pierces the transversus abdominis muscle and continues anteriorly around the body between the transversus abdominis and internal oblique muscles. Above the iliac crest, a **lateral cutaneous branch** pierces the internal and external oblique muscles to supply the posterolateral gluteal skin (Fig. 4.162; see also Fig. 3.19).

The remaining part of the iliohypogastric nerve (the **anterior cutaneous branch**) continues in an anterior direction, piercing the internal oblique just medial to the anterior superior iliac spine as it continues in an obliquely downward and medial direction. Becoming cutaneous, just above the superficial inguinal ring, after piercing the aponeurosis of the external oblique, it distributes to the skin in the pubic region (Fig. 4.162). Throughout its course, it also supplies branches to the abdominal musculature.

Ilioinguinal nerve

The ilioinguinal nerve is smaller than, and inferior to, the iliohypogastric nerve as it crosses the quadratus lumborum

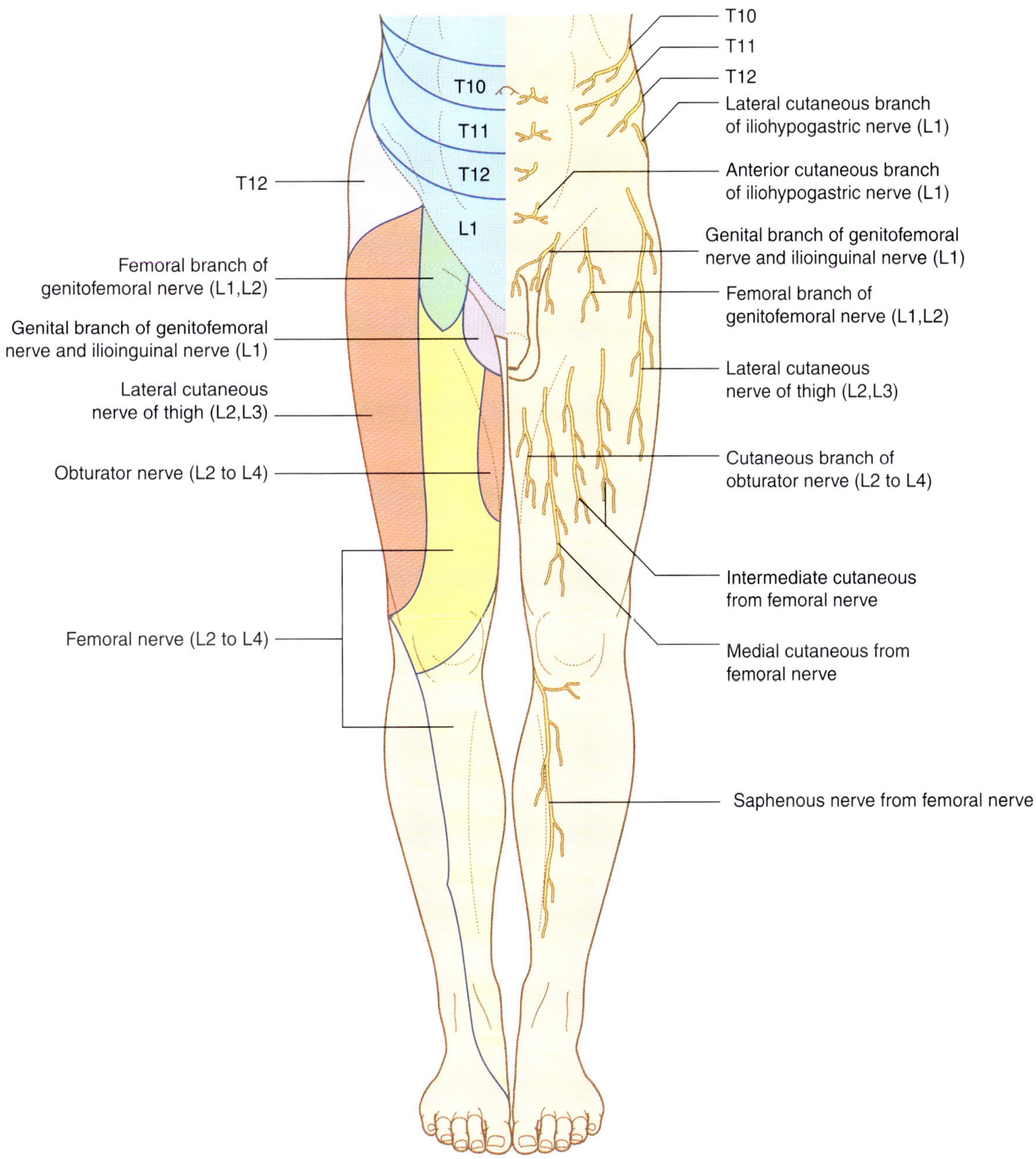

Fig. 4.162 Cutaneous distribution of the nerves from the lumbar plexus.

muscle. Its course is more oblique than that of the iliohypogastric nerve, and it usually crosses part of the iliacus muscle on its way to the iliac crest. Near the anterior end of the iliac crest, it pierces the transversus abdominis muscle, and then pierces the internal oblique muscle and enters the inguinal canal (Fig. 4.37).

The ilioinguinal nerve emerges through the superficial inguinal ring, along with the spermatic cord, and provides cutaneous innervation to the upper medial thigh, the root of the penis, and the anterior surface of the scrotum in men, or the mons pubis and labium majus in women (Fig. 4.162). Throughout its course, it also supplies branches to the abdominal musculature.

Genitofemoral nerve (L1 and L2)

The genitofemoral nerve arises from the anterior rami of nerves L1 and L2 (Fig. 4.160). It passes downward in the substance of the psoas major muscle until it emerges on the anterior surface of the psoas major. It then descends on the surface of the muscle, in a retroperitoneal position, passing posterior to the ureter. It eventually divides into genital and femoral branches (Fig. 4.161).

The **genital branch** continues downward and enters the inguinal canal through the deep inguinal ring. It continues through the canal and

- In men, innervates the cremasteric muscle and terminates on the skin in the upper anterior part of the scrotum.
- In women, accompanies the round ligament of the uterus and terminates on the skin of the mons pubis and labium majus.

The **femoral branch** descends on the lateral side of the external iliac artery and passes posterior to the inguinal ligament, entering the femoral sheath lateral to the femoral artery. It pierces the anterior layer of the femoral sheath and the fascia lata to supply the skin of the upper anterior thigh (Fig. 4.162).

Lateral cutaneous nerve of the thigh (L2 and L3)

The lateral cutaneous nerve of the thigh arises from the anterior rami of nerves L2 and L3 (Fig. 4.160). It emerges from the lateral border of the psoas major muscle, and passes obliquely downward across the iliacus muscle toward the anterior superior iliac spine (Fig. 4.162). It passes posterior to the inguinal ligament and enters the thigh.

The lateral cutaneous nerve of the thigh supplies the skin on the anterior and lateral thigh to the level of the knee (Fig. 4.162).

Obturator nerve (L2 to L4)

The obturator nerve arises from the anterior rami of nerves L2 to L4 (Fig. 4.160). It descends in the psoas major muscle, emerging from its medial side near the pelvic brim (Fig. 4.161).

The obturator nerve continues posterior to the common iliac vessels, passes across the lateral wall of the pelvic cavity, and enters the obturator canal, through which the obturator nerve gains access to the medial compartment of the thigh.

In the area of the obturator canal, the obturator nerve divides into **anterior** and **posterior branches**. On entering the medial compartment of the thigh, the two branches are separated by the obturator externus and adductor brevis muscles (Fig. 3.60). Throughout their course through the medial compartment, these two branches supply:

- Articular branches to the hip joint
- Muscular branches to the obturator externus, pectineus, adductor longus, gracilis, adductor brevis, and adductor magnus muscles
- Cutaneous branches to the medial aspect of the thigh (Fig. 4.162)
- In association with the saphenous nerve, cutaneous branches to the medial aspect of the upper part of the leg and articular branches to the knee joint

Femoral nerve (L2 to L4)

The femoral nerve arises from the anterior rami of nerves L2 to L4 (Fig. 4.160). It descends through the substance of the psoas major muscle, emerging from the lower lateral border of the psoas major (Fig. 4.161). Continuing its descent, the femoral nerve lies between the lateral border of the psoas major and the anterior surface of the iliacus muscle. It is deep to the iliacus fascia and lateral to the femoral artery as it passes posterior to the inguinal ligament and enters the anterior compartment of the thigh. Upon entering the thigh, it immediately divides into multiple branches.

Cutaneous branches of the femoral nerve include:

- Medial and intermediate cutaneous nerves supplying the skin on the anterior surface of the thigh
- The saphenous nerve supplying the skin on the medial surface of the leg (Fig. 4.162)

Muscular branches innervate the iliacus, pectineus, sartorius, rectus femoris, vastus medialis, vastus intermedius, and vastus lateralis muscles. Articular branches supply the hip and knee joints.

SURFACE ANATOMY

Abdomen surface anatomy

Visualization of the position of abdominal viscera is fundamental to a physical examination. Some of these viscera or their parts can be felt by palpating through the abdominal wall. Surface features can be used to establish the positions of deep structures.

Defining the surface projection of the abdomen

Palpable landmarks can be used to delineate the extent of the abdomen on the surface of the body. These landmarks are

- The costal margin above
- The pubic tubercle, anterior superior iliac spine, and iliac crest below (Fig. 4.163)

The costal margin is readily palpable and separates the abdominal wall from the thoracic wall.

A line between the anterior superior iliac spine and the pubic tubercle marks the position of the inguinal ligament, which separates the anterior abdominal wall above from the thigh of the lower limb below.

The iliac crest separates the posterolateral abdominal wall from the gluteal region of the lower limb.

The upper part of the abdominal cavity projects above the costal margin to the diaphragm, and therefore abdominal viscera in this region of the abdomen are protected by the thoracic wall.

The level of the diaphragm varies during the breathing cycle. The dome of the diaphragm on the right can reach as high as the fourth costal cartilage during forced expiration.

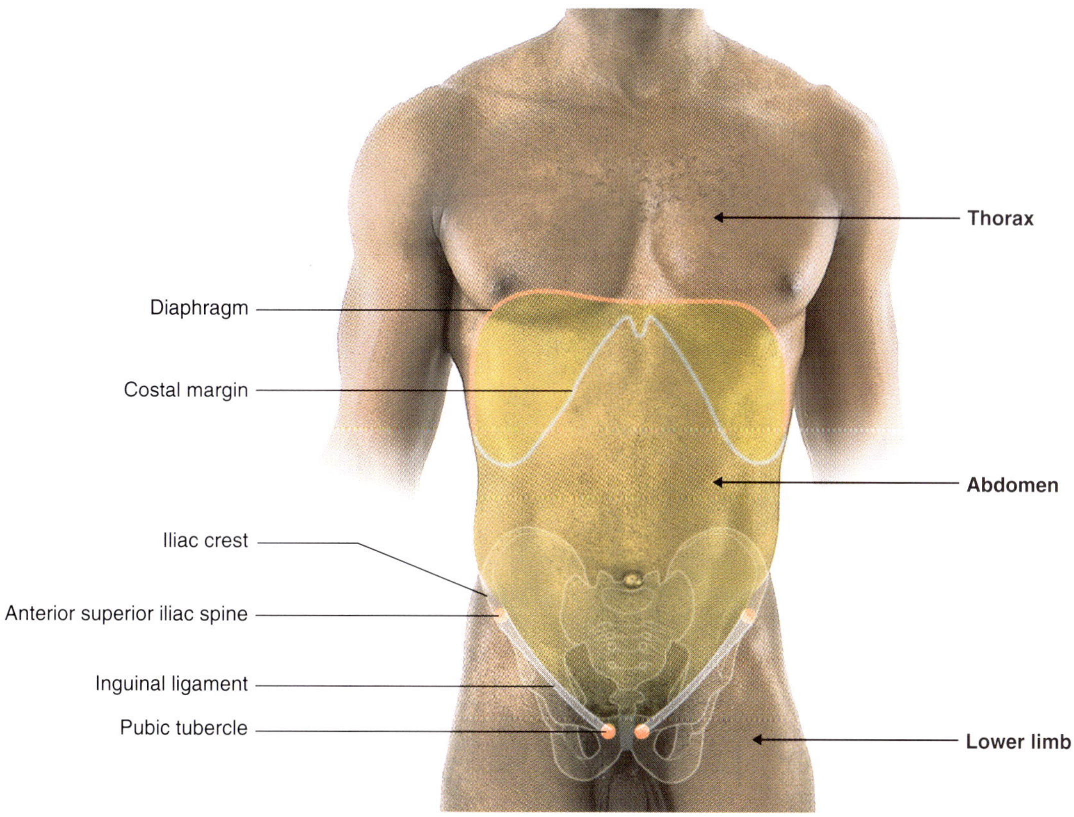

Fig. 4.163 Interior view of the abdominal region of a man. Palpable bony landmarks, the inguinal ligament, and the position of the diaphragm are indicated.

How to find the superficial inguinal ring

The superficial inguinal ring is an elongate triangular defect in the aponeurosis of the external oblique (Fig. 4.164). It lies in the lower medial aspect of the anterior abdominal wall and is the external opening of the inguinal canal. The inguinal canal and superficial inguinal ring are larger in men than in women:

- In men, structures that pass between the abdomen and the testis pass through the inguinal canal and superficial inguinal ring.

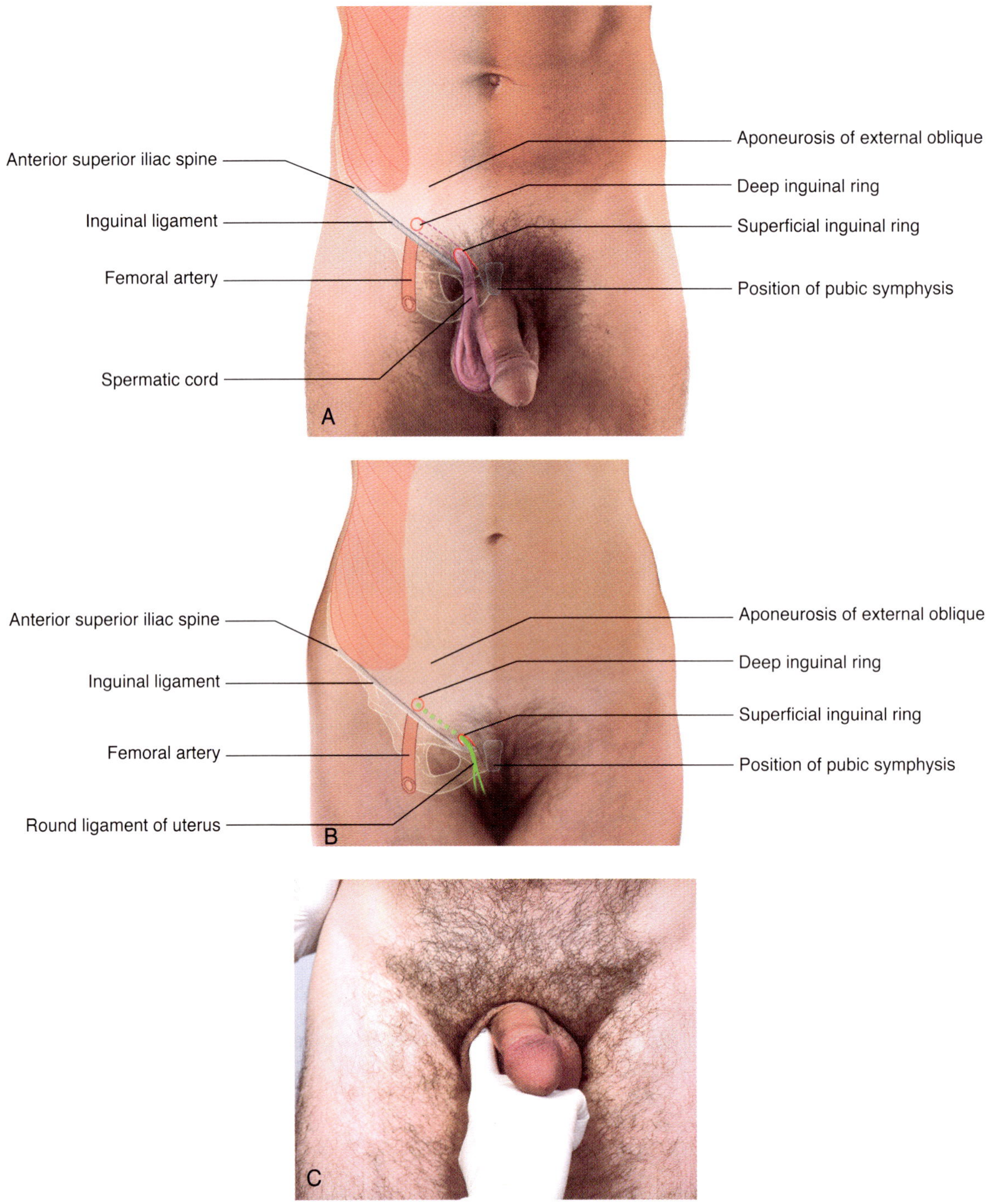

Fig. 4.164 Groin. **(A)** In a man. **(B)** In a woman. **(C)** Examination of the superficial inguinal ring and related regions of the inguinal canal in a man.

- In women, the round ligament of the uterus passes through the inguinal canal and superficial inguinal ring to merge with connective tissue of the labium majus.

The superficial inguinal ring is superior to the pubic crest and pubic tubercle and to the medial end of the inguinal ligament:

- In men, the superficial inguinal ring can be easily located by following the spermatic cord superiorly from the root of the scrotum to the lower abdominal wall where the external spermatic fascia of the spermatic cord is continuous with the margins of the superficial inguinal ring.
- In women, the pubic tubercle can be palpated and the ring is superior and lateral to it.

The deep inguinal ring, which is the internal opening to the inguinal canal, lies superior to the inguinal ligament, midway between the anterior superior iliac spine and pubic symphysis. The pulse of the femoral artery can be felt in the same position but deep to the inguinal ligament.

Because the superficial inguinal ring is the site where inguinal hernias appear, particularly in men, this ring and related parts of the inguinal canal are often evaluated during physical examination.

How to determine lumbar vertebral levels

Lumbar vertebral levels are useful for visualizing the positions of viscera and major blood vessels. The approximate positions of the lumbar vertebrae can be established using palpable or visible landmarks (Fig. 4.165):

- A horizontal plane passes through the medial ends of the ninth costal cartilages and the body of the LI vertebra—this transpyloric plane cuts through the body midway between the suprasternal (jugular) notch and the pubic symphysis.

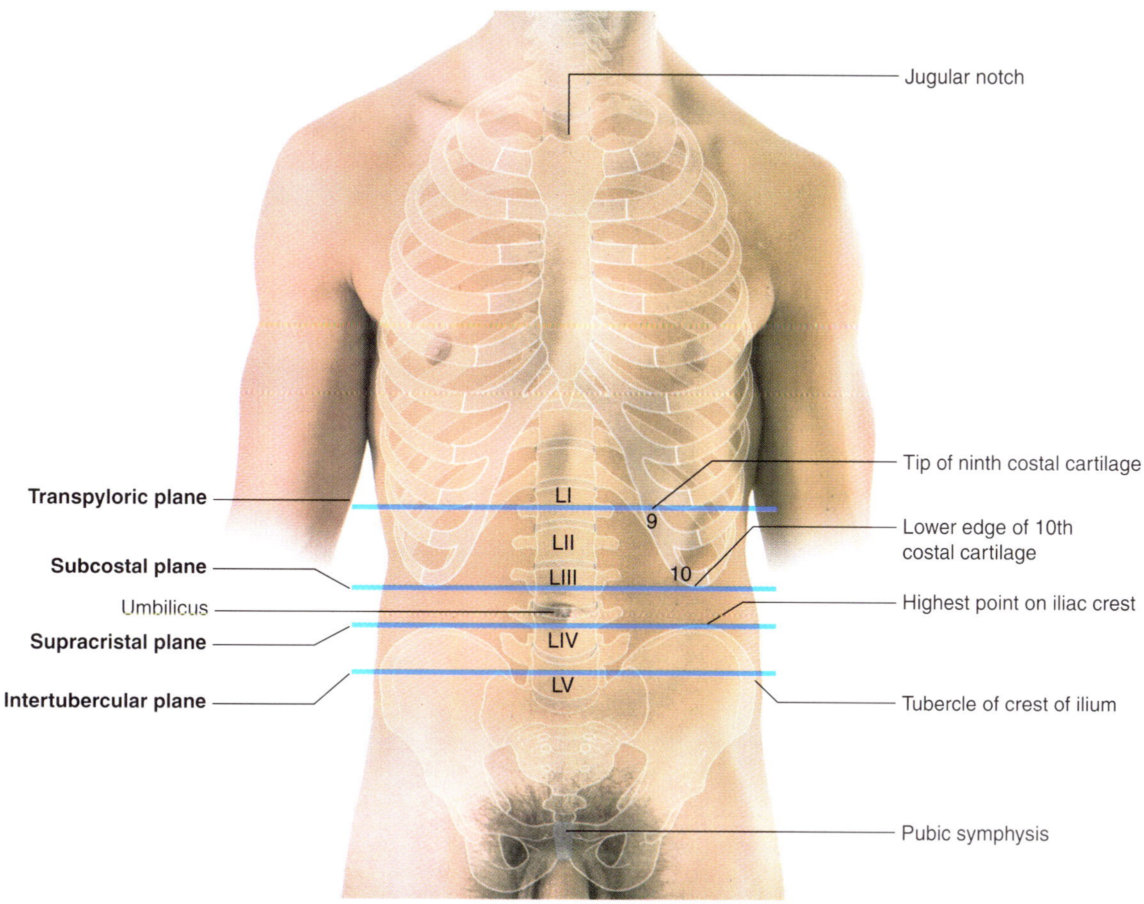

Fig. 4.165 Landmarks used for establishing the positions of lumbar vertebrae are indicated. Anterior view of the abdominal region of a man.

- A horizontal plane passes through the lower edge of the costal margin (10th costal cartilage) and the body of the LIII vertebra—the umbilicus is normally on a horizontal plane that passes through the disc between the LIII and LIV vertebrae.
- A horizontal plane (supracristal plane) through the highest point on the iliac crest passes through the spine and body of the LIV vertebra.
- A plane through the tubercles of the crest of the ilium passes through the body of the LV vertebra.

Visualizing structures at the LI vertebral level

The LI vertebral level is marked by the transpyloric plane, which cuts transversely through the body midway between the jugular notch and pubic symphysis, and through the tips of the ninth costal cartilages (Fig. 4.166). At this level are the following:

- The beginning and upper limit of the end of the duodenum
- The hila of the kidneys
- The neck of the pancreas
- The origin of the superior mesenteric artery from the aorta

The left and right colic flexures also are close to this level (Fig. 4.83).

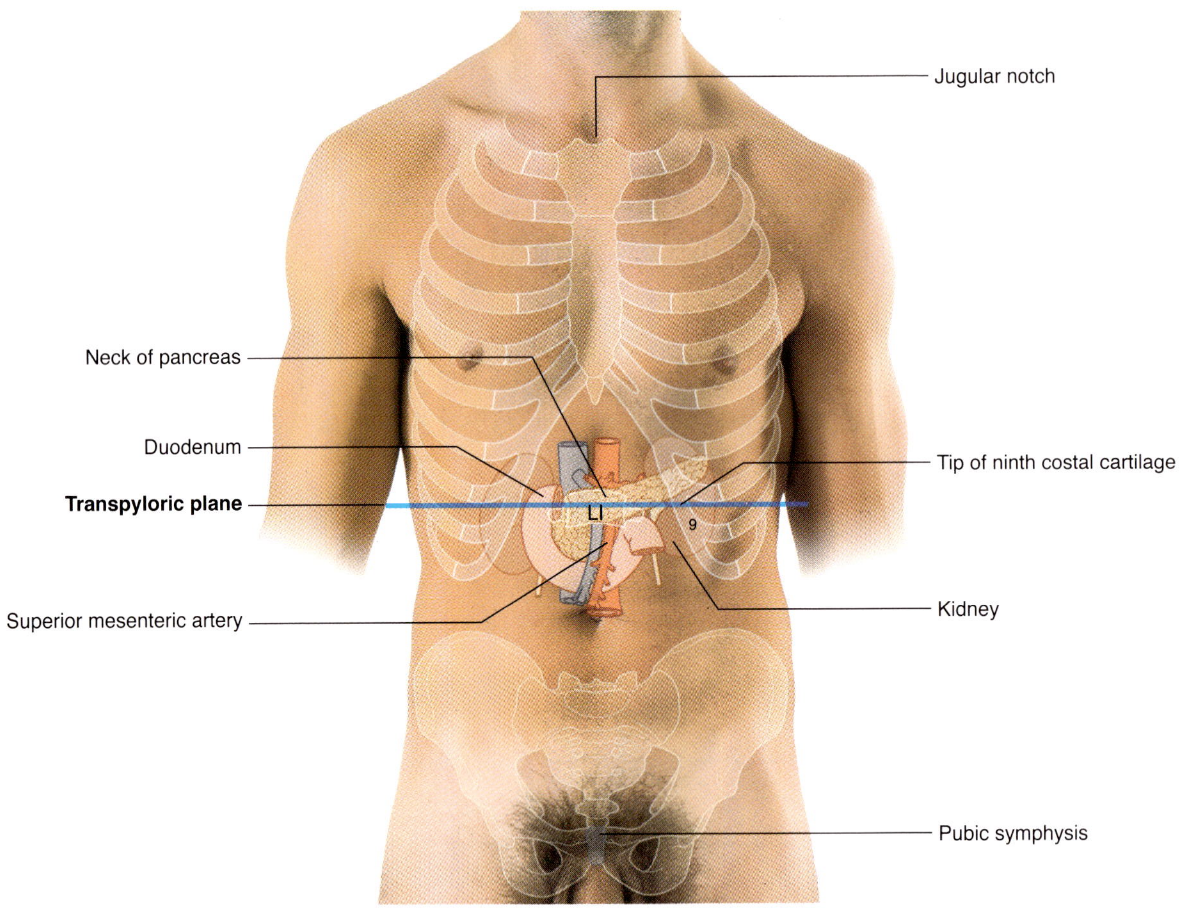

Fig. 4.166 LI vertebral level and the important viscera associated with this level. Anterior view of the abdominal region of a man.

Visualizing the position of major blood vessels

Each of the following vertebral levels in the abdomen is related to the origin of major blood vessels (Fig. 4.167):

- The celiac trunk originates from the aorta at the upper border of the LI vertebra.
- The superior mesenteric artery originates at the lower border of the LI vertebra.
- The renal arteries originate at approximately the LII vertebra.
- The inferior mesenteric artery originates at the LIII vertebra.
- The aorta bifurcates into the right and left common iliac arteries at the level of the LIV vertebra.
- The left and right common iliac veins join to form the inferior vena cava at the LV vertebral level.

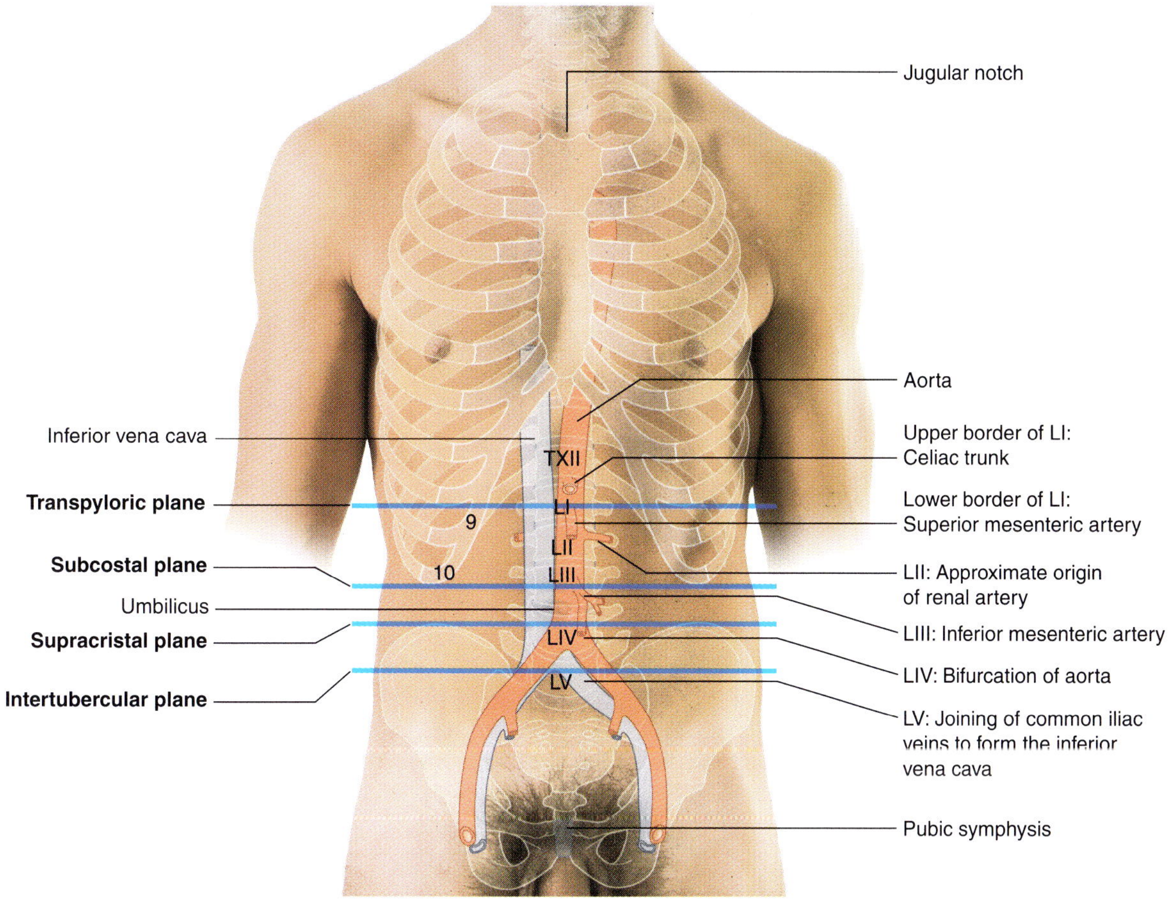

Fig. 4.167 Major vessels projected onto the body's surface. Anterior view of the abdominal region of a man.

Using abdominal quadrants to locate major viscera

The abdomen can be divided into quadrants by a vertical median plane and a horizontal transumbilical plane, which passes through the umbilicus (Fig. 4.168):

- The liver and gallbladder are in the right upper quadrant.
- The stomach and spleen are in the left upper quadrant.
- The cecum and appendix are in the right lower quadrant.
- The end of the descending colon and sigmoid colon are in the left lower quadrant.

Most of the liver is under the right dome of the diaphragm and is deep to the lower thoracic wall. The inferior margin of the liver can be palpated descending below the right costal margin when a patient is asked to inhale deeply. On deep inspiration, the edge of the liver can be felt "slipping" under the palpating fingers placed under the costal margin.

A common surface projection of the appendix is McBurney's point, which is one-third of the way up along a line from the right anterior superior iliac spine to the umbilicus.

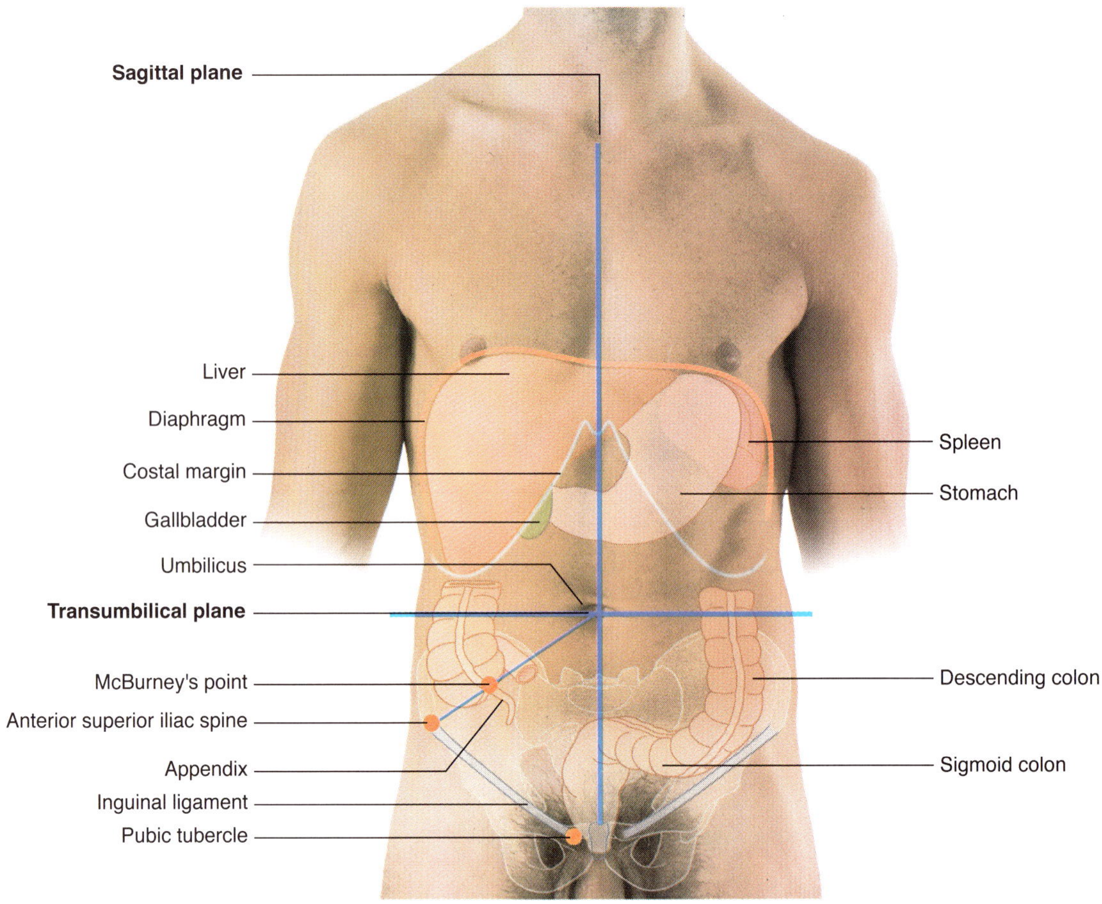

Fig. 4.168 Abdominal quadrants and the positions of major viscera. Anterior view of a man.

Defining surface regions to which pain from the gut is referred

The abdomen can be divided into nine regions by a midclavicular sagittal plane on each side and by the subcostal and intertubercular planes, which pass through the body transversely (Fig. 4.169). These planes separate the abdomen into:

- Three central regions (epigastric, umbilical, pubic)
- Three regions on each side (hypochondrium, flank, groin)

Pain from the abdominal part of the foregut is referred to the epigastric region, pain from the midgut is referred to the umbilical region, and pain from the hindgut is referred to the pubic region.

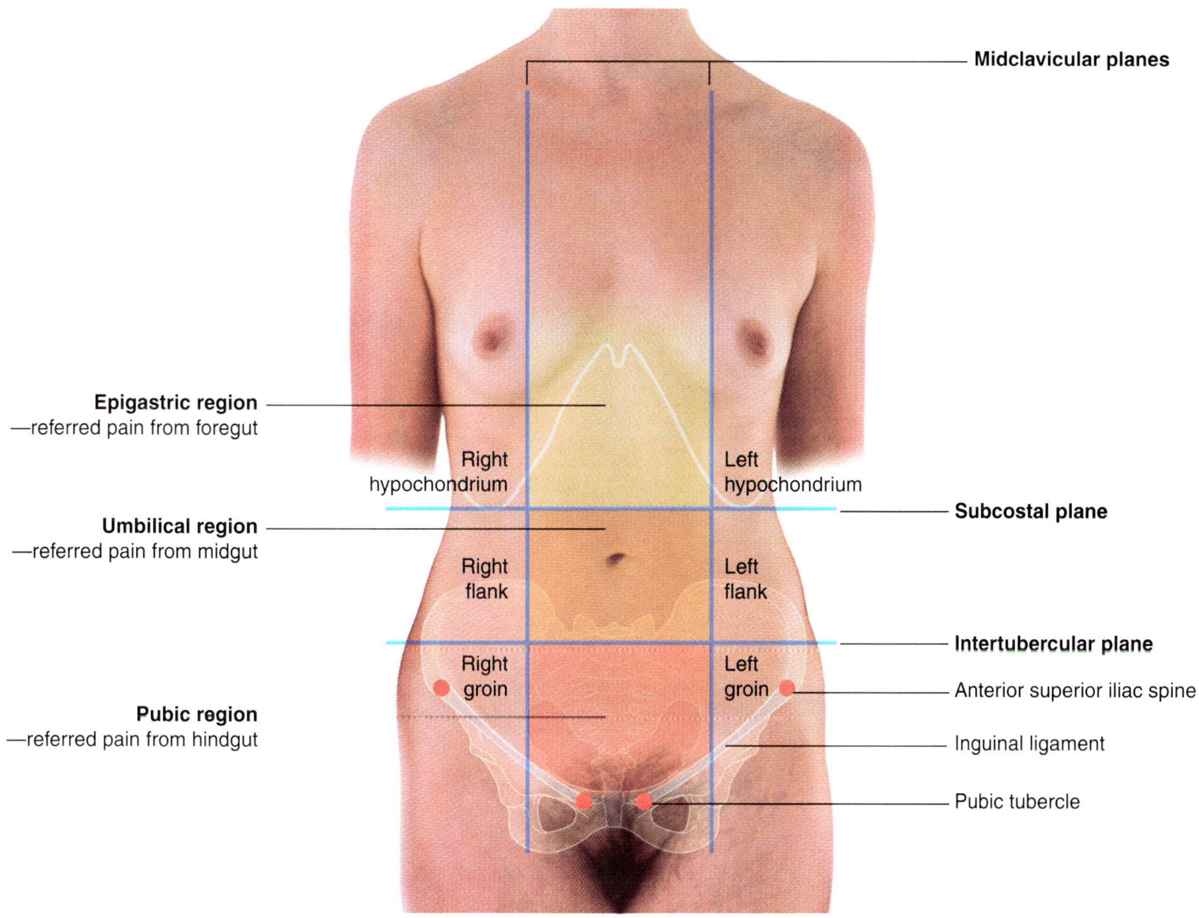

Fig. 4.169 The nine regions of the abdomen. Anterior view of a woman.

Where to find the kidneys

The kidneys project onto the back on either side of the midline and are related to the lower ribs (Fig. 4.170):

- The left kidney is a little higher than the right and reaches as high as rib XI.
- The superior pole of the right kidney reaches only as high as the 11th intercostal space.

The lower poles of the kidneys are located around the level of the disc between the LIII and LIV vertebrae. The hila of the kidneys and the beginnings of the ureters are at approximately the LI vertebra.

The ureters descend vertically anterior to the tips of the transverse processes of the lower lumbar vertebrae and enter the pelvis.

Where to find the spleen

The spleen projects onto the left side and back in the area of ribs IX to XI (Fig. 4.171). The long axis of the spleen follows the contour of rib X and extends from the superior pole of the left kidney to just posterior to the midaxillary line.

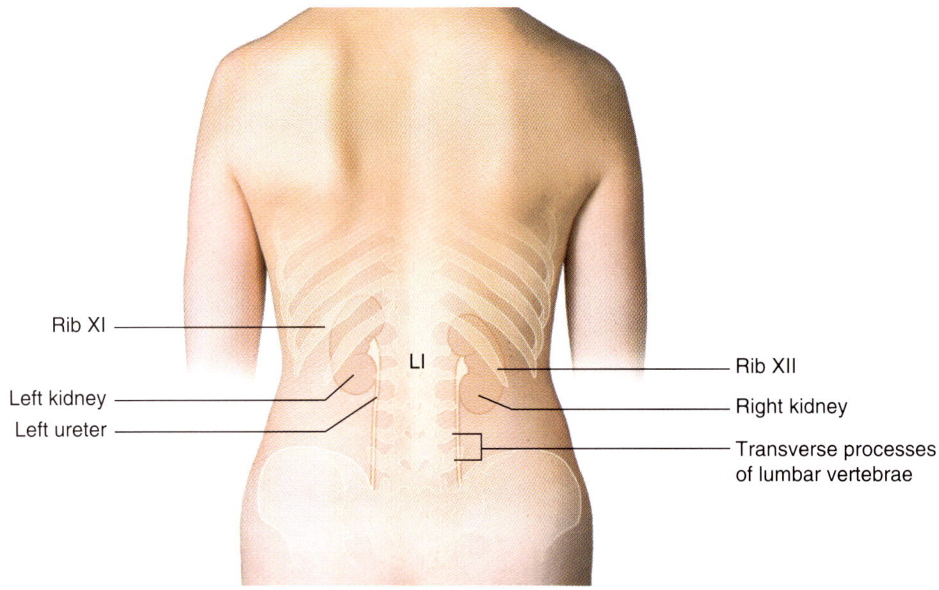

Fig. 4.170 Surface projection of the kidneys and ureters. Posterior view of the abdominal region of a woman.

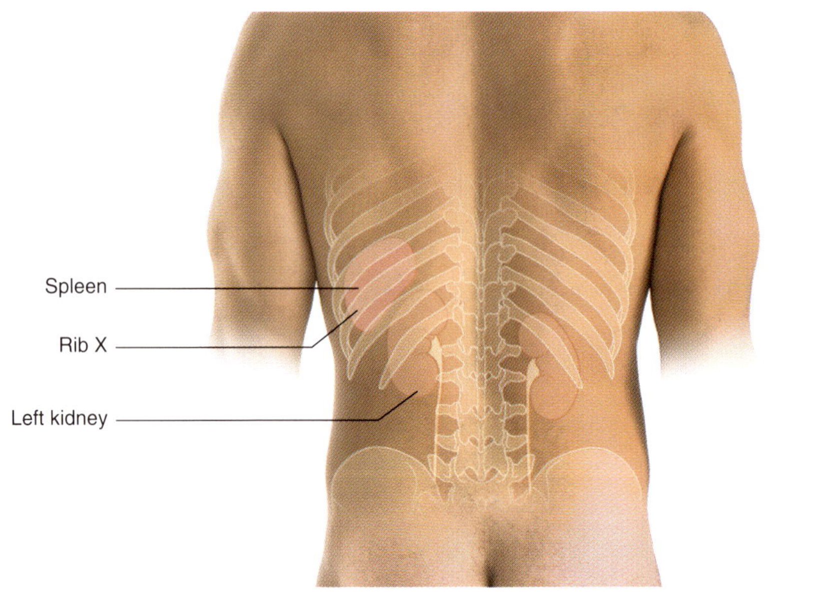

Fig. 4.171 Surface projection of the spleen. Posterior view of a man.

Clinical cases

Case 1

TRAUMATIC RUPTURE OF THE DIAPHRAGM

A 45-year-old man had mild epigastric pain, and a diagnosis of esophageal reflux was made. He was given appropriate medication, which worked well. However, at the time of the initial consultation, the family practitioner requested a chest radiograph, which demonstrated a prominent hump on the left side of the diaphragm and old rib fractures.

The patient was recalled for further questioning.

He was extremely pleased with the treatment he had been given for his gastroesophageal reflux, but was concerned about being recalled for further history and examination. During the interview, he revealed that he had previously been involved in a motorcycle accident and had undergone a laparotomy for a "rupture." The patient did not recall what operation was performed, but was assured at the time that the operation was a great success.

The patient is likely to have undergone a splenectomy.

In any patient who has had severe blunt abdominal trauma (such as that caused by a motorcycle accident), lower left-sided rib fractures are an extremely important sign of appreciable trauma.

A review of the patient's old notes revealed that at the time of the injury, the spleen was removed surgically, but it was not appreciated that there was a small rupture of the dome of the left hemidiaphragm. The patient gradually developed a hernia through which bowel could enter, producing the "hump" on the diaphragm seen on the chest radiograph.

Because this injury occurred many years ago and the patient has been asymptomatic, it is unlikely that the patient will come to any harm and was counseled.

Case 2

CHRONIC THROMBOSIS OF THE INFERIOR VENA CAVA

A medical student was asked to inspect the abdomen of two patients. In the first patient, he noted irregular veins radiating from the umbilicus. In the second patient, he noted irregular veins over the anterior abdominal wall. The direction of the flow of blood in the veins coursed in a caudal to cranial direction, from the groin to the chest. He was asked to explain his findings and determine the significance of these features.

In the first patient, the veins were draining radially away from the periumbilical region. In normal individuals, enlarged veins do not radiate from the umbilicus. In patients with portal hypertension, the portal venous pressure is increased as a result of hepatic disease. Small collateral paraumbilical veins open up around the obliterated umbilical vein. These veins pass through the umbilicus and drain onto the anterior abdominal wall, forming a portosystemic anastomosis. The eventual diagnosis for this patient was cirrhosis of the liver.

The finding of veins draining in a caudocranial direction on the anterior abdominal wall in the second patient is not typical for veins on the anterior abdominal wall. When veins are so prominent, it usually implies that there is an obstruction to the normal route of venous drainage and an alternative route has been taken. Typically, blood from the lower limbs and the retroperitoneal organs drains into the inferior vena cava and from here to the right atrium of the heart. This patient had a chronic thrombosis of the inferior vena cava, preventing blood from returning to the heart by the "usual" route.

Blood from the lower limbs and the pelvis may drain via a series of collateral vessels, some of which include the superficial and inferior epigastric veins. The former runs in the superficial fascia. These anastomose with the superior, superficial, and deep epigastric venous systems to drain into the lateral thoracic and internal thoracic veins, which in turn drain into the brachiocephalic veins and the superior vena cava.

After the initial inferior vena cava thrombosis, the veins of the anterior abdominal wall and other collateral pathways hypertrophy to accommodate the increase in blood flow.

Case 3

LIVER BIOPSY IN PATIENTS WITH SUSPECTED LIVER CIRRHOSIS

A 55-year-old man developed severe jaundice and a massively distended abdomen. A diagnosis of cirrhosis of the liver was made, and further confirmatory tests demonstrated that the patient had significant ascites (free fluid within the peritoneal cavity). A liver biopsy was necessary to confirm the cirrhosis, but there was some debate about how this biopsy should be obtained (Fig. 4.172**).**

In patients with cirrhosis, it is important to determine the extent of the cirrhosis and the etiology.

History, examination, and blood tests are useful and are supported by complex radiological investigations. To begin treatment and determine the prognosis, a sample of liver tissue must be obtained. However, there are important issues to consider when taking a liver biopsy from a patient with suspected cirrhosis.

One issue is liver function.

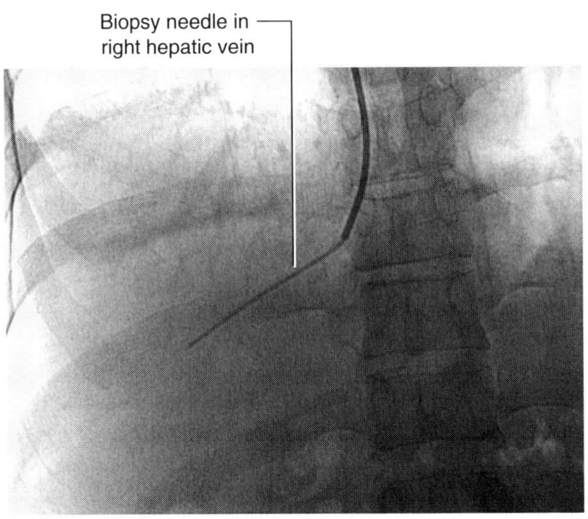

Fig. 4.172 Transjugular liver biopsy needle in the right hepatic vein. Radiograph.

The liver function of patients with suspected liver disease is poor, as demonstrated by the patient's jaundice—an inability to conjugate bilirubin. Importantly, because some liver products are blood-clotting factors involved in the clotting cascade, the blood-clotting ability of patients with severe liver disease is significantly impaired. These patients therefore have a high risk of bleeding.

Another issue is the presence of ascites.

Normally, the liver rests against the lateral and anterior abdominal walls. This direct contact can be useful for care after a liver biopsy has been obtained. After the procedure, the patient lies over the region where the biopsy has been obtained and the weight of the liver stems any localized bleeding. When patients have significant ascites, the liver cannot be compressed against the walls of the abdomen and blood may pour freely into the ascitic fluid.

The patient has ascites, so another approach for a liver biopsy must be considered.

The patient was referred to the radiology department for a transjugular liver biopsy.

The skin around the jugular vein in the neck was anesthetized. Access was obtained through insertion of a needle and a guidewire. The guidewire was advanced through the right internal jugular vein and into the right brachiocephalic vein. It entered the superior vena cava, was passed along the posterior wall of the atrium, and entered the superior aspect of the inferior vena cava. A catheter was inserted over the wire and directed into the right hepatic vein. Using a series of dilators, the vein was enlarged and a biopsy needle was placed over the wire and into the right hepatic vein. The liver was biopsied through the right hepatic vein and the biopsy sample was removed. A simple suture was used to close the internal jugular vein in the neck, and minor compression stemmed any blood flow.

Assuming that the biopsy needle does not penetrate the liver capsule, it is not important how much the patient bleeds from the liver, because this bleeding will enter the hepatic vein and is immediately returned to the circulation.

Case 4

HODGKIN'S LYMPHOMA

A 30-year-old man had a diffuse and poorly defined epigastric mass. Further examination revealed asymmetrical scrotal enlargement.

As part of her differential diagnosis, the resident considered the possibility that the man had testicular cancer with regional abdominal paraaortic (lateral aortic or lumbar) nodal involvement.

A primary testicular neoplasm is the most common tumor in men between the ages of 25 and 34 years and accounts for between 1% and 2% of all malignancies in men. A family history of testicular cancer and maldescent of the testis are strong predisposing factors.

Spread of the tumor is typically to the lymph node chains that drain the testes.

The testes develop from structures adjacent to the renal vessels in the upper abdomen, between the transversalis fascia and the peritoneum. They normally migrate through the inguinal canals into the scrotum just before birth. The testes take with them their arterial supply, their venous drainage, their nerve supply, and their lymphatics.

A CT scan revealed a paraaortic lymph node mass in the upper abdomen and enlarged lymph nodes throughout the internal and common iliac lymph node chains.

Assuming the scrotal mass was a carcinoma of the testes, which would normally drain into the lateral aortic (lumbar) nodes in the upper abdomen, it would be very unusual for iliac lymphadenopathy to be present.

Further examination of the scrotal mass was required.

A transillumination test of the scrotum on the affected side was positive. An ultrasound scan revealed normal right and left testes and a large fluid collection around the right testis. A diagnosis of a right-sided hydrocele was made.

Scrotal masses are common in young males, and determining the exact anatomical site of the scrotal mass is of utmost clinical importance. Any mass that arises from the testis should be investigated to exclude testicular cancer. Masses that arise from the epididymis and scrotal lesions, such as fluid (hydrocele) or hernias, are also clinically important but are not malignant.

The ultrasound scan revealed fluid surrounding the testis, which is diagnostic of a hydrocele. Simple cysts arising from and around the epididymis (epididymal cysts) can be easily defined.

A diagnosis of lymphoma was suspected.

Lymphoma is a malignant disease of lymph nodes. Most lymphomas are divided into two specific types, namely Hodgkin's lymphoma and non-Hodgkin's lymphoma. If caught early, the prognosis following radical chemotherapy is excellent.

The patient underwent a biopsy, which was performed from the posterior approach. He was placed in the prone position in the CT scanner. A fine needle with a special cutting device was used to obtain a lymph node sample. A left-sided approach was used because the inferior vena cava is on the right side and the nodes were in the paraaortic regions (i.e., the biopsy needle would have to pass between the inferior vena cava and the aorta from a posterior approach, which is difficult). The skin was anesthetized using local anesthetic at the lateral border of the quadratus lumborum muscle. The needle was angled at approximately 45° within the quadratus lumborum muscle and entered the retroperitoneum to lie beside the left-sided paraaortic lymph nodes. Because this procedure is performed using CT guidance, the operator can advance the needle slowly, taking care not to "hit" other retroperitoneal structures.

A good biopsy was obtained and the diagnosis was Hodgkin's lymphoma. The patient underwent chemotherapy and 2 years later was in full remission and was leading an active life.

Case 5

INGUINAL HERNIA

A 35-year-old man had a soft mass approximately 3 cm in diameter in the right scrotum. The diagnosis was a right indirect inguinal hernia.

What were the examination findings?

The mass was not tender and the physician was not able to "get above it." The testes were felt separate from the mass, and a transillumination test (in which a bright light is placed behind the scrotum and the scrotal sac is viewed from the front) was negative. (A positive test occurs when the light penetrates through the scrotum.)

When the patient stood up, a positive cough "impulse" was felt within the mass.

After careful and delicate maneuvering, the mass could be massaged into the inguinal canal, so being emptied from the scrotum. When the massaging hand was removed, the mass recurred in the scrotum.

An indirect inguinal hernia enters the inguinal canal through the deep inguinal ring. It passes through the inguinal canal to exit through the superficial inguinal ring in the aponeurosis of the external oblique muscle. The neck of the hernial sac lies superior and medial to the pubic tubercle and enters into the scrotum within the spermatic cord.

A direct inguinal hernia passes directly through the posterior wall of the inguinal canal. It does not pass down the inguinal canal. If large enough, it may pass through the superficial inguinal ring and into the scrotum.

Case 6

URETERIC STONE

A 25-year-old man developed severe pain in the left lower quadrant of his abdomen. The pain was diffuse and relatively constant but did ease for short periods of time. On direct questioning, the patient indicated that the pain was in the inguinal region and radiated posteriorly into his left infrascapular region (loin). A urine dipstick was positive for blood (hematuria).

A diagnosis of a ureteric stone (calculus) was made.

The patient initially had infrascapular pain, which later radiated to the left groin. This was related to the passage of the ureteric stone along the ureter.

The origin of the pain relates to ureteral distention.

A series of peristaltic waves along the ureter transport urine along the length of the ureter from the kidney to the bladder. As the ureteric stone obstructs the kidney, the ureter becomes distended, resulting in pain. The peristaltic waves are superimposed upon the distention, resulting in periods of exacerbation and periods of relief.

The pain is referred.

The visceral afferent (sensory) nerve fibers from the ureter pass into the spinal cord, entering the first and second lumbar segments of the spinal cord. Pain is thus referred to cutaneous regions innervated by somatic sensory nerves from the same spinal cord levels.

The patient was investigated by a CT scan.

Traditionally, patients are investigated with a plain radiograph to look for a radiopaque stone (90% of renal stones are radiopaque).

An ultrasound scan may be useful to assess for pelvicaliceal dilatation and may reveal stones at the pelviureteral junction or the vesicoureteric junction. Ultrasound is also valuable for assessing other causes of obstruction (e.g., tumors at and around the ureteric orifices in the bladder).

Usually an intravenous urogram would be carried out to enable assessment of the upper urinary tract and precise location of the stone.

Not infrequently, CT scans of the abdomen are also obtained. These scans not only give information about the kidneys, ureters, and bladder but also show the position of the stone and other associated pathology.

If this patient's infrascapular pain was on the right and predominantly within the right lower abdomen, appendicitis would also have to be excluded. A CT scan would enable differentiation of appendicitis and urinary colic.

Case 7

INTRAABDOMINAL ABSCESS

A 27-year-old woman was admitted to the surgical ward with appendicitis. She underwent an appendectomy. It was noted at operation that the appendix had perforated and there was pus within the abdominal cavity. The appendix was removed and the stump tied. The abdomen was washed out with warm saline solution. The patient initially made an uneventful recovery, but by day 7 she had become unwell, with pain over her right shoulder and spiking temperatures.

This patient had developed an intraabdominal abscess.

Any operation on the bowel may result in peritoneal contamination with fecal contents and fecal flora. This may not be appreciated at the time of the operation.

Over the postoperative period, an inflammatory reaction ensued and an abscess developed filled with pus. Typically, the observation chart revealed a "swinging" pyrexia (fever).

The most common sites for abscess to develop are the pelvis and the hepatorenal recess.

When a patient is in the supine position, the lowest points in the abdominal and pelvic cavities are the posterior superior aspect of the peritoneal cavity (the hepatorenal recess) and, in women, the rectouterine pouch (pouch of Douglas).

The shoulder pain suggested that the abscess was in the hepatorenal recess and that the pain was referred from the diaphragm.

The motor and sensory innervation of the diaphragm is from nerves C3 to C5. The somatic pain sensation from the parietal peritoneum covering the undersurface of the diaphragm is carried into the spinal cord by the phrenic nerve (C3 to C5) and is interpreted by the brain as coming from skin over the shoulder—a region supplied by other somatic sensory nerves entering the same levels of the spinal cord as those from the diaphragm.

A chest radiograph demonstrated elevation of the right hemidiaphragm.

This elevation of the right hemidiaphragm was due to the pus tracking from the hepatorenal space around the lateral and anterior aspect of the liver to reach the top of the liver in a subphrenic position. An ultrasound scan demonstrated this collection of fluid. The abscess cavity could be clearly seen by placing the ultrasound probe between ribs XI and XII. The inferior border of the right lower lobe lies at rib X in the midaxillary line. When the probe is placed between ribs XI and XII, the ultrasound waves pass between the intercostal muscles and the parietal pleura laterally on the chest wall, and continue through the parietal pleura overlying the diaphragm into the cavity of the abscess, which lies below the diaphragm.

Drainage was not by an intercostal route. Instead, using CT guidance and local anesthesia, a subcostal drain was established and 1 L of pus was removed (Fig. 4.173). It is important to bear in mind that placing a drain through the pleural cavity into the abdominal cavity effectively allows intraabdominal pus to pass into the thoracic cavity, and that this may produce an empyema (pus in the pleural space).

The patient made a slow and uneventful recovery.

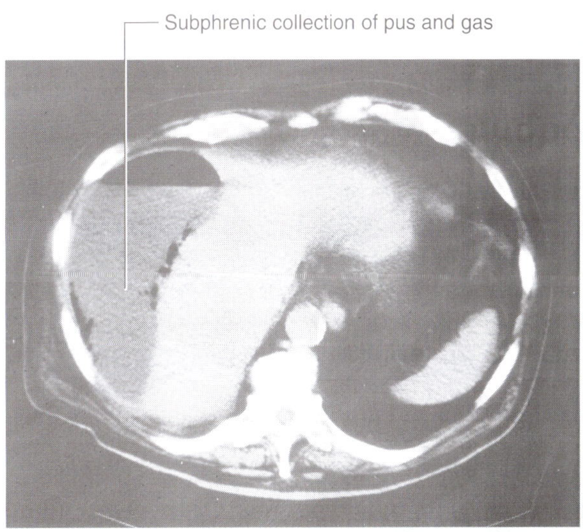

Fig. 4.173 Subphrenic collection of pus and gas. Computed tomogram in the axial plane.

Case 8

COMPLICATIONS OF AN ABDOMINOPERINEAL RESECTION

A 45-year-old man developed a low-grade rectal carcinoma just above the anorectal margin. He underwent an abdominoperineal resection of the tumor and was left with a left lower abdominal colostomy (which is described below). Unfortunately, the man's wife left him for a number of reasons, including lack of sexual desire. He "turned to drink" and over the ensuing years developed cirrhosis. He was brought into the emergency room with severe bleeding from enlarged veins around his colostomy. An emergency transjugular intrahepatic portosystemic shunt was created, which stopped all bleeding (Fig. 4.174 and 4.175)**. He is now doing well in a rehabilitation program.**

A colostomy was necessary because of the low site of the tumor.

Carcinoma of the colon and rectum usually develops in older patients, but some people get tumors early in life. Most tumors develop from benign polyps, which undergo malignant change. As the malignancy develops, it invades through the wall of the bowel and then metastasizes to local lymphatics. The tumor extends within the wall for a few centimeters above and below its origin. Lymphatic spread is to local and regional lymph nodes and then to the preaortic lymph node chain. These drain eventually into the thoracic duct.

When this man was assessed for surgery, the tumor was so close to the anal margin that resection of the sphincters was necessary to be certain that the tumor margins were clear. The bowel cannot be joined to the anus without sphincters because the patient would be fecally incontinent. At surgery, the tumor was excised, including the locoregional lymph node chains and the peritumoral fat around the rectum.

The free end of the sigmoid colon was brought through a hole in the anterior abdominal wall. The bowel was then carefully sutured to the anterior abdominal wall to allow placement of a bag to collect the feces. This is a colostomy.

Contrary to their usual immediate negative reaction to having a bag on the anterior abdominal wall, most patients cope extremely well, especially if they have been cured of cancer.

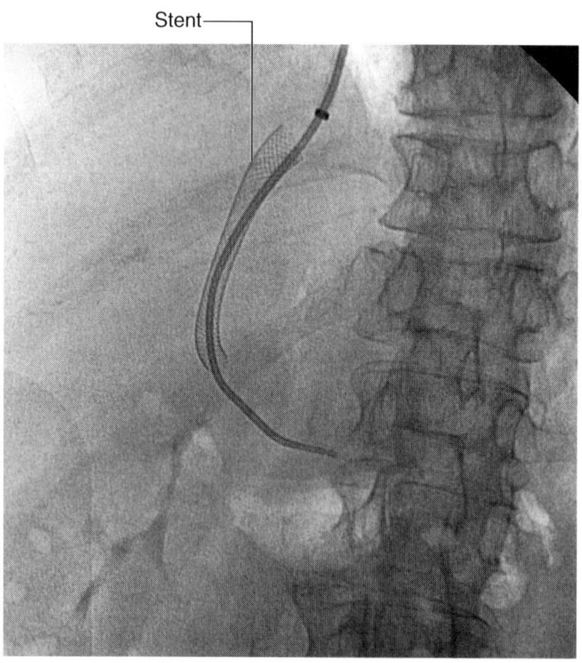

Fig. 4.174 Position of a transjugular intrahepatic portosystemic shunt stent. Radiograph.

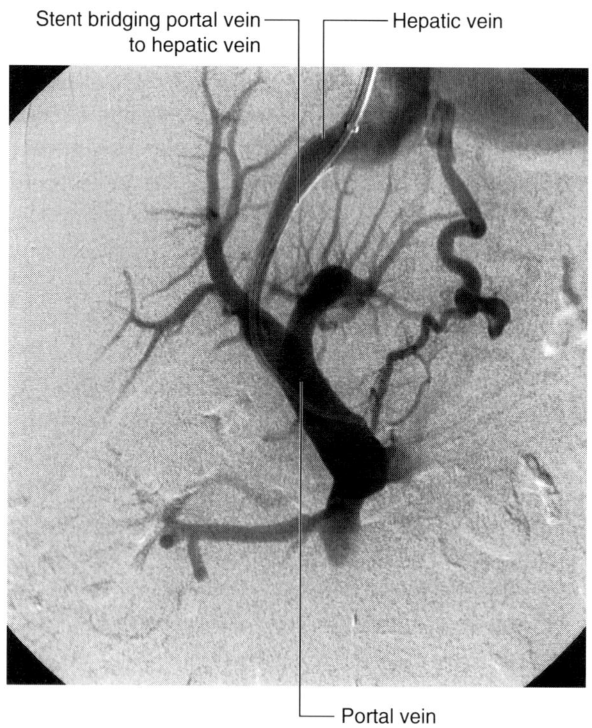

Fig. 4.175 Functioning transjugular intrahepatic portosystemic shunt. Venogram.

Case 8 *(continued)*

This patient's pelvic nerves were damaged. The radical pelvic surgical dissection damaged the pelvic parasympathetic nerve supply necessary for erection of the penis. Unfortunately, this was not well explained to the patient, which in some part led to the failure of his relationship. With any radical surgery in the pelvis, the nerves that supply the penis or clitoris may be damaged, so interfering with sexual function.

This patient was bleeding from stomal varices.

As he developed a serious drinking problem, his liver became cirrhotic and this damaged the normal liver architecture. This in turn increased the blood pressure in the portal vein (**portal hypertension**).

In patients with portal hypertension, small anastomoses develop between the veins of the portal system and the veins of the systemic circulation. These portosystemic anastomoses are usually of little consequence; however, at the gastroesophageal junction, they lie in a submucosal and mucosal position and are subject to trauma. Torrential hemorrhage may occur from even minor trauma, and death may ensue following blood loss. These varices require urgent treatment, which includes injecting sclerosant substances, banding, and even surgical ligation.

Fortunately, most of the other portosystemic anastomoses are of relatively little consequence. In patients with colostomies, small veins may develop between the veins of the large bowel (portal system drainage) and cutaneous veins on the anterior abdominal wall (systemic veins). If these veins become enlarged because of portal hypertension, they are subject to trauma as feces are passed through the colostomy. Torrential hemorrhage may ensue if they are damaged.

A procedure was carried out to lower the portal pressure.

To reduce the pressure in the portal vein in this patient, several surgical procedures were considered. These included connecting the side of the portal vein onto the inferior vena cava (**portacaval shunt**) and connecting the splenic vein onto the renal vein (a **splenorenal shunt**). These procedures, however, require a large abdominal incision and are extremely complex. As an alternative, it was decided to create a transjugular intrahepatic portosystemic shunt.

Creating a **transjugular intrahepatic portosystemic shunt** also called TIPPS is a relatively new technique that may be carried out under local anesthesia. Using a right internal jugular approach, a long needle is placed through the internal jugular vein, the superior vena cava, and the right atrium, into the inferior vena cava. The right hepatic vein is cannulated and, with special steering wires, a needle is passed through the hepatic substance directly into the right branch of the portal vein. A small balloon is passed over the wire and through the hepatic substance and is inflated. After the balloon has been removed, a metallic stent (a flexible wire tube) is placed across this tract in the liver to keep it open. Blood now freely flows from the portal vein into the right hepatic vein, creating a portosystemic shunt.

As a result of this procedure, the pressure in this patient's portal system is lower and similar to that of the systemic venous system, so reducing the potential for bleeding at the portosystemic anastomoses (i.e., the colostomy).

Case 9

CARCINOMA OF THE HEAD OF THE PANCREAS

A 52-year-old woman visited her family physician with complaints of increasing lethargy and vomiting. The physician examined her and noted that compared to previous visits, she had lost significant weight. She was also jaundiced, and on examination of the abdomen, a well-defined 10-cm rounded mass was palpable below the liver edge in the right upper quadrant (Fig. 4.176**).**

The clinical diagnosis was carcinoma of the head of the pancreas.

It is difficult to appreciate how such a precise diagnosis can be made clinically when only three clinical signs have been described.

The patient's obstruction was in the distal bile duct.

When a patient has jaundice, the causes are excessive breakdown of red blood cells (prehepatic), hepatic failure (hepatic jaundice), and posthepatic causes, which include obstruction along the length of the biliary tree.

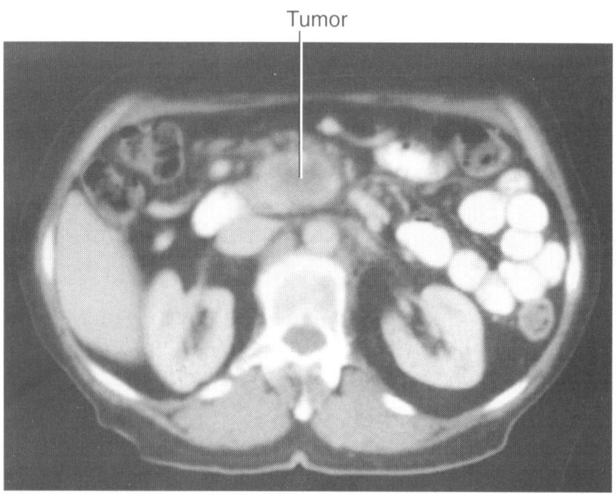

Fig. 4.176 Tumor in the head of the pancreas. Computed tomogram in the axial plane.

The patient had a mass in her right upper quadrant that was palpable below the liver; this was the gallbladder.

In healthy individuals, the gallbladder is not palpable. An expanded gallbladder indicates obstruction either within the cystic duct or below the level of the end of the cystic duct (i.e., the bile duct).

The patient's vomiting was related to the position of the tumor.

It is not uncommon for vomiting and weight loss (cachexia) to occur in patients with a malignant disease. The head of the pancreas lies within the curve of the duodenum, primarily adjacent to the descending part of the duodenum. Any tumor mass in the region of the head of the pancreas is likely to expand and may encase and invade the duodenum. Unfortunately, in this patient's case, this happened, producing almost complete obstruction. Further discussion with the patient revealed that she was vomiting relatively undigested food soon after each meal.

A CT scan demonstrated further complications.

In the region of the head and neck of the pancreas are complex anatomical structures, which may be involved with a malignant process. The CT scan confirmed a mass in the region of the head of the pancreas, which had invaded the descending part of the duodenum. The mass extended into the neck of the pancreas and had blocked the distal part of the bile duct and the pancreatic duct. Posteriorly, the mass had directly invaded the portal venous confluence of the splenic and superior mesenteric veins, producing a series of gastric, splenic, and small bowel varices.

This patient underwent palliative chemotherapy, but died 7 months later.

Case 10

OBSTRUCTION OF THE INFERIOR VENA CAVA

A 62-year-old man came to the emergency department with swelling of both legs and a large left varicocele (enlarged and engorged varicose veins around the left testis and within the left pampiniform plexus of veins).

The patient was known to have a left renal cell carcinoma and was due to have this operated on the following week.

Anatomically, it is possible to link all of the findings with the renal cell carcinoma by knowing the usual mode of spread of the tumor.

Renal cell carcinoma tends to grow steadily and predictably. Typically, when the tumor is less than 3–4 cm, it remains confined to the kidney. Large tumors have the propensity to grow into the renal vein, the inferior vena cava and the right atrium and through the heart into the pulmonary artery.

The tumor grew into the left renal vein.

As the tumor grew into the left renal vein, it blocked off all tributaries draining into that vein, the largest of which is the left testicular vein. This blockage of the left testicular vein caused a dilation of the veins around the left testis (a varicocele occurred).

The swollen legs were accounted for by obstruction of the inferior vena cava.

The tumor grew along the renal vein and into the inferior vena cava toward the heart. Renal tumors can grow rapidly; in this case, the tumor grew rapidly into the inferior vena cava, occluding it. This increased the pressure in the leg veins, resulting in swelling and pitting edema of the ankles.

The patient unfortunately died on the operating table.

In this patient's case, a "tongue" of tumor grew into the inferior vena cava. At the time of surgery, the initial dissection mobilized the kidney on its vascular pedicle; however, a large portion of tumor became detached in the inferior vena cava. The tumor embolus passed through the right atrium and right ventricle and occluded the pulmonary artery. This could not be cleared at the time of surgery, and the patient succumbed.

Case 11

DIVERTICULAR DISEASE

A 65-year-old businessman came to the emergency department with severe lower abdominal pain that was predominantly central and left sided. He had pain radiating into the left loin, and he also noticed he was passing gas and fecal debris as he urinated.

A CT scan of his abdomen and pelvis was performed (Fig. 4.177).

The CT scan demonstrated a collection of fluid (likely a pelvic abscess) in the left iliac fossa. Associated with this collection of fluid was significant bowel wall thickening of the sigmoid colon and multiple small diverticula arising throughout the sigmoid colon. Gas was present in the urinary bladder. An obstruction was noted in the left ureter and the left pelvicalyceal system.

The patient underwent an urgent operation.

As the surgeons entered into the abdominal cavity through a midline incision, they noted that tissues in the left iliac fossa were significantly inflamed. The surgeon used his hand to mobilize the sigmoid colon and entered a cavity in which

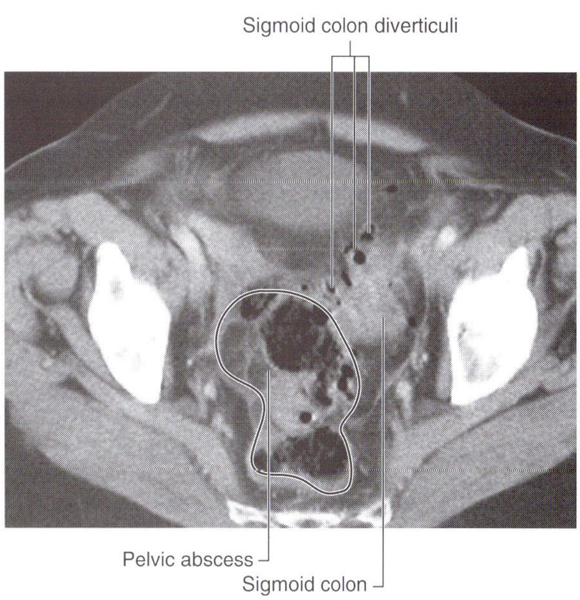

Fig. 4.177 A computed tomogram, in the axial plane, of the pelvis demonstrates a loop of sigmoid colon with numerous diverticula and a large abscess in the pelvic cavity.

Continued

Case 11 *(continued)*

there was a collection of pus as indicated on the CT scan. The pus was washed out and drained. The sigmoid colon was remarkably thickened and inflamed and stuck to the superior surface of the urinary bladder. Careful finger dissection revealed a small perforation in the superior surface of the urinary bladder, allowing the passage of fecal material and gas into the bladder and producing the patient's symptoms of pneumaturia and fecaluria. The sigmoid colon was resected. The rectal stump was oversewn and the descending colon was passed through the anterior abdominal wall to form a colostomy. The bladder was catheterized and the small hole in the dome of the bladder was oversewn.

The patient had a difficult postoperative period in the intensive care unit where he remained pyrexial and septic. The colostomy began to function well.

An ultrasound was performed and demonstrated the continued dilatation in the left kidney, and the patient underwent a nephrostomy.

Under ultrasound guidance, a drainage catheter was placed into the renal pelvis through the renal cortex on the left. A significant amount of pus was drained initially; however, after 24 hours urine passed freely.

The likely cause for the obstruction was the inflammation around the distal ureter on the left. It is also possible that a small ureteric perforation occurred, allowing bacteria to enter the urinary tract.

The patient made a further uneventful recovery with resumption of normal renal function and left the hospital.

On return to the surgeon in the outpatient clinic some weeks later, the patient did not wish to continue with his colostomy and bag. Further to discussion, surgery was planned to "rejoin" the ends of the colon.

At operation, the colostomy was "taken down" and the rectal stump was identified. There was, however, a significant gap between the bowel ends. To enable the bowel to be sutured, the descending colon was mobilized from the posterior abdominal wall. An anastomosis was performed and the patient left the hospital 1 week later and currently remains well.

Case 12

ENDOLEAK AFTER ENDOVASCULAR REPAIR OF ABDOMINAL AORTIC ANEURYSM

A 72-year-old man was brought to the emergency department with an abdominal aortic aneurysm (an expansion of the infrarenal abdominal aorta). The aneurysm measured 10 cm, and after discussion with the patient a repair was scheduled.

The surgical and endovascular treatment options were explained to the patient.

Treatment of abdominal aortic aneurysms has been, for many years, an operative procedure where the dilatation (ballooning) of the aorta is resected and a graft is sewn into position. A modern option is to place a graft to line the aneurysm from within the artery (endovascular aneurysm repair). In this technique, the surgeon dissects the femoral artery and makes a small hole in it. The graft is compressed within a catheter and the catheter is passed through the femoral artery and the iliac arterial system into the distal abdominal aorta. The graft can then be released inside the aorta, effectively relining it to prevent further expansion of the aneurysm.

Occasionally, the relined aneurysm may continue to enlarge after the endovascular graft has been placed and the cause needs to be identified.

A Doppler ultrasound investigation of the abdomen and a CT scan revealed there was flow between the endovascular lining and the wall of the aneurysm.

The likely sources for this bleeding were assessed.

The graft usually begins below the level of the renal arteries and divides into two limbs that end in the common iliac arteries. The aneurysm may continue to be fed from any vessels between the graft and the aneurysm wall. These vessels can include the lumbar arteries and the inferior mesenteric artery. Interestingly, blood usually flows from the abdominal aorta into the inferior mesenteric artery and the lumbar arteries; however, with the changes in flow dynamics with the graft in place, blood may flow in the opposite direction through these branches, thereby leading to enlargement of the aneurysm.

Blood flow was from the superior mesenteric artery into the aneurysm sac.

Case 12 *(continued)*

Above the level of the graft, the superior mesenteric artery arises normally. From the right colic and middle colic branches, a marginal branch around the colon anastomoses, in the region of the splenic flexure, with marginal branches from the inferior mesenteric artery (this can become a hypertrophied vessel known as the marginal artery of Drummond). In this situation, blood passed retrogradely into the inferior mesenteric artery, filling the aneurysm and allowing it to remain pressurized and expand.

The inferior mesenteric artery was ligated **laparoscopically** and the aneurysm failed to expand further. Over the ensuing 6 months, the aneurysm contracted. The patient remains fit and healthy, with two small scars in the groin.

Case 13

METASTATIC LESIONS IN THE LIVER

A 44-year-old woman had been recently diagnosed with melanoma on a toe and underwent a series of investigations.

Melanoma (properly called malignant melanoma) can be an aggressive form of skin cancer that spreads to lymph nodes and multiple other organs throughout the body. The malignant potential is dependent upon its cellular configuration and also the depth of its penetration through the skin.

The patient developed malignant melanoma in the foot, which spread to the lymph nodes of the groin. The inguinal lymph nodes were resected; however, it was noted on follow-up imaging that the patient had developed two metastatic lesions within the right lobe of the liver.

Surgeons and physicians considered the possibility of removing these lesions.

A CT scan was performed that demonstrated the lesions within segments V and VI of the liver (Fig. 4.178).

The segmental anatomy of the liver is important because it enables the surgical planning for resection.

The surgery was undertaken and involved identifying the portal vein and the confluence of the right and left hepatic ducts. The liver was divided in the imaginary principal plane of the middle hepatic vein. The right hepatic duct and biliary radicals were ligated and the right liver was successfully resected.

The segments remaining included the left lobe of the liver.

The patient underwent a surgical resection of segments V, VI, VII, and VIII. The remaining segments included IVa, IVb, I, II, and III. It is important to remember that the traditional lobes of the liver do not correlate with the hepatic volume. The traditional left lobe of the liver contains only segments II and III. The right lobe of the liver contains segments IV, V, VI, VII, and VIII. Hence, cross-sectional imaging is important when planning surgical segmental resection.

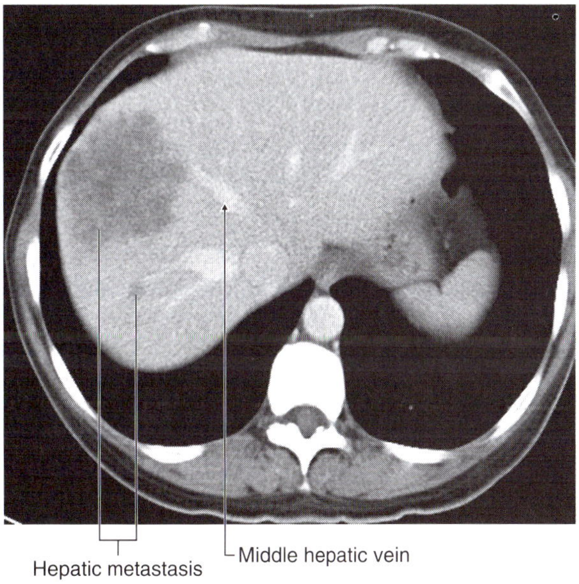

Fig. 4.178 This postcontrast computed tomogram, in the axial plane, demonstrates two metastases situated within the right lobe of the liver. The left lobe of the liver is clear. The larger of the two metastases is situated to the right of the middle hepatic vein, which lies in the principal plane of the liver dividing the left and right sides of the liver.

5

Pelvis and Perineum

ADDITIONAL LEARNING RESOURCES for Chapter 5, *Pelvis and Perineum,* on MedEnact (www.MedEnact.com):

- Multiple Choice Questions
- Short Questions—these are questions requiring short responses
- Medical Clinical Case Studies
  Pelvic fracture
  Rectovaginal fistula

FREE Online Anatomy Self-Study Course

- Anatomy modules 18 through 22

Conceptual overview

Competency: The first-year medical students should be able to apply their knowledge of the anatomy of the abdominal walls and abdominal viscera to explain the anatomical basis of common clinical conditions and procedures.

SET INDUCTION—CASE SCENARIO 1: PROSTATE CANCER

A 78-year-old male complained of lower back pain. A plain X-ray revealed a radiopaque shadow in the lumbar vertebrae. A diagnosis of prostatic cancer with metastatic spread to the vertebrae was suspected. Knowledge of the anatomy of the prostate and its venous drainage is needed to diagnose this case.

REMEMBER [Recall Facts]	OUTLINE 1. CONCEPTUAL OVERVIEW AND PELVIC REGION 1 (MALE)—LEARNING OBJECTIVES [By the end of this section, the student should be able to:] DEMONSTRATE AND ANALYZE RELATIONSHIPS [Identify structures in a Prosected Specimen or Figure]			EVALUATE [Explain Concepts]
	Level I	**Level II**	**Level III**	

1. Explain briefly the component parts of pelvic region and its relationship to other regions
2. Describe in detail the anatomy of anal canal and add a note on the anal sphincters
3. Describe the extent, embryological origin, internal features, sphincters, blood supply, lymphatic drainage, nerve supply and applied anatomy of the anal canal
4. Describe in detail the gross anatomy of urinary bladder
5. Describe in detail the location, coverings, and interior of prostate gland and add a note on the zones of prostate
6. Explain the course of ductus deferens
7. Describe the lymphatic drainage of pelvic and perineal organs
8. Describe the anatomy of testis and explain the clinical significance of blood supply to testis in relation to torsion and varicocele
	■ Pelvis wall muscles
	■ Obturator internus
	■ Levator ani
	■ Pelvis diaphragm:
	  ■ Levator ani
	  ■ Coccygeus
	■ **Rectum:**
	  ■ Location, extent, curvatures
	  ■ Houston's valves, important relations
	■ **Anal canal:**
	  ■ Interior, pectinate line
	  ■ Anal columns, anal valves
	  ■ Anal sinuses, anal sphincters
	  ■ Pelvis course of ureter in male
	■ **Urinary bladder:**
	  ■ Location, shape, parts
	  ■ Surfaces, trigone
	  ■ Ureteric and urethral openings
	  ■ Rectovesical pouch
	  ■ Important relations
	■ Parts of male urethra
	■ **Prostate gland:**
	  ■ Location, coverings
	  ■ Parts, surfaces,
	  ■ Prostatic urethra, lobes
	■ Testis
	■ Ductus deferens
	■ Seminal vesicle
		■ Internal iliac artery and vein
		■ Branches of anterior division
		■ Branches of posterior division
		■ Lumbosacral trunk (L4 and L5)
		■ Anterior rami of S1, S2, S3 forming sacral plexus
		■ Obturator nerve
		■ Rectum:
		  ■ Anorectal junction and angle
			■ Median sacral artery
			■ Superior and inferior hypogastric plexus
			■ Pelvic splanchnic
			■ Anterior rami of S4, S5, and co forming coccygeal plexus
			■ Ganglion impar
			■ Anococcygeal ligament
				■ Pelvic measurements
				■ Formation and functions of the pelvic diaphragm
				■ Autonomic nerve supply to the pelvic viscera
				■ Trigone of the urinary bladder
				■ Nerve supply of the urinary bladder
				■ Course of male urethra
				■ Lobes of the prostate
				■ Prostatic venous plexus
				■ Importance of pectinate line

EARLY CLINICAL EXPOSURE [Apply Anatomical knowledge]	
Surgical Anatomy/ Pathology/ Trauma	**Imaging/ Surface Anatomy**
■ Bladder catheterization ■ Cystitis ■ Bladder calculi ■ Benign hypertrophy of prostate ■ Carcinoma of the prostate ■ Prostatectomy ■ Stricture of the urethra ■ Rupture of the urethra ■ Carcinoma of the rectum ■ Hemorrhoids ■ Anal fissures ■ Perianal abscesses, anal fistulae ■ Digital rectal examination	■ Cystoscopy

PROBLEM SOLVING/ CLINICAL CASES [Interpret]
■ Pelvic kidney ■ Left common iliac vein obstruction (May–Thurner syndrome) ■ Reason for majority of varicoceles being on the left side

GENERAL DESCRIPTION

The pelvis and perineum are interrelated regions associated with the pelvic bones and terminal parts of the vertebral column. The bony pelvis is divided into two regions:

- The superior region related to upper parts of the pelvic bones and lower lumbar vertebrae is the **false pelvis** (**greater pelvis**) and is generally considered part of the abdomen (Fig. 5.1).
- The **true pelvis** (**lesser pelvis**) is related to the inferior parts of the pelvic bones, sacrum, and coccyx, and has an inlet and an outlet. It encloses the pelvic cavity above and the perineum below.

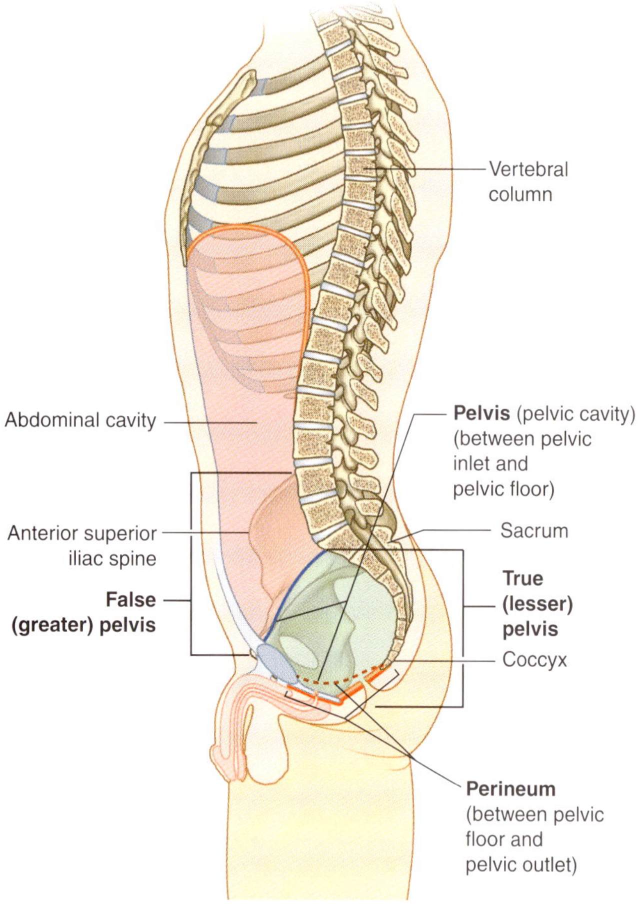

Fig. 5.1 Pelvis and perineum.

The bowl-shaped **pelvic cavity** (pelvis) consists of the pelvic inlet, walls, and pelvic floor. This cavity is continuous superiorly with the abdominal cavity and contains elements of the urinary, gastrointestinal, and reproductive systems.

The perineum (Fig. 5.1) is inferior to the floor of the pelvic cavity; its inferior boundary forms the **pelvic outlet**. The perineum contains the external genitalia and external openings of the genitourinary and gastrointestinal systems.

FUNCTIONS

Contains and supports the bladder, rectum, anal canal, and reproductive tracts

Within the pelvic cavity, the bladder is positioned anteriorly and the rectum posteriorly in the midline.

As it fills, the bladder expands superiorly into the abdomen. It is supported by adjacent elements of the pelvic bone and by the pelvic floor. The urethra passes through the pelvic floor to the perineum, where, in women, it opens externally (Fig. 5.2A) and in men it enters the base of the penis (Fig. 5.2B).

Continuous with the sigmoid colon at the level of vertebra SIII, the rectum terminates at the anal canal, which penetrates the pelvic floor to open into the perineum. The anal canal is angled posteriorly on the rectum. This flexure is maintained by muscles of the pelvic floor and is relaxed during defecation. A skeletal muscle sphincter is associated with the anal canal and the urethra as each passes through the pelvic floor.

The pelvic cavity contains most of the reproductive tract in women and part of the reproductive tract in men.

- In women, the vagina penetrates the pelvic floor and connects with the uterus in the pelvic cavity. The uterus is positioned between the rectum and the bladder. A uterine (fallopian) tube extends laterally on each side toward the pelvic wall to open near the ovary.
- In men, the pelvic cavity contains the site of connection between the urinary and reproductive tracts. It also contains major glands associated with the reproductive system—the prostate and two seminal vesicles.

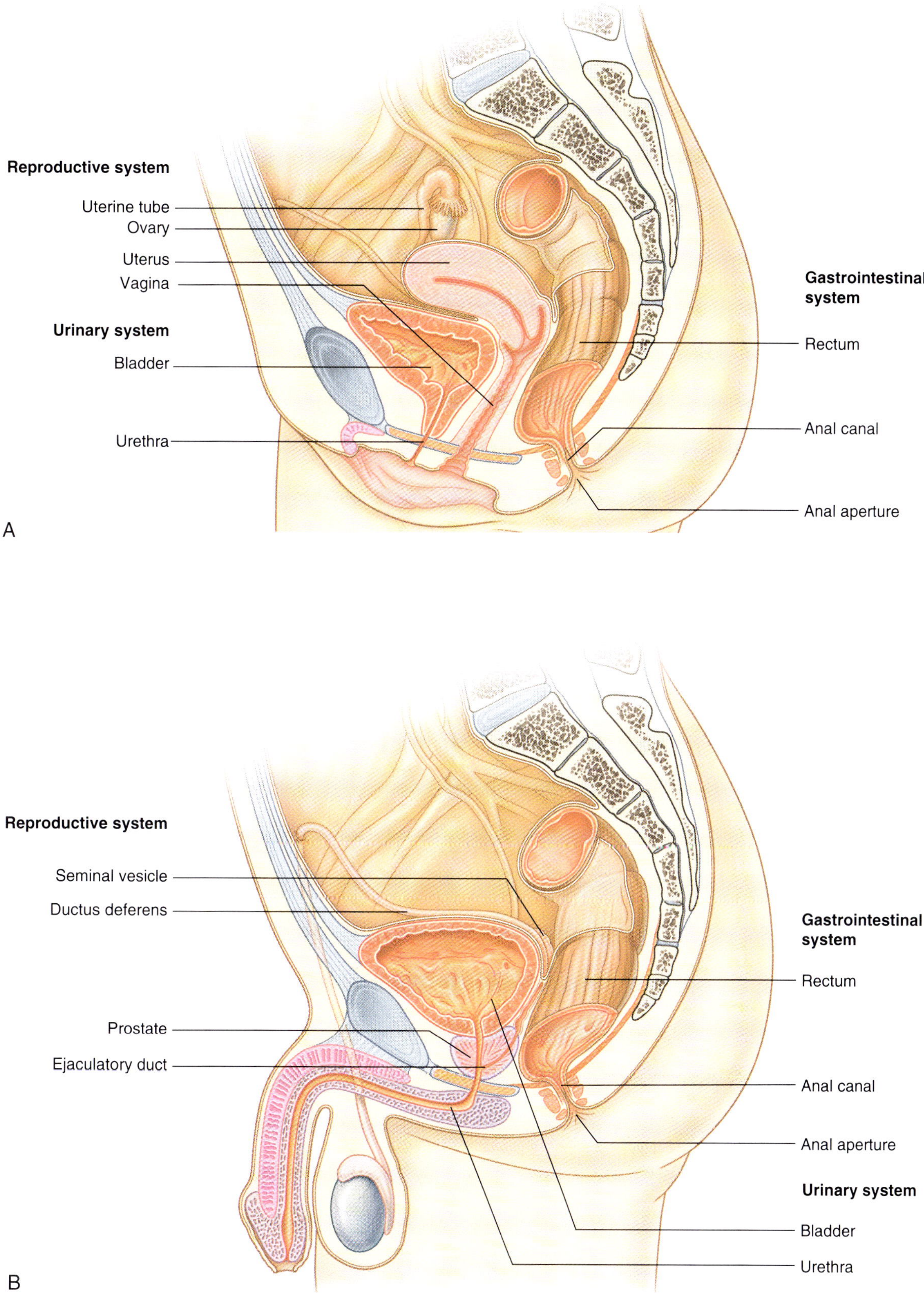

Fig. 5.2 The pelvis and perineum contain and support terminal parts of the gastrointestinal, urinary, and reproductive systems. **(A)** In women. **(B)** In men.

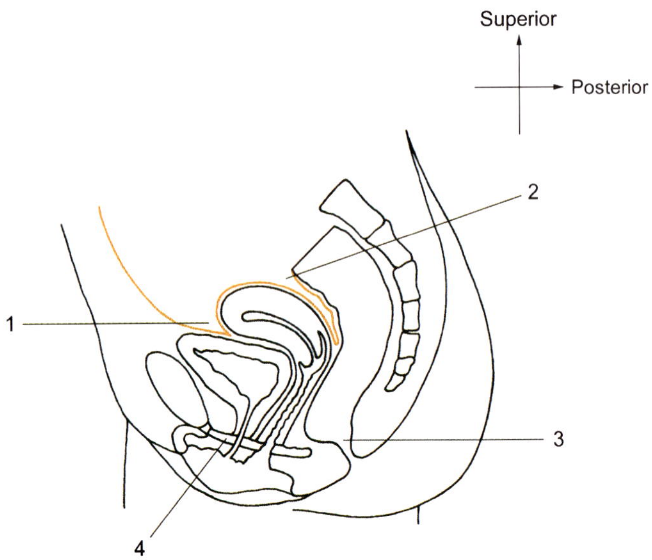

LD Fig. 5.2A.1 Outline of sagittal section of female pelvis.

Questions

5.2A.1.A Name the structures indicated by the labels.

5.2A.1.B Name the structure located in the space between the anal canal, vagina, and perineal skin.

5.2A.1.C Will a plane at the level of the ischial spines, third piece of sacrum, and the middle of the pubic symphysis pass through the cervix?

Answers

5.2A.1.A The structures indicated by the labels are the

1. Uterovesical pouch
2. Rectouterine pouch
3. Junction of rectum and anal canal
4. Urogenital diaphragm

5.2A.1.B

The structure located in the space between the anal canal, vagina, and perineal skin is the perineal body.

5.2A.1.C

Yes, a plane at the level of the ischial spines, third piece of sacrum, and the middle of the pubic symphysis will pass through the cervix.

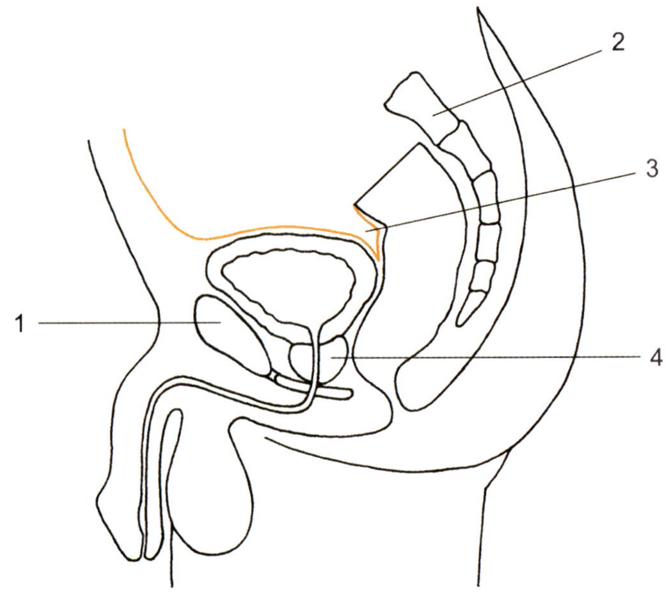

LD Fig. 5.2B.1 Outline of sagittal section of male pelvis.

Questions

5.2B.1.A Name the structures indicated by the labels.

5.2B.1.B Will a testis be seen in a midline section?

Answers

5.2B.1.A The structures indicated by the labels are the

1. Pubic symphysis
2. Sacrum
3. Rectovesical pouch
4. Prostate

5.2B.1.B

No, the testis will not be seen in a midline section.

Anchors the roots of the external genitalia

In both genders, the roots of the external genitalia, the clitoris and the penis, are firmly anchored to:

- The bony margin of the anterior half of the pelvic outlet
- A thick, fibrous, perineal membrane, which fills the area (Fig. 5.3)

The roots of the external genitalia consist of erectile (vascular) tissues and associated skeletal muscles.

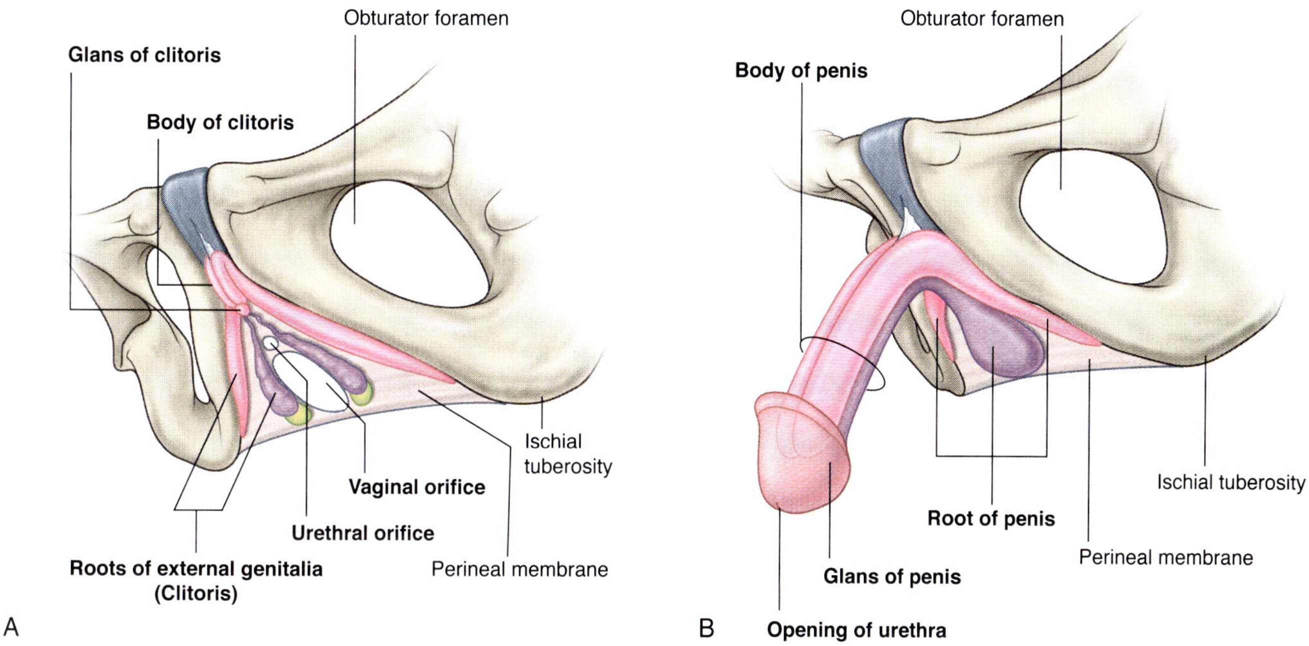

Fig. 5.3 The perineum contains and anchors the roots of the external genitalia. **(A)** In women. **(B)** In men.

COMPONENT PARTS

Pelvic inlet

The pelvic inlet is somewhat heart shaped and completely ringed by bone (Fig. 5.4). Posteriorly, the inlet is bordered by the body of vertebra SI, which projects into the inlet as the sacral **promontory**. On each side of this vertebra, wing-like transverse processes called the **alae** (**wings**) contribute to the margin of the pelvic inlet. Laterally, a prominent rim on the pelvic bone continues the boundary of the inlet forward to the pubic symphysis, where the two pelvic bones are joined in the midline.

Structures pass between the pelvic cavity and the abdomen through the pelvic inlet.

During childbirth, the fetus passes through the pelvic inlet from the abdomen, into which the uterus had expanded during pregnancy, and then passes through the pelvic outlet.

Pelvic walls

The walls of the true pelvis consist predominantly of bone, muscle, and ligaments, with the sacrum, coccyx, and inferior half of the pelvic bones forming much of them.

Two ligaments, the **sacrospinous** and the **sacrotuberous ligaments**, are important architectural elements of the walls because they link each pelvic bone to the sacrum and coccyx (Fig. 5.5A). These ligaments also convert two notches on the pelvic bones—the **greater** and **lesser sciatic notches**—into foramina on the lateral pelvic walls.

Completing the walls are the **obturator internus** and **piriformis** muscles (Fig. 5.5B), which arise in the pelvis and exit through the sciatic foramina to act on the hip joint.

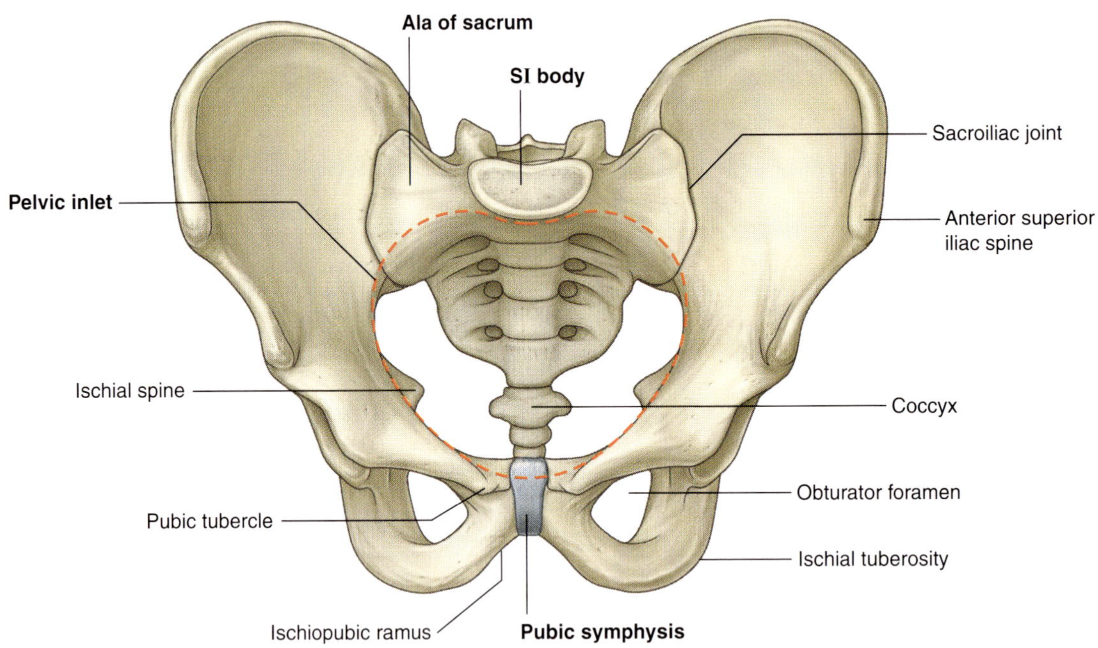

Fig. 5.4 Pelvic inlet.

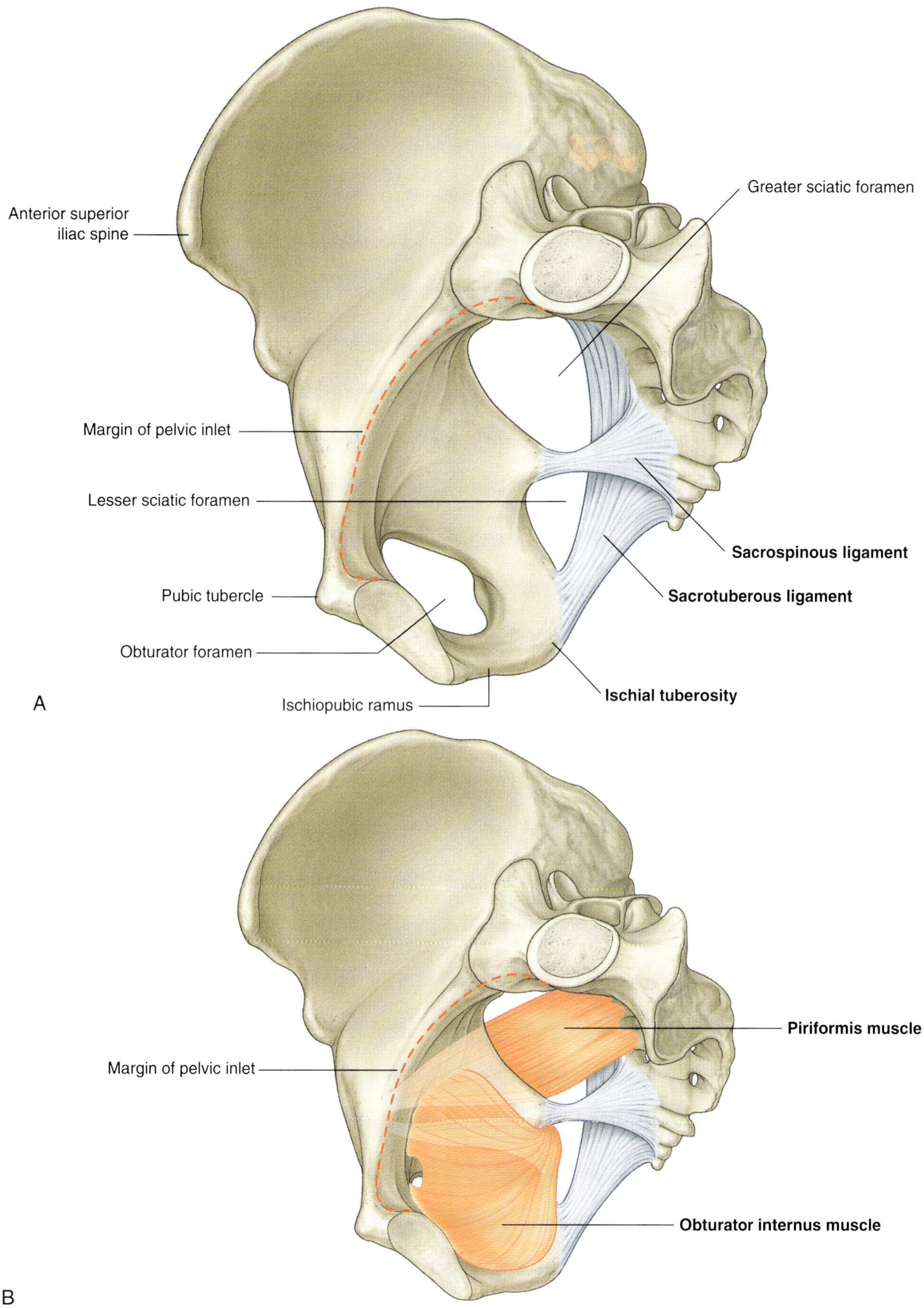

Fig. 5.5 Pelvic walls. **(A)** Bones and ligaments of the pelvic walls. **(B)** Muscles of the pelvic walls.

Pelvic outlet

The diamond-shaped pelvic outlet is formed by both bone and ligaments (Fig. 5.6). It is limited anteriorly in the midline by the pubic symphysis.

On each side, the inferior margin of the pelvic bone projects posteriorly and laterally from the pubic symphysis to end in a prominent tuberosity, the **ischial tuberosity**. Together, these elements construct the pubic arch, which forms the margin of the anterior half of the pelvic outlet. The sacrotuberous ligament continues this margin posteriorly from the ischial tuberosity to the coccyx and sacrum. The pubic symphysis, ischial tuberosities, and coccyx can all be palpated.

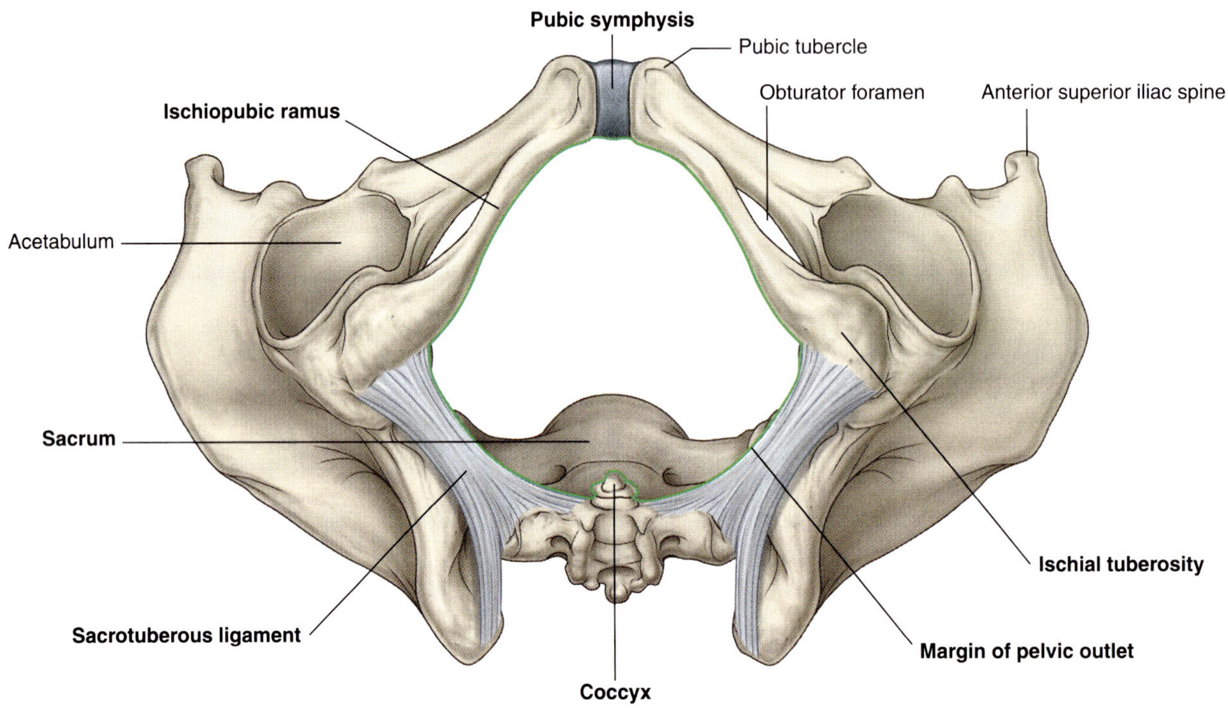

Fig. 5.6 Pelvic outlet.

Pelvic floor

The pelvic floor, which separates the pelvic cavity from the perineum, is formed by muscles and fascia (Fig. 5.7).

Two **levator ani** muscles attach peripherally to the pelvic walls and join each other at the midline by a connective tissue raphe. Together they are the largest components of the bowl- or funnel-shaped structure known as the **pelvic diaphragm**, which is completed posteriorly by the **coccygeus muscles**. The latter muscle overlies the sacrospinous ligament and passes between the margins of the sacrum and the coccyx and a prominent spine on the pelvic bone, the **ischial spine** (Figs 5.5A and 5.7).

The pelvic diaphragm forms most of the pelvic floor and in its anterior regions contains a U-shaped defect, which is associated with elements of the urogenital system (see Fig. 5.56A).

The anal canal passes from the pelvis to the perineum through a posterior circular orifice in the pelvic diaphragm.

The pelvic floor is supported anteriorly by:

- The perineal membrane
- Muscles in the **deep perineal pouch**

The **perineal membrane** is a thick, triangular fascial sheet that fills the space between the rami of the pubic arch, and has a free posterior border (Fig. 5.7). The deep perineal pouch is a narrow region superior to the perineal membrane.

The margins of the U-shaped defect in the pelvic diaphragm merge into the walls of the associated viscera and with muscles in the deep perineal pouch below.

The vagina and the urethra penetrate the pelvic floor to pass from the pelvic cavity to the perineum.

Pelvic cavity

The pelvic cavity is lined by peritoneum continuous with the peritoneum of the abdominal cavity that drapes over the superior aspects of the pelvic viscera, but in most regions, does not reach the pelvic floor (Fig. 5.8A).

The pelvic viscera are located in the midline of the pelvic cavity. The bladder is anterior and the rectum is posterior. In women, the uterus lies between the bladder and rectum (Fig. 5.8B). Other structures, such as vessels and nerves, lie deep to the peritoneum in association with the pelvic walls and on either side of the pelvic viscera.

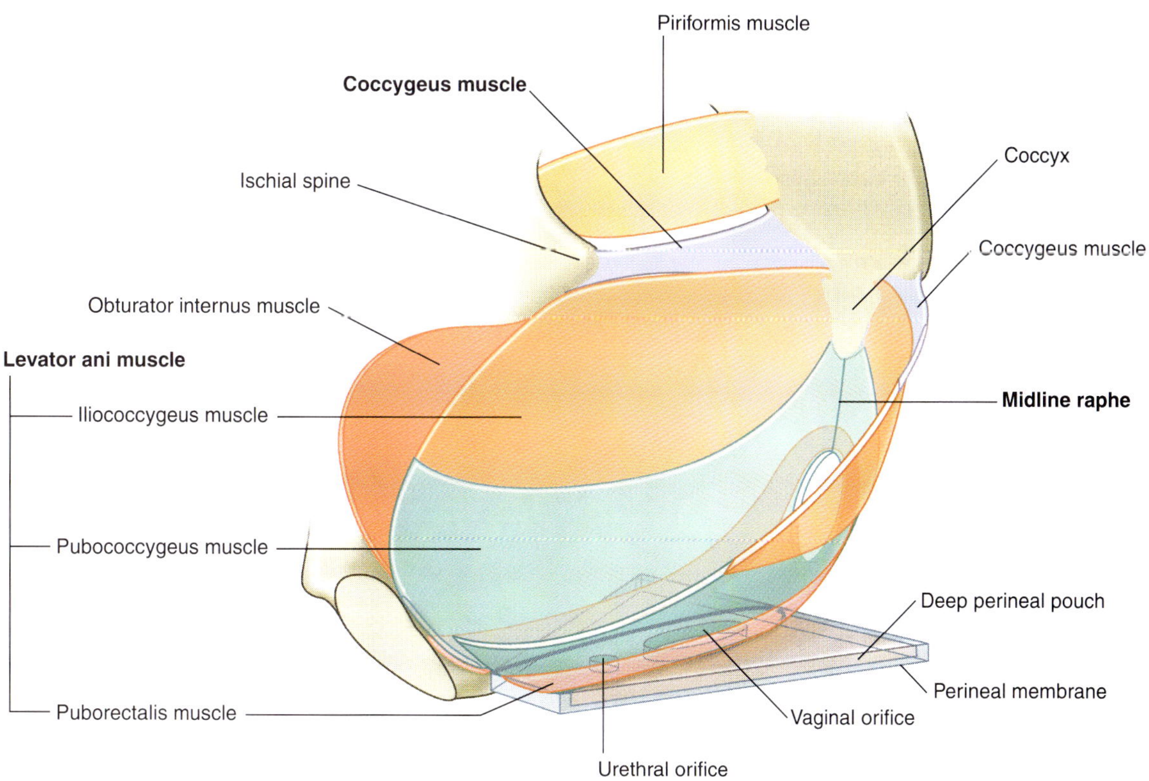

Fig. 5.7 Pelvic floor.

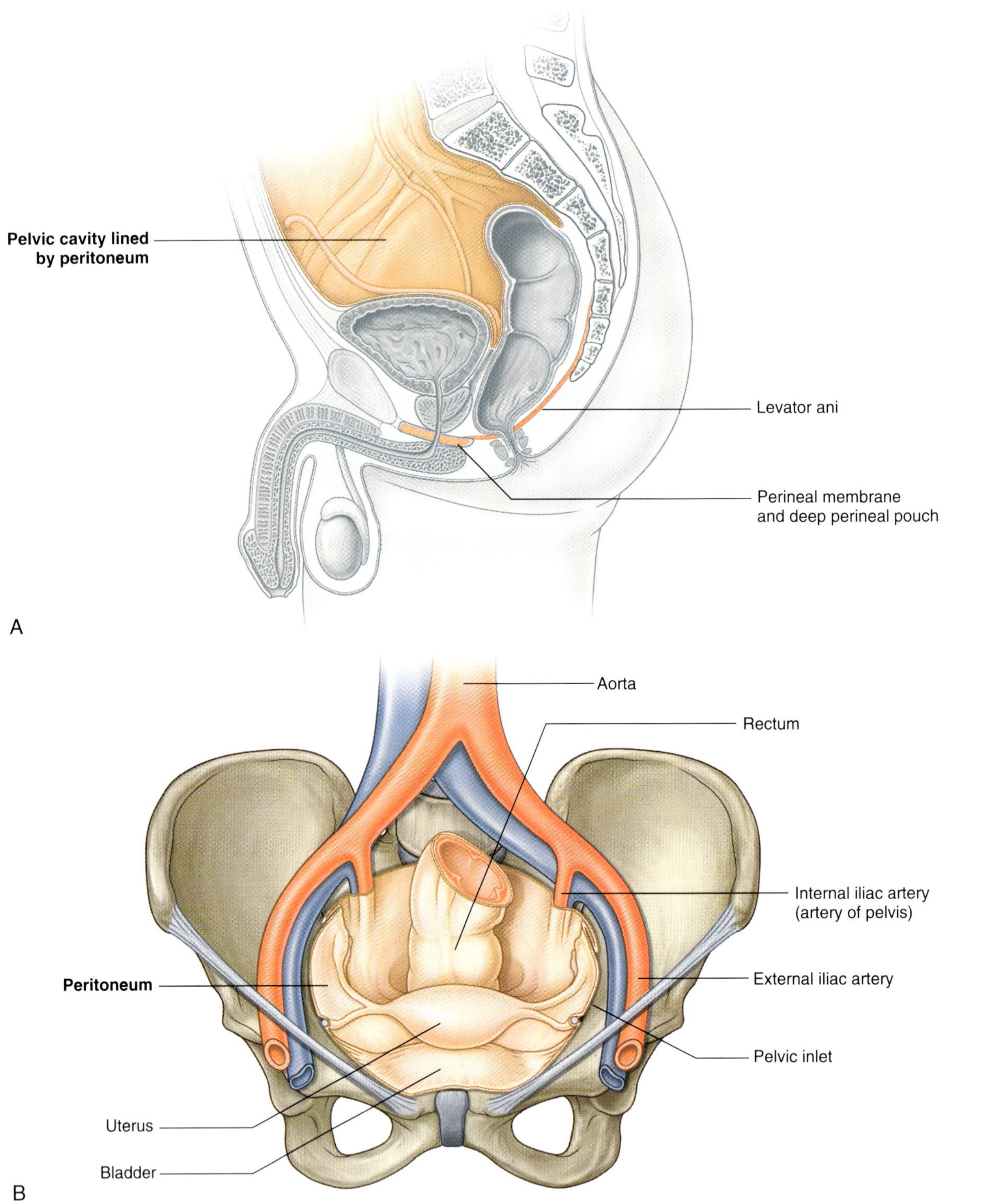

Fig. 5.8 Pelvic cavity and peritoneum. **(A)** In men (sagittal section). **(B)** In women (anterior view).

Perineum

The perineum lies inferior to the pelvic floor between the lower limbs (Fig. 5.9). Its margin is formed by the pelvic outlet. An imaginary line between the ischial tuberosities divides the perineum into two triangular regions.

- Anteriorly, the **urogenital triangle** contains the roots of the external genitalia and, in women, the openings of the urethra and the vagina (Fig. 5.9A). In men, the distal part of the urethra is enclosed by erectile tissues and opens at the end of the penis (Fig. 5.9B).
- Posteriorly, the **anal triangle** contains the anal aperture.

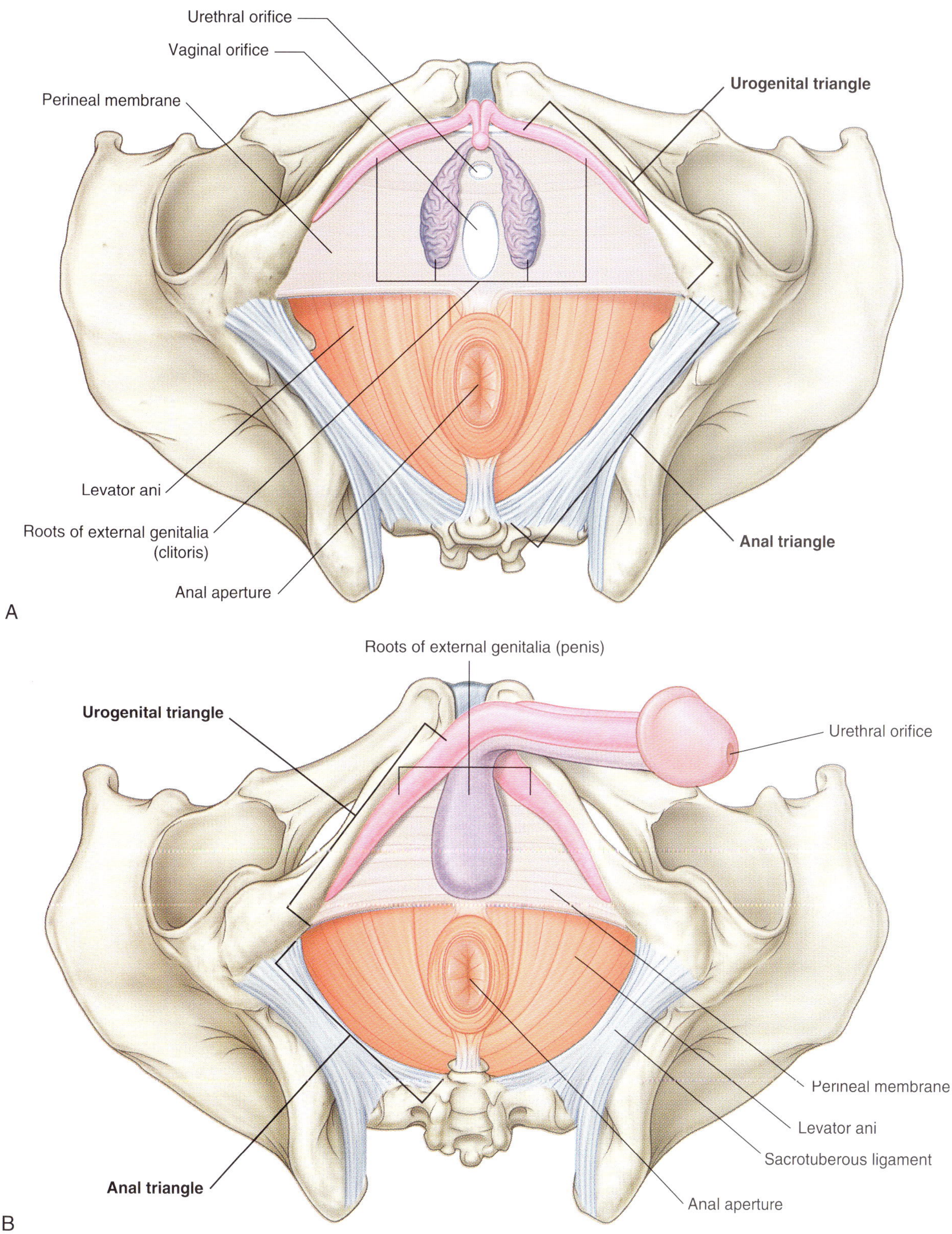

Fig. 5.9 Perineum, consisting of the urogenital and anal triangles. **(A)** In women. **(B)** In men.

RELATIONSHIP TO OTHER REGIONS

Abdomen

The cavity of the true pelvis is continuous with the abdominal cavity at the pelvic inlet (Figs 5.4 and 5.10A). All structures passing between the pelvic cavity and abdomen, including major vessels, nerves, and lymphatics, as well as the sigmoid colon and ureters, pass via the inlet. In men, the ductus deferens on each side passes through the anterior abdominal wall and over the inlet to enter the pelvic cavity. In women, ovarian vessels, nerves, and lymphatics pass through the inlet to reach the ovaries, which lie on each side just inferior to the pelvic inlet.

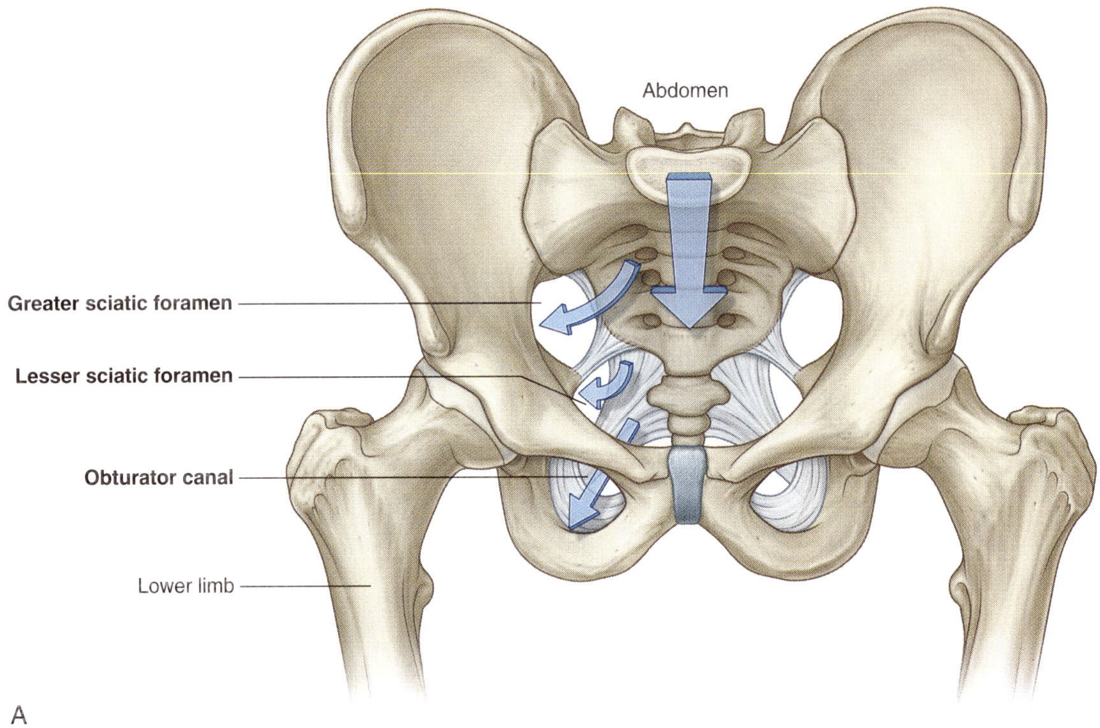

Fig. 5.10 Areas of communication between the true pelvis and other regions. **(A)** Between the true pelvis, abdomen, and lower limb.

Lower limb

Three apertures in the pelvic wall communicate with the lower limb (Fig. 5.10A):

- The obturator canal
- The greater sciatic foramen
- The lesser sciatic foramen

The obturator canal forms a passageway between the pelvic cavity and the adductor region of the thigh, and is formed in the superior aspect of the obturator foramen, between bone, a connective tissue membrane, and muscles that almost fill the foramen.

The lesser sciatic foramen, which lies inferior to the pelvic floor, provides communication between the gluteal region and the perineum (Fig. 5.10B).

The pelvic cavity also communicates directly with the perineum through a small gap between the pubic symphysis and the perineal membrane (Fig. 5.10B).

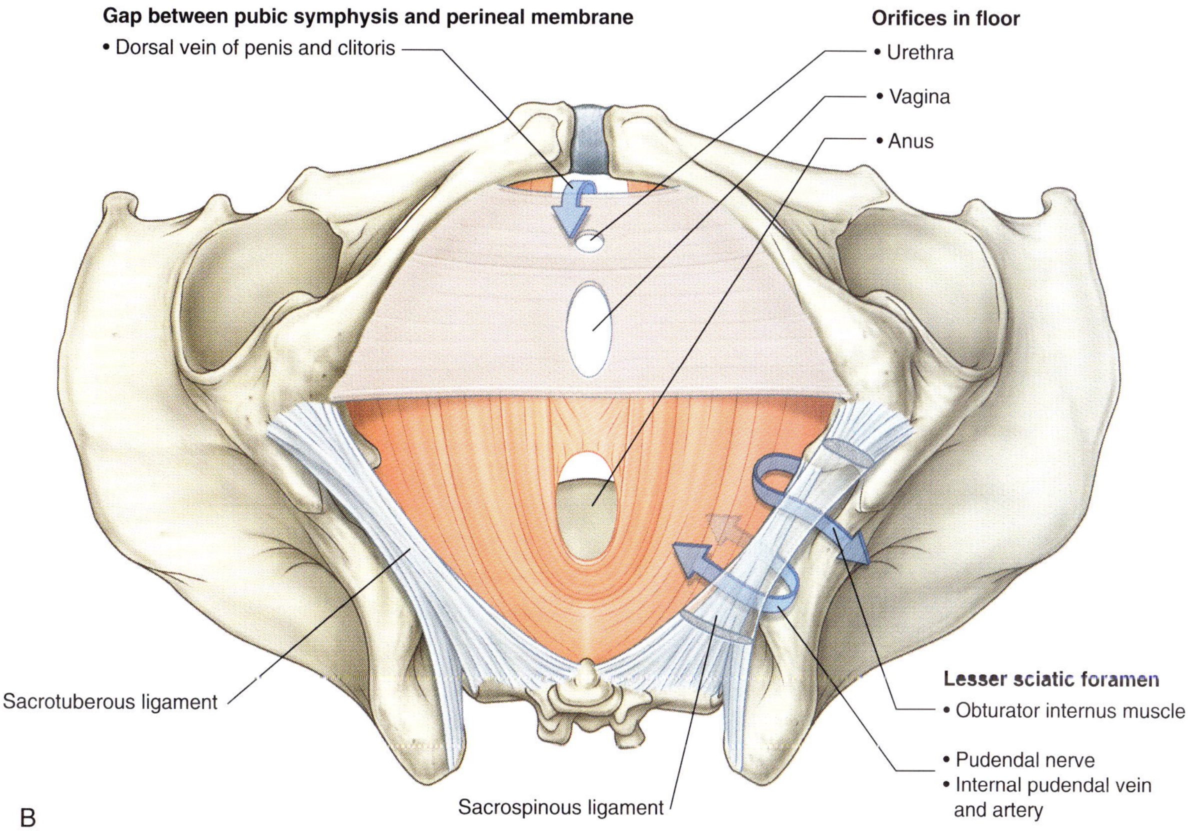

Fig. 5.10, cont'd (B) Between the perineum and other regions.

KEY FEATURES

The pelvic cavity projects posteriorly

In the anatomical position, the anterior superior iliac spines and the superior edge of the pubic symphysis lie in the same vertical plane (Fig. 5.11). Consequently, the pelvic inlet is angled 50°–60° forward relative to the horizontal plane, and the pelvic cavity projects posteriorly from the abdominal cavity.

Meanwhile, the urogenital part of the pelvic outlet (the pubic arch) is oriented in a nearly horizontal plane, whereas the posterior part of the outlet is positioned more vertically. The urogenital triangle of the perineum therefore faces inferiorly, while the anal triangle faces more posteriorly.

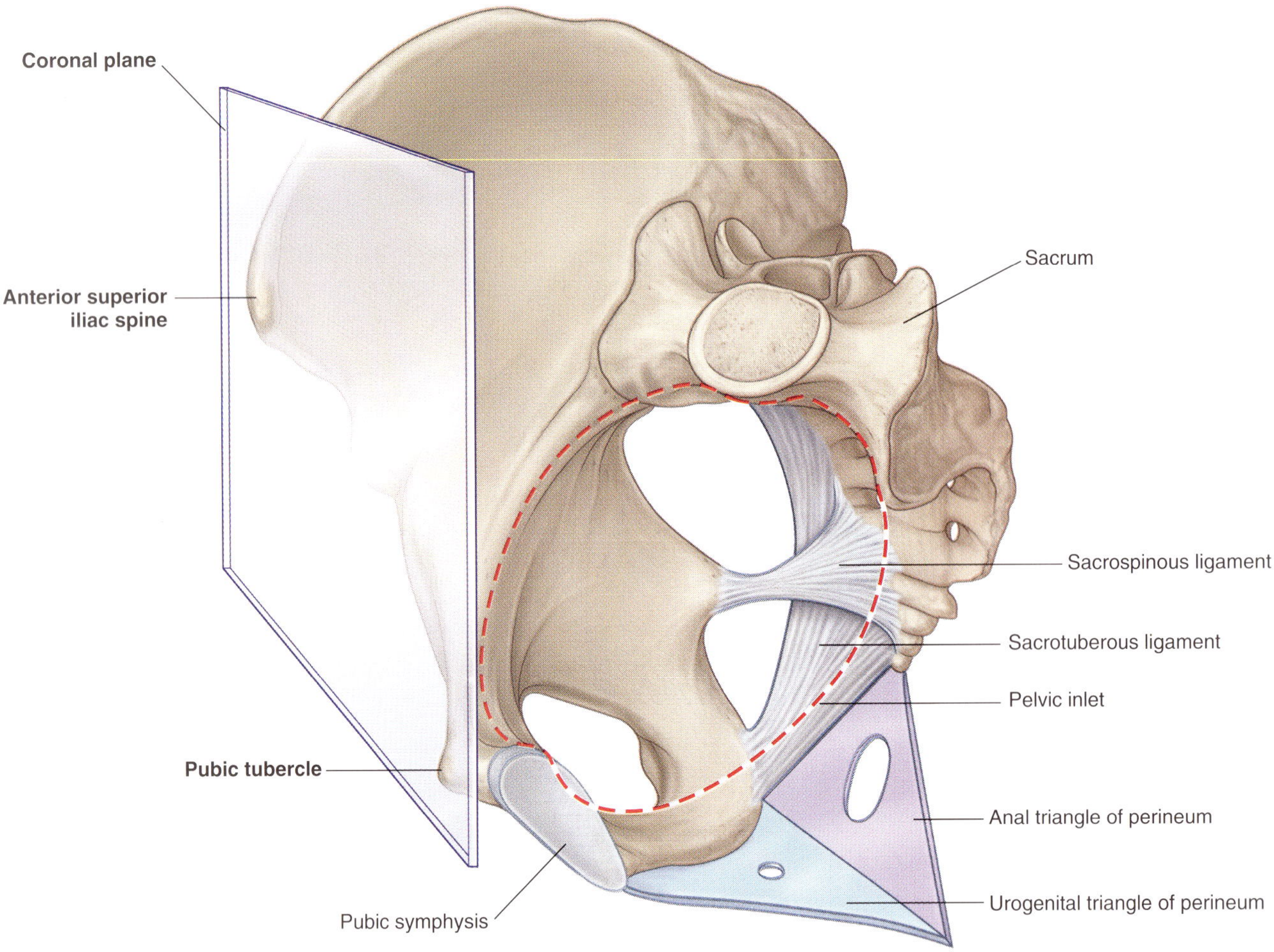

Fig. 5.11 Orientation of the pelvis and pelvic cavity in the anatomical position.

Important structures cross the ureters in the pelvic cavity

The ureters drain the kidneys, course down the posterior abdominal wall, and cross the pelvic inlet to enter the pelvic cavity. They continue inferiorly along the lateral pelvic wall and ultimately connect with the base of the bladder.

An important structure crosses the ureters in the pelvic cavity in both men and women—in women, the uterine artery crosses over the ureter, passing superior to it, to reach the lateral part of the cervix of the uterus (Fig. 5.12A). The ureter may be inadvertently injured when clamping the uterine artery here. In men, the ductus deferens crosses over the ureter just posterior to the bladder (Fig. 5.12B).

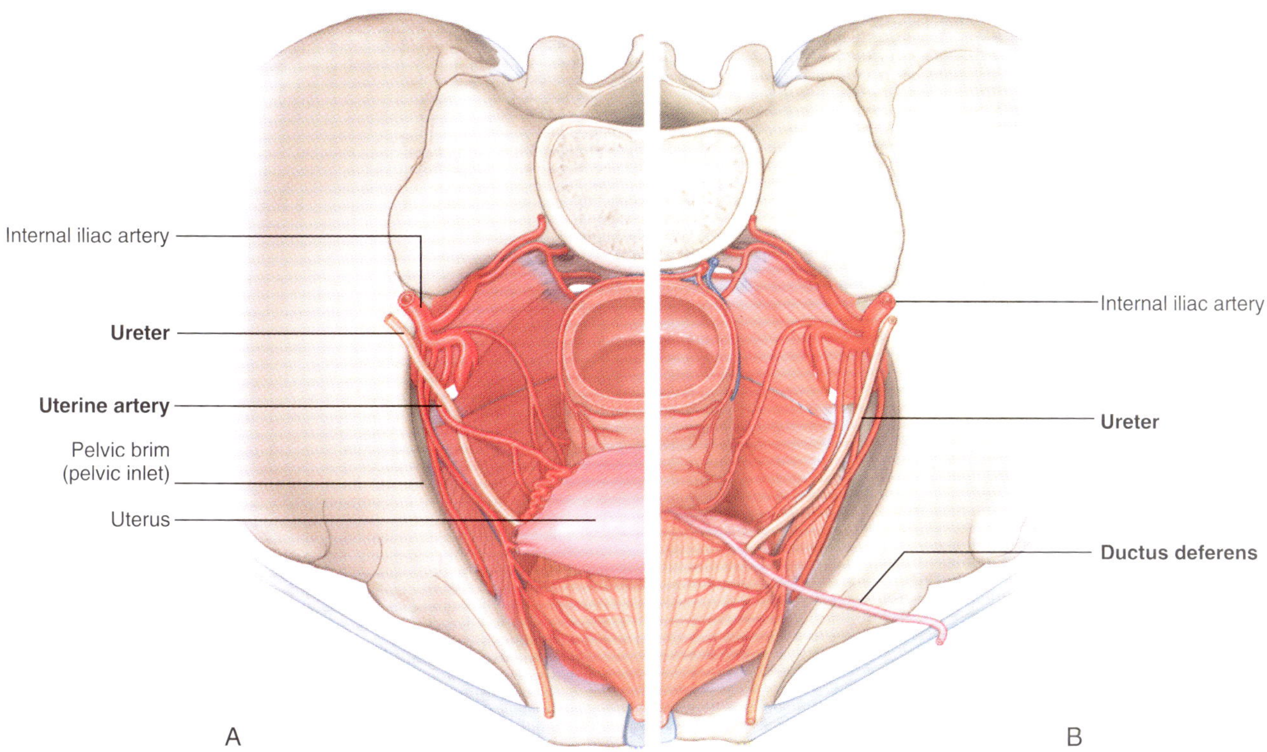

Fig. 5.12 Structures that cross the ureters in the pelvic cavity. **(A)** In women. **(B)** In men.

The prostate in men and the uterus in women are anterior to the rectum

In men, the prostate gland is situated immediately anterior to the rectum, just above the pelvic floor (Fig. 5.13). It can be felt by digital palpation during a rectal examination.

In both sexes, the anal canal and the lower rectum also can be evaluated during a rectal examination by a clinician. In women, the cervix and lower part of the body of the uterus also are palpable. However, these structures can more easily be palpated with a bimanual examination where the index and middle fingers of a clinician's hand are placed in the vagina and the other hand is placed on the lower anterior abdominal wall. The organs are felt between the two hands. This bimanual technique can also be used to examine the ovaries and uterine tubes.

The perineum is innervated by sacral spinal cord segments

Dermatomes of the perineum in both men and women are from spinal cord levels S3 to S5, except for the anterior regions, which tend to be innervated by spinal cord level L1 by nerves associated with the abdominal wall (Fig. 5.14). Dermatomes of L2 to S2 are predominantly in the lower limb.

Most of the skeletal muscles contained in the perineum and the pelvic floor, including the external anal sphincter and external urethral sphincter, are innervated by spinal cord levels S2 to S4.

Much of the somatic motor and sensory innervation of the perineum is provided by the pudendal nerve from spinal cord levels S2 to S4.

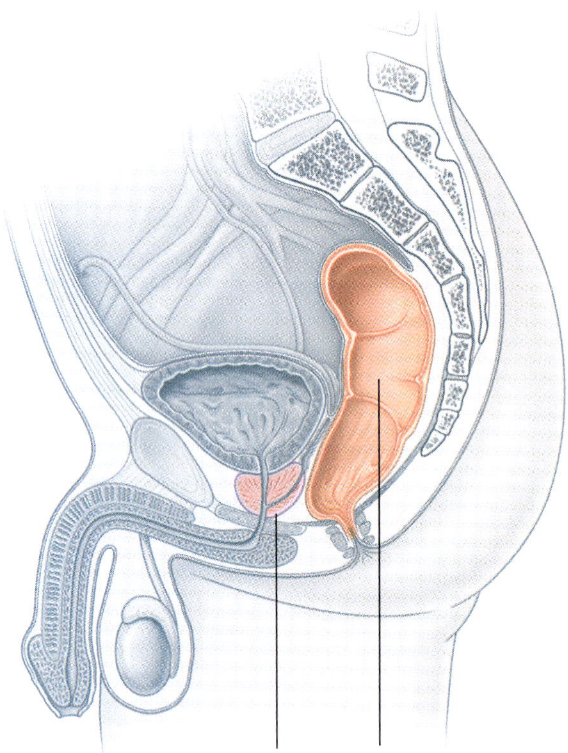

Fig. 5.13 Position of the prostate gland.

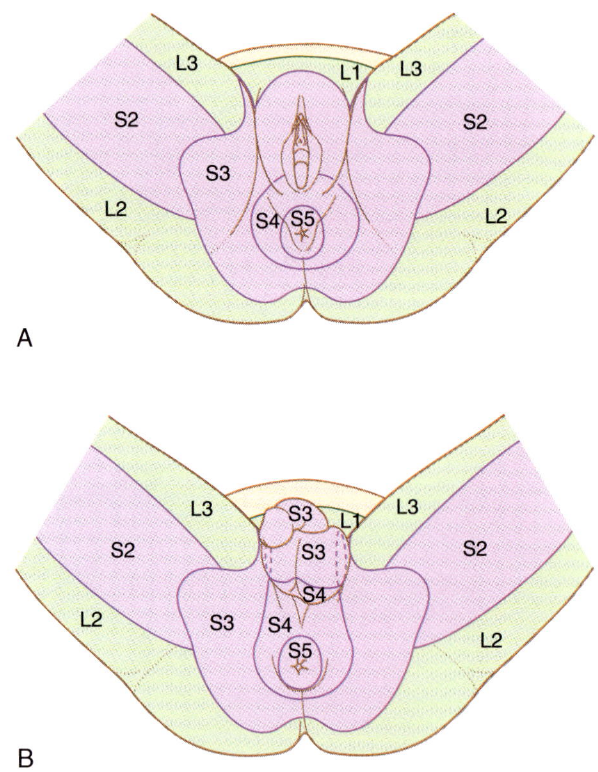

Fig. 5.14 Dermatomes of the perineum. **(A)** In women. **(B)** In men.

Nerves are related to bone

The **pudendal nerve** is the major nerve of the perineum and is directly associated with the ischial spine of the pelvis (Fig. 5.15). On each side of the body, these spines and the attached sacrospinous ligaments separate the greater sciatic foramina from the lesser sciatic foramina on the lateral pelvic wall.

The pudendal nerve leaves the pelvic cavity through the greater sciatic foramen and then immediately enters the perineum inferior to the pelvic floor by passing around the ischial spine and through the lesser sciatic foramen (Fig. 5.15). The ischial spine can be palpated transvaginally in women and is the landmark for administering a pudendal nerve block.

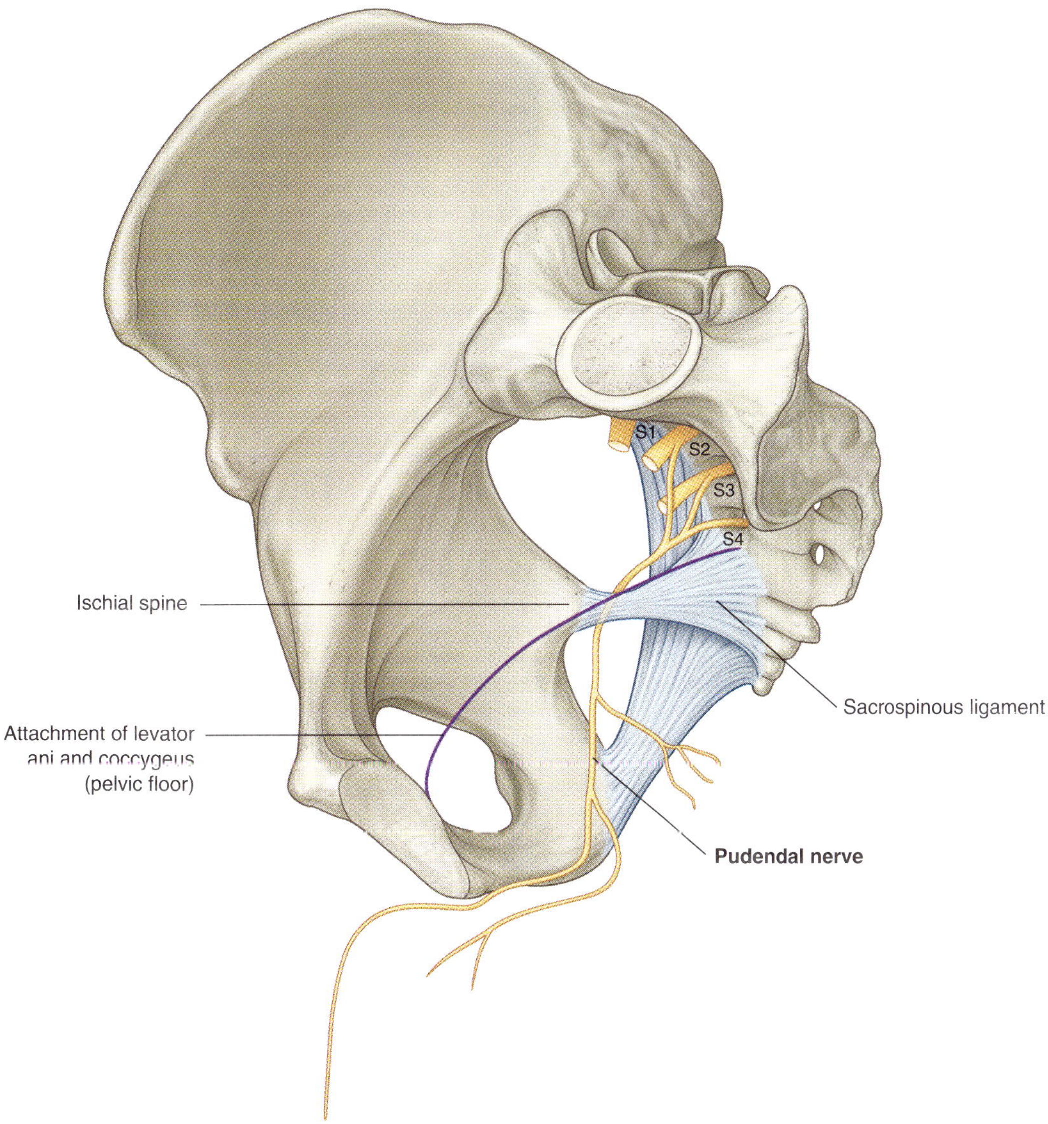

Fig. 5.15 Pudendal nerve.

Parasympathetic innervation from spinal cord levels S2 to S4 controls erection

The parasympathetic innervation from spinal cord levels S2 to S4 controls genital erection in both women and men (Fig. 5.16). On each side, preganglionic parasympathetic nerves leave the anterior rami of the sacral spinal nerves and enter the **inferior hypogastric plexus** (pelvic plexus) on the lateral pelvic wall.

The two inferior hypogastric plexuses are inferior extensions of the abdominal prevertebral plexus that forms on the posterior abdominal wall in association with the abdominal aorta. Nerves derived from these plexuses penetrate the pelvic floor to innervate the erectile tissues of the clitoris in women and the penis in men.

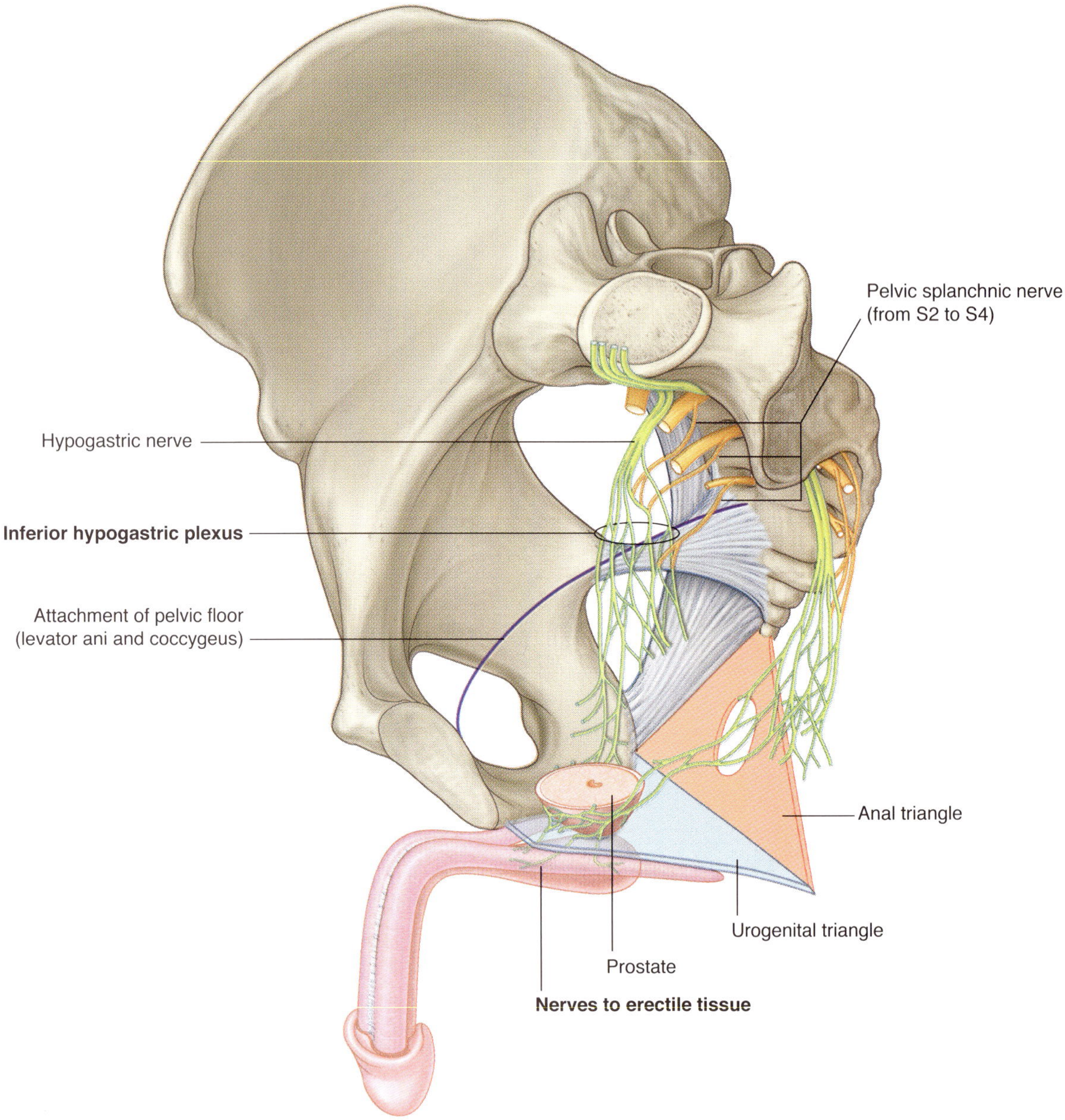

Fig. 5.16 Pelvic splanchnic nerve from spinal levels S2 to S4 controls erection.

Muscles and fascia of the pelvic floor and perineum intersect at the perineal body

Structures of the pelvic floor intersect with structures in the perineum at the **perineal body** (Fig. 5.17). This poorly defined fibromuscular node lies at the center of the perineum, approximately midway between the two ischial tuberosities. Converging at the perineal body are

- The levator ani muscles of the pelvic diaphragm
- Muscles in the urogenital and anal triangles of the perineum, including the skeletal muscle sphincters associated with the urethra, vagina, and anus

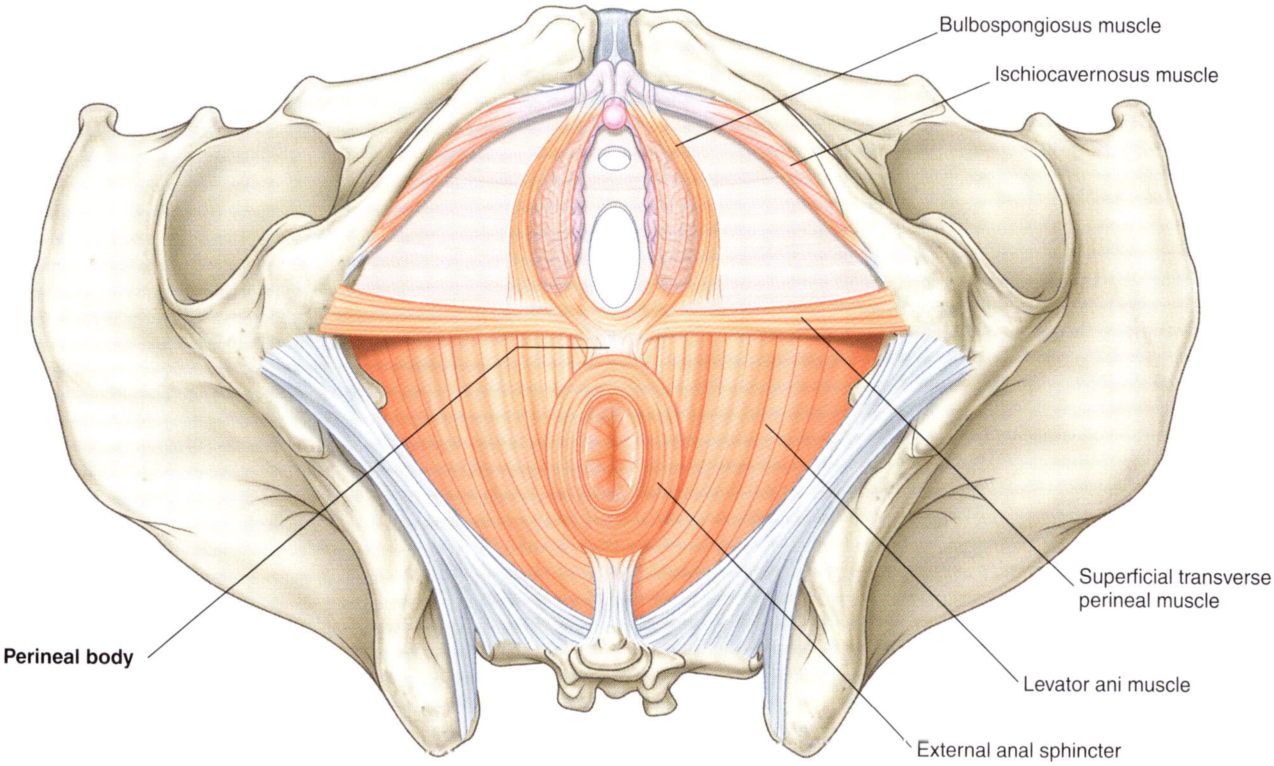

Fig. 5.17 Perineal body.

The course of the urethra is different in men and women

In women, the urethra is short and passes inferiorly from the bladder through the pelvic floor and opens directly into the perineum (Fig. 5.18A).

In men, the urethra passes through the prostate before coursing through the deep perineal pouch and perineal membrane and then becomes enclosed within the erectile tissues of the penis before opening at the end of the penis (Fig. 5.18B). The penile part of the male urethra has two angles:

- The more important of these is a fixed angle where the urethra bends anteriorly in the root of the penis after passing through the perineal membrane.
- Another angle occurs distally where the unattached part of the penis curves inferiorly—when the penis is erect, this second angle disappears.

It is important to consider the different courses of the urethra in men and women when catheterizing patients and when evaluating perineal injuries and pelvic pathology.

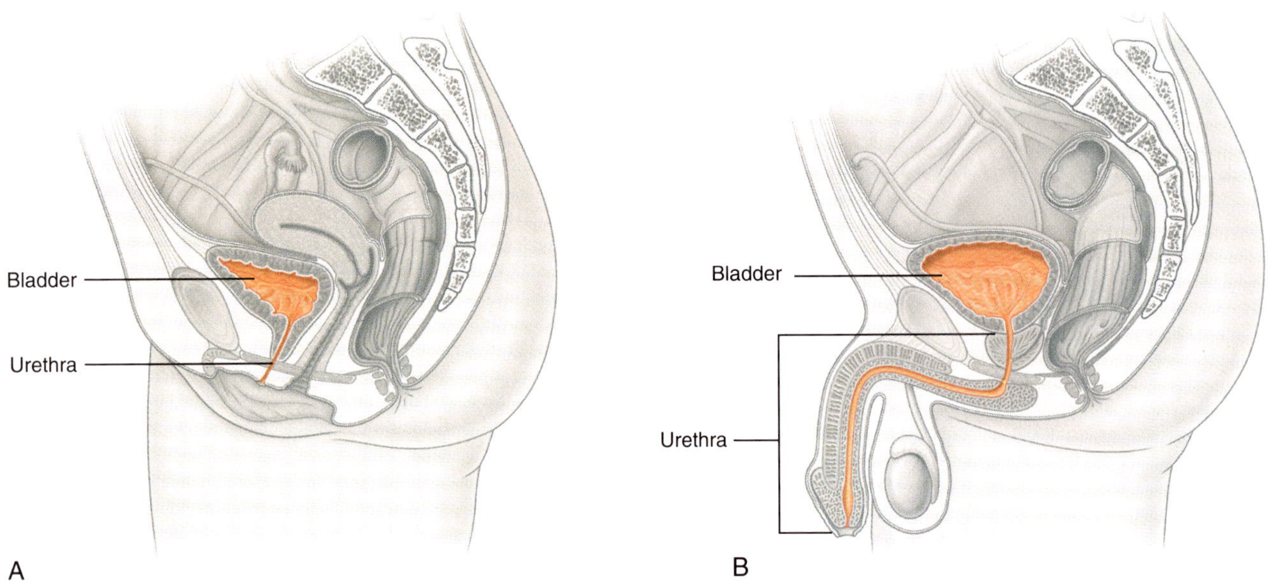

Fig. 5.18 Course of the urethra. **(A)** In women. **(B)** In men.

Regional anatomy

The pelvis is the region of the body surrounded by the pelvic bones and the inferior elements of the vertebral column. It is divided into two major regions: the superior region is the false (greater) pelvis and is part of the abdominal cavity; the inferior region is the true (lesser) pelvis, which encloses the pelvic cavity.

The bowl-shaped pelvic cavity is continuous above with the abdominal cavity. The rim of the pelvic cavity (the pelvic inlet) is completely encircled by bone (Fig. 5.4). The pelvic floor is a fibromuscular structure separating the pelvic cavity above from the perineum below (see Figs 5.59 and 5.68).

The perineum is inferior to the pelvic floor and its margin is formed by the pelvic outlet (Fig. 5.6). The perineum contains:

- The terminal openings of the gastrointestinal and urinary systems
- The external opening of the reproductive tract
- The roots of the external genitalia

PELVIS

Bones

The bones of the pelvis consist of the right and left pelvic (hip) bones, the sacrum, and the coccyx. The sacrum articulates superiorly with vertebra LV at the lumbosacral joint. The pelvic bones articulate posteriorly with the sacrum at the sacroiliac joints and with each other anteriorly at the pubic symphysis.

Pelvic bone

The pelvic bone is irregular in shape and has two major parts separated by an oblique line on the medial surface of the bone (Fig. 5.19A):

- The pelvic bone above this line represents the lateral wall of the false pelvis, which is part of the abdominal cavity.
- The pelvic bone below this line represents the lateral wall of the true pelvis, which contains the pelvic cavity.

The linea terminalis is the lower two-thirds of this line and contributes to the margin of the pelvic inlet (see Fig. 5.28).

The lateral surface of the pelvic bone has a large articular socket, the **acetabulum**, which, together with the head of the femur, forms the hip joint (Fig. 5.19B).

Inferior to the acetabulum is the large **obturator foramen**, most of which is closed by a flat connective tissue membrane, the **obturator membrane**. A small obturator canal remains open superiorly between the membrane and adjacent bone, providing a route of communication between the lower limb and the pelvic cavity.

The posterior margin of the bone is marked by two notches separated by the **ischial spine**:

- The **greater sciatic notch**
- The **lesser sciatic notch**

The posterior margin terminates inferiorly as the large **ischial tuberosity**.

The irregular anterior margin of the pelvic bone is marked by the **anterior superior iliac spine**, the **anterior inferior iliac spine**, and the **pubic tubercle**.

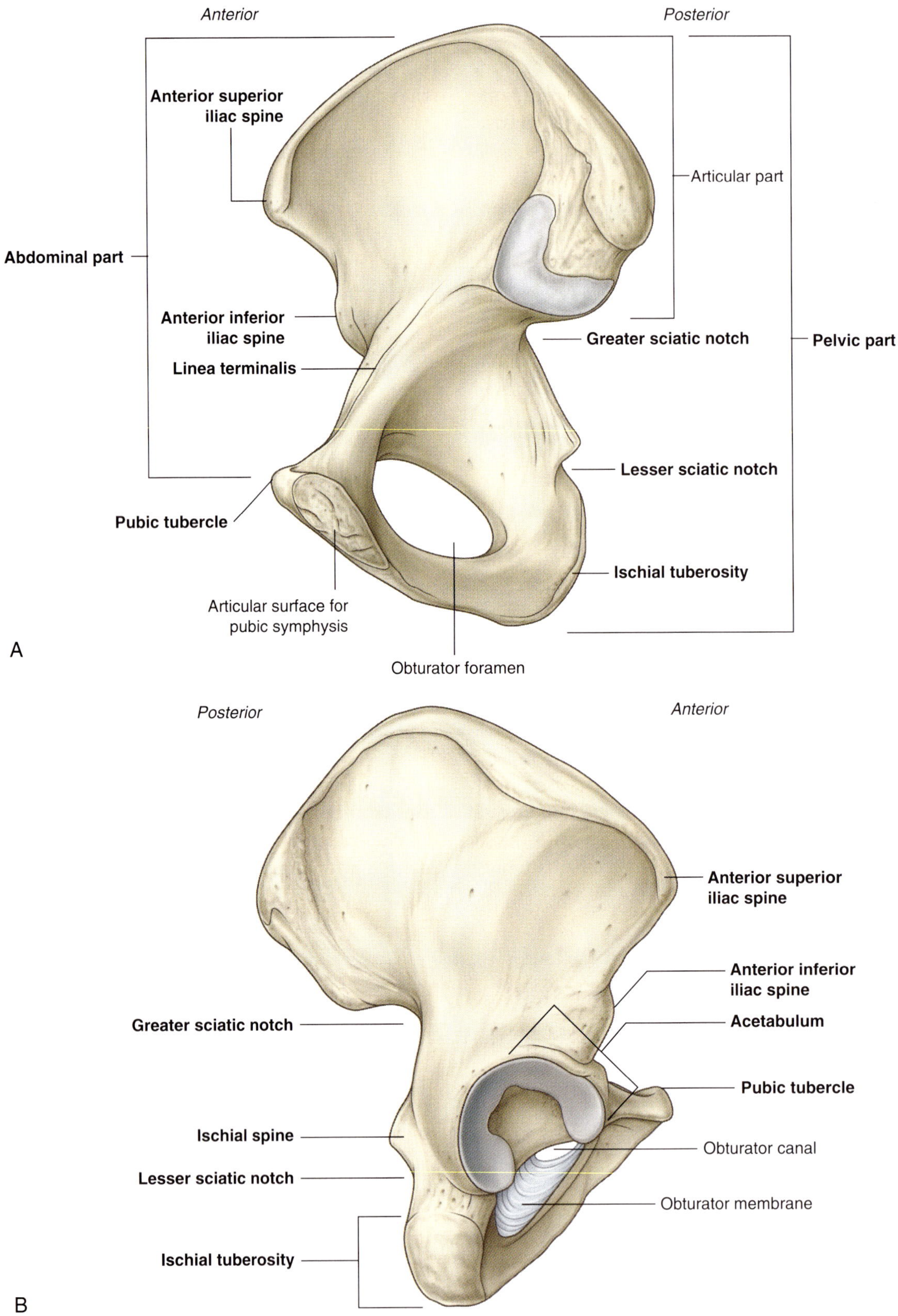

Fig. 5.19 Right pelvic bone. **(A)** Medial view. **(B)** Lateral view.

Components of the pelvic bone

Each pelvic bone is formed by three elements: the ilium, pubis, and ischium. At birth, these bones are connected by cartilage in the area of the acetabulum; later, at between 16 and 18 years of age, they fuse into a single bone (Fig. 5.20).

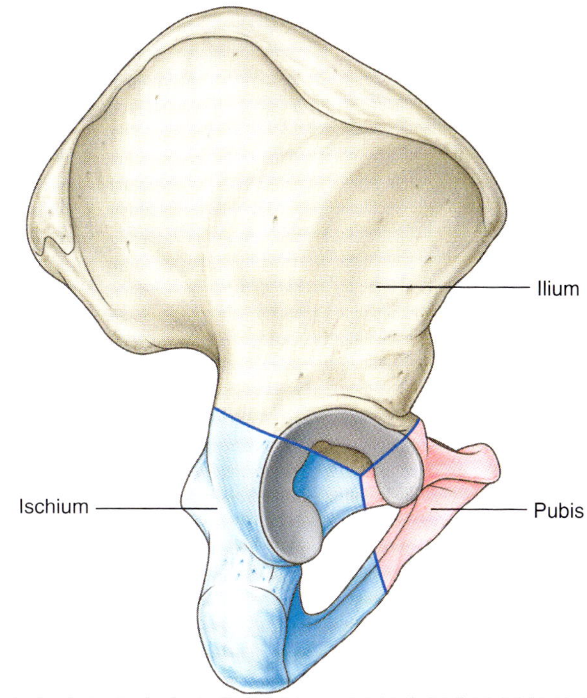

Fig. 5.20 Ilium, ischium, and pubis.

Ilium

Of the three components of the pelvic bone, the **ilium** is the most superior in position.

The ilium is separated into upper and lower parts by a ridge on the medial surface (Fig. 5.21A).

- Posteriorly, the ridge is sharp and lies immediately superior to the surface of the bone that articulates with the sacrum. This sacral surface has a large L-shaped facet for articulating with the sacrum and an expanded, posterior roughened area for the attachment of the strong ligaments that support the sacroiliac joint (Fig. 5.21).
- Anteriorly, the ridge separating the upper and lower parts of the ilium is rounded and termed the **arcuate line**.

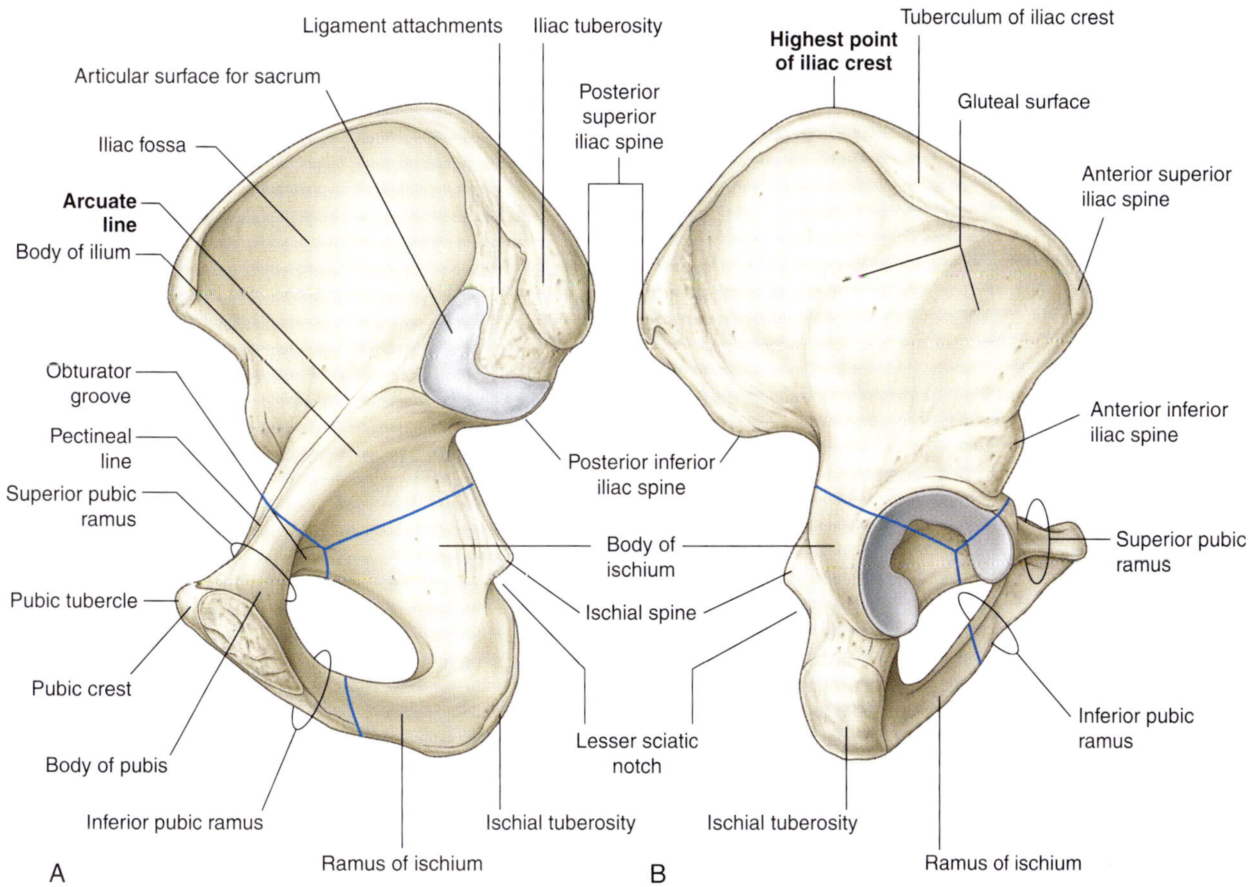

Fig. 5.21 Components of the pelvic bone. **(A)** Medial surface. **(B)** Lateral surface.

The arcuate line forms part of the linea terminalis and the pelvic brim.

The portion of the ilium lying inferior to the arcuate line is the pelvic part of the ilium and contributes to the wall of the lesser or true pelvis.

The upper part of the ilium expands to form a flat, fan-shaped "wing," which provides bony support for the lower abdomen, or false pelvis. This part of the ilium provides attachment for muscles functionally associated with the lower limb. The anteromedial surface of the wing is concave and forms the **iliac fossa**. The external (gluteal) surface of the wing is marked by lines and roughened areas and is related to the gluteal region of the lower limb (Fig. 5.21B).

The entire superior margin of the ilium is thickened to form a prominent crest (the **iliac crest**), which is the site of attachment for muscles and fascia of the abdomen, back, and lower limb and terminates anteriorly as the **anterior superior iliac spine** and posteriorly as the **posterior superior iliac spine**.

A prominent tubercle, the **tuberculum of the iliac crest**, projects laterally near the anterior end of the crest; the posterior end of the crest thickens to form the **iliac tuberosity**.

Inferior to the anterior superior iliac spine of the crest, on the anterior margin of the ilium, is a rounded protuberance called the **anterior inferior iliac spine**. This structure serves as the point of attachment for the rectus femoris muscle of the anterior compartment of the thigh and the iliofemoral ligament associated with the hip joint. A less prominent **posterior inferior iliac spine** occurs along the posterior border of the sacral surface of the ilium, where the bone angles forward to form the superior margin of the greater sciatic notch.

Early clinical exposure

Bone marrow biopsy

In certain diseases (e.g., leukemia), a sample of bone marrow must be obtained to assess the stage and severity of the problem. The iliac crest is often used for such bone marrow biopsies. The iliac crest lies close to the surface and is easily palpated.

A bone marrow biopsy is performed by injecting anesthetic in the skin and passing a cutting needle through the cortical bone of the iliac crest. The bone marrow is aspirated and viewed under a microscope. Samples of cortical bone can also be obtained in this way to provide information about bone metabolism.

Pubis

The anterior and inferior part of the pelvic bone is the **pubis** (Fig. 5.21). It has a body and two arms (rami).

- The **body** is flattened dorsoventrally and articulates with the body of the pubic bone on the other side at the **pubic symphysis**. The body has a rounded pubic crest on its superior surface that ends laterally as the prominent **pubic tubercle**.
- The **superior pubic ramus** projects posterolaterally from the body and joins with the ilium and ischium at its base, which is positioned toward the acetabulum. The sharp superior margin of this triangular surface is termed the **pecten pubis** (**pectineal line**), which forms part of the linea terminalis of the pelvic bone and the pelvic inlet. Anteriorly, this line is continuous with the **pubic crest**, which also is part of the linea terminalis and pelvic inlet. The **superior pubic ramus** is marked on its inferior surface by the **obturator groove**, which forms the upper margin of the obturator canal.
- The inferior ramus projects laterally and inferiorly to join with the ramus of the ischium.

Ischium

The ischium is the posterior and inferior part of the pelvic bone (Fig. 5.21). It has:

- A large body that projects superiorly to join with the ilium and the superior ramus of the pubis
- A ramus that projects anteriorly to join with the inferior ramus of the pubis

The posterior margin of the bone is marked by a prominent **ischial spine** that separates the lesser sciatic notch, below, from the greater sciatic notch, above.

The most prominent feature of the ischium is a large tuberosity (the **ischial tuberosity**) on the posteroinferior aspect of the bone. This tuberosity is an important site for the attachment of lower limb muscles and for supporting the body when sitting.

Sacrum

The sacrum, which has the appearance of an inverted triangle, is formed by the fusion of the five sacral vertebrae (Fig. 5.22). The base of the sacrum articulates with vertebra LV, and its apex articulates with the coccyx. Each of the lateral surfaces of the bone bears a large L-shaped facet for articulation with the ilium of the pelvic bone. Posterior to the facet is a large roughened area for the attachment of ligaments that support the sacroiliac joint. The superior surface of the sacrum is characterized by the superior

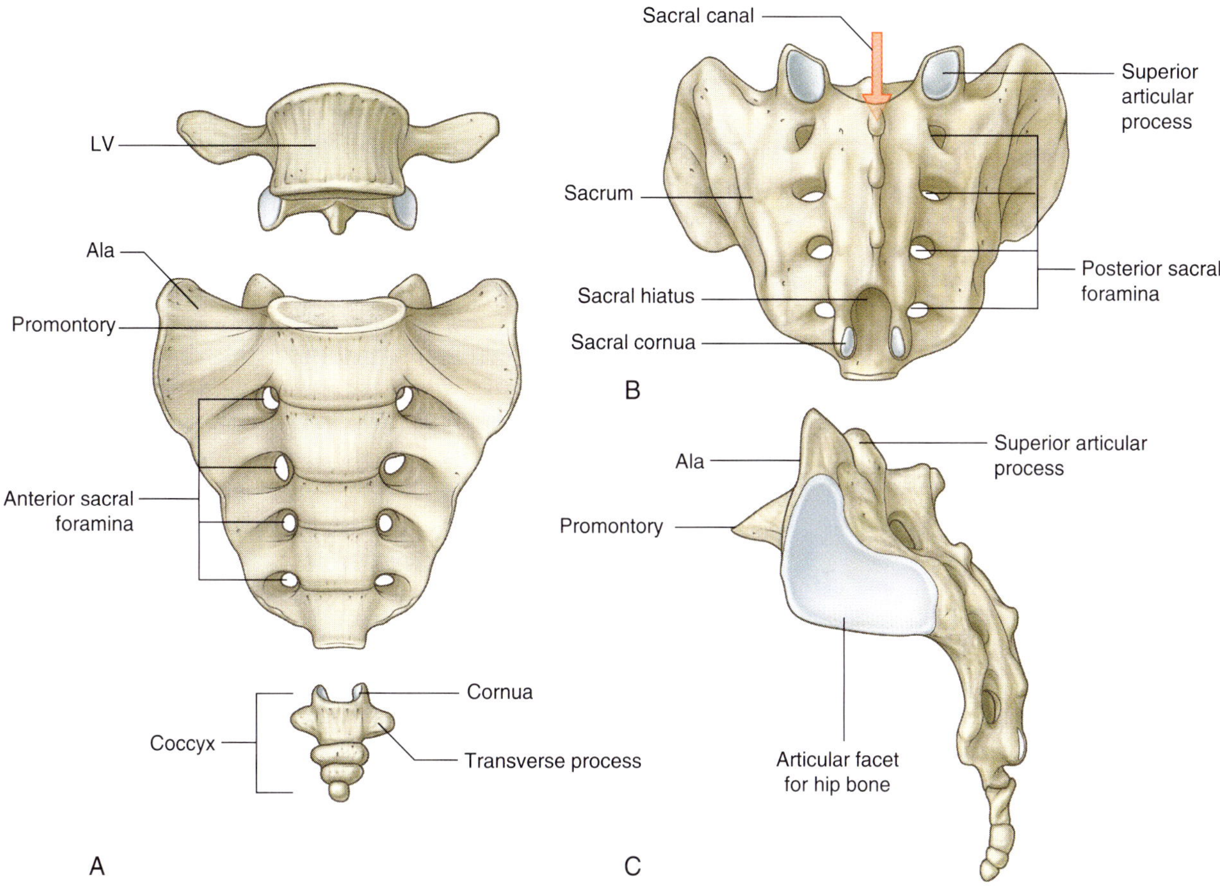

Fig. 5.22 Sacrum and coccyx. **(A)** Anterior view. **(B)** Posterior view. **(C)** Lateral view.

aspect of the body of vertebra SI and is flanked on each side by an expanded wing-like transverse process termed the **ala**. The anterior edge of the vertebral body projects forward as the **promontory**. The anterior surface of the sacrum is concave; the posterior surface is convex. Because the transverse processes of adjacent sacral vertebrae fuse lateral to the position of the intervertebral foramina and lateral to the bifurcation of spinal nerves into posterior and anterior rami, the posterior and anterior rami of spinal nerves S1 to S4 emerge from the sacrum through separate foramina. There are four pairs of **anterior sacral foramina** on the anterior surface of the sacrum for anterior rami, and four pairs of **posterior sacral foramina** on the posterior surface for the posterior rami. The **sacral canal** is a continuation of the vertebral canal that terminates as the **sacral hiatus**.

Coccyx

The small terminal part of the vertebral column is the coccyx, which consists of four fused coccygeal vertebrae (Fig. 5.22) and, like the sacrum, has the shape of an inverted triangle. The base of the coccyx is directed superiorly. The superior surface bears a facet for articulation with the sacrum and two **horns**, or **cornua**, one on each side, that project upward to articulate or fuse with similar downward-projecting cornua from the sacrum. These processes are modified superior and inferior articular processes that are present on other vertebrae. Each lateral surface of the coccyx has a small rudimentary transverse process, extending from the first coccygeal vertebra. Vertebral arches are absent from coccygeal vertebrae; therefore, no bony vertebral canal is present in the coccyx.

Early clinical exposure

Pelvic fracture

The pelvis can be viewed as a series of anatomical rings. There are three bony rings and four fibro-osseous rings. The major bony pelvic ring consists of parts of the sacrum, ilium, and pubis, which forms the pelvic inlet. Two smaller subsidiary rings are the obturator foramina. The greater and lesser sciatic foramina formed by the greater and lesser sciatic notches and the sacrospinous and sacrotuberous ligaments form the four fibro-osseous rings. The rings, which are predominantly bony (i.e., the pelvic inlet and the obturator foramina), are brittle rings. It is not possible to break one side of the ring without breaking the other side of the ring, which in clinical terms means that if a fracture is demonstrated on one side, a second fracture should always be suspected.

Fractures of the pelvis may occur in isolation; however, they usually occur in trauma patients and warrant special mention.

Owing to the large bony surfaces of the pelvis, a fracture produces an area of bone that **can bleed** significantly. A large hematoma may be produced, which can compress organs such as the bladder and the ureters. This blood loss may occur rapidly, reducing the circulating blood volume and, unless this is replaced, the patient will become hypovolemic and shock will develop.

Pelvic fractures may also disrupt the contents of the pelvis, leading to urethral disruption, potential bowel rupture, and nerve damage.

Joints

Lumbosacral joints

The sacrum articulates superiorly with the lumbar part of the vertebral column. The lumbosacral joints are formed between vertebra LV and the sacrum and consist of:

- The two **zygapophysial joints**, which occur between adjacent inferior and superior articular processes.
- An intervertebral disc that joins the bodies of vertebrae LV and SI (Fig. 5.23A).

These joints are similar to those between other vertebrae, with the exception that the sacrum is angled posteriorly on vertebra LV. As a result, the anterior part of the intervertebral disc between the two bones is thicker than the posterior part.

The lumbosacral joints are reinforced by strong iliolumbar and lumbosacral ligaments that extend from the expanded transverse processes of vertebra LV to the ilium and the sacrum, respectively (Fig. 5.23B).

Sacroiliac joints

The sacroiliac joints transmit forces from the lower limbs to the vertebral column. They are synovial joints between the L-shaped articular facets on the lateral surfaces of the sacrum and similar facets on the iliac parts of the pelvic bones (Fig. 5.24A). The joint surfaces have an irregular contour and interlock to resist movement. The joints often

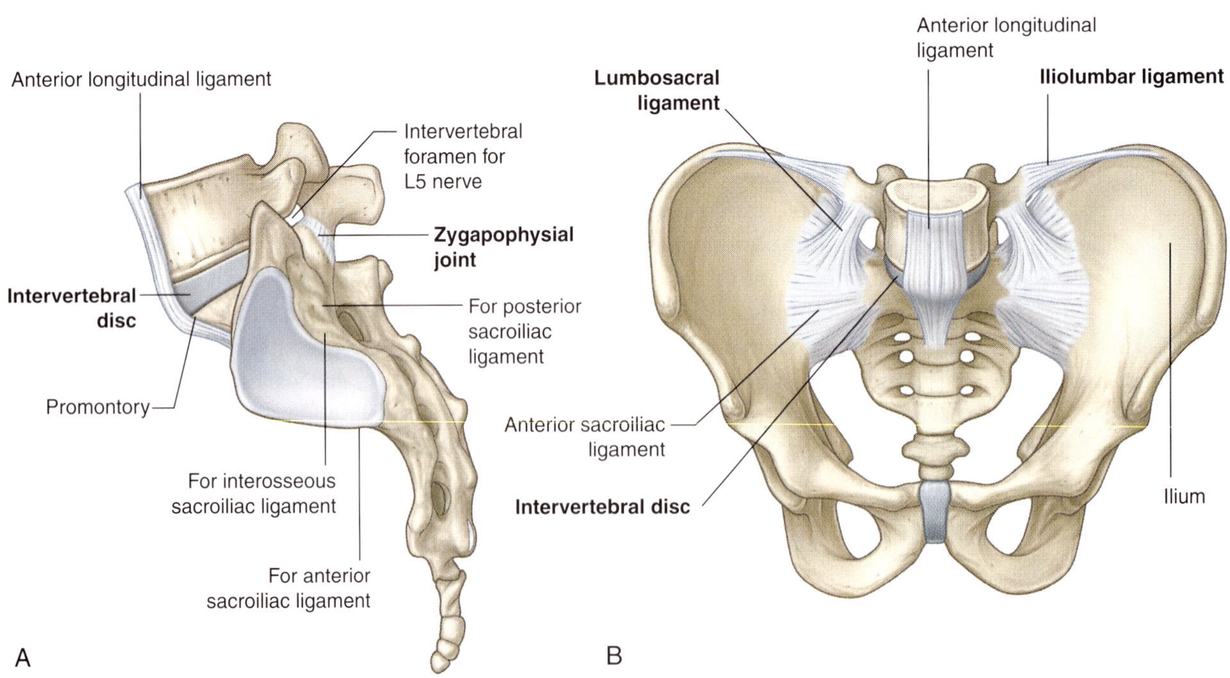

Fig. 5.23 Lumbosacral joints and associated ligaments. **(A)** Lateral view. **(B)** Anterior view.

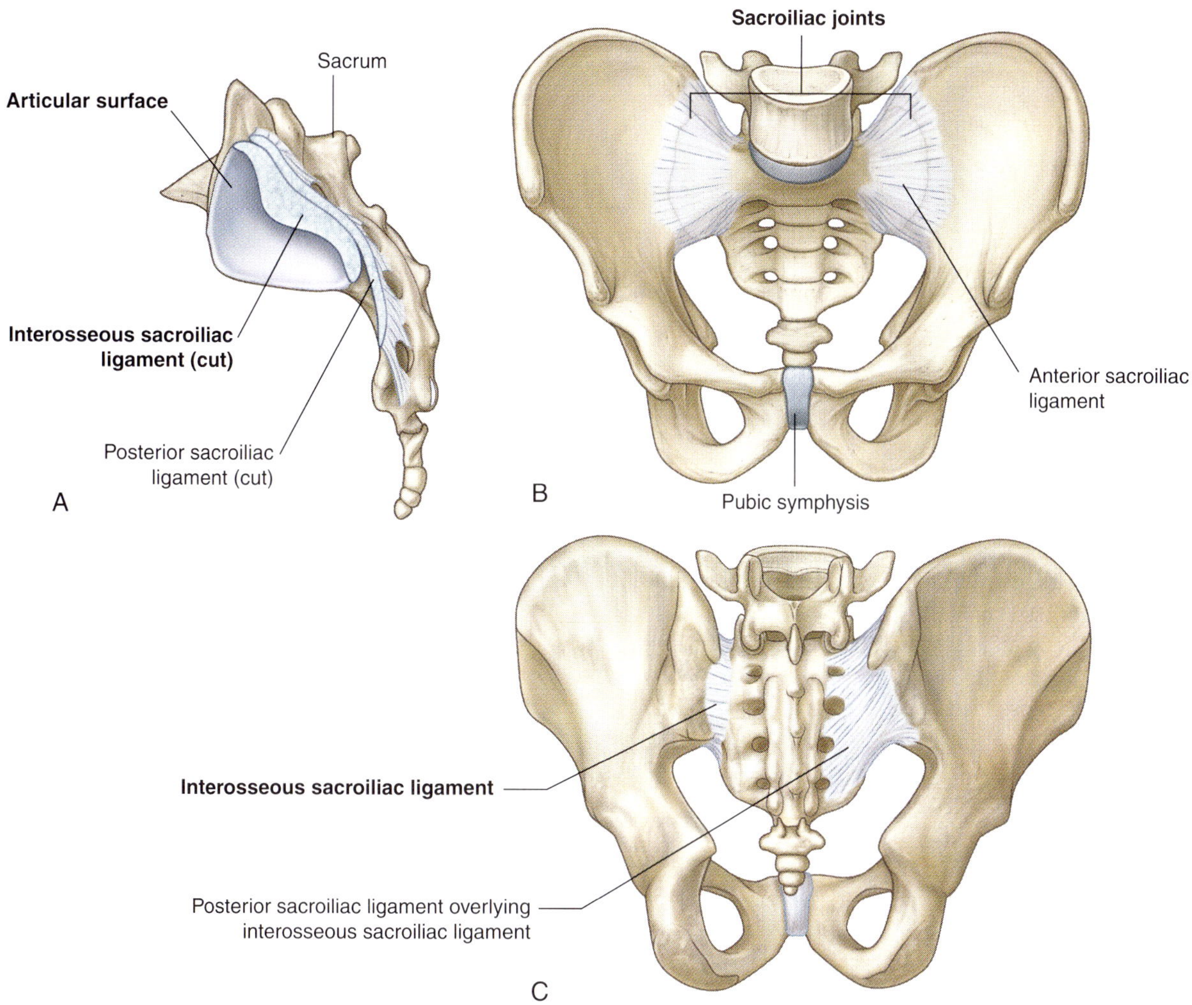

Fig. 5.24 Sacroiliac joints and associated ligaments. **(A)** Lateral view. **(B)** Anterior view. **(C)** Posterior view.

become fibrous with age and may become completely ossified.

Each sacroiliac joint is stabilized by three ligaments:

- The **anterior sacroiliac ligament**, which is a thickening of the fibrous membrane of the joint capsule and runs anteriorly and inferiorly to the joint (Fig. 5.24B)
- The **interosseous sacroiliac ligament**, which is the largest, strongest ligament of the three, and is positioned immediately posterosuperior to the joint and attaches to adjacent expansive roughened areas on the ilium and sacrum, thereby filling the gap between the two bones (Fig. 5.24A and C)
- The **posterior sacroiliac ligament**, which covers the interosseous sacroiliac ligament (Fig. 5.24C)

Pubic symphysis joint

The pubic symphysis lies anteriorly between the adjacent surfaces of the pubic bones (Fig. 5.25). Each of the joint's surfaces is covered by hyaline cartilage and is linked across the midline to adjacent surfaces by fibrocartilage. The joint is surrounded by interwoven layers of collagen fibers and the two major ligaments associated with it are

- The **superior pubic ligament**, located above the joint
- The **inferior pubic ligament**, located below it

Early clinical exposure

Common problems with the sacroiliac joints

The sacroiliac joints have both fibrous and synovial components, and as with many weight-bearing joints, degenerative changes may occur and cause pain and discomfort in the sacroiliac region. In addition, disorders associated with the major histocompatibility complex antigen HLA-B27, such as rheumatoid arthritis, psoriasis, and inflammatory bowel disease, can produce specific inflammatory changes within these joints.

Orientation

In the anatomical position, the pelvis is oriented so that the front edge of the top of the pubic symphysis and the anterior superior iliac spines lie in the same vertical plane (Fig. 5.26). As a consequence, the pelvic inlet, which marks the entrance to the pelvic cavity, is tilted to face anteriorly, and the bodies of the pubic bones and the pubic arch are positioned in a nearly horizontal plane facing the ground.

Differences between men and women

The pelves of women and men differ in a number of ways, many of which have to do with the passing of a baby through a woman's pelvic cavity during childbirth. The differences in the pelvic inlet, pelvic cavity, and pelvic outlet may be explained by observing the sequence of the passage of the fetal head during parturition along the axis of birth canal (obstetric axis). The largest diameter of the fetal head passes through the transverse diameter of the pelvic inlet, the diagonal diameter of the pelvic

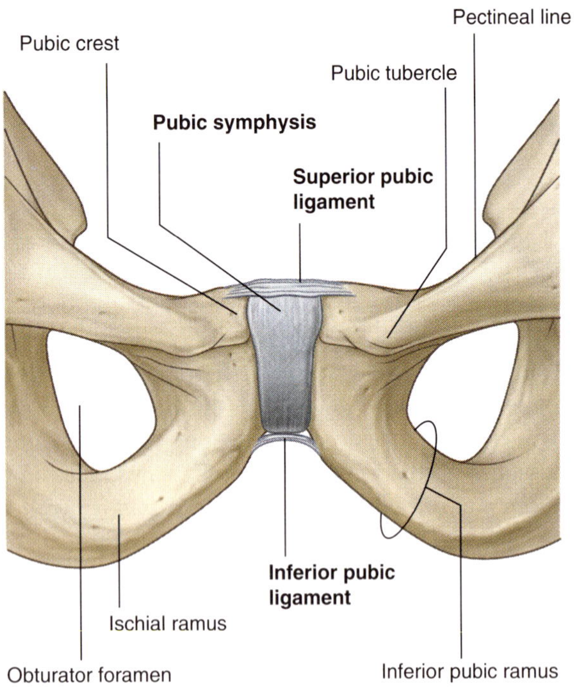

Fig. 5.25 Pubic symphysis and associated ligaments.

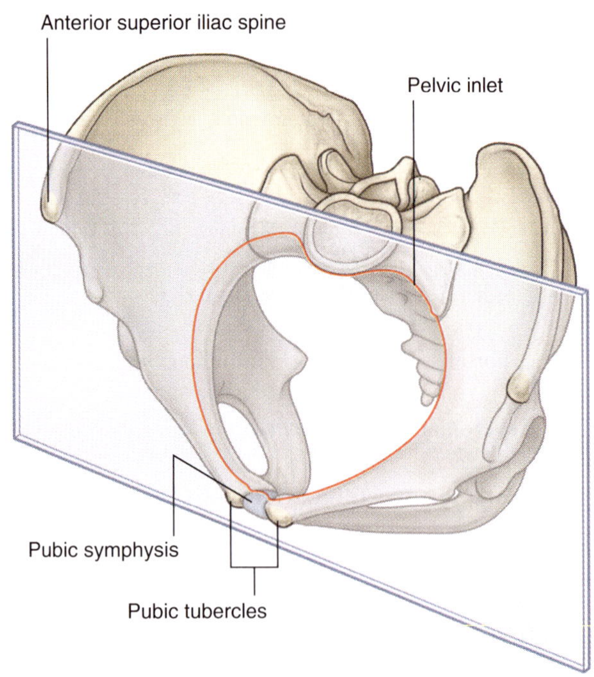

Fig. 5.26 Orientation of the pelvis (anatomical position).

cavity, and the anteroposterior diameter of the pelvic outlet.

- The **pelvic inlet** in women is circular (Fig. 5.27A) compared with the heart-shaped pelvic inlet (Fig. 5.27B) in men. The more circular shape is partly caused by the less distinct promontory and broader alae in women. The width of each ala is usually more than the maximum width of the body of the S1 vertebra in women (the opposite is true in men). Pelves are classified into four types based on various features including the shape of the pelvic inlet. Initially, during development, the anteroposterior diameter of the pelvic inlet is more than the transverse diameter (**anthropoid pelvis**). Later in development, the anteroposterior and transverse diameters of the pelvic inlet become equal, the pelvic inlet is heart shaped (wider posteriorly), is present in both genders before puberty, and is the predominant type present in men (**android pelvis**). In women, after puberty, the pelvic inlet becomes circular (due to an increase in the transverse diameter anteriorly), the transverse diameter of the pelvic inlet may be slightly more than the anteroposterior diameter **(gynecoid pelvis)**. The transverse diameter of the pelvic inlet may be much more than the anteroposterior diameter (**platypelloid pelvis**). All types of pelves are found in women, and only about 50% of women have a gynecoid pelvis. The majority of pelves are of mixed types. The **obstetric conjugate**, which is 10 cm or more, is the distance between the sacral promontory and the thickest part of the body of the pubis.

Pelvic cavity: The pelvic cavity is vertically shorter and more cylindrical in women, whereas it is vertically longer and more conical in males. The ischial spines generally do not project as far medially into the pelvic cavity in women as they do in men. The interspinous diameter, which is 10 cm or more, is at the level of the ischial spines and is the smallest diameter of the true pelvis. The plane of least pelvic dimensions (obstetric outlet) is bounded laterally by the ischial spines, anteriorly by the lower border of the pubic symphysis and posteriorly by the lower end of the sacrum. The anatomical outlet is at the level of the ischial tuberosities.

- The distance from the lower margin of the pubic symphysis to the sacral promontory is the **diagonal conjugate** which is 11.5 cm or more. During per vaginal examination, the sacral promontory cannot be palpated normally. If the sacral promontory can be palpated, it indicates a contracted pelvis. The distance from the superior margin of the pubic symphysis to the sacral promontory is the **true conjugate** which can be measured in an X-ray. The distance from the anterior margin of the acetabulum to the pubic symphysis is more than the diameter of the acetabulum in women, whereas it is usually equal in men. The diameter of the acetabulum is usually more in men than in women. The **sacral index** is the maximum width to the maximum straight length of the sacrum multiplied by 100. It is 115 in women and 105 in men. The angle at the greater sciatic notch is about 74.4° in females and 54.4° in males, which is due to the greater backward sacral tilt in females. The ischiopubic ramus bears a rough everted area for attachment of the root of the penis or clitoris, which is more distinct in men. The preauricular sulcus (a vertical

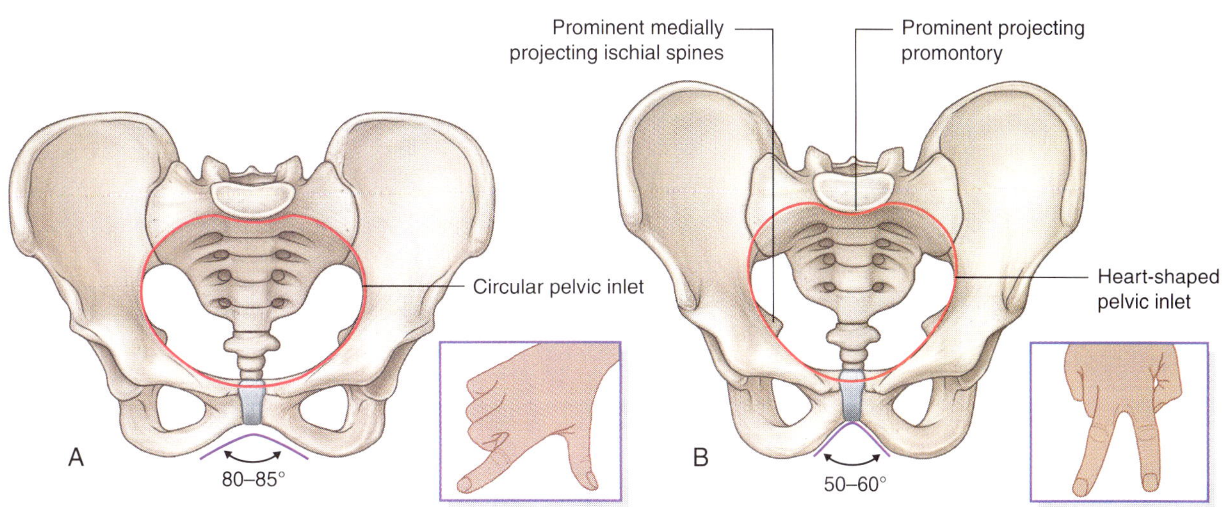

Fig. 5.27 Structure of the bony pelvis. **(A)** In women. **(B)** In men. The angle formed by the pubic arch can be approximated by the angle between the thumb and index finger for women and the angle between the index finger and middle finger for men as shown in the insets.

groove on the ilium anterior to the sacroiliac joint) is seen more commonly and is more defined in women, compared with men. The angle at the pubic arch is larger in women (80–85°) than it is in men (50–60°). This difference may be very apparent in a bony pelvis.

True pelvis

The true pelvis is cylindrical and has an inlet, a wall, and an outlet. The inlet is open, whereas the pelvic floor closes the outlet and separates the pelvic cavity, above, from the perineum, below.

Pelvic inlet

The pelvic inlet is the circular opening between the abdominal cavity and the pelvic cavity through which structures traverse between the abdomen and pelvic cavity. It is completely surrounded by bones and joints (Fig. 5.28). The promontory of the sacrum protrudes into the inlet, forming its posterior margin in the midline. On each side of the promontory, the margin is formed by the alae of the sacrum. The margin of the pelvic inlet then crosses the sacroiliac joint and continues along the linea terminalis (i.e., the arcuate line, the pecten pubis or pectineal line, and the pubic crest) to the pubic symphysis.

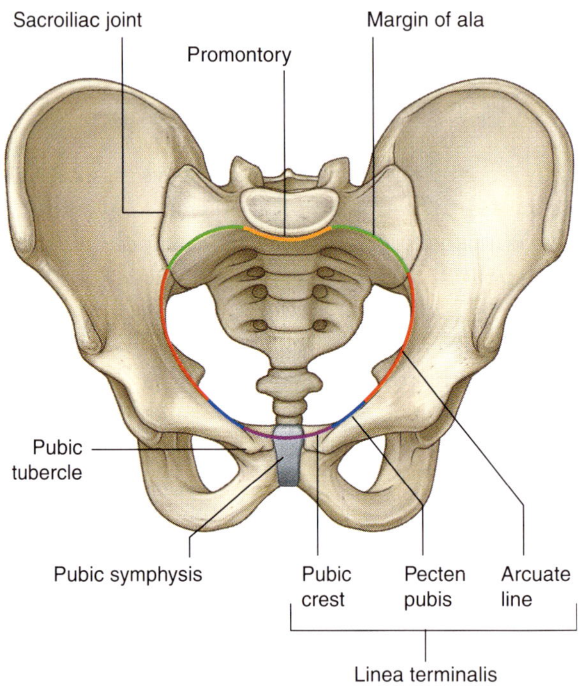

Fig. 5.28 Pelvic inlet.

Pelvic wall

The walls of the pelvic cavity consist of the sacrum, the coccyx, the pelvic bones inferior to the linea terminalis, two ligaments, and two muscles.

Ligaments of the pelvic wall

The sacrospinous and sacrotuberous ligaments (Fig. 5.29A) are major components of the lateral pelvic walls that help define the apertures between the pelvic cavity and adjacent regions through which structures pass.

- The smaller of the two, the sacrospinous ligament, is triangular, with its apex attached to the ischial spine and its base attached to the related margins of the sacrum and the coccyx.
- The sacrotuberous ligament is also triangular and is superficial to the sacrospinous ligament. Its base has a broad attachment that extends from the posterior superior iliac spine of the pelvic bone, along the dorsal aspect and the lateral margin of the sacrum, and onto the dorsolateral surface of the coccyx. Laterally, the apex of the ligament is attached to the medial margin of the ischial tuberosity.

These ligaments stabilize the sacrum on the pelvic bones by resisting the upward tilting of the inferior aspect of the sacrum (Fig. 5.29B). They also convert the greater and lesser sciatic notches of the pelvic bone into foramina (Fig. 5.29A and B).

- The **greater sciatic foramen** lies superior to the sacrospinous ligament and the ischial spine.
- The **lesser sciatic foramen** lies inferior to the ischial spine and sacrospinous ligament between the sacrospinous and sacrotuberous ligaments.

Muscles of the pelvic wall

Two muscles, the obturator internus and the piriformis, contribute to the lateral walls of the pelvic cavity. These muscles originate in the pelvic cavity but attach peripherally to the femur.

Obturator internus

The obturator internus is a flat, fan-shaped muscle that originates from the deep surface of the obturator membrane and from associated regions of the pelvic bone that surround the obturator foramen (Fig. 5.30; Table 5.1).

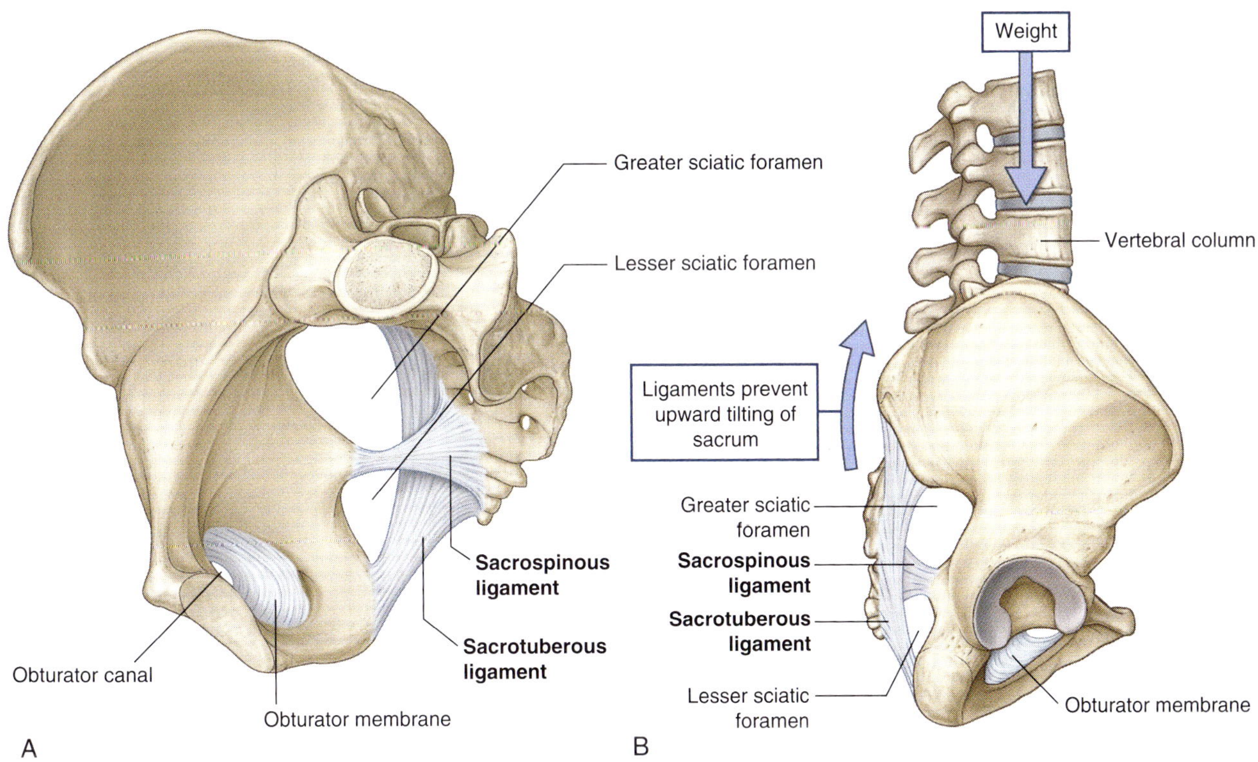

Fig. 5.29 Sacrospinous and sacrotuberous ligaments. **(A)** Medial view of right side of pelvis. **(B)** Function of the ligaments.

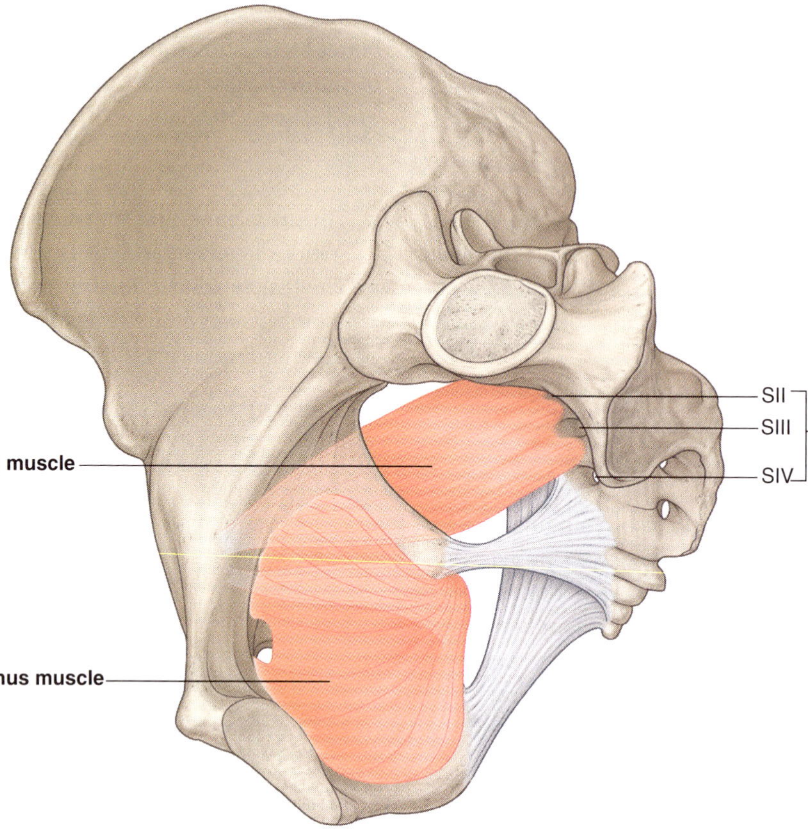

Fig. 5.30 Obturator internus and piriformis muscles (medial view of right side of pelvis).

Table 5.1 Muscles of the pelvic walls

Muscle	Origin	Insertion	Innervation	Function
Obturator internus	Anterolateral wall of true pelvis (deep surface of obturator membrane and surrounding bone)	Medial surface of greater trochanter of femur	Nerve to obturator internus **L5, SI**	Lateral rotation of the extended hip joint; abduction of flexed hip
Piriformis	Anterior surface of sacrum between anterior sacral foramina	Medial side of superior border of greater trochanter of femur	Branches from **SI** and **S2**	Lateral rotation of the extended hip joint; abduction of flexed hip

The muscle fibers of the obturator internus converge to form a tendon that leaves the pelvic cavity through the lesser sciatic foramen, makes a 90° bend around the ischium between the ischial spine and ischial tuberosity, and then passes posterior to the hip joint to insert on the greater trochanter of the femur.

The obturator internus forms a large part of the anterolateral wall of the pelvic cavity.

Piriformis

The piriformis is triangular and originates in the bridges of bone between the four anterior sacral foramina. It passes laterally through the greater sciatic foramen, crosses the posterosuperior aspect of the hip joint, and inserts on the greater trochanter of the femur above the insertion of the obturator internus muscle (Fig. 5.30; Table 5.1).

A large part of the posterolateral wall of the pelvic cavity is formed by the piriformis. In addition, this muscle separates the greater sciatic foramen into **two regions**, one above the muscle and one below. Vessels and nerves coursing between the pelvic cavity and the gluteal region pass through these two regions.

Apertures in the pelvic wall

Each lateral pelvic wall has three major apertures through which structures pass between the pelvic cavity and other regions:

- The obturator canal
- The greater sciatic foramen
- The lesser sciatic foramen

Obturator canal

At the top of the obturator foramen is the obturator canal, which is bordered by the obturator membrane, the associated obturator muscles, and the superior pubic ramus (Fig. 5.31). The obturator nerve and vessels pass from the pelvic cavity to the thigh through this canal.

Greater sciatic foramen

The greater sciatic foramen is a major route of communication between the pelvic cavity and the lower limb (Fig. 5.31). It is formed by the greater sciatic notch in the pelvic bone, the sacrotuberous and the sacrospinous ligaments, and the spine of the ischium.

The piriformis muscle passes through the greater sciatic foramen, dividing it into two parts.

- The superior gluteal nerves and vessels pass through the foramen above the piriformis.
- Passing through the foramen below the piriformis are the inferior gluteal nerves and vessels, the sciatic nerve, the pudendal nerve, the internal pudendal vessels, the posterior femoral cutaneous nerves, and the nerves to the obturator internus and quadratus femoris muscles.

Lesser sciatic foramen

The lesser sciatic foramen is formed by the lesser sciatic notch of the pelvic bone, the ischial spine, the sacrospinous ligament, and the sacrotuberous ligament (Fig. 5.31). The tendon of the obturator internus muscle passes through this foramen to enter the gluteal region of the lower limb.

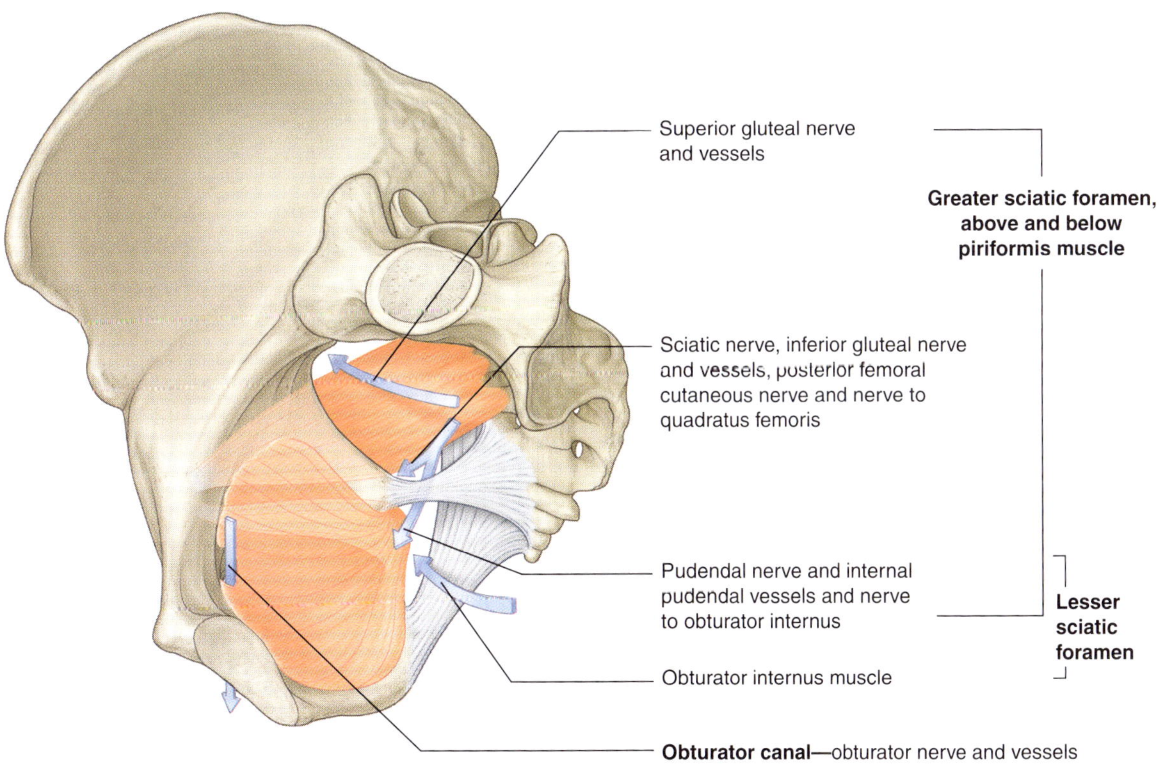

Fig. 5.31 Apertures in the pelvic wall.

Because the lesser sciatic foramen is positioned below the attachment of the pelvic floor, it acts as a route of communication between the perineum and the gluteal region. The pudendal nerve and internal pudendal vessels pass between the pelvic cavity (above the pelvic floor) and the perineum (below the pelvic floor), by first passing out of the pelvic cavity through the greater sciatic foramen and then looping around the ischial spine and sacrospinous ligament to pass through the lesser sciatic foramen to enter the perineum.

Pelvic outlet

The pelvic outlet is diamond shaped, with the anterior part of the diamond defined predominantly by bone and the posterior part mainly by ligaments (Fig. 5.32). In the midline anteriorly, the boundary of the pelvic outlet is the pubic symphysis. Extending laterally and posteriorly, the boundary on each side is the inferior border of the body of the pubis, the inferior ramus of the pubis, the ramus of the ischium, and the ischial tuberosity. Together, the elements on both sides form the pubic arch.

From the ischial tuberosities, the boundaries continue posteriorly and medially along the sacrotuberous ligament on both sides to the coccyx.

Terminal parts of the urinary and gastrointestinal tracts and the vagina pass through the pelvic outlet.

The area enclosed by the boundaries of the pelvic outlet and below the pelvic floor is the **perineum**.

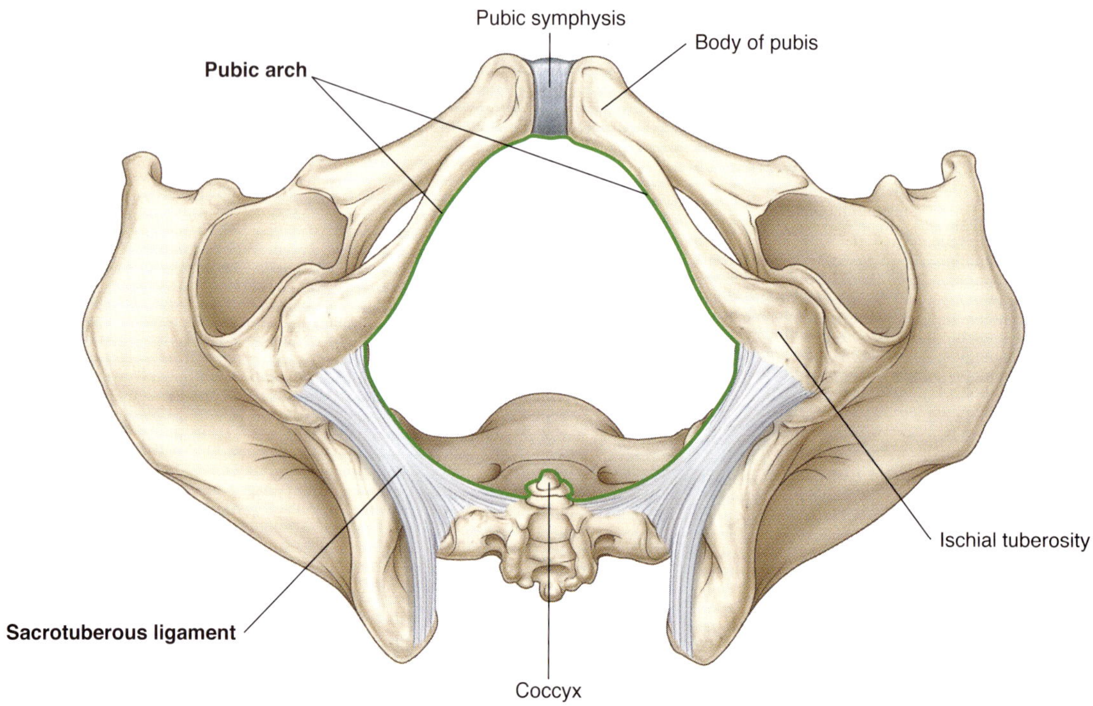

Fig. 5.32 Pelvic outlet.

Early clinical exposure

Pelvic measurements in obstetrics

Transverse and sagittal measurements of a woman's pelvic inlet and outlet can help in predicting the likelihood of a successful vaginal delivery. These measurements include:

- The sagittal inlet (between the promontory and the top of the pubic symphysis)
- The maximum transverse diameter of the inlet
- The bispinous diameter (the distance between ischial spines)
- The sagittal outlet (the distance between the tip of the coccyx and the inferior margin of the pubic symphysis)

These measurements can be obtained using magnetic resonance imaging, which carries no radiation risk for the fetus or mother (Fig. 5.33).

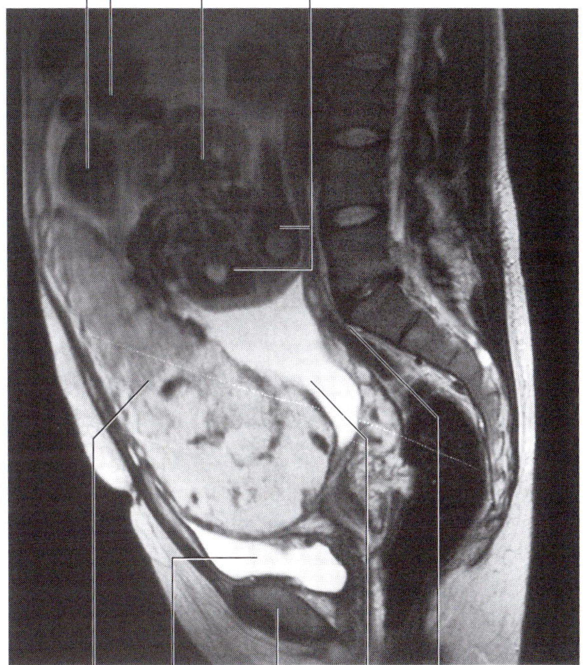

Fig. 5.33 Sagittal T2-weighted magnetic resonance image of the lower abdomen and pelvis of a pregnant woman.

Pelvic floor

The pelvic floor is formed by the pelvic diaphragm. The pelvic diaphragm is formed by the levator ani and the coccygeus muscles from both sides. The pelvic floor separates the pelvic cavity, above, from the perineum, below.

The pelvic diaphragm

The pelvic diaphragm is the muscular part of the pelvic floor. Shaped like a bowl or funnel and attached superiorly to the pelvic walls, it consists of the levator ani and the coccygeus muscles (Fig. 5.34 A; Table 5.2).

The pelvic diaphragm's circular line of attachment to the cylindrical pelvic wall passes, on each side, between the greater sciatic foramen and the lesser sciatic foramen. Thus:

- The greater sciatic foramen is situated above the level of the pelvic floor and is a route of communication between the pelvic cavity and the gluteal region of the lower limb.
- The lesser sciatic foramen is situated below the pelvic floor, providing a route of communication between the gluteal region of the lower limb and the perineum.

Levator ani.

The two levator ani muscles originate from each side of the pelvic wall, course medially and inferiorly, and join together in the midline. The attachment to the pelvic wall follows the circular contour of the wall and includes:

- The posterior aspect of the body of the pubic bone
- A linear thickening called the **tendinous arch**, of the fascia covering the obturator internus muscle
- The spine of the ischium

In the midline, the muscles blend together posterior to the vagina in women and around the anal aperture in both sexes. Posterior to the anal aperture, the muscles come together as a ligament or raphe called the **anococcygeal ligament** (**anococcygeal body**) and attaches to the coccyx.

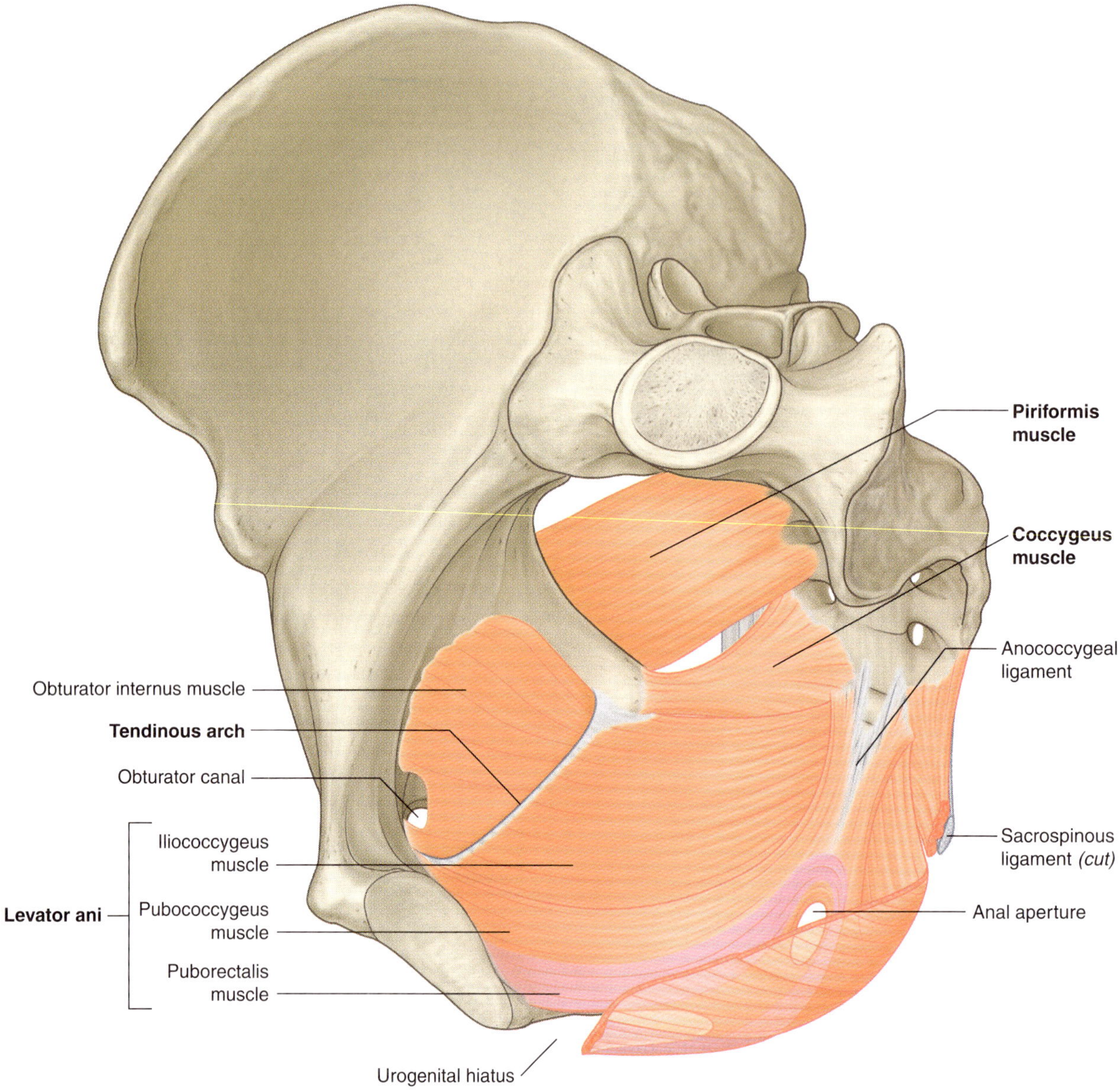

Fig. 5.34 (A) Pelvic diaphragm.

Table 5.2 Muscles of the pelvic diaphragm

Muscle	Origin	Insertion	Innervation	Function
Levator ani	In a line around the pelvic wall beginning on the posterior aspect of the pubic bone and extending across the obturator internus muscle as a tendinous arch (thickening of the obturator internus fascia) to the ischial spine	The anterior part is attached to the superior surface of the perineal membrane; the posterior part meets its partner on the other side at the perineal body, around the anal canal, and along the anococcygeal ligament	Branches direct from the anterior ramus of S4, and by the inferior rectal branch of the pudendal nerve (S2 to S4)	Contributes to the formation of the pelvic floor, which supports the pelvic viscera; maintains an angle between the rectum and anal canal; reinforces the external anal sphincter and, in women, functions as a vaginal sphincter
Coccygeus	Ischial spine and pelvic surface of the sacrospinous ligament	Lateral margin of coccyx and related border of sacrum	Branches from the anterior rami of S3 and S4	Contributes to the formation of the pelvic floor, which supports the pelvic viscera; pulls coccyx forward after defecation

Anteriorly, the muscles are separated by a U-shaped defect or gap termed the **urogenital hiatus**. The margins of this hiatus merge with the walls of the associated viscera and with muscles in the deep perineal pouch below. The hiatus allows the urethra (in both men and women), and the vagina (in women), to pass through the pelvic diaphragm (Fig. 5.34A).

The levator ani muscles include three collections of muscle fibers, based on site of origin and relationship to viscera in the midline: the pubococcygeus, the puborectalis, and the iliococcygeus muscles.

- The **pubococcygeus** originates from the body of the pubis and courses posteriorly to attach along the midline as far back as the coccyx. This part of the muscle is further subdivided on the basis of association with structures in the midline into the **puboprostaticus (levator prostatae)**, the **pubovaginalis**, and the **puboanalis muscles**.
- A second major collection of muscle fibers, the **puborectalis** portion of the levator ani muscles, originates, in association with the pubococcygeus muscle, from the pubis and passes inferiorly on each side to form a sling around the terminal part of the gastrointestinal tract. This muscular sling maintains an angle or flexure, called the **perineal flexure**, at the anorectal junction. This angle functions as part of the mechanism that keeps the end of the gastrointestinal system closed.
- The final part of the levator ani muscle is the **iliococcygeus**. This part of the muscle originates from the fascia that covers the obturator internus muscle. It joins the same muscle on the other side in the midline to form a ligament or raphe that extends from the anal aperture to the coccyx.

The levator ani muscles help support the pelvic viscera and maintain closure of the rectum and vagina. They are innervated directly by branches from the anterior ramus of S4 and by branches of the pudendal nerve (S2 to S4).

Early clinical exposure

Defecation

At the beginning of defecation, closure of the larynx stabilizes the diaphragm and intraabdominal pressure is increased by contraction of abdominal wall muscles. As defecation proceeds, the puborectalis muscle surrounding the anorectal junction relaxes, which straightens the anorectal angle. Both the internal and the external anal sphincters also relax to allow feces to move through the anal canal. Normally, the puborectal sling maintains an angle of about 90° between the rectum and the anal canal and acts as a "pinch valve" to prevent defecation. When the puborectalis muscle relaxes, the anorectal angle increases to about 130°–140°.

The fatty tissue of the ischioanal fossa allows for changes in the position and size of the anal canal and anus during defecation. During evacuation, the anorectal junction moves down and back and the pelvic floor usually descends slightly.

During defecation, the circular muscles of the rectal wall undergo a wave of contraction to push feces toward the anus. As feces emerge from the anus, the longitudinal muscles of the rectum and levator ani bring the anal canal back up, the feces are expelled, and the anus and rectum return to their normal positions.

A magnetic resonance defecating proctogram is a fairly new imaging technique that allows assessment of different phases of defecation, including rectal function and behavior of the pelvic floor musculature during this process. It is useful in detecting pelvic organ abnormal descent/prolapse during dynamic scanning and potential formation of cystocele or rectocele (Fig. 5.34B).

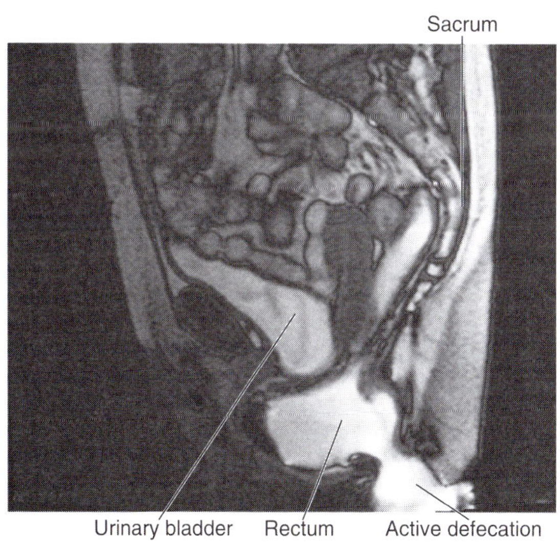

Fig. 5.34 (B) MRI defecating proctogram in sagittal plane showing active defecation.

Coccygeus

The two coccygeus muscles, one on each side, are triangular and overlie the sacrospinous ligaments; together they complete the posterior part of the pelvic diaphragm (Fig. 5.34A; Table 5.2). They are attached, by their apices, to the tips of the ischial spines and, by their bases, to the lateral margins of the coccyx and adjacent margins of the sacrum.

These coccygeus muscles are innervated by branches from the anterior rami of S3 and S4 and participate in supporting the posterior aspect of the pelvic floor.

The perineal membrane and deep perineal pouch

The **perineal membrane** is a thick fascial, triangular structure attached to the bony framework of the pubic arch (Fig. 5.35A). It is oriented in the horizontal plane and has a free posterior margin. Anteriorly, there is a small gap (blue arrow in Fig. 5.35A) between the membrane and the **inferior pubic ligament** (a ligament associated with the pubic symphysis).

The perineal membrane is related above to a thin space called the **deep perineal pouch** (**deep perineal space**) (Fig. 5.35B), which contains a layer of skeletal muscle and various neurovascular elements.

The deep perineal pouch is open above and is not separated from more superior structures by a distinct layer of fascia. The parts of the perineal membrane and structures in the deep perineal pouch, enclosed by the urogenital hiatus above, therefore contribute to the pelvic floor and support elements of the urogenital system in the pelvic cavity, even though the perineal membrane and deep perineal pouch are usually considered parts of the perineum.

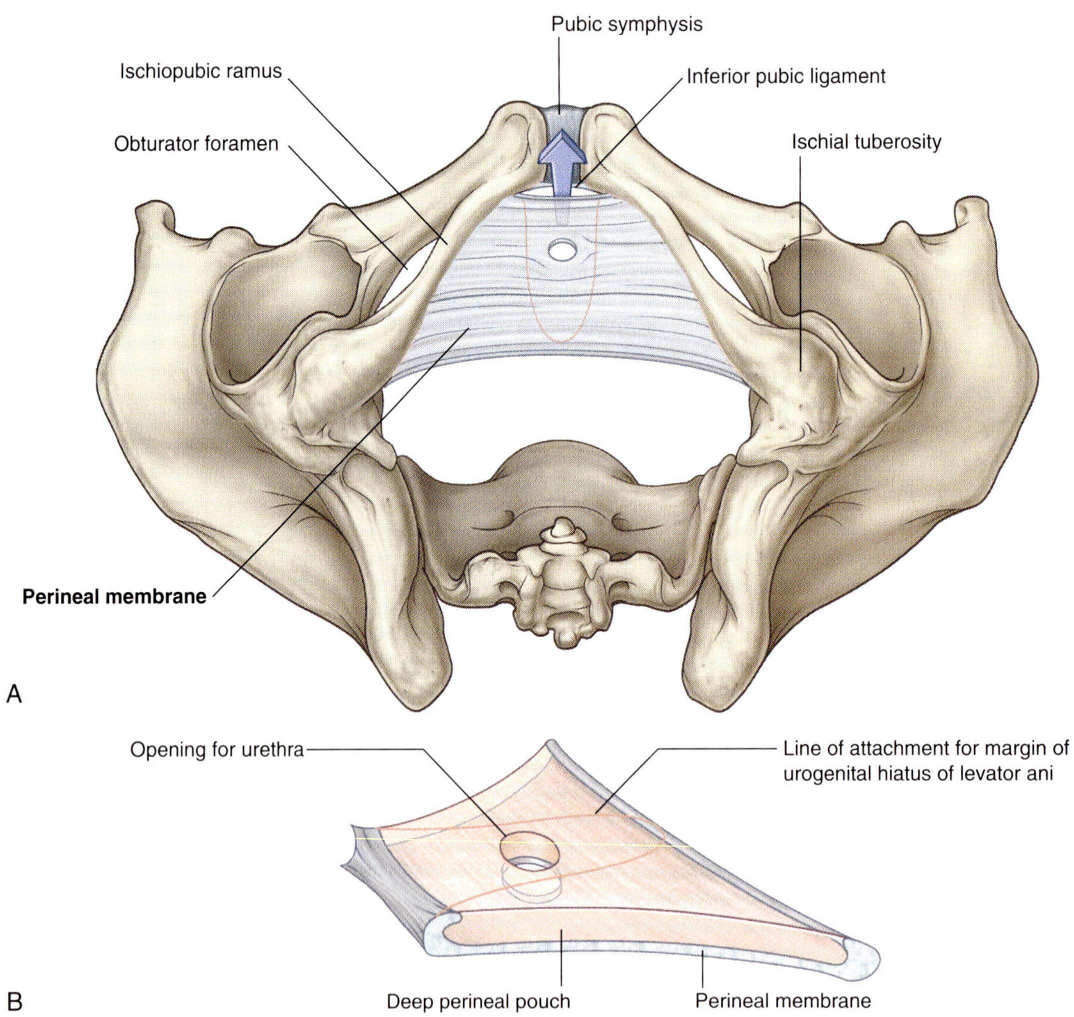

Fig. 5.35 Perineal membrane and deep perineal pouch. **(A)** Inferior view. **(B)** Superolateral view. Perineal membrane and deep perineal pouch.

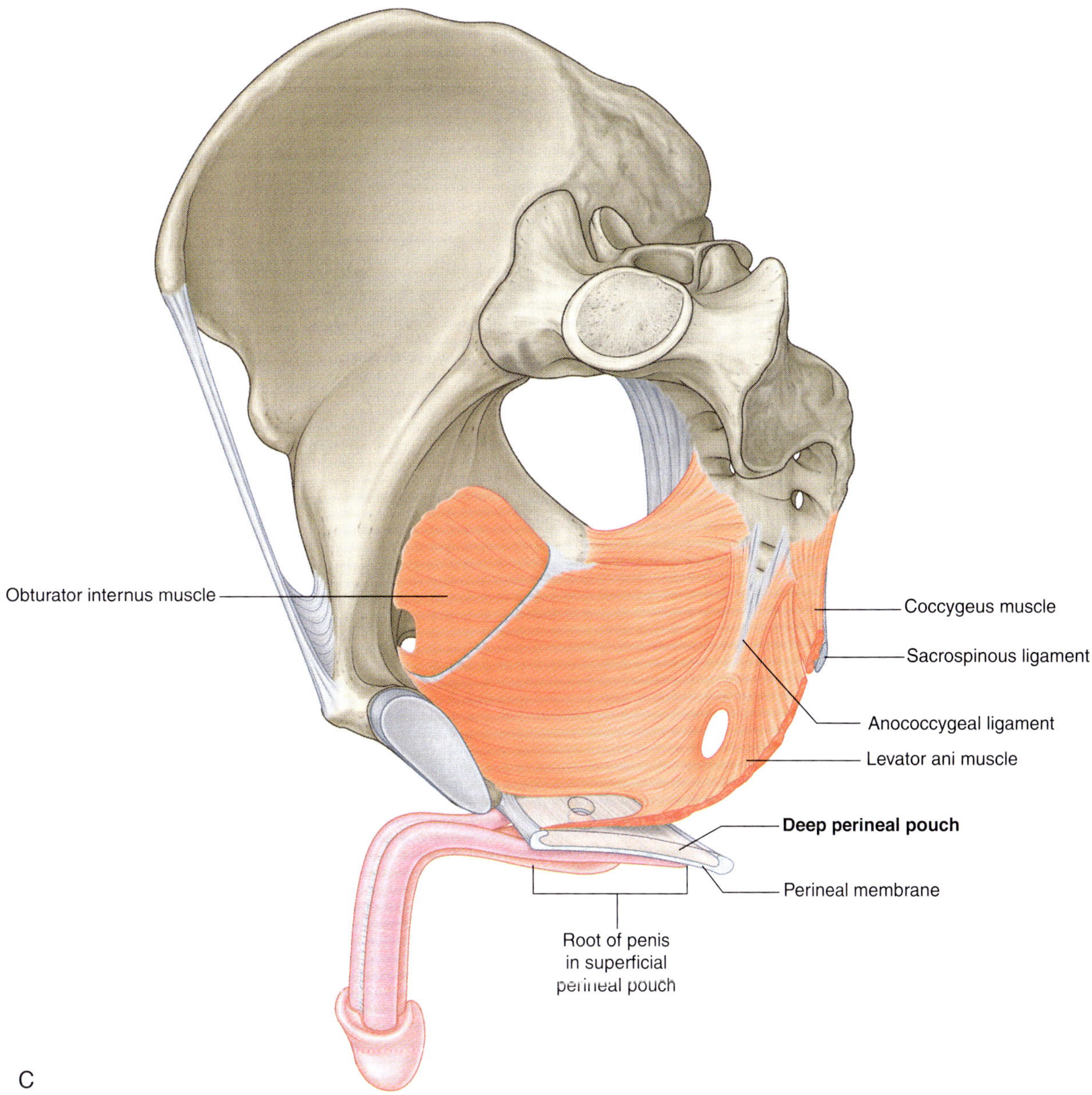

Fig. 5.35, cont'd (C) Medial view.

The perineal membrane and adjacent pubic arch provide attachment for the roots of the external genitalia and the muscles associated with them (Fig. 5.35C).

The urethra penetrates vertically through a circular hiatus in the perineal membrane as it passes from the pelvic cavity, above, to the perineum, below. In women, the vagina also passes through a hiatus in the perineal membrane just posterior to the urethral hiatus.

Within the deep perineal pouch, a sheet of skeletal muscle functions as a sphincter, mainly for the urethra, and as a stabilizer of the posterior edge of the perineal membrane (Fig. 5.36; Table 5.3).

- Anteriorly, a group of muscle fibers surround the urethra and collectively form the **external urethral sphincter**.

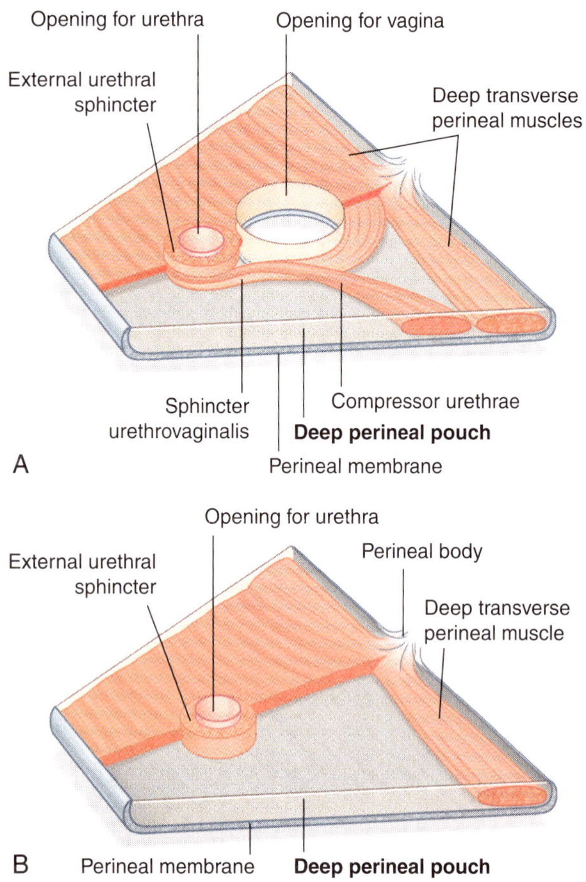

Fig. 5.36 Muscles in the deep perineal pouch. **(A)** In women. **(B)** In men.

- Two additional groups of muscle fibers are associated with the urethra and vagina in women. One group forms the **sphincter urethrovaginalis**, which surrounds the urethra and vagina as a unit. The second group forms the **compressor urethrae**, on each side, which originate from the ischiopubic rami and meet anterior to the urethra. Together with the external urethral sphincter, the sphincter urethrovaginalis and compressor urethrae facilitate closing of the urethra.
- In both men and women, a **deep transverse perineal muscle** on each side parallels the free margin of the perineal membrane and joins with its partner at the midline. These muscles are thought to stabilize the position of the perineal body, which is a midline structure along the posterior edge of the perineal membrane.

Perineal body

The perineal body is an ill-defined but important connective tissue structure into which muscles of the pelvic floor and the perineum attach (Figs 5.36A and B, 5.37, and 5.38C). It is positioned in the midline along the posterior border of the perineal membrane, to which it attaches. The posterior end of the urogenital hiatus in the levator ani muscles is also connected to it.

The deep transverse perineal muscles intersect at the perineal body; in women, the sphincter urethrovaginalis also attaches to the perineal body. Other muscles that connect to the perineal body include the external anal sphincter, the superficial transverse perineal muscles, and the bulbospongiosus muscles of the perineum (Fig. 5.71).

Table 5.3 Muscles within the deep perineal pouch

Muscle	Origin	Insertion	Innervation	Function
External urethral sphincter	From the inferior ramus of the pubis on each side and adjacent walls of the deep perineal pouch	Surrounds membranous part of urethra	Perineal branches of the pudendal nerve (S2 to S4)	Compresses the membranous urethra; relaxes during micturition
Deep transverse perineal	Medial aspect of ischial ramus	Perineal body	Perineal branches of the pudendal nerve (S2 to S4)	Stabilizes the position of the perineal body
Compressor urethrae (in women only)	Ischiopubic ramus on each side	Blends with partner on other side anterior to the urethra	Perineal branches of the pudendal nerve (S2 to S4)	Functions as an accessory sphincter of the urethra
Sphincter urethrovagin alis (in women only)	Perineal body	Passes forward lateral to the vagina to blend with partner on other side anterior to the urethra	Perineal branches of the pudendal nerve (S2 to S4)	Functions as an accessory sphincter of the urethra (also may facilitate closing the vagina)

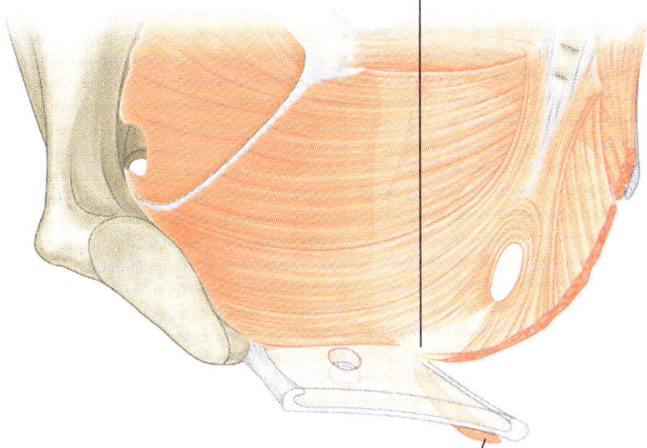

Fig. 5.37 Perineal body.

Early clinical exposure

Episiotomy

During childbirth, the perineal body may be stretched and torn. Traditionally, it was felt that if a perineal tear is likely, the obstetrician may proceed with an episiotomy. This is a procedure in which an incision is made in the perineal body to allow the head of the fetus to pass through the vagina. There are two types of episiotomies: a median episiotomy cuts through the perineal body, while a mediolateral episiotomy is an incision 45° from the midline. The maternal benefits of this procedure have been thought to be less traumatic to the perineum and to result in decreased pelvic floor dysfunction after childbirth. However, more recent evidence suggests that an episiotomy should not be performed routinely. Review of data has failed to show a decrease in pelvic floor damage with routine use of episiotomies.

Viscera

The pelvic viscera include parts of the gastrointestinal system, the urinary system, and the reproductive system. The viscera are arranged in the midline, from front to back; the neurovascular supply is through branches that pass medially from vessels and nerves associated with the pelvic walls.

Gastrointestinal system

Pelvic parts of the gastrointestinal system consist mainly of the rectum and the anal canal, although the terminal part of the sigmoid colon is also in the pelvic cavity (Fig. 5.38).

Rectum

The **rectum** is continuous:

- Above, with the sigmoid colon at about the level of vertebra SIII, and below, with the anal canal as this

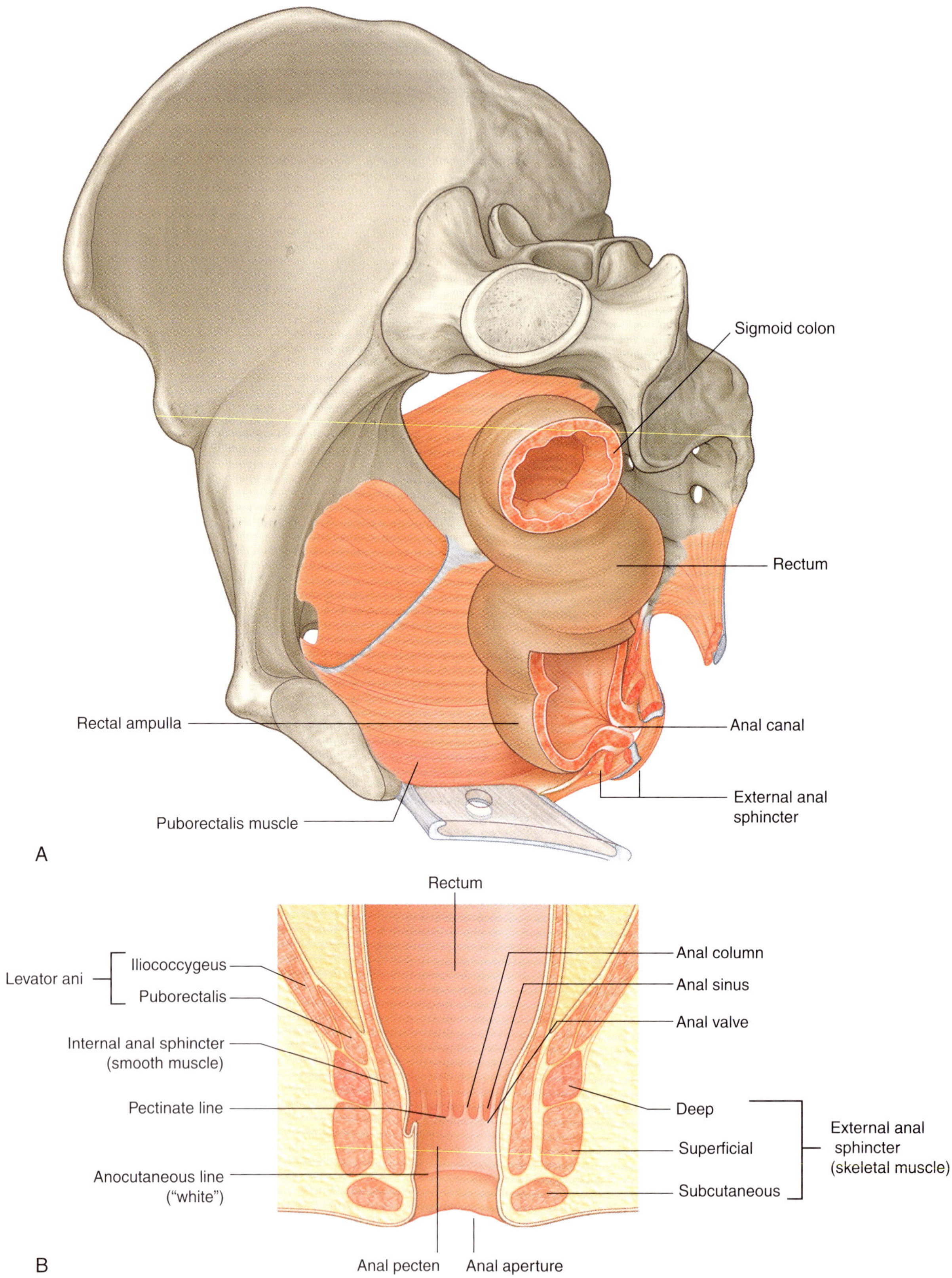

Fig. 5.38 Rectum and anal canal. **(A)** Left pelvic bone removed. **(B)** Longitudinal section.

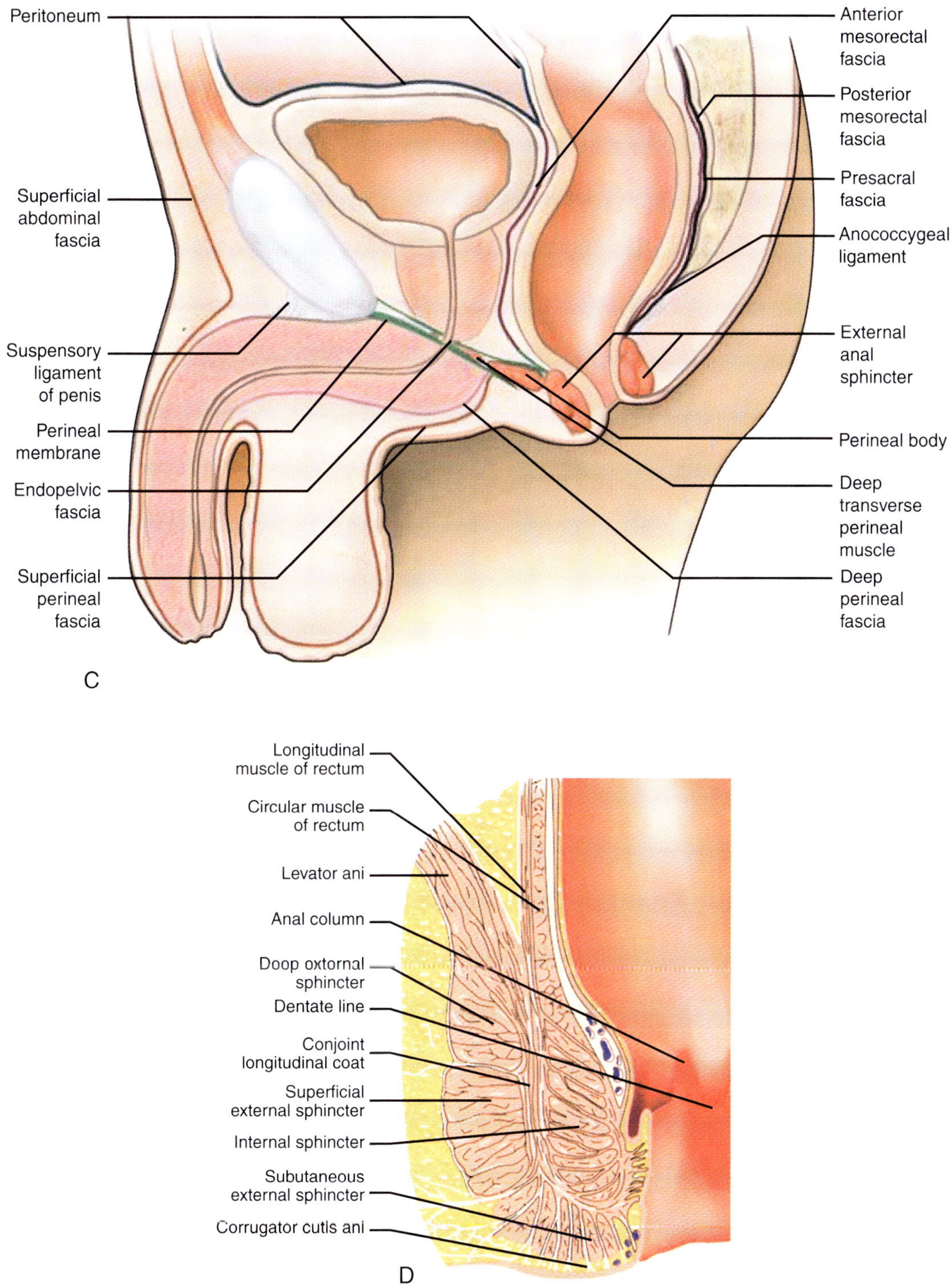

Fig. 5.38, cont'd (C) Fascia of the rectum. **(D)** Sphincters of the anal canal. *Source:* **(C)** http://clinicalgate.com/true-pelvis-pelvic-floor-and-perineum/; **(D)** http://jumed14.weebly.com/uploads/5/8/7/5/58753271/anatomy-of-the-rectum-and-anus-student-version.pdf

structure penetrates the pelvic floor and passes through the perineum to end as the anus. The anorectal angle corresponds to the anorectal junction.

The rectum, the most posterior element of the pelvic viscera, is immediately anterior to, and follows the concave contour of the sacrum.

The anorectal junction is pulled forward (perineal flexure) by the action of the puborectalis part of the levator ani muscle, so the anal canal moves in a posterior direction as it passes inferiorly through the pelvic floor.

In addition to conforming to the general curvature of the sacrum in the anteroposterior plane, the rectum has three lateral curvatures; the upper and lower curvatures are convex to the right and the middle curvature to the left. These lateral curves of the rectum correspond on the intraluminal aspect to the rectal valves or valves of Houston. There are usually three rectal valves (two on the left and one on the right). The middle rectal valve, known as the fold of Kohlrausch, is very prominent (see Fig. 5.66).

The lower part of the rectum is expanded to form the **rectal ampulla**. Finally, unlike the colon, the rectum lacks distinct taeniae coli muscles, omental appendices, and sacculations (haustra of the colon).

The upper third of the rectum is covered by peritoneum anteriorly and laterally while the middle third is covered by peritoneum only on its anterior aspect. The lower third of the rectum is extraperitoneal.

The **relations of the rectum** are as follows: Posteriorly are the median sacral vessels, superior and middle rectal vessels, (see Fig. 5.66A) sympathetic trunk, ganglion impar (see Fig. 5.61), pelvic splanchnic nerves (Fig. 5.59), pirformis, sacral plexus, coccygeal plexus, sacrum and coccyx; laterally are the peritoneum (see Fig. 5.53), obturator internus, obturator internus fascia, levator ani, coccygeus; anteriorly, in women are the recto-uterine pouch (of Douglas) and posterior fornix of the vagina (see Fig. 5.58A); anteriorly, in men are the rectovesical pouch, prostate, urinary bladder and seminal vesicle (the last three are separated from the rectum by the rectoprostatic fascia or Denonvilliers' fascia).

Fascia of the rectum: The fat surrounding the rectum is enclosed in a fascial envelope known as the mesorectum which is derived from the dorsal mesentery (Fig. 5.38C). The contents of the mesorectum include the superior rectal artery and its branches, superior rectal vein and its tributaries, lymphatics and fat. The mesorectal fascia is separated posteriorly from the presacral fascia (fascia of Waldeyer) that covers the presacral veins, sacrum, coccyx, and middle sacral artery. The relatively avascular "holy plane" of rectal surgery (or perimesorectal plane) is located between the mesorectum and the parietal presacral fascia. Posterior to this plane is the presacral venous plexuses, which is at risk during rectal surgery. The distal condensation of mesorectal fascia form lateral ligaments that contain middle rectal vessels. The anterior condensation of mesorectal fascia forms the membranous rectoprostatic fascia or fascia of Denonvilliers, between the rectum and prostate, that is well defined in men (see Fig. 5.58B). During rectal surgery, Denonvilliers' fascia together with the rectum is separated from the seminal vesicle in men and from the vagina in women.

Early clinical exposure

Digital rectal examination

A digital rectal examination (DRE) is performed by placing the gloved and lubricated index finger into the rectum through the anus. The anal mucosa can be palpated for abnormal masses, and in women, the posterior wall of the vagina and the cervix can be palpated. In men, the prostate can be evaluated for any areas of hardness, extraneous nodules or masses.

In many instances, the DRE may be followed by proctoscopy or colonoscopy. An ultrasound probe may be placed into the rectum to assess the gynecological structures in females and the prostate in the male before performing a prostatic biopsy.

A DRE also allows detection of fresh or altered blood in the rectum in patients with acute gastrointestinal bleeding or chronic anemia.

Anal canal

The **anal canal** begins at the terminal end of the rectal ampulla where it narrows at the pelvic floor. It terminates as the anus at the anal verge after passing through the perineum. As it passes through the pelvic floor, the anal canal is surrounded along its entire length by the internal and external anal sphincters, which normally keep it closed.

The lining of the anal canal bears a number of characteristic structural features that reflect the approximate position of the anococcygeal membrane in the fetus (which closes the terminal end of the developing gastrointestinal system in the fetus) and the transition from gastrointestinal mucosa to skin in the adult (Fig. 5.38B).

- The upper part of the anal canal is lined by mucosa similar to that lining the rectum and is distinguished by a number of longitudinally oriented folds known as **anal columns (columns of Morgagni)**, which are united inferiorly by crescentic folds termed **anal valves**. Superior to each valve is a depression termed an **anal sinus, where anal glands open**. The anal valves together form a circle around the anal canal at a location known as the **pectinate line**, or **dentate line** which marks the approximate position of the anal membrane in the fetus.

- Inferior to the pectinate line is a transition zone known as the **anal pecten**, which is lined by nonkeratinized stratified squamous epithelium. The anal pecten ends inferiorly at the **anocutaneous line** ("white line"), or where the lining of the anal canal becomes true skin. The pectinate line is a "watershed area," and the features which differ above and below the pectinate line are given below with the contrasting details mentioned in the brackets after each feature: **epithelium** (simple columnar—stratified squamous); **arterial supply** (superior rectal artery—middle and inferior rectal arteries); **venous drainage** (portal circulation via superior rectal vein—systemic circulation via middle and inferior rectal veins); **lymphatics** (internal iliac nodes—inguinal lymph nodes); **nerve supply (a**utonomic fibers via parasympathetic and sympathetics—somatic fibers via the inferior rectal nerve); and **development** (primitive rectum, from endoderm—anal pit, from ectoderm).

The anal sphincter complex includes the internal and external anal sphincters separated by the conjoint longitudinal muscle (Fig. 5.38D). The internal anal sphincter is the inner thickened circular muscle of the large intestine which is innervated by autonomic nerves. The external anal sphincter is formed by striated muscle with deep, superficial, and subcutaneous parts. The deep part merges with the puborectalis sling posteriorly. The superficial part is attached to the perineal body anteriorly and anococcygeal ligament posteriorly. The subcutaneous part is circular. The external anal sphincter is innervated by the inferior rectal nerve and by the perineal branch of the fourth sacral nerve. The conjoint longitudinal muscle lies between the internal and external anal sphincters. It is a continuation of the longitudinal muscle of rectum. At its distal aspect, its fibers pass in different directions: fibers that pass inferolaterally traverse the distal external anal sphincter and insert into the perianal skin, forming the corrugators cutis ani muscle; fibers that pass inferomedially through the internal sphincter to form subepithelial smooth muscle fibers called Treitz's muscle or muscularis submucosa ani; and fibers that pass medially to the intersphincteric groove, which is palpable in the living at the lower end of the internal sphincter. The attachment of the submucosal muscle is dense at the pectinate line and known as the mucosal suspensory ligament of Parks. The tone of the external anal sphincter can be assessed during DRE when the patient is asked to squeeze the examining finger to test for the function of S4 spinal segment.

Early clinical exposure

Carcinoma of the colon and rectum

Carcinoma of the colon and rectum (colorectum) is a common and often lethal disease. Recent advances in surgery, radiotherapy, and chemotherapy have only slightly improved 5-year survival rates.

The biological behavior of tumors of the colon and rectum is relatively predictable. Most of the tumors develop from benign polyps, some of which undergo malignant change. The overall prognosis is related to:

- The degree of tumor penetration through the bowel wall
- The presence or absence of lymphatic dissemination
- The presence or absence of systemic metastases

Given the position of the colon and rectum in the abdominopelvic cavity and its proximity to other organs, it is extremely important to accurately stage colorectal tumors: a tumor in the pelvis, for example, could invade the uterus or bladder.

Assessing whether spread has occurred usually involves computed tomography (assessment for distal metastases) and magnetic resonance imaging (local staging). Endoscopic ultrasound (EUS) is also used in some instances for local staging of rectal cancer.

Urinary system

The pelvic parts of the urinary system consist of the terminal parts of the ureters, the bladder, and the proximal part of the urethra (Fig. 5.39).

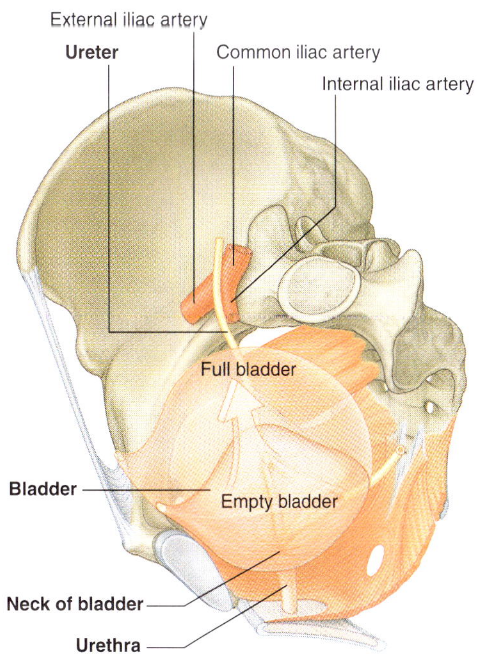

Fig. 5.39 Pelvic parts of the urinary system.

Ureters

The ureters enter the pelvic cavity from the abdomen by passing through the pelvic inlet. On each side, the ureter crosses the pelvic inlet and enters the pelvic cavity in the area anterior to the bifurcation of the common iliac artery. From this point, it continues along the pelvic wall and floor to join the base of the bladder.

In the pelvis, the ureter is crossed by:

- The ductus deferens in men
- The uterine artery in women

Early clinical exposure

Iatrogenic injury of the ureters

Ureters can be injured during various surgeries within the abdomen and pelvis as they lie close to the dissection planes. The most common surgeries that can result in ureteric injury are total abdominal hysterectomy and bilateral salpingo-oophorectomy (removal of the uterus, fallopian tubes, and ovaries), laparoscopic vaginal hysterectomy, laparoscopic anterior resection of the rectum, and open left hemicolectomy. At increased risk of ureteric injury are patients with a bulky tumor (uterine, colonic, rectal) and those with a history of previous operations or pelvic irradiation, all of which make dissection of tissues more difficult. During surgery, the ureter can be crushed, cut open, devascularized, or avulsed. It can also be injured during cryoablation or electric cauterization to control intraoperative bleeding. Ureters can also undergo trauma during the course of ureteroscopy, a procedure where a small endoscope is introduced through the urethra and urinary bladder into one of the ureters to treat stones or tumors of the ureter (usually due to a tear or electrocauterization).

Ureteric injury leads to high morbidity due to infection and in most severe cases to renal impairment. The prognosis is improved when the diagnosis is made intraoperatively and the ureter is repaired immediately. Delayed diagnosis leads to urine leakage and contamination of the abdominal and pelvic cavity, development of sepsis, and in the case of injury near the vagina, a ureterovaginal fistula can develop. When the diagnosis is made postoperatively, sometimes diversion of urine flow is required and percutaneous nephrostomy is performed.

Bladder

The bladder is the most anterior element of the pelvic viscera. Although it is entirely situated in the pelvic cavity when empty, it expands superiorly into the abdominal cavity when full (Fig. 5.39).

The empty bladder is shaped like a three-sided pyramid that has tipped over to lie on one of its margins (Fig. 5.40A). It has an apex, a base, a superior surface, and two inferolateral surfaces.

- The **apex** of the bladder is directed toward the top of the pubic symphysis; a structure known as the **median umbilical ligament** (a remnant of the embryological urachus that contributes to the formation of the bladder) continues from it superiorly up the anterior abdominal wall to the umbilicus.
- The **base** of the bladder (or posterior surface of the bladder) is shaped like an inverted triangle and faces posteroinferiorly. The two ureters enter the bladder at each of the upper corners of the base, and the urethra drains inferiorly from the lower corner of the base.
- Inside the bladder, the mucosal lining on the base of the bladder is smooth and firmly attached to the underlying smooth muscle coat of the wall—unlike elsewhere in the bladder where the mucosa is folded and loosely attached to the wall. The smooth triangular area between the openings of the ureters and urethra on the inside of the bladder is known as the **trigone** (Fig. 5.40B). The muscle fibers between the two ureteric orifices form a fold, the interureteric ridge. Behind the internal urethral orifice a raised fold, called the uvula, may be present due to an enlarged transition zone (or median lobe) of the prostate. The interior of the bladder may be visualized using a cystoscope. The **inferolateral surfaces** of the bladder are cradled between the levator ani muscles of the pelvic diaphragm and the adjacent obturator internus muscles above the attachment of the pelvic diaphragm. The inferolateral surfaces meet at the anterior border, which is related to the retropubic space. The superior surface is slightly domed when the bladder is empty; it balloons upward in the extraperitoneal space as the bladder fills and strips the peritoneum off the anterior abdominal wall. If the urethra is obstructed, a catheter may be passed into the urinary bladder without entering the peritoneal cavity (suprapubic catheterization).

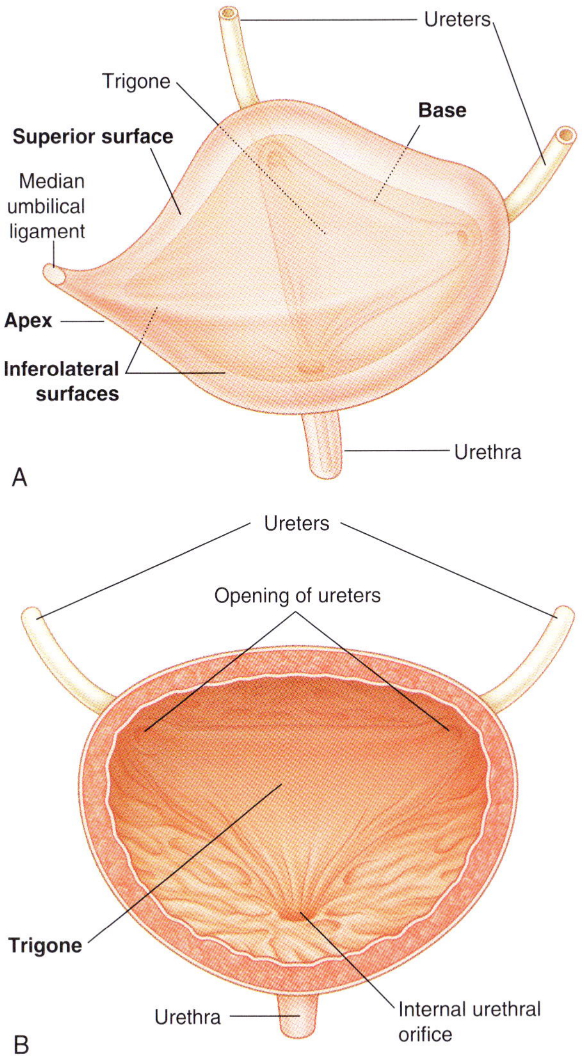

Fig. 5.40 Bladder. **(A)** Superolateral view. **(B)** The trigone. Anterior view with the anterior part of the bladder cut away.

Neck of bladder

The neck of the bladder surrounds the origin of the urethra at the point where the two inferolateral surfaces and the base intersect.

The neck is the most inferior part of the bladder and also the most "fixed" part. It is anchored into position by a pair of tough fibromuscular bands, which connect the neck and pelvic part of the urethra to the posteroinferior aspect of each pubic bone.

- In women, these fibromuscular bands are termed **pubovesical ligaments** (Fig. 5.41A). Together with the perineal membrane and associated muscles, the levator ani muscles, and the pubic bones, these ligaments help support the bladder, and prevent it from prolapsing through the vagina.
- In men, the paired fibromuscular bands are known as **puboprostatic ligaments** because they blend with the fibrous capsule of the prostate, which surrounds the neck of the bladder and adjacent part of the urethra (Fig. 5.41B).

Although the bladder is considered to be pelvic in the adult, it has a higher position in children. At birth, the bladder is almost entirely abdominal; the urethra begins approximately at the upper margin of the pubic symphysis. With age, the bladder descends until after puberty when it assumes the adult position.

The blood supply of the urinary bladder includes the arterial supply by the superior vesical artery, inferior vesical artery (in men) and the vaginal artery (in women). The venous drainage is by the vesical venous plexus, which drains into the internal iliac vein.

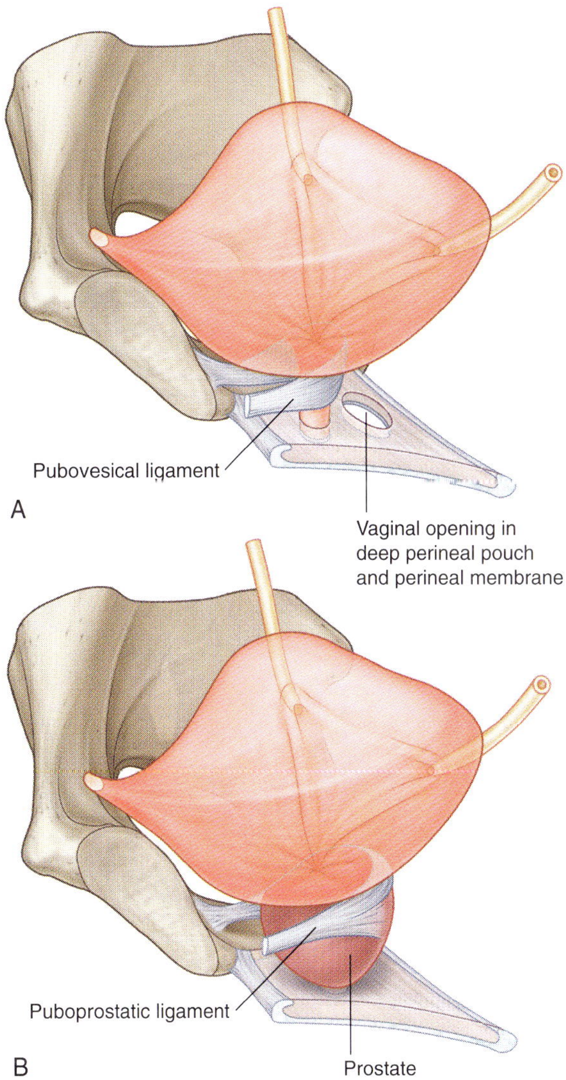

Fig. 5.41 Ligaments that anchor the neck of the bladder and pelvic part of the urethra to the pelvic bones. **(A)** In women. **(B)** In men.

The nerve supply of the urinary bladder includes visceral sensory fibers which pass along with the parasympathetics, visceral motor fibers to make the detrusor contract pass from S2 to S4 spinal segments via the pelvic splanchnic nerves and inferior hypogastric plexus to ganglia near the wall of the urinary bladder. Visceral motor fibers to the internal urethral sphincter pass from T11 to L3 spinal segments via lumbar splanchnic nerves to ganglia in the hypogastric plexuses (see Figs 1.47 and 1.48). Voluntary fibers to the external urethral sphincter pass from S2 to S4 spinal segments via the pudendal nerve.

Early clinical exposure

Bladder stones

In some patients, small calculi (stones) form in the kidneys. These may pass down the ureter, causing ureteric obstruction, and into the bladder (Fig. 5.42), where insoluble salts further precipitate on these small calculi to form larger calculi. Often, these patients develop (or may already have) problems with bladder emptying, which leaves residual urine in the bladder. This urine may become infected, which alters the pH of the urine, permitting further precipitation of insoluble salts.

If small enough, the stones may be removed via a transurethral route using specialized instruments. If the stones are too big, it may be necessary to make a suprapubic incision and enter the bladder retroperitoneally to remove them.

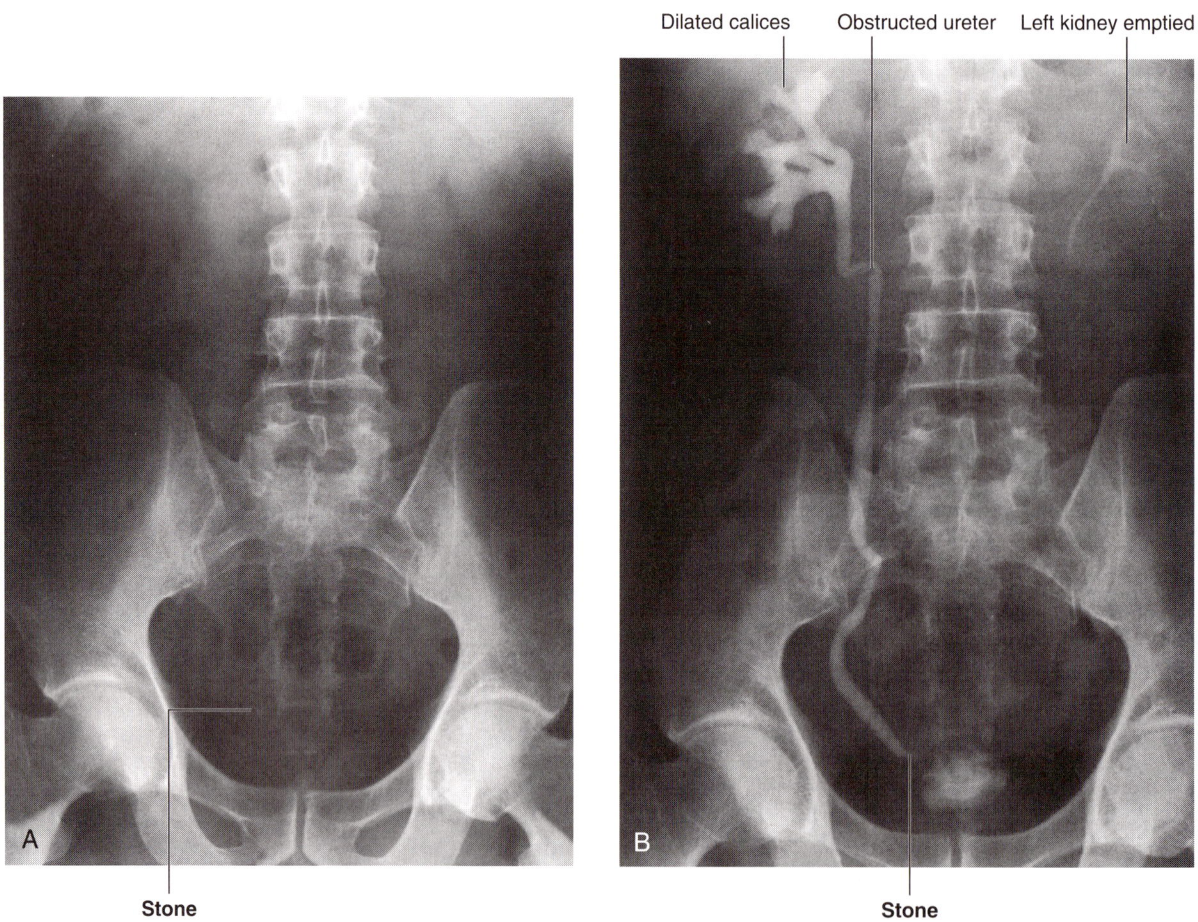

Fig. 5.42 Intravenous urogram demonstrating a stone in the lower portion of the ureter. **(A)** Control radiograph. **(B)** Intravenous urogram, postmicturition.

Early clinical exposure

Suprapubic catheterization

In certain instances, it is necessary to catheterize the bladder through the anterior abdominal wall. For example, when the prostate is markedly enlarged and it is impossible to pass a urethral catheter, a suprapubic catheter may be placed.

The bladder is a retroperitoneal structure and when full lies adjacent to the anterior abdominal wall. Ultrasound visualization of the bladder may be useful in assessing the size of this structure and, importantly, differentiating this structure from other potential abdominal masses.

The procedure of suprapubic catheterization is straightforward and involves the passage of a small catheter on a needle in the midline approximately 2 cm above the pubic symphysis. The catheter passes easily into the bladder without compromise of other structures and permits free drainage.

Early clinical exposure

Bladder cancer

Bladder cancer (Fig. 5.43) is the most common tumor of the urinary tract and is usually a disease of the sixth and seventh decades, although there is an increasing trend for younger patients to develop this disease.

Approximately one-third of bladder tumors are multifocal; fortunately, two-thirds are superficial tumors and amenable to local treatment.

Bladder tumors may spread through the bladder wall and invade local structures, including the rectum, uterus (in women), and lateral walls of the pelvic cavity. Prostatic involvement is not uncommon in male patients. The disease spreads via the internal iliac lymph nodes. Spread to distant metastatic sites rarely includes the lung.

Large bladder tumors may produce complications, including invasion and obstruction of the ureters. Ureteric obstruction can then obstruct the kidneys and induce kidney failure. Moreover, bladder tumors can invade other structures of the pelvic cavity.

Treatment for early-stage tumors includes local resection with preservation of the bladder. Diffuse tumors may be treated with local chemotherapy; more extensive tumors may require radical surgical removal of the bladder (cystectomy) and, in men, the prostate (prostatectomy). Bladder reconstruction (formation of so-called neobladder) is performed in patients after cystectomy using part of a bowel, most commonly the ileum.

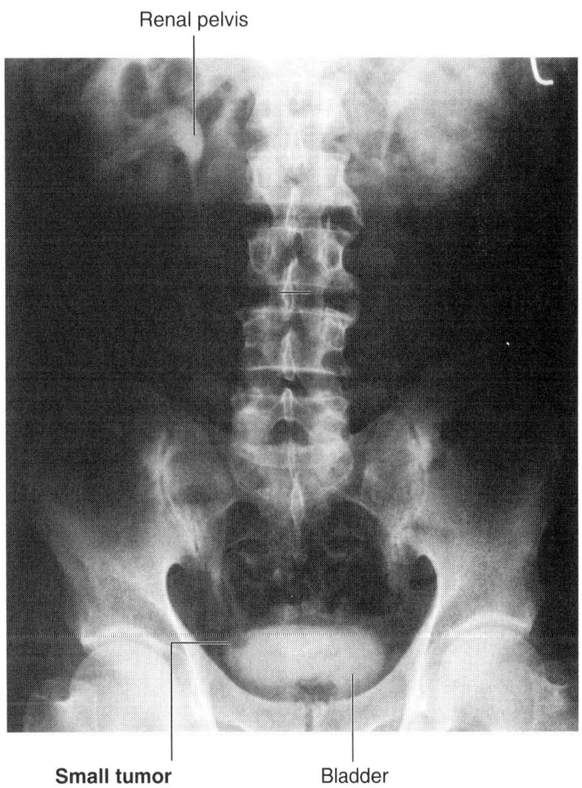

Fig. 5.43 Intravenous urogram demonstrating a small tumor in the wall of the bladder.

Urethra

The urethra begins at the base of the bladder and ends with an external opening in the perineum. The paths taken by the urethra differ significantly in women and men.

In women

In women, the urethra is short, being about 4 cm long. It travels a slightly curved course as it passes inferiorly through the pelvic floor into the perineum, where it passes through the deep perineal pouch and perineal membrane before opening in the vestibule that lies between the labia minora (Fig. 5.44A).

The urethral opening is anterior to the vaginal opening in the vestibule. The inferior aspect of the urethra is bound to the anterior surface of the vagina. Two small paraurethral mucous glands (**Skene's glands**) are associated with the lower end of the urethra. Each drains via a duct that opens onto the lateral margin of the external urethral orifice.

In men

In men, the urethra is long, about 20 cm, and bends twice along its course (Fig. 5.44B). Beginning at the base of the bladder and passing inferiorly through the prostate, it passes through the deep perineal pouch and perineal membrane and immediately enters the root of the penis. As the urethra exits the deep perineal pouch, it bends forward to course anteriorly in the root of the penis. When the penis is flaccid, the urethra makes another bend, this time inferiorly, when passing from the root to the body of the penis. During erection, the bend between the root and body of the penis disappears.

The urethra in men is divided into preprostatic, prostatic, membranous, and spongy parts.

Preprostatic part

The preprostatic part of the urethra is about 1 cm long, extends from the base of the bladder to the prostate, and is associated with a circular cuff of smooth muscle fibers (the **internal urethral sphincter**). Contraction of this sphincter prevents retrograde movement of semen into the bladder during ejaculation.

Prostatic part

The prostatic part of the urethra (Fig. 5.44C) is 3–4 cm long and is surrounded by the prostate. In this region, the lumen of the urethra is marked by a longitudinal midline fold of mucosa (the **urethral crest**). The depression on

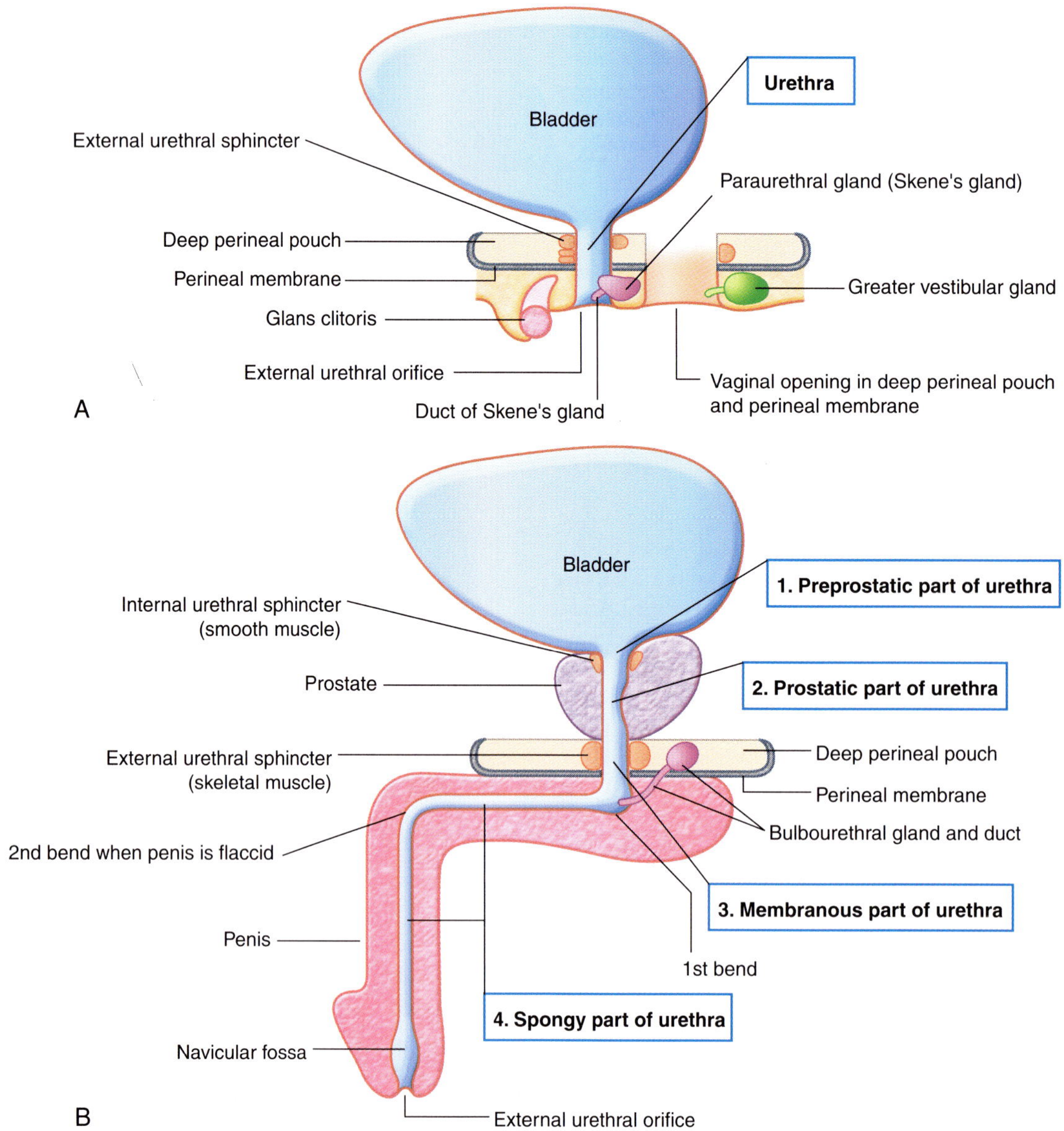

Fig. 5.44 Urethra. **(A)** In women. **(B)** In men.

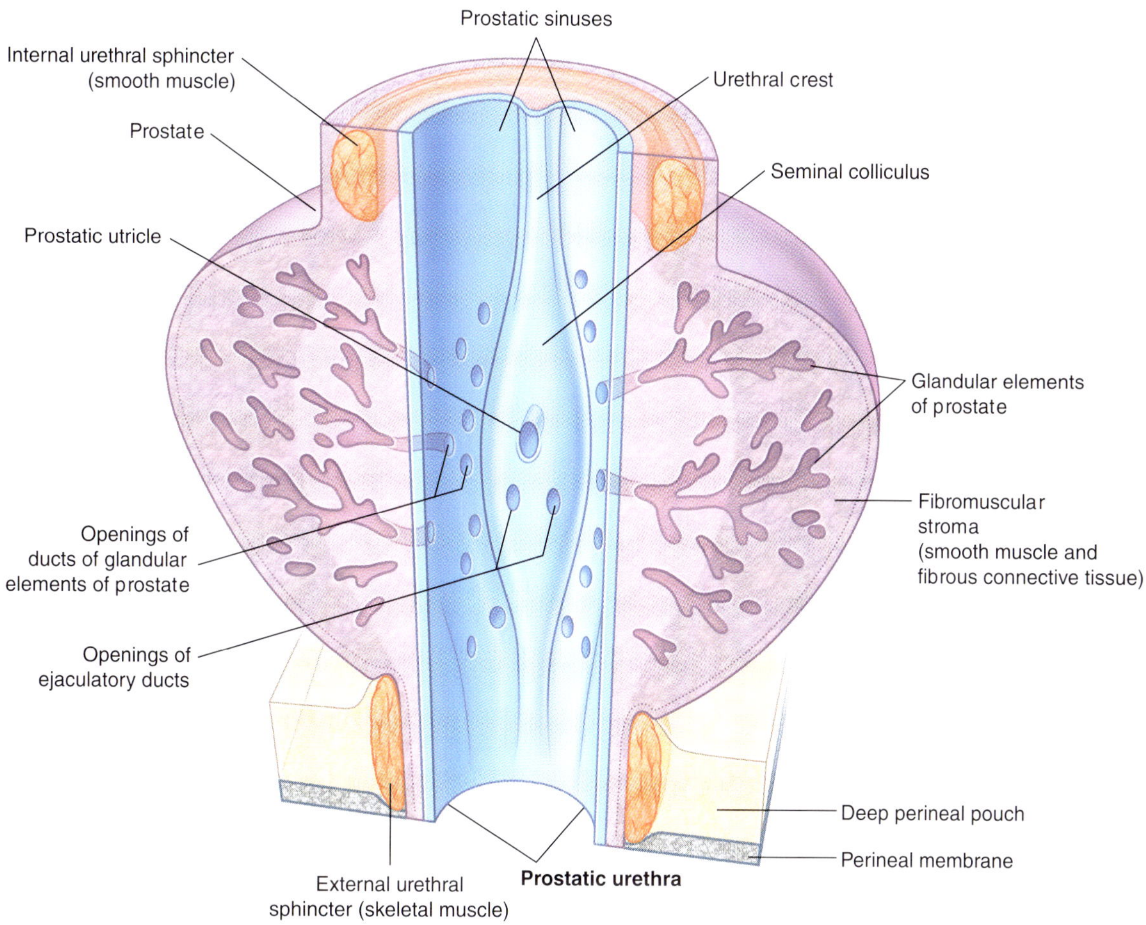

Fig. 5.44, cont'd (C) Prostatic part of the urethra in men.

each side of the crest is the **prostatic sinus**; the ducts of the prostate empty into these two sinuses.

Midway along its length, the urethral crest is enlarged to form a somewhat circular elevation (the seminal colliculus). In men, the seminal colliculus is used to determine the position of the prostate gland during transurethral transection of the prostate.

A small blind-ended pouch—the **prostatic utricle** (thought to be the homologue of the uterus in women)—opens onto the center of the seminal colliculus. On each side of the prostatic utricle is the opening of the ejaculatory duct of the male reproductive system. Therefore, the connection between the urinary and reproductive tracts in men occurs in the prostatic part of the urethra.

Membranous part

The membranous part of the urethra is narrow and passes through the deep perineal pouch (Fig. 5.44B). During its transit through this pouch, the urethra, in both men and women, is surrounded by skeletal muscle of the **external urethral sphincter**.

Spongy urethra

The spongy urethra is surrounded by erectile tissue (the **corpus spongiosum**) of the penis. It is enlarged to form a bulb at the base of the penis and again at the end of the penis to form the **navicular fossa** (Fig. 5.44B). The two bulbourethral glands in the deep perineal pouch are part of the male reproductive system and open into the bulb of the spongy urethra. The external urethral orifice is the sagittal slit at the end of the penis.

Early clinical exposure

Bladder infection

The relatively short length of the urethra in women makes them more susceptible than men to bladder infection. The primary symptom of urinary tract infection in women is usually inflammation of the bladder (cystitis). The infection can be controlled in most instances by oral antibiotics and resolves without complication. In children under 1 year of age, infection from the bladder may spread via the ureters to the kidneys, where it can produce renal damage and ultimately lead to renal failure. Early diagnosis and treatment are necessary.

Early clinical exposure

Urethral catheterization

Urethral catheterization is often performed to drain urine from a patient's bladder when the patient is unable to micturate. When inserting urinary catheters, it is important to appreciate the gender anatomy of the patient.

In men:

- The spongy urethra is surrounded by the erectile tissue of the bulb of the penis immediately inferior to the deep perineal pouch. The wall of this short segment of urethra is relatively thin and angles superiorly to pass through the deep perineal pouch; at this position, the urethra is vulnerable to damage, notably during cystoscopy.
- The membranous part of the urethra runs superiorly as it passes through the deep perineal pouch.
- The prostatic part of the urethra takes a slight concave curve anteriorly as it passes through the prostate gland.

In women, it is much simpler to pass catheters and cystoscopes because the urethra is short and straight. Urine may therefore be readily drained from a distended bladder without significant concern for urethral rupture.

Occasionally, it is impossible to pass any form of instrumentation through the urethra to drain the bladder, usually because there is a urethral stricture or prostatic enlargement. In such cases, an ultrasound of the lower abdomen will demonstrate a full bladder (Fig. 5.45) behind the anterior abdominal wall. A suprapubic catheter may be inserted into the bladder with minimal trauma through a small incision under local anesthetic.

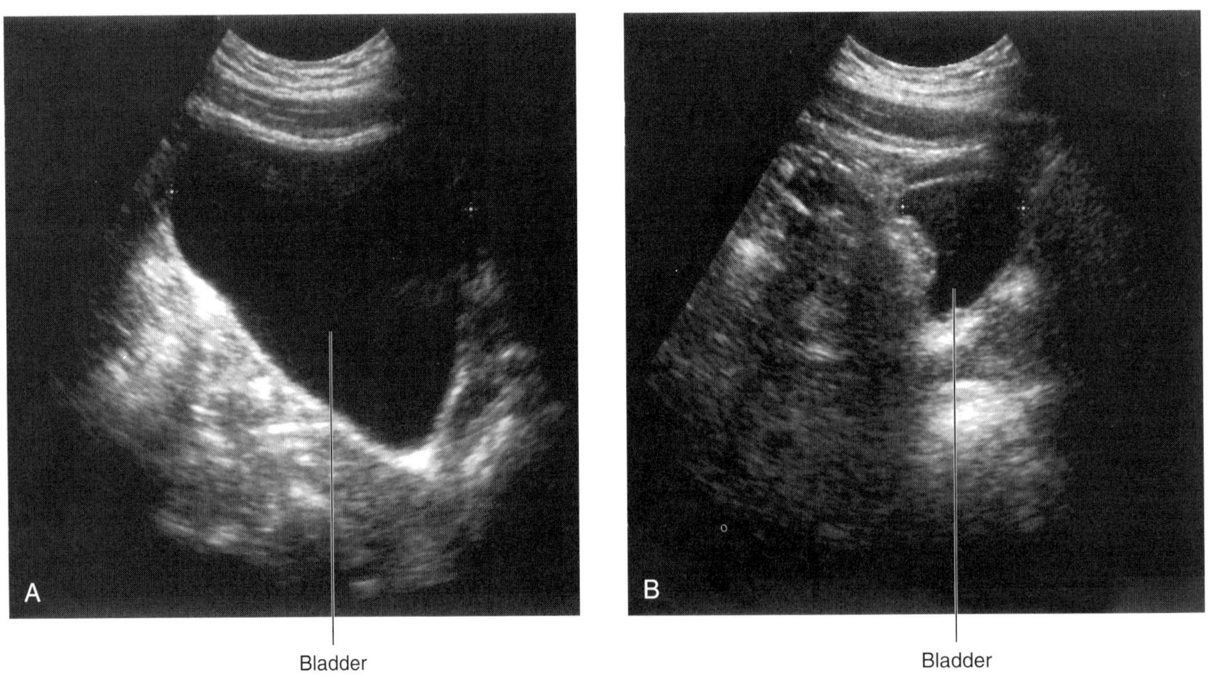

Fig. 5.45 Ultrasound demonstrating the bladder. **(A)** Full bladder. **(B)** Postmicturition bladder.

Reproductive system

In men

The reproductive system in men has components in the abdomen, pelvis, and perineum (Fig. 5.46A). The major components are a testis, epididymis, ductus deferens, and ejaculatory duct on each side, and the urethra and penis in the midline. In addition, three types of accessory glands are associated with the system:

- A single prostate
- A pair of seminal vesicles
- A pair of bulbourethral glands

The design of the reproductive system in men is basically a series of ducts and tubules. The arrangement of parts and linkage to the urinary tract reflects its embryological development.

Testes

The **testes** originally develop high on the posterior abdominal wall and then descend, normally before birth, through the inguinal canal in the anterior abdominal wall and into the scrotum of the perineum. During descent, the testes carry their vessels, lymphatics, and nerves, as well as their principal drainage ducts, the **ductus deferens** (**vas deferens**) with them. The lymph drainage of the testes is therefore to the lateral aortic or lumbar nodes and preaortic nodes in the abdomen, and not to the inguinal or pelvic lymph nodes.

Each ellipsoid-shaped testis is enclosed within the end of an elongated musculofascial pouch, which is continuous with the anterior abdominal wall and projects into the scrotum. The **spermatic cord** is the tube-shaped connection between the pouch in the scrotum and the abdominal wall.

The sides and anterior aspect of the testis are covered by a closed sac of peritoneum (the **tunica vaginalis**), which originally connected to the abdominal cavity. Normally after testicular descent, the connection closes, leaving a fibrous remnant.

Each testis (Fig. 5.46B) is composed of seminiferous tubules and interstitial tissue surrounded by a thick connective tissue capsule (the **tunica albuginea**). Spermatozoa are produced by the seminiferous tubules. The 400–600 highly coiled seminiferous tubules are modified at each end to become straight tubules, which connect to a collecting chamber (the **rete testis**) in a thick, vertically oriented linear wedge of connective tissue (the **mediastinum testis**), projecting from the capsule into the posterior aspect of the gonad. Approximately 12–20 **efferent ductules** originate from the upper end of the rete testis, penetrate the capsule, and connect with the epididymis. The testis has two free surfaces, the medial and the lateral, and two borders, the anterior and the posterior. The posterior border has a superior portion that is related to the head of the epididymis, and an inferior portion that is related to the body and tail of the epididymis. A space between testis and the body of the epididymis, called the sinus of the epididymis has an opening which is directed laterally. The vas deferens is located medial to the posterior border of the testis.

The right testis, in most cases, is at a higher level than the left. Occasionally, the right testis is lower in total situs inversus

Early clinical exposure

Testicular tumors

Tumors of the testis account for a small percentage of malignancies in men. However, they generally occur in younger patients (between 20 and 40 years of age). When diagnosed at an early stage, most of these tumors are curable by surgery and chemotherapy.

Early diagnosis of testicular tumor is extremely important. Abnormal lumps can be detected by palpation, and diagnosis can be made using ultrasound. Simple ultrasound scanning can reveal the extent of the local tumor, usually at an early stage.

Surgical removal of the malignant testis is often carried out using an inguinal approach. The testis is not usually removed through a scrotal incision, because it is possible to spread tumor cells into the subcutaneous tissues of the scrotum, which has a different lymphatic drainage than the testis.

Cancer from the right testis may spread via lymph vessels to lymph nodes at the angle between the right renal vein and the inferior vena cava and to the precaval nodes at the aortic bifurcation. However, cancer from the left testis may spread to paraaortic nodes and preaortic nodes.

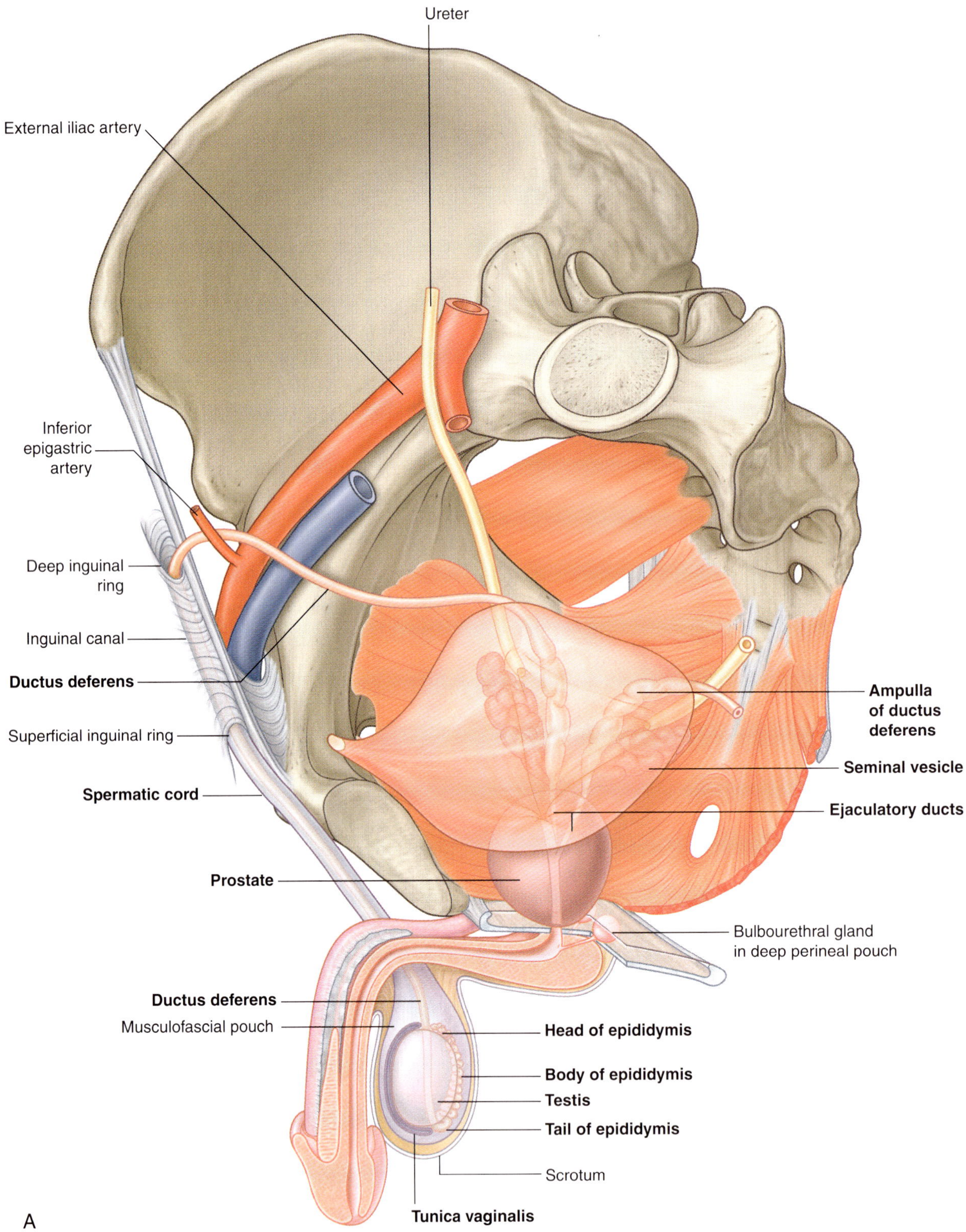

Fig. 5.46 Reproductive system in men. **(A)** Overview.

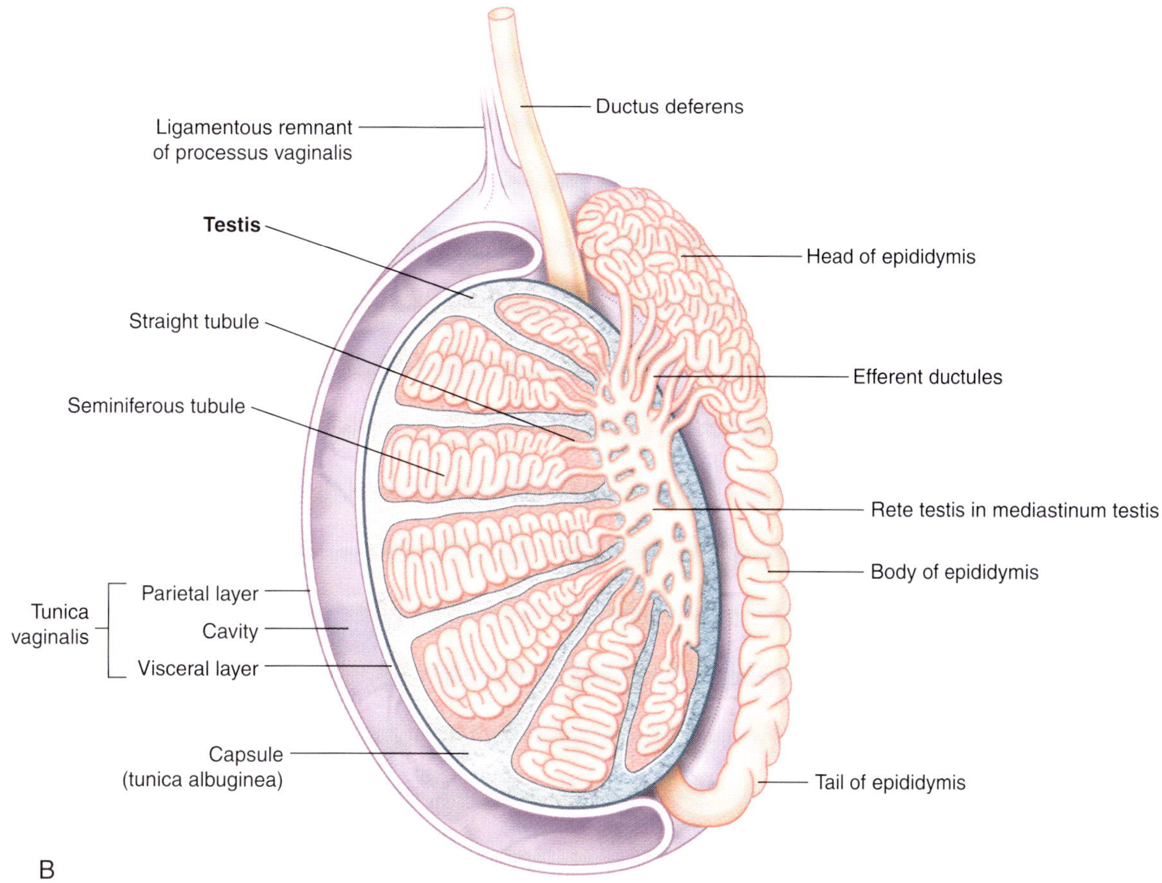

Fig. 5.46, cont'd (B) Testis and surrounding structures.

Early clinical exposure

Ectopic testes

Interrupted descent of testis leads to an empty scrotal sac and abnormal location of the testis, which can lie anywhere along the usual route of descent. Most commonly, the testis is present in the inguinal canal, where it can be palpated. This condition is usually diagnosed at birth or within the first year of life. A higher incidence of ectopic (undescended) testis occurs in premature births (30%) than in term births (3–5%). Normally, the ectopic testis can complete its descent within the first 3 months after a child is born; therefore, watchful waiting is recommended for the first couple of months. A specialist referral is usually made at 6 months if the testis is still absent from the scrotal sac. It is crucial to make the diagnosis early so that an appropriate management plan can be initiated to avoid or reduce the risk of complications such as testicular malignancy, subfertility or infertility, testicular torsion, and inguinal hernia (due to patent processus vaginalis). If surgical correction is required, the ectopic testis is moved from the inguinal canal into the scrotum (orchiopexy). During mobilization of the testis, dissection of tissues must be performed carefully to avoid injuring the ilioinguinal nerve adjacent to the spermatic cord. At the time of orchiopexy, the patent processus vaginalis is closed and any inguinal hernia, if present, is repaired.

Epididymis

The **epididymis** courses along the posterolateral side of the testis (Fig. 5.46B). It has two distinct components:

- The **efferent ductules**, which form an enlarged coiled mass that sits on the posterior superior pole of the testis and forms the **head of the epididymis**
- The **true epididymis**, which is a single, long coiled duct into which the efferent ductules all drain, and which continues inferiorly along the posterolateral margin of the testis as the **body of the epididymis** and enlarges to form the **tail of the epididymis** at the inferior pole of the testis

During passage through the epididymis, spermatozoa acquire the ability to move and fertilize an egg. The epididymis also stores spermatozoa until ejaculation. The end of the epididymis is continuous with the ductus deferens.

Ductus deferens

The ductus deferens is a long muscular duct that transports spermatozoa from the tail of the epididymis in the scrotum to the ejaculatory duct in the pelvic cavity (Fig. 5.46A). It ascends in the scrotum as a component of the spermatic cord and passes through the inguinal canal in the anterior abdominal wall.

After passing through the deep inguinal ring, the ductus deferens bends medially around the lateral side of the inferior epigastric artery and crosses the external iliac artery and the external iliac vein at the pelvic inlet to enter the pelvic cavity.

The duct descends medially on the pelvic wall, deep to the peritoneum, and crosses the ureter posterior to the bladder. It continues inferomedially along the base of the bladder, anterior to the rectum, almost to the midline, where it is joined by the duct of the seminal vesicle to form the ejaculatory duct.

Between the ureter and ejaculatory duct, the ductus deferens expands to form the ampulla of the ductus deferens. The ejaculatory duct penetrates through the prostate gland to connect with the prostatic urethra.

Early clinical exposure

Vasectomy

The ductus deferens transports spermatozoa from the tail of the epididymis in the scrotum to the ejaculatory duct in the pelvic cavity. Because it has a thick smooth muscle wall, it can be easily palpated in the spermatic cord between the testes and the superficial inguinal ring. Also, because it can be accessed through skin and superficial fascia, it is amenable to surgical dissection and surgical division. When this is carried out bilaterally (vasectomy), the patient is rendered sterile—this is a useful method for male contraception.

Seminal vesicle

Each **seminal vesicle** is an accessory gland of the male reproductive system that develops as a blind-ended tubular outgrowth from the ductus deferens (Fig. 5.46A). The tube is coiled with numerous pocket-like outgrowths and is encapsulated by connective tissue to form an elongate structure situated between the bladder and rectum. The gland is immediately lateral to and follows the course of the ductus deferens at the base of the bladder.

The duct of the seminal vesicle joins the ductus deferens to form the **ejaculatory duct** (Fig. 5.47). Secretions from the seminal vesicle contribute significantly to the volume of the ejaculate (semen).

Prostate

The **prostate** is an unpaired accessory structure of the male reproductive system that surrounds the urethra in the pelvic cavity (Figs 5.46A and 5.47). The three zones of the prostate are the peripheral zone (the subcapsular part that surrounds the distal urethra); the central zone (that surrounds the ejaculatory ducts); and the transitional zone (or transition zone, which surrounds the proximal part of the urethra). There is an anterior fibromuscular stroma, which is nonglandular. The contemporary description of prostatic zones is based on the location of the zones and their histology and embryology. The lobes of the prostate are the anterior lobe (anterior to the urethra), posterior lobe (posterior to the urethra and inferior to the ejaculatory ducts), median lobe (between the urethra and the ejaculatory ducts), and the lateral lobes (lateral to the urethra). The lobes are not apparent in a section of the prostate. The prostate lies immediately inferior to the bladder, posterior to the pubic symphysis, and anterior to the rectum.

The prostate is shaped like an inverted rounded cone with a larger base, which is continuous above with the neck of the bladder, and a narrower apex, which rests below on the pelvic floor. The inferolateral surfaces of the prostate are in contact with the levator ani muscles that together cradle the prostate between them. The anterior surface is related to the retropubic space. The posterior surface is related to the rectum, with the rectovesical septum (Denonvilliers' fascia) between them. The prostate drains into the prostatic plexus which mainly drains into the internal iliac vein (see Fig. 5.66). The prostatic plexus communicates with the internal vertebral venous plexus (of Batson). Hence, cancer from the prostate often spreads to vertebrae, and occasionally to the skull.

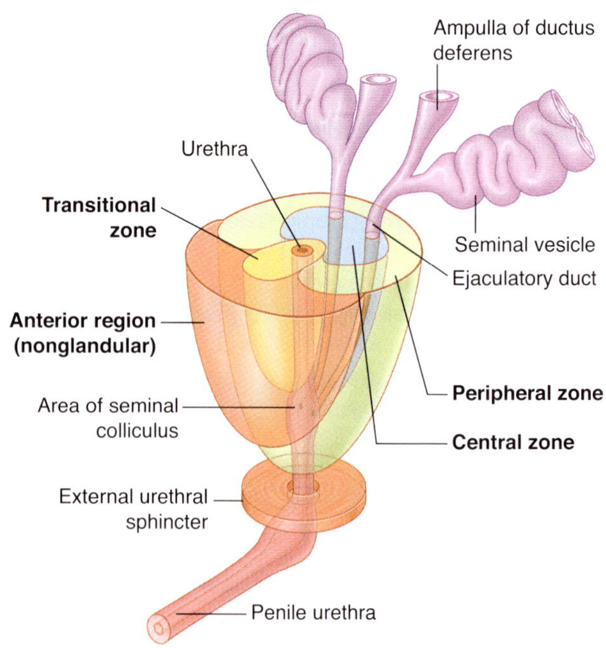

Fig. 5.47 The prostate gland. Zonal anatomy.

Early clinical exposure

Prostate problems

Prostate cancer is one of the most commonly diagnosed malignancies in men, and often the disease is advanced at diagnosis. Prostate cancer typically occurs in the peripheral zone of the prostate (see Fig. 5.47) and is relatively asymptomatic. In many cases, it is diagnosed by a DRE (Fig. 5.48A) and by blood tests, which include serum acid phosphatase and serum prostate-specific antigen (PSA). In rectal exams, the tumorous prostate feels "rock" hard. The diagnosis is usually made by obtaining a number of biopsies of the prostate. Ultrasound is used during the biopsy procedure to image the prostate for the purpose of taking measurements and for needle placement.

Benign prostatic hypertrophy is a disease of the prostate that occurs with increasing age in most men (Fig. 5.48B). It generally involves the more central zone (median lobe) of the prostate (see Fig. 5.47), which gradually enlarge. The prostate feels "bulky" on DRE. Owing to the more central hypertrophic change of the prostate, the urethra is compressed, and a urinary outflow obstruction develops in a number of patients. With time, the bladder may become hypertrophied in response to the urinary outflow obstruction. In some male patients, the obstruction becomes so severe that urine cannot be passed and transurethral or suprapubic catheterization is necessary. Despite being a benign disease, benign prostatic hypertrophy can therefore have a marked effect on the daily lives of many patients.

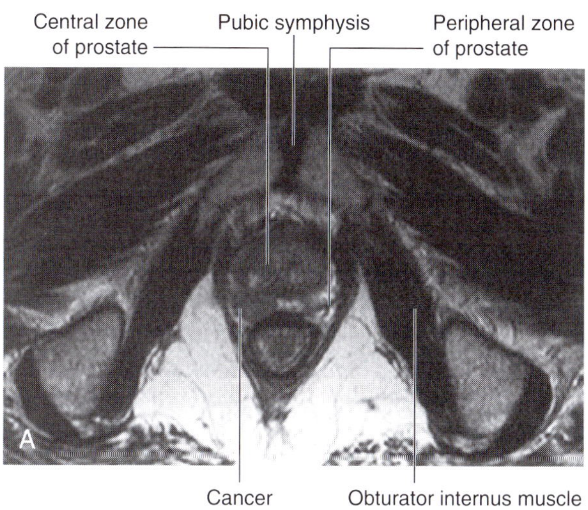

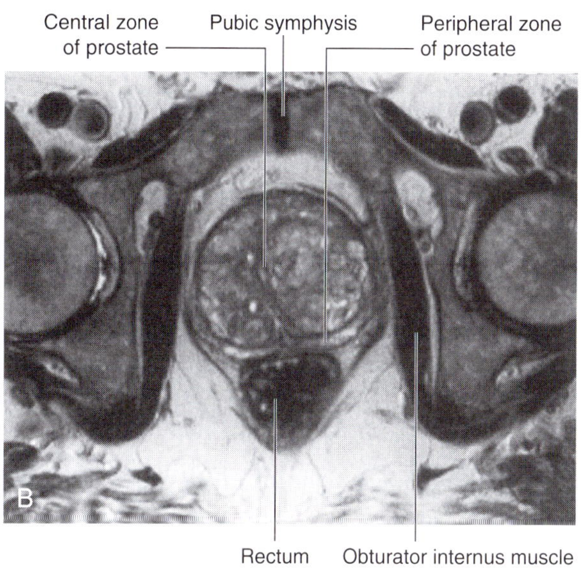

Fig. 5.48 Axial T2-weighted magnetic resonance images of prostate problems. **(A)** A small prostatic cancer in the peripheral zone of a normal-sized prostate. **(B)** Benign prostatic hypertrophy.

Bulbourethral glands

The **bulbourethral glands** (see Fig. 5.46A), one on each side, are small, pea-shaped mucous glands situated within the deep perineal pouch. They are lateral to the membranous part of the urethra. The duct from each gland passes inferomedially through the **perineal membrane**, to open into the bulb of the spongy urethra at the root of the penis.

Together with small glands positioned along the length of the spongy urethra, the bulbourethral glands contribute to lubrication of the urethra and the pre-ejaculatory emission from the penis.

In women

SET INDUCTION—CASE SCENARIO 2: URINARY TRACT INFECTION

A 26-year-old woman came to the gynecology department with complaints of lower abdominal pain and fever for 7 days. On questioning, it was found that her urine was blood-stained and this was associated with pain while passing urine and not related to her menstrual cycles. A diagnosis of urinary tract infection was made. Knowledge of the anatomy of the female urethra is needed to diagnose this case.

The reproductive tract in women is contained mainly in the pelvic cavity and perineum, although during pregnancy, the uterus expands into the abdominal cavity. Major components of the system consist of:

- An ovary on each side
- A uterus, vagina, and clitoris in the midline (Fig. 5.49)

In addition, a pair of accessory glands (the **greater vestibular glands**) is associated with the tract.

<table>
<tr><th rowspan="2">REMEMBER
[Recall Facts]</th><th colspan="3">OUTLINE 2. PELVIS REGION 2
(FEMALE)—LEARNING OBJECTIVES
[By the end of this section, the student should be able to:]</th><th colspan="2" rowspan="2">EVALUATE
[Explain Concepts]</th></tr>
<tr><th colspan="3">DEMONSTRATE AND ANALYZE RELATIONSHIPS
[Identify structures in a Prosected Specimen or Figure]</th></tr>
<tr><td rowspan="6">1. Describe the relations of urinary bladder in both male and females
2. Describe the position and parts, relations, blood supply, development and supports of the uterus
3. Describe the relations of rectum in females
4. Describe the pelvic course of ureter in females</td><td>Level I</td><td>Level II</td><td>Level III</td><td colspan="2">■ Anteversion and anteflexion of the uterus
■ Supports of the uterus
■ Rectouterine pouch and its importance
■ Blood supply of the uterus
■ Parts of the broad ligament</td></tr>
<tr><td rowspan="5">■ Urinary bladder:
  ■ Relations in female
■ Female urethra
■ Rectum and anal canal relations in female
■ Uterus:
  ■ Location, parts
  ■ Axes, surfaces
  ■ Uterine cavity
  ■ Uterovesical pouch
  ■ Rectouterine pouch
  ■ Important relations
■ Vagina with fornices
■ Pelvic part of the ureter
■ Broad ligament and its parts
■ Uterine tube
■ Ovary
■ Uterine artery</td><td rowspan="5">■ Ligament of the ovary
■ Round ligament of the uterus
■ Ovarian artery</td><td rowspan="5">■ Ovarian fossa</td><th colspan="2">EARLY CLINICAL EXPOSURE
[Apply Anatomical Knowledge]</th></tr>
<tr><th>Surgical Anatomy/ Pathology/ Trauma</th><th>Imaging/ Surface Anatomy</th></tr>
<tr><td>■ Prolapse of the uterus
■ Tumors of the uterus
■ Hysterectomy
■ Tubal pregnancy
■ Tubectomy
■ Tumors of the ovary
■ Vaginal examination
■ Culdocentesis
■ Importance of the pouch of Douglas</td><td>■ Hysterosalpingogram</td></tr>
<tr><th colspan="2">PROBLEM SOLVING/
CLINICAL CASES
[Interpret]</th></tr>
<tr><td colspan="2">■ Iatrogenic ureteric injury
■ Ectopic pregnancy
■ Uterine tumor
■ Uterine fibroid</td></tr>
</table>

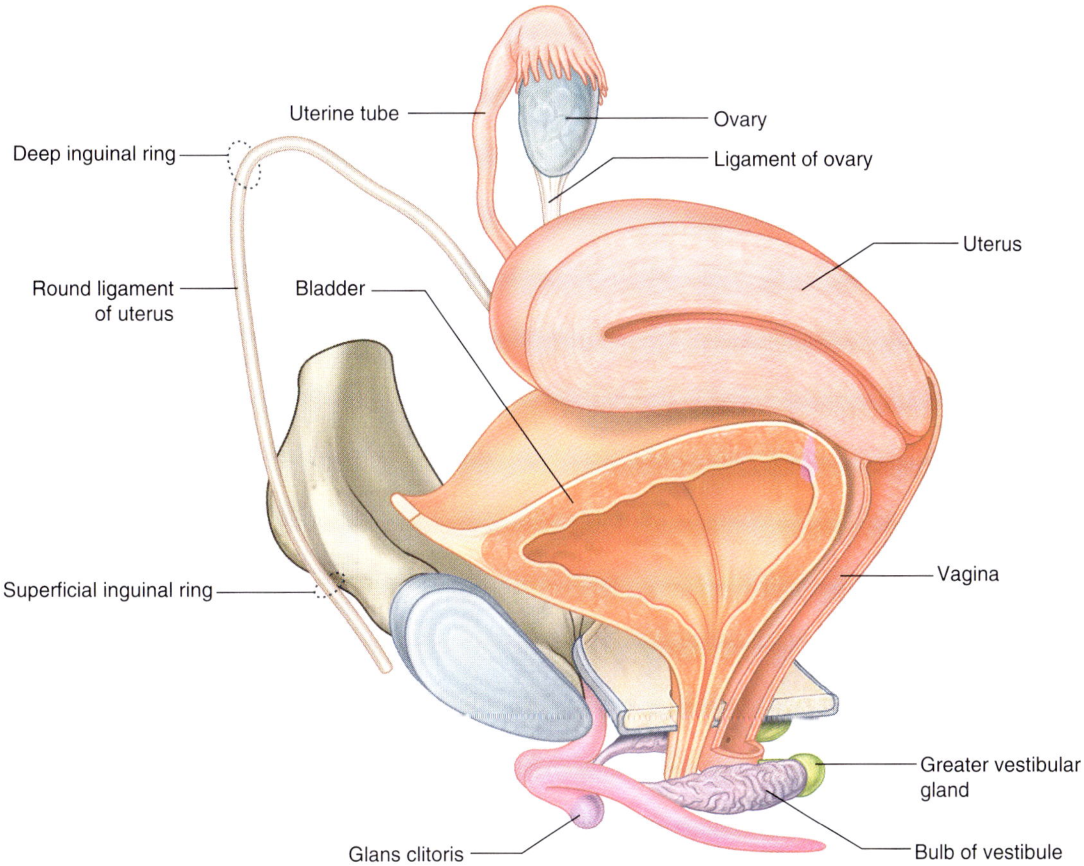

Fig. 5.49 Reproductive system in women.

Ovaries

Like the testes in men, the **ovaries** develop high on the posterior abdominal wall and then descend before birth, bringing with them their vessels, lymphatics, and nerves. Unlike the testes, the ovaries do not migrate through the inguinal canal into the perineum, but stop short and assume a position on the lateral wall of the pelvic cavity (Fig. 5.50).

The ovaries are the sites of egg production (oogenesis). Mature eggs are ovulated into the peritoneal cavity and normally directed into the adjacent openings of the uterine tubes by cilia on the ends of the uterine tubes.

The ovaries lie adjacent to the lateral pelvic wall just inferior to the pelvic inlet in the ovarian fossa. The ovarian fossa is bounded superiorly by the external iliac vessels, inferiorly by the levator ani, anteriorly by the mesovarium, broad ligament, ovarian vessels and obliterated umbilical vein, posteriorly by the ureter and internal iliac vessels, medially by ligament of the ovary and laterally by the obturator nerve and vessels. Each of the two almond-shaped ovaries is about 3 cm long and is suspended by a mesentery (the **mesovarium**) that is a posterior extension of the broad ligament (see Fig. 5.58).

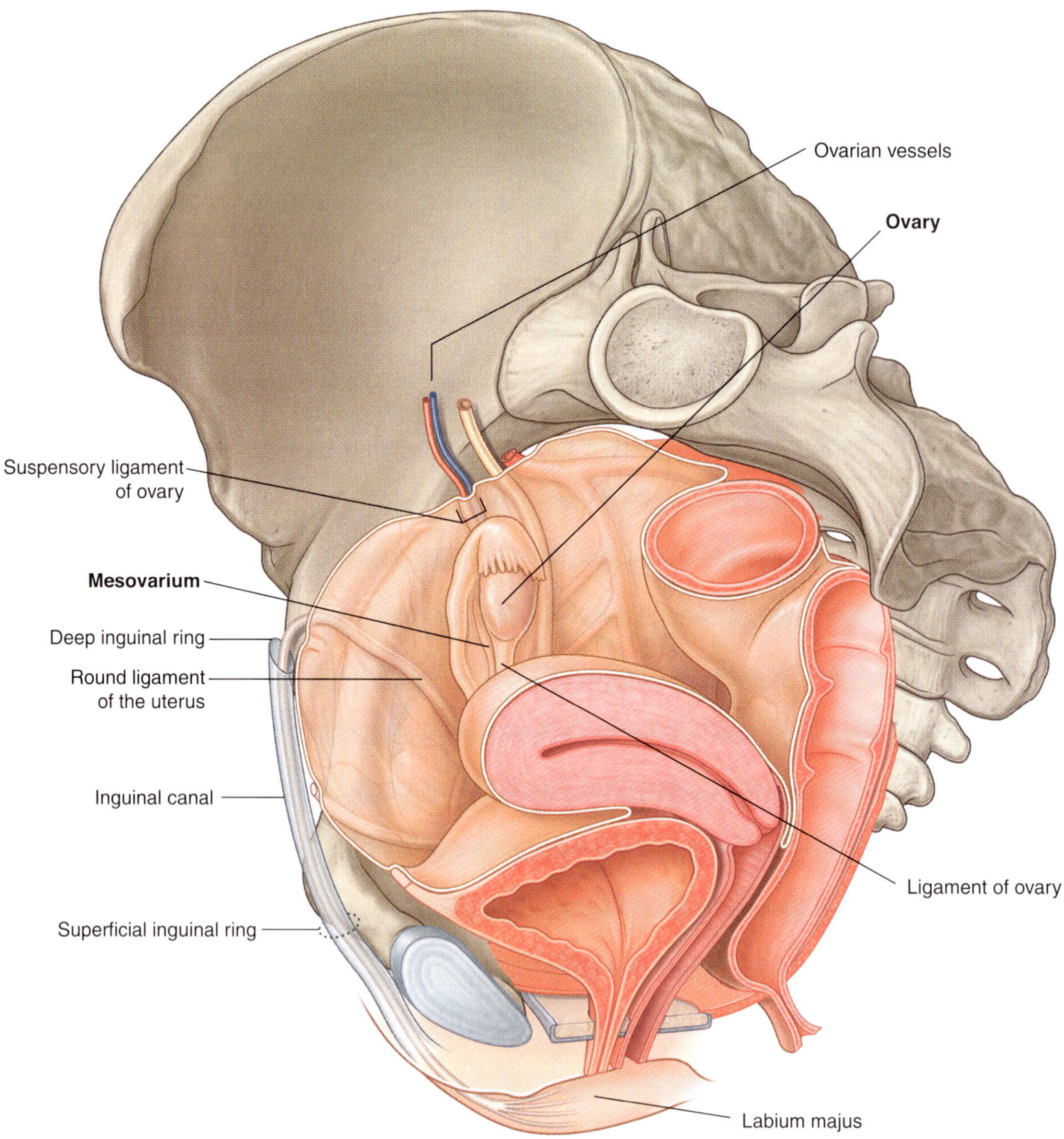

Fig. 5.50 Ovaries and broad ligament.

Early clinical exposure

Ovarian cancer

Ovarian cancer remains one of the major challenges in oncology. The ovaries contain numerous cell types, all of which can undergo malignant change and require different imaging and treatment protocols and ultimately have different prognoses.

Ovarian tumors most commonly originate from the surface epithelium that covers the ovary and is continuous at a sharp transition zone with the peritoneum of the mesovarium.

Many factors have been linked with the development of ovarian tumors, including a strong family history.

Ovarian cancer may occur at any age, but more typically it occurs in older women.

Cancer of the ovaries may spread via the blood and lymphatics, and frequently metastasizes directly into the peritoneal cavity. Such direct peritoneal cavity spread allows the passage of tumor cells along the paracolic gutters and over the liver from where this disease may disseminate easily. Unfortunately, many patients already have metastatic and diffuse disease (Fig. 5.51) at the time of diagnosis.

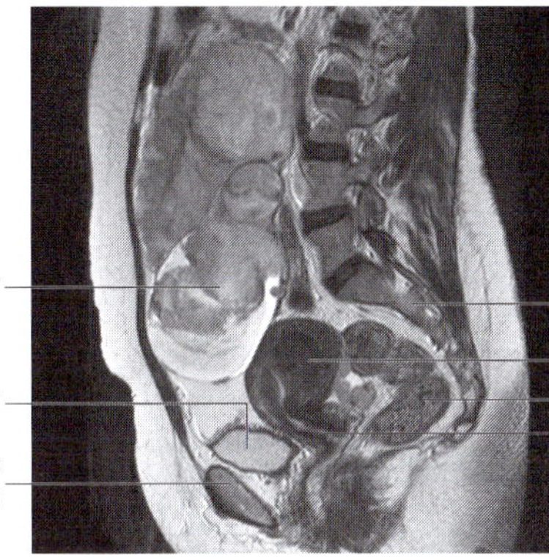

Fig. 5.51 Sagittal magnetic resonance image demonstrating ovarian cancer.

Early clinical exposure

Imaging the ovary

The ovaries can be visualized using ultrasound. If the patient drinks enough water, the bladder becomes enlarged and full. This fluid-filled cavity provides an excellent acoustic window, behind which the uterus and ovaries may be identified by transabdominal scanning with ultrasound. This technique also allows obstetricians and technicians to view a fetus and record its growth throughout pregnancy.

Some patients are not suitable for transabdominal scanning, in which case a probe may be passed into the vagina, permitting close visualization of the uterus, the contents of the rectouterine pouch (pouch of Douglas), and the ovaries. The ovaries can also be visualized laparoscopically.

Uterus

The **uterus** is a thick-walled muscular organ in the midline between the bladder and rectum (see Fig. 5.50). It consists of a fundus, body and a cervix, and inferiorly it joins the vagina (Fig. 5.52). Superiorly, uterine tubes project laterally from the uterus and open into the peritoneal cavity immediately adjacent to the ovaries.

The body of the uterus is flattened anteroposteriorly. Above the level of origin of the uterine tubes (Fig. 5.52), the rounded superior end is the **fundus of the uterus**. The cavity of the body of the uterus is a narrow slit, when viewed laterally, and is shaped like an inverted triangle, when viewed anteriorly. Each of the superior corners of the cavity is continuous with the lumen of a uterine tube; the inferior corner is continuous with the central canal of the cervix. The cervix is the lower, cylindrical part. The junction of the body and the cervix is the isthmus. Here, the peritoneum reflects from the surface of the uterus onto the urinary bladder.

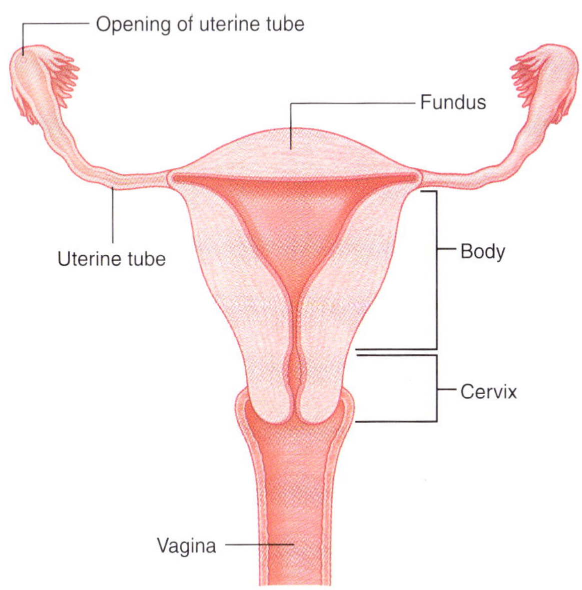

Fig. 5.52 Uterus. Anterior view. The anterior halves of the uterus and vagina have been cut away.

Implantation of the blastocyst normally occurs in the body of the uterus. During pregnancy, the uterus dramatically expands superiorly into the abdominal cavity.

Early clinical exposure

Hysterectomy

A hysterectomy is the surgical removal of the uterus. This is usually complete excision of the body, fundus, and cervix of the uterus, though occasionally the cervix may be left in situ. In some instances, the uterine (fallopian) tubes and ovaries are removed as well. This procedure is called a total abdominal hysterectomy and bilateral salpingo-oophorectomy.

Hysterectomy, oophorectomy, and salpingo-oophorectomy may be performed in patients who have reproductive malignancy, such as uterine, cervical, and ovarian cancers. Other indications include a strong family history of reproductive disorders, endometriosis, and excessive bleeding. Occasionally, the uterus may need to be removed postpartum because of excessive postpartum bleeding.

A hysterectomy is performed through a transverse suprapubic incision (Pfannenstiel's incision). During the procedure, tremendous care is taken to identify the distal ureters and to ligate the nearby uterine arteries without damage to the ureters.

Uterine tubes

The **uterine tubes** extend from each side of the superior end of the body of the uterus to the lateral pelvic wall and are enclosed within the upper margins of the mesosalpinx portions of the broad ligaments (see p. 664). Because the ovaries are suspended from the posterior aspect of the broad ligaments, the uterine tubes pass superiorly over, and terminate laterally to, the ovaries.

Each uterine tube has an expanded trumpet-shaped end (the **infundibulum**), which curves around the superolateral pole of the related ovary (Fig. 5.53). The margin of the infundibulum is rimmed with small finger-like projections termed **fimbriae**. The lumen of the uterine tube opens into the peritoneal cavity at the narrowed end of the infundibulum. Medial to the infundibulum, the tube expands to form the **ampulla** and then narrows to form the **isthmus**, before joining with the body of the uterus.

The fimbriated infundibulum facilitates the collection of ovulated eggs from the ovary. Fertilization normally occurs in the ampulla.

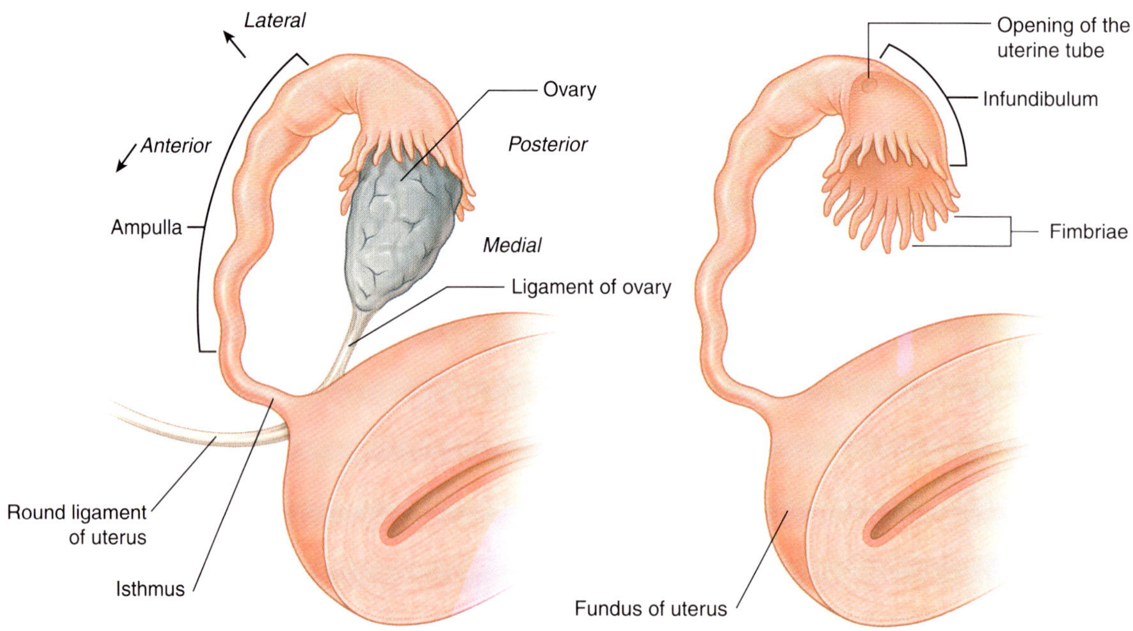

Fig. 5.53 Uterine tubes.

Early clinical exposure

Tubal ligation

After ovulation, the unfertilized egg is gathered by the fimbriae of the uterine tube. The egg passes into the uterine tube where it is normally fertilized in the ampulla. The zygote then begins development and passes into the uterine cavity where it implants in the uterine wall.

A simple and effective method of birth control is to surgically ligate (clip) the uterine tubes, preventing spermatozoa from reaching ova. This simple short procedure is performed under general anesthetic. A small laparoscope is passed into the peritoneal cavity and special equipment is used to identify the tubes.

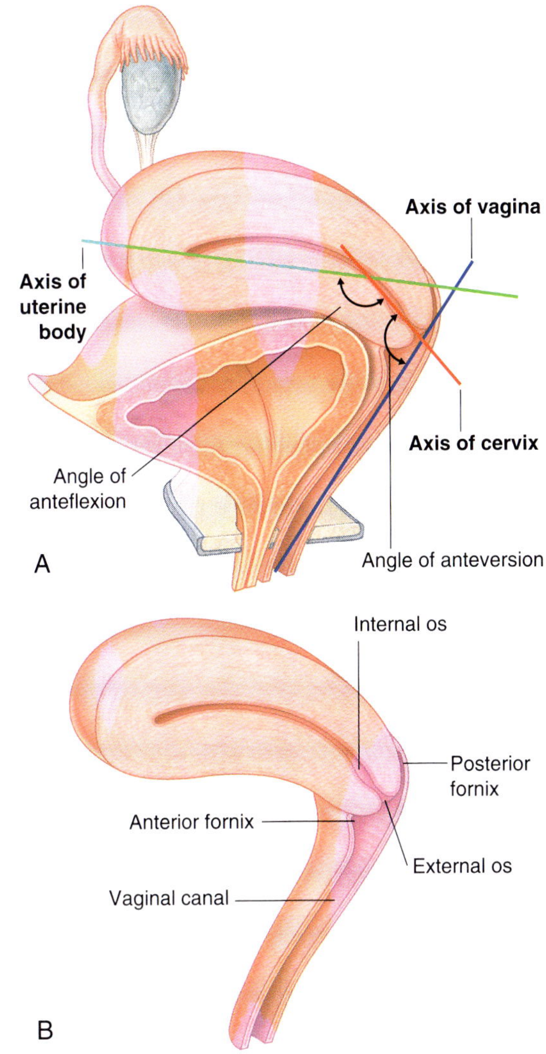

Fig. 5.54 Uterus and vagina. **(A)** Angles of anteflexion and anteversion. **(B)** The cervix protrudes into the vagina.

Cervix

The **cervix** forms the inferior part of the uterus and is shaped like a short, broad cylinder with a narrow central channel. The body of the uterus normally arches forward (anteflexed on the cervix) over the superior surface of the emptied bladder (Fig. 5.54A). In addition, the cervix is angled forward (anteverted) on the vagina so that the inferior end of the cervix projects into the upper anterior aspect of the vagina. Because the end of the cervix is dome shaped, it bulges into the vagina, and a gutter, or fornix, is formed around the margin of the cervix where it joins the vaginal wall (Fig. 5.54B). The tubular central canal of the cervix opens, below, as the **external os**, into the vaginal cavity and, above, as the **internal os**, into the uterine cavity. The normal position of the uterus, of anteflexion and anteversion helps to prevent prolapse of the uterus through the vagina.

The **supports of the uterus** include primary supports—muscular or active supports (the pelvic diaphragm, perineal body, and the urogenital diaphragm), ligaments (transverse cervical ligament or cardinal ligament or Mackenrodt's ligament, uterosacral ligament, pubocervical ligament, round ligament), and the uterine axis of anteflexion and anteversion; and secondary supports—peritoneal ligaments (broad ligament, uterovesical fold of peritoneum, and rectouterine fold of peritoneum).

Early clinical exposure

Carcinoma of the cervix and uterus

Carcinoma of the cervix (Fig. 5.55) and uterus is a common disease in women. Diagnosis is by inspection, cytology (examination of the cervical cells), imaging, biopsy, and dilatation and curettage (D&C) of the uterus.

Carcinoma of the cervix and uterus may be treated by local resection, removal of the uterus (hysterectomy), and adjuvant chemotherapy. The tumor spreads via lymphatics to the internal and common iliac lymph nodes.

Many countries have introduced screening programs for cervical cancer where women are regularly called for smear tests. The age of women included in the screening population varies depending on the country.

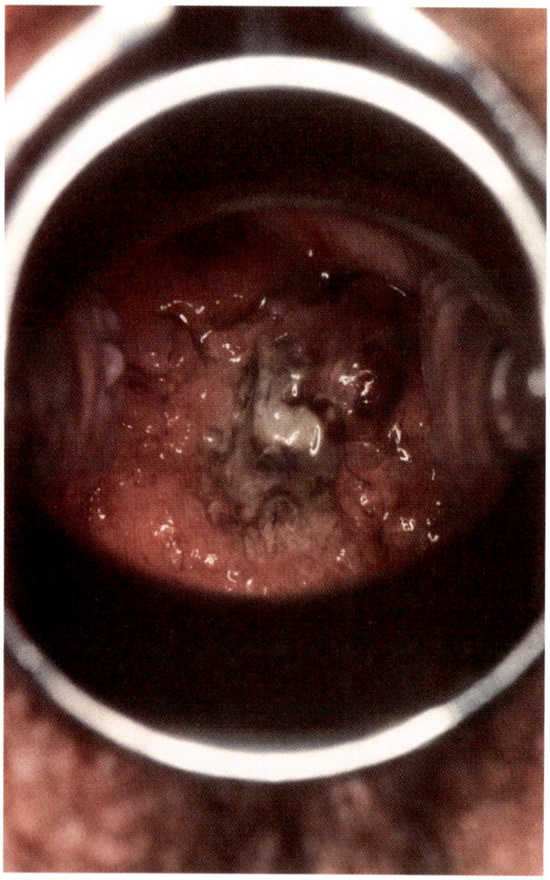

Fig. 5.55 Picture taken through a speculum inserted into the vagina demonstrating cervical cancer (see Fig. 5.83E on p. 707 for a view of the normal cervix).

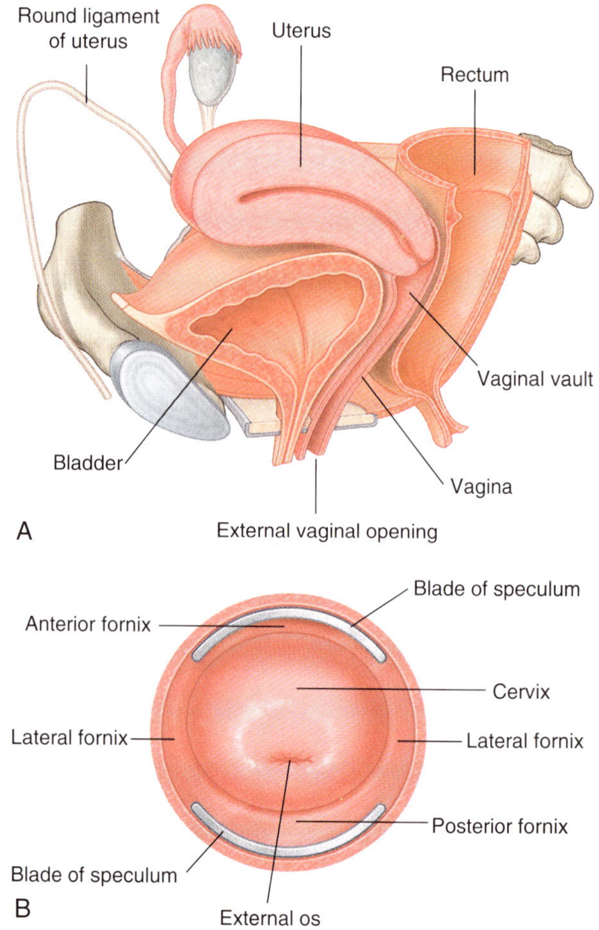

Fig. 5.56 Vagina. **(A)** Left half of pelvis cut away. **(B)** Vaginal fornices and cervix as viewed through a speculum.

Vagina

The **vagina** is the copulatory organ in women. It is a distensible fibromuscular tube that extends from the perineum through the pelvic floor and into the pelvic cavity (Fig. 5.56A). The internal end of the canal is enlarged to form a region called the **vaginal vault**.

The anterior wall of the vagina is related to the base of the bladder and to the urethra; in fact, the urethra is embedded in, or fused to, the anterior vaginal wall.

Posteriorly, the vagina is related principally to the rectum.

Inferiorly, the vagina opens into the vestibule of the perineum immediately posterior to the external opening of the urethra. From its external opening (the **introitus**), the vagina courses posterosuperiorly through the perineal membrane and into the pelvic cavity, where it is attached by its anterior wall to the circular margin of the cervix.

The **vaginal fornix** is the recess formed between the margin of the cervix and the vaginal wall. Based on position, the fornix is subdivided into a posterior fornix, an anterior fornix, and two lateral fornices (see Fig. 5.54 and 5.56A).

The vaginal canal is normally collapsed so that the anterior wall is in contact with the posterior wall. By using a speculum to open the vaginal canal, a physician can see the domed inferior end of the cervix, the vaginal fornices, and the external os of the cervical canal in a patient (Fig. 5.56B).

During intercourse, semen is deposited in the vaginal vault. Spermatozoa make their way into the external os of the cervical canal, pass through the cervical canal into the uterine cavity, and then continue through the uterine cavity into the uterine tubes where fertilization normally occurs in the ampulla.

Early clinical exposure

The rectouterine pouch

The rectouterine pouch (**pouch of Douglas**) is an extremely important clinical region situated between the rectum and uterus. When the patient is in the supine position, the rectouterine pouch is the lowest portion of the abdominopelvic cavity and is a site where infection and fluids typically collect. It is impossible to palpate this region transabdominally, but it can be examined by transvaginal and transrectal digital palpation. If an abscess is suspected, it may be drained through the vagina or the rectum without necessitating transabdominal surgery.

Fascia

Fascia in the pelvic cavity lines the pelvic walls, surrounds the bases of the pelvic viscera, and forms sheaths around blood vessels and nerves that course medially from the pelvic walls to reach the viscera in the midline. This pelvic fascia is a continuation of the extraperitoneal connective tissue layer found in the abdomen.

In women

In women, a **rectovaginal septum** separates the posterior surface of the vagina from the rectum (Fig. 5.57A). Condensations of fascia form ligaments that extend from the cervix to the anterior (**pubocervical ligament**), lateral (**transverse cervical** or **cardinal ligament**), and posterior (**uterosacral ligament**) pelvic walls (Fig. 5.57A). These ligaments, together with the perineal membrane, the levator ani muscles, and the perineal body, are thought to stabilize the uterus in the pelvic cavity. The most important of these ligaments are the transverse cervical or cardinal ligaments, which extend laterally from each side of the cervix and vaginal vault to the related pelvic wall.

In men

In men, a condensation of fascia around the anterior and lateral region of the prostate (**prostatic fascia**) contains and surrounds the prostatic plexus of veins and is continuous posteriorly with the **rectovesical septum**, which separates the posterior surface of the prostate and base of the bladder from the rectum (Fig. 5.57B).

Peritoneum

The peritoneum of the pelvis is continuous at the pelvic inlet with the peritoneum of the abdomen. In the pelvis, the peritoneum drapes over the pelvic viscera in the midline, forming:

- Pouches between adjacent viscera
- Folds and ligaments between viscera and pelvic walls

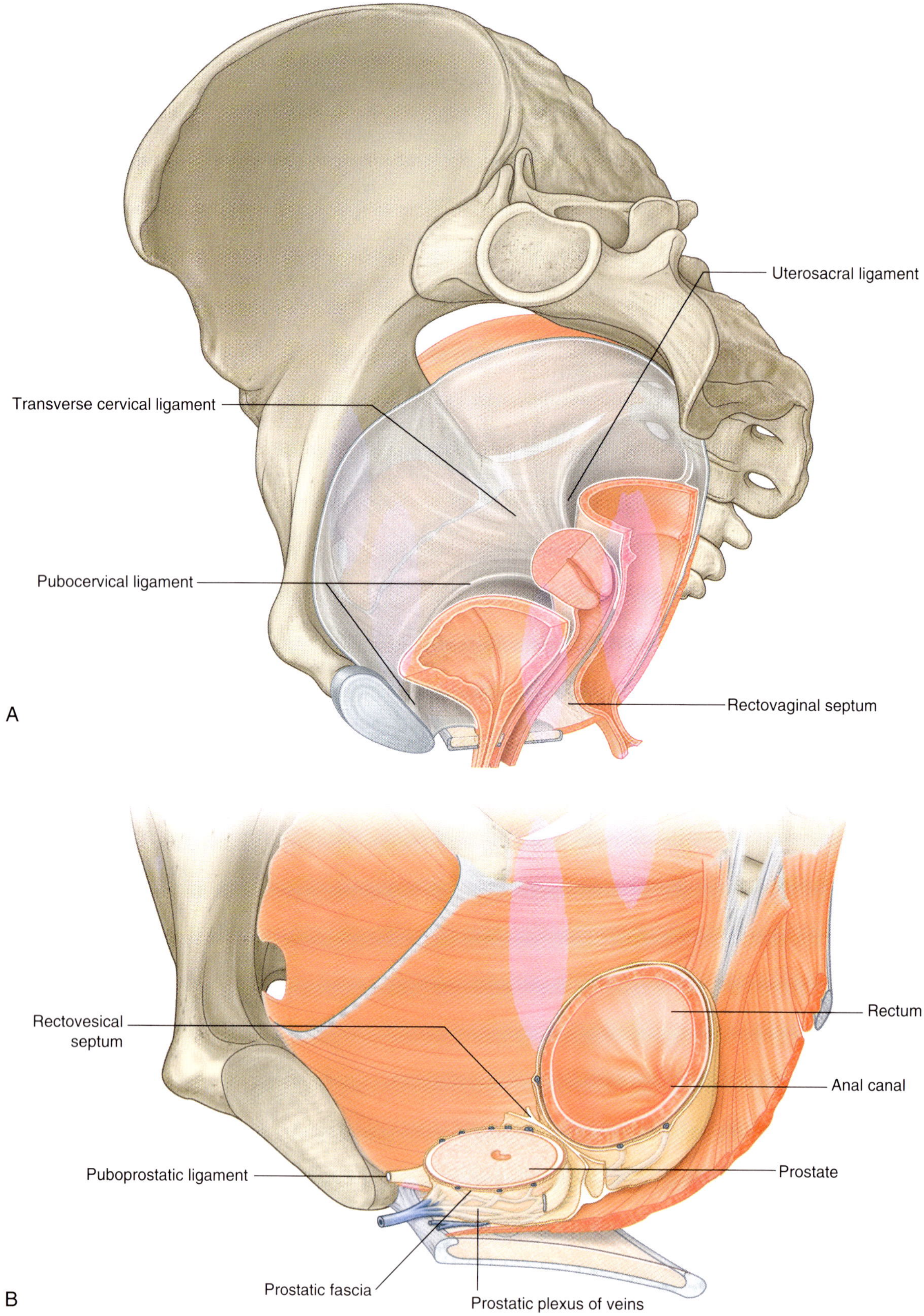

Fig. 5.57 Pelvic fascia. **(A)** In women. **(B)** In men.

Anteriorly, median and medial umbilical folds of peritoneum cover the embryological remnants of the urachus and umbilical arteries, respectively (Fig. 5.58). These folds ascend out of the pelvis and onto the anterior abdominal wall. Posteriorly, peritoneum drapes over the anterior and lateral aspects of the upper third of the rectum, but only the anterior surface of the middle third of the rectum is covered by peritoneum; the lower third of the rectum is not covered at all.

In women

In women, the uterus lies between the bladder and rectum, and the uterine tubes extend from the superior aspect of the uterus to the lateral pelvic walls (Fig. 5.58A). As a consequence, a shallow **vesicouterine pouch** occurs anteriorly, between the bladder and uterus, and a deep **rectouterine pouch** (pouch of Douglas) occurs posteriorly, between the uterus and rectum. In addition, a large fold of peritoneum (the broad ligament), with a uterine tube enclosed in its superior margin and an ovary attached posteriorly, is located on each side of the uterus and extends to the lateral pelvic walls.

In the midline, the peritoneum descends over the posterior surface of the uterus and cervix and onto the vaginal wall adjacent to the posterior vaginal fornix. It then reflects onto the anterior and lateral walls of the rectum. The deep pouch of peritoneum formed between the anterior surface of the rectum and posterior surfaces of the uterus, cervix, and vagina is the rectouterine pouch. A sharp sickle-shaped ridge of peritoneum (**rectouterine fold**) occurs on each side near the base of the rectouterine pouch. The **rectouterine folds** overlie the **uterosacral ligaments**, which are condensations of pelvic fascia that extend from the cervix to the posterolateral pelvic walls.

Broad ligament

The **broad ligament** is a sheet-like fold of peritoneum, oriented in the coronal plane that runs from the lateral pelvic wall to the uterus, and encloses the uterine tube in its superior margin and suspends the ovary from its posterior aspect (Fig. 5.58A). The uterine arteries cross the ureters at the base of the broad ligaments, and the ligament of the ovary and round ligament of the uterus are enclosed within the parts of the broad ligament related to the ovary and uterus, respectively. The broad ligament has three parts:

- The mesometrium, the largest part of the broad ligament, which extends from the lateral pelvic walls to the body of the uterus
- The mesosalpinx, the most superior part of the broad ligament, which suspends the uterine tube in the pelvic cavity
- The mesovarium, a posterior extension of the broad ligament, which attaches to the ovary

The peritoneum of the mesovarium becomes firmly attached to the ovary as the surface epithelium of the ovary. The ovaries are positioned with their long axis in the vertical plane. The ovarian vessels, nerves, and lymphatics enter the superior pole of the ovary from a lateral position and are covered by another raised fold of peritoneum, which with the structures it contains forms the **suspensory ligament of the ovary** (**infundibulopelvic ligament**).

The inferior pole of the ovary is attached to a fibromuscular band of tissue (the **ligament of the ovary**), which courses medially in the margin of the mesovarium to the uterus and then continues anterolaterally as the **round ligament of the uterus** (Fig. 5.58A). The round ligament of the uterus passes over the pelvic inlet to reach the deep inguinal ring and then courses through the inguinal canal to end in connective tissue related to the labium majus in the perineum. Both the ligament of the ovary and the round ligament of the uterus are remnants of the gubernaculum, which attaches the gonad to the labioscrotal swellings in the embryo.

In men

In men, the visceral peritoneum drapes over the top of the bladder onto the superior poles of the seminal vesicles and then reflects onto the anterior and lateral surfaces of the rectum (Fig. 5.58B). A **rectovesical pouch** occurs between the bladder and rectum.

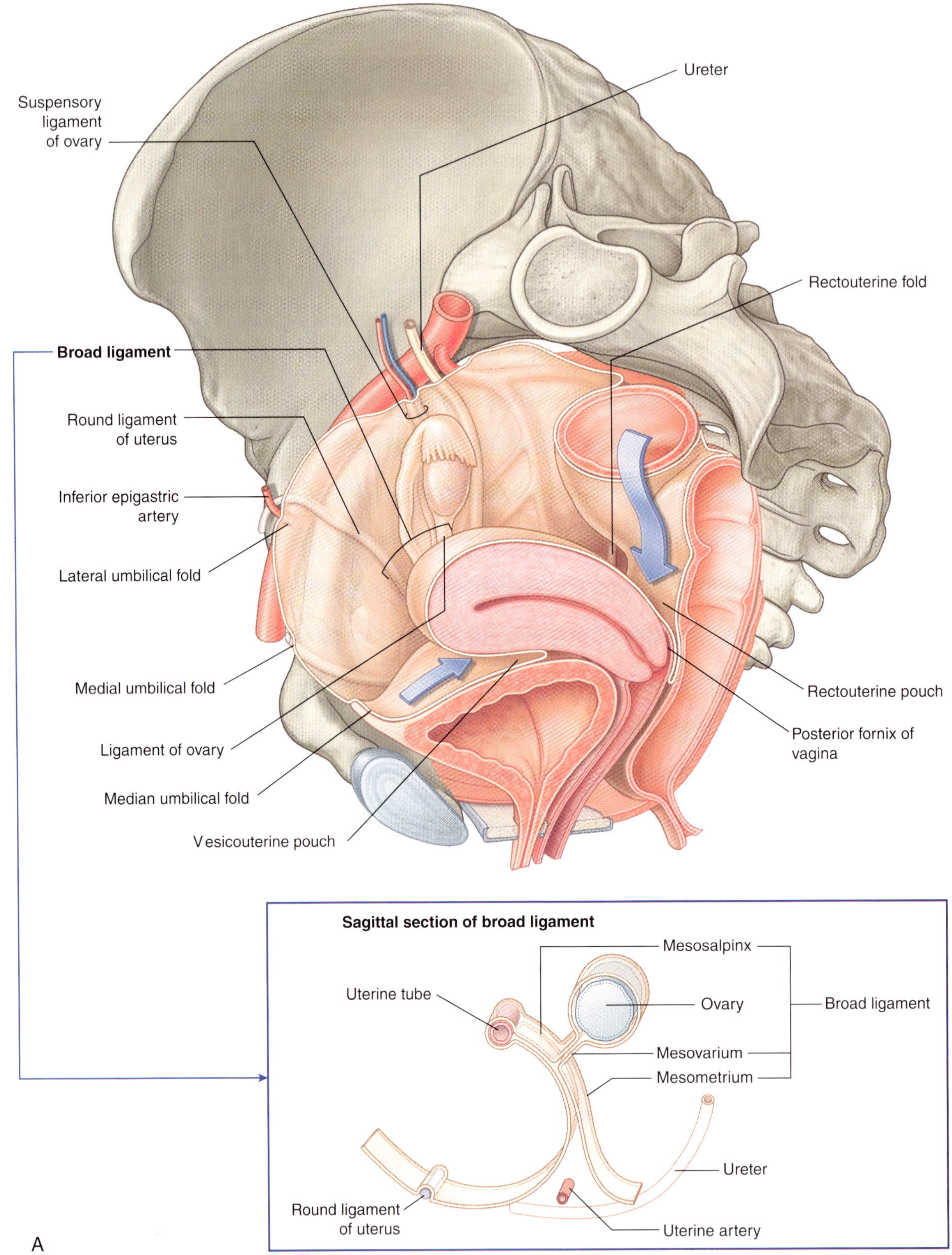

Fig. 5.58 Peritoneum in the pelvis. **(A)** In women.

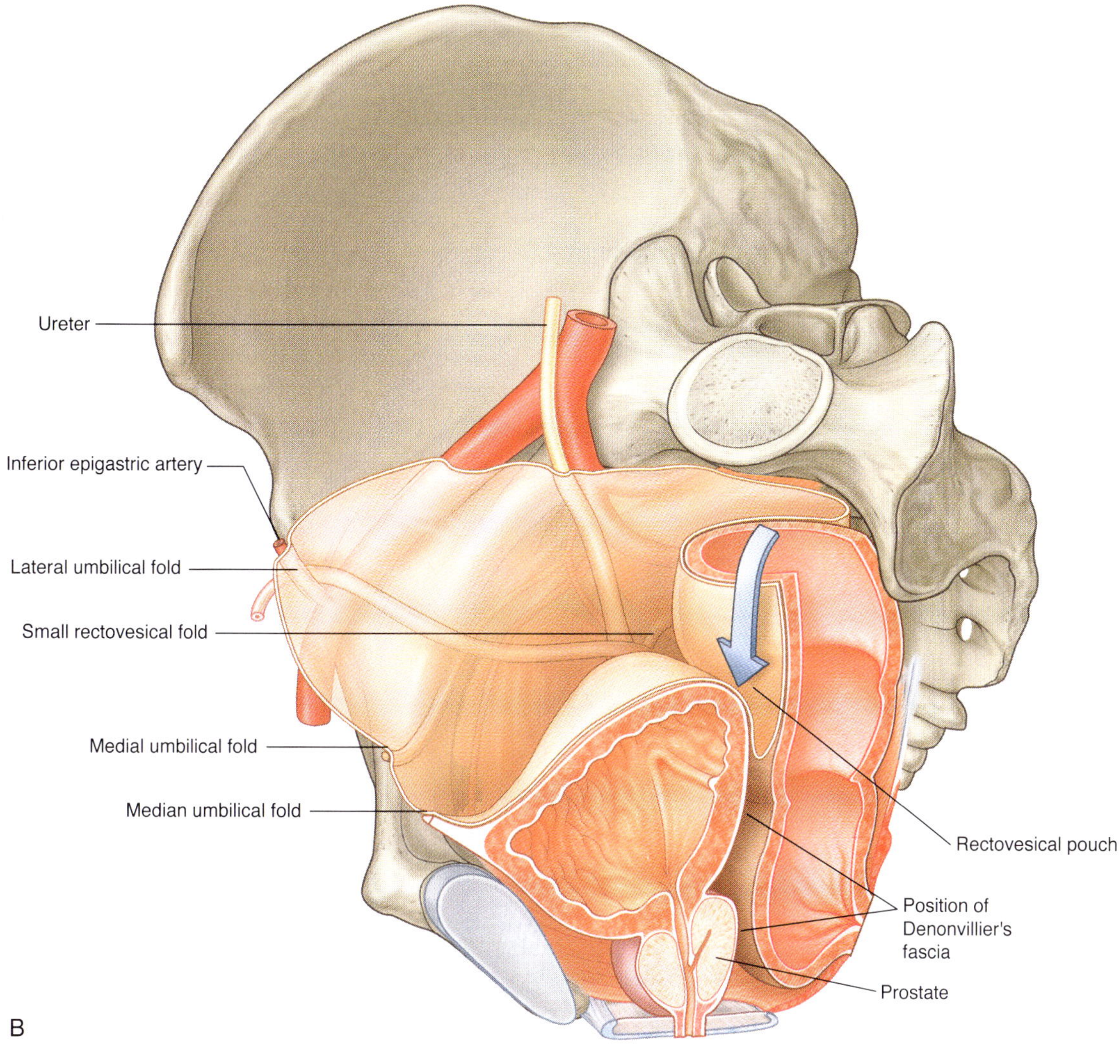

Fig. 5.58, cont'd (B) In men.

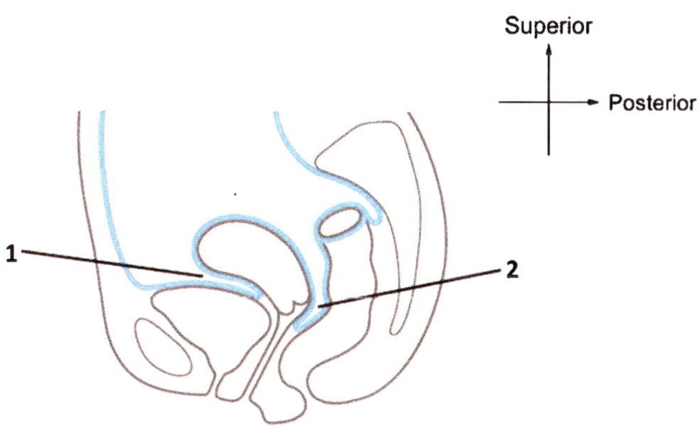

LD Fig. 5.58A.1 Outline of peritoneum in the female pelvis

Question

LD Fig. 5.58A.1.A Name the areas indicated by the pointers, and list the structures related to these areas.

Answer

The areas indicated and the structures related to each area are

1—uterovesical pouch: inferiorly is the urinary bladder, and superiorly is the uterus.

2—rectouterine pouch: anteriorly is the vagina and uterus, and posteriorly is the rectum.

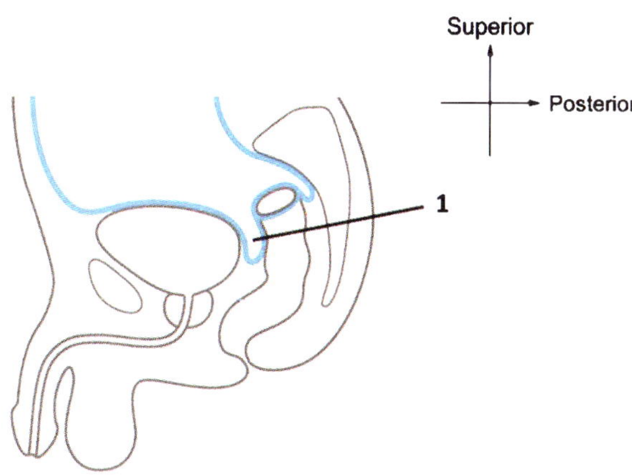

LD Fig. 5.58B.1 Outline of peritoneum in the male pelvis.

Question

LD Fig. 5.58B.1.A Name the area indicated by the pointer labeled 1 and list the structures related to these areas.

Answer

The area indicated is the rectovesical pouch and the structures related to it are the urinary bladder anteriorly and the rectum posteriorly.

Nerves

Somatic plexuses

Sacral and coccygeal plexuses

The sacral and coccygeal plexuses are situated on the posterolateral wall of the pelvic cavity and generally occur in the plane between the muscles and blood vessels. They are formed by the ventral rami of S1 to Co, with a significant contribution from L4 and L5, which enter the pelvis from the lumbar plexus (Fig. 5.59). Nerves from these mainly somatic plexuses contribute to the innervation of the lower limb and muscles of the pelvis and perineum. Cutaneous branches supply skin over the medial side of the foot, the posterior aspect of the lower limb, and most of the perineum.

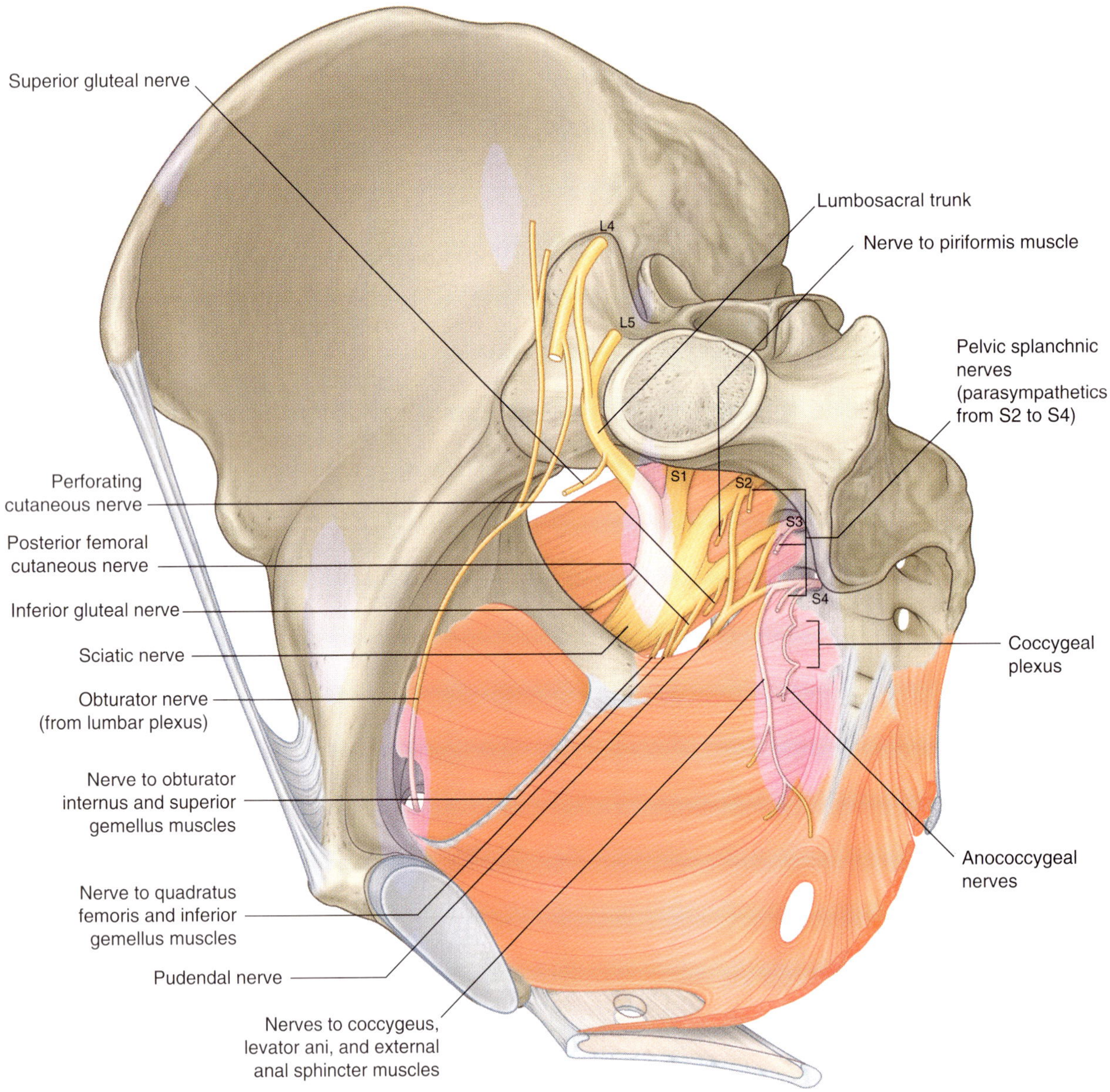

Fig. 5.59 Sacral and coccygeal plexuses.

Sacral plexus

The sacral plexus on each side is formed by the anterior rami of S1 to S3, and the lumbosacral trunk (L4 and L5) (Fig. 5.60). It has two terminal branches, the sciatic nerve and the pudendal nerve. The plexus is formed in relation to the anterior surface of the piriformis muscle, which is part of the posterolateral pelvic wall. Sacral contributions to the plexus pass out of the anterior sacral foramina and course laterally and inferiorly on the pelvic wall. The lumbosacral trunk, consisting of part of the anterior ramus of L4 and all of the anterior ramus of L5, courses vertically into the pelvic cavity from the abdomen by passing immediately anterior to the sacroiliac joint.

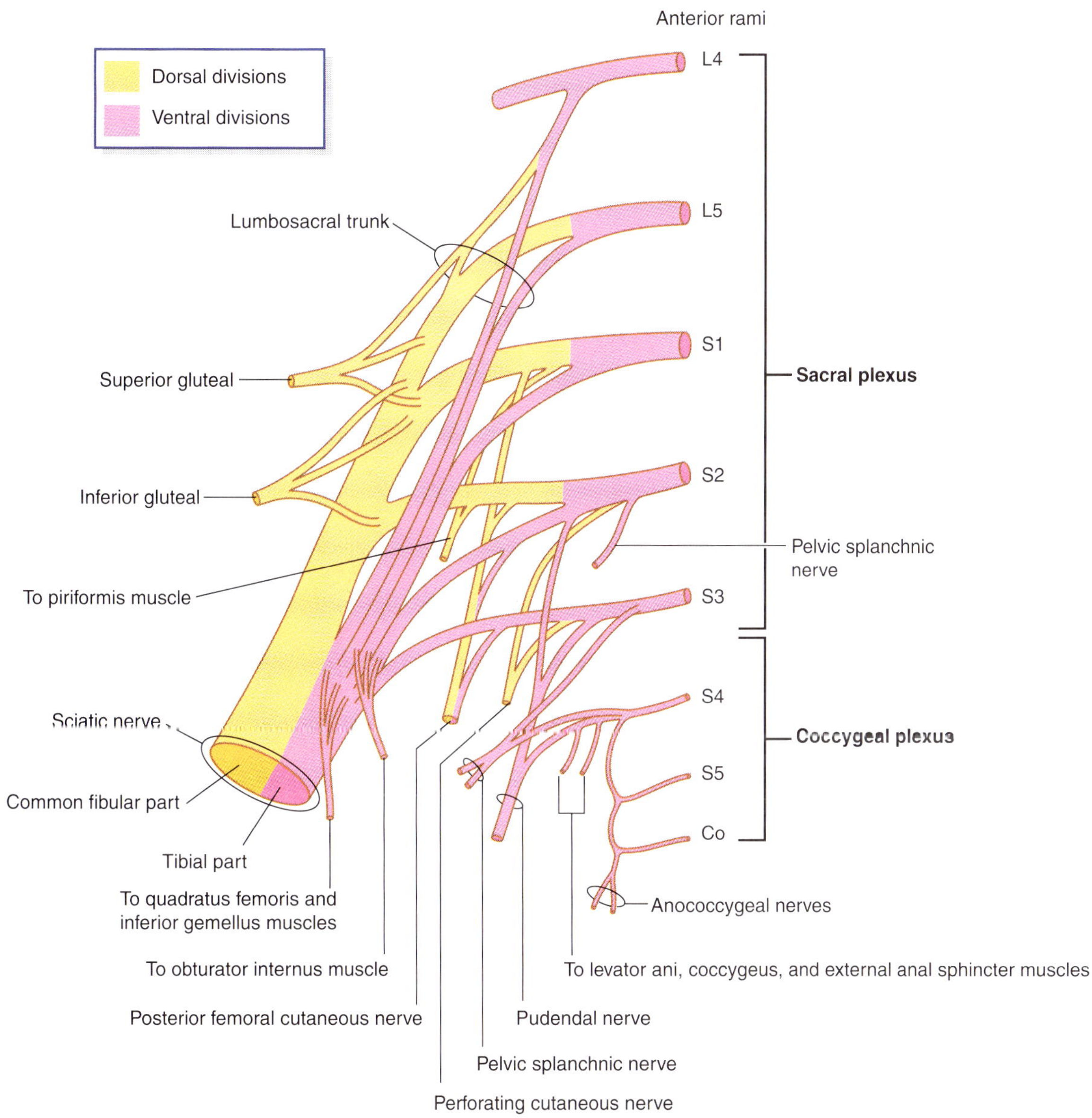

Fig. 5.60 Components and branches of the sacral and coccygeal plexuses.

Gray rami communicantes from ganglia of the sympathetic trunk connect with each of the anterior rami and carry postganglionic sympathetic fibers destined for the periphery to the somatic nerves (Fig. 5.61). In addition, special visceral nerves (**pelvic splanchnic nerves**) originating from S2 to S4 deliver preganglionic parasympathetic fibers to the pelvic part of the prevertebral plexus (Figs 5.59 and 5.60).

Each anterior ramus has ventral and dorsal divisions that combine with similar divisions from other levels to form terminal nerves (Fig. 5.60). The anterior ramus of S4 has only a ventral division.

Branches of the sacral plexus include the sciatic nerve and gluteal nerves, which are major nerves of the lower limb, and the pudendal nerve, which is the nerve of the perineum (Table 5.4). Numerous smaller branches supply the pelvic wall, floor, and lower limb.

Most nerves originating from the sacral plexus leave the pelvic cavity by passing through the greater sciatic

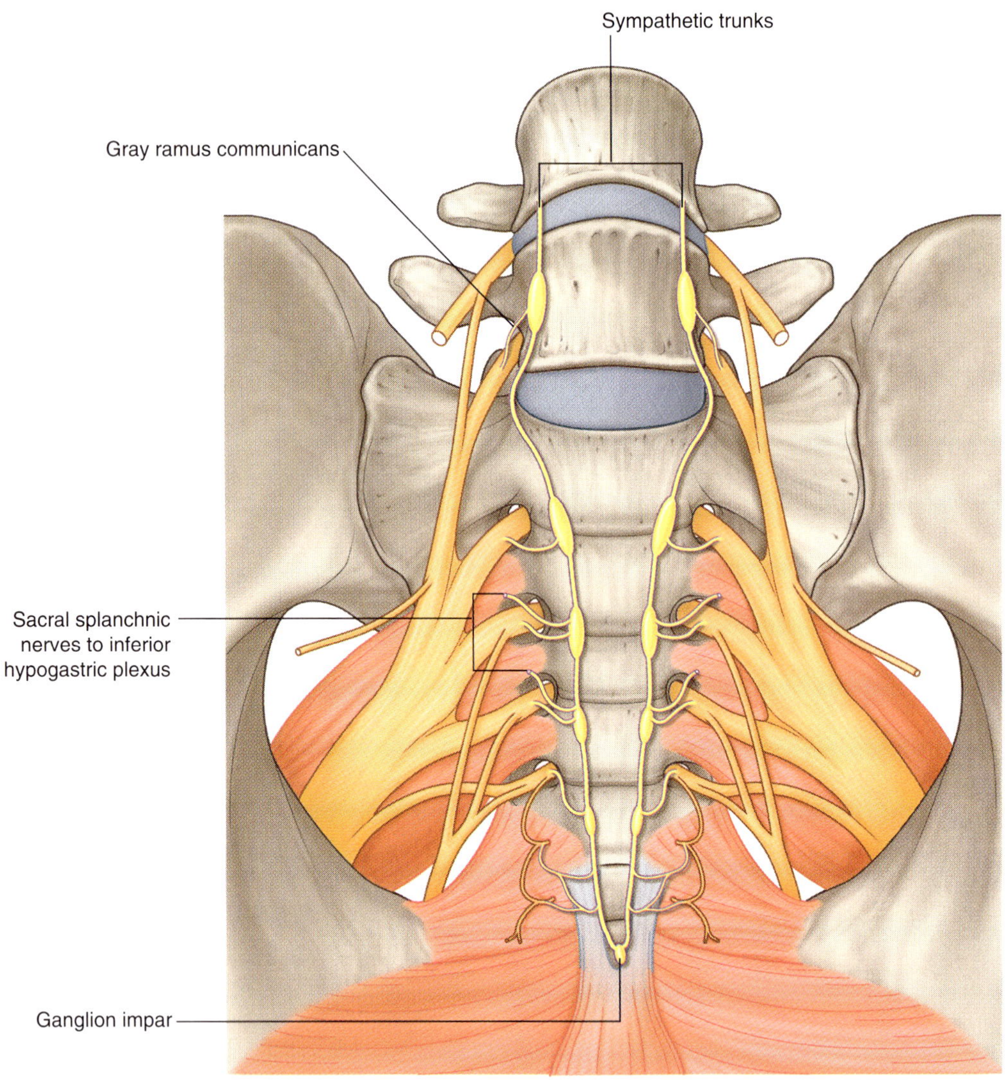

Fig. 5.61 Sympathetic trunks in the pelvis.

Table 5.4 Branches of the sacral and coccygeal plexuses (spinal segments in parentheses do not consistently participate)

Branch	Spinal segments	Function
SACRAL PLEXUS		
Sciatic 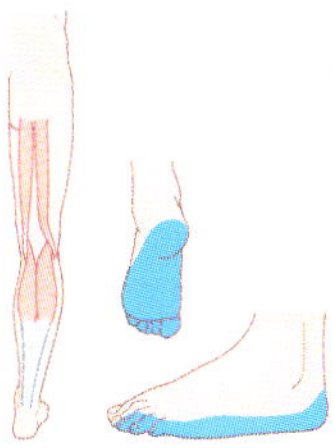 Tibial part	L4 to S3	**Motor function** All muscles in the posterior or hamstring compartment of the thigh (including the hamstring part of the adductor magnus) except for the short head of the biceps All muscles in the posterior compartment of the leg All muscles in the sole of the foot **Sensory (cutaneous) function** Skin on posterolateral and lateral surfaces of foot and sole of foot
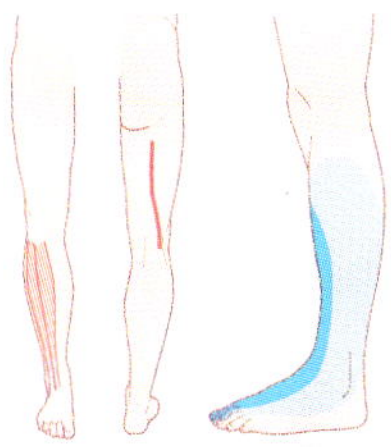 Common fibular part	L4 to S2	**Motor function** Short head of biceps in the posterior compartment of the thigh All muscles in the anterior and lateral compartments of the leg Extensor digitorum brevis in the foot (also contributes to the supply of the first dorsal interosseous muscle) **Sensory (cutaneous) function** Skin on the anterolateral surface of the leg and dorsal surface of the foot
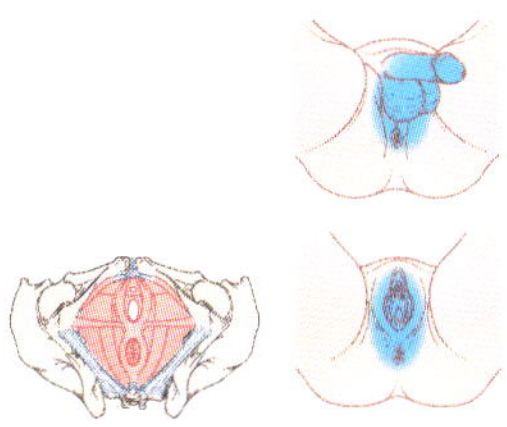 **Pudendal**	S2 to S4	**Motor function** Skeletal muscles in the perineum including the external urethral and anal sphincters and levator ani (overlaps in supply of the levator ani and external sphincter with branches directly from ventral division of S4) **Sensory (cutaneous) function** Most skin of the perineum. Penis and clitoris
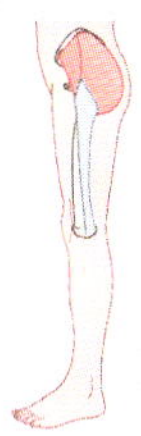 **Superior gluteal**	L4 to S1	**Motor function** Gluteus medius, gluteus minimus, and tensor fasciae latae
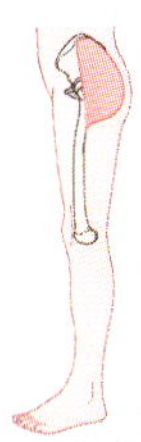 **Inferior gluteal**	L5 to S2	**Motor function** Gluteus maximus
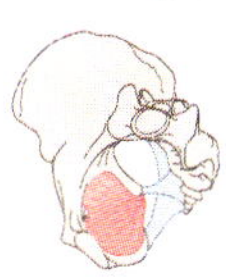 **Nerve to obturator internus and superior gemellus**	L5 to S2	**Motor function** Obturator internus and superior gemellus

Continued

Table 5.4 Branches of the sacral and coccygeal plexuses (spinal segments in parentheses do not consistently participate)—cont'd

Branch		
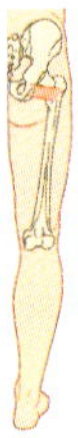 **Nerve to quadratus femoris and inferior gemellus**	L4 to S1	**Motor function** Quadratus femoris and inferior gemellus
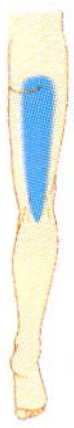 **Posterior femoral cutaneous (posterior cutaneous nerve of thigh)**	S1, S3	**Sensory(cutaneous)function** Skin on the posterior aspect of the thigh
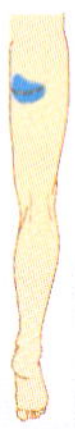 Perforating cutaneous	S2, S3	**Sensory (cutaneous) function** Skin over gluteal fold (overlaps with posterior femoral cutaneous)
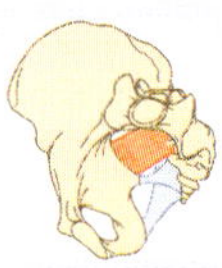 **Nerve to piriformis**	S1, S2	**Motor function** Piriformis muscle
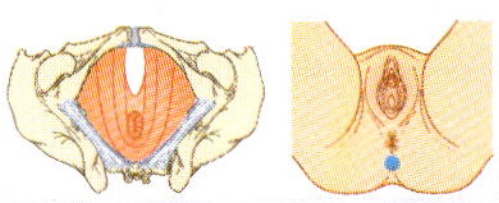 **Nerves to levator ani, coccygeus, and external anal sphincter**	S4	**Motor function** Levator ani, coccygeus, and external anal sphincter (overlaps with pudendal nerve) **Sensory (cutaneous) function** Small patch of skin between anus and coccyx
Pelvic splanchnic nerves	S2, S3 (4)	**Motor (visceral) function** Visceral motor (preganglionic parasympathetic) to pelvic part of prevertebral plexus Stimulate erection, modulate mobility in gastrointestinal system distal to the left colic flexure, inhibitory to internal urethral sphincter **Sensory (visceral) function** Visceral afferents (that follow the parasympathetics) from pelvic viscera and distal parts of colon; pain from cervix and possibly from bladder and proximal urethra
COCCYGEAL PLEXUS		
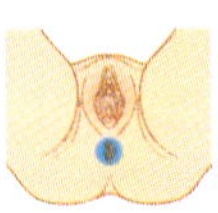 **Anococcygeal nerves**	S4 to Co	**Sensory (cutaneous) function** Perianal skin

foramen inferior to the piriformis muscle, and enter the gluteal region of the lower limb. Other nerves leave the pelvic cavity using different routes; a few nerves do not leave the pelvic cavity and course directly into the muscles in the pelvic cavity. Finally, two nerves that leave the pelvic cavity through the greater sciatic foramen loop around the ischial spine and sacrospinous ligament and pass medially through the lesser sciatic foramen to supply structures in the perineum and lateral pelvic wall.

Sciatic nerve

The **sciatic nerve** is the largest nerve of the body and carries contributions from L4 to S3 (Figs 5.59 and 5.60). It:

- Forms on the anterior surface of the piriformis muscle and leaves the pelvic cavity through the greater sciatic foramen inferior to the piriformis.
- Passes through the gluteal region into the thigh, where it divides into its two major branches, the common fibular nerve (common peroneal nerve) and the tibial nerve—dorsal divisions of L4, L5, S1, and S2 are carried in the common fibular part of the nerve and the ventral divisions of L4, L5, S1, S2, and S3 are carried in the tibial part.
- Innervates muscles in the posterior compartment of the thigh and muscles in the leg and foot.
- Carries sensory fibers from the skin of the foot and lateral leg.

Pudendal nerve

The **pudendal nerve** forms anteriorly to the lower part of the piriformis muscle from ventral divisions of S2 to S4 (Figs 5.59 and 5.60). It:

- Leaves the pelvic cavity through the greater sciatic foramen, inferior to the piriformis muscle, and enters the gluteal region.
- Courses into the perineum by immediately passing around the sacrospinous ligament, where the ligament joins the ischial spine, and through the lesser sciatic foramen (this course takes the nerve out of the pelvic cavity, around the peripheral attachment of the pelvic floor, and into the perineum).
- Is accompanied throughout its course by the internal pudendal vessels.
- Innervates skin and skeletal muscles of the perineum, including the external anal and external urethral sphincters (Flowchart 5.1).

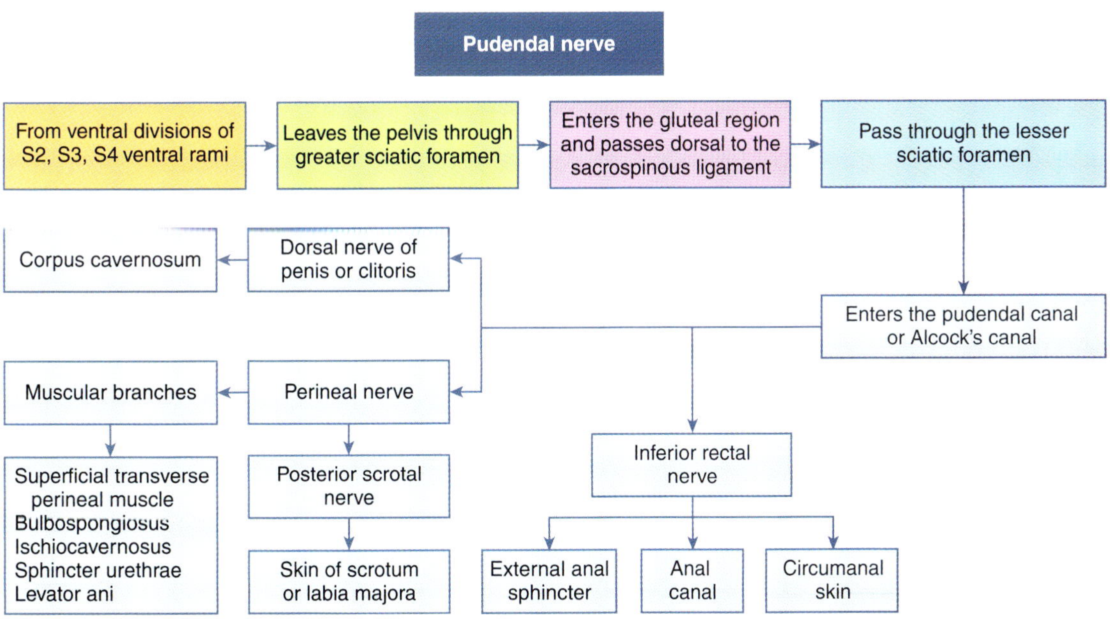

Flowchart 5.1 Pudendal nerve.

Early clinical exposure

Pudendal block

Pudendal block anesthesia is performed to relieve the pain associated with childbirth. Although the use of this procedure is less common since the widespread adoption of epidural anesthesia, it provides an excellent option for women who have a contraindication to neuraxial anesthesia (e.g., spinal anatomy, low platelets, too close to delivery). Pudendal blocks are also used for certain types of chronic pelvic pain and in some rectal or urological procedures. The injection is usually given where the pudendal nerve crosses the lateral aspect of the sacrospinous ligament near its attachment to the ischial spine. During childbirth, a finger inserted into the vagina can palpate the ischial spine. The needle is passed transcutaneously to the medial aspect of the ischial spine and around the sacrospinous ligament. Infiltration is performed and the perineum is anesthetized. Pudendal nerve blocks can also be performed with imaging guidance (using fluoroscopy, computed tomography, or ultrasound) to localize the nerve rather than relying purely on anatomical landmarks.

Other branches of the sacral plexus

Other branches of the sacral plexus include:

- Motor branches to muscles of the gluteal region, pelvic wall, and pelvic floor (superior and inferior gluteal nerves, nerve to obturator internus and superior gemellus, nerve to quadratus femoris and inferior gemellus, nerve to piriformis, nerves to levator ani).
- Sensory nerves to skin over the inferior gluteal region and posterior aspects of the thigh and upper leg (perforating cutaneous nerve and posterior cutaneous nerve of the thigh) (Figs 5.59 and 5.60).

The **superior gluteal nerve**, formed by branches from the dorsal divisions of L4 to S1, leaves the pelvic cavity through the greater sciatic foramen superior to the piriformis muscle and supplies muscles in the gluteal region—**gluteus medius**, **gluteus minimus**, and **tensor fasciae latae (tensor of fascia lata) muscles**.

The **inferior gluteal nerve**, formed by branches from the dorsal divisions of L5 to S2, leaves the pelvic cavity through the greater sciatic foramen inferior to the piriformis muscle and supplies the **gluteus maximus**, the largest muscle in the gluteal region.

Both superior and inferior gluteal nerves are accompanied by corresponding arteries.

The **nerve to the obturator internus** and the associated **superior gemellus** muscle originates from the ventral divisions of L5 to S2 and leaves the pelvic cavity through the greater sciatic foramen inferior to the piriformis muscle. Like the pudendal nerve, it passes around the ischial spine and through the lesser sciatic foramen to enter the perineum and supply the obturator internus muscle from the medial side of the muscle, inferior to the attachment of the levator ani muscle.

The **nerve to the quadratus femoris** muscle and the **inferior gemellus** muscle, and the **posterior cutaneous nerve of the thigh (posterior femoral cutaneous nerve)** also leave the pelvic cavity through the greater sciatic foramen inferior to the piriformis muscle and course to muscles and skin, respectively, in the lower limb.

Unlike most of the other nerves originating from the sacral plexus, which leave the pelvic cavity through the greater sciatic foramen either above or below the piriformis muscle, the **perforating cutaneous nerve** leaves the pelvic cavity by penetrating directly through the sacrotuberous ligament and then courses to skin over the inferior aspect of the buttocks.

The **nerve to the piriformis** and a number of small nerves to the levator ani and coccygeus muscles originate from the sacral plexus and pass directly into their target muscles without leaving the pelvic cavity.

The **obturator nerve** (L2 to L4) is a branch of the lumbar plexus. It passes inferiorly along the posterior abdominal wall within the psoas muscle, emerges from the medial surface of the psoas, passes posteriorly to the common iliac artery and medially to the internal iliac artery at the pelvic inlet, and then courses along the lateral pelvic wall. It leaves the pelvic cavity by traveling through the obturator canal and supplies the adductor region of the thigh.

Coccygeal plexus

The small coccygeal plexus has a minor contribution from S4 and is formed mainly by the anterior rami of S5 and Co, which originate inferiorly to the pelvic floor. They penetrate the coccygeus muscle to enter the pelvic cavity and join with the anterior ramus of S4 to form a single trunk, from which small **anococcygeal nerves** originate (Table 5.4). These nerves penetrate the muscle and the overlying sacrospinous and sacrotuberous ligaments and pass superficially to innervate skin in the anal triangle of the perineum.

Visceral plexuses

Paravertebral sympathetic chain

The paravertebral part of the visceral nervous system is represented in the pelvis by the inferior ends of the sympathetic trunks (Fig. 5.62A). Each trunk enters the pelvic cavity from the abdomen by passing over the ala of the sacrum medially to the lumbosacral trunks and posteriorly to the iliac vessels. The trunks course inferiorly along the anterior surface of the sacrum, where they are positioned medially to the anterior sacral foramina. Four ganglia occur along each trunk. Anteriorly to the coccyx, the two trunks join to form a single small terminal ganglion (the **ganglion impar**).

The principal function of the sympathetic trunks in the pelvis is to deliver postganglionic sympathetic fibers to the anterior rami of sacral nerves for distribution to the periphery, mainly to parts of the lower limb and perineum. This is accomplished by gray rami communicantes, which connect the trunks to the sacral anterior rami.

In addition to gray rami communicantes, other branches (the **sacral splanchnic nerves**) join and contribute to the pelvic part of the prevertebral plexus associated with innervating pelvic viscera (Fig. 5.62A).

Pelvic extensions of the prevertebral plexus

The pelvic parts of the prevertebral plexus carry sympathetic, parasympathetic, and visceral afferent fibers (Fig. 5.62A). Pelvic parts of the plexus are associated with innervating pelvic viscera and erectile tissues of the perineum.

The prevertebral plexus enters the pelvis as two **hypogastric nerves**, one on each side, that cross the pelvic inlet medially to the internal iliac vessels (Fig. 5.62A).

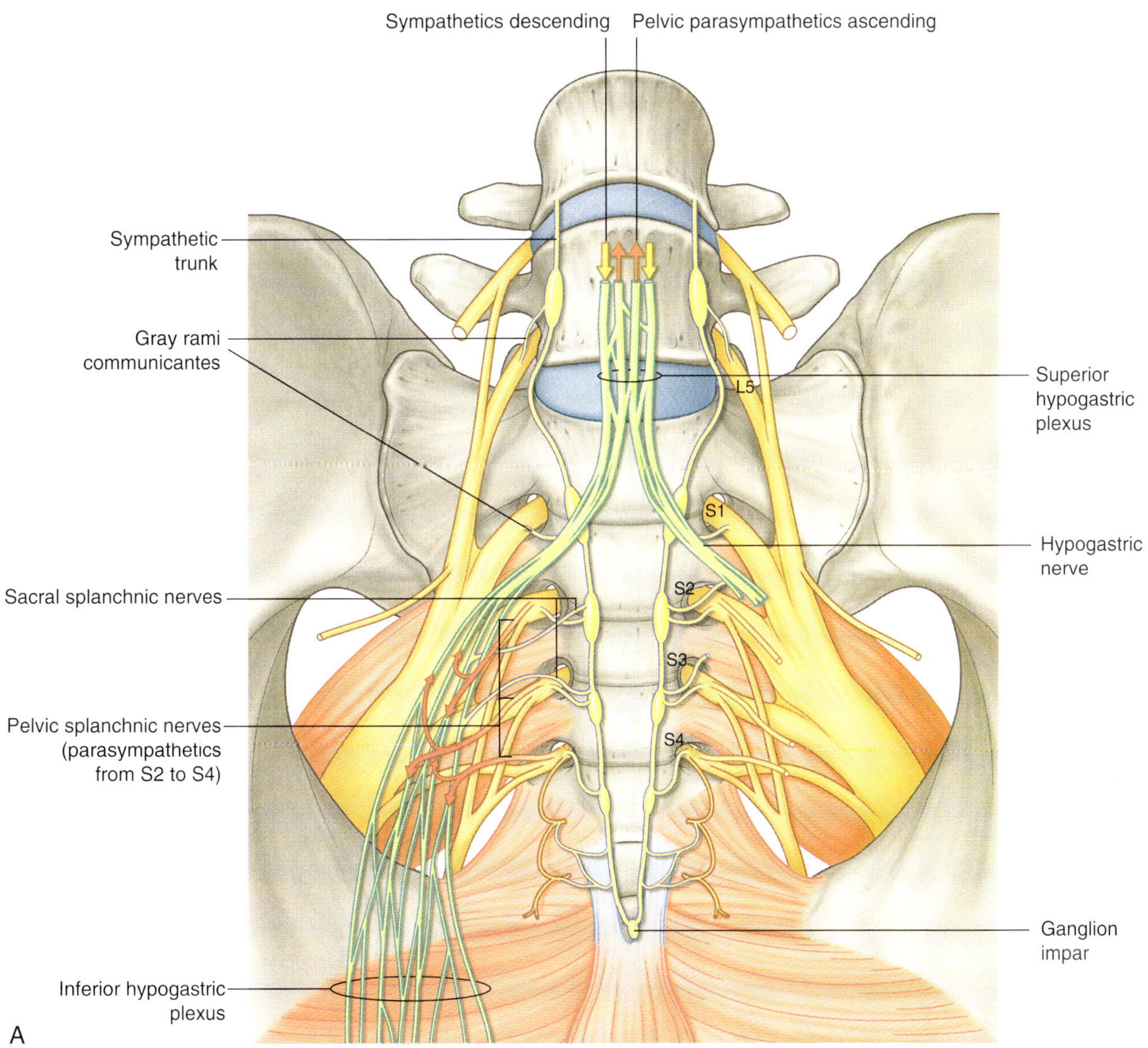

Fig. 5.62 Pelvic extensions of the prevertebral plexus. **(A)** Anterior view.

Continued

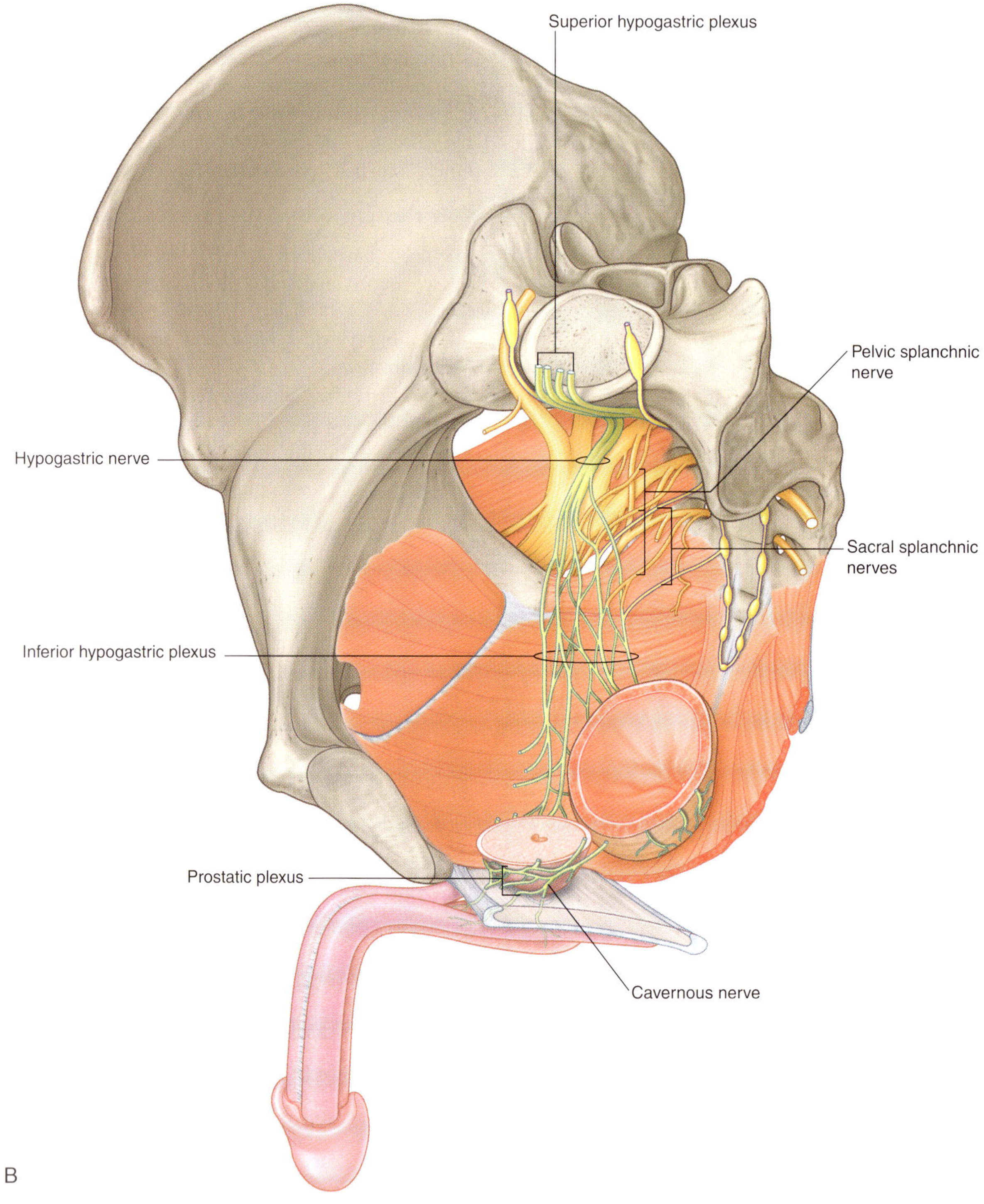

Fig. 5.62, cont'd (B) Anteromedial view of right side of plexus.

The hypogastric nerves are formed by the separation of the fibers in the **superior hypogastric plexus**, into right and left bundles. The superior hypogastric plexus is situated anterior to vertebra LV between the promontory of the sacrum and the bifurcation of the aorta.

When the hypogastric nerves are joined by pelvic splanchnic nerves carrying preganglionic parasympathetic fibers from S2 to S4, the **pelvic plexuses** (**inferior hypogastric plexuses**) are formed (Fig. 5.62). The inferior hypogastric plexuses, one on each side, course in an inferior direction around the pelvic walls, medially to major vessels and somatic nerves. They give origin to the following subsidiary plexuses, which innervate the pelvic viscera:

- The rectal plexus
- The uterovaginal plexus
- The prostatic plexus
- The vesical plexus

Terminal branches of the inferior hypogastric plexuses penetrate and pass through the deep perineal pouch and innervate erectile tissues of the penis and the clitoris in the perineum (Fig. 5.62B). In men, these nerves, called **cavernous nerves**, are extensions of the prostatic plexus. The pattern of distribution of similar nerves in women is not entirely clear, but they are likely extensions of the uterovaginal plexus.

Sympathetic fibers

Sympathetic fibers enter the inferior hypogastric plexuses from the hypogastric nerves and from branches (sacral splanchnic nerves) of the upper sacral parts of the sympathetic trunks (Fig. 5.62A). Ultimately, these nerves are derived from preganglionic fibers that leave the spinal cord in the anterior roots, mainly of T10 to L2. These fibers:

- Innervate blood vessels.
- Cause contraction of smooth muscle in the internal urethral sphincter in men and the internal anal sphincters in both men and women.
- Cause smooth muscle contraction associated with the reproductive tract and with the accessory glands of the reproductive system.
- Are important in moving secretions from the epididymis and associated glands into the urethra to form semen during ejaculation.

Parasympathetic fibers

Parasympathetic fibers enter the pelvic plexus in pelvic splanchnic nerves that originate from spinal cord levels S2 to S4 (Fig. 5.62A). They:

- Are generally vasodilatory.
- Stimulate bladder contraction.
- Stimulate erection.
- Modulate activity of the enteric nervous system of the colon distal to the left colic flexure (in addition to pelvic viscera, some of the fibers from the pelvic plexus course superiorly in the prevertebral plexus, or as separate nerves, and pass into the inferior mesenteric plexus of the abdomen).

Visceral afferent fibers

Visceral afferent fibers follow the course of the sympathetic and parasympathetic fibers to the spinal cord. Afferent fibers that enter the cord in lower thoracic levels and lumbar levels with sympathetic fibers generally carry pain; however, pain fibers from the cervix and some pain fibers from the bladder and urethra may accompany parasympathetic nerves to sacral levels of the spinal cord.

Early clinical exposure

Prostatectomy and impotence

It may be necessary to perform radical surgery to cure cancer of the prostate. To do this, the prostate and its attachments around the base of the bladder, including the seminal vesicles, must be removed en masse. Parts of the inferior hypogastric plexus in this region give rise to nerves that innervate the erectile tissues of the penis. Impotence may occur if these nerves cannot be or are not preserved during removal of the prostate.

For the same reasons, women may experience sexual dysfunction if similar nerves are damaged during pelvic surgery, for example, during a total hysterectomy.

Early clinical exposure

Robotic prostatectomy

This is a new and innovative way of performing radical prostatectomy in patients with prostate cancer. The patient is placed on an operating table near a so-called patient unit consisting of a high-resolution camera and three arms containing microsurgical instruments. The surgeon operates the robot from a computer console and views the surgical field on a monitor as magnified 3D images. The operator usually makes a number of incisions between 1 and 2 cm wide through which the camera and surgical instruments are inserted into the pelvis. The surgeon's hand movements are filtered and translated by the robot into very fine and precise movements of the microtools. This markedly increases the precision of prostate removal and reduces the risk of nerve damage and potential development of postsurgical erectile dysfunction.

Blood vessels

Arteries

The major artery of the pelvis and perineum is the internal iliac artery on each side (Fig. 5.63). In addition to providing a blood supply to most of the pelvic viscera, pelvic walls and floor, and structures in the perineum, including erectile tissues of the clitoris and the penis, this artery gives rise to branches that follow nerves into the gluteal region of the lower limb. Other vessels that originate in the abdomen and contribute to the supply of pelvic structures include the median sacral artery and, in women, the ovarian arteries.

Internal iliac artery

The internal iliac artery originates from the common iliac artery on each side, approximately at the level of the

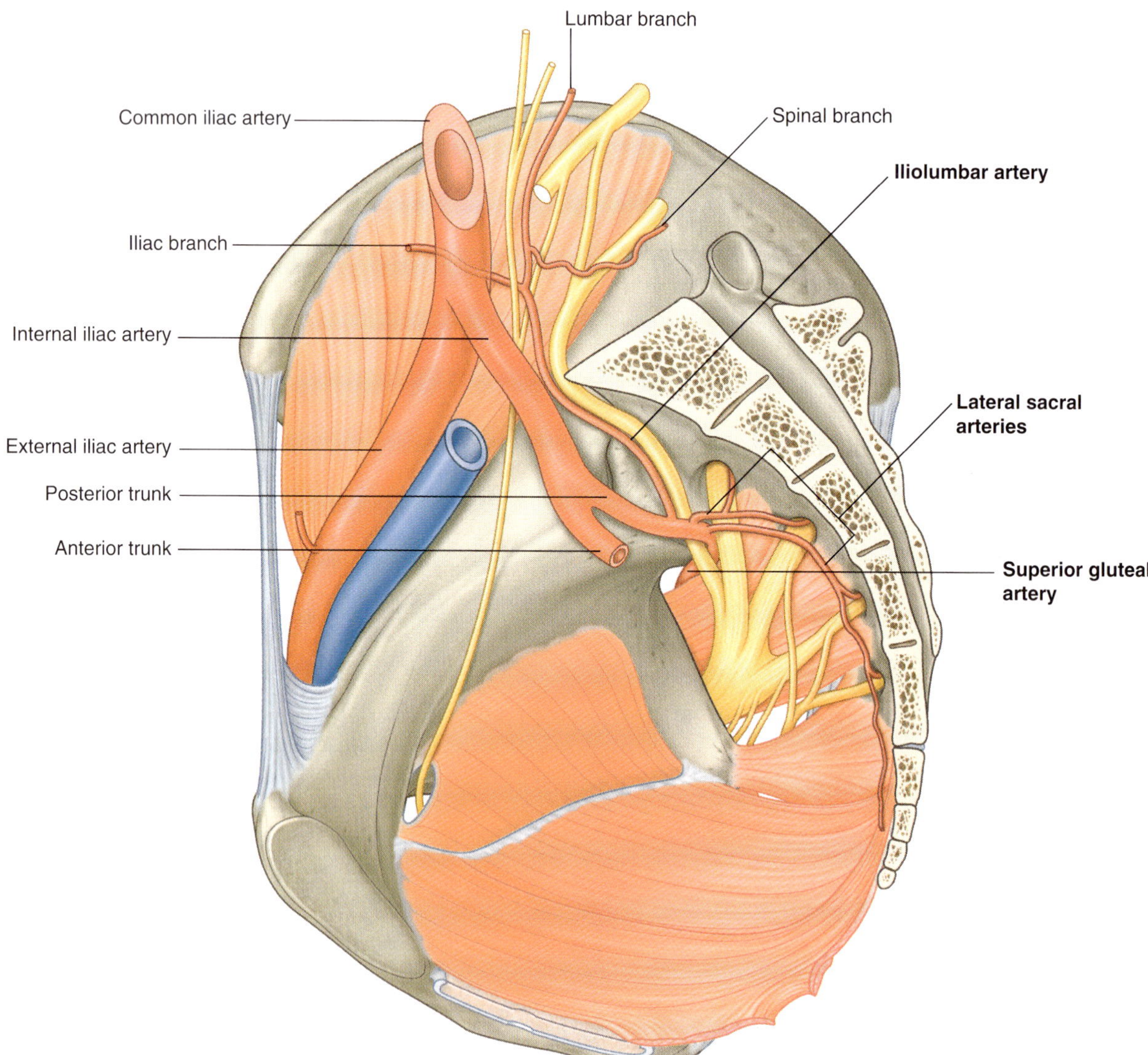

Fig. 5.63 Branches of the posterior trunk of the internal iliac artery.

intervertebral disc between LV and SI, and lies anteromedial to the sacroiliac joint (Fig. 5.63). The vessel courses inferiorly over the pelvic inlet and then divides into anterior and posterior trunks at the level of the superior border of the greater sciatic foramen. Branches from the posterior trunk contribute to the supply of the lower posterior abdominal wall, the posterior pelvic wall, and the gluteal region. Branches from the anterior trunk supply the pelvic viscera, the perineum, the gluteal region, the adductor region of the thigh, and, in the fetus, the placenta.

Posterior trunk

Branches of the posterior trunk of the internal iliac artery are the iliolumbar artery, the lateral sacral artery, and the superior gluteal artery (Fig. 5.63).

- The **iliolumbar artery** ascends laterally back out of the pelvic inlet and divides into a lumbar branch and an iliac branch. The lumbar branch contributes to the supply of the posterior abdominal wall, psoas and quadratus lumborum muscles, and cauda equina, via a small spinal branch that passes through the intervertebral foramen between LV and SI. The iliac branch passes laterally into the iliac fossa to supply muscle and bone.
- The **lateral sacral arteries**, usually two, originate from the posterior division of the internal iliac artery and course medially and inferiorly along the posterior pelvic wall. They give rise to branches that pass into the anterior sacral foramina to supply related bone and soft tissues, structures in the vertebral (sacral) canal, and skin and muscle posterior to the sacrum.
- The **superior gluteal artery** is the largest branch of the internal iliac artery and is the terminal continuation of the posterior trunk. It courses posteriorly, usually passing between the lumbosacral trunk and anterior ramus of S1, to leave the pelvic cavity through the greater sciatic foramen above the piriformis muscle and enter the gluteal region of the lower limb. This vessel makes a substantial contribution to the blood supply of muscles and skin in the gluteal region and also supplies branches to adjacent muscles and bones of the pelvic walls.

Anterior trunk

Branches of the anterior trunk of the internal iliac artery include the superior vesical artery, the umbilical artery, the inferior vesical artery, the middle rectal artery, the uterine artery, the vaginal artery, the obturator artery, the internal pudendal artery, and the inferior gluteal artery (Fig. 5.64).

- The first branch of the anterior trunk is the **umbilical artery**, which gives origin to the superior vesical artery and then travels forward just inferior to the margin of the pelvic inlet. Anteriorly, the vessel leaves the pelvic cavity and ascends on the internal aspect of the anterior abdominal wall to reach the umbilicus. In the fetus, the umbilical artery is large and carries blood from the fetus to the placenta. After birth, the vessel closes distally to the origin of the superior vesical artery and eventually becomes a solid fibrous cord. On the anterior abdominal wall, the cord raises a fold of peritoneum termed the **medial umbilical fold**. The fibrous remnant of the umbilical artery itself is the **medial umbilical ligament**.
- The **superior vesical artery** normally originates from the root of the umbilical artery and courses medially and inferiorly to supply the superior aspect of the bladder and distal parts of the ureter. In men, it also may give rise to an artery that supplies the ductus deferens.
- The **inferior vesical artery** occurs in men and supplies branches to the bladder, ureter, seminal vesicle, and prostate. The **vaginal artery** in women is the equivalent of the inferior vesical artery in men and, descending to the vagina, supplies branches to the vagina and to adjacent parts of the bladder and rectum.
- The **middle rectal artery** courses medially to supply the rectum. The vessel anastomoses with the superior rectal artery, which originates from the inferior mesenteric artery in the abdomen, and the inferior rectal artery, which originates from the internal pudendal artery in the perineum.
- The **obturator artery** courses anteriorly along the pelvic wall and leaves the pelvic cavity via the obturator canal. Together with the obturator nerve, above, and obturator vein, below, it enters and supplies the adductor region of the thigh.
- The **internal pudendal artery** courses inferiorly from its origin in the anterior trunk and leaves the pelvic cavity through the greater sciatic foramen inferior to the piriformis muscle. In association with the pudendal nerve on its medial side, the vessel passes laterally to the ischial spine and then through the lesser sciatic foramen to enter the perineum. The internal pudendal artery is the main artery of the perineum. Among the structures it supplies are the erectile tissues of the clitoris and the penis.
- The **inferior gluteal artery** is a large terminal branch of the anterior trunk of the internal iliac artery. It passes between the anterior rami S1 and S2 or S2 and S3 of the sacral plexus and leaves the pelvic cavity through the greater sciatic foramen inferior to the piriformis muscle. It enters and contributes to the blood supply of the gluteal region and anastomoses with a network of vessels around the hip joint.

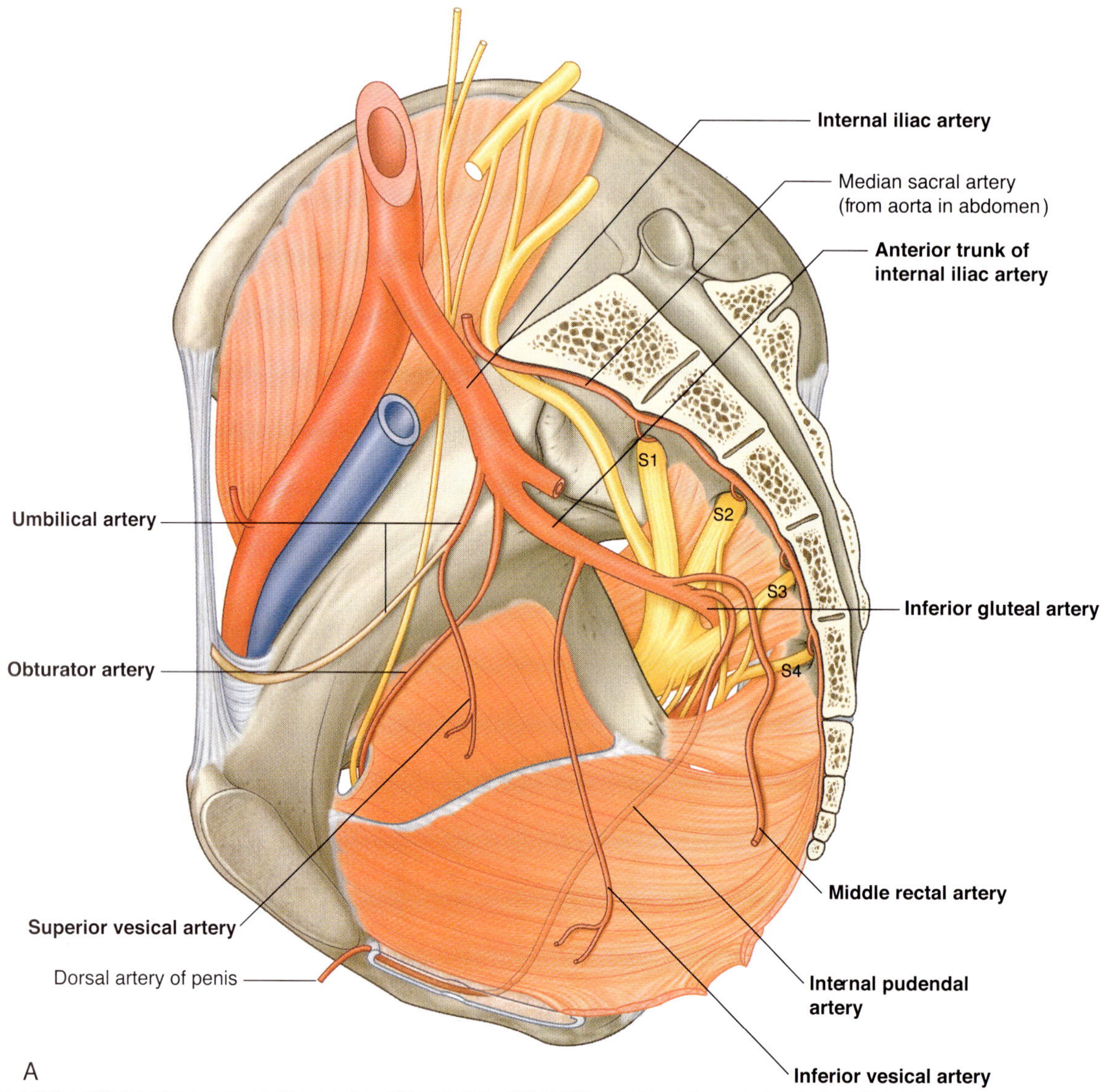

Fig. 5.64 Branches of the anterior trunk of the internal iliac artery. **(A)** Male.

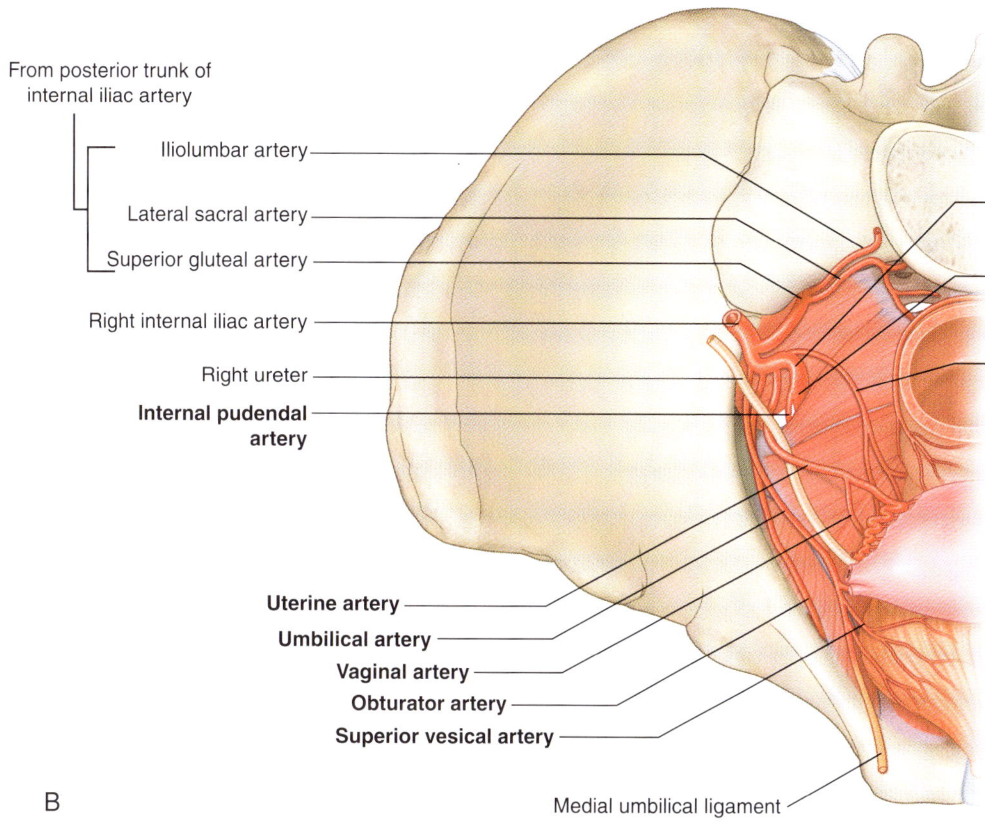

Fig. 5.64, cont'd (B) Female.

- The **uterine artery** in women courses medially and anteriorly in the base of the broad ligament to reach the cervix (Figs 5.64B and 5.65). Along its course, the vessel crosses the ureter and passes superiorly to the lateral vaginal fornix. Once the vessel reaches the cervix, it ascends along the lateral margin of the uterus to reach the uterine tube, where it curves laterally and anastomoses with the ovarian artery. The uterine artery is the major blood supply to the uterus and enlarges significantly during pregnancy. Through anastomoses with other arteries, the vessel contributes to the blood supply of the ovary and vagina as well.

Ovarian arteries

In women, the gonadal (ovarian) vessels originate from the abdominal aorta and then descend to cross the pelvic inlet and supply the ovaries. They anastomose with terminal parts of the uterine arteries (Fig. 5.65). On each side, the vessels travel in the **suspensory ligament of the ovary** (the **infundibulopelvic ligament**) as they cross the pelvic inlet to the ovary. Branches pass through the mesovarium to reach the ovary and through the mesometrium of the broad ligament to anastomose with the uterine artery. The ovarian arteries enlarge significantly during pregnancy to augment the uterine blood supply.

Median sacral artery

The median sacral artery (Figs 5.64A and 5.65) originates from the posterior surface of the aorta just superior to the aortic bifurcation at vertebral level LIV in the abdomen. It descends in the midline, crosses the pelvic inlet, and then courses along the anterior surface of the sacrum and coccyx. It gives rise to the last pair of lumbar arteries and to branches that anastomose with the iliolumbar and lateral sacral arteries.

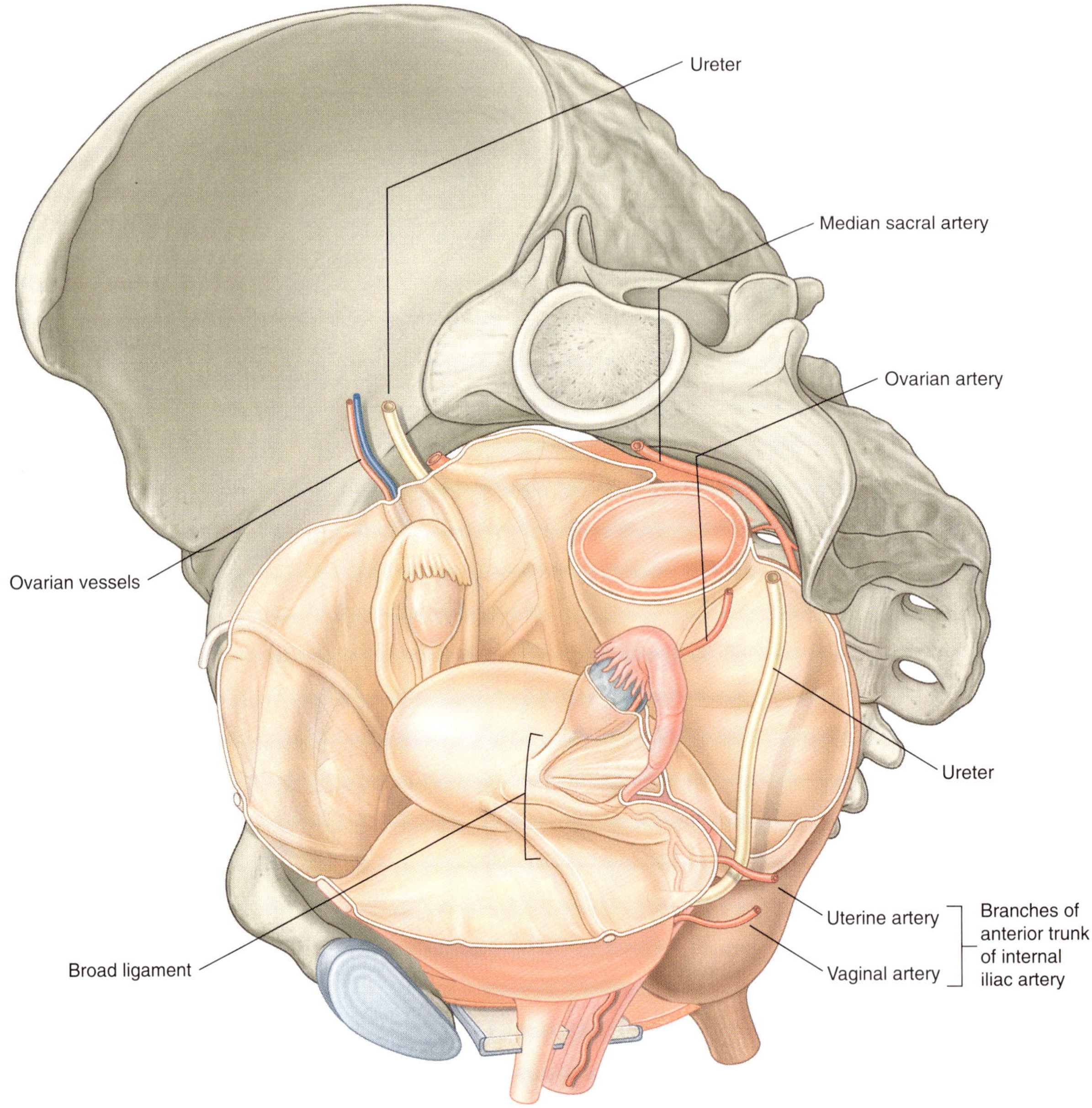

Fig. 5.65 Uterine and vaginal arteries.

Veins

Pelvic veins follow the course of all branches of the internal iliac artery except for the umbilical artery and the iliolumbar artery (Fig. 5.66A). On each side, the veins drain into internal iliac veins, which leave the pelvic cavity to join common iliac veins situated just superior and lateral to the pelvic inlet.

Within the pelvic cavity, extensive interconnected venous plexuses are associated with the surfaces of the viscera (bladder, rectum, prostate, uterus, and vagina). Together, these plexuses form the pelvic plexus of veins. The part of the venous plexus surrounding the rectum and anal canal drains via superior rectal veins (tributaries of inferior mesenteric veins) into the hepatic portal system, and via middle and inferior rectal veins into the caval system. This pelvic plexus is an important portacaval shunt when the hepatic portal system is blocked (Fig. 5.66B).

The inferior part of the rectal plexus around the anal canal has two parts, an internal and an external. The internal rectal plexus is in connective tissue between the internal anal sphincter and the epithelium lining the canal. This plexus connects superiorly with longitudinally arranged branches of the superior rectal vein that lie one in each anal column. When enlarged, these branches form internal hemorrhoids, which originate above the pectinate line and are covered by colonic mucosa. The external rectal

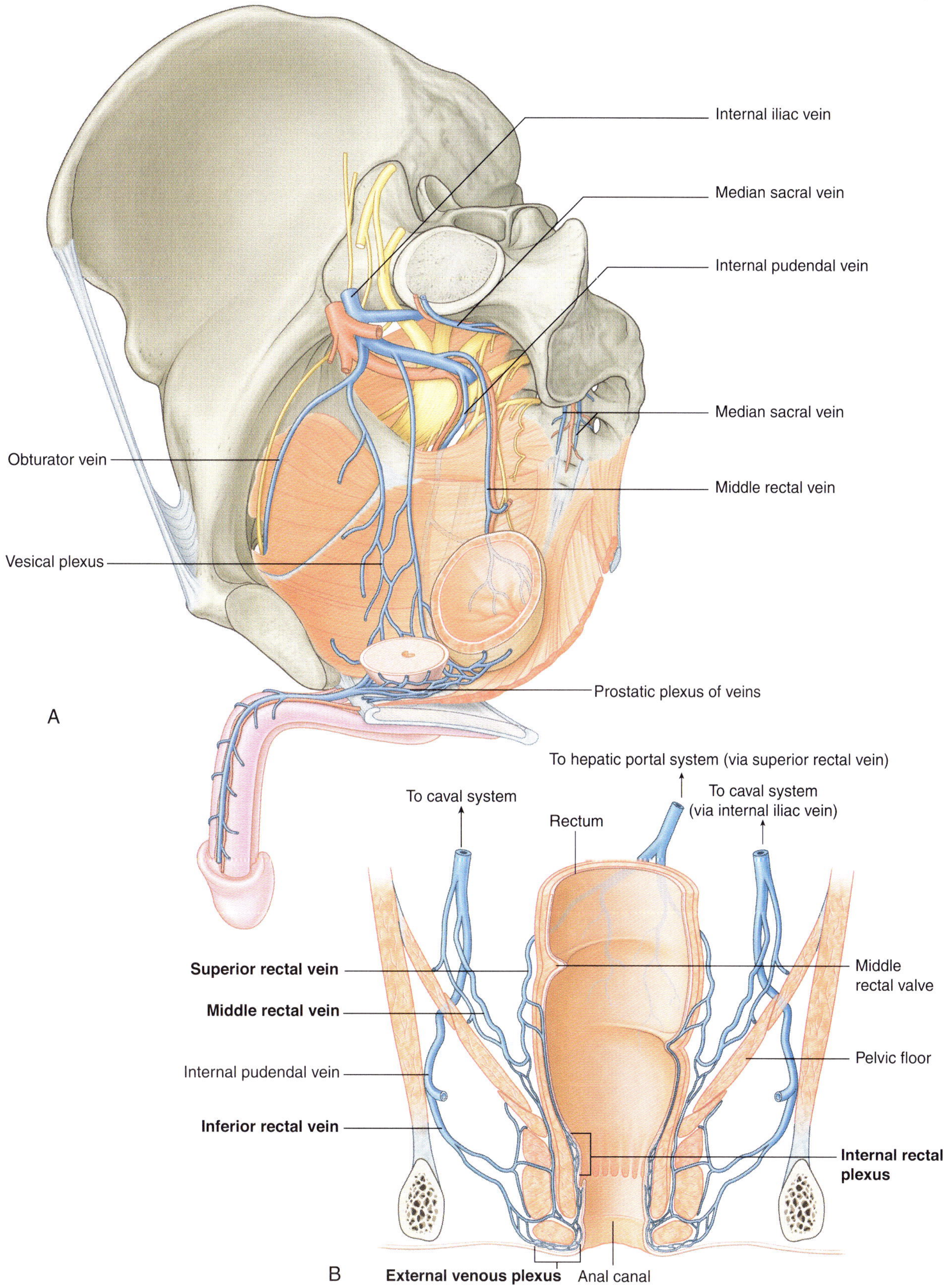

Fig. 5.66 Pelvic veins. **(A)** In a man with the left side of the pelvis and most of the viscera removed. **(B)** Veins associated with the rectum and anal canal.

plexus circles the external anal sphincter and is subcutaneous. Enlargement of vessels in the external rectal plexus results in external hemorrhoids.

The single **deep dorsal vein** that drains erectile tissues of the clitoris and the penis does not follow branches of the internal pudendal artery into the pelvic cavity. Instead, this vein passes directly into the pelvic cavity through a gap formed between the arcuate pubic ligament and the anterior margin of the perineal membrane. The vein joins the prostatic plexus of veins in men and the vesical (bladder) plexus of veins in women. (Superficial veins that drain the skin of the penis and corresponding regions of the clitoris drain into the external pudendal veins, which are tributaries of the great saphenous vein in the thigh.)

In addition to tributaries of the internal iliac vein, median sacral veins and ovarian veins parallel the courses of the median sacral artery and ovarian artery, respectively, and leave the pelvic cavity to join veins in the abdomen:

- The **median sacral veins** coalesce to form a single vein that joins either the left common iliac vein or the junction of the two common iliac veins to form the inferior vena cava.
- The **ovarian veins** follow the course of the corresponding arteries; on the left, they join the left renal vein and, on the right, they join the inferior vena cava in the abdomen.

Lymphatics

Lymphatics from most pelvic viscera drain mainly into lymph nodes distributed along the internal iliac and external iliac arteries and their associated branches (Fig. 5.67), which drain into nodes associated with the common iliac arteries and then into the lateral aortic or lumbar nodes associated with the lateral surfaces of the abdominal aorta. In turn, these lateral aortic or lumbar nodes drain into the lumbar trunks, which continue to the origin of the thoracic duct at approximately vertebral level TXII.

Lymphatics from the ovaries and related parts of the uterus and uterine tubes leave the pelvic cavity superiorly and drain, via vessels that accompany the ovarian arteries, directly into lateral aortic or lumbar nodes and, in some cases, into the preaortic nodes on the anterior surface of the aorta.

In addition to draining pelvic viscera, nodes along the internal iliac artery also receive drainage from the gluteal region of the lower limb and from deep areas of the perineum.

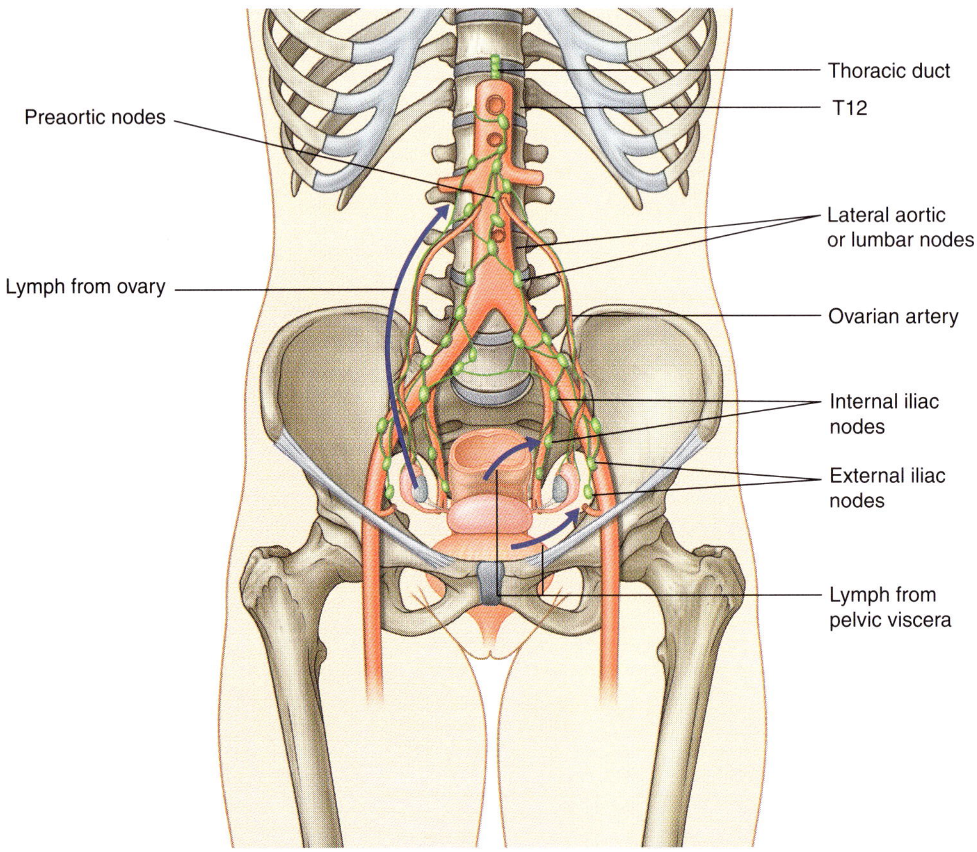

Fig. 5.67 Pelvic lymphatics.

PERINEUM

SET INDUCTION—CASE SCENARIO 3: EPISIOTOMY

A 32-year-old woman needed a forceps delivery due to delayed labor. An episiotomy was also done to widen the vaginal opening. Knowledge of the anatomy of the perineum is needed to manage this case.

<table>
<tr><th rowspan="2">REMEMBER
[Recall Facts]</th><th colspan="3">OUTLINE 3. PERINEUM—LEARNING OBJECTIVES
[By the end of this section, the student should be able to:]</th><th colspan="2" rowspan="2">EVALUATE
[Explain Concepts]</th></tr>
<tr><th colspan="3">DEMONSTRATE AND ANALYZE RELATIONSHIPS
[Identify structures in a Prosected Specimen or Figure]</th></tr>
<tr><td rowspan="7">1. Explain the boundaries of pelvic outlet and the divisions of the perineum
2. Describe the boundaries and contents of superficial perineal pouch
3. Describe the boundaries and contents of deep perineal pouch
4. Describe the course and distribution of pudendal nerve
5. Describe the boundaries and contents of ischiorectal fossa
6. Describe the innervation and mechanism involved in the erection of cavernous tissue and emission in males</td><td>Level I</td><td>Level II</td><td>Level III</td><td colspan="2" rowspan="2">■ Divisions of perineum
■ Arrangement of fascia in the urogenital triangle
■ Structures piercing the perineal membrane
■ Importance of perineal body
■ Formation and contents of pudendal canal
■ Course and branches of pudendal nerve and internal pudendal artery</td></tr>
<tr><td rowspan="6">■ Perineal body—location
■ Colles fascia
■ Fat in ischiorectal fossa
■ Boundaries and contents of the superficial perineal pouch
■ Boundaries and contents of ischiorectal fossa
■ Pudendal canal and its contents
■ Perineal membrane
■ Boundaries and contents of deep perineal pouch</td><td rowspan="6">Pudendal nerve</td><td rowspan="6">■ Internal pudendal artery and its branches</td></tr>
<tr><th colspan="2">EARLY CLINICAL EXPOSURE
[Apply Anatomical Knowledge]</th></tr>
<tr><th>Surgical Anatomy/ Pathology/ Trauma</th><th>Imaging/ Surface Anatomy</th></tr>
<tr><td>■ Ischiorectal abscess
■ Hiatus of Schwalbe and ischiorectal hernia
■ Episiotomy
■ Pudendal nerve block
■ Urethral rupture</td><td></td></tr>
<tr><th colspan="2">PROBLEM SOLVING/ CLINICAL CASES
[Interpret]</th></tr>
<tr><td colspan="2">■ Ischioanal abscess</td></tr>
</table>

The perineum is a diamond-shaped region positioned inferiorly to the pelvic floor between the thighs. Its peripheral boundary is the pelvic outlet; its ceiling is the pelvic diaphragm (the levator ani and coccygeus muscles); and its narrow lateral walls are formed by the walls of the pelvic cavity below the attachment of the levator ani muscle (Fig. 5.68A).

The perineum is divided into an anterior urogenital triangle and a posterior anal triangle.

- The urogenital triangle is associated with the openings of the urinary systems and the reproductive systems and functions to anchor the external genitalia.
- The anal triangle contains the anus and the external anal sphincter.

The pudendal nerve (S2 to S4) and the internal pudendal artery are the major nerve and artery of the region.

Borders and ceiling

The margin of the perineum is marked by the inferior border of the pubic symphysis at its anterior point, the tip of the coccyx at its posterior point, and the ischial tuberosities at each of the lateral points (Fig. 5.68A). The lateral margins are formed by the ischiopubic rami anteriorly and by the sacrotuberous ligaments posteriorly. The pubic symphysis, the ischial tuberosities, and the coccyx can be palpated on the patient.

The perineum is divided into two triangles by an imaginary line between the two ischial tuberosities (Fig. 5.68A). Anterior to the line is the urogenital triangle and posterior to the line is the anal triangle. Significantly, the two triangles are not in the same plane. In the anatomical position, the urogenital triangle is oriented in the horizontal plane, whereas the anal triangle is tilted upward at the transtubercular line so that it faces more posteriorly.

The roof of the perineum is formed mainly by the levator ani muscles that separate the pelvic cavity, above, from the perineum, below. These muscles, one on each side, form a cone- or funnel-shaped pelvic diaphragm, with the anal aperture at its inferior apex in the anal triangle.

Anteriorly, in the **urogenital triangle**, a U-shaped defect in the muscles, the **urogenital hiatus**, allows the passage of the urethra and vagina.

Perineal membrane and deep perineal pouch

The perineal membrane (see pp. 634–636) is a thick fibrous sheet that fills the urogenital triangle (Fig. 5.68B). It has a free posterior border, which is anchored in the midline to the perineal body and is attached laterally to the pubic arch. Immediately superior to the perineal membrane is a thin region termed the deep perineal pouch, containing a layer of skeletal muscle and neurovascular tissues. Among the skeletal muscles in the pouch (see p. 636, Fig. 5.36) is the external urethral sphincter.

The perineal membrane and deep perineal pouch provide support for the external genitalia, which are attached to its inferior surface. Also, the parts of the perineal membrane and deep perineal pouch inferior to the urogenital hiatus in the levator ani provide support for the pelvic viscera, above.

The urethra leaves the pelvic cavity and enters the perineum by passing through the deep perineal pouch and perineal membrane. In women, the vagina also passes through these structures posterior to the urethra.

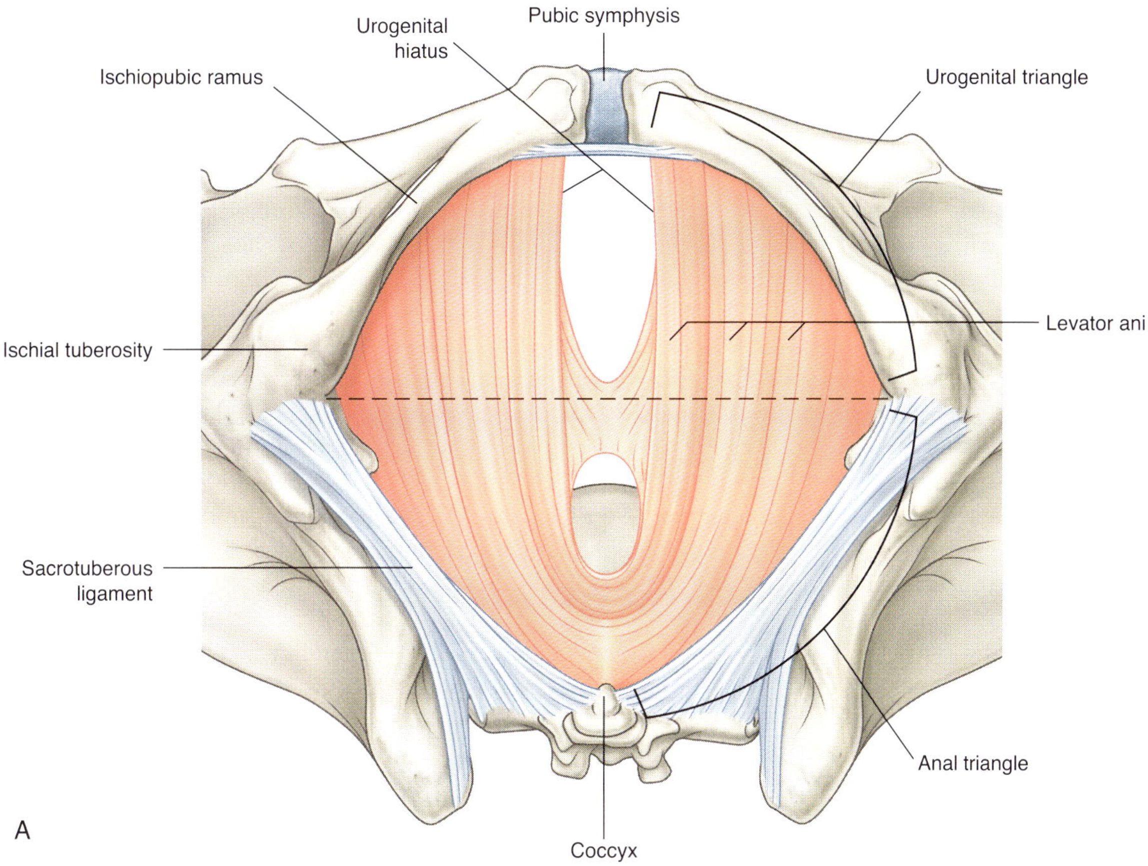

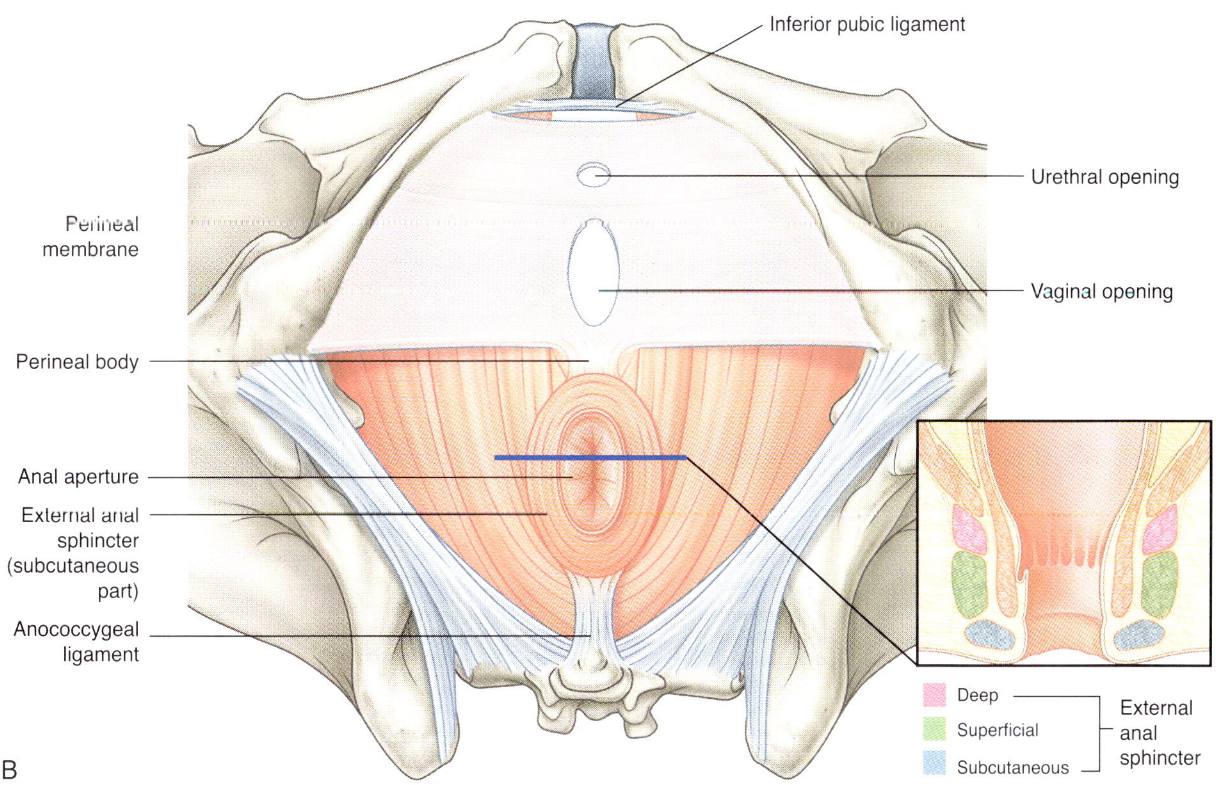

Fig. 5.68 Borders and roof of the perineum. **(A)** Boundaries of the perineum. **(B)** Perineal membrane.

Ischioanal fossae and their anterior recesses

Because the levator ani muscles course medially from their origin on the lateral pelvic walls, above, to the anal aperture and urogenital hiatus, below, inverted wedge-shaped gutters occur between the levator ani muscles and adjacent pelvic walls as the two structures diverge inferiorly (Fig. 5.69). In the anal triangle, these gutters, one on each side of the anal aperture, are termed **ischioanal fossae**. The lateral wall of each fossa is formed mainly by the ischium, obturator internus muscle, and sacrotuberous ligament. The medial wall is the levator ani muscle. The medial and lateral walls converge superiorly where the levator ani muscle attaches to the fascia overlying the obturator internus muscle. The ischioanal fossae allow movement of the pelvic diaphragm and expansion of the anal canal during defecation.

The ischioanal fossae of the anal triangle are continuous anteriorly with recesses that project into the urogenital triangle superior to the deep perineal pouch. These anterior recesses of the ischioanal fossae are shaped like three-sided pyramids that have been tipped onto one of their sides (Fig. 5.69C). The apex of each pyramid is closed and points anteriorly toward the pubis. The base is open and continuous posteriorly with its related ischioanal fossa. The inferior wall of each pyramid is the deep perineal pouch. The superomedial wall is the levator ani muscle, and the superolateral wall is formed mainly by the obturator internus muscle. The ischioanal fossae and their anterior recesses are normally filled with fat.

Early clinical exposure

Abscesses in the ischioanal fossae

The anal mucosa is particularly vulnerable to injury and may be easily torn by hard feces. Occasionally, patients develop inflammation and infection of the anal canal (sinuses or crypts). This infection can spread between the sphincters, producing intersphincteric fistulas. The infection can spread superiorly into the pelvic cavity or laterally into the ischioanal fossae.

Anal triangle

The anal triangle of the perineum faces posteroinferiorly and is defined laterally by the medial margins of the sacrotuberous ligaments, anteriorly by a horizontal line between the two ischial tuberosities, and posteriorly by the coccyx. The ceiling of the anal triangle is the pelvic diaphragm, which is formed by the levator ani and coccygeus muscles. The anal aperture occurs centrally in the anal triangle and is related on either side to an ischioanal fossa. The major muscle in the anal triangle is the external anal sphincter.

The **external anal sphincter**, which surrounds the anal canal, is formed by skeletal muscle and consists of three parts—deep, superficial, and subcutaneous—arranged sequentially along the canal from superior to inferior (Fig. 5.68B; Table 5.5). The deep part is a thick ring-shaped muscle that circles the upper part of the anal canal and blends with the fibers of the levator ani muscle. The superficial part also surrounds the anal canal, but is anchored anteriorly to the perineal body and posteriorly to the coccyx and anococcygeal ligament. The subcutaneous part is a horizontally flattened disc of muscle that surrounds the anal aperture just beneath the skin. The external anal sphincter is innervated by inferior rectal branches of the pudendal nerve and by branches directly from the anterior ramus of S4.

Early clinical exposure

Hemorrhoids

A hemorrhoid is an engorgement of the venous plexus at or inside the anal sphincter. It is a common complaint and has prevalence of approximately 4% in the USA. Hemorrhoids have a slight genetic predisposition; however, straining during bowel movements, obesity, and sedentary lifestyle can also produce hemorrhoids. The symptoms include irritation, pain, and swelling. Hemorrhoids occurring at the anal verge (distal boundary of the anal canal) are typically called external hemorrhoids. Internal hemorrhoids occur inside the rectum and have a tendency to bleed. Prolapsed hemorrhoids are internal hemorrhoids that pass outside the anal canal and form lumps, which may undergo thrombosis and become painful.

There are many treatments for hemorrhoids, which include ligation above the pectinate (dentate) line using simple rubber bands or surgical excision. Surgery to this region is not without complications and care must be taken to preserve the internal anal sphincter.

In the back of every physician's mind is the concern that the rectal bleeding or symptoms may not be attributable to hemorrhoids. Therefore, excluding a tumor within the bowel is as important as treating the hemorrhoids.

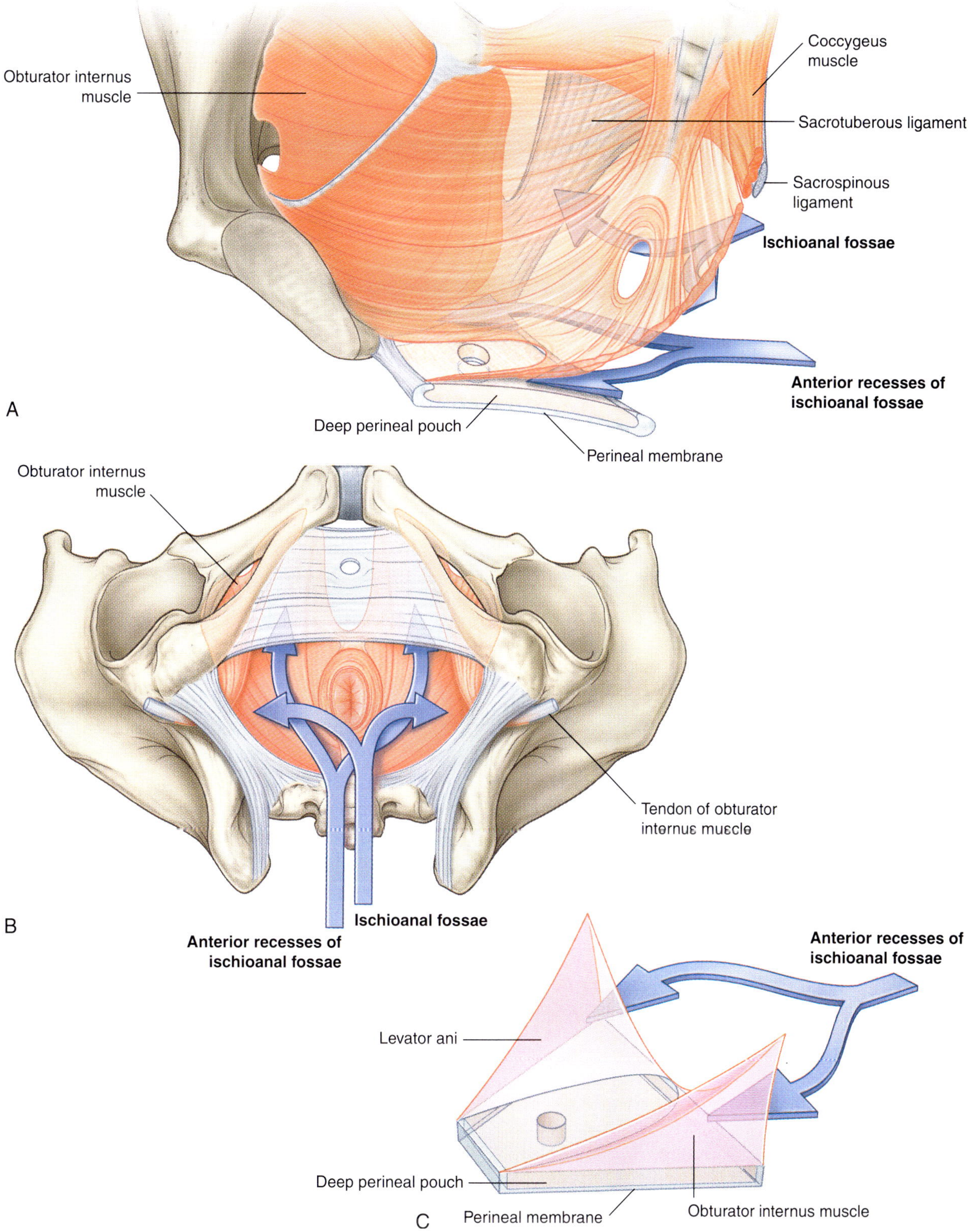

Fig. 5.69 Ischioanal fossae and their anterior recesses. **(A)** Anterolateral view with left pelvic wall removed. **(B)** Inferior view. **(C)** Anterolateral view with pelvic walls and diaphragm removed.

Table 5.5 Muscles of the anal triangle

Muscles	Origin	Insertion	Innervation	Function
EXTERNAL ANAL SPHINCTER				
Deep part	Surrounds superior aspect of anal canal		Pudendal nerve (S2 and S3) and branches directly from S4	Closes anal canal
Superficial part	Surrounds lower part of anal canal	Anchored to perineal body and anococcygeal body		
Subcutaneous part	Surrounds anal aperture			

Urogenital triangle

The urogenital triangle of the perineum is the anterior half of the perineum and is oriented in the horizontal plane. It contains the roots of the external genitalia (Fig. 5.70) and the openings of the urogenital system.

The urogenital triangle is defined:

- Laterally by the ischiopubic rami,
- Posteriorly by an imaginary line between the ischial tuberosities.
- Anteriorly by the inferior margin of the pubic symphysis.

As with the anal triangle, the roof or ceiling of the urogenital triangle is the levator ani muscle.

Unlike the anal triangle, the urogenital triangle contains a strong fibromuscular support platform, the perineal membrane and deep perineal pouch (see pp. 634–636), which is attached to the pubic arch.

Anterior extensions of the ischioanal fossae occur between the deep perineal pouch and the levator ani muscle on each side.

Between the perineal membrane and the membranous layer of superficial fascia is the **superficial perineal pouch**. The principal structures in this pouch are the erectile tissues of the penis and clitoris and associated skeletal muscles.

Structures in the superficial perineal pouch

The superficial perineal pouch contains:

- Erectile structures that join together to form the penis in men and the clitoris in women.
- Skeletal muscles that are associated mainly with parts of the erectile structures attached to the perineal membrane and adjacent bone.

Each erectile structure consists of a central core of expandable vascular tissue and its surrounding connective tissue capsule.

Erectile tissues

Two sets of erectile structures join to form the penis and the clitoris.

A pair of cylindrically shaped **corpora cavernosa**, one on each side of the urogenital triangle, is anchored by their proximal ends to the pubic arch. These attached parts are often termed the **crura** (from the Latin for "legs") of the clitoris or the penis. The distal ends of the corpora, which are not attached to bone, form the body of the clitoris in women and the dorsal parts of the body of the penis in men.

The second set of erectile tissues surrounds the openings of the urogenital system.

- In women, a pair of erectile structures, termed the **bulbs of the vestibule**, are situated, one on each side, at the vaginal opening and are firmly anchored to the perineal membrane (Fig. 5.70A). Small bands of erectile tissues connect the anterior ends of these bulbs to a single, small, pea-shaped erectile mass, the **glans clitoris**, which is positioned in the midline at the end of the body of the clitoris and anterior to the opening of the urethra.
- In men, a single large erectile mass, the **corpus spongiosum**, is the structural equivalent to the bulbs of the vestibule, the glans clitoris, and the interconnecting bands of erectile tissues in women (Fig. 5.70B). The corpus spongiosum is anchored at its base to the perineal membrane. Its proximal end, which is not attached, forms the ventral part of the body of the penis and expands over the end of the body of the penis to form the glans penis. This pattern in men results from the absence of a vaginal opening and from the fusion of structures across the midline during embryological development. As the originally paired erectile structures fuse, they enclose the urethral opening and form an additional channel that ultimately becomes most of the penile part of the urethra. As a consequence of this fusion and growth in men, the urethra is enclosed by the corpus spongiosum and opens at the end of the penis.

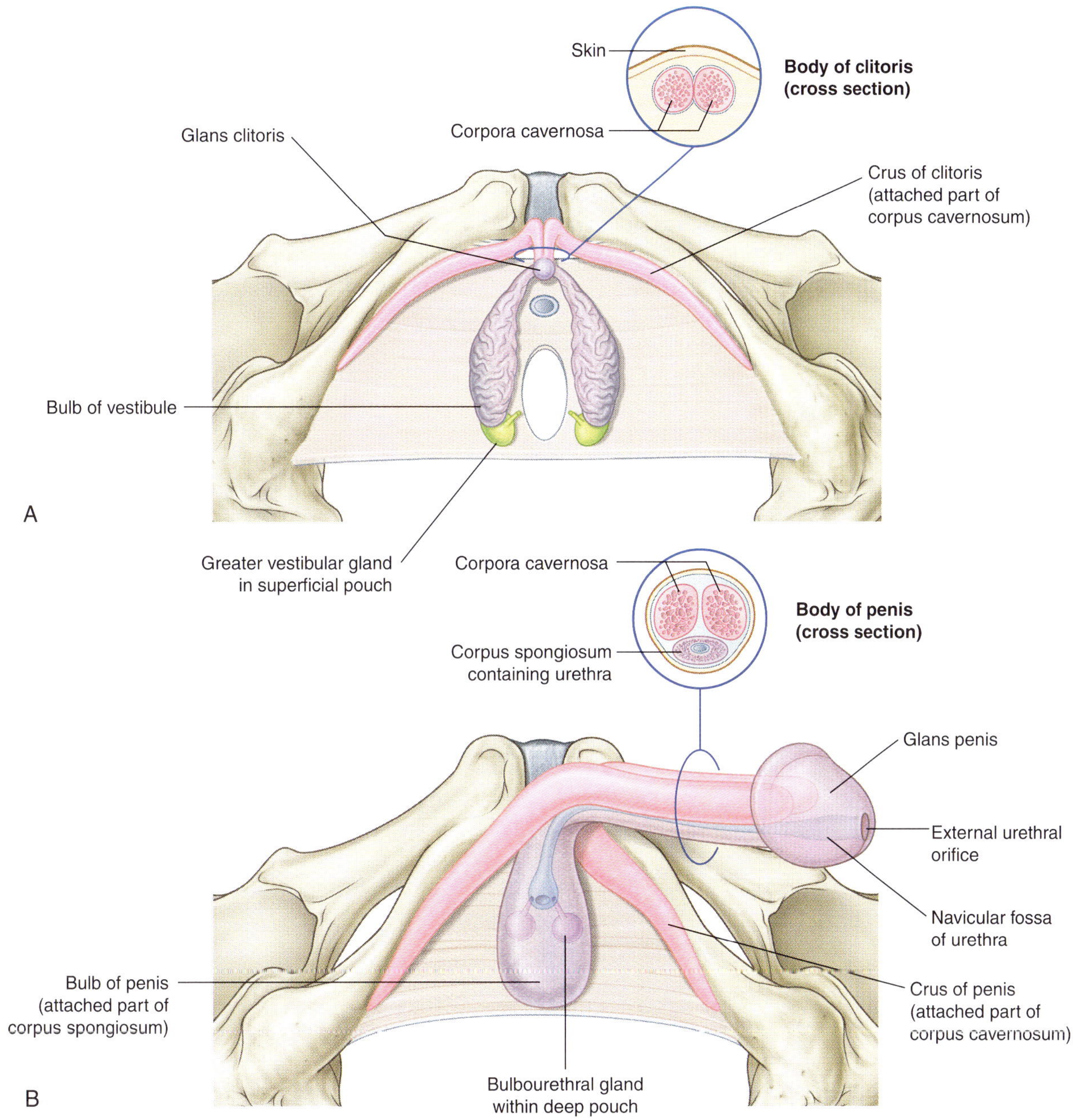

Fig. 5.70 Erectile tissues of clitoris and penis. **(A)** Clitoris. **(B)** Penis.

This is unlike the situation in women, where the urethra is not enclosed by erectile tissue of the clitoris and opens directly into the vestibule of the perineum.

Clitoris

The clitoris is composed of two corpora cavernosa and the **glans clitoris** (Fig. 5.70A). As in the penis, it has an attached part (root) and a free part (body).

- Unlike the root of the penis, the **root of the clitoris** technically consists only of the two crura. (Although the bulbs of the vestibule are attached to the glans clitoris by thin bands of erectile tissue, they are not included in the attached part of the clitoris.)
- The **body of the clitoris**, which is formed only by the unattached parts of the two corpora cavernosa, angles posteriorly and is embedded in the connective tissues of the perineum.

The body of the clitoris is supported by a suspensory ligament that attaches superiorly to the pubic symphysis. The glans clitoris is attached to the distal end of the body and is connected to the bulbs of the vestibule by small bands of erectile tissue. The glans clitoris is exposed in the perineum and the body of the clitoris can be palpated through skin.

Penis

The penis is composed mainly of the two corpora cavernosa and the single corpus spongiosum, which contains the urethra (Fig. 5.70B.) As in the clitoris, it has an attached part (root) and a free part (body):

- The **root of the penis** consists of the two crura, which are proximal parts of the corpora cavernosa attached to the pubic arch, and the **bulb of the penis**, which is the proximal part of the corpus spongiosum anchored to the perineal membrane.
- The **body of the penis**, which is covered entirely by skin, is formed by the tethering of the two proximal free parts of the corpora cavernosa and the related free part of the corpus spongiosum.

The base of the body of the penis is supported by two ligaments: the **suspensory ligament of the penis** (attached superiorly to the pubic symphysis) and the more superficially positioned **fundiform ligament of the penis** (attached above to the linea alba of the anterior abdominal wall and split below into two bands that pass on each side of the penis and unite inferiorly).

Because the anatomical position of the penis is erect, the paired corpora are defined as dorsal in the body of the penis and the single corpus spongiosum as ventral, even though the positions are reversed in the nonerect (flaccid) penis.

The corpus spongiosum expands to form the head of the penis (**glans penis**) over the distal ends of the corpora cavernosa (Fig. 5.70B).

Erection

Erection of the penis and clitoris is a vascular event generated by parasympathetic fibers carried in pelvic splanchnic nerves from the anterior rami of S2 to S4, which enter the inferior hypogastric part of the prevertebral plexus and ultimately pass through the deep perineal pouch and perineal membrane to innervate the erectile tissues. Stimulation of these nerves causes specific arteries in the erectile tissues to relax. This allows blood to fill the tissues, causing the penis and clitoris to become erect.

Arteries supplying the penis and clitoris are branches of the internal pudendal artery; branches of the pudendal nerve (S2 to S4) carry general sensory nerves from the penis and clitoris.

Greater vestibular glands

The greater vestibular glands (**Bartholin's glands**) are seen in women. They are small, pea-shaped mucous glands that lie posterior to the bulbs of the vestibule on each side of the vaginal opening and are the female homologues of the bulbourethral glands in men (Fig. 5.70). However, the bulbourethral glands are located within the deep perineal pouch, whereas the greater vestibular glands are in the superficial perineal pouch.

The duct of each greater vestibular gland opens into the vestibule of the perineum along the posterolateral margin of the vaginal opening.

Like the bulbourethral glands in men, the greater vestibular glands produce secretion during sexual arousal.

Muscles

The superficial perineal pouch contains three pairs of muscles: the ischiocavernosus, bulbospongiosus, and superficial transverse perineal muscles (Fig. 5.71; Table 5.6). Two of these three pairs of muscles are associated with the roots of the penis and clitoris; the other pair is associated with the perineal body.

Ischiocavernosus

The two **ischiocavernosus muscles** cover the crura of the penis and clitoris (Fig. 5.71). Each muscle is anchored to the medial margin of the ischial tuberosity and related ischial ramus and passes forward to attach to the sides and inferior surface of the related crus, and forces blood from the crus into the body of the erect penis and clitoris.

Bulbospongiosus

The two **bulbospongiosus muscles** are associated mainly with the bulbs of the vestibule in women and with the attached part of the corpus spongiosum in men (Fig. 5.71).

In women, each bulbospongiosus muscle is anchored posteriorly to the perineal body and courses anterolaterally over the inferior surface of the related greater vestibular gland and the bulb of the vestibule to attach to the surface of the bulb and to the perineal membrane (Fig. 5.71A). Other fibers course anterolaterally to blend with the fibers of the ischiocavernosus muscle, and still others travel anteriorly and arch over the body of the clitoris.

In men, the bulbospongiosus muscles are joined in the midline to a raphe on the inferior surface of the bulb of the penis. The raphe is anchored posteriorly to the perineal body. Muscle fibers course anterolaterally, on each side, from the raphe and perineal body to cover each side of the bulb of the penis and attach to the perineal membrane and connective tissue of the bulb. Others extend anterolaterally

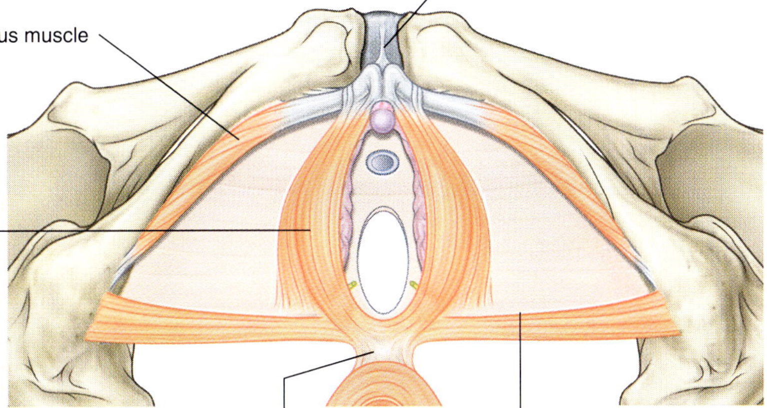

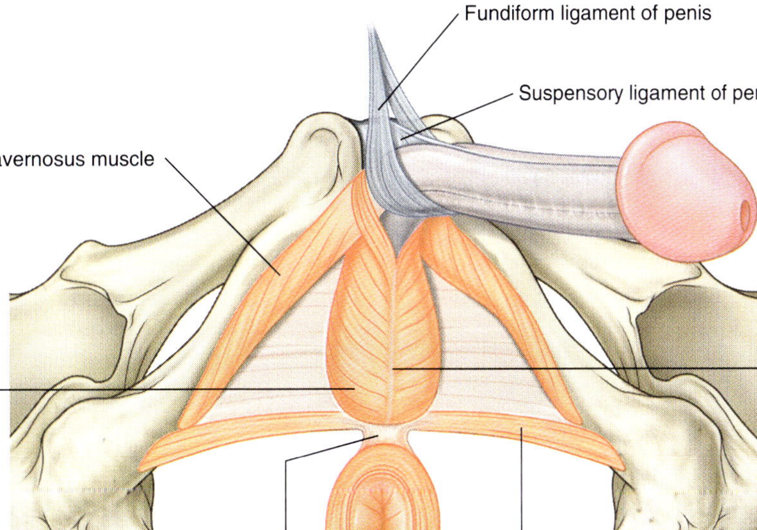

Fig. 5.71 Muscles in the superficial perineal pouch. **(A)** In women. **(B)** In men.

Table 5.6 Muscles of the superficial perineal pouch

Muscles	Origin	Insertion	Innervation	Function
Ischiocavernosus	Ischial tuberosity and ramus	Crus of penis and clitoris	Pudendal nerve (S2 to S4)	Move blood from crura into the body of the erect penis and clitoris
Bulbospongiosus	In women: perineal body In men: perineal body, midline raphe	In women: bulb of vestibule, perineal membrane, body of clitoris, and corpus cavernosum In men: bulbospongiosus, perineal membrane, corpus cavernosum	Pudendal nerve (S2 to S4)	Move blood from attached parts of the clitoris and penis into the glans In men: removal of residual urine from urethra after urination; pulsatile emission of semen during ejaculation
Superficial transverse perineal	Ischial tuberosity and ramus	Perineal body	Pudendal nerve (S2 to S4)	Stabilize the perineal body

to associate with the crura and attach anteriorly to the ischiocavernosus muscles.

In both men and women, the bulbospongiosus muscles compress attached parts of the erect corpus spongiosum and bulbs of the vestibule and force blood into more distal regions, mainly the glans. In men, the bulbospongiosus muscles have two additional functions:

- They facilitate emptying of the bulbous part of the penile urethra following urination (micturition).
- Their reflex contraction during ejaculation is responsible for the pulsatile emission of semen from the penis.

Early clinical exposure

Emission and ejaculation of semen

- In men, emission is the formation of semen, and ejaculation is the expulsion of semen from the penis.
- Although erection of the penis is a vascular event generated by parasympathetic nerves from spinal levels S2 to S4, the formation of semen in the urethra is caused by the contraction of smooth muscle of the ducts and glands of the reproductive system that is innervated by the sympathetic part of the visceral nervous system. Ejaculation of semen from the penis is through the action of skeletal muscles innervated by somatic motor nerves.
- Smooth muscle in the duct system of the male reproductive tract and in the accessory glands is innervated by sympathetic fibers from the lower thoracic and upper lumbar spinal levels (T12, L1, L2). The fibers pass into the prevertebral plexus and are then distributed to target tissues. Semen is formed as luminal contents from the ducts (epididymis, ductus deferens, ampulla of the ductus deferens) and glands (prostate, seminal vesicles) are moved into the urethra at the base of the penis by the contraction of smooth muscle in the walls of the structures.
- Pulsatile emission of semen from the penis is generated by the reflex contraction of the bulbospongiosus muscle that forces semen from the base of the penis and out of the external urethral meatus. Bulbospongiosus muscle is innervated by somatic motor fibers carried in the pudendal nerve (S2 to S4). Contraction of the internal urethral sphincter and periurethral smooth muscle, innervated by the sympathetic part of the visceral nervous system, prevents retrograde ejaculation into the bladder.

Early clinical exposure

Erectile dysfunction

Erectile dysfunction (ED) is a complex condition in which men are unable to initiate or maintain penile erection. When this affects erections during sleep, and with self-stimulation as well as with a partner, vascular and/or nerve impairment is present. This generalized type of ED increases with age and is recognized as a risk factor for coronary artery disease. It is frequently associated with cardiovascular disease, diabetes, and neurological conditions including Parkinson's disease, spinal cord injuries, multiple sclerosis, and as nerve damage from pelvic surgeries or radiation for pelvic malignancies. Low testosterone states can impair erections and consistently prevent sleep-induced erections. Medications including serotonin reuptake inhibitors (SSRIs), thiazides, and antiandrogens can also underlie ED. When only partnered erections are problematic, psychological factors underlie the dysfunction—the normal erections from sleep confirming healthy vascular and neurological function. Most cases of ED are multifactorial in etiology, and all markedly lessen quality of life and a person's well-being and can lead to depression and low self-esteem as well as emotional and social isolation.

Delayed (or absent) ejaculation can result from nerve damage in conditions such as diabetes, Parkinson's disease, spinal cord injuries, multiple sclerosis, complications after major pelvic surgeries, and pelvic irradiation. Ejaculation is absent after radical prostatectomy for prostate cancer (which also removes the seminal vesicles), but orgasm is still possible as the spared pudendal nerve is a mixed nerve containing the peripheral autonomic and somatic fibers necessary for orgasm. SSRIs, neuroleptics, alcohol, and recreational drugs (marijuana, cocaine, and heroin) often delay orgasm and therefore ejaculation, as in health the two occur together (even though the nerves involved are different).

Because erectile tissues in the clitoris have similar innervation and blood supply as the penis, vulvar swelling is likely compromised by the same conditions that cause ED in men. However, it appears that this is a rare cause of female sexual dysfunction. Reduced clitoral swelling is rarely symptomatic. Note that phosphodiesterase type 5 (PDE5) inhibitors (sildenafil) do not improve female sexual dysfunction even in conditions such as diabetes. Research confirms that otherwise healthy women with complaints of low sexual arousal have a physiologically normal increase in genital congestion in response to visual sexual stimuli, even though they do not find the stimuli mentally sexually arousing. Loss of genital sexual sensitivity from somatic nerve damage from multiple sclerosis or diabetes can be highly symptomatic and preclude orgasm. Medications preventing orgasm in men can also affect women.

Superficial transverse perineal muscles

The paired **superficial transverse perineal muscles** follow a course parallel to the posterior margin of the inferior surface of the perineal membrane (Fig. 5.71). These flat band-shaped muscles, which are attached to ischial tuberosities and rami, extend medially to the perineal body in the midline and stabilize the perineal body.

Superficial features of the external genitalia

In women

In women, the clitoris and vestibular apparatus, together with a number of skin and tissue folds, form the **vulva** (Fig. 5.72). On either side of the midline are two thin folds of skin termed the **labia minora**. The region enclosed between them, and into which the urethra and vagina open, is the **vestibule**. Anteriorly, the labia minora each bifurcate, forming a medial and a lateral fold. The medial folds unite to form the **frenulum of the clitoris**, that joins the glans clitoris. The lateral folds unite ventrally over the glans clitoris and the body of the clitoris to form the **prepuce of the clitoris** (hood). The body of the clitoris extends posteriorly from the glans clitoris and is palpable deep to the prepuce and related skin. Posterior to the vestibule, the labia minora unite, forming a small transverse fold, the **frenulum of the labia minora** (the **fourchette**).

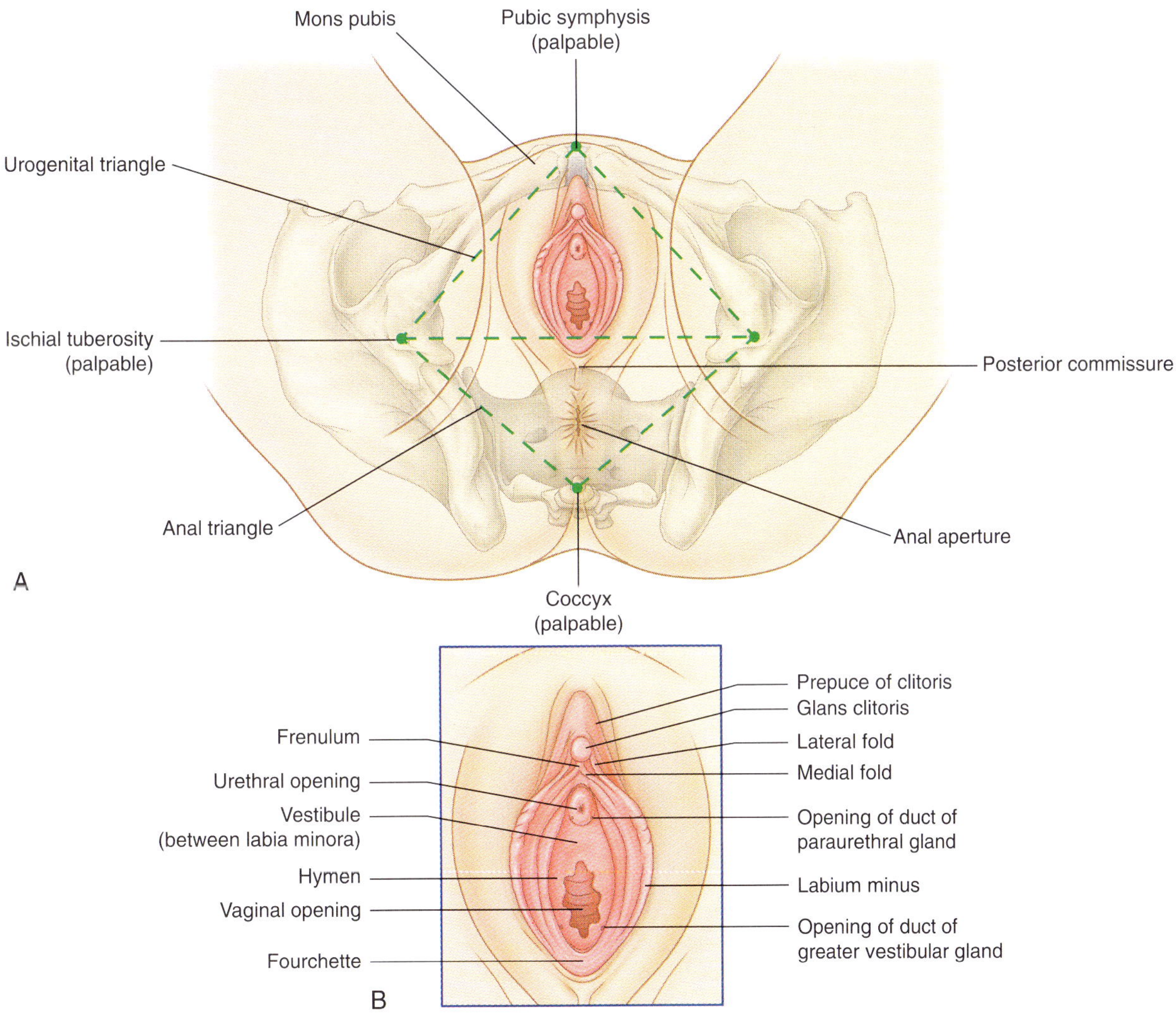

Fig. 5.72 Superficial features of the perineum in women. **(A)** Overview. **(B)** Close-up of external genitalia.

Within the vestibule, the vaginal orifice is surrounded to varying degrees by a ring-like fold of membrane, the **hymen**, which may have a small central perforation or may completely close the vaginal opening. Following rupture of the hymen (resulting from first sexual intercourse or injury), irregular remnants of the hymen fringe the vaginal opening.

The orifices of the urethra and the vagina are associated with the openings of glands. The ducts of the paraurethral glands (**Skene's glands**) open into the vestibule, one on each side of the lateral margin of the urethra. The ducts of the greater vestibular glands (Bartholin's glands) open adjacent to the posterolateral margin of the vaginal opening in the crease between the vaginal orifice and remnants of the hymen.

Lateral to the labia minora are two broad folds, the **labia majora**, which unite anteriorly to form the mons pubis. The **mons pubis** overlies the inferior aspect of the pubic symphysis and is anterior to the vestibule and the clitoris. Posteriorly, the labia majora do not unite and are separated by a depression termed the **posterior commissure**, which overlies the position of the perineal body.

In men

Superficial components of the genital organs in men consist of the scrotum and the penis (Fig. 5.73). The **scrotum** is the male homologue of the labia majora in women. In the fetus, labioscrotal swellings fuse across the midline, resulting in a single scrotum into which the testes and their associated musculofascial coverings, blood vessels, nerves, lymphatics, and drainage ducts descend from the abdomen. The remnant of the line of fusion between the labioscrotal swellings in the fetus is visible on the skin of the scrotum as a longitudinal midline **raphe** that extends from the anus, over the scrotal sac, and onto the inferior aspect of the body of the penis.

The **penis** consists of a root and body. The attached root of the penis is palpable posterior to the scrotum in the urogenital triangle of the perineum. The pendulous part of the

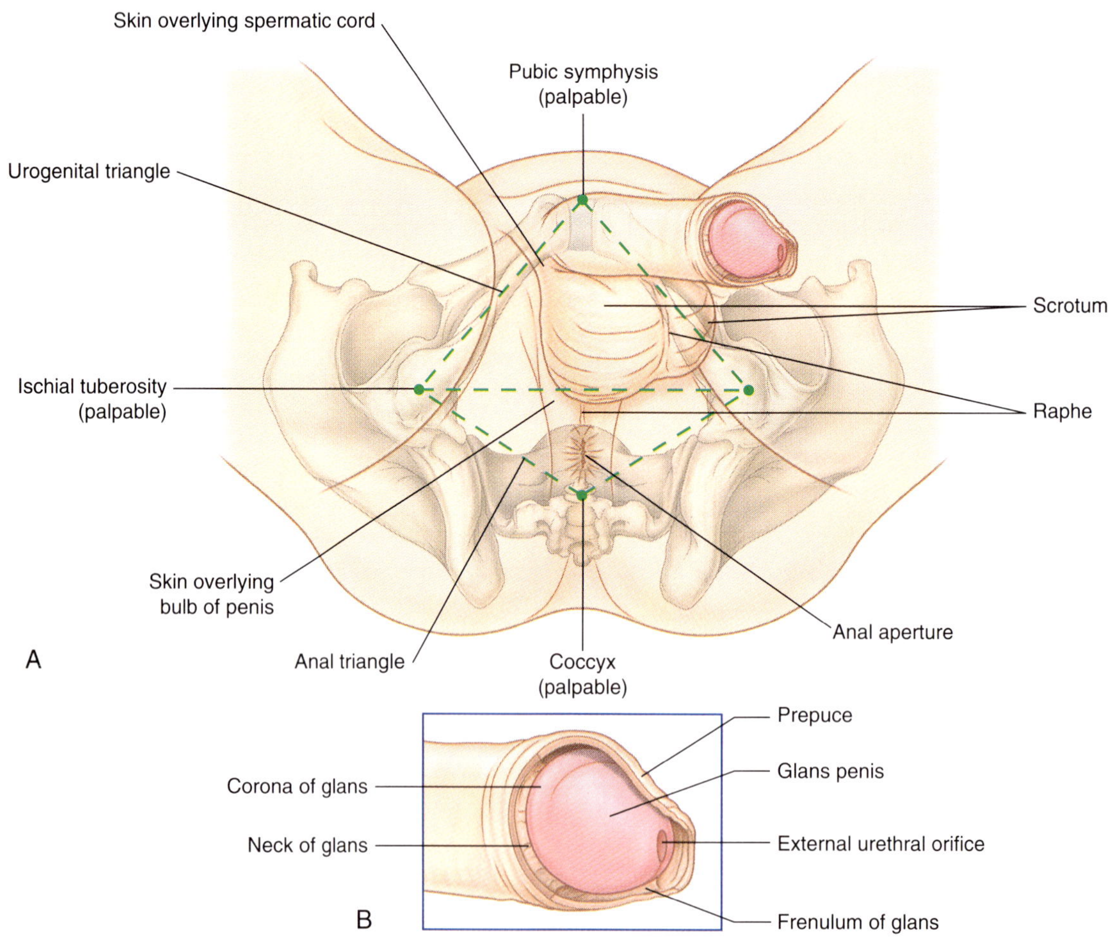

Fig. 5.73 Superficial features of the perineum in men. **(A)** Overview. **(B)** Close-up of external genitalia.

penis (body of penis) is entirely covered by skin; the tip of the body is covered by the glans penis.

The external urethral orifice is a sagittal slit, normally positioned at the tip of the glans. The inferior margin of the urethral orifice is continuous with a midline **raphe of the penis**, which represents a line of fusion formed in the glans as the urethra develops in the fetus. The base of this raphe is continuous with the **frenulum** of the glans, which is a median fold of skin that attaches the glans to more loosely attached skin proximal to the glans. The base of the glans is expanded to form a raised circular margin (the **corona of the glans**); the two lateral ends of the corona join inferiorly at the midline raphe of the glans. The depression posterior to the corona is the neck of the glans. Normally, a fold of skin at the neck of the glans is continuous anteriorly with thin skin that tightly adheres to the glans and posteriorly with thicker skin loosely attached to the body. This fold, known as the prepuce, extends forward to cover the glans. The prepuce is removed during male circumcision, leaving the glans exposed.

Superficial fascia of the urogenital triangle

The superficial fascia of the urogenital triangle is continuous with similar fascia on the anterior abdominal wall.

As with the superficial fascia of the abdominal wall, the perineal fascia has a membranous layer on its deep surface. This membranous layer (**Colles' fascia**) is attached:

- Posteriorly to the perineal membrane and therefore does not extend into the anal triangle (Fig. 5.74).
- To the ischiopubic rami that form the lateral borders of the urogenital triangle and therefore does not extend into the thigh (Fig. 5.74).

It defines the external limits of the superficial perineal pouch, lines the scrotum or labia, and extends around the body of the penis and clitoris.

Anteriorly, the membranous layer of fascia is continuous over the pubic symphysis and pubic bones with the membranous layer of fascia on the anterior abdominal wall. In the lower lateral abdominal wall, the membranous layer of abdominal fascia is attached to the deep fascia of the thigh just inferior to the inguinal ligament.

Because the membranous layer of fascia encloses the superficial perineal pouch and continues up the anterior abdominal wall, fluids or infectious materials that accumulate in the pouch can track out of the perineum and onto the lower abdominal wall. This material will not track into the anal triangle or the thigh because the fascia fuses with deep tissues at the borders of these regions.

Early clinical exposure

Urethral rupture

Urethral rupture may occur at a series of well-defined anatomical points.

The commonest injury is a rupture of the proximal spongy urethra below the perineal membrane. The urethra is usually torn when structures of the perineum are caught between a hard object (e.g., a steel beam or crossbar of a bicycle) and the inferior pubic arch. Urine escapes through the rupture into the superficial perineal pouch and descends into the scrotum and up onto the anterior abdominal wall deep to the superficial fascia.

In association with severe pelvic fractures, urethral rupture may occur at the prostatomembranous junction above the deep perineal pouch. The urine will extravasate into the true pelvis.

The worst and most serious urethral rupture is related to serious pelvic injuries where there is complete disruption of the puboprostatic ligaments. The prostate is dislocated superiorly not only by the ligamentous disruption but also by the extensive hematoma formed within the true pelvis. The diagnosis can be made by palpating the elevated prostate during a DRE.

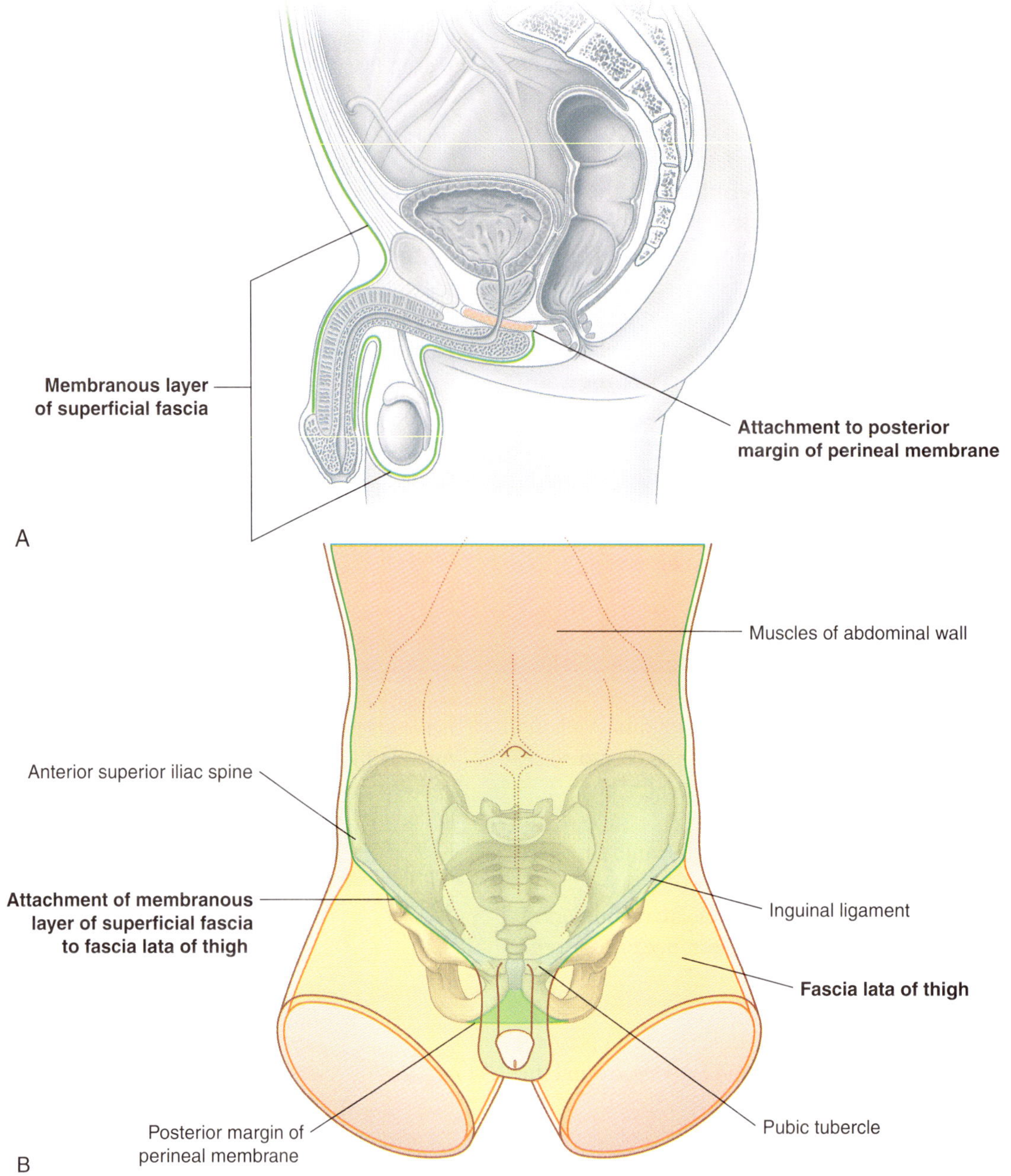

Fig. 5.74 Superficial fascia. **(A)** Lateral view. **(B)** Anterior view.

Somatic nerves

Pudendal nerve

The major somatic nerve of the perineum is the pudendal nerve. This nerve originates from the sacral plexus and carries fibers from spinal cord levels S2 to S4. It leaves the pelvic cavity through the greater sciatic foramen inferior to the piriformis muscle, passes around the sacrospinous ligament, and then enters the anal triangle of the perineum by passing medially through the lesser sciatic foramen. As it enters and courses through the perineum, it travels along the lateral wall of the ischioanal fossa in the **pudendal canal**, which is a tubular compartment formed in the fascia that covers the obturator internus muscle. This pudendal canal also contains the internal pudendal artery and accompanying veins.

The pudendal nerve (Fig. 5.75) has three major terminal branches—the inferior rectal and perineal nerves and the dorsal nerve of the penis or clitoris—which are

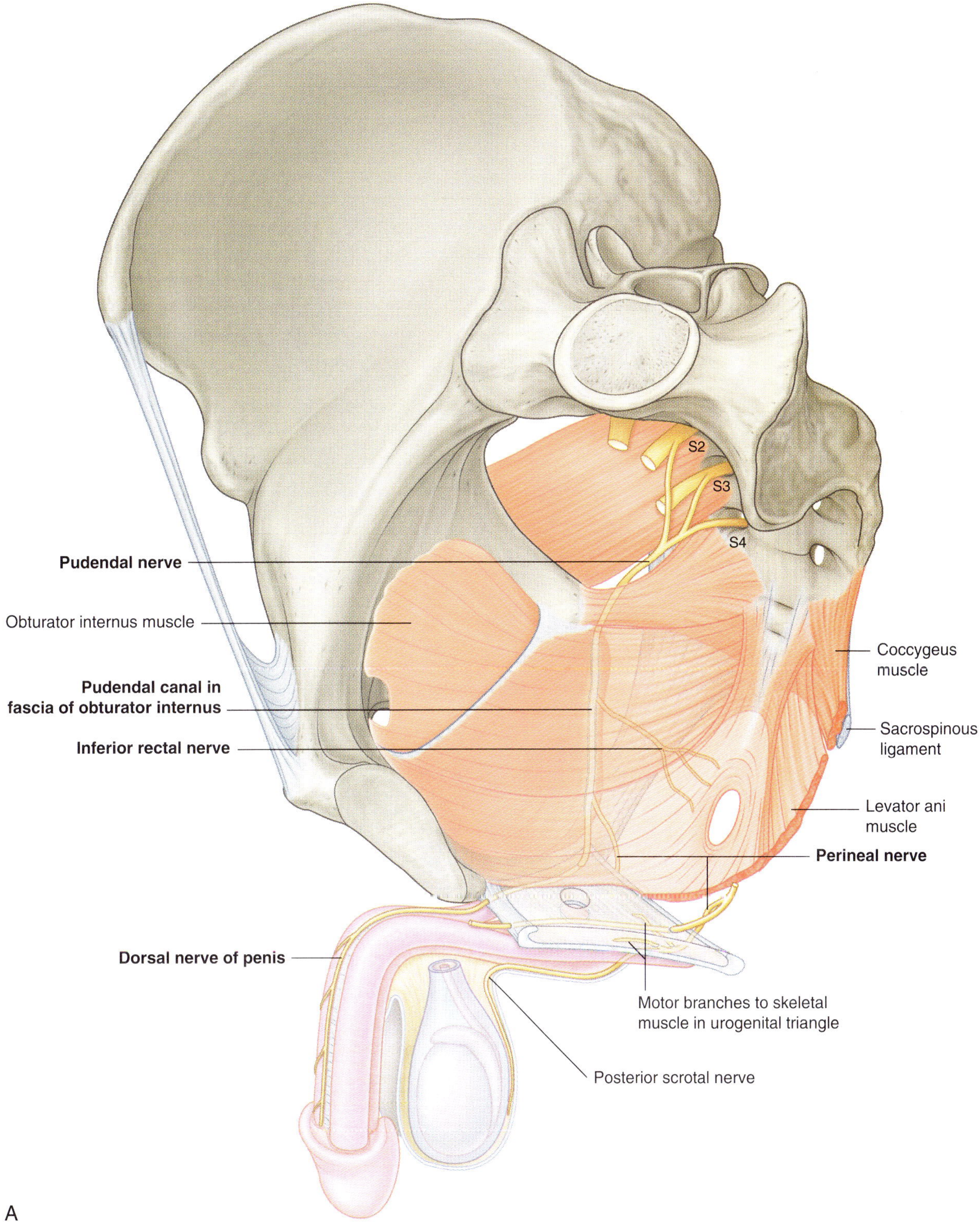

Fig. 5.75 Pudendal nerve. **(A)** In men.

Continued

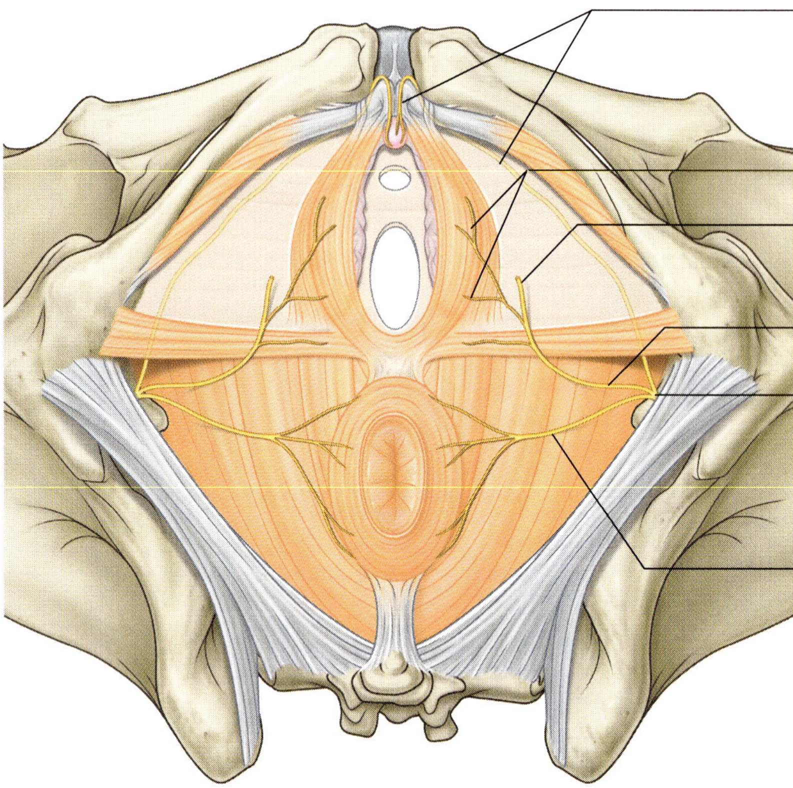

Fig. 5.75, cont'd (B) In women.

accompanied by branches of the internal pudendal artery (Fig. 5.76).

- The **inferior rectal nerve** is often multiple, penetrates through the fascia of the pudendal canal, and courses medially across the ischioanal fossa to innervate the external anal sphincter and related regions of the levator ani muscles. The nerve is also general sensory for the skin of the anal triangle.
- The **perineal nerve** passes into the urogenital triangle and gives rise to motor and cutaneous branches. The motor branches supply skeletal muscles in the superficial and deep perineal pouches. The largest of the sensory branches is the posterior scrotal nerve in men and the posterior labial nerve in women.
- The **dorsal nerve of the penis** and **clitoris** enters the deep perineal pouch (Fig. 5.75). It passes along the lateral margin of the pouch and then exits by passing inferiorly through the perineal membrane in a position just inferior to the pubic symphysis where it meets the body of the clitoris or the penis. It courses along the dorsal surface of the body to reach the glans. The dorsal nerve is sensory to the penis and clitoris, particularly to the glans.

Other somatic nerves

Other somatic nerves that enter the perineum are mainly sensory and include branches of the ilio-inguinal, genitofemoral, posterior femoral cutaneous, and anococcygeal nerves.

Visceral nerves

Visceral nerves enter the perineum by two routes:

- Those to the skin, which consist mainly of postganglionic sympathetics, are delivered into the region along the pudendal nerve. These fibers join the pudendal nerve from gray rami communicantes that connect pelvic parts of the sympathetic trunks to the anterior rami of the sacral spinal nerves (see p. 667 and Fig. 5.61).
- Those to erectile tissues enter the region mainly by passing through the deep perineal pouch from the inferior hypogastric plexus in the pelvic cavity (see p. 675 and Fig. 5.62B). The fibers that stimulate erection are parasympathetic fibers, which enter the inferior hypogastric plexus via pelvic splanchnic nerves from spinal cord levels of S2 to S4 (see Fig. 5.62A and B).

Blood vessels

Arteries

The most significant artery of the perineum is the internal pudendal artery (Fig. 5.76). Other arteries entering the area include the external pudendal, the testicular, and the cremasteric arteries.

Internal pudendal artery

The **internal pudendal artery** originates as a branch of the anterior trunk of the internal iliac artery in the pelvis (Fig. 5.76). Along with the pudendal nerve, it leaves the pelvis through the greater sciatic foramen inferior to the piriformis muscle. It passes around the ischial spine, where the artery lies lateral to the nerve, enters the perineum by coursing through the lesser sciatic foramen, and accompanies the pudendal nerve in the pudendal canal on the lateral wall of the ischioanal fossa.

The branches of the internal pudendal artery are similar to those of the pudendal nerve in the perineum and include the inferior rectal and perineal arteries, and branches to the erectile tissues of the penis and clitoris (Fig. 5.76).

Inferior rectal arteries

One or more **inferior rectal arteries** originate from the internal pudendal artery in the anal triangle and cross the ischioanal fossa medially to branch and supply muscle and related skin (Fig. 5.76). They anastomose with middle and superior rectal arteries from the internal iliac artery and the inferior mesenteric artery, respectively, to form a network of vessels that supply the rectum and anal canal.

Perineal artery.

The **perineal artery** originates near the anterior end of the pudendal canal and gives off a transverse perineal branch, and a posterior scrotal or labial artery to surrounding tissues and skin (Fig. 5.76).

Terminal part of the internal pudendal artery.

The terminal part of the internal pudendal artery accompanies the dorsal nerve of the penis or clitoris into the deep perineal pouch and supplies branches to the tissues in the deep perineal pouch and erectile tissues.

Branches that supply the erectile tissues in men include the artery to the bulb of the penis, the urethral artery, the deep artery of the penis, and the dorsal artery of the penis (Fig. 5.76).

- The **artery of the bulb of the penis** has a branch that supplies the bulbourethral gland and then penetrates the perineal membrane to supply the corpus spongiosum.
- A **urethral artery** also penetrates the perineal membrane and supplies the penile urethra and surrounding erectile tissue to the glans.
- Near the anterior margin of the deep perineal pouch, the internal pudendal artery bifurcates into two terminal branches. A **deep artery of the penis** penetrates the perineal membrane to enter the crus and supply the crus and corpus cavernosum of the body. The **dorsal artery of the penis** penetrates the anterior margin of the perineal membrane to meet the dorsal surface of the body of the penis. The vessel courses along the dorsal surface of the penis, medial to the dorsal nerve, and supplies the glans penis and superficial tissues of the penis; it also anastomoses with branches of the deep artery of the penis and the urethral artery.

Branches that supply the erectile tissues in women are similar to those in men.

- **Arteries of the bulb of the vestibule** supply the bulb of the vestibule and related vagina.
- **Deep arteries of the clitoris** supply the crura and corpus cavernosum of the body.
- **Dorsal arteries of the clitoris** supply surrounding tissues and the glans.

External pudendal arteries.

The **external pudendal arteries** consist of a superficial vessel and a deep vessel, which originate in the femoral artery in the thigh. They course medially to enter the perineum anteriorly and supply related skin of the penis and scrotum or the clitoris and labia majora.

Testicular and cremasteric arteries.

In men, the **testicular arteries** originate from the abdominal aorta and descend into the scrotum through the inguinal canal to supply the testes. Also, **cremasteric arteries**, which originate from the inferior epigastric branch of the external iliac artery, accompany the spermatic cord into the scrotum.

In women, small cremasteric arteries follow the round ligament of the uterus through the inguinal canal.

Veins

Veins in the perineum generally accompany the arteries and join the **internal pudendal veins** that connect with the **internal iliac vein** in the pelvis (Fig. 5.77). The exception is the **deep dorsal vein of the penis or clitoris** that drains mainly the glans and the corpora cavernosa. The deep dorsal vein courses along the midline between the dorsal arteries on each side of the body of the penis or

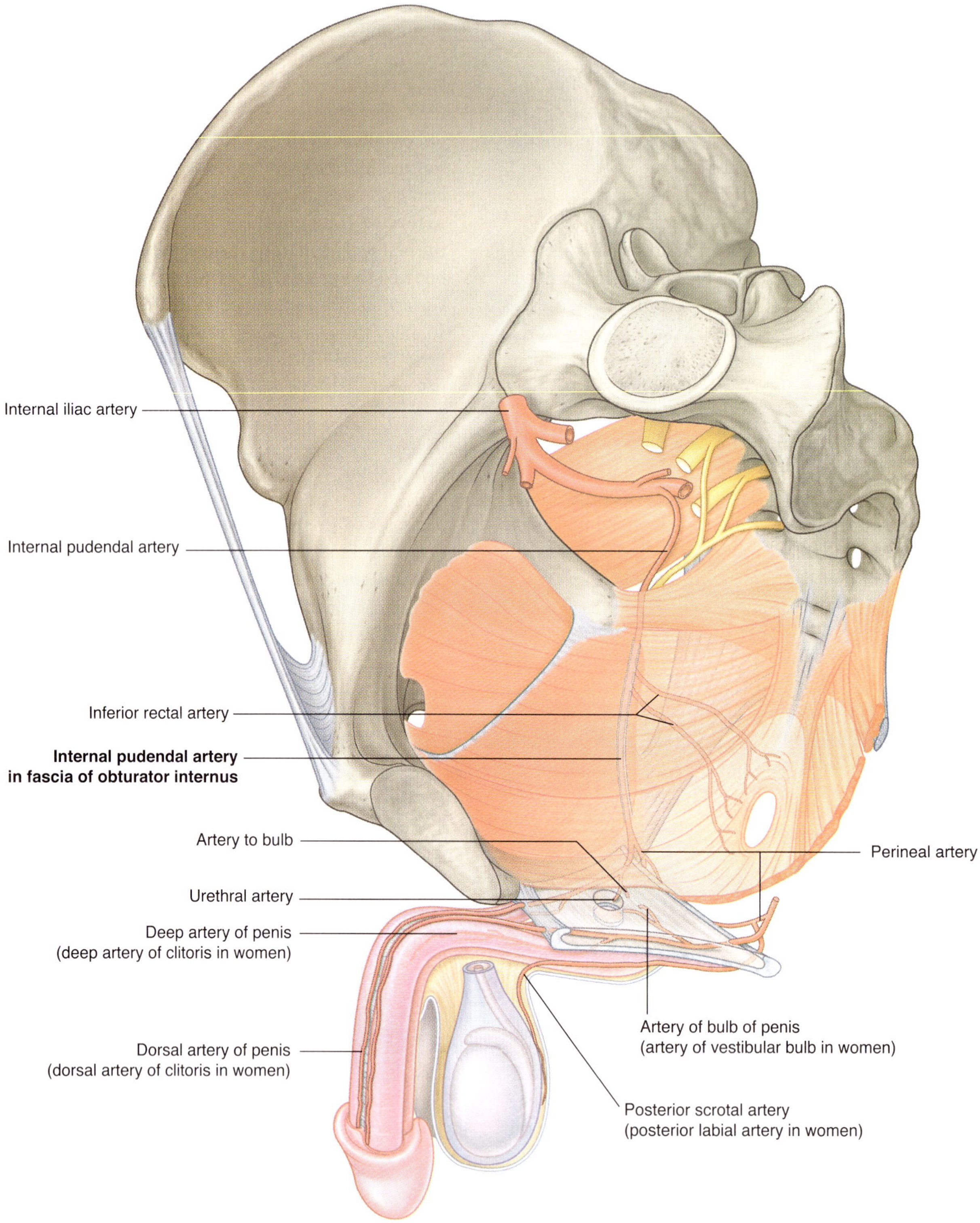

Fig. 5.76 Arteries in the perineum.

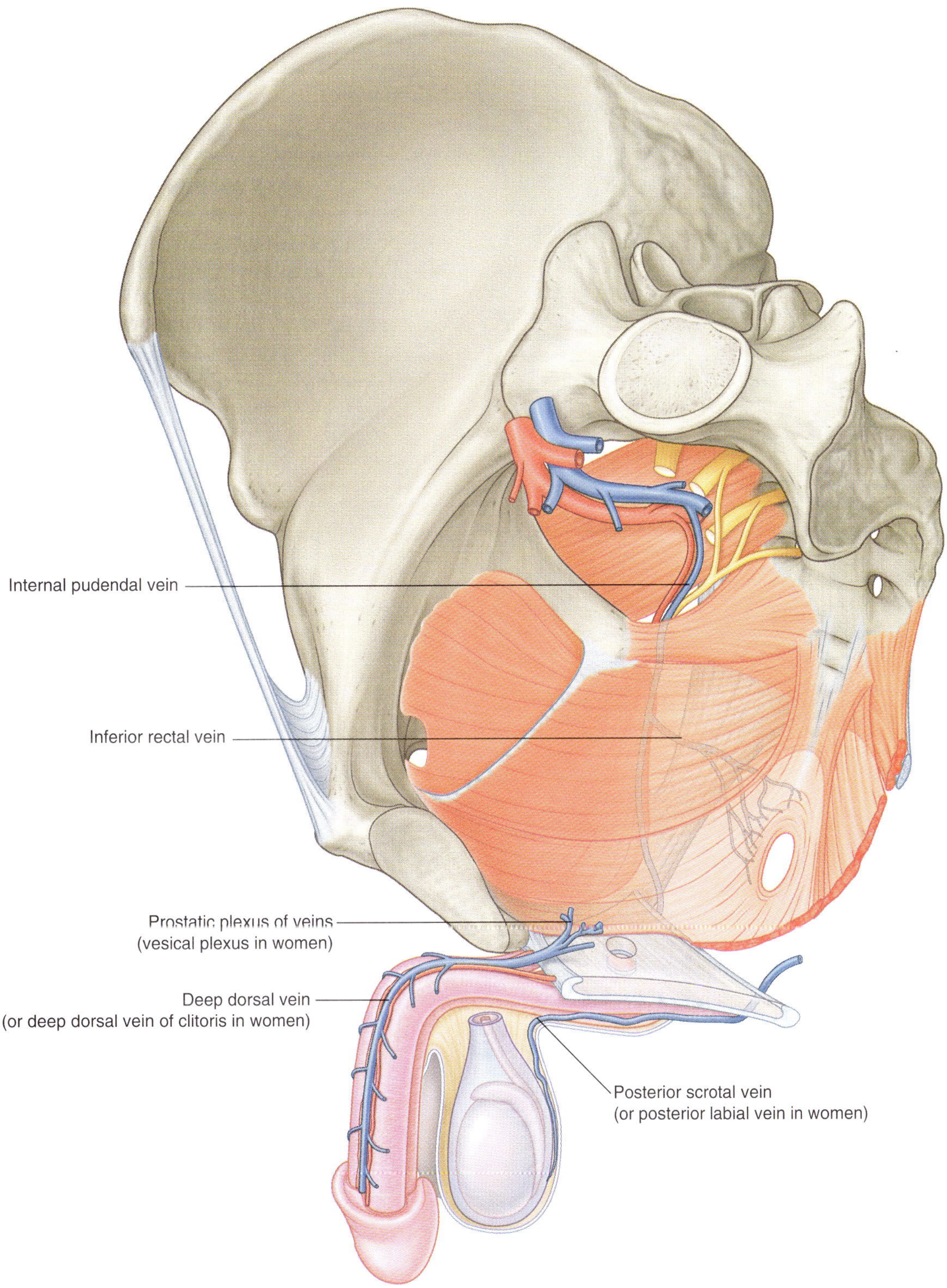

Fig. 5.77 Perineal veins.

clitoris, passes though the gap between the inferior pubic ligament and the deep perineal pouch, and connects with the plexus of veins surrounding the prostate in men or bladder in women.

External pudendal veins, which drain anterior parts of the labia majora or the scrotum and overlap with the area of drainage of the internal pudendal veins, connect with the femoral vein in the thigh. Superficial dorsal veins of the penis or clitoris that drain skin are tributaries of the external pudendal veins.

Lymphatics

Lymphatic vessels from deep parts of the perineum accompany the internal pudendal blood vessels and drain mainly into **internal iliac nodes** in the pelvis.

Lymphatic channels from superficial tissues of the penis or the clitoris accompany the superficial external pudendal blood vessels and drain mainly into **superficial inguinal nodes**, as do lymphatic channels from the scrotum or labia majora (Fig. 5.78). The glans penis, glans clitoris, labia minora, and terminal inferior end of the vagina drain into **deep inguinal nodes** and **external iliac nodes**.

Lymphatics from the testes drain via channels that ascend in the spermatic cord, pass through the inguinal canal, and course up the posterior abdominal wall to connect directly with lateral aortic or lumbar nodes and preaortic nodes around the aorta, at approximately vertebral levels LI and LII. Therefore, disease from the testes tracks superiorly to nodes high in the posterior abdominal wall and not to inguinal or iliac nodes.

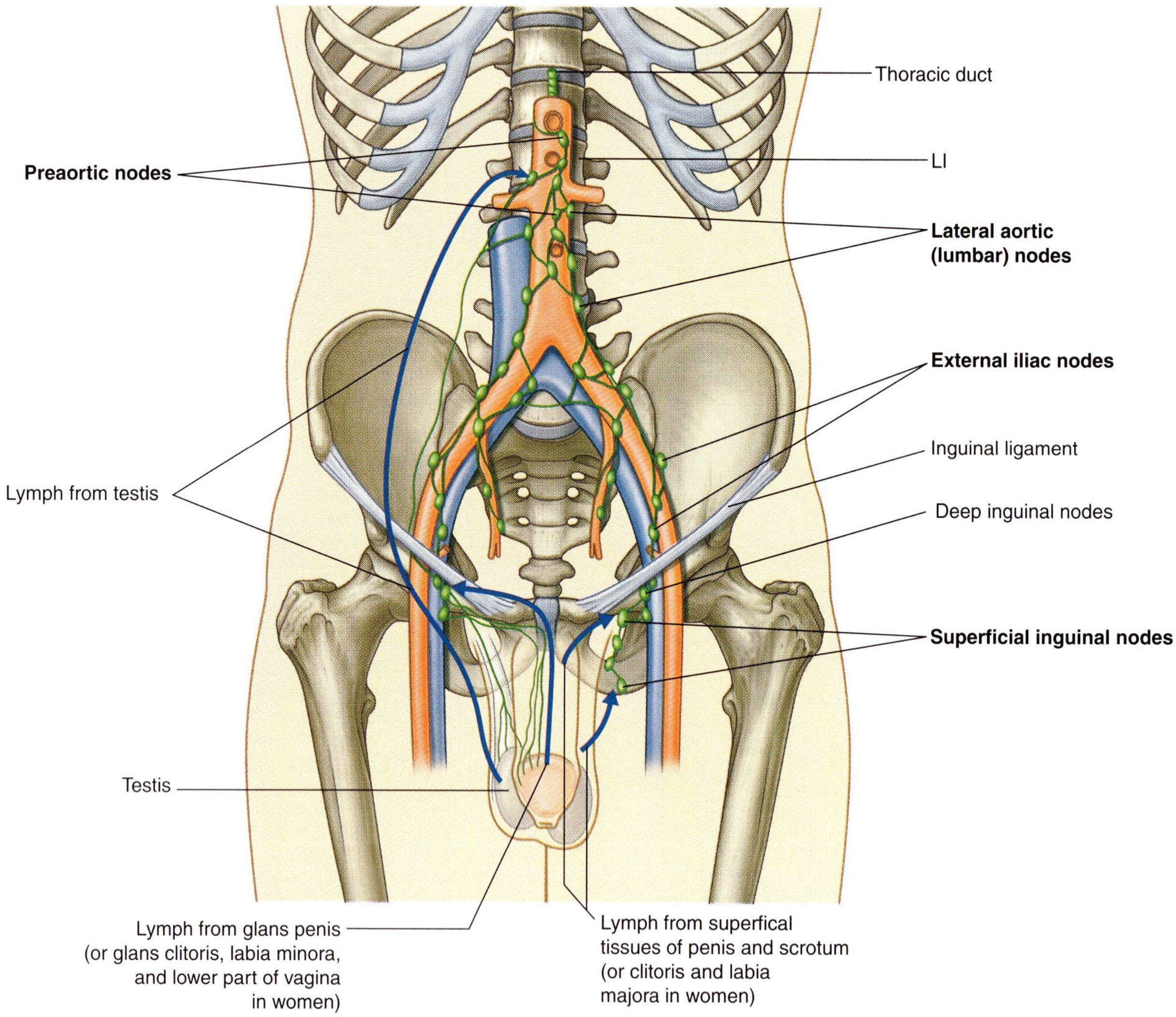

Fig. 5.78 Lymphatic drainage of the perineum.

Surface anatomy

Surface anatomy of the pelvis and perineum

Palpable bony features of the pelvis are used as landmarks for:

- Locating soft tissue structures
- Visualizing the orientation of the pelvic inlet
- Defining the margins of the perineum

The ability to recognize the normal appearance of structures in the perineum is an essential part of a physical examination.

In women, the cervix can be visualized directly by opening the vaginal canal using a speculum.

In men, the size and texture of the prostate in the pelvic cavity can be assessed by digital palpation through the anal aperture.

Orientation of the pelvis and perineum in the anatomical position

In the anatomical position, the anterior superior iliac spines and the anterior superior edge of the pubic symphysis lie in the same vertical plane. The pelvic inlet faces anterosuperiorly. The urogenital triangle of the perineum is oriented in an almost horizontal plane and faces inferiorly, whereas the anal triangle is more vertical and faces posteriorly (Figs 5.79 and 5.80).

How to define the margins of the perineum

The pubic symphysis, ischial tuberosities, and tip of the sacrum are palpable on patients and can be used to define the boundaries of the perineum. This is best done with patients lying on their backs with their thighs flexed and abducted in the lithotomy position (Fig. 5.81).

- The ischial tuberosities are palpable on each side as large bony masses near the crease of skin (gluteal fold) between the thigh and gluteal region. They mark the lateral corners of the diamond-shaped perineum.
- The tip of the coccyx is palpable in the midline posterior to the anal aperture and marks the most posterior limit of the perineum.
- The anterior limit of the perineum is the pubic symphysis. In women, this is palpable in the midline deep to the mons pubis. In men, the pubic symphysis is palpable immediately superior to where the body of the penis joins the lower abdominal wall.

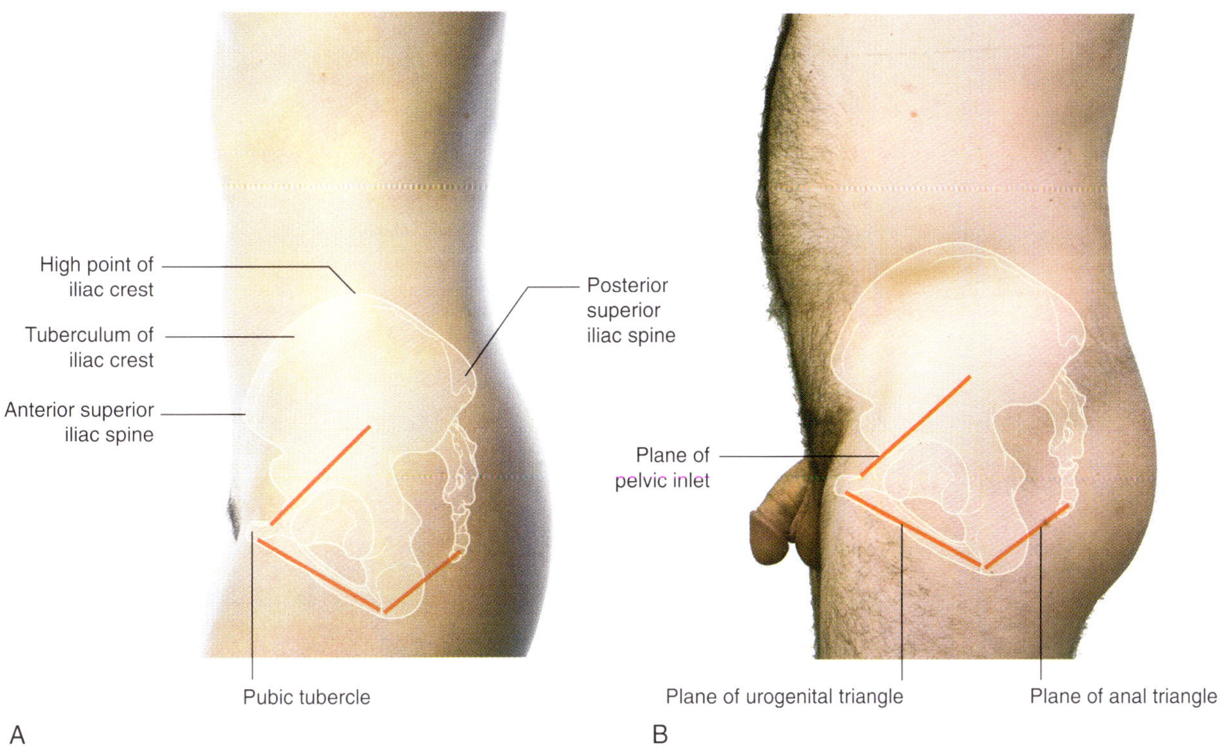

Fig. 5.79 Lateral view of the pelvic area with the position of the skeletal features indicated. The orientation of the pelvic inlet, urogenital triangle, and anal triangle is also shown. **(A)** In a woman. **(B)** In a man.

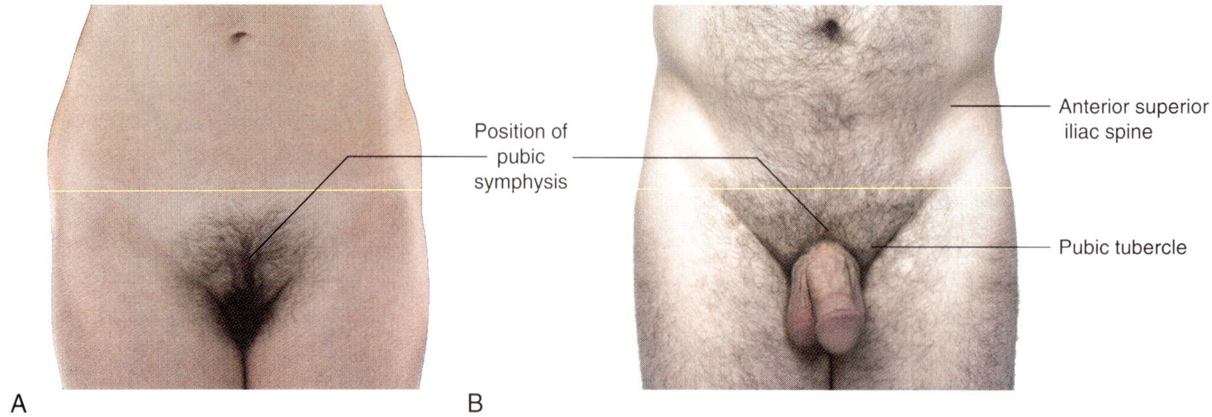

Fig. 5.80 Anterior view of the pelvic area. (**A**) In a woman showing the position of the pubic symphysis. (**B**) In a man showing the position of the pubic tubercle, pubic symphysis, and anterior superior iliac spine.

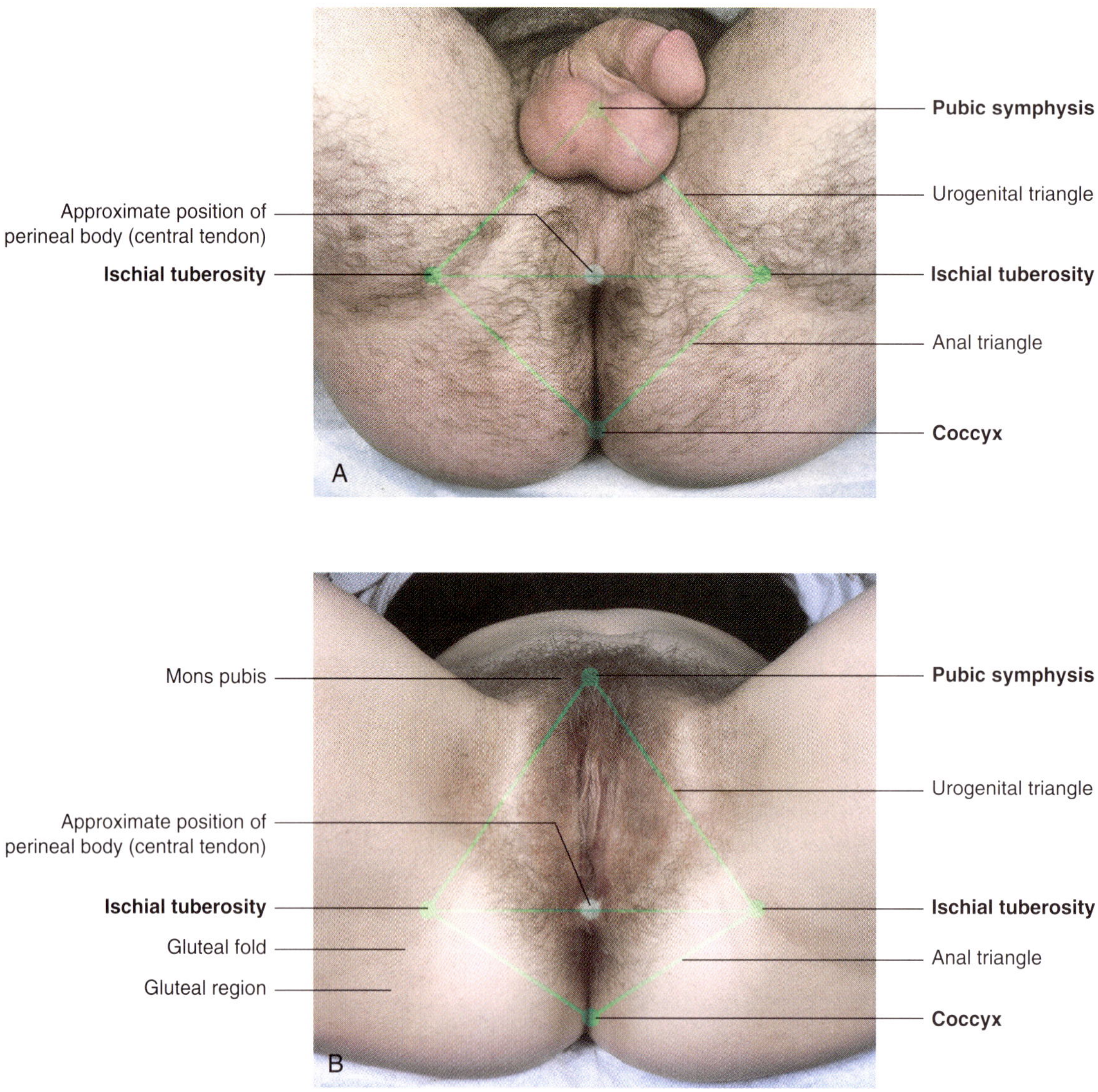

Fig. 5.81 Inferior view of the perineum in the lithotomy position. Boundaries, subdivisions, and palpable landmarks are indicated. **(A)** In a man. **(B)** In a woman.

Imaginary lines that join the ischial tuberosities with the pubic symphysis in front, and with the tip of the coccyx behind, outline the diamond-shaped perineum. An additional line between the ischial tuberosities divides the perineum into two triangles, the urogenital triangle anteriorly and anal triangle posteriorly. This line also approximates the position of the posterior margin of the perineal membrane. The midpoint of this line marks the location of the perineal body or central tendon of the perineum.

Identification of structures in the anal triangle

The anal triangle is the posterior half of the perineum. The base of the triangle faces anteriorly and is an imaginary line joining the two ischial tuberosities. The apex of the triangle is the tip of the coccyx; the lateral margins can be approximated by lines joining the coccyx to the ischial tuberosities. In both women and men, the major feature of the anal triangle is the anal aperture in the center of the triangle. Fat fills the ischioanal fossa on each side of the anal aperture (Fig. 5.82).

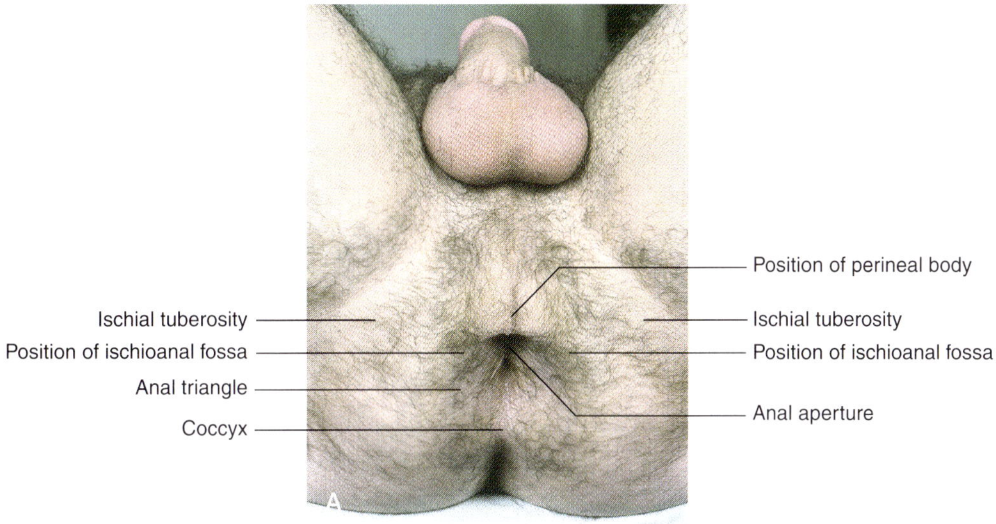

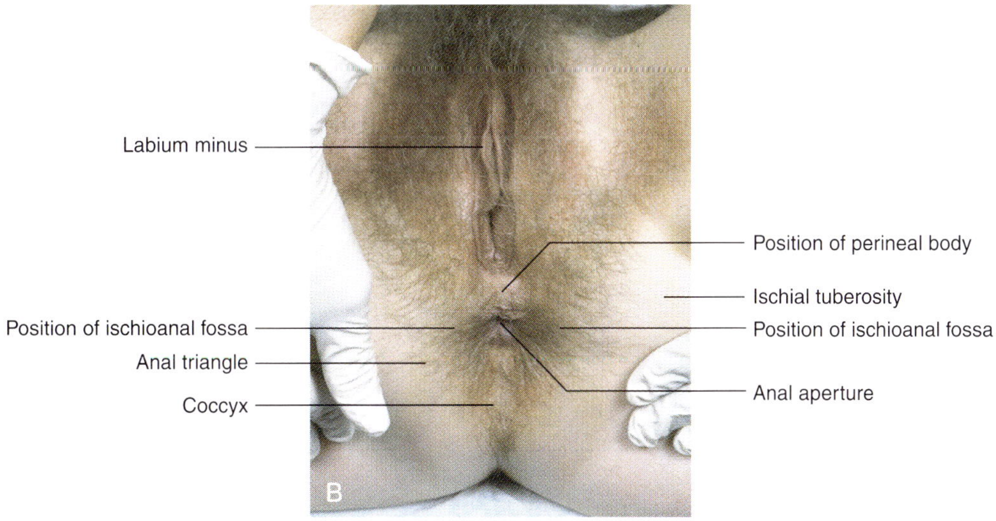

Fig. 5.82 Anal triangle with the anal aperture and position of the ischioanal fossae indicated. **(A)** In a man. **(B)** In a woman.

Identification of structures in the urogenital triangle of women

The urogenital triangle is the anterior half of the perineum. The base of the triangle faces posteriorly and is an imaginary line joining the two ischial tuberosities. The apex of the triangle is the pubic symphysis. The lateral margins can be approximated by lines joining the pubic symphysis to the ischial tuberosities. These lines overlie the ischiopubic rami, which can be felt on deep palpation.

In women, the major contents of the urogenital triangle are the clitoris, the vestibule, and skin folds that together form the vulva (Fig. 5.83A and B).

Two thin skin folds, the labia minora, enclose between them a space termed the vestibule into which the vagina and the urethra open (Fig. 5.83C). Gentle lateral traction on the labia minora opens the vestibule and reveals a soft tissue mound on which the urethra opens. The paraurethral (Skene's) glands, one on each side, open into the skin crease between the urethra and the labia minora (Fig. 5.83D).

Posterior to the urethra is the vaginal opening. The vaginal opening (introitus) is ringed by remnants of the hymen that originally closes the vaginal orifice and is usually ruptured during the first sexual intercourse. The ducts of the greater vestibular (Bartholin's) glands, one on each

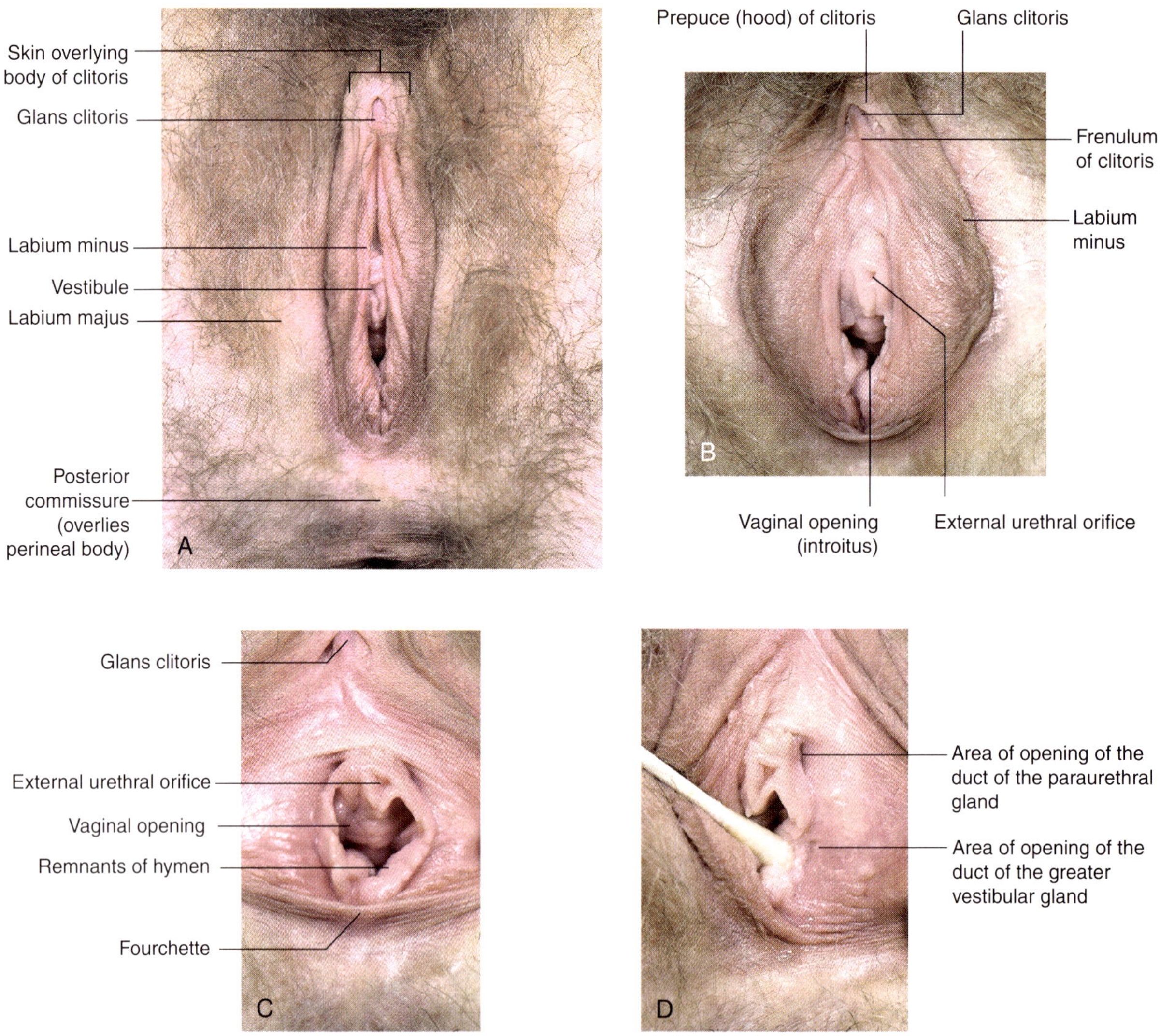

Fig. 5.83 Structures in the urogenital triangle of a woman. **(A)** Inferior view of the urogenital triangle of a woman with major features indicated. **(B)** Inferior view of the vestibule. The labia minora have been pulled apart to open the vestibule. Also indicated are the glans clitoris, the clitoral hood, and the frenulum of the clitoris. **(C)** Inferior view of the vestibule showing the urethral and vaginal orifices and the hymen. The labia minora have been pulled further apart than in Fig. 5.83B. **(D)** Inferior view of the vestibule with the left labium minus pulled to the side to show the regions of the vestibule into which the greater vestibular and paraurethral glands open.

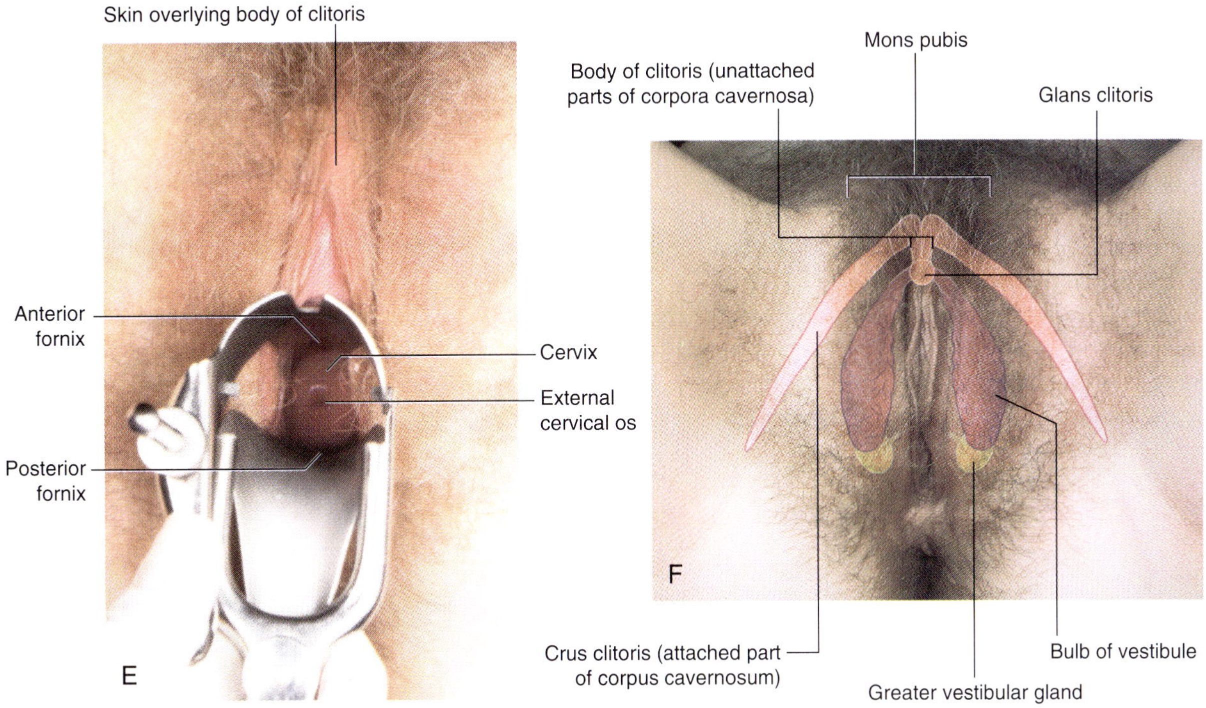

Fig. 5.83, cont'd (E) View through the vaginal canal of the cervix. **(F)** Inferior view of the urogenital triangle of a woman with the erectile tissues of the clitoris and vestibule and the greater vestibular glands indicated with overlays.

side, open into the skin crease between the hymen and the adjacent labium minus (Fig. 5.83D).

The labia minora each bifurcate anteriorly into medial and lateral folds. The medial folds unite at the midline to form the frenulum of the clitoris. The larger lateral folds also unite across the midline to form the clitoral hood or prepuce that covers the glans clitoris and distal parts of the body of the clitoris. Posterior to the vaginal orifice, the labia minora join, forming a transverse skin fold (the fourchette).

The labia majora are broad folds positioned lateral to the labia minora. They come together in front to form the mons pubis, which overlies the inferior aspect of the pubic symphysis. The posterior ends of the labia majora are separated by a depression termed the posterior commissure, which overlies the position of the perineal body.

The cervix is visible when the vaginal canal is opened with a speculum (Fig. 5.83E). The external cervical os opens onto the surface of the dome-shaped cervix. A recess or gutter, termed the fornix, occurs between the cervix and the vaginal wall and is further subdivided, based on location, into anterior, posterior, and lateral fornices.

The roots of the clitoris occur deep to surface features of the perineum and are attached to the ischiopubic rami and the perineal membrane.

The bulbs of the vestibule (Fig. 5.83F), composed of erectile tissues, lie deep to the labia minora on either side of the vestibule. These erectile masses are continuous, via thin bands of erectile tissues, with the glans clitoris, which is visible under the clitoral hood. The greater vestibular glands occur posterior to the bulbs of the vestibule on either side of the vaginal orifice.

The crura of the clitoris are attached, one on each side, to the ischiopubic rami. Each crus is formed by the attached part of the corpus cavernosum. Anteriorly, these erectile corpora detach from bone, curve posteroinferiorly, and unite to form the body of the clitoris.

The body of the clitoris underlies the ridge of skin immediately anterior to the clitoral hood (prepuce). The glans clitoris is positioned at the end of the body of the clitoris.

Identification of structures in the urogenital triangle of men

In men, the urogenital triangle contains the root of the penis. The testes and associated structures, although they migrate into the scrotum from the abdomen, are generally evaluated with the penis during a physical examination.

The scrotum in men is homologous to the labia majora in women. Each oval testis is readily palpable through the skin of the scrotum (Fig. 5.84A). Posterolateral to the testis is an elongated mass of tissue, often visible as a raised ridge that contains lymphatics and blood vessels of the testis, and the epididymis and ductus deferens. A midline raphe (Fig. 5.84B) is visible on the skin separating left and right sides of the scrotum. In some individuals, this raphe is prominent and extends from the anal aperture, over the scrotum and along the ventral surface of the body of the penis, to the frenulum of the glans.

The root of the penis is formed by the attached parts of the corpus spongiosum and the corpora cavernosa. The corpus spongiosum is attached to the perineal membrane and can be easily palpated as a large mass anterior to the perineal body. This mass, which is covered by the bulbospongiosus muscles, is the bulb of penis.

The corpus spongiosum detaches from the perineal membrane anteriorly, becomes the ventral part of the body of the penis (shaft of penis), and eventually terminates as the expanded glans penis (Fig. 5.84C and D).

The crura of the penis, one crus on each side, are the attached parts of the corpora cavernosa and are anchored to the ischiopubic rami (Fig. 5.84E). The corpora cavernosa are unattached anteriorly and become the paired erectile masses that form the dorsal part of the body of the penis. The glans penis caps the anterior ends of the corpora cavernosa.

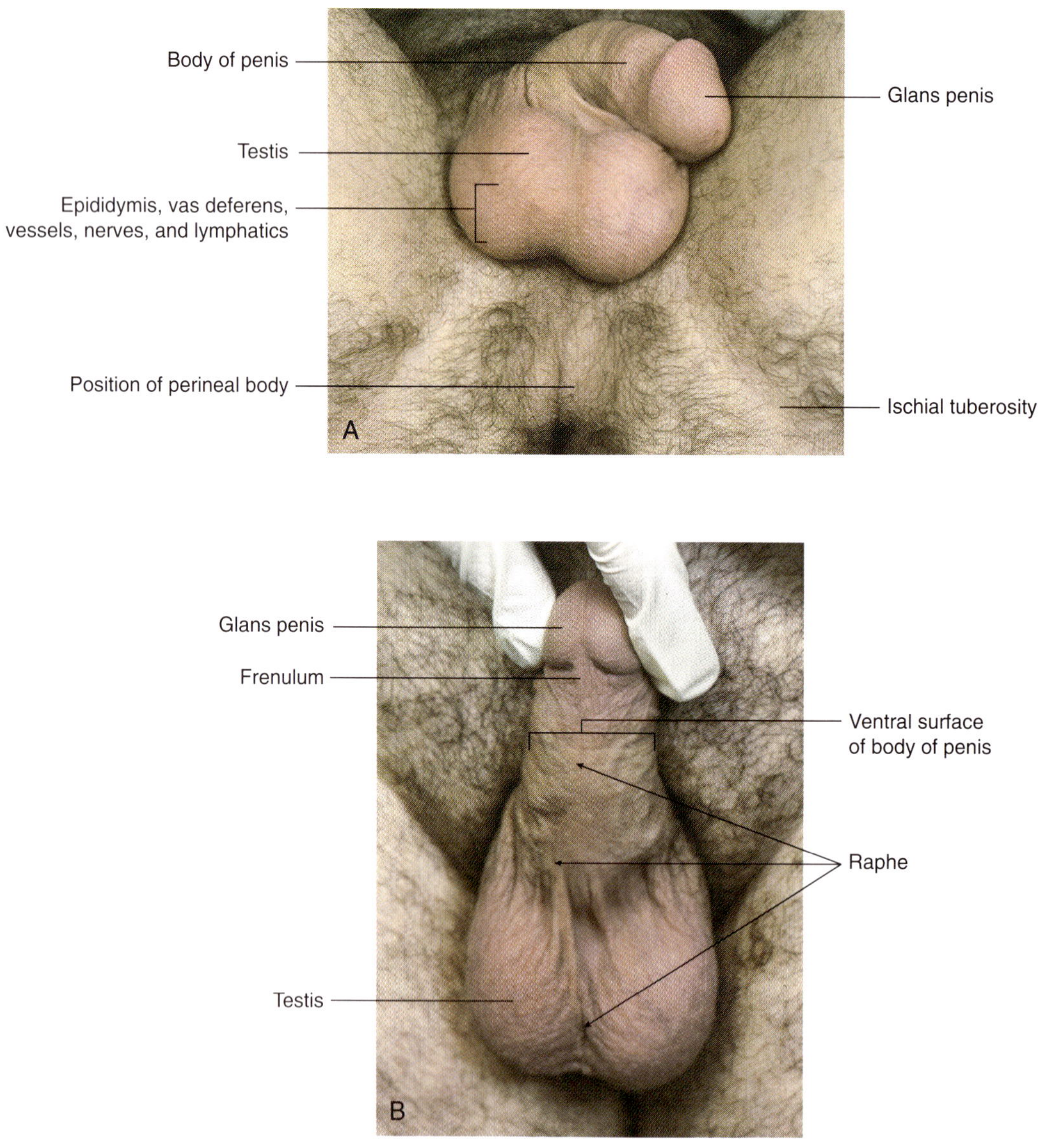

Fig. 5.84 Structures in the urogenital triangle of a man. **(A)** Inferior view. **(B)** Ventral surface of the body of the penis.

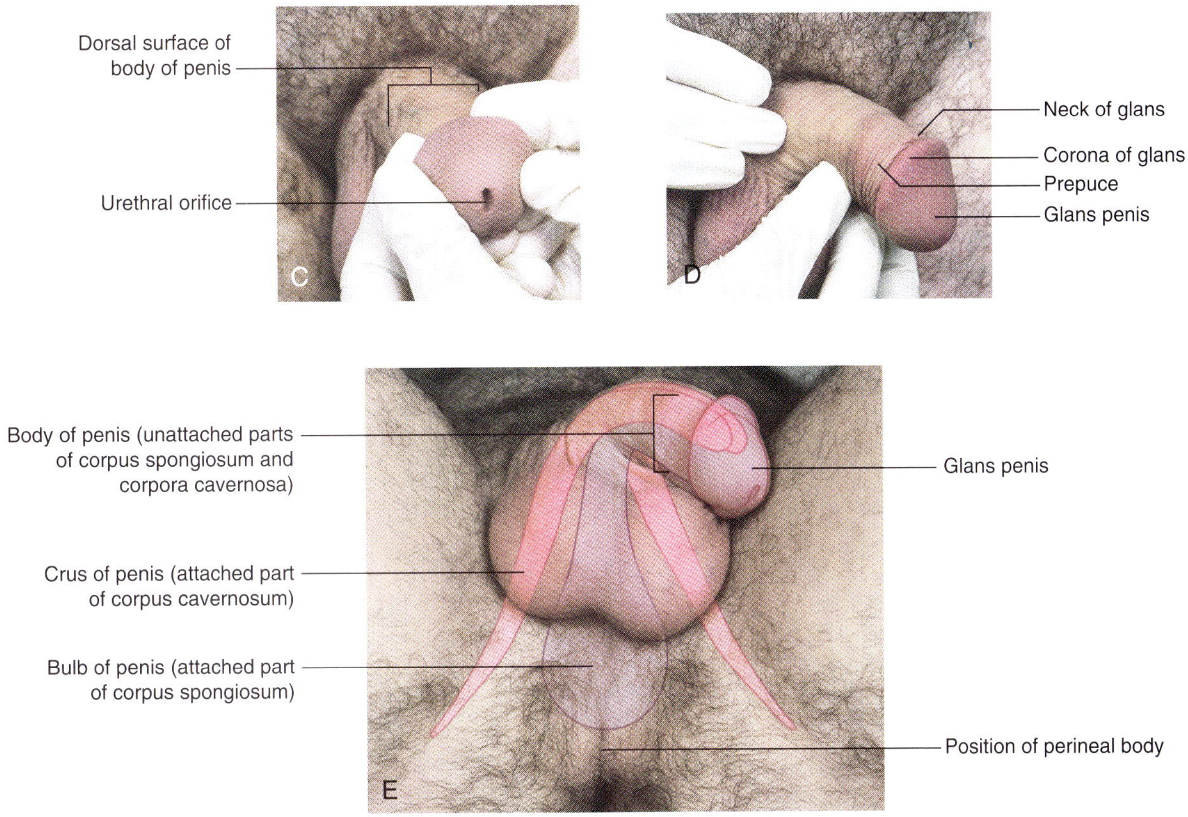

Fig. 5.84, cont'd (C) Anterior view of the glans penis showing the urethral opening. **(D)** Lateral view of the body of the penis and glans. **(E)**. Inferior view of the urogenital triangle of a man with the erectile tissues of the penis indicated with overlays.

Clinical cases

Case 1

VARICOCELE

A 25-year-old man visited his family physician because he had a "dragging feeling" in the left side of his scrotum. He was otherwise healthy and had no other symptoms. During examination, the physician palpated the left testis, which was normal, although he noted soft nodular swelling around the superior aspect of the testes and the epididymis. In his clinical notes, he described these findings as a "bag of worms" (Fig. 5.85)**. The bag of worms was a varicocele.**

The venous drainage of the testis is via the pampiniform plexus of veins that runs within the spermatic cord. A varicocele is a collection of dilated veins that arise from the pampiniform plexus. In many ways, they are similar to varicose veins that develop in the legs. Typically, the patient complains of a dragging feeling in the scrotum and around the testis, which is usually worse toward the end of the day.

The family physician recommended surgical treatment, with a recommendation for surgery through an inguinal incision.

A simple surgical technique divides the skin around the inguinal ligament. The aponeurosis of the external oblique muscle is divided in the anterior abdominal wall to display the spermatic cord. Careful inspection of the spermatic cord reveals the veins, which are surgically ligated.

Another option is to embolize the varicocele.

In this technique, a small catheter is placed via the right femoral vein. The catheter is advanced along the external iliac vein and the common iliac vein and into the inferior vena cava. The catheter is then positioned in the left renal vein, and a venogram is performed to demonstrate the origin of the left testicular vein. The catheter is advanced down the left testicular vein into the veins of the inguinal canal and the pampiniform plexus. Metal coils to occlude the vessels are injected, and the catheter is withdrawn.

The patient asked how blood would drain from the testis after the operation.

Although the major veins of the testis had been occluded, small collateral veins running within the scrotum and around the outer aspect of the spermatic cord permitted drainage without recurrence of the varicocele.

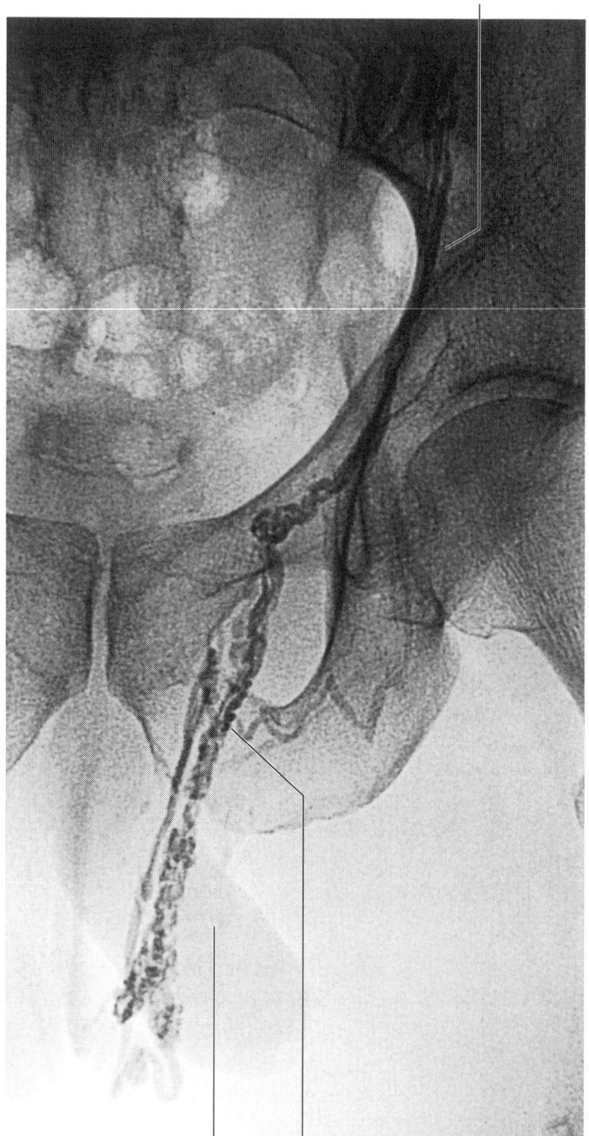

Fig. 5.85 Left testicular venogram demonstrating the pampiniform plexus of veins.

Case 2

SCIATIC NERVE COMPRESSION

A young man developed pain in his right gluteal region, in the posterior aspect of the thigh and around the posterior and lateral aspects of the leg. On further questioning, he reported that the pain also radiated over the lateral part of the foot, particularly around the lateral malleolus.

The areas of pain correspond to dermatomes L4 to S3 nerves.

Over the following weeks, the patient began to develop muscular weakness, predominantly footdrop.

These findings are consistent with loss of the motor function and sensory change in the common fibular nerve, which is a branch of the sciatic nerve in the lower limb.

A computed tomography (CT) scan of the abdomen and pelvis revealed a mass in the posterior aspect of the right side of the pelvis. The mass was anterior to the piriformis muscle and adjacent to the rectum.

On the anterior belly of the piriformis muscle, the sciatic nerve is formed from the roots of L4 to S3 nerves. The mass in the patient's pelvis compressed this nerve, producing his sensory and motor dysfunction.

During surgery, the mass was found to be a benign nerve tumor and was excised. This patient had no long-standing neurological deficit.

Case 3

PELVIC KIDNEY

A young woman visited her family practitioner because she had mild upper abdominal pain. An ultrasound demonstrated gallstones within the gallbladder, which explained the patient's pain. However, when the technician assessed the pelvis, she noted a mass behind the bladder, which had sonographic findings similar to a kidney (Fig. 5.86).

What did the sonographer do next? Having demonstrated this pelvic mass behind the bladder, the sonographer assessed both kidneys. The patient had a normal right kidney. However, the left kidney could not be found in its usual place. The technician diagnosed a pelvic kidney.

A pelvic kidney can be explained by the embryology. The kidneys develop from a complex series of structures that originate adjacent to the bladder within the fetal pelvis. As development proceeds and the functions of the various parts of the developing kidneys change, they attain a superior position in the upper abdomen adjacent to the abdominal aorta and inferior vena cava, on the posterior abdominal wall. A developmental arrest or complication may prevent the kidney from obtaining its usual position. Fortunately, it is unusual for patients to have any symptoms relating to a pelvic kidney.

This patient had no symptoms attributable to the pelvic kidney and she was discharged.

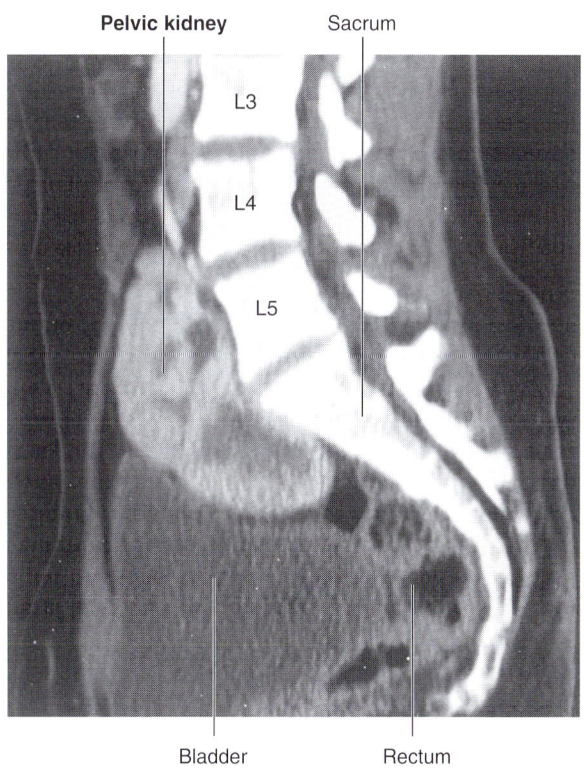

Fig. 5.86 Sagittal computed tomogram demonstrating a pelvic kidney.

Case 4

LEFT COMMON ILIAC ARTERY OBSTRUCTION

A 65-year-old man was examined by a surgical intern because he had a history of buttock pain and impotence. On examination, he had a reduced peripheral pulse on the left foot compared to the right. On direct questioning, the patient revealed that he experienced severe left-sided buttock pain after walking 100 yards. After a short period of rest, he could walk another 100 yards before the same symptoms recurred. He also noticed that over the past year he was unable to obtain an erection. He smoked heavily and was not on any drugs or treatment.

The pain in the left buttock is ischemic in nature. He gives a typical history relating to lack of blood flow to the muscles. A similar finding is present when muscular branches of the femoral artery are occluded or stenosed. Such patients develop similar (ischemic) pain in the calf muscles called intermittent claudication.

How does the blood get to the gluteal muscles?

Blood arrives at the aortic bifurcation and then passes into the common iliac arteries, which divide into the internal and external iliac vessels. The internal iliac artery then divides into anterior and posterior divisions, which in turn give rise to vessels that leave the pelvis by passing through the greater sciatic foramen and supply the gluteal muscles. The internal pudendal artery also arises from the anterior division of the internal iliac artery and supplies the penis.

The patient's symptoms occur on the left side, suggesting that an obstruction exists on that side only.

Because the patient's symptoms occur on the left side only, the lesion is likely in the left common iliac artery (Fig. 5.87) and is preventing blood flow into the external and internal iliac arteries on the left side.

"How will I be treated?" asked the patient.

The patient was asked to stop smoking and begin regular exercise. Other treatment options include unblocking the lesion by ballooning the blockage to reopen the vessels or by a surgical bypass graft.

Stopping smoking and regular exercise improved the patient's walking distance. The patient underwent the less invasive procedure of ballooning the vessel (angioplasty) and as a result he was able to walk unhindered and to have an erection.

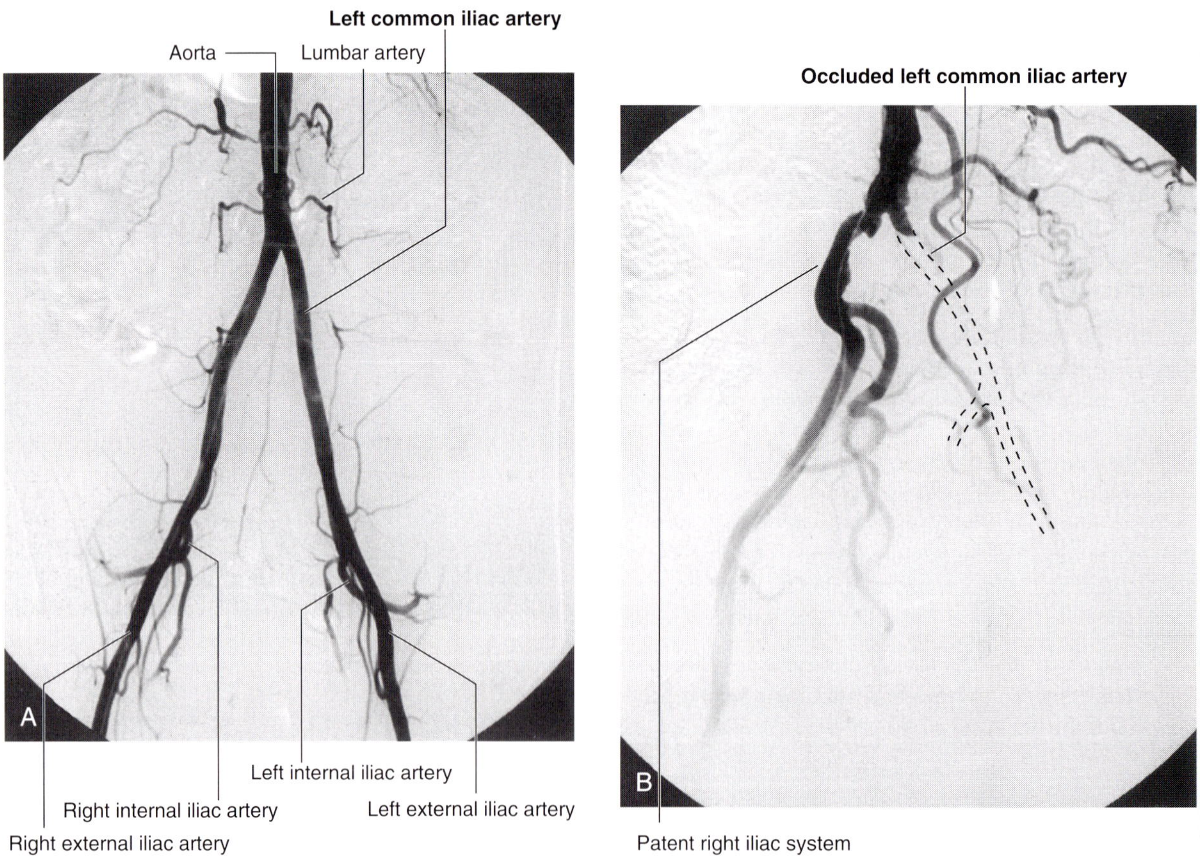

Fig. 5.87 Digital subtraction aortoiliac angiogram. **(A)** Normal circulation pattern. **(B)** Occluded left common iliac artery.

Case 5

IATROGENIC URETERIC INJURY

A 50-year-old woman was admitted to hospital for surgical resection of the uterus (hysterectomy) for cancer. The surgeon was also going to remove all the pelvic lymph nodes and carry out a bilateral salpingo-oophorectomy (removal of uterine tubes and ovaries). The patient was prepared for this procedure and underwent routine surgery. Twenty-five hours after surgery, it was noted that the patient had passed no urine and her abdomen was expanding. An ultrasound scan demonstrated a considerable amount of fluid within the abdomen. Fluid withdrawn from the abdomen was tested and found to be urine.

It was postulated that this patient's ureters had been damaged during the surgery.

The pelvic part of the ureter courses posteroinferiorly and external to the parietal peritoneum on the lateral wall of the pelvis anterior to the internal iliac artery. It continues in its course to a point approximately 2 cm superior to the ischial spine and then passes anteromedially and superior to the levator ani muscles. Importantly, the ureter closely adheres to the peritoneum. The only structure that passes between the ureter and the peritoneum in men is the ductus deferens. In women, however, as the ureter descends on the pelvic wall, it passes under the uterine artery. The ureter continues close to the lateral fornix of the vagina, especially on the left, and enters the posterosuperior angle of the bladder. It was at this point that the ureter was inadvertently damaged.

Knowing the anatomy and recognizing the possibility of ureteric damage enabled the surgeons to reestablish continuity of the ureter surgically. The patient was hospitalized a few days longer than expected and made an uneventful recovery.

Case 6

ECTOPIC PREGNANCY

A 25-year-old woman was admitted to the emergency department with a complaint of pain in her right iliac fossa. The pain had developed rapidly over approximately 40 minutes and was associated with cramps and vomiting. The surgical intern made an initial diagnosis of appendicitis.

The typical history for appendicitis is a central abdominal, colicky (intermittent waxing and waning) pain, which over a period of hours localizes to become a constant pain in the right iliac fossa. The central colicky pain is typical for a poorly localized visceral type of pain. As the parietal peritoneum becomes inflamed, the pain becomes localized. Although this patient does have right iliac fossa pain, the history is not typical for appendicitis (although it must be remembered that patients may not always have a classical history for appendicitis).

The surgical intern asked a more senior colleague for an opinion.

The senior colleague considered other anatomical structures that lie within the right iliac fossa as a potential cause of pain. These include the appendix, the cecum, and the small bowel. Musculoskeletal pain and referred pain could also be potential causes. In women, pain may also arise from the ovary, fallopian tube, and uterus. In a young patient, diseases of these organs are rare. Infection and pelvic inflammatory disease may occur in the younger patient and need to be considered.

The patient gave no history of these disorders.

Upon further questioning, however, the patient revealed that her last menstrual period was 6 weeks before this examination. The senior physician realized that a potential cause of the abdominal pain was a pregnancy outside the uterus (ectopic pregnancy). The patient was rushed for an abdominal ultrasound, which revealed no fetus or sac in the uterus. She was also noted to have a positive pregnancy test. The patient underwent surgery and was found to have a ruptured fallopian tube caused by an ectopic pregnancy.

Whenever a patient has apparent pelvic pain, it is important to consider the gender-related anatomical differences. Ectopic pregnancy should always be considered in women of childbearing age.

Case 7

UTERINE TUMOR

A 35-year-old woman visited her family practitioner because she had a "bloating" feeling and an increase in abdominal girth. The family practitioner examined the lower abdomen, which revealed a mass that extended from the superior pubic rami to the level of the umbilicus. The superior margin of the mass was easily palpated, but the inferior margin appeared to be less well defined.

This patient has a pelvic mass.

When examining a patient in the supine position, the observer should uncover the whole of the abdomen.

Inspection revealed a bulge in the lower abdomen to the level of the umbilicus. Palpation revealed a hard and slightly irregular mass with well-defined superior and lateral borders and a less well-defined inferior border, giving the impression that the mass continued into the pelvis. The lesion was dull to percussion. Auscultation did not reveal any abnormal sounds.

The doctor pondered which structures this mass may be arising from. When examining the pelvis, it is important to remember the sex differences. Common to both men and women are the rectum, bowel, bladder, and musculature. Certain pathological states are also common to both sexes, including the development of pelvic abscesses and fluid collections.

In men, the prostate cannot be palpated transabdominally, and it is extremely rare for it to enlarge to such an extent in benign diseases. Aggressive prostate cancer can spread throughout the whole of the pelvis, although this is often associated with bowel obstruction and severe bladder symptoms.

In women, a number of organs can develop large masses, including the ovaries (solid and cystic tumors), the embryological remnants within the broad ligaments, and the uterus (pregnancy and fibroids).

The physician asked further questions.

It is always important to establish whether the patient is pregnant (occasionally, pregnancy may come as a surprise to the patient).

This patient's pregnancy test was negative. After the patient emptied her bladder, there was no change in the mass. The physician thought the mass might be a common benign tumor of the uterus (fibroid). To establish the diagnosis, he obtained an ultrasound scan of the pelvis, which confirmed that the mass stemmed from the uterus.

The patient was referred to a gynecologist, and after a long discussion regarding her symptomatology, fertility, and risks, the surgeon and the patient agreed that a hysterectomy (surgical removal of the uterus) would be an appropriate course of therapy.

The patient sought a series of opinions from other gynecologists, all of whom agreed that surgery was the appropriate option.

The fibroid was removed without any complications.

Case 8

UTERINE FIBROIDS

A 52-year-old woman was referred to a gynecologist. Magnetic resonance imaging (MRI) indicated the presence of uterine fibroids. After a long discussion regarding her symptomatology, fertility, and risks, she was offered the choice between hysterectomy (surgical removal of the uterus) and uterine artery embolization.

A uterine artery embolization is a procedure where an interventional radiologist uses a catheter to inject small particles into the uterine arteries. This reduces the blood supply to the fibroids and causes them to shrink.

The patient opted for the uterine artery embolization.

An MRI performed 6 months after the embolization procedure showed a favorable reduction in the size of the uterine fibroids (Fig. 5.88).

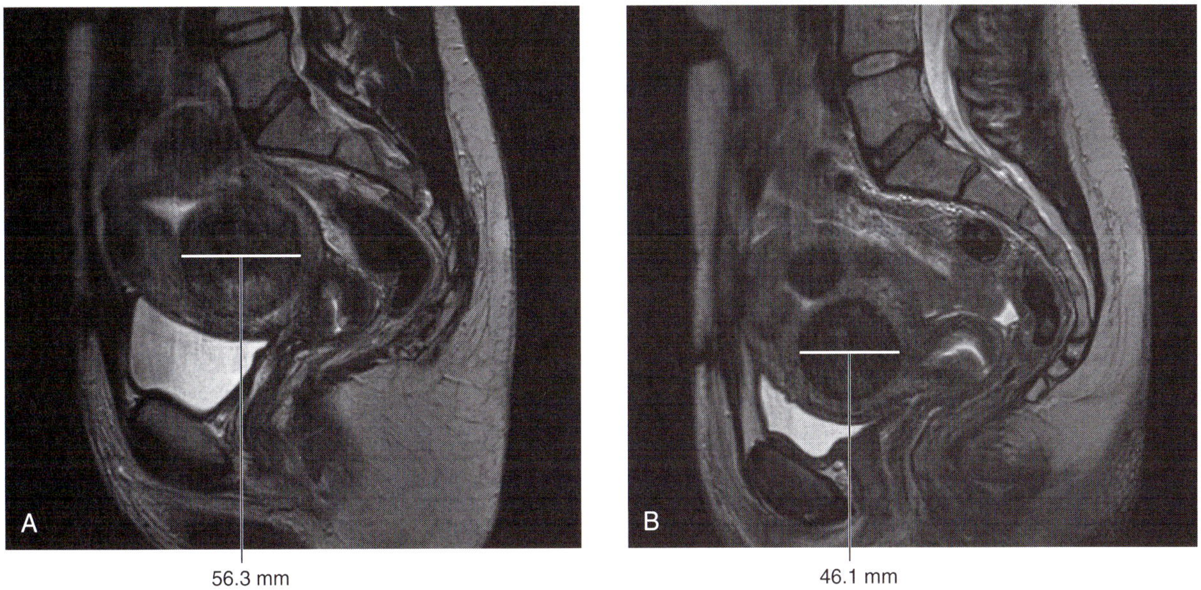

Fig. 5.88 Sagittal MRI of the pelvic cavity. **(A)** Measurement of a fibroid before the uterine artery embolization. **(B)** Measurement of a fibroid 6 months after the embolization. The size of the fibroid has decreased.

Case 9

OVARIAN TORSION

A 19-year-old woman presented to the emergency department with a 36-hour history of lower abdominal pain that was sharp and initially intermittent, later becoming constant and severe. The patient also reported feeling nauseated and vomited once in the ER. She did not have diarrhea and had opened her bowels normally 8 hours before admission. She had no symptoms of dysuria. She was afebrile, slightly tachycardic at 95/min, and had a normal blood pressure. Blood results showed mild leukocytosis of 11.6×10^9/L and normal renal and liver function tests. She reported being sexually active with a long-term partner. She was never pregnant, and the urine pregnancy test on admission was negative.

On physical examination, there was tenderness in the right iliac fossa with guarding. On vaginal examination, a tender mass in the right adnexal region was felt. The patient subsequently underwent a transvaginal ultrasound examination for evaluation of adnexal pathology. The scan showed a markedly enlarged right ovary measuring up to 8 cm in long axis with echogenic stroma and peripherally distributed follicles. There was no internal vascularity when color Doppler was applied. A small amount of free fluid was seen in the pouch of Douglas. The diagnosis of ovarian torsion was made.

Ovarian torsion is the twisting of an ovary on its suspensory ligament, which contains arterial, venous, and lymphatic vessels (forming so-called vascular pedicle), leading to a compromised blood supply. Initially, the venous and lymphatic circulation is compromised, resulting in ovarian edema and enlargement. The arterial flow is maintained longer due to thicker and less compressible arterial walls. Prolonged torsion leads to increased internal ovarian pressure that eventually results in arterial thrombosis, ischemia of the ovarian tissue, and necrosis. If the correct diagnosis and treatment are delayed, the patient may develop generalized sepsis.

The symptoms are nonspecific, making the diagnosis of ovarian torsion challenging. There is often no significant past medical history.

At surgery, the right ovary was hemorrhagic and necrotic with the pedicle twisted 360°. The left ovary was normal in appearance. Right-sided salpingo-oophorectomy was performed, and histopathological examination confirmed completely necrotic ovary without any residual normal ovarian tissue. The patient made a quick recovery after surgical intervention.

Ovarian torsion is encountered in women of all ages, but those of reproductive age have much higher prevalence. Torsion of a normal ovary is uncommon and is seen more frequently in adolescent population, with elongated pelvic ligaments, fallopian tube spasm, or more mobile fallopian tubes or mesosalpinx cited as contributing factors.

Index

C

Index

N

O

P

Index

W

X

Y

Z